PEDIATRICS

A PRIMARY CARE

APPROACH

A SAUNDERS TEXT

PEDIATRICS

A PRIMARY CARE

APPROACH

SECOND EDITION

CAROL D. BERKOWITZ, M.D.

Professor of Clinical Pediatrics
University of California Los Angeles School of Medicine
Los Angeles, California

Executive Vice Chair
Department of Pediatrics
Harbor-UCLA Medical Center
Torrance, California

SAUNDERS
An Imprint of Elsevier Science

SAUNDERS
An Imprint of Elsevier Science

The Curtis Center
Independence Square West
Philadelphia, Pennsylvania 19106

Library of Congress Cataloging-in-Publication Data

Pediatrics : a primary care approach / [edited by] Carol D. Berkowitz.—2nd
ed.

p.   ;   cm.

Includes bibliographical references and index.

ISBN 0–7216–8183–2

1. Pediatrics. I. Berkowitz, Carol D.
   [DNLM: 1. Pediatrics.   2. Primary Health Care.   WS 200 P3733 2000]

RJ45 B43 2000

618.92—dc21   99–049760

Pediatrics: A Primary Care Approach, 2nd Edition   ISBN 0–7216–8183–2

Permissions may be sought directly from Elsevier's Health Sciences Rights Department in Philadelphia,
USA: phone: (+1)215-238-7869, fax: (+1)215-238-2239, e-mail: healthpermissions@elsevier.com. You may also
complete your request on-line via the Elsevier Science homepage (http://www.elsevier.com), by selecting
'Customer Support' and then 'Obtaining Permissions'.

Printed in China

Last digit is the print number: 9   8   7   6   5   4   3   2

PREFACE

Primary care continues to be the foundation of pediatrics. The incorporation of psychosocial issues into every pediatric evaluation ensures that the entire health care of the child is being addressed. In this second edition, we continue our commitment to providing a comprehensive overview of the most common issues confronting pediatricians. Based on the very valuable feedback we received from pediatric clerkship and residency program directors, we decided to expand this edition to include nine new chapters. We'd personally like to take this opportunity to thank these individuals for their valuable advice and, as noted in our first edition, we would like to thank our own families for their support and our patients and their families for all they have taught us. Additional thanks to Ellie Berkowitz for her assistance with the illustrations and Sally Montoya for her secretarial and coordination skills. The authors appreciate the advice and help of Anne-Marie Shaw, Becky Heinz-Baxter, and Carol Vartanian at W.B. Saunders.

CAROL D. BERKOWITZ

CONTRIBUTORS

SUDHIR K. ANAND, M.D.

Professor of Clinical Pediatrics, University of California Los Angeles School of Medicine, Los Angeles, California; Chief, Division of Pediatric Nephrology, Harbor–UCLA Medical Center, Torrance, California

Fluid and Electrolyte Disturbances; Acute Renal Failure; Hypertension; Urinary Tract Infections

JILL M. BAREN, M.D.

Assistant Professor of Emergency Medicine and Pediatrics, Department of Emergency Medicine, University of Pennsylvania School of Medicine, Philadelphia, Pennsylvania; Attending Physician, Emergency Department, The Hospital of the University of Pennsylvania and The Children's Hospital of Philadelphia, Philadelphia, Pennsylvania

Approach to the Traumatized Child; Abdominal Trauma; Head Trauma

CAROL D. BERKOWITZ, M.D.

Professor of Clinical Pediatrics, University of California Los Angeles School of Medicine, Los Angeles, California; Executive Vice Chair, Department of Pediatrics, Harbor–UCLA Medical Center, Torrance, California

Caring for Twins; Circumcision; Sibling Rivalry; Toilet Training; Discipline; Fears and Phobias; Thumb Sucking and Other Habits; Enuresis; Encopresis; SIDS and ALTE; Craniofacial Anomalies; Vomiting; Diarrhea; Constipation; Abdominal Pain; Jaundice; Papulosquamous Eruptions; Maculopapular Rashes; Physical Abuse; Child Sexual Abuse; Failure to Thrive; Infants of Substance-Abusing Mothers; Divorce; Violence; Pediatric HIV

IRIS WAGMAN BOROWSKY, M.D., Ph.D.

Assistant Professor of Pediatrics, Division of General Pediatrics and Adolescent Health, University of Minnesota, Minneapolis, Minnesota

Telephone Management; Gifted Children; Injury Prevention; Attention Deficit/Hyperactivity Disorder

PAMELYN CLOSE, M.D., M.P.H.

Associate Professor, Pediatric Hematology-Oncology, University of California Los Angeles School of Medicine, Los Angeles, California; Clinical Director, Division of Pediatric Hematology-Oncology, Harbor–UCLA Medical Center, Torrance, California

Anemia; Bleeding Disorders; Lymphadenopathy; Cancer in Children

PAMELA S. COHEN, M.D.

Adjunct Professor, Pediatrics, New York University Medical Center, New York, New York; Associate Director, Clinical Pharmacology/Oncology, Novartis Pharmaceutical Corporation, East Hanover, New Jersey

Anemia; Bleeding Disorders; Lymphadenopathy; Cancer in Children

CARLO DI LORENZO, M.D.

Associate Professor of Pediatrics, University of Pittsburgh School of Medicine, Pittsburgh, Pennsylvania; Director, Pediatric Gastrointestinal Motility Center, Children's Hospital of Pittsburgh; Pittsburgh, Pennsylvania

Gastroesophageal Reflux; Gastrointestinal Bleeding

ROBIN WINKLER DOROSHOW, M.D.
Clinical Professor of Pediatrics, University of California Los Angeles School of Medicine, Los Angeles, California; Pediatric Cardiologist, Long Beach Memorial Heart Institute, Long Beach, California

Heart Murmurs; Cyanosis in the Newborn; Congestive Heart Failure

HELEN DUPLESSIS, M.D., M.P.H.
Assistant Clinical Professor, Department of Pediatrics, University of California Los Angeles School of Medicine, Los Angeles, California; Attending staff, Division of General and Emergency Pediatrics, Harbor–UCLA Medical Center, Torrance, California

Diabetes Mellitus; Chronic Lung Disease; Osteomyelitis; Juvenile Rheumatoid Arthritis

ELIZABETH A. EDGERTON, M.D., M.P.H.
Assistant Professor, Department of Pediatrics, University of California Los Angeles School of Medicine, Los Angeles, California; Director of Community Pediatrics, Co-Director of Childhood Injury Prevention Center, Harbor–UCLA Medical Center, Torrance, California

Principles of Pediatric Therapeutics; Syncope; Diabetes Mellitus; Chronic Lung Disease; Osteomyelitis; Juvenile Rheumatoid Arthritis

GEETA GROVER, M.D.
Assistant Clinical Professor of Pediatrics, Harbor–UCLA Medical Center, University of California Los Angeles School of Medicine, Los Angeles, California; Attending Physician, Children's Hospital of Orange County, Orange, California

Talking to Parents; Talking to Children; Nutritional Needs; Sleep: Normal Patterns and Common Disorders; Dental Care; Normal Development and Developmental Assessment; Language Development: Speech and Hearing Assessment; Immunizations; Crying and Colic; Temper Tantrums; Breath-Holding Spells; Fever and Bacteremia; Common Oral Lesions; Strabismus; Infections of the Eye; Excessive Tearing; Developmental Hip Dysplasia; Rotational Problems of the Lower Extremity: In-Toeing and Out-Toeing; Angular Deformities of the Lower Extremity: Bow Legs and Knock Knees; Orthopedic Injuries and Growing Pains; Evaluation of Limp; Musculoskeletal Disorders of the Neck and Back; Disorders of the Hair and Scalp; Diaper Dermatitis

KENNETH R. HUFF, M.D.
Associate Professor of Pediatrics and Neurology, University of California Los Angeles, Los Angeles, California; Chief, Division of Neurology, Department of Pediatrics, Harbor–UCLA Medical Center, Torrance, California

Febrile Seizures; Increased Intracranial Pressure; Hypotonia; Headaches; Tics; Seizures and Epilepsy

STANLEY H. INKELIS, M.D.
Professor of Pediatrics, University of California Los Angeles School of Medicine, Los Angeles, California; Attending staff, Division of General and Emergency Pediatrics, Harbor–UCLA Medical Center, Torrance, California

Sore Throat; Nosebleeds; Neck Masses

ELAINE S. KAMIL, M.D.
Clinical Professor of Pediatrics, University of California Los Angeles School of Medicine, Los Angeles, California; Associate Director, Pediatric Nephrology and Transplant Immunology, Cedars-Sinai Medical Center, Los Angeles, California

Hematuria; Proteinuria; Nephrotic Syndrome

CHARLOTTE W. LEWIS, M.D., R.D.
Robert Wood Johnson Clinical Scholar, University of Washington, Seattle, Washington; Acting Instructor, Department of Pediatrics, University of Washington, Seattle, Washington

Fluid and Electrolyte Disturbances; Childhood Obesity

JULIE E. NOBLE, M.D.
Associate Clinical Professor of Pediatrics, University of California Los Angeles School of Medicine, Los Angeles, California; Director, Pediatric Managed Care, Director, Low Risk Nursery, Harbor–UCLA Medical Center, Torrance, California

Primary Care: Introduction; Approach to the Dysmorphic Child; Allergic Disease; Cough; Inguinal Lumps and Bumps

CHERYL P. SANCHEZ, M.D.
Assistant Professor of Pediatrics, University of Wisconsin Medical School, Pediatrics, Madison, Wisconsin

Chronic Renal Failure

ISIDRO B. SALUSKY, M.D.
Professor of Pediatrics, University of California Los Angeles School of Medicine, Los Angeles, California; Director, Pediatric Dialysis Program, Program Director, General Clinical Research Center, University of California Los Angeles, Los Angeles, California

Chronic Renal Failure

JAMES S. SEIDEL, M.D., Ph.D.
Professor of Pediatrics, University of California Los Angeles School of Medicine, Los Angeles, California; Chief, Division of General and Emergency Pediatrics, Harbor–UCLA Medical Center, Torrance, California

Respiratory Distress; Stridor and Croup; Wheezing and Asthma

MONICA SIFUENTES, M.D.
Associate Professor of Clinical Pediatrics, University of California Los Angeles School of Medicine, Los Angeles, California; Program Director, Harbor–UCLA Medical Center, Torrance, California

Talking to Adolescents; Neonatal Examination and Nursery Visit; Screening in Newborns; Health Maintenance in Older Children and Adolescents; Well Child Care for Children with Trisomy 21; Well Child Care for Preterm Infants; Needs of Children With Physical and Sensory Disabilities; Reproductive Health; Fostering Self-Esteem; Otitis Media; Hearing Impairments; Ambiguous Genitalia; Vaginitis; Sexually Transmitted Diseases; Menstrual Disorders; Disorders of the Breast; Sports-Related Injuries; Hepatitis; Acne; Vesicular Exanthems; Substance Abuse; Eating Disorders; Adolescent Depression and Suicide

ERIC A. VASILIAUSKAS, M.D.
Assistant Clinical Professor of Pediatrics and Medicine, University of California Los Angeles School of Medicine, Los Angeles, California; Associate Clinical Director, Cedars-Sinai Inflammatory Bowel Disease Center, Department of Medicine and Pediatrics, Divisions of Gastroenterology and Pediatric Gastroenterology and Nutrition, Cedars-Sinai Medical Center, Los Angeles, California

Gastrointestinal Bleeding

KELLY D. YOUNG, M.D.
Assistant Clinical Professor of Pediatrics, University of California Los Angeles School of Medicine, Los Angeles, California; Harbor–UCLA Medical Center, Torrance, California

Shock; Ingestions: Diagnosis and Management

CONTENTS

SECTION I

PRIMARY CARE: SKILLS AND CONCEPTS

SECTION II

HEALTH MAINTENANCE AND ANTICIPATORY GUIDANCE

S E C T I O N   I I I

ACUTE AND EMERGENT PROBLEMS

SECTION IV

HEAD, NECK, AND RESPIRATORY SYSTEM

S E C T I O N   V

HEMATOLOGIC DISORDERS

S E C T I O N   VI

CARDIOVASCULAR SYSTEM

SECTION VII

GENITOURINARY DISORDERS

SECTION VIII

ORTHOPEDIC DISORDERS

SECTION IX

GASTROINTESTINAL DISORDERS

SECTION X

NEUROLOGIC DISORDERS

SECTION XI

DERMATOLOGIC DISORDERS

SECTION XII

THE NEW MORBIDITY

S E C T I O N   X I I I

Chronic Diseases of Childhood and Adolescence

SECTION I

PRIMARY CARE: SKILLS AND CONCEPTS

CHAPTER 1

PRIMARY CARE: INTRODUCTION

Julie E. Noble, M.D.

Primary care is defined as the comprehensive health care that patients receive from the same health care provider over a longitudinal period of time. The term was first used in the 1960s in response to the abundance of subspecialists and lack of generalists among practicing physicians. It is generally accepted that primary care physicians include pediatricians, family physicians, and internists. In 1966, the Millis Committee Report to the AMA on graduate medical education recognized the importance of primary care and recommended a national commitment to educating primary care physicians. Primary care was further defined in 1974 by Charney and Alpert, who separated it into component parts: first contact, longitudinal care, family orientation, and integration of comprehensive care. In order to understand the depth of primary care, the component parts should be explored.

First contact occurs when a patient arrives for medical care at the office of a primary care physician. The visit includes an intake history, complete physical examination, and an assessment of problems with treatment (if indicated). Of great importance is the establishment of the physician-patient relationship. Physicians become the primary medical resource and counselors to these patients and their families and the first contacts when successive medical problems arise.

Longitudinal care, the second component of primary care, implies continuity of care over a period of time. Physicians assume responsibility for issues concerning both health and illness. In pediatrics, such care involves monitoring growth and development, following school progress, screening for commonly found disorders, making psychosocial assessments, promoting health, and preventing illness with immunization and safety counseling programs.

Family orientation is the third component of primary care. Patients must be viewed in the context of their environment and family. Otherwise, practitioners cannot adequately care for patients. In pediatrics, a child's problems become the family's, and the family's prob-

lems become the child's. This has become increasingly apparent with the emergence of problems of poverty, drug use, HIV exposure, teenage pregnancy, and gang involvement that have overtaken the pediatric population. The psychosocial forces in a particular child's life are intricately interwoven, and their assessment is an essential component of the primary care of that child.

As pediatric medical problems become more complex, many health and educational resources may be utilized to supplement care. Primary care physicians integrate and coordinate these services in the best interest of patients, thus providing **integration of comprehensive care,** the fourth component of primary care. Working with social service agencies, home care providers, educational agencies, and government agencies, physicians can use multiple resources for the benefit of patients. Understanding the resources of the community is an important part of a primary physician's education.

When patients select a primary care provider, they have identified a medical "home." That home incorporates the physical, psychological, and social aspects of individual patients into comprehensive health care services, thus meeting the needs of the whole person. To make that home work for patients, geographic and financial accessibility are key elements. The most important aspect of a home is that it is a place where patients feel "cared for."

SUBSPECIALIST CARE

Medical knowledge and technology have made amazing advancements in the past several decades. Total knowledge of all fields is impossible for individual physicians. As a result, the role of the subspecialist physician has developed as an adjunct to that of the primary care physician. Primary care physicians seek subspecialist consultation when the suspected or known disease process is unusual or complicated, when it demands specialized technology, or when they have

1

little experience with the disease. Generally, subspecialists evaluate patients and concentrate on the organ system or disease process in their area of expertise.

Primary care physicians can use a subspecialist for either a consultation or referral. When initiating a consultation, primary physicians send patients for advice. Consulting physicians assess the patients with a history and physical examination, focusing on their specialty. They then recommend possible additional laboratory tests, offer a diagnosis and treatment plan, and send the patients back to their primary care physicians for coordination of further care.

Use of the subspecialist is termed **secondary care.** For example, an 8-year-old girl with weight loss and persistent abdominal pain has an upper GI x-ray series that reveals a duodenal ulcer. She is sent by her primary care physician to a pediatric gastroenterologist for **consultation,** with a request for an endoscopy to allow definitive diagnosis and up-to-date management guidelines. The girl then returns to the primary care physician with recommendations for treatment and further care.

Primary care physicians can also generate a referral to a subspecialist, which differs from a consultation. A **referral** requests that the subspecialist assume complete care of the patient. This transfer of a patient to a tertiary care site establishes a subspecialist as the coordinator of further health care for the patient. For example, a 4-year-old boy with recurrent fevers, hepatosplenomegaly, and blasts on peripheral blood smear is referred to a pediatric oncologist for diagnosis, the latest treatment, and ongoing medical care.

When requesting advice from subspecialists, whether on a consultative or referral basis, primary care physicians should outline specific questions with a probable diagnosis to be addressed by the subspecialist. For example, a consultation requesting evaluation of a child with hematuria is inappropriate. The primary care physician should perform a basic diagnostic evaluation and should make the most likely diagnosis. The child can then be referred appropriately. A child diagnosed with nephritis should be sent to a pediatric nephrologist, whereas a child diagnosed with Wilms' tumor should be sent to a pediatric oncologist.

When primary care physicians and subspecialists function cooperatively and offer the three levels of care (primary, referral, and consultative), patients receive the highest quality medical care. However, the number of generalist physicians declined over the last several decades as the number of subspecialist physicians rose excessively. This imbalance of physician supply resulted in a decreased accessibility to primary medical care by underserved populations and an overuse of subspecialists by patients. In general, care provided by subspecialists is characterized as being more expensive and procedure-driven. Laboratory studies are ordered with increased frequency by subspecialists, further inflating the cost of medical care. If patients have no longitudinal health care and see multiple providers, repeat laboratory studies are often ordered. Primary care is believed to deliver more cost-effective, improved medical care. With the spiraling cost of medical care, there continues to be a nationwide movement to produce more primary care physicians. However, it should be remembered that the role of the subspecialist is an essential supplement to the primary care physician when managing complicated disease. A balance between generalists and subspecialists needs to be maintained in the education process.

LABORATORY TESTS

For most conditions, the diagnosis is revealed by the history and physical examination in over 95% of cases. Thus, good communication skills are a basic tenet of primary care. Patients' complaints often concern unnecessary laboratory tests, which increase the cost of medical care and the prescription of unnecessary medications. To lessen these problems, the primary care physician should use laboratory tests and medications discriminately, recognizing their value as well as their potential iatrogenic effects.

In primary care, laboratory tests should be used to help confirm a condition suspected on the basis of the history or physical examination or diagnose a condition that may not be apparent after a thorough history and physical assessment. In pediatrics, especially, the value of each test result should be weighed against the inconvenience, discomfort, and possible side effects in children. Tests can be used as screening tools to prevent disease or to identify a disease early so that treatment can begin and symptoms can be minimized. Laboratory studies can provide a variety of other information, including data to establish a diagnosis, knowledge necessary to select therapy or to monitor a disease, and information about the risk of future disease. Organ function, metabolic activity, and nutritional status can also be assessed, and evidence of neoplastic or infectious disease can be provided. In addition, laboratory studies can be used to identify infectious and therapeutic agents or poisons.

Screening laboratory tests are used when the incidence of an unsuspected condition is high enough in a general population to justify the expense of the test. (See Chapter 8, Screening in Newborns.) Subclinical conditions such as anemia, lead poisoning, and hypercholesterolemia are part of some health maintenance assessments.

Physicians must remember that there is variability in test results and that laboratory error can occur. Laboratory results should always be viewed in the context of the patient. The sensitivity of a test, the ability of the test to detect low levels, and the specificity of a test for the substance being measured must also be considered by the physician when evaluating a test result.

COST CONTAINMENT

In recent years, cost containment for medical care has become a primary economic concern in the United States. Health care costs are increasing at rates well above inflation. Currently there is a national movement to decrease the financial burden of the cost of medical care. Traditional medicine has operated on a fee-for-service basis; that is, if a physician saw a patient, the physician would be reimbursed for services provided. Some have suggested that this plan has given physicians a financial incentive to generate more services and see patients more than is necessary.

Many alternative ways to run the business of medicine are gradually infiltrating the medical care arena. One of the more popular alternatives is **managed care,** which replaces traditional insurance programs with a system that integrates financing with appropriate case-managed health care for its enrollees. It relies on a monthly capitation fee for each enrollee in the plan, which contracts with selected physicians and hospitals to furnish comprehensive health services. Cost containment depends on control of services provided. That control is provided through physician selection, financial incentives for physicians, and monitoring and utilization review of services provided. Preventive health issues and patient education are important services that keep the enrolled population healthy. Each member of the managed care organization is supplied with a primary care physician to ensure comprehensive longitudinal care. This physician serves as a gatekeeper for initial contact, restricting subspecialist referrals to only appropriate cases. Each member also has a case manager, who may be the physician or a nurse, to coordinate services and provide individual patients with a health care plan.

Managed care organizations vary in structure. The managed care organizations may be **health maintenance organizations (HMOs),** groups that offer coverage of health services for a fixed premium either from a group, network, or staff model, or **individual practice associations (IPAs),** which contract with physicians who provide health care from their offices. Individual HMOs may function on a for-profit or not-for-profit basis. Managed care plans may also be **preferred provider organizations (PPOs),** where the program contracts with providers for services, usually on a discounted fee-for-service basis. These organizations have proliferated in recent years with an associated decrease in the number of solo practitioners.

Utilization review, the review of the appropriateness of health care services, and the development of practice guidelines for physicians to decrease variability and cost in disease treatment are essential elements of managed health care. These elements impose greater control over physicians as they decide medical management of individual cases. This organizational model tends to view disease on a population-based approach and may not ensure the best care for the individual.

Goals of managed care include not only cost containment but the reduction of fragmented and duplicative care for patients. Currently many patients see several different providers for the same illness and inappropriately utilize the emergency room for minor illnesses. A designated primary care physician should eliminate these problems. In the past decade enrollment in HMOs in the United States has more than tripled. No data clearly indicate whether managed care is resulting in

medical cost savings, however, and it remains to be seen whether managed care is the answer for the health care crisis in the United States. Controlling HMOs and ensuring appropriate patient care in a time of emphasis on cost containment have generated a new government bureaucracy. Each state is now passing legislation to regulate the administration of HMOs as well as the medical care delivered.

The issue of cost containment has also spawned additional movements toward shorter hospital stays and outpatient management of diseases that used to be treated in the hospital. Improved technology now allows many surgical conditions that a few years ago required hospital stays of several days to be performed on an outpatient basis, with the patient discharged hours after the procedure. Gallbladder surgery is an example of this new management. Other conditions, such as sepsis and treatment of osteomyelitis, have also moved to the outpatient arena as treatments have advanced. The development of oral rehydration therapy now allows patients with dehydration to be treated as outpatients, without intravenous therapy, eliminating the possible complications associated with intravenous access. Even respirator care in chronically ill patients can be done in the home setting. Medical advances are increasing the value of outpatient care and the importance of primary care physicians in supplying and coordinating care.

CHALLENGES FOR THE FUTURE

The many changes in health care delivery have expanded the role of the physician as a health care provider to include being a fiscal overseer. For many physicians, such a change has been frustrating and has challenged the basic principles of medical ethics, particularly professionalism. The key to maintaining one's role as the health care provider is to ask, whose interests are being served by any decision? The answer should always be, the patient's.

Focusing on patient interest above self-interest is essential for both the physician and the entire health care industry.

Selected Readings

American Association of Medical Colleges. Policy on the generalist physician. Academic Medicine 68:1–6, 1993.

Alpert, J. J. Primary care: the future for pediatric education. Pediatrics 86:653–659, 1990.

Arkans, H. D. Pediatric perspective on the changing healthcare delivery system. Pediatr. Ann. 27:205–208, 1998.

Iglehart, J. K. The American health care system: managed care. N. Engl. J. Med. 327:742–747, 1992.

Kassi, J. P. Managing care—should we adopt a new ethic? N. Engl. J. Med. 339:397–398, 1998.

Noe, D. A., and R. C. Rock. Laboratory Medicine: The Selection and Interpretation of Clinical Laboratory Studies. Baltimore, Williams & Wilkins, 1994.

Sia, C. C. J. The medical home: pediatric practice and child advocacy in the 1990s. Pediatrics 90:419–423, 1992.

Starfield, B. Primary Care. Concept, Evaluation, and Policy. New York, Oxford University Press, 1992.

CHAPTER 2

TALKING TO PARENTS

Geeta Grover, M.D.

H_x An 8-month-old boy with a 1-week history of cough and runny nose and a 2-day history of vomiting, diarrhea, and fever, with temperature of 101° F (38.3° C), is evaluated in the emergency department. The mother is very concerned because her son's appetite has decreased and he has been waking up several times at night for the last 2 days.

A nurse interrupts and says that paramedics are bringing a 5-year-old trauma victim to the emergency department. The appearance of the 8-month-old child is quickly assessed; he seems active and alert. Bilateral otitis media is diagnosed. Before leaving the examination room the physician says to the mother: "Your son has a viral syndrome and infection in his ears. I am going to prescribe an antibiotic that you can begin giving him today. Give him Tylenol as needed for the fever. Don't worry about his vomiting and diarrhea; just make sure that he drinks plenty of liquids and don't give him milk or milk products for a few days. Bring him back here or to his regular doctor if his fever persists, he doesn't eat, he has too much vomiting or diarrhea, he looks lethargic, or if he isn't better in 2 days."

Questions

1. Did this mother receive more information than she can be reasonably expected to remember?
2. Did the physician address the mother's concerns sufficiently?
3. Was the mother given a chance to acknowledge that she had understood the diagnosis and treatment plan?
4. What are some barriers to effective doctor-patient communication?
5. How does the setting itself influence communication?

Effective communication in the pediatric setting involves the exchange of information between physicians, parents, and children. In addition, observing the interaction between parents and children gives physicians an opportunity to assess parenting skills and the dynamics of the parent-child relationship. The communication needs of both parents and children are quite different; this makes the exchange of information challenging. Parental concerns should be addressed in a sensitive, empathetic, and nonjudgmental manner. A nonthreatening, pleasant demeanor and age-appropriate language help facilitate communication with children (see Chapter 3, Talking to Children).

Pediatrics encompasses not only the traditional medical model of diagnosis and treatment of disease but also maintenance of the health and well-being of children through longitudinal care and the establishment of ongoing relationships between physicians and families. Personal relationships between physicians and families create an atmosphere in which information can be exchanged openly. The pediatrician's role in such relationships is to not only diagnose and treat, but also to listen, advise, guide, and teach.

The doctor-patient relationship is truly a privilege. Patients entrust physicians with their innermost thoughts and feelings, allow them to touch private parts of their bodies, and then trust them to perform invasive procedures or administer medications. Mutual respect is essential for the development of a healthy relationship between physicians, parents, and children. Through practice and continued awareness of interpersonal abilities, physicians can develop good communication skills. All physicians eventually develop their own personal interviewing and examination style. What seems awkward and difficult at first soon becomes routine and even enjoyable as physicians become more comfortable with patients.

PARENTAL CONCERNS

Parents' preconceived ideas and concerns regarding their children's illnesses can greatly influence the exchange of information between physicians and patients. At health maintenance or well child care visits, it is important for pediatricians to address the nonmedical and psychosocial concerns of parents, such as their children's development, nutrition, and growth. Often these questions stem from discussions with other parents or information received through the media. Although such concerns may seem trivial to pediatricians, they may be extremely important to parents. In addition to addressing the needs of the child, the health maintenance visit also gives the pediatrician an opportunity to assess and address parental needs. Parental depression, substance abuse, family violence, or marital discord can all have profound effects on children's health and development. When evaluating children brought in for illness, it is important to ask parents what concerns them the most. Parental fears may be much different than medical concerns. Failure to give parents the opportunity to ask questions or to address these concerns in a sensitive manner may lead to dissatisfaction and poor communication.

THE PEDIATRIC INTERVIEW

Pediatric interviews are conducted in a variety of settings for many different reasons. The first interaction between the physician and parents may be during the prenatal interview before the birth of the child, in the hospital following the delivery, or in the doctor's office during the well baby visit. Later, the physician may see children in the office for regular health maintenance visits or in the office, emergency department, or hospital for an acute illness.

The specific clinical situation dictates the information that needs to be gathered and the appropriate interviewing techniques. During the prenatal visit, physicians should discuss common concerns and anxieties about the new baby with prospective parents. In addition, parents have an opportunity to interview physicians and evaluate their offices and staffs.

In the emergency setting, physicians must elicit pertinent information needed to make decisions regarding management within a short period of time. Absence of long-term relationships can make communication in the emergency department particularly challenging. Focused, closed-ended questions should be used primarily. The periodic health maintenance visit is at the opposite end of this spectrum. Here the use of broad, open-ended questions is more appropriate; closed-ended questions should be used as needed for clarification.

COMMUNICATION GUIDELINES

Overall principles, applicable regardless of the setting, include interacting with the child and family in a professional yet sensitive and nonjudgmental manner. Common courtesies, such as knocking before entering the room, dressing and behaving in a professional manner, introducing oneself, and addressing parents and children by their preferred names, are always appreciated and welcomed. Taking a few moments to socialize with families develops a more personal relationship that may allow more open conversation about sensitive and emotional issues.

The medical visit may be divided into three parts: the interview, the physical examination, and the concluding remarks. Examples of doctor-parent and doctor-child communications for each of these components are given in Table 2–1.

The Interview

The goal of the interview is to ascertain the chief complaint and determine the appropriate medical history. The interview usually begins with open-ended questions to give parents and children an opportunity to discuss their concerns and outline their agenda for the visit. Not uncommonly, the real reason for the visit may not be disclosed until the family believes the physician is trustworthy and honest. Once the issues have been laid out, closed-ended questions can be used to clarify and further define the information presented. It often becomes necessary to guide the interview, especially when parents have several broad issues on their agenda for that visit and time does not permit their discussion.

Physicians should gently acknowledge parental concerns and define time limitations. These actions allow physicians to focus on the most salient issues of that

TABLE 2–1.   Communication Guidelines and Techniques

Techniques	Examples
The Interview	
Open-ended questions	"How is Susie?"
Closed-ended questions	"Does she have a cough?"
Repetition of important phrases	"She has had a high fever for four days now?"
Clarification	"What do you mean by 'Susie was acting funny'?"
Pauses and silent periods	
Limit medical jargon	"Susie has an ear infection" vs. "Susie has otitis media"
Guide the interview	"Right now I am most interested in hearing about the symptoms of this illness"
Be aware of nonverbal communication	Use eye contact and phrases such as "I see"
Acknowledge parental concerns	"Worrying about hearing loss is understandable"
Empathize	"A fever of 104° F can be very frightening"
Remember common courtesies	Knock before entering
Recognize personal limitations	"I am not an expert in this area. I would like to consult with a colleague"
Summarize	"So she has had fever for four days but the rash and cough began one week ago?"
The Physical Examination	
Show consideration for the child	"It's OK to be afraid"
Inform	"That took me some time, but her heart sounds normal"
Explain procedures	"You may feel a little uncomfortable during the rectal examination"
Avoid exclamations	"Wow! I have never seen anything like this"
Concluding Remarks	
Provide closure	"Our time is over today. May we discuss this at the next visit?"
Minimize discharge instructions	
Be specific	"I am going to treat her with amoxicillin" vs. "I'll prescribe an antibiotic"
Compliment	"You're doing a great job"
Confirm parental understanding	"Please repeat for me Susie's diagnosis and treatment instructions"

visit. Physicians should limit their use of medical jargon (scientific terms) and be aware of nonverbal communication. Practitioners should empathize with parents; this makes them feel that their situation is truly understood even if physicians can do very little to help them. Pauses and silent periods should be used, especially when discussing emotionally difficult issues, to convey to parents and children that their physician cares enough to listen. Physicians should not underrate their own knowledge, but at the same time they should recognize their limitations and use consultants appropriately. Finally, physicians' understanding of the chief complaint and history should be summarized so parents have an opportunity to clarify points of disagreement.

The Physical Examination

Parents keenly observe physicians' interactions with their children during the examination. It is an important time for physicians to build a therapeutic relationship with children (see Chapter 3, Talking to Children). The transition between the history and physical examination can be made by briefly telling children and parents what to expect during the examination. Practitioners should show consideration for children's fears. Clinicians often find it helpful to speak to families at periodic intervals during the examination regarding their observations. Prolonged periods of silence as the doctor listens or palpates may be anxiety-provoking for families. Physicians should be sure to explain any procedures that either they or their staff are going to perform at a level that is appropriate for both parents and children. In addition, physicians should try to avoid exclamations or comments to themselves during the examination (e.g., "Wow, that's some murmur!"), which may be alarming to families.

Concluding Remarks

This portion of the visit, which is all too easy to rush through, is extremely important. Closure can be provided by either summarizing the diagnosis or outlining plans for the following visit. Parents should be asked to participate by acknowledging closure and helping to develop a management plan. It is important to assess parental readiness for knowledge (especially in emotionally difficult situations) and keep family resources and limitations in mind. Discharge instructions should be minimized; physicians should be specific and the number of diagnoses, medications, and "PRN" instructions (indications for seeking medical advice such as "return PRN for high fever") should be limited. When complicated discharge instructions are given, additional physician time may be required to ensure parental understanding. Complimenting parents on their care of their children can boost their self-esteem and confidence and may minimize calls and questions. Parental understanding should be confirmed; parents should be asked to repeat the diagnosis and treatment plan. Simply asking parents if they have understood is not enough, because parents often say "yes" out of respect for the physician's time or embarrassment that they have not understood what has been said. For example, the physician could say, "I want to be sure that I've spoken clearly enough. Please repeat for me [child's name] diagnosis and treatment instructions."

BARRIERS TO EFFECTIVE COMMUNICATION

Barriers to effective communication may be divided into systems barriers and interpersonal barriers (Table 2–2). The primary systems barriers are the setting itself and lack of continuity of care. Because of access problems within the health care system (i.e., lack of health insurance coverage), many children receive only episodic care from different physicians in acute care clinics or emergency departments. Without the benefit of long-term relationships, doctor-patient communication may suffer.

Interpersonal barriers include physician time constraints, frequent interruptions, and cultural insensitivity. Frequent interruptions or apparent impatience on

TABLE 2–2.   Barriers to Effective Communication

Systems Barriers	Examples
Lack of continuity of care	Episodic care that is primarily illness driven
The setting itself	Emergency departments and acute care clinics
Interpersonal Barriers	
Physician time constraints	Appearing impatient or preoccupied
Frequent interruptions	
Cultural insensitivity	Suggesting treatments that are not acceptable within the family's belief systems

the part of physicians conveys to parents and children that either they do not care or they are too busy for them. Language differences may pose a significant barrier depending on the region in which physicians practice. Ideally, physicians themselves should be able to speak to parents and children. If translators must be used, children should not play this role, if possible, because this places them in an awkward situation. Parents of other patients should not be used because this violates patients' privacy. Physicians should be sensitive to cultural differences (e.g., gender issues, views on illness, folk remedies, and beliefs). Suggesting treatments that are not culturally acceptable or are contrary to folk wisdom simply decreases compliance with prescribed treatment plans. For example, many Eastern cultures believe in the concept of "hot" and "cold" foods and illnesses. Suggesting to a mother that she feed primarily "hot" foods to a child she believes to have an illness that is also "hot" may not be acceptable to her. Such information is rarely volunteered and must be elicited through sensitive patient interviewing.

Case Resolution

The doctor-patient interaction presented in the case history illustrates several of the points discussed here. The physician did not acknowledge parental concerns or make sure that the mother had understood the diagnosis and treatment plan. The mother was presented with more information than she could have reasonably been asked to remember. This interaction could have been improved (1) if the physician conveyed to the mother that her concerns were appreciated and (2) then reassured her that her child was going to be all right. Furthermore, the physician could have told the mother the name and dosage schedule of the antibiotic to be prescribed and limited the number of PRN instructions.

Selected Readings

American Academy of Pediatrics. Guidelines for Health Supervision III. Elk Grove Village, IL, American Academy of Pediatrics, 1997.

Bernzweig, J., et al. Gender differences in physician-patient communication. Arch. Pediatr. Adolesc. Med. 151:586–591, 1997.

Grover, G., C. D. Berkowitz, and R. J. Lewis. Parental recall after a visit to the emergency department. Clin. Pediatr. 33:194–201, 1994.

Korsch, B. M., B. F. Freemon, and V. F. Negrete. Practical implications of doctor-patient interaction analysis for pediatric practice. Am. J. Dis. Child. 12:110–114, 1971.

McMahon, S. R., M. E. Rimsza, and R. C. Bay. Parents can dose liquid medication accurately. Pediatrics. 100:330–333, 1997.

Regalado, M. G., and N. Halfon. Parenting: issues for the pediatrician. Pediatr. Ann. 27:31–37, 1998.

Stein, M. T. Interviewing in a pediatric setting. In Dixon, S. D., and M. T. Stein. Encounters with Children: Pediatric Behavior and Development, 2nd ed. Chicago, Mosby-Year Book, 1992.

Wissow, L. S., D. L. Roter, and M. E. H. Wilson. Pediatrician interview style and mother's disclosure of psychosocial issues. Pediatrics 93:289–295, 1994.

Young, K. T., K. Davis, C. Schoen, and S. Parker. Listening to parents: a national survey of parents with young children. Arch. Pediatr. Adolesc. Med. 152:255–262, 1998.

CHAPTER 3

TALKING TO CHILDREN

Geeta Grover, M.D.

H$_x$ The moment you walk into the examination room, the 2-year-old girl begins to cry and scream uncontrollably. She clings to her mother and turns her face away. The mother appears embarrassed and states that her daughter reacts to all physicians this way. After reassuring the mother that you have received such welcomes before, you sit down at a comfortable distance from the girl and her mother. You smile at the girl and compliment her on her dress, but she does not seem to be interested in interacting with you at this point. You begin your interview with the mother and try not to look at the girl. Out of the corner of your eye, you see that her crying is easing a bit and that she is looking at you very carefully. Without moving from your chair, you hand her your stethoscope with a clip-on toy teddy bear attached to it. She accepts it hesitantly and begins to examine it as you and the mother continue talking.

Questions

1. How does children's age influence their understanding of health and illness?
2. Should physicians speak directly with children about their illnesses?
3. At what age can children begin to communicate with physicians about their illnesses?
4. How can positioning and placement of children in the examination room affect the overall tone and quality of the visit?

Effective doctor-patient communication, which is difficult enough when patients are adults, becomes even more challenging when patients are children. In pediatrics, interviewing involves balancing the needs of both parents and children. Whereas parents may be more focused on issues pertaining to disease, treatment, or aspects of parenting, children look to physicians with different needs and concerns, depending on their age. To have a meaningful and satisfying exchange with children, pediatricians must take into account chil-

dren's developmental maturity and how this affects their concepts of health and illness. As children grow and develop, their understanding of health and illness increases.

DEVELOPMENTAL APPROACH TO COMMUNICATING WITH CHILDREN

An appreciation of the cognitive stages of development helps pediatricians develop a healthy relationship with their patients by allowing them to communicate with the children in an age-appropriate manner. Piaget defined four stages of cognitive development, which occur in the same sequence but not at the same rate in all children (Table 3–1). Children in the sensorimotor stage (birth–2 years of age) experience the world and act through sensations and motor acts. They are developing the concepts of object permanence, causality, and spatial relationships. Children in the preoperational stage (2–6 years) understand reality only from their own viewpoint. As egocentric thinkers, they are unable to separate internal from external reality, and fantasy play is important. School-age children (6–11 years) are capable of concrete operational thinking. These children can reason through problems that relate to real objects. Older children (>11 years) have the

TABLE 3–1.   Piaget's Stages of Cognitive Development

Age*	Stage	Characteristics
Birth–2 yr	Sensorimotor	Experiences world through sensations and motor acts
2–6 yr	Preoperational	Egocentric thinking; imitation and fantasy play
6–11 yr	Concrete operational	Mental processes only as they relate to real objects
>11 yr	Formal operations	Capacity for abstract thought

*Approximate ages.

TABLE 3–2. Children's Concepts of Illness

Age	Concept of Illness	Example
2–6 yr	**Preoperational** Phenomenism Contagion	How do people get colds? "From the sun" "When someone else gets near them"
7–10 yr	**Concrete Operational** Contamination	How do people get colds? "You're outside without a hat and you start sneezing. Your head would get cold—the cold would touch it—and then it would go all over your body"
	Internalization	"In winter, people breathe in too much air into their nose and it blocks up the nose"
>11 yr	**Formal Operations** Physiologic Psychophysiologic	How do people get colds? "They come from viruses, I guess" How do people get a heart attack? "It can come from being all nerve-racked. You worry too much, and the tension can affect your heart"

Modified and reproduced, with permission, from Bibace, R., and M.E. Walsh. Development of children's concepts of illness. Pediatrics 66:912–917, 1980.

capacity for abstract thought, which defines the stage of formal operations.

An appreciation of how children's cognitive development affects their understanding of illness and pain aids physicians in developing therapeutic relationships. Bibace and colleagues have outlined a developmental approach to children's understanding of illness: Children's explanations of illness are classified into six categories consistent with Piaget's cognitive developmental stages. Children 2–6 years of age view illness as caused by external factors near the body (phenomenism and contagion). Young children engage in so-called magical thinking; proximity alone provides the link between cause and illness. Children 7–10 years of age should be able to differentiate between self and nonself. At this stage they begin to understand that although illness may be caused by some factor outside the body, illness itself is located inside the body (contamination and internalization). Children over 11 years of age understand physiologic and psychophysiologic explanations for illness (Table 3–2).

A similar developmental sequence applies to children's understanding of pain. Gaffney and Dunne have outlined a developmental approach to this understanding. Younger children may attribute pain to punishment for some transgression or wrongdoing on their part. They may not understand the relationship between pain and illness (e.g., "pain is something in my tummy"). Children with concrete operational thought can appreciate that pain and illness are related, but they may have no clear understanding of the causation of pain (e.g., "pain is a feeling you get when you are sick"). Older children and adolescents begin to understand the complex physical and psychological components of pain. For example, they realize that although the bone in the arm is broken, pain is ultimately felt in the head (e.g., "pain goes up some nerves from the broken bone in my arm to my head").

GUIDELINES FOR DOCTOR-CHILD COMMUNICATION

Successful communication with children depends not only on spoken words but also nonverbal cues and the environment itself. A pleasant, child-friendly environment with bright colors, wall decorations, and toys helps make children feel more comfortable. Health care practitioners should be sincere, because children are extremely sensitive to nonverbal cues. Pediatricians should take a few minutes to enjoy children; this not only gives children a chance to evaluate their physicians, but also allows clinicians to begin assessing areas of development. A general principle of the pediatric examination is to begin with the least invasive portions of the examination (e.g., heart, lungs, abdomen) and save the most invasive for last (e.g., oropharynx, ears). Pediatricians should maintain their self-control in difficult situations. If they approach their limit, they should step outside for a few minutes or ask someone for assistance. Overall guidelines for communicating with children are provided in Table 3–3. Age-specific guidelines are outlined below.

Birth to Six Months

Examination of children of this age is usually pleasant. Although verbal interaction is limited, it is important to play with children, hold them, and talk to them. By watching physicians interact with their children, new parents have an opportunity to learn how to behave with their infants. Infants have not yet developed a fear of strangers and can usually be easily examined either in parents' arms or on the examination table.

Seven Months to Three Years

This is perhaps the most challenging age group with regard to developing rapport and performing examinations. After entering the examination room, pediatricians should take a few moments to converse or play with children. Such actions help put children at ease and allow them to get to know their doctors. Children who are 1–2 years of age will probably busy themselves, exploring the room during the history taking. By acknowledging them periodically, physicians build rapport that will help later during the examination. Two- to three-year-old children are usually very apprehensive of the examination. Physicians should get down to chil-

TABLE 3–3. Physician-Child Communication

Do's	Don't's
Provide a pleasant environment	Limit the child's participation
Pay attention to nonverbal cues	Threaten the child
Be sincere and honest	Compare the child to others
Enjoy the child	Get into power struggles
Speak age appropriately	
Get down to the child's eye level	
Examine from least to most invasive	
Respect the child's privacy	
Maintain self-control	
Have a sense of humor	

dren's eye level when speaking to them. Reassurances such as, "You're not going to get any shots today," can help alleviate their fears. Because stranger anxiety has developed, physicians should try to do as much of the examination as possible with children in parents' laps. Distractions such as stethoscope toys, flashing penlights, or keys may be helpful.

Three to Six Years

Children's expressive capabilities are growing at tremendous rates during this period. Children can usually be engaged in conversation. They should be given repeated opportunities for participation, but they should not feel pressured to take part. Children may doubt physicians' true intentions and will probably only speak once their comfort level has been achieved. Children should be involved; they can be asked simple questions regarding their illness (e.g., "where does it hurt?"). In addition, children should be given some control during the examination (e.g., "should I look in your mouth next or your ears?"), and they should be allowed to handle physicians' equipment. Knowing what to expect next and having some control over the examination can help to decrease fear and increase cooperation.

Seven to Eleven Years

Examination of children in this age group can be rewarding. Physicians should make a point to speak directly with children and not just to parents concerning the chief complaint and history. Children can usually provide a good history regarding their illness, although their concept of time may be misleading. For example, a "long, long time" may mean hours, days, or months, and parents need to clarify this. Children should be asked about school, friends, and favorite activities. Answers to such questions give physicians an idea of children's social and emotional well-being, which may be affecting their physical health. Physicians sometimes overlook children's need for privacy at this age. Drapes should be used appropriately during the examination, and physicians should be sensitive to the presence of other children or adults in the room.

Physicians should begin to involve older children in the management of their illness. Children's understanding of their illness and its management should be assessed (e.g., children with asthma could be asked "What is this inhaler for? When are you going to use it? Show me how."). Children should be given an opportunity to express their fears and anxieties, and these concerns should be discussed (e.g., "Asthma can be scary, especially when you can't catch your breath. Have you ever felt like that? Tell me about it."). Children should be involved in the management of their illness, which allows them to develop a sense of responsibility for their own health and medical care.

Over Twelve Years

Communication with adolescents is discussed in detail in Chapter 4, Talking to Adolescents.

BARRIERS TO EFFECTIVE COMMUNICATION WITH CHILDREN

The manner in which adults speak to children is influenced by what they think children can understand. Clinicians tend to overestimate the understanding capabilities of younger children and underestimate those of older children. Lack of appreciation for the cognitive sophistication of children may lead to frustration for all involved. Younger children are presented with information they may not be able to comprehend, and older children may feel frustrated because they are being spoken to in a childlike manner.

Another potential barrier in communicating with children is limiting their participation. Physicians tend to elicit information from children but exclude them from diagnostic and management information. Older children want to know about their illness and are capable of learning about management.

All physicians have been frustrated or pushed to the limit at one time or another when working with children. In such situations, practitioners should remember that children are probably not trying to irritate physicians on purpose. Crying or lack of cooperation generally stems from fear or a sense of lack of control over the situation. Pediatricians should avoid taking part in a battle over power or control with children. Threatening remarks (e.g., "If you're not good, I'll have to give you a shot") or comparisons between children (e.g., "Your brother is younger than you, and he didn't cry") not only are ineffective but may make the situation worse. A clear perspective, empathy, and a sense of humor are much more useful.

Case Resolution

In the case presented in the opening scenario, you learn from the mother that her daughter has been in good health. The mother has brought in the child for a routine health maintenance visit. You assess that her development is normal and that her immunizations are up-to-date. As you and the mother talk, the child appears more relaxed and less frightened. She begins to respond to your questions and cooperate with the examination, but she chooses to remain on her mother's lap.

Selected Readings

Bibace, R., and M. E. Walsh. Development of children's concepts of illness. Pediatrics 66:912–917, 1980.

Gaffney, A., and E. A. Dunne. Developmental aspects of children's definitions of pain. Pain 26:105–117, 1986.

Ginsburg, H., and S. Opper. Piaget's Theory of Intellectual Development, 3rd ed. Englewood Cliffs, NJ, Prentice-Hall, 1988.

Lewis, C. C., R. H. Pantell, and L. Sharp. Increasing patient knowledge, satisfaction, and involvement: randomized trial of a communication intervention. Pediatrics 88:351–358, 1991.

McGrath, P. J., and K. D. Craig. Developmental and psychological factors in children's pain. Pediatr. Clin. North Am. 36:823–836, 1989.

Perrin, E. C., and P. S. Gerrity. There's a demon in your belly: children's understanding of illness. Pediatrics 67:841–849, 1981.

Perrin, E. C., and J. M. Perrin. Clinicians' assessments of children's understanding of illness. Am. J. Dis. Child. 137:874–878, 1983.

Van Dulmen, A. M. Children's contributions to pediatric outpatient encounters. Pediatrics 102:563–568, 1998.

TALKING TO ADOLESCENTS

Monica Sifuentes, M.D.

Hx This is a first-time visit for a quiet, shy, adolescent girl who is accompanied by her mother. The mother is concerned because her daughter's grades have been dropping, and she has been fatigued and irritable. The mother reports no new activities or recent changes in the family's schedule and no new stressors at home. Both parents are employed, the girl has the same friends she has always had, and her siblings are currently doing well academically. The girl is healthy and has never been hospitalized.

After the mother leaves the room, the girl is interviewed alone.

Questions

1. When interviewing adolescents, what is the significance of identifying their stage of development?
2. What are important areas to cover in the adolescent interview?
3. What issues of confidentiality and competence need to be discussed with adolescents before conducting the interview?
4. When should information be disclosed to others, despite issues of confidentiality?

Adolescence is a time of unique change. Unlike other periods in life when individuals have at least some knowledge or experience to guide them, adolescence is stereotypically characterized by feelings of physical awkwardness, emotional turmoil, and social isolation. Unfortunately, the teenage years are dreaded by most parents, who often feel ill equipped to handle the wide range of children's responses. So instead of "taking the bull by the horns," parents choose the route of quiet observation. They fully intend to "be there" for their children but wait to be approached. Hence, many adolescents do not have the guidance or advice of parents during the teenage years and prefer to spend their time alone or in the company of friends or acquaintances. Most adolescents pass through this period uneventfully. In fact, many individuals go through this period gladly, finally being permitted to drive a car or go out on a date.

Physicians must use a different approach when interviewing adolescents, since information must come directly from the teenager, rather than the parents. Unlike an interview with a younger pediatric patient, the adolescent interview should focus on several psychosocial issues that may be uncomfortable to discuss with the parent present. Each teenager should, therefore, be interviewed alone. The goal of the interview is the discovery of any problems that might interfere with a relatively smooth passage through adolescence.

STAGES OF ADOLESCENCE

Adolescents are stereotypically labeled as difficult, complex, time-consuming patients with problems or complaints that lead to uninteresting diagnoses. In addition, they are often accompanied by overbearing, demanding parents, or sometimes no parents at all.

The quality and quantity of information obtained during the medical and psychosocial interview can be greatly enhanced by taking developmental milestones into consideration. Adolescence can be divided into three developmental stages: early, middle, and late (Table 4–1). For example, interest in discussing long-term educational goals varies depending on the age of the adolescent. Most 18-year-olds are prepared to discuss college plans, specific vocational interests, and employment opportunities. In contrast, 12-year-olds are still anchored in the concreteness of early adolescence and often are ill prepared to discuss higher education. School experiences are much more important to this age group and should therefore be the focus of discussion. Peer pressure is most prominent during middle adolescence; 14-year-olds with friends who smoke cigarettes and drink beer probably use the same illicit materials.

Knowledge of these differences allows interviewers to more clearly explain instructions and diagnoses to teenagers. For example, 19-year-olds can better understand the effects of untreated or recurrent chlamydia cervicitis on long-term fertility than 13-year-olds. This is not to say that physicians should not tell sexually active 13-year-olds with chlamydia about these possible effects, but they should use more concrete wording and repeat the information at future visits. Age guidelines

TABLE 4–1. Developmental Milestones During Adolescence

	Early Adolescence (11–13 years)	Middle Adolescence (14–16 years)	Late Adolescence (17–21 years)
Thought processes	Concrete	± Abstract	Abstract
Parental supervision	+	±	−
Risk-taking behavior	+	±	−
Peer pressure	±	++	+

Modified from March, C.A., and M.S. Jay. Adolescents in the emergency department: an overview. Adolesc. Med. State Art Rev. 4:1, 1993.

are not rigid, however, and each interview should be individually tailored to the particular adolescent and the circumstances surrounding the visit.

ISSUES OF CONFIDENTIALITY AND COMPETENCE

The discussion of **confidentiality** can be approached in two ways. Each method has distinct advantages as well as disadvantages. Interviewers should use the approach that they find most comfortable; this allows conversation to flow more naturally.

The first approach involves informing adolescents at the beginning of the interview that most issues discussed are held in confidence and will not be repeated to anyone. Exceptions are suicidal or homicidal behavior and sexual or physical abuse. In any of these instances, other professionals are told of the disclosed information, and parents may ultimately find out. The advantages to this approach are that discussion of these "logistics" at the beginning of the interview is less awkward, and the ground rules are clear from the start. This contributes to an atmosphere of trust and honesty. The disadvantage is possible inhibition of adolescents who are unsure about disclosing particular incidents (e.g., those concerning sexual abuse); some teenagers are now almost certain not to share this information for fear of involving other professionals or family members. Interviewers should be nonjudgmental, reassuring, and patient in order to reduce the possibility of such an occurrence.

The second, less popular approach to the discussion of confidentiality involves informing adolescents at the end of the interview or when and if one of the exceptions to maintaining confidentiality arises. Proponents of this approach argue that adolescents tend to respond more honestly to questions when they do not believe physicians will inform others, including their parents or legal guardians. Physicians have a legal responsibility, however, to report sexual and physical abuse; in cases of suicidal or homicidal behavior, it is in the patient's best interest to inform other professionals of this disclosure. The disadvantage to this method is that these issues often arise at very emotional times during the interview, and it is difficult to interrupt the patient to discuss mandated reporting. If physicians wait until the end of the interview to inform adolescents about mandated reporting, however, patients may leave the office feeling deceived and probably will not return for future visits. Most health care providers prefer to inform adolescents at the onset of the interview about confidentiality with the hope that it contributes to the development of a trusting relationship.

Assessments of adolescents' ability to make health-related decisions is another important aspect of the interview. **Competence** is the ability to understand the significance of information and assess the alternatives and consequences sufficiently to then identify a preference. Various factors besides age must be considered such as level of maturity, intelligence, degree of independence, and presence of any chronic illness. This last factor is included because adolescents with chronic conditions have presumably already participated in decisions regarding their health care. Regardless, it may be difficult to assess competence from just one visit. It may not even be necessary to make that assessment emergently, except in certain cases such as pregnancy.

Although it is imperative to interview adolescents alone, every attempt should be made to involve parents in all health-related decisions. Although specific state laws allow physicians to treat minors in emergent situations and in cases of suspected venereal disease without parents' consent, physicians should urge adolescents to inform their parents of any problems disclosed during the interview. The ultimate decision rests with the adolescent. Physicians can offer to help, however, adolescents discuss delicate issues with parents by role-playing or by sitting in on the adolescent-parent conversation.

PSYCHOSOCIAL REVIEW OF SYSTEMS

A major part of the adolescent interview involves taking an adequate psychosocial history. The approach known by the acronym **HEADSSS** (**h**ome environment, **e**mployment and education, **a**ctivities, **d**rugs, **s**exual activity/sexuality, **s**uicide and depression, **s**afety) allows interviewers to evaluate the critical areas in adolescents' lives that may contribute to a less than optimal environment for normal growth and development (Questions Box). Questions about sexuality must be asked in a nondirected, nonjudgmental fashion, giving adolescents time to respond. This information is useful to assess risks for conditions such as HIV. In addition, an inquiry about both sexual and physical abuse is indicated during this part of the interview.

ISSUES THAT NEED IMMEDIATE ATTENTION

Many issues discussed during the psychosocial interview can be a source of anxiety for adolescents. Certain problems must be taken more seriously than others, and may demand immediate attention. Suicidal ideation, with or without a previous attempt, definitely requires a more in-depth analysis of the gravity of the problem. Physicians should make sure that adolescents feel they can make a verbal contract to call someone if they feel like hurting themselves. Mental health professionals should help assess these situations. Other issues that require immediate attention include possible danger to others, possible or confirmed pregnancy, and sexual or physical abuse.

CONCLUDING THE INTERVIEW

The adolescent interview should be conducted at a time when adolescents are relatively healthy and the interviewer has set aside time for a thorough discussion. All topics need not be addressed at one visit. Issues that arise at one visit can be readdressed at the next visit. The number of appointments needed to solve a particular problem is unlimited.

At the end of each visit, the interview should be summarized; any difficult topics should be mentioned, and the issue of confidentiality should be reviewed.

Questions: Talking to Adolescents: HEADSSS

H: Home environment
- With whom does the adolescent live?
- Have there been any recent changes in the living situation?
- How are things between parents at home?
- Are the parents employed?
- How does the adolescent get along with siblings?

E: Employment and education
- Is the adolescent currently in school?
- What are his or her favorite subjects?
- How is the adolescent performing academically?
- Has the adolescent ever been truant or expelled from school?
- Are the adolescent's friends attending school?
- What are the adolescent's future education/employment goals?

A: Activities
- What does the adolescent do in his or her spare time?
- What does the adolescent do for fun? Is the adolescent ever bored?
- With whom does the adolescent spend time?

D: Drugs
- Has the adolescent ever used any illicit drugs? Has the adolescent ever used tobacco? What about steroids? Alcohol?
- Is the adolescent still using these drugs? Are friends using or selling any drugs? Is someone in the family using drugs?

S: Sexual activity/sexuality
- What is the adolescent's sexual orientation?
- Is the adolescent sexually active?
  - If so, what was the age of the adolescent's sexual debut?
  - How many sexual partners has the adolescent had in his or her lifetime?
  - Does the adolescent have a history of STDs?
  - Does the adolescent (or the partner) use condoms?
  - Does the adolescent (or the partner) use other methods of contraception?
- Does the adolescent have a history of sexual or physical abuse?

S: Suicide/depression
- Is the adolescent ever sad or tearful? Tired and unmotivated?
- Has the adolescent ever felt that life is not worth living or ever thought of or tried to hurt himself or herself? More importantly, does the adolescent have a suicide plan or access to a firearm?

S: Safety
- Does the adolescent use a seat belt and bicycle helmet?
- Does the adolescent participate in high-risk situations?
- Is there a firearm in the adolescent's home? If so, does the adolescent know about firearm safety?

For more detailed information, see the reference by Goldenring and Cohen.

Adolescents should then be asked to identify a person whom they can trust or confide in should any problems arise before the next visit. In some instances, this issue may already have been addressed. Adolescents should also be given the opportunity to express any other concerns not covered in the interview and ask questions that may have arisen during the interview.

Physicians should frankly inform adolescents about any significant risk factors or risk-taking behaviors that have been identified. In addition, physicians should give adolescents positive feedback for strengths and accomplishments identified during the interview and acknowledge that things are going well. They should tell adolescents about available resources such as teen hotlines and offer follow-up visits or other opportunities to talk.

Case Resolution

The adolescent in the case history should first be informed about confidentiality and the specific exceptions to maintaining it. Nonthreatening topics such as home life, school, and outside activities should first be explored, followed by questions regarding sexuality, sexual activity, and illicit drug use. Suicidal behavior or depression and safety issues should also be reviewed.

Selected Readings

Alderman, E. M., and A. R. Fleischman. Should adolescents make their own health-care choices? Contemp. Pediatr. 10:65–82, 1993.

Council on Scientific Affairs, American Medical Association. Confidential health services for adolescents. J.A.M.A. 268:1420–1424, 1993.

Coupey, S. M. Interviewing adolescents. Pediatr. Clin. North Am. 44:1349–1364, 1997.

Ehrman, W. G., and S. C. Matson. Approach to assessing adolescents on serious or sensitive issues. Pediatr. Clin. North Am. 45:189–204, 1998.

English, A. Treating adolescents: legal and ethical considerations. Med. Clin. North Am. 74:1097, 1990.

Epner, J. E., P. B. Levenberg, and M. E. Schoeny. Primary care providers' responsiveness to health-risk behaviors reported by adolescent patients. Arch. Pediatr. Adol. Med. 152:774–780, 1998.

Goldenring, J. M., and E. Cohen. Getting into adolescent heads. Contemp. Pediatr. 5:75–90, 1988.

Schuster, M. A., R. M. Bell, L. P. Peterson, and D. E. Kanouse. Communication between adolescents and physicians about sexual behavior and risk prevention. Arch. Pediatr. Adolesc. Med. 150:906–913, 1996.

CHAPTER 5

TELEPHONE MANAGEMENT

Iris Wagman Borowsky, M.D., Ph.D.

H_x The mother of an otherwise healthy 10-month-old girl calls and tells you that her daughter has a fever. The girl's rectal temperature has been 103–104° F (39.4–40.0° C) for the past 2 days. Although she is cranky with the fever, she plays normally after receiving acetaminophen. The girl is eating well and has no runny nose, cough, vomiting, diarrhea, or rash.

Questions

1. How do telephone and face-to-face encounters between physicians and patients differ?
2. What are some general guidelines for effective doctor-patient communication over the telephone?
3. What historical information is necessary for appropriate telephone management?
4. What points are important to cover in home treatment advice?

Parents frequently call their pediatricians seeking medical advice about their children. It is estimated that pediatricians spend over 25% of their total practice time engaged in "telephone medicine." Telephone medicine serves two purposes: (1) it provides a service and (2) it controls costs and overcrowding by reducing unnecessary visits to the office and emergency department. Most calls concern upper respiratory symptoms, fever, rash, trauma, or GI complaints—the same problems most commonly seen in the office.

Telephone management of illnesses differs in that it requires pediatricians to give advice based on history alone and precludes the opportunity to see the child, much less do a careful physical examination. For example, a practitioner in the emergency department who does not know the patient or family may choose to see the child if questions about the child's general health or the feasibility of continued contact with the family arise. On the other hand, a primary care physician who knows the patient and family and can follow the child's progress by telephone may advise home management for a child with a similar history. Pediatric practice settings, whether in an emergency department or primary care office, should have an organized approach to telephone care. In addition to physicians, nurse practitioners, and physician's assistants, telephone care systems may include trained and supervised nurses and nonmedical office staff using protocols.

TELEPHONE COMMUNICATION SKILLS

Parents commonly call their pediatricians because they are worried about their child. The friendly voice of a health care worker who is ready to lend an ear goes a long way toward reassuring an anxious parent. Calls should begin with a "verbal handshake." Staff should identify themselves and the place where the call is received and offer to help. They should learn the caller's name, his or her relationship to the child, and the child's name and gender; these names, as well as the child's gender, should be used in the conversation, thereby creating a more personal atmosphere.

Telephone calls for medical advice are often received in busy environments such as emergency departments or clinics where patients are waiting to be seen. It is easy to be abrupt under these circumstances and not give complete attention to callers. If calls are not emergencies, practitioners can take the caller's telephone number and return the call as soon as possible. If callers do not feel that their concerns have been fully acknowledged, they are likely to feel dissatisfied, even if they are given sound advice. Furthermore, research on doctor-patient relationships suggests that lack of friendliness or warmth in the doctor-patient relationship and patient dissatisfaction are associated with noncompliance with medical advice. Interestingly, studies show that the length of a patient visit does not correlate with patient satisfaction. Telephone encounters do not necessarily have to be lengthy; the average length of a call is reported to be 3–5 minutes, depending on the setting. Calls must be pleasant, however, and they must address callers' concerns. Open-ended questions such as "Tell me about your child's illness" or "Are there any other symptoms?" are useful at the beginning of a call because they give callers an opportunity to explain the situation without interruptions.

Establishing rapport over the telephone is more difficult than in person because the practitioner is limited to verbal communication. In face-to-face encounters, physicians can use words as well as means of nonverbal communication such as facial expressions, eye contact, gesturing, and touch to convey warmth and empathy. Practitioners should use various aspects of **verbal communication** to convey sincere interest in callers' concerns, and they should pay attention to these verbal cues in callers. Many components of verbal communication, in addition to words themselves, including vocal expression, pace, articulation, tone, volume, and pauses, affect telephone interactions. Health care professionals should speak clearly and use vocabulary that callers understand; **medical jargon should be avoided.** A friendly yet respectful tone and a calm, professional manner should be maintained.

Careful listening is crucial to obtaining the information necessary to make medical decisions over the telephone. One of the major goals of health care professionals is to recognize and respond to callers' main concerns and expectations. This can be difficult, because most callers do not specifically tell their major concerns to their physicians. Researchers have found the following questions useful in the identification of parents' chief concerns: "What worries you the most about [use child's name] illness?" and "Why does that worry you?"

For callers who ramble, health care professionals may need to focus the conversation. Asking the question "What can I do to help?" should clarify the reason for the call. If information needs to be verified, practitioners can summarize what they have heard and ask if they have understood correctly.

Angry callers may elicit defensive or confrontational behavior from health care professionals. Responding to anger with arguments, however, is time-consuming, stressful, and pointless. Practitioners should be warm and understanding so that callers who want to discuss their feelings are comfortable. Acknowledging anger may encourage open discussion and problem-solving (e.g., "You sound upset. Is there anything I can do to help?"). Empathizing with callers (e.g., "I don't blame you for being upset," "That must have been very frustrating") may also help.

Practitioners can build confidence in callers by complimenting them on the way they have handled things so far (e.g., "You did the right thing by giving [child's name] Tylenol and a lukewarm sponge bath for the fever. That is exactly what I would have done" or "I'm glad that you called about this"). They may even be able to offer reassurance to parents who are not managing their child's illness correctly by commenting that many parents try the same treatment. A different treatment approach can then be suggested.

Before the end of the conversation, callers can be given an opportunity to ask questions and encouraged to call again if additional problems occur.

TELEPHONE HISTORY TAKING

How much history should be obtained over the telephone? Enough information should be gathered to make an appropriate decision. Questions should be directed at **determining whether an emergency exists** and **making a diagnosis.** For example, if the mother of a 20-day-old girl reports that her daughter has a temperature of 102° F (38.9° C), the infant must be seen immediately. If diarrhea is the chief complaint, some additional information would be helpful before giving advice (e.g., "How many bowel movements did the girl have in the last 24 hours? Is there any blood in the diarrhea? Does she have a fever? Is she drinking less than usual? Is there any decrease in urine output?"). An

older child with the same chief complaint of fever may be safely managed at home, depending on the answers to other questions about additional symptoms.

Pediatricians typically follow an organized approach to history taking for acute care visits that includes the chief complaint, history of present illness, pertinent review of systems, medical history, and family and social history. A similarly **organized framework** should be used to obtain a history over the telephone (Questions Box). Specific questions should then be asked to clarify the child's condition and obtain all the information necessary to make a good decision. A child's medical history may affect a practitioner's management of the current problem. For example, knowing that a child who has been exposed to chickenpox has asthma and is receiving steroids or has leukemia is crucial in providing the appropriate telephone advice.

Practitioners can refer to several texts on pediatric telephone decision making (see Selected Readings). These books outline protocols for common chief complaints to serve as guides for history taking and management over the telephone. The most efficient way to provide such medical advice is to obtain critical information that affects decisions about diagnosis and management instead of asking all possible questions. For example, with a child who is vomiting or has diarrhea, the state of hydration is critical; with a cough, the occurrence of breathing difficulty; and with head trauma, loss of consciousness. Methods of teaching telephone management skills include role playing, listening to mock calls by "simulated" mothers, and reviewing tapes of actual calls.

Because most childhood illnesses are mild and self-limited, evaluation of the safety of medical advice obtained over the telephone requires large samples to detect poor outcomes associated with mismanagement. Research has described a "wellness bias" in which practitioners, who primarily see patients with mild, self-limited illnesses, may downplay the severity of reported symptoms and choose the most benign diagnostic possibility. This bias may be more pronounced in a telephone encounter, where the physician cannot see the child. One study reported telephone encounters in which physicians seemed to make a decision early in the conversation and then "shut out" additional information that should have led to the consideration of more serious diagnoses. The safest approach is to always have a high index of suspicion for a serious condition. Questions can then be asked to confirm or dispel those suspicions.

Questions: Telephone Management

- How old is the child?
- What is the child's chief problem? What are the child's symptoms?
- How long has the child had these symptoms?
- How is the child acting?
- Does the child have any chronic illnesses?
- Is the child taking any medications?
- What is the caller most worried about?

TELEPHONE ADVICE

Pediatricians should formulate an **assessment and management plan** based on the child's history. If the situation is an emergency, this should be explained to the caller, and appropriate follow-up plans should be made (i.e., sending an ambulance for life-threatening conditions such as respiratory depression or uncontrollable bleeding, advising the caller to bring the child by car to the emergency department or physician's office within a specified amount of time for potentially dangerous complaints, such as right lower quadrant pain or possible fracture). If the call is not an emergency, then health care professionals must decide if and when the child should be seen by a physician and the appropriate home treatment.

Research shows that parents need and expect to receive an explanation of their child's illness. Practitioners should clearly state what the child's illness seems to be, what probably caused it, and what the parents can expect (e.g., length of time that the child is likely to be sick, additional symptoms that may appear).

Before giving any treatment advice, health care professionals should ask callers the following questions: "What have you done so far?," "Have you given the child any medications?," and "How is this treatment working?" If the therapy appears appropriate, callers should be complimented and encouraged to continue the treatment. The regimen should be modified as indicated. Instructions for home treatment should be clear and as easy to implement as possible. If the instructions are complicated or lengthy, callers may want to write them down. When prescribing medication, ask if the child has any known drug allergies, and give the dose, frequency of administration, and information about possible side effects. Practitioners should verify that the caller can follow the telephone advice (e.g., a parent has a thermometer and knows how to use it). If pediatricians plan to check up on children by telephone, they should confirm that callers (or relatives or neighbors) have a telephone and record the number.

Practitioners should confirm that callers understand the information and instructions and agree with the plan. Asking questions such as "What questions do you have?" encourages callers to raise uncertainties and ask for needed clarification. Most importantly, if the decision is to manage at home, callers should always receive specific instructions about when to call back (e.g., child has fever for more than 2 days, irritability, decreased urination). Parents who seem unduly anxious or uncomfortable with home treatment should be given the opportunity to have their child seen by a physician.

DOCUMENTATION

All calls for medical advice should be documented in a telephone log book or the child's medical record, for both medical reasons (e.g., better follow-up, improved continuity of care) and legal purposes. The form used for documentation should include the date and time of the call; the name, identity, and telephone number of the caller; the name and age of the child; the chief complaint; other symptoms; possible diagnoses; advice given; and the name of the person who took the call.

Case Resolution

In the case history at the beginning of this chapter, the pediatrician learns several facts that lead to the recommendation that the child be seen that day (the next day if the call is made at night). These facts include the child's age, the height and duration of the fever, and lack of any symptoms of localized infection.

Selected Readings

Baker, R. C., and B. D. Schmitt. Pediatric Telephone Advice. Philadelphia, Lippincott-Raven, 1998.

Benjamin, J. T. Pediatric resident's telephone triage experience: relevant to general pediatric practice? Arch. Pediatr. Adoles. Med. 151:1254–1257, 1997.

Brown, J. L. Pediatric Telephone Medicine: Principles, Triage and Advice, 2nd ed. Philadelphia, J.B. Lippincott, 1994.

Katz, H. P. Telephone Medicine: Triage and Training—A Handbook for Primary Health Care Professionals. Philadelphia, F. A. Davis, 1990.

Kosower, E., S. H. Inkelis, and J. S. Seidel. Telephone T.A.L.K.: a telephone communication program. Pediatr. Emerg. Care 7:76–79, 1991.

Pert, J. C., T. W. Furth, and H. P. Katz. A 10-year experience in pediatric after-hours telecommunications. Curr. Opin. Pediatr. 8:181–187, 1996.

Sebring, R. H., and M. Gueco. Quality improvement: an ACQIP exercise on telephone advice. Pediatr. Rev. 18:103–106, 1997.

Studdiford, J. S., K. N. Panitch, D. A. Snyderman, and M. E. Pharr. The telephone in primary care. Prim. Care Clin. Off. Pract. 23:83–102, 1996.

Wheeler, S. Q., and J. H. Windt. Telephone Triage: Theory, Practice, and Protocol Development. Albany, NY, Delmar, 1993.

CHAPTER 6

PRINCIPLES OF PEDIATRIC THERAPEUTICS

Elizabeth A. Edgerton, M.D., M.P.H.

Hx An 18-month-old girl who has had a cough, runny nose, and fever for 2 days is brought to your clinic for evaluation. The previous night, she awoke from sleep crying and pulling at her ear. Her brother has also been suffering from a cold. The patient has no other symptoms. Her mother states that she has a history of previous ear infections; the most recent occurred 2 months ago. The last time the patient took amoxicillin, she broke out in hives. Otherwise, the patient has no significant past medical history. The family is especially concerned about their daughter's illness and the need for medication because they are leaving on a camping trip tomorrow. In addition, the mother wants a medication that will treat the cough, since the family will be sleeping in the same tent.

On physical examination, the patient is febrile and has clear rhinorrhea. The ear examination reveals a red, bulging, nonmobile tympanic membrane in one ear, while the other ear appears normal. The remainder of the examination is benign.

Questions

1. How does one determine the most appropriate medication for a patient's condition?
2. How does one deal with the expectation of the family for a medication?
3. How does a history of a previous reaction to a medication influence decision-making?
4. How do factors such as school, work, and family plans affect the choice of medication?
5. What resources are available to obtain information on therapeutic effectiveness, costs, side effects, and interactions?

The use of medications, both prescription and over-the-counter, is common in pediatrics. Antibiotics are the most common medications prescribed, and as many as 50% of 3-year-olds take some over-the-counter medication. Since 1962, the Food and Drug Administration (FDA) has required drugs to be proven safe and effective before they can be marketed. Unfortunately, research in the area of pediatric therapeutics has lagged behind that of adult medicine. Only 25% of the drugs currently marketed in the United States can be advertised as safe and effective for the pediatric population. This does not mean that the other 75% of drugs are unsafe for children but that their use in children is based on studies of adult use. The consequences of not fully studying the clinical effectiveness and safety profile of therapeutics in the pediatric population can lead to potentially harmful outcomes. Examples include vaginal cancer associated with *in utero* exposure to diethylstilbestrol, aplastic anemia with chloramphenicol use, kernicterus with sulfonamide use in neonates, and retinopathy of prematurity with oxygen use in premature infants. The physiologic and drug elimination mechanisms in infants and children are frequently different from those in adults and can produce significant differences in drug toxicity.

In pediatrics, many diseases affect only a small number of patients, making it difficult to study the effectiveness of a therapeutic agent. Often a drug has been proven effective in adults, but appropriate studies have not been conducted in children. When a drug has an actual or potential benefit for a child but has not been approved by the FDA for pediatric use, it is known as a "therapeutic orphan." FDA regulations regarding the safety and effectiveness of a medication for pediatric use often lag behind clinical experience; therefore, the physician must rely on results from adult studies to decide whether or not medication is appropriate for a sick child. The physician must balance the benefits of a medication for a child with a serious illness with the potential risks of using a medication that has not been fully evaluated in pediatrics. The FDA is attempting to improve this situation by providing incentives for developing and studying drugs for rare diseases, and by adopting guidelines for studying the effect of patient age on the safety and effectiveness of medications. In addition, researchers are now required to justify their exclusion of study subjects on the basis of their age.

PRINCIPLES OF THERAPEUTICS

A drug or therapeutic can be defined as any substance that is ingested, absorbed, or injected that alters the body's function. This includes over-the-counter medications, homeopathic substances, illicit substances, and prescription drugs. Each drug has a different safety profile and level of regulation, depending on its category. The most regulated and standardized drugs are those prescribed by a physician. Homeopathic substances often lack any standardization, safety testing, and regulation; and, of course, illicit drugs such as heroin and cocaine receive no quality testing at all.

Choosing the most appropriate therapeutic is a complex process, involving a number of factors physicians must consider (Table 6–1).

Patient Characteristics

The **age** of a patient affects how a medication is absorbed, distributed, and excreted. For example, because their gastrointestinal tract, kidneys, and liver are not fully developed, neonates might not absorb oral

---

TABLE 6–1.   Factors in Choosing the Appropriate Therapeutic

Patient Characteristics Age Past medical history Allergies Use of other medications	**Safety Profile** Therapeutic index Food and drug interactions
Diagnosis	**Patient Compliance** Taste Understanding of purpose of drug Storage Side effects
Cost-effectiveness Drug availability Generic drug availability	

---

medications as effectively as older infants, and the half-lives of medications requiring renal or hepatic excretion might be longer in newborns than in adolescents. It is essential, therefore, to consult a drug reference that indicates age-appropriate routes and doses.

Patients' past medical history and **present medical conditions** influence the choice of drug or route of administration because of their impact on the effectiveness or toxicity of a drug. For example, children with short bowel syndrome can have difficulty absorbing oral medications, depending on which portion of the bowel was removed. Children with mental retardation who are given CNS-altering medications can be difficult to monitor for changes in mental status. In addition, children with glucose-6-phosphate dehydrogenase (G6PD) deficiency can suffer from drug-induced hemolytic anemia when given certain drugs, such as sulfonamides. Malnourished children are at greater risk for drug toxicity because their lower serum albumin levels affect the binding of certain drugs, leading to an increased amount of free drug in circulation compared with that in well-nourished children. These examples are not exhaustive of medical conditions that can alter the effect of a medication but rather illustrate the diverse issues that need to be considered.

Before prescribing any medication, physicians should question patients and their families about any previous reactions to drugs and obtain detailed information about the symptoms and medications involved in these reactions. **Drug allergies** are those reactions that have an immunologic basis. Of the four types of immune mechanisms associated with drug allergies, IgE-mediated reactions are of greatest concern because they can result in anaphylaxis, a life-threatening condition. Adverse reactions can be idiosyncratic or non-immune-mediated. A side effect is an expected but undesirable consequence of taking the medication. Families often will attribute any symptom the patient suffered while taking a medication to a drug allergy. It is therefore important to know which side effects are associated with a medication in order to determine whether an allergy is present or not. Any medication that has been associated with an allergic reaction (e.g., skin eruptions, swelling, urticaria, respiratory difficulty) in a given patient should not be used again without consulting a specialist.

Finally, knowing what **other medications** a patient is taking can affect the choice of therapeutic. The mechanism of metabolism of one drug can affect the metab-olism of another. Drug metabolism is divided into two types: **phase I reactions** include oxidation, reduction, and hydrolysis; and **phase II reactions** entail adding subgroups to a drug. Other drugs can affect reactions in either type of metabolism. For example, the cytochrome P-450 system is involved in many aspects of oxidation. The enzyme activity of this system can be induced or inhibited by one drug and as a result increase or decrease the rate of metabolism of a second drug. Drugs that can inhibit the P-450 system include cimetidine and erythromycin, and inducers include phenobarbital and phenytoin. All these drugs are commonly used in the pediatric population. While drug interactions are not a contraindication to the use of a therapeutic, the dose and serum levels of a drug may need to be closely monitored when the patient is taking a medication that has a potential interaction. Drug interactions are listed in the medication's package label insert, *Physicians' Desk Reference (PDR)*, and in clinical pharmacology textbooks. Pharmacists may serve as consultants to physicians caring for children taking multiple medications.

Diagnosis

Once a condition or diagnosis has been defined, it is important to choose the most appropriate therapeutic. Choosing the appropriate medication depends on understanding the condition being treated as well as the specifics of that condition for each age group. Commonly, a patient has an infection that requires treatment with an antibiotic specific to the organism causing the infection. For a patient diagnosed with a group A streptococcal pharyngitis, a gram-positive organism, penicillin G, penicillin V, erythromycin, or a first-generation cephalosporin are all acceptable choices. Although tetracycline and sulfonamides can be effective in treating patients with gram-positive infections, tetracycline is contraindicated in young children, and sulfonamides do not eradicate the group A streptococcal infection even though they can be effective in preventing recurrence of infection. The duration of treatment for a child can be different than for adults. For example, in treating urinary tract infections (UTIs), trimethoprim-sulfamethoxazole is used for both children and adults. While adults with a simple UTI may receive only a 1- to 3-day course of treatment, children receive 7–10 days of treatment because of the high recurrence of infection that has been observed with a shorter duration of treatment.

Cost-effectiveness

Cost-effectiveness is defined as the best outcome per unit cost. The outcome is the treatment of a condition or alleviation of a symptom; the cost includes the price of the medication and the time spent by the physician and family. For instance, one drug may cost less but be less effective, so that, in the long run, it costs more to the patient in return visits to the doctor. Many physicians practice in settings where the pharmacy (known as a formulary) provides only a limited selection of medications for each condition. Thus, the physician's choice of a cost-effective drug might depend on which drugs are available in the formulary and the efficacy of those drugs in treating the condition. In addition, many families have limited insurance coverage for prescriptions and may have to incur the total cost of a medication. Thus, an appropriate drug choice could be influenced by the out-of-pocket cost to the family. The perceived cost-effectiveness of a therapeutic is different for each situation and depends on the external factors affecting the physician and the family.

Safety Profile

The safety profile of a medication is the balance between its benefits and its potential risks. The risks can be dependent on the duration of treatment, dose, or interactions with other medications. Using the **therapeutic index** is one way to quantify the risk associated with a specific dose. The therapeutic index is the difference between the dose that provides a desired effect and the dose that provides an undesired effect. For example, a medication with a wide therapeutic index is one in which a desired effect is achieved with a dose much lower than that required to produce a toxic effect. In general, a medication with a wide therapeutic index, such as acetaminophen, is considered safer than a medication with a narrow therapeutic index. The higher the morbidity and mortality associated with a condition, the smaller the accepted therapeutic index can be.

Food-drug interactions and **drug-drug interactions** are other risks that can be anticipated. These are best delineated in pharmacologic reference books. There are also risks that are independent of the dose of the therapeutic called **idiosyncratic effects**. These are unexpected and usually unpreventable risks associated with a medication.

Patient Compliance

Patient compliance is dependent upon the convenience of administering and taking the medication, the patient's and caregiver's comprehension of the medication's purpose, and the discomfort caused by side effects.

Since children are dependent on their caregivers to administer medication, it is crucial that caregivers know why the drug has been prescribed, how it must be dispensed, and why it must be given for the specified length of time. For instance, if caregivers don't understand the need for completing the course of medication in order for it to be effective, they might administer it only until the symptoms resolve. In order to ensure accurate dosing, physicians should show how to dispense the medication and then ask caregivers to repeat the procedure. Such a simple intervention can make an important difference in obtaining compliance, which will ultimately influence the effectiveness of the medication.

The taste and texture of a medication is also an important consideration in pediatrics. Children may not be able to understand the importance of taking a medication and may refuse to take it because they don't like its taste. Physicians should know the taste and consistency of the medications and be prepared to suggest ways of hiding the bad taste. Drugs used in adult populations are often not available in pleasant-tasting suspension formulas; therefore, pills or bad-tasting suspensions might need to be blended into food before children will take them.

DRUG DOSING

Most medications used in the adult population are based on a standard dose for individuals regardless of age or size. In pediatrics, a patient's size and metabolism vary with age such that dosing is usually based on body size. Either the weight of the patient or body surface area can be used to determine a drug dose. When a drug dose is determined by weight, it represents a proportion of the adult dose; when a child reaches adult weight, the dosing is changed to a standard dose. This usually occurs when the patient approaches 40–50 kg. Body surface area is more commonly used for drugs with a narrow therapeutic index such as chemotherapy medications.

Once a drug is identified, the appropriate dosing schedule must be determined. Dosing guidelines can be presented as a total dose per 24 hours or as an amount per dose. Usually a range is given per unit weight, and then the physician must determine the amount of medication based on the concentration of the therapeutic agent. An example for dosing acetaminophen for a 1-year-old child is given in Box 6–1.

BOX 6–1.   Dosing

A 1-year-old is suffering from a fever, and the family wants to know how much acetaminophen to give their child. She weighs 11.2 kg. The recommended dose of acetaminophen is 10–15 mg/kg. Acetaminophen drops are sold in a concentration of 80 mg/0.8 mL, and the suspension is sold in a concentration of 160 mg/5 mL.

1. Determine the amount of medication needed by multiplying the weight of the child by the recommended dose.

$$11.2 \text{ kg} \times 10 \text{ mg/kg} = 112 \text{ mg acetaminophen}$$

2. Determine the volume of medication based on the concentration of acetaminophen to be used. Either the dropper or the suspension can be used.

$$\text{Dosing volume} = (\text{amount of medication}) \div (\text{concentration of medication})$$

Dropper:

$$\text{Dosing volume} = 112 \text{ mg} \div 80 \text{ mg/0.8 mL}$$
$$= (112 \times 0.8)/80$$
$$= 1.12 \text{ mL}$$

(This can be rounded off to 1.2 mL, equivalent to 1.5 droppers.)

Suspension:

$$\text{Dosing volume} = 112 \text{ mg} \div 160 \text{ mg/5 mL}$$
$$= (112 \times 5)/160$$
$$= 3.5 \text{ mL}$$

The family should be instructed to give their daughter either 1.2 mL using the drops or 3.5 mL of acetaminophen suspension by mouth every 4–6 hours as needed for fever.

THERAPEUTIC REFERENCES

Various resources provide information on drug uses, dosing, side effects, and costs. The *Physicians' Desk Reference* is a comprehensive listing of FDA-approved prescription and commonly used over-the-counter drugs that provides a description of the drug, pharmacology, indications and contraindications, adverse reactions, drug interactions, and manufacturer name. The *Medical Letter* is a periodical that reviews drugs, citing current research on risks and benefits, as well as cost comparisons of newly released drugs with those already approved for similar indications. Pocket manuals that are specific to pediatrics include the *Pediatric Drug Handbook* and *Harriet Lane Manual*. Both of these references provide pediatrics-specific dosing guidelines and are updated every few years.

Case Resolution

After obtaining the history and performing a physical examination, the pediatrician determines that the patient has an ear infection. Many antibiotics are effective for treating an ear infection, so the question is, which one to choose? According to the principles of prescribing, an antibiotic that treats the organisms causing the ear infection is needed. This could be amoxicillin, trimethoprim-sulfamethoxazole, erythromycin with sulfisoxazole, azithromycin, or a second-generation cephalosporin. The patient's history of an allergic reaction to amoxicillin and the family not having access to a refrigerator rule out the use of amoxicillin or a second-generation cephalosporin. Of the remaining options, erythromycin with sulfisoxazole is the least convenient because it requires dosing four times a day, whereas trimethoprim-sulfamethoxazole and azithromycin require dosing twice a day and once a day, respectively. Azithromycin would be the best choice except that the family's insurance does not cover prescriptions. Being a newer drug, azithromycin is several times more expensive than trimethoprim-sulfamethoxazole.

In this situation, trimethoprim-sulfamethoxazole is the best choice to treat the patient's ear infection. It requires only twice a day dosing, is pleasant tasting, does not need refrigeration, and is relatively inexpensive. The family needs to be told that the cough should improve with the treatment of the infection and that it is important to complete the course of antibiotics in order to treat the infection rather than the symptoms. While this case illustrates several obvious and straightforward constraints, it is important to emphasize that choosing an appropriate medication is dependent on both the intrinsic needs of the patient and extrinsic factors that can affect compliance and ultimately the effectiveness of the medication.

Selected Readings

Berlin, C. M. Advances in pediatric pharmacology and toxicology. *In* Barness, L. A., et al. Advances in Pediatrics. St. Louis, Mosby-Year Book. Adv. Pediatr. 43:545–574, 1997.

Choice of antimicrobial drugs. Med. Lett. Drugs Ther. 40(1023), 1998.

Katzung, B. G. Basic and Clinical Pharmacology, 6th ed., Stamford, CT, Appleton & Lange, 1995.

McMahon, S. R., M. E. Rimsza, and R. C. Bay. Parents can dose liquid medication accurately. Pediatrics 100:330–333, 1997.

Nightingale, C. H., and R. Quintiliani. Cost of oral antibiotic therapy. Pharmacotherapy 17(2):302–307, 1997.

Papp, C. M. Drug therapy. *In* Hay, W. W., et al. Current Pediatric Diagnosis and Treatment, 13th ed., Stamford, CT, Appleton & Lange, 1997, pp. 1116–1123.

Peter, G. (ed.). 1997 Red Book: Report of the Committee on Infectious Diseases, 24th ed. Elk Grove Village, IL: American Academy of Pediatrics, 1997.

Rane, A. Drug disposition and action in infants and children. *In* Yaffee, S. J., and J. V. Aranda (eds.). Pediatric Pharmacology: Therapeutic Principles in Practice, 2nd ed. Philadelphia, W. B. Saunders, 1992, pp. 10–21.

Yaffee, S. J., and J. V. Aranda. Introduction and historical perspectives. *In* Yaffee, S. J., and J. V. Aranda (eds.). Pediatric Pharmacology: Therapeutic Principles in Practice, 2nd ed. Philadelphia, W. B. Saunders, 1992, pp. 3–9.

CHAPTER 7

NEONATAL EXAMINATION AND NURSERY VISIT

Monica Sifuentes, M.D.

Hx You are performing a discharge examination on a 1-day-old infant, who was born at 39 weeks' gestation to a 28-year-old healthy primigravida via normal vaginal delivery. There were no complications. The infant weighed 7 lb, 1 oz (3200 g) and was 19.7 inches (50 cm) long at birth. The mother received prenatal care beginning at 10 weeks' gestation; had no prenatal problems, including infections; and used no drugs, alcohol, or tobacco during the pregnancy. Her blood type is O positive. She is negative for the hepatitis B surface antigen and nonreactive for syphilis. The father is also healthy.

On physical examination, the infant is average size-for-gestational-age with a length and head circumference in the 50th percentile. Aside from small bilateral subconjunctival hemorrhages, the rest of the physical examination is entirely normal.

Questions

1. What parts of the maternal history are important to review before performing the infant's physical examination?
2. What aspects of the physical examination of newborns are essential to explain to parents?
3. What physical findings mandate a more extensive work-up prior to discharge?
4. What are important points to cover with parents at the discharge examination of a normal term newborn?
5. What laboratory studies, if any, should be performed prior to discharge?

The purpose of the newborn nursery visit is to answer the question foremost in a parent's mind: "Is the baby normal?" By performing a physical examination in the parents' presence during the infant's first 24 hours of life, pediatricians can play a major role in allaying parental anxiety. In addition, medical problems that the newborn may experience in this important transitional period to extrauterine life may be detected. Treatment can be initiated, if necessary, before discharge from the nursery.

PEDIATRIC PRENATAL VISIT

Ideally, the pediatrician has spoken with the parents at a prenatal visit before meeting them in the hospital. This meeting provides a time when the parents are able to interview the physician as well as the rest of the office staff regarding general policies and procedures for well child appointments, sick visits, and contacting the physician after hours. It also is a time to discuss what will take place at the hospital and explain the role of allied health professionals (e.g., lactation specialists) in the overall care of the mother and newborn. For pediatricians and other health care practitioners, the prenatal visit is a time to gather vital medical information regarding the current pregnancy, inquire about any problems with previous deliveries, and review any pertinent family history. In addition, it is important that physicians be sensitive to cultural rituals or ceremonies surrounding the birth of an infant and inquire about any specific familial preferences before delivery. Whether the infant is born at a birthing center or in the more traditional hospital setting, arrangements should be made to accommodate the wishes of the family. The prenatal visit also allows physicians to assess any psychosocial issues that may negatively influence initial maternal-infant bonding, such as maternal drug use, paternal uninvolvement, or the absence of a supportive social network. Other issues such as breast-feeding, circumcision, and child passenger safety can also be introduced.

NEONATAL NURSERY VISIT

The timing of the newborn visit and its length depend on several factors, including the type of delivery (vaginal delivery or cesarean section), the history of prenatal care, and the occurrence of any perinatal complications, such as severe, prolonged bradycardia or meconium aspiration. These complications may warrant early neonatal examination in the nursery. Other reasons for a more lengthy initial visit include suspected congenital anomalies (e.g., congenital heart disease, hydronephrosis) as noted on prenatal fetal ultrasound, a history of prematurity, the presence of maternal fever or sepsis, ABO or Rh incompatibility, and any evidence of infant drug withdrawal.

EVALUATION

Perinatal History

The prenatal history and results of maternal laboratory tests, such as blood type, RPR status, and chlamydial and gonococcal cultures, should be noted (Questions Box). Perinatal events should then be reviewed before performing the physical examination of the neonate. This review helps the physician focus the examination on findings consistent with the maternal history. The occurrence of any unusual circumstances surrounding the delivery must also be explained to the parents at this time. They may have been very puzzled by a sudden change in plans such as the need for an emergent cesarean section. It is also important to be prepared to discuss the medical implications of such events and to address any concerns the parents have about the newborn infant.

Physical Examination

Every attempt should be made to perform the neonatal physical examination at the bedside. This gives the physician an opportunity to meet with parents and gives parents a chance to have all their initial questions answered immediately. In certain circumstances, such as when the infant is premature or when the mother is particularly exhausted postpartum, an initial bedside

---

Questions: Neonatal Examination

- Did the mother receive prenatal care? If so, since what month of gestation?
- Were all prenatal studies normal?
- Does either parent have a history of STDs, such as syphilis, gonorrhea, or herpes?
- Does either parent have a history of alcohol, tobacco, or illicit drug use?
- Did the mother take any prescribed or over-the-counter medications routinely during pregnancy?
- Did the mother have any complications, such as bleeding or decreased fetal movement, during the pregnancy?
- Is the mother planning to breast-feed?
- Does the neonate have any siblings? If so, what are their ages?
- Is anyone available to help with the new baby or siblings?

---

examination may be impossible to perform. In any event, physicians or other health care providers should speak to parents about the results once the examination has been completed.

The neonatal examination should be performed with the infant completely unclothed and the infant's body temperature maintained. A search for congenital anomalies is the priority. The infant's birth weight, length, and head circumference should be plotted; physicians should keep in mind that these measurements are often made in the delivery room and may be subject to error. Temperature, respiratory rate, and heart rate should be reviewed via the nursery record.

The infant's overall appearance should be noted, particularly for the presence of any dysmorphic features. Physicians should determine whether the infant looks normal or has any abnormal facial features such as low set ears and widely spaced eyes.

Skin

The presence and location of any rashes or birthmarks should be carefully described and pointed out to the parents; the particular location of the lesion may aid in its diagnosis. Skin color should also be noted, such as the presence of jaundice or blue-black macules called mongolian spots.

Head

Head size and shape, including the size of the fontanelle and the position of the sutures, should be evaluated. A cephalohematoma, which is a subperiosteal bleed that does not cross the suture line, appears as a unilateral lump on the side of the head and can be quite disfiguring. This should be differentiated from a caput succedaneum, which occurs at the crown of the head crossing the midline, and can be indented by pressure. Both conditions occur commonly, and resolve spontaneously (but are often a source of concern to parents).

Eyes

The eyes should be evaluated for subconjunctival hemorrhages, extraocular movements, and the presence of red reflexes. Any difficulty in obtaining a red reflex should be taken seriously, because conditions such as congenital cataracts are important to diagnose early in life.

Ears

The placement, size, and shape of the pinnae should be noted as well, along with any preauricular pits or appendages. The presence of a significant auricular abnormality suggests an associated renal anomaly.

Nose

The nose should be checked carefully for patency. Choanal atresia is an important condition to rule out, because infants are obligate nose breathers until 3 months of age.

Mouth

The oropharynx should be examined closely for any defects in the hard or soft palate. A bifid uvula may indicate a submucosal defect of the soft palate that may be difficult to appreciate without palpation (see Chapter 50, Craniofacial Anomalies). Common normal findings in the oropharynx, including Epstein's pearls located at the midline on the hard palate and epithelial cysts along the gum line, should also be noted. Loose natal teeth should be removed to prevent the possibility of aspiration (see Chapter 51, Common Oral Lesions).

Chest

The neck should be palpated for sternocleidomastoid hematomas and the clavicles for fractures, especially in infants who are large-for-gestational-age. Chest wall deformities such as a pectus excavatum should be noted. The presence of breast buds and supernumerary nipples are of no clinical consequence, although widely spaced nipples suggest Turner's syndrome.

Heart

Cardiac murmurs should be appreciated and documented. The presence of a murmur does not always indicate complex congenital heart disease, however. Each case should be evaluated on an individual basis, and advice from specialists in pediatric cardiology should be sought as necessary. Equal and symmetric pulses should also be palpated in all extremities.

Abdomen

The abdomen should be palpated for any masses or organomegaly (e.g., polycystic kidneys, hepatosplenomegaly) that warrant further investigation.

Genitalia

In female neonates, the labia majora are often swollen, making an examination of the hymen difficult, but clitoral size should be noted. Parents should be told that a physiologic vaginal discharge and the presence later of a pink or blood-tinged discharge are a normal neonatal response to maternal estrogen withdrawal. In uncircumcised male infants, it is imperative that the foreskin be retracted sufficiently to reveal the location of the urethra. A testicular examination can rule out hydroceles, inguinal hernias, and cryptorchidism.

Skeleton

The Ortolani test is performed to evaluate the newborn for developmental dysplasia of the hip. The "clunk" felt when performing the examination is the relocation of the femoral head of the affected hip in the joint capsule. In contrast, a "click" may indicate normal perinatal ligament laxity. The spine should be palpated completely to the sacrum. Sacral defects, deep sacral pits, or sacral tufts of hair warrant an investigation for such conditions as spina bifida occulta. Fingers and toes should be counted. The feet may be turned inward, outward, or up and should be gently moved to a normal position to assure flexibility.

Neurologic Examination

Primitive reflexes such as the Moro, rooting, grasp, and stepping reflexes are a primary component of the neonatal neurologic examination. In addition, tone, sensation, and deep tendon reflexes should be evaluated. Tone can be assessed by holding the infant upright below the shoulder girdle or by observing the crying infant; all extremities should be in the flexed position.

Normal findings of the nursery physical examination are summarized in Table 7–1. Emergent findings that must be addressed immediately when noted at the initial nursery examination include evidence of hydrocephalus, a ductal dependent cardiac lesion, a diaphragmatic hernia, an abdominal mass, or a possible chromosomal abnormality such as trisomy 13 or trisomy 18. The physical conditions associated with trisomy 21 are rarely life-threatening, although its suspicion does warrant a careful examination and evaluation for cardiac and abdominal anomalies (see Chapter 19, Well Child Care for Children With Trisomy 21).

Laboratory Tests

The only laboratory test required of all newborns prior to discharge from the nursery is the newborn screening heel stick for inheritable conditions such as phenylketonuria and hypothyroidism. Mandated neonatal screening varies by state and depends on the prevalence of a particular disease in a given region (see Chapter 8, Screening in Newborns).

Other laboratory tests that are often performed include a serum glucose, especially in lethargic, poly-

---

TABLE 7–1. Common Physical Findings in Newborns

Skin
Milia, erythema toxicum, salmon patch, nevus flammeus, hemangiomas, mongolian spots, lanugo (body hair)
Head
Cephalohematoma, caput succedaneum
Face
Swollen overall appearance
Eyes
Swollen eyelids, subconjunctival hemorrhages
Ears
Preauricular appendages/pits, folded pinnae
Nose
Flattened nose, milia over bridge
Mouth and Throat
Epstein's pearls, epithelial pearls, natal teeth, shortened frenulum
Chest
Supernumerary nipples, breast buds, galactorrhea, pectus excavatum or carinatum
Genitalia
Females: swollen labia, hymenal tags, vaginal discharge
Males: hydrocele, undescended testicle (palpated in inguinal canal)
Hips
Click
Extremities
Feet turned up, in, or out, but malleable
Neurologic Examination
Primitive reflexes: Moro, grasp, rooting, stepping

cythemic, or jittery infants, and a hematocrit in jaundiced or ruddy-appearing newborns. In cases of ABO or Rh incompatibility, a serum bilirubin and a Coombs' test are often necessary to obtain, after confirming the maternal and infant blood types.

Although not routinely performed at this time, newborn hearing screening may also be done prior to discharge from the hospital. Screening studies include an automated auditory brainstem response, otoacoustic emission testing, or conventional auditory brainstem response.

Imaging Studies

Routine x-rays are not indicated in neonates whose newborn examination is normal or who have minor abnormalities such as pectus excavatum. Vertebral x-rays are appropriate in the neonate with a deep sacral pit or sacral tuft of hair for the diagnosis of spina bifida occulta. Clavicular x-rays are indicated if swelling or pain is located in the clavicular area or if an asymmetric Moro reflex is elicited. A chest x-ray and ECG are warranted for a significant murmur. A renal ultrasound is appropriate in the infant with significant ear deformities. More extensive studies are necessary if an emergent physical finding is discovered.

MANAGEMENT

The administration of intramuscular vitamin K and the application of ophthalmic ointment or silver nitrate in the newborn's eyes is universal. Because of the possibility of maternal infection with HIV, many institutions are reevaluating the timing of the vitamin K administration. They are waiting until all maternal blood is washed from the infant before giving the injection. The infant is then kept in the transitional nursery in an isolette for the initial few hours following delivery to ensure the maintenance of an adequate body temperature and stable vital signs. Serum glucose is often monitored as well.

If desired, the circumcision is usually performed on the day of discharge (see Chapter 10, Circumcision). Local anesthesia is now universally recommended for the procedure, but its use remains at the discretion of the physician and parents. Following the procedure, the parents are instructed to leave the gauze or Plastibell in place. It will fall off spontaneously. Petroleum ointment may also be placed on the corona of the penis to prevent its sticking to the diaper. The physician should be notified if excessive bleeding or oozing occurs (e.g., soaking of the diaper with blood) after discharge from the nursery.

DISCHARGE PLANNING/COUNSELING

Before the infant is discharged to home, physicians should discuss normal variants found on the physical examination with parents. Abnormal physical findings

and their relevance should also be explained. If any further studies were performed other than routine neonatal screening, parents should also be informed of the results.

Other topics that should be covered at the bedside include breast-feeding versus bottle feeding, sleeping and elimination patterns in the newborn, umbilical cord care, bathing the newborn, and safety issues such as car seats and sleeping position. In addition, the timing of the first dose of the hepatitis B vaccine should be discussed. It can be administered prior to hospital discharge or at the first follow-up visit. Guidelines regarding when to call the office or emergency department should also be addressed. These include a rectal fever of 100.4° F (38.0° C), respiratory distress, irritability, lethargy, decreased feeding, and evidence of dehydration. Parents should be encouraged to call the physician's office about any concern they may have, especially if they are first-time parents, and to trust their own instincts. A follow-up visit should be arranged for 1–3 weeks after discharge, or sooner if the newborn is sent home at less than 48 hours or is breast-feeding.

Case Resolution

In the case presented at the beginning of the chapter, the parents should be told that the weight, length, and head circumference are all normal. The subconjunctival hemorrhages should be shown to the parents and their self-limited nature explained. Routine neonatal screening, feeding, sleeping, elimination, bathing, and safety should be reviewed. Prior to discharge, the infant should receive the hepatitis B vaccine. A follow-up appointment should be made for 1–3 weeks of age.

Selected Readings

American Academy of Pediatrics, Committee on Fetus and Newborn. Hospital stay for healthy term newborns. Pediatrics 96:788–790, 1995.

American Academy of Pediatrics, Committee on Psychosocial Aspects of Child and Family Health. The prenatal visit. Pediatrics 97:141–142, 1996.

American Academy of Pediatrics, Vitamin K Ad Hoc Task Force. Controversies concerning vitamin K and the newborn. Pediatrics 91:1001–1003, 1993.

American Academy of Pediatrics and the American College of Obstetricians and Gynecologists. Guidelines for Perinatal Care, 4th ed. Elk Grove, IL, American Academy of Pediatrics, 1997.

Britton, J. R., H. L. Britton, and S. A. Beebe. Early discharge of the term newborn: a continued dilemma. Pediatrics 94:291–295, 1994.

Hurt, H. Early discharge for newborns–when is it safe? Contemp. Pediatr. 11:68–88, 1994.

Kessel, J., and R. M. Ward. Congenital malformations presenting during the neonatal period. Clin. Perinatol. 25:351–369, 1998.

Mehl, A. L., and V. Thomson. Newborn hearing screening: the great omission. Pediatrics 101:E4, 1998.

Schmitt, B. D. Characteristics of newborn babies. In Your Child's Health, 2nd ed. New York, Bantam Books, 1991.

Schmitt, B. D. The first weeks at home with your new baby. In Your Child's Health, 2nd ed. New York, Bantam Books, 1991.

Vasiloudes, P., J. G. Morelli, and W. L. Weston. A guide to rashes in newborns. Contemp. Pediatr. 14:156–167, 1997.

CHAPTER 8

SCREENING IN NEWBORNS

Monica Sifuentes, M.D.

H$_x$ A 6-day-old infant is brought to the office by the parents because of an abnormal neonatal screening test for galactosemia. The family recently moved to the area. The parents report that their daughter has been doing well. Initially she seemed a bit sleepy, but she is now taking short naps during the day and waking every 2–3 hours at night for feedings. The infant is breast-fed, with occasional formula supplementation. She wets seven to eight diapers per day and has had normal, soft, seedy stools since birth.

The infant, the product of a 39-week gestation, was born via normal spontaneous vaginal delivery to a 28-year-old gravida II para II woman in good health. The mother received appropriate prenatal care beginning at 14 weeks' gestation and had no problems during the pregnancy. She reportedly used no alcohol, drugs, or medications, and the results of all prenatal laboratory tests were normal. At birth the infant weighed 6 lb, 13 oz (3100 g) and was 19 inches (48.25 cm) long. She was discharged 18 hours later at the parents' insistence.

The family history is unremarkable. The 4-year-old sibling is healthy and developmentally normal.

The infant's current weight is 6 lb, 6 oz (2900 g). The physical examination is entirely within normal limits.

Questions

1. What are the proposed benefits of newborn screening?
2. What newborn screening tests are most commonly performed?
3. How are results of newborn screening tests reported to physicians?
4. What measures should be taken when results of newborn screening tests are abnormal?
5. What are the most common causes of false-positive and false-negative tests?

Newborn screening programs were initially developed over 30 years ago. The goal was early identification of specific metabolic disorders in newborn infants; the hope was prevention, or at least amelioration, of known catastrophic outcomes associated with the delayed treatment of these conditions. Neonatal screening for multiple metabolic disorders is now routine. All 50 states in the United States require newborn screening for phenylketonuria and congenital hypothyroidism. In addition, screening tests for over 50 other disorders are now available.

Each state requires newborn screening for different conditions. The incidence of a specific disorder, the availability of effective treatment for the condition, and the financial advantages of providing early diagnosis and treatment all influence state requirements. For example, in a state where the African-American popu-

lation is large, screening for hemoglobinopathies such as sickle cell anemia is particularly useful.

Primary care physicians must participate in the standard screening program of the state in which they practice. Because all neonates must be screened and certain conditions may be life-threatening in the newborn period, it behooves pediatricians and other health care practitioners to become familiar with all aspects of the state-mandated program that affects them. Table 8–1 lists the conditions for which most states require neonatal screening.

Some newborn tests may not be state-mandated. Anonymous samples may be collected and analyzed for purely epidemiologic reasons or in conjunction with a research protocol. These results are never reported to the families or physicians. For example, random newborn screening tests may be used to determine the prevalence of HIV within a given community.

NEWBORN SCREENING PRACTICES

Parental Education and Informed Consent

The AAP recommends that all infants have a blood specimen taken for newborn screening before discharge from the nursery. All parents should therefore be informed of the state screening program either at the prenatal visit or during the initial newborn examination. Written materials that explain the screening program may be useful. Health care providers are responsible for educating parents regarding the method for obtaining the blood specimen, the risks and benefits of the screening tests, the conditions to be screened, and the implications of positive results. It is important to tell parents that positive results do not necessarily mean that their infant has a particular disorder; the results must be repeated and confirmed by more sensitive methods. In addition, parents should know that disorders in some children are missed either because of sampling errors, faulty testing, or inadequate accumulation of the abnormal metabolite at the time of testing.

Legal requirements for obtaining signed informed consent differ from state to state. Theoretically, all parents have given informed consent if practitioners have discussed the state-mandated program with them and they have agreed to participate. Although consenting parents are not required to sign any forms, parental refusal is important to document on newborns' charts regardless of state laws. Primary care practitioners must be particularly alert for signs and symptoms of undiagnosed metabolic disorders in children who have not been screened for these conditions.

TABLE 8–1.   Neonatal Screening Tests Mandated by Most States in the United States

Disorders and Incidence*	No. of States	Symptoms Without Treatment	Special Considerations
Congenital hypothyroidism 1:3600–5000	50	Mental retardation, poor growth, constipation, poor appetite	Late onset of disorder in 10% of cases
Phenylketonuria (PKU) 1:10,000–25,000	50	Mental retardation, seizures, eczema	Neonatal symptoms usually absent
Galactosemia 1:60,000–80,000	45	Lethargy, feeding intolerance, vomiting, jaundice, hepatomegaly, sepsis, seizures, cataracts	Approximately 25% of unrecognized infants develop sepsis (usually *Escherichia coli*) by week 1–2 of life
Hemoglobinopathies (sickle cell disease; 1:400 African-Americans)	42	Anemia, sepsis, vaso-occlusive crisis, osteomyelitis	Clinical diagnosis is rarely made before 1 year of age if disorder not identified by newborn screening
Maple syrup urine disease 1:250,000–300,000	23	Feeding intolerance, vomiting, lethargy, severe ketoacidosis, coma, death	Death within first 2 weeks of life is not uncommon; characteristic urine odor of maple syrup or curry

*Other disorders screened for by some states: Homocystinuria (1:50,000–200,000), 21 states; biotinidase deficiency (1:40,000–70,000), 16; congenital adrenal hyperplasia (21-OH deficiency) (1:12,000), 13; tyrosinemia (<1:400,000), 7; cystic fibrosis (1:2000) (whites), 3; toxoplasmosis (1:500), 3.

Modified and reproduced, with permission, from Clayton, E.W. Newborn screening: legal requirements and beyond. Contemp. Pediatr. 10:35, 1993, and Buist, N.R.M., and J.M. Tuerck. The practitioner's role in newborn screening. Pediatr. Clin. North Am. 39:202–203, 1992.

Specimen Collection and Handling

Proper specimen collection and handling are essential components of a successful screening program because they may influence the results. The Committee on Genetics of the AAP has published specific guidelines regarding timing of the test, type of blood specimens that are acceptable, indications for rescreening, and influence of treatments such as transfusions and dialysis.

Recommendations concerning **timing of the test** stipulate that all newborns be screened before discharge from the nursery as close to the time of discharge as possible, and before day seven of life. If the test is performed before infants are 24 hours old (as in the case of early discharges), the test should be repeated at 1–2 weeks of age.

An adequate **blood specimen** can often be obtained from a heel stick. Cord blood is unacceptable for routine newborn screening because specific metabolites measured in certain tests such as phenylalanine (used to test for phenylketonuria) do not accumulate until after birth when infants have been on a normal protein diet. One drop of blood may be sufficient. Only 3 µL are needed for each disk on the filter paper, but the sample must

saturate the paper evenly. The use of needles and glass capillary tubes for blood collection is discouraged because they may cause hemolysis or microtears in the filter paper. The specimens must be individually air dried in a horizontal position, thus avoiding contamination and excessive exposure to heat. They should be mailed to the laboratory within 24 hours of collection.

Rescreening is currently mandated only for newborns who are less than 24 hours old (early discharges). Retesting should occur before 2 weeks of age. Infants who appear symptomatic for a metabolic disorder should be definitively tested, even if initial screening results are normal. Reports indicate that initial screening tests for congenital hypothyroidism are normal in 6–12% of patients who have the disease.

If possible, blood samples should be obtained prior to any transfusions or dialysis. Otherwise, screening tests should still be performed as outlined above, and arrangements should be made to have them repeated at an appropriate time (i.e., at 2–3 months of age).

Other specific circumstances must also be taken into consideration when performing newborn screening tests, including prematurity, illness, hyperalimentation therapy, and antibiotic administration. Premature infants may have a low T_4 level consistent with their gestational age. Studies have reported that ill infants exposed to topical iodinated antiseptic agents can have transient hypothyroidism as well. Hyperalimentation may influence the measurement of certain amino acids. Parenteral antibiotics may inhibit the growth of bacteria used in some assays. As with transfusions and dialysis, initial specimens should still be obtained. Results should be interpreted cautiously, however, and often tests must be repeated.

Inadequate specimen collection and handling can lead to test inaccuracies, delays in reporting results to physicians, and unnecessary repetition of screening tests. Therefore, all individuals who are involved in the newborn screening process should adhere strictly to the procedures discussed above.

Reporting of Results

In most states, all results of neonatal screening tests, whether normal or abnormal, are reported to the physician of record. Normal results are mailed to the physician for placement in the patient's medical record. Abnormal results are usually reported by telephone or letter, depending on the significance of the abnormality. Results are also sent to the hospital where the infant was born for inclusion in the medical record. The physician of record is responsible for contacting the parents regarding the need for confirmatory testing. If a newborn is no longer under the care of this physician or if the family cannot be located, state and local public health departments can be called on to assist in the search for the infant and family.

Diagnostic and Therapeutic Considerations

All abnormal results, whether borderline or clearly significant, should be repeated and evaluated by primary care physicians. In addition, a complete physical examination should be performed. Depending on the nature of the suspected disorder, initiation of treatment before repeat laboratory results are known may be appropriate. For example, prophylactic antibiotics should be administered if sickle cell anemia is suspected. After confirmatory results have been received, the treatment can be modified or halted. The ultimate decision for the initiation of early treatment, however, lies with practitioners.

Potentially life-threatening conditions in the newborn period such as galactosemia, maple syrup urine disease, and congenital adrenal hyperplasia are particularly important to evaluate and treat emergently. Depending on the clinical picture, the suspected disorder, and the experience of the practitioner, telephone consultation with a specialist or immediate referral to a regional medical center may be necessary.

If the confirmed disorder is inherited, such as cystic fibrosis or sickle cell disease, the siblings of affected infants should be carefully evaluated. Laboratory tests may be required in some instances. Families should be offered reproductive counseling for future pregnancies, in addition to written information about the newly diagnosed condition.

THE FUTURE OF NEWBORN SCREENING PROGRAMS

Future screening programs will probably become more sophisticated as the inherited pattern or defect associated with particular conditions is better defined using DNA technology. The polymerase chain reaction, which amplifies a specific area of DNA, has already been applied to studies concerning the early detection of several important viral infections such as HIV and herpes simplex. This method has also proved to be particularly helpful in screening certain families who are known to have a specific mutation. At present, the cost and labor intensiveness of this technology preclude its use for general newborn screening purposes.

Other conditions for which DNA sampling could be helpful exist, such as screening for the development of diabetes mellitus. Current trials of newborns and children at risk for this disorder suggest the presence of specific genetic and immunologic markers that could help predict diabetes. Screening at birth for illnesses like diabetes, however, is controversial since limited preventive options are available at this time.

No single program for screening, identification, and treatment of metabolic disorders is ideal. The decision to add metabolic disorders to existing state-mandated newborn screening programs is a complicated issue. Three questions must be asked. What is the expected effect of early intervention on the patient's outcome? Could identification of this disorder lead to increased availability of medical and educational resources for affected infants and their families? What are the broader public health consequences of undiagnosed, untreated infectious conditions (e.g., unrecognized maternal HIV infection)? Pediatricians should be involved in decisions concerning the addition of new disorders to existing newborn screening programs because they are key players in the implementation of these programs.

Case Resolution

The infant should be examined carefully for any stigmata of a metabolic condition such as hepatomegaly, lethargy, irritability, or poor weight gain. She should be placed on a soy formula until the definitive test results are returned. The mother can pump her breasts to maintain her supply of milk, pending the results of the repeat test. With early diagnosis and treatment, the infant's outcome is excellent.

Selected Readings

American Academy of Pediatrics, Committee on Genetics. Issues in newborn screening. Pediatrics 89:345–349, 1992.

American Academy of Pediatrics, Committee on Genetics. Newborn screening fact sheets. Pediatrics 98:473–476, 1996.

American Academy of Pediatrics, Section on Endocrinology and Committee on Genetics, American Thyroid Association Committee on Public Health. Newborn screening for congenital hypothyroidism. Pediatrics 91:1203–1209, 1993.

Buist, N. R. M., and J. M. Tuerck. The practitioner's role in newborn screening. Pediatr. Clin. North Am. 39:199–211, 1992.

Clayton, E. W. Issues in state newborn screening programs. Pediatrics 90:641–646, 1992.

Clayton, E. W. Newborn screening: legal requirements and beyond. Contemp. Pediatr. 10:34–46, 1993.

Hiller, E. H., G. Landenburger, and M. R. Natowicz. Public participation in medical policy-making and the status of consumer autonomy: the example of newborn-screening programs in the United States. Am. J. Public Health 87:1280–1288, 1997.

Irons, M. Screening for metabolic disorders. Pediatr. Clin. North Am. 40:1073–1085, 1993.

Listernick, R., L. Frisone, and B. L. Silverman. Delayed diagnosis of infants with abnormal neonatal screens. J.A.M.A. 267:1095–1099, 1992.

Sinai, L. N., S. C. Kim, B. Casey, and J. A. Pinto-Martin. Phenylketonuria screening: effect of early newborn discharge. Pediatrics 96:605–608, 1995.

CHAPTER 9

CARING FOR TWINS

Carol D. Berkowitz, M.D.

H$_x$ An expectant mother visits you. She has been advised by her obstetrician that ultrasound shows she is pregnant with twins. She asks about care of twins and what special considerations she should keep in mind as she looks forward to the delivery. In particular, she is concerned about the feeding schedule and whether she will be able to breast-feed.

Questions

1. What is the incidence of multiple births?
2. What is the difference between fraternal and identical twins?
3. What major medical problems may affect twins?
4. What developmental and behavioral problems are associated with raising twins?

Counseling the mother of twins is a unique opportunity for pediatricians. In the past, twins were often not diagnosed before delivery. With the advent of ultrasound, the diagnosis is made prenatally in over 90% of cases. Many societies have been fascinated with twins, and many myths and superstitions surround their birth. Some people believe that a mother of twins must have been unfaithful to her husband because a father cannot sire two children. Native Americans of the Iroquois tribe believed that one twin was good and the other was evil. To prevent the recurrence of twins, the Khoikhain remove one of the father's testicles.

Part of the fascination with twins relates to the concern about being able to tell them apart. Mark Twain wrote, "My twin and I got mixed up in the bath when we were only two weeks old, and one was drowned, but we never knew which." Researchers have noted marked differences in temperament and responsiveness of twins. Twins are different, and maintaining the individuality of each twin is important both for the parents and for the health care provider.

Parents of twins often have many questions that concern their care, but they rarely pose them to health care providers. In one study in which 18 out of 29 mothers breast-fed their twins, only three received information about breast-feeding from their physicians. One mother had been told by her obstetrician that she could not breast-feed her twins. Physicians should become knowledgeable about caring for twins. They can help the parents of twins with problems related to feeding, sleeping, and behavior.

EPIDEMIOLOGY

The overall natural incidence of twin births is about 1 in 87. Twins account for just slightly more than 1% of all births, and 20% of infants born under 30 weeks' gestation are twins. The average incidence of monozygotic or identical twins, which is the same for all women regardless of race and age, is about 1 in 250 births. The incidence of dizygotic or fraternal twins varies among different groups. In the United States it is 0.6 per 100 in Caucasians and 0.9 per 100 in African Americans. The occurrence of dizygotic twins may be inherited recessively in some families. The likelihood of dizygotic twins is believed to be higher in low socioeconomic classes and in mothers between the ages of 35 and 40. In older mothers the incidence is 10-fold that of teenage mothers. Births of twins increase after the fifth pregnancy, the use of oral contraceptives, and the use of fertility drugs. After the use of such drugs, twin births reportedly occur in up to 50% of cases.

The incidence of multiple births has increased dramatically. Between 1980 and 1995, twin births have increased by 42% in the United States, and "higher order multiples" (triplets, quadruplets, etc.) by 272%. Contributing factors include the use of ovulation-stimulating drugs (e.g., Clomid); *in vitro* fertilization, in which multiple eggs may be placed in the uterus; and the trend for delay in starting a family. Maternal age of 35 years or above is associated with increased gonadotropin production and the release by the ovary of multiple eggs, increasing the chance of multiple births.

PATHOPHYSIOLOGY

Monozygotic twins result from the splitting of a single egg. They may share a placenta (monochorionic and monoamniotic) (Fig. 9–1A and 1B). When splitting occurs early (after several cell divisions of the zygote), each fetus develops its own chorion and amnion, leading to dichorionic and diamniotic placentas. Dizygotic twins result from two eggs, and each egg is fertilized by a different sperm. Dizygotic twins have two placentas (Fig. 9–1C). Although these placentas may fuse together like two pancakes, they are always dichorionic and diamniotic (Fig. 9–1D).

Following the birth, it is important to determine whether twins are monozygotic or dizygotic. About 50% of families specifically request this information. If transplantation becomes a concern, this knowledge is also significant. Monozygotic twins have a higher incidence of malformations. Different sex twins are almost always dizygotic, although monozygotic twins of

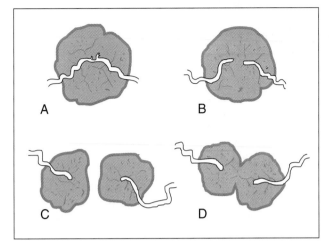

FIGURE 9–1. Variations in placentas in twin births.
A. Monochorionic, monoamniotic placenta, cords close together.
B. Monochorionic, monoamniotic placenta, cords further apart.
C. Dichorionic, diamniotic placentas, separate.
D. Dichorionic, diamniotic placentas, fused.

different sexes have been reported in the literature. This occurs when one twin loses a Y chromosome and becomes a phenotypic female with Turner's Syndrome (XO). Occasionally the male twin may be XXY and have Klinefelter's syndrome.

To determine whether twins are monozygotic or dizygotic, a number of procedures can be undertaken. Visual or pathologic examination of the placenta is helpful. About two-thirds of monozygotic twins have a common chorion and share one placenta. Finding a single chorion usually means the twins are monozygotic, unless the placentas of dizygotic twins have fused together (see above). Examination of hair whorls, iris patterns, ear configuration, eye color, dental morphology, and fingerprint patterns may give a clue to the type of twinning. Laboratory evaluation to determine the nature of twinning begins with human leukocyte antigen (HLA) testing. The HLA genes are on chromosome 6. Dizygotic twins have a 20% chance of having the same HLA type. If the HLA types are the same, the next step involves testing blood group types. If the blood group types are the same, enzyme and protein analysis should be undertaken. Enzymes, such as phosphoglucomutase, and proteins, such as haptoglobin and transferrin, should be evaluated. Agreement in all these areas suggests that the twins are monozygotic.

DIFFERENTIAL DIAGNOSIS

Diagnosing twins is not difficult, but physicians should be aware that twins may have problems.

Perinatal Complications

The perinatal mortality of monozygotic twins is eight times that of singletons and four times that of dizygotic twins as a result of many factors, including small size and prematurity. Twins have a mean gestational age of 262 days, as opposed to 280 days for singletons. The mean gestational age for monozygotic twins is less than

for dizygotic twins. In addition, hydramnios is 16 times more likely to occur in twin pregnancies. Other perinatal complications associated with twin births include pregnancy-induced hypertension, placenta previa, antepartum hemorrhage, prolapse of the cord, abnormal presentation, and uterine inertia. In 41% of twin pregnancies, both twins are delivered by vertex presentation. In 37% of births, one twin is breech, and in 8%, both twins are breech.

Congenital Malformations

Monozygotic twins have a higher incidence of congenital malformations. Anomalies that have been reported with increased incidence include anencephaly and spina bifida, holoprosencephaly, VATERL, (vertebral defects, imperforate anus, tracheoesophageal fistula, renal dysplasia, and limb defects), sirenomelia (mermaidlike extremity), and extrophy of the cloaca. In addition to malformations, twins may suffer from deformations secondary to crowding. Growth in twins tends to be normal until 30–34 weeks, when the combined weight of twins reaches 8 lb, 13 oz (4 kg).

Postnatal Complications

Smaller twins have an increased incidence of hypoglycemia. Twin-to-twin transfusions, which may account for persistent growth differences, are seen in 10–15% of monochorional pregnancies. Artery-to-vein shunts result in one twin transfusing the other, and this may be diagnosed prenatally by ultrasound of the placenta, which shows one sac with oligohydramnios and the other sac with polyhydramnios. Artery-to-artery shunts and vein-to-vein shunts can also be anticipated by ultrasound and result in twin-to-twin transfusions.

EVALUATION

History

A general medical history should be obtained, including a history of the pregnancy. Any specific medical complaints should also be addressed (Questions Box).

Physical Examination

The initial evaluation of newly born twins involves assessment of gestational age and determination of the presence of any medical problems or anomalies (see Chapter 7, Neonatal Examination). Older twins should

---

Questions: Caring for Twins

- Did the mother have any problems during the pregnancy?
- How long did the pregnancy last?
- Did the mother take any medications, including fertility drugs?
- Did either twin have any problem after the delivery or in the newborn nursery?
- Which was twin A (first-born twin) and which was twin B (second-born twin)?

undergo health maintenance visits where routine as well as specific complaints are addressed.

Laboratory Tests

The twins should be assessed in the newborn period for the presence of anemia or polycythemia with a hemoglobin determination. Hypoglycemia may occur in the newborn period and can be assessed with a rapid test, such as glucometer testing or a serum glucose. If the twins are premature, they may have many of the problems seen in preterm infants, such as respiratory distress syndrome and necrotizing enterocolitis.

Older twins should receive an appropriate evaluation for age, with a specific focus on any behavioral concerns.

MANAGEMENT

The focus of the management of twins involves counseling the mother about issues related to routine care. Mothers often care for two or more children at the same time, but twins are two children who are developmentally and chronologically at the same point in time. Baby care books that specifically deal with birthing and raising twins are available in libraries and bookstores. In addition, *Twins Magazine* (800-821-5533), which is published bimonthly, contains pertinent articles and lists organizations to help parents of twins.

Feeding is a major issue. Breast-feeding is both physically and emotionally possible. Wet nurses have fed up to six infants at a time, and the difficulty appears more with timing and positioning of the infants rather than with the supply of milk. Some suggestions about breast-feeding twins follow.

1. Feed both infants at the same time, with one on each breast. The infants may be put in a number of positions. The mother can be sitting and cradling one infant while holding the other infant like a football. Alternatively, the mother may cradle both infants, so that they are lying over one another, or she may have both infants under her arms in a football position. Both infants may not be hungry at the same time, however, which may present a problem.

2. Feed the infants at different times. The mother breast-feeds one infant and then the other. The mother starts with the more vigorous feeder. This approach may pose a problem; both infants may be hungry at the same time.

3. Breast-feed one infant and bottle-feed the other, which gives the mother a free hand. Bottle-feeding presents certain difficulties too, primarily cost.

Research shows that mothers who bottle-feed their twins use powder rather than concentrated formula and wean their infants from formula earlier than is recommended. Breast-feeding mothers tend to breast-feed their infants longer for economic reasons. One problem with formula feeding concerns storage, that is, making up enough formula and having enough room to keep a supply of milk. It is suggested that a half-day supply be prepared to reduce the needed storage space. Another suggestion involves the use of plastic-bag nursers because they take up less room. Some physicians recommend sticking to a feeding schedule for twins. A mother can let the first infant feed on demand but wake up the second one when the first one is done. Eighty percent of parents of twins acknowledge that they prop the bottle instead of holding it, and they should be counseled about this.

Twin infants on solid foods may be given two meals a day instead of three. Putting strained baby food in the bottle to facilitate feeding is also an option. Most parents of twins use one dish and one spoon and feed both infants at the same time using this technique.

Sleeping is also a consideration. Many parents use one crib with a partition, but the twins may disturb one another. A play pen is bigger and provides more room. Twins on apnea monitors should not sleep next to each other, however, because their wires can become entangled. Twin strollers, which are available in different types, are useful. Some strollers have seats adjacent to each other, but sometimes these are too wide to fit through a doorway. Other strollers have the infants facing each other, which may be a problem because of fighting.

Children should have separate dressers, clothing areas, and toys. Diapers are also an issue. Disposable diapers are more convenient, but the cost is high. Diaper services are less expensive, and many parents choose to use cloth diapers and rinse them out themselves. Toilet training is reportedly easier with some twins because one twin learns from the other.

It is important to counsel parents about **car seats.** Parents who cannot afford the cost of two car seats may resort to placing one twin in the car seat and the other on the seat of the car, a dangerous practice that is illegal in all states in the United States. Parents should be advised about the need for car seats for both infants. Consideration can be given to renting car seats.

Bathing should be done separately in the interest of safety.

Having twins is a **financial hardship** for some families. Some mothers must leave work 2–3 months before delivery because of their large size. Prematurity necessitates prolonged hospitalization. Physicians should consider whether a discount should be given if twins are seen at the same time.

Maternal fatigue is another important issue. One mother said that her physician should be aware that she felt like a zombie because she was not getting enough sleep. Physicians frequently recommend that mothers rest when infants rest. With twins, however, this is rarely possible because of the so-called "ping-pong" effect. While one infant sleeps, the other gets up, and as soon as the second one falls asleep, the first one is up again.

Help from fathers is variable in families with twins. Physicians should check with mothers about how much help they are receiving from husbands. If help is not forthcoming, they should schedule a family meeting at 1 month. It is also important to suggest that mothers of twins obtain outside aid, including help from high school students after school and family members.

Lastly, **maintenance of individuality** for twins may be challenging. Researchers suggest that mothers can bond to only one infant at a time, a concept called monotropy. For this reason, twins are often dressed alike and given similar names. This may facilitate the bonding process. To help with individual development, physicians are encouraged to examine each child individually. Physicians should attempt to distinguish the twins from one another independent of parental reminders. Twins should not be referred to as "the twins" but by their respective names. As twins get older, issues related to classrooms and birthday parties frequently arise, and they should be consulted concerning their preferences. It is often recommended that twins be in different classrooms and that they be allowed to have individual birthday parties and gifts. (Some twins comment on their disappointment at receiving the same present for birthdays and holidays. There is no surprise in opening gifts if the other twin opened a gift first.)

PROGNOSIS

Although twins have a higher incidence of perinatal problems, appropriate anticipatory guidance and routine health maintenance result in normal growth and development.

Case Resolution

The mother in the case scenario is advised that breast-feeding is not only possible but recommended. She is told about the options for timing and positioning of the infants. The issues of family history and child passenger safety are also discussed.

Selected Readings

Baldwin, V. J. Pathology of Multiple Pregnancy. New York, Springer-Verlag, 1994.

Becker, P. G. Counseling families with twins: birth to 3 years of age. Pediatr. Rev. 8:81–86, 1986.

Blickstein, I., and M. Lancet. The growth discordant twin. Obstet. Gynecol. Surv. 43:509–515, 1988.

Dungy, C. I., L. Cooper, and D. Wacker. Behavioral problems and twins. J. Dev. Behav. Pediatr. 14:336–339, 1993.

Grether, J. K., B. K. Nelson, and S. K. Cummings. Twinning and cerebral palsy: experience in four northern California counties, births 1983 through 1985. Pediatrics 92:854–858, 1993.

Noble, E. Having Twins, 2nd ed. Boston, Houghton Mifflin, 1991.

Taffel, S. M. Health and demographic characteristics of twin births: United States, 1988. National Center for Health Statistics. Vital Health Statistics 21(50), 1992.

CHAPTER 10

CIRCUMCISION

Carol D. Berkowitz, M.D.

H_x An expectant mother visits you prenatally. She talks about circumcision in addition to issues relating to breast-feeding and car passenger safety. Her husband is circumcised. She is unclear about the medical indications for circumcision and asks your opinion about circumcision in the newborn period.

Questions

1. What are the benefits of circumcision in neonates?
2. What are the indications for circumcision in older children?
3. What are the techniques used to perform circumcision?
4. What are the complications of circumcision?

Male circumcision, a procedure in which the foreskin of the penis is removed, has been performed for over 4000 years. It is routinely performed in certain groups, most notably among Jewish and Muslim people. In many other cultures (e.g., Abyssinian, Australian [aborigine], Polynesian), circumcision is presumably performed to facilitate intercourse. Circumcision can be viewed as a ritual procedure, but its role as a medical one is open to greater controversy.

The benefits of male circumcision have been debated for years. Over the past 20 years, even the American Academy of Pediatrics has changed its official position on the medical indication for circumcision. Disadvantages of routine circumcision in infants concern cost effectiveness and the risk of complications. The procedure is sometimes viewed as an archaic and maiming ritual. Female circumcision, which may involve clitorectomy or resection and closure of the labia minor or majora, is infrequently practiced in Western culture and is not discussed here. There are no medical benefits attributable to female circumcision.

Circumcision in newborns has been performed in a routine and preventive manner, much the same way immunizations are administered. Primary care physicians should be aware of the risks and benefits of the procedure to be able to counsel parents and make referrals to consultants when certain medical conditions arise.

EPIDEMIOLOGY

The prevalence of circumcision, a procedure that became increasingly popular in the United States in the 1950s and 1960s, once ranged from 69–97% depending on cultural mores. Changing cultural patterns have resulted in a lower frequency of circumcision. In recent years the prevalence has decreased to about 59%. The prevalence of circumcision in Australia is reported to be 70%; in Canada, 48%; and in the United Kingdom, 24%. Circumcision is the second most common surgical procedure after vasectomy in males. It is the most commonly performed operation in children.

A reported 10% of uncircumcised males ultimately require circumcision as adults because of complications of phimosis and balanitis. Uncircumcised males with diabetes are particularly prone to these complications.

PATHOPHYSIOLOGY

In uncircumcised males, the foreskin adheres to the glans until about the age of 6 years. This adhesiveness, or crusting, may be controlled by androgens. A gradual, normal lysing of the adhesive bands connecting the foreskin to the underportion of the glans then occurs. Nonphysiologic phimosis occurs as a result of scarring of the preputial wing. Lysing of adhesions in an effort to treat the phimosis usually leads to further adhesions. If the foreskin is retracted and remains in that position, paraphimosis develops.

BENEFITS

It has been stated that circumcision facilitates penile hygiene by removing the foreskin, which may serve as a repository for bacteria, smegma, and dirt. Retractability of the foreskin increases with age (Table 10–1), and thus penile hygiene is easier to achieve in older children. The term **phimosis** refers to inability to retract the foreskin. In male infants beyond the newborn period, phimosis is the major indication for circumcision. Phimosis is normal in children up to about 6 years of age but is nonphysiologic if urination results in ballooning of the foreskin, regardless of age. When the retracted foreskin acts as a tourniquet in the midshaft of the penis, **paraphimosis** occurs, preventing the return of lymphatic flow. Paraphimosis is believed to be iatrogenic or matratrogenic, that is, related to the mother's retracting

TABLE 10–1.	Retractability of the Foreskin in Boys (by Age)
Age	Percentage With Retractable Foreskin
Birth	4%
6 mo	15%
1 yr	50%
3 yr	80%
6 yr	90%

the foreskin. In the past, mothers were advised to retract the foreskin in an effort to lyse adhesions. This is no longer routinely recommended because adhesions are thought to be normal.

Balanitis, or inflammation of the glans, is not uncommon in young infants. It is frequently associated with *Candida* infection, and the glans is swollen and erythematous. Posthitis, or inflammation of the foreskin, is also often secondary to *Candida* infection. Other organisms, including gram-negative microbes, may be associated with balanitis. The presence of recurrent balanitis is an indication for circumcision. In older males, indications for circumcision include phimosis, paraphimosis, balanitis, posthitis, and balanoposthitis.

Bacterial colonization of the skin also leads to possible balanitis and posthitis. Group B streptococci, which bind to the foreskin of adults, causing balanitis, may be transmitted sexually. The incidence of STDs, particularly herpes and condyloma acuminatum, is increased in uncircumcised men.

Penile cancer, which is reported in 0.7 to 0.9 per 100,000 men in the United States, is also thought to be related to lack of circumcision of the penis. Only a few isolated cases of cancer of the penis occur in circumcised men. The lifetime risk of penile cancer is 1 in 500 in uncircumcised males compared to 1 in 50,000 to 1 in 12 million in circumcised men. In the last 45 years, 11,000 men have died from penile cancer. The reported mortality of penile cancer is 25%. This type of cancer appears to be associated with infection with human papillomavirus types 16 and 18. Whether lack of circumcision, poor hygiene, or the presence of STDs is responsible for the increased incidence of penile carcinoma is unclear.

Cervical carcinoma among the partners of uncircumcised men has been reported with increased incidence. Human papillomavirus types 16 and 18 are believed to play a role here. Herpes simplex virus type II has also been linked with cervical cancer. The link between uncircumcised males and cervical carcinoma is inconclusive.

Urinary tract infections (UTIs) reportedly occur ten times more often in uncircumcised male infants than in circumcised infants. In young uncircumcised boys, UTIs are directly related to colonization of the foreskin with urotoxic organisms. Pyronephritogenic, fimbriated *Escherichia coli* bind to the inner lining of the foreskin within the first few days of life. Other bacteria preferentially bind to this mucosal surface, including fimbriated strains of *Proteus mirabilis* and nonfimbriated *Pseudomonas, Klebsiella,* and *Serratia* species. The incidence of

---

TABLE 10–2.   Complications Associated With Circumcision

Bleeding	Inclusion cysts
Infection	Penile lymphedema
Repeat circumcision	Urethrocutaneous fistulae
Phimosis	Penile cyanosis
Skin bridges	Penile necrosis
Urinary retention	Wound dehiscence
Meatitis	

UTIs has increased as the rate of circumcision has decreased. In addition, complications associated with UTIs, particularly bacteremia, meningitis, and subsequent death, have occurred.

RISKS

The risks related to circumcision are related to complications from the procedure. These are listed in Table 10–2 and discussed in Management.

PARENT COUNSELING

Parents of Newborns

In the newborn period, proper counseling of the parents, including a discussion of the risks and benefits of circumcision, is important. Opposition to neonatal circumcision cite psychological trauma to neonates from so painful a procedure. Newer techniques involve sedation or local anesthesia to minimize this effect. Parents should be informed about the benefits of circumcision, including a reduction in occurrence of UTIs, STDs, and cancer of the penis and cervix. Problems related to the foreskin itself, such as phimosis, paraphimosis, posthitis, and balanitis, should also be discussed.

It is appropriate to tell parents that boys who are not circumcised in the neonatal period may need to be circumcised later in life. In addition, parents should be told that approximately 10% of circumcised neonates require a second circumcision. Parents should be informed about the risks associated with circumcision in newborns, which are discussed in greater detail in the following text. In older individuals, risks include hemorrhage, infection, and injuries to the penis and urethra.

Research has shown that parents are more influenced by friends than by physicians regarding their ultimate decision about circumcision. Counseling during the second trimester of pregnancy results in no change in parents' decision about circumcision. A survey of physician attitudes, conducted in 1979, showed that 41% recommended routine circumcision, 15% did not, and 38% had no recommendations (no answers: 5%).

Parents of Older Infants

The need for circumcision in young male infants who present with UTIs is problematic. The evaluation usually tries to determine the existence of other predisposing conditions that could lead to the UTI. Investigators disagree on the need for circumcision following the initial UTI in uncircumcised boys. No clear-cut evidence indicates that circumcision at this time decreases the incidence of future UTIs, so the decision is parental rather than medical. In older children who present with phimosis, paraphimosis, balanitis, or balanoposthitis, circumcision is usually recommended to prevent recurrences of these problems. Medical management, including the use of topical steroids for phimosis, may obviate the need for surgery in some children. Such treatment involves the daily external application of betamethasone 0.05% cream from the foreskin tip to the corona glandis for 4–6 weeks. A history including the duration of symptoms and whether the child has had similar episodes in the past helps formulate the appropriate management.

MANAGEMENT

The medical attitude toward circumcision has changed over the last 40 years, with an initial inclination toward circumcision, followed by a move away from circumcision. The present position on circumcision as described by the Task Force on Circumcision of the AAP suggests that newborn circumcision has potential medical benefits and advantages as well as disadvantages and risks. In recent years, the benefit of neonatal circumcision in diminishing the incidence of UTIs has been acknowledged. When circumcision is considered, the benefits and risks should be explained to the parents, and informed consent should be obtained. Parents should be advised that the frequency with which third-party payers reimburse for circumcisions, particularly for routine circumcisions in the newborn period, has decreased.

Contraindications

Circumcisions should only be performed in completely healthy neonates. Contraindications to circumcision are well defined. Any abnormalities of the penis, such as hypospadias, absence of any portion of the foreskin, or chordee, preclude circumcision. Prematurity is a contraindication. Circumcision should be delayed in premature infants until they are ready for discharge. A family history of bleeding diatheses is also a contraindication to circumcision. Infants from such families should be assessed for evidence of coagulation problems. If these are present, circumcision should not be carried out. Infants with meningomyelocele should also not be circumcised because it is easier to fit such boys with an external collecting device if they are uncircumcised.

Circumcision Procedure

Numerous techniques are used to perform circumcisions. These procedures may involve clamp techniques with Gomco, Mogen, or Plastibell clamps. Any of these techniques is believed to give comparable results in the hands of trained, experienced operators. Formal surgical excision may also be carried out, usually in older children and adults. Three guidelines should be followed to decrease the incidence of complications: (1) marking of the coronal sulcus in ink, (2) dilation of the prepucial wing, and (3) retraction of the foreskin so that the urethral meatus is visualized. This prevents cutting the meatus. Electrocautery should never be used in conjunction with metal clamps because of the danger of extensive injury.

Appropriate anesthesia in newborns undergoing circumcision is now considered the standard of care. The pain and stress of circumcision is evidenced by changes in infant state and behavior. Local anesthesia may be carried out with a dorsal penile nerve block (DPNB) using 1% lidocaine without epinephrine in a dose of 3–4 mg per kg. Alternatively, topical application of lidocaine-prilocaine cream (EMLA) is effacious and safe in preventing pain in neonatal circumcision. Oral sucrose solution on a pacifier also reduces pain and its associated stress, but to a lesser extent than DPNB or EMLA. Neonatal circumcision without attention to pain relief is no longer accepted.

Complications

A number of complications are associated with circumcision in newborns (see Table 10–2). The most common complication is **bleeding,** which may occur in 0.1–35% of cases. This wide variation may reflect differences in method, technique, and skill. Bleeding can usually be controlled using local pressure, with 1:1000 adrenaline-soaked gauze or with the use of other topical agents such as Surgicel. The second most frequently seen complication is **infection,** reported in up to 8% of circumcised infants. Neonatal sepsis may occur secondary to infections following circumcision. Plastibell clamps, which are associated with a higher incidence of infection than Gomco clamps, generally require intravenous antibiotics. Gomco-related infections usually respond to local treatment with hydrogen peroxide and 3% hexachlorophene.

In addition, true **phimosis** may occur if removal of the foreskin is insufficient. If the foreskin is inadequately freed up from the inner prepucial epithelium, a concealed penis, with the shaft retracted backwards into the abdominal wall, may develop. **Skin bridges** may form between the glans and the shaft, leading to accumulation of smegma or the tethering of the erect penis. Most postcircumcision adhesions are reported to resolve at the time of puberty with the onset of masturbation or sexual activity.

In the immediate postsurgical period, urinary retention may occur secondary to tight surgical bandages. Meatitis and meatal ulcers, believed to be caused by irritation from ammonia, are also reported in 8–31% of circumcised males. Inclusion cysts that represent implantation of smegma are also seen. Additional injuries following circumcision may include penile lymphedema, urethrocutaneous fistulae secondary to misplaced sutures, penile cyanosis secondary to tight Plastibell clamps, and penile necrosis. Wound dehiscence, which involves separation of the penile skin from the mucous membrane, and denudation of the penile shaft may occur more frequently with Gomco than Plastibell clamps.

Case Resolution

In the case history at the beginning of this chapter, the risks and benefits of circumcision should be discussed with the mother. The father should be encouraged to participate in the decision-making process.

If the parents elect not to have their son circumcised, they should be instructed on the appropriate care of the uncircumcised penis, which involves gentle external washing without retraction of the foreskin.

Selected Readings

Anderson, G. Circumcision. Pediatr. Ann. 18:205–213, 1989.

Anderson, J. E., and K. A. Anderson. What to tell parents about circumcision. Contemp. Pediatr. 16:87–103, 1999.

Herschel, M., B. Khoshnood, C. Ellman, N. Maydew, and R. Mittendorf. Neonatal circumcision: Randomized trial of a sucrose pacifier for pain control. Arch. Pediatr. Adolesc. Med. 152:279–284, 1998.

Howard, C. R., F. M. Howard, L. C. Garfunkel, E. A. de Blieck, and M. Weitzman. Neonatal circumcision and pain relief: Current training practices. Pediatrics 101:423–428, 1998.

Langer, J. C., and D. E. Coplen. Circumcision and pediatric disorders of the penis. Pediatr. Clin. North Am. 45:801–812, 1998.

Larsen, G. L., and S. D. Williams. Postneonatal circumcision: population profile. Pediatrics 85:808–812, 1990.

Poland, P. L. The questions of routine neonatal circumcision. N. Engl. J. Med. 322:1312–1315, 1990.

Report of the Task Force on Circumcision. Circumcision policy statement. American Academy of Pediatrics. Pediatrics 103:686–693, 1999.

Ryan, C. A., and N. N. Finer. Changing attitudes and practices regarding local analgesia for newborn circumcision. Pediatrics 94:230–233, 1994.

Schoen, E. J. Circumcision updated–indicated? (Commentary.) Pediatrics 92:860–861, 1993.

Schoen, E. J. The status of circumcision of newborns. N. Engl. J. Med. 322:1308–1312, 1990.

Taddio, A., et al. Efficacy and safety of lidocaine-prilocaine cream for pain during circumcision. N. Engl. J. Med. 336:1197–1201, 1997.

Weiss, G. N. Prophylactic neonatal surgery and infectious diseases. Pediatr. Infect. Dis. J. 16:727–734, 1997.

Wiswell, T. E. Circumcision circumspection. N. Engl. J. Med. 336:1244–1245, 1997.

Wiswell, T. E., and H. L. Tencer. Circumcision in children beyond the neonatal period. Pediatrics 92:791–793, 1993.

CHAPTER 11

NUTRITIONAL NEEDS

Geeta Grover, M.D.

H$_x$ At a routine health maintenance visit, a mother asks if she may begin giving her 4-month-old daughter solid foods. The infant is taking about 4–5 ounces of formula every 3–4 hours during the day (about 32 oz per day) and sleeps from 12 PM to 5 AM without awakening for a feeding. Her birth weight was 7 pounds, and her present weight and height (13 pounds and 25 inches, respectively) are at the 50th percentile for age. The physical examination, including developmental assessment, is within normal limits.

Questions

1. What are some of the parameters that may be used to decide when infants are ready to begin taking solid foods?
2. Up to what age are breast milk or infant formulas alone considered to be adequate intake for infants?
3. At what age do infants double their birth weight? At what age do they triple their birth weight?
4. What problems are associated with the early introduction of solid foods?

Good nutrition is essential for normal growth and development. The physician plays an important role not only in assessing the growth of children from infancy through adolescence but also in counseling parents regarding the nutritional needs of maturing children. The primary care physician should be knowledgeable about key nutritional concepts in children, including growth patterns and nutritional requirements of normal children and how they vary with age; feeding patterns of infants and children; assessment of nutritional status; and common feeding and nutritional disorders.

GROWTH PATTERNS AND NUTRITIONAL REQUIREMENTS OF NORMAL CHILDREN

Monitoring the growth and nutritional status of infants and children is an integral component of well child care. The average normal expected increases in weight, height, and head circumference for the first several years of life are listed in Table 11–1.

The energy and nutritional requirements of children vary with age. Postnatal growth is most rapid during the first 6–12 months of life. Hence, caloric and protein needs are very high at this time. The average daily energy and protein needs of children from birth to 18 years of age are presented in Table 11–2.

On average, newborns weigh 7.7 lb (3.5 kg), are about 20 inches (50 cm) long, and have a head circumference of 14 inches (35 cm). They lose about 5–10% of their birth weight during the first several days of life and usually regain this weight by the age of 10–14 days. During the first several months of life, weight gain serves as an important indicator of children's general well being. Failure to gain weight during this time may be a clue to a wide variety of problems, ranging from underfeeding to malabsorption. Newborns gain about 30 g/day (roughly 1% of their birth weight per day) for the first 3 months of life, and about 10–20 g/day for the rest of the first year. Infants double their birth weight by 6 months of age and triple their birth weight by 12 months of age. On average, children weigh about 10 kg at one year of age, 20 kg at 5 years of age, and 30 kg at 10 years of age. A rough rule of thumb that can be used to estimate the expected weight of a child based on age is

$$2 \times (\text{age in years}) + 10 = \text{weight (kg)}$$

FEEDING PATTERNS OF INFANTS AND CHILDREN

Liquid Foods

Breast milk or one of the several iron-fortified infant formulas provides complete nutrition for infants during the first 4–6 months of life. During the first month or two of life, infants take about 2–3 ounces of formula (approximately 10 minutes on each breast) every 2–3 hours.

Because breast milk is more easily digested than formula, it passes out of the stomach in 1½ hours. Formula may take up to 4 hours. Therefore, during the first 4–6 weeks of life, breast-fed infants want to feed more frequently (8–12 times in 24 hours) than formula-fed infants (6–8 times in 24 hours), with an increased number of nighttime feedings as well. By about 3–5 months of age, breast-fed and bottle-fed infants do not differ in the number of nighttime feedings, although some breast-fed infants continue to awaken out of habit.

Most infants 6 months of age or less consume about 4–5 ounces per feeding every 4–5 hours. Under routine circumstances, breast milk is preferred to infant formulas because it has emotional, nutritional, and immunologic advantages. Breast-feeding allows infants and mothers to develop a unique relationship that can be emotionally satisfying.

The composition of breast milk varies over time. Colostrum, the first milk produced after delivery, is high in protein, immunoglobulins, and secretory IgA. Colostrum gradually changes to mature milk 7–10 days after delivery. The nutrient content of human milk of mothers who deliver preterm compared to those who deliver at term may vary considerably. Individual assessment may

TABLE 11–1. Normal Expected Increase in Weight, Height, and Head Circumference of Infants and Children

Normal Weight Gain in Children

Age	Expected Weight Increase
0–3 mo	25–35 g/day
3–6 mo	12–21 g/day
6–12 mo	10–13 g/day
1–6 yr	5–8 g/day
7–10 yr	5–11 g/day

Normal Height Increase in Children

Age	Expected Height Increase
0–12 mo	10 in/yr (25 cm/yr)
13–24 mo	5 in/yr (12.5 cm/yr)
2 yr–puberty	2.5 in/yr (6.25 cm/yr)

Normal Increase in Head Circumference

Age	Expected Increase in Head Circumference
0–3 mo	2 cm/mo
4–6 mo	1 cm/mo
7–12 mo	½ cm/mo
Total increase:	12 cm in the first year

be necessary to determine the appropriateness of breast milk for preterm infants.

Nutritionally, breast milk is uniquely tailored to meet the specific needs of human infants. Human milk provides approximately 20 kcal/oz, the same as routine infant formulas. Table 11–3 compares the composition of human milk and several infant formulas. Human milk has relatively low amounts of protein when compared to cow's milk (1% vs. 3%), yet the levels are sufficient to provide for satisfactory growth of infants.

Qualitative differences also make human milk more desirable. The casein-to-whey ratio in human milk is about 40:60, making it easier to digest than most infant formulas, which tend to have higher casein-to-whey ratios. Fat is the primary source of calories in human milk. The fat in cow's milk, which contains primarily saturated fatty acids, is not as well digested by infants as human milk fat, which is predominately composed of polyunsaturated fats. Lactose is the major carbohydrate of both human and cow's milk, but it is present in higher concentrations in human milk.

Human milk from well-nourished women should provide adequate amounts of all vitamins and other micronutrients. However, vitamin K, vitamin D, iron, and fluoride are not present in sufficient quantities to satisfy all nutritional needs over a prolonged period, and supplementation should be considered. The AAP recommends that all newborns receive a prophylactic dose of 0.5–1 mg of parenteral vitamin K in the immediate newborn period to help prevent bleeding disorders.

TABLE 11–2. Energy and Protein Needs of Children

Age (yr)	Calories (kcal/kg/d)	Protein (g/kg/d)
0–1	90–120	2.5–3.0
1–7	75–90	1.5–2.5
7–12	60–75	1.5–2.5
12–18	30–60	1.0–1.5

Even though the vitamin D content of human milk is low compared to cow's milk, infants of healthy mothers have generally not been observed to develop rickets if there is sufficient exposure to sunlight. The newborn requires about one minute of exposure to sunlight on the face to produce enough vitamin D. Rarely, exclusively breast-fed infants may require 400 IU per day of vitamin D supplementation, especially if exposure to sunlight is limited, to prevent rickets. Although human milk contains less iron than iron-fortified formulas (fortified to about 12 mg/L of iron), the bioavailability of the iron in human milk is greater. Breast-fed infants do not need iron supplementation until the sixth month of life. Exclusively breast-fed infants and infants who are fed ready-to-eat formulas or formulas prepared with bottled water should all receive supplementation with 0.25 mg of fluoride per day starting at 6 months of age (see Chapter 13, Dental Care).

Human milk has several immunologic advantages, which are both allergy-protective and infection-protective, over standard cow milk-based formulas. Its allergy-protective characteristics are attributed, in part, to the decreased intestinal permeability associated with human milk compared to standard formulas. The host defense factors present in human milk include immunoglobulins, complement, and cellular components (e.g., macrophages, neutrophils, lymphocytes). Studies have shown that the incidences of both viral and bacterial illnesses are lower in exclusively breast-fed infants compared to their formula-fed peers.

Breast-feeding is the recommended method of infant feeding during the first 6 months of life, but it is not always possible and is occasionally contraindicated. Although maternal infection is usually not a contraindication to breast-feeding, maternal HIV infection is one exception to this recommendation in the United States. This is not necessarily true, however, in many developing countries, where the risk of death during the first year of life without breast-feeding is greater than the risk of HIV infection. Antibiotics are generally safe during breast-feeding, but certain other drugs are contraindicated (Table 11–4).

Solid Foods

Supplemental foods may be added to infants' diets between the ages of 4–6 months. Solid foods should be introduced as soon as infants require the additional calories and are developmentally mature (e.g., infant can sit and support the head). Early introduction of solid foods has been associated with an increased incidence of food allergy and may contribute to overeating and obesity. Factors that indicate infants may be ready for solid foods include (1) current weight twice that of birth weight, or about 13 pounds; (2) consumption of more than 32 ounces of formula per day; (3) frequent feeding (regularly more than 8–10 times per day or more often than every 3 hours); and (4) persistent unsatisfaction due to hunger.

The quantity of formula should be limited to no more than 32 ounces to allow for the introduction of solid foods. An iron-fortified infant cereal, most commonly

TABLE 11–3. Composition of Breast Milk and Select Infant Formulas (Calories: 20 kcal/oz)

Formula	Protein	Carbohydrate	Fat
Human milk (mature)	40% casein and 60% whey	Lactose	Human milk fat
Cow's milk	80% casein and 20% whey	Lactose	Butterfat
Enfamil 20	Nonfat cow's milk and whey	Lactose	Palm olein, soy, coconut, and high-oleic sunflower oils
Isomil	Soy protein and methionine	Corn syrup and sucrose	Soy and coconut oils
Nutramigen	Casein hydrolysate, and cystine, tyrosine, tryptophan	Corn syrup solids and cornstarch	Palm olein, soy, coconut, and high-oleic sunflower oils
Pregestimil	Casein hydrolysate, and cystine, tyrosine, tryptophan	Corn syrup solids, modified tapioca starch, and dextrose	MCT, corn, high-oleic safflower and soy oils
ProSobee	Soy protein and methionine	Corn syrup solids	Palm olein, soy, coconut, and high-oleic sunflower oil
Similac 20	Nonfat cow's milk and whey	Lactose	High-oleic safflower, coconut, and soy oils

Abbreviation: MCT, medium-chain triglycerides.

rice cereal, is usually the first solid food offered to infants. Other single-grained cereals, such as barley cereal or oatmeal, are also appropriate early supplemental foods. Fruits and vegetables may be introduced within a few weeks. The order is not as important as the need to add only one new food at a time—no more than one to two new foods per week. Meats may be introduced after 6 months of age.

Although commercially prepared infant juices are an important source of vitamin C for infants and may provide a smooth transition to solid foods, excessive juice intake may be associated with diarrhea and growth

failure. About 2 ounces of apple juice can be given at 4–6 months of age. This can be gradually increased to about 4 ounces per day. Once infants have accepted the juice, a small quantity of cereal can be added to it and offered to infants with a spoon. Solid foods should not be mixed in the bottle; caregivers should wait until the infant can accept spoon feedings. It is not unusual for infants to reject their first several spoonfuls of cereal, because the tastes and textures are new. If they refuse the feeding, it should be stopped. Solid foods should be reintroduced in one week.

Precooked infant cereals, such as rice cereal, can be mixed with a variety of liquids, including breast milk, formula, infant fruit juices, or water. Initially, the cereal should be mixed to a thinner consistency (e.g., about 1 tablespoon of cereal to 2 oz of liquid), and once infants have accepted the new taste and texture, the mixture should gradually be worked to a thicker consistency. By about 7–8 months of age, infants should be taking 4–6 tablespoons of cereal mixed with enough liquid to give the mixture the consistency of mustard. Mixed cereal grains may be introduced to older infants.

A wide variety of commercially prepared baby foods designed to be developmentally appropriate and labeled by stage (i.e., first-, second-, third-stage) are available. The jars of different stages contain the amount of food that an infant at a given age should be able to eat at one sitting. This is not always the case, however, and opened jars of baby food may safely be stored in the refrigerator for 2–3 days. Infants should not be fed directly from the jar, because saliva on the spoon mixes with the remaining food and digests it, causing it to liquefy. Vegetables and meats may be offered at room temperature but should be warmed slightly for greater palatability. Fruits and desserts may be at room or refrigerator temperature.

First-stage foods, for infants 4–6 months of age, include strained infant juices, single-grain cereals, and puréed fruits and vegetables, such as bananas, carrots, and peas. These foods contain no egg, milk, wheat, or citrus, to which some infants may be sensitive. Second-stage foods, for infants from about 6–9 months of age, are smooth, mixed-ingredient foods, such as mixed vegetables, or meat dinners, such as chicken noodle. Third-stage foods, or junior foods, are for infants about 9–10 months of age who can sit well without support,

TABLE 11–4. Drugs and Breast-feeding

Contraindicated	Avoid or Use With Great Caution	Probably Safe But Use With Caution
Antineoplastic agents	Anthroquinolones (laxatives)	Anesthetics
Amphetamine	Aspirin	Acetaminophen
Bromocriptine	Atropine	Aldomet
Clemastine	Birth control pills	Antibiotics (not tetracycline)
Cimetidine	Bromides	
Chloramphenicol	Calciferol	Antithyroids (not methimazole)
Cocaine	Cascara	
Cyclophosphamide	Danthron	Antiepileptics
Cyclosporine	Dihydrotachysterol	Antihistamines*
Diethylstilbestrol	Estrogens	Antihypertensives/ cardiovascular agents
Doxorubicin	Ethanol	
Ergots	Metoclopramide	Bishydroxycoumarin
Gold salts	Metronidazole	Chlorpromazine*
Heroin	Narcotics	Codeine*
Immunosuppressants	Phenobarbital*	Digoxin
Iodides	Primidone	Dilantin
Lithium	Psychotropic drugs	Diuretics
Meprobamate	Reserpine	Furosemide
Methimazole	Salicylazosulfapyridine (sulfasalizine)	Haloperidol*
Methamphetamine		Hydralazine
Nicotine (smoking)		Indomethacin
Phencyclidine (PCP)		Methadone*
Phenindione		Muscle relaxants
Radiopharmaceuticals		Prednisone
Tetracycline		Propranolol
Thiouracil		Propylthiouracil
		Sedatives
		Theophylline
		Vitamins
		Warfarin

*Watch for sedation.
Reproduced, with permission, from Behrman, R.E., (ed.). Nelson Textbook of Pediatrics, 14th ed. Philadelphia, W.B. Saunders, 1992, p. 428.

have some teeth, and have begun self-feeding. These more coarsely textured foods contain a wider variety of nutrients, such as vegetable and meat dinner combinations. Finger foods, such as crackers, cheese wedges, or cookies, can also be introduced by 9–10 months of age, once infants have developed a pincer grasp. Most infants are eating the same meals as the rest of the family (table foods) by about one year of age. Foods that can easily be aspirated, such as raw carrots, nuts, and hard candies, should be avoided, however, until children are over 4 years of age.

Baby foods can be prepared at home as long as they are finely puréed or strained and contain enough liquid to make them easy for infants to swallow. One danger of preparing foods at home is that sugar, salt, or spices can be easily added to make foods palatable to adults. These ingredients are not necessary for infants. In addition, home-grown, home-prepared vegetables may be contaminated with high levels of nitrates (e.g., due to contaminated well water) and nitrites (e.g., in vegetables such as carrots, beets, and spinach). Nitrates and nitrites have been implicated in the development of methemoglobinemia, especially in infants under 6 months of age. Methemoglobinemia decreases the oxygen-carrying capacity of the blood, leading to anoxic injury and death.

Weaning from the breast or bottle to a cup usually occurs at 6–12 months of age but may be delayed up to 18 months of age in some children. Homogenized, vitamin D–fortified cow's milk may be given at 12 months of age. Skim milk or lowfat milk (2% milk fat) should not be given before 2 years of age.

DIET OF CHILDREN AND ADOLESCENTS

The caloric and protein needs of children decrease in the second year of life, paralleling the decrease in growth rate during this time. Milk intake also decreases, and may drop to 16 ounces per day by 24–36 months of age. Except for increased caloric requirements, the diet of school-age children and adolescents should be similar to that of normal adults. Evidence that foods eaten during childhood may have long-lasting effects on adult health is increasing, and it is important that children develop healthy eating habits early in life. Atherosclerosis, osteoporosis, and obesity are some of the diseases that may have their beginnings during childhood.

ASSESSMENT OF NUTRITIONAL STATUS IN INFANTS AND CHILDREN

History

Nutritional assessment begins with a complete dietary history. The dietary assessment should emphasize the quantity, quality, and variety of foods in the diet. Any special or restricted dietary habits should be noted (e.g., vegetarian diet). A 3-day food record listing the types and quantities of food eaten throughout the day can be very helpful in evaluating the dietary history.

In addition, the child's routine medical, family, and social history all may influence nutritional status. For example, the economic status of families may affect the variety and type of foods that they may be able to purchase, and the level of education of parents influences their ability to understand the concepts of a healthy diet. Poverty and ignorance regarding nutritional needs are among the most common reasons for malnutrition in children. Family access to food can be estimated by asking parents about how often the family skips meals during the average month.

Physical Examination

Height, weight, and head circumference should be measured routinely and plotted on a longitudinal basis on appropriate growth curves. Changes in the rate of growth over time are more useful than a single measurement in time in the assessment of nutritional problems. Calculation of the height age (age for which the child's height is at the 50th percentile), weight age (age for which the child's weight is at the 50th percentile), and ideal weight for actual height may be useful when deviations from normal are noted.

In addition to the overall impression regarding nutritional status, certain findings on physical examination may be characteristic of particular nutritional disorders. The evaluation of the hair, skin, eyes, lips and oral mucosa, dentition, and musculoskeletal system should be emphasized, because the examination of these areas is most likely to show the effects of malnutrition. Muscle wasting, hepatosplenomegaly, skeletal deformities, decayed teeth, rough dry skin, easily pluckable hair, and irritability may all be clues to inadequate nutrition (Table 11–5).

Laboratory Tests

Suspected malnutrition or nutrition-related disorders, based on history and physical examination, can be further investigated with laboratory studies. Tests that may be used in the evaluation of anemia, one of the most common nutrition-related disorders seen in children, include a CBC, reticulocyte count, serum iron, ferritin, and total iron-binding capacity. Investigation of suspected malnutrition begins with an assessment of protein status, with measures of indicators such as serum albumin, total protein, and prealbumin. Liver function tests and a lipid profile may also be useful in the evaluation of suspected malnutrition. Screening tests that may be used in the evaluation of failure to thrive (FTT) include thyroid function studies, urinalysis, and bone age. More specific tests, such as serum vitamin levels (e.g., folate or vitamin B_{12} levels in suspected malabsorption) or hormone assays (e.g., growth hormone levels in the evaluation of FTT), may be obtained in certain instances.

COMMON FEEDING AND NUTRITIONAL PROBLEMS OF CHILDHOOD

Several GI problems have been attributed to diet. A small amount of spitting up is seen in the majority of children, especially during the first 6 months of life.

TABLE 11–5. Physical Signs of Nutritional Deficiency Disorders

System	Sign	Deficiency
General appearance	Reduced weight for height	Calories
Skin/hair	Pallor	Anemias (iron, B_{12}, vitamin E, folate, and copper)
	Edema	Protein, thiamine
	Nasolabial seborrhea	Calories, protein, vitamin B_6
	Dermatitis	Riboflavin, essential fatty acids, biotin
	Photosensitivity dermatitis	Niacin
	Acrodermatitis	Zinc
	Follicular hyperkeratosis (sandpaperlike)	Vitamin A
	Depigmented skin	Calories, protein
	Purpura	Vitamins C, K
	Scrotal, vulval dermatitis	Riboflavin
	Alopecia	Zinc, biotin, protein
	Depigmented, dull hair	Protein, calories, copper
Subcutaneous tissue	Decreased	Calories
Eye (vision)	Adaptation to dark	Vitamins A, E, zinc
	Color discrimination	Vitamin A
	Bitot spots, xerophthalmia, keratomalacia	Vitamin A
	Conjunctival pallor	Nutritional anemias
	Fundal capillary microaneurysms	Vitamin C
Face, mouth, neck	Angular stomatitis	Riboflavin, iron
	Cheilosis	Vitamins B_6, niacin, riboflavin
	Bleeding gums	Vitamins C, K
	Atrophic papillae	Riboflavin, iron, niacin
	Smooth tongue	Iron
	Red tongue (glossitis)	Vitamins B_6, B_{12}, niacin, riboflavin, folate
	Parotid swelling	Protein
	Caries	Fluoride
	Anosmia	Vitamins A, B_{12}, zinc
	Hypogeusia	Vitamin A, zinc
	Goiter	Iodine
Cardiovascular	Heart failure	Thiamine, selenium, nutritional anemias
Genital	Hypogonadism	Zinc
Skeletal	Costochondral beading	Vitamins D, C
	Subperiosteal hemorrhage	Vitamin C, copper
	Cranial bossing	Vitamin D
	Wide fontanelle	Vitamin D
	Epiphyseal enlargement	Vitamin D
	Craniotabes	Vitamin D, calcium
	Tender bones	Vitamin C
	Tender calves	Thiamine, selenium
	Spoon-shaped nails (koilonychia)	Iron
	Transverse nail lines	Protein
Neurologic	Sensory, motor neuropathy	Thiamine, vitamins E, B_6, B_{12}
	Ataxia, areflexia	Vitamin E
	Ophthalmoplegia	Vitamin E, thiamine
	Tetany	Vitamin D, Ca^{++}, Mg^{++}
	Retardation	Iodine, niacin
	Dementia, delirium	Vitamin E, niacin, thiamine

Reproduced, with permission, from Behrman, R.E., and R.M. Kleigman (eds.). Nelson's Essentials of Pediatrics, 2nd ed. Philadelphia, W.B. Saunders, 1994.

However, vomiting can be a sign of several disorders, ranging from viral GI tract infections to more severe illnesses such as pyloric stenosis, urinary tract infection, and GI obstruction (see Chapter 86, Vomiting). Constipation, which is seen more commonly in formula-fed than breast-fed infants, may be due to insufficient fluid intake (see Chapter 90, Constipation). The simple addition of 4–6 ounces of water to an infants' diet or temporary use of apple or prune juice may solve the problem. Enemas and suppositories should not be recommended routinely.

Chronic nonspecific diarrhea of childhood, or "toddler's diarrhea," may be seen in infants and children 6 months to 5 years of age with low dietary fat intake and excessive fruit juice consumption (see Chapter 89, Diarrhea). Failure to absorb sugars, especially sorbitol and fructose, can lead to an osmotic diarrhea.

Underfeeding or a diet that is not nutritionally balanced may result in FTT (see Chapter 106, Failure to Thrive). The opposite problem, obesity, is one of the most common nutritional problems of children in the United States (see Chapter 110, Childhood Obesity). The prevalence of this condition in children 6–11 years of age is estimated to be about 20–25%. Finally, the eating disorders, anorexia nervosa and bulimia, are estimated to affect about 1 in 100 adolescent females 16–18 years of age (see Chapter 109, Eating Disorders).

Nutritional disorders include malnutrition and deficiencies of vitamins and minerals. Table 11–5 lists the characteristics of various vitamin and mineral deficiencies. Anemia is one of the most common nutrition-related problems seen in children. Malnutrition is one of the leading causes of childhood morbidity and mortality worldwide. Although primary protein-calorie malnutrition (PCM) is rare in most parts of the United States, surveys conducted on pediatric wards have demonstrated that about one third of pediatric inpatients with chronic disease have evidence of some degree of PCM. The most common deficits were weight for height below 90% of standard (i.e., evidence of acute malnutrition) and height for age less than 95% of standard (i.e., evidence of chronic malnutrition). The two forms of PCM are marasmus (severe caloric depletion) and kwashiorkor (inadequate protein intake). Untreated PCM can result in impaired growth, poor intellectual development, and impaired immune functioning.

Case Resolution

The infant described in the case history is probably ready to begin some solid foods because she is consuming 32 ounces of formula per day and continues to be hungry. In addition, she has reached a weight of 13 pounds and has almost doubled her birth weight. The mother is counseled to begin feeding her daughter a single-grain infant cereal mixed with either formula or juice. (The cereal should be fed by spoon, not given in a bottle.) Within a few weeks, once the infant is taking the cereal well, other first foods such as fruits and vegetables may be introduced.

Selected Readings

Balint, J. P. Physical findings in nutritional deficiencies. Pediatr. Clin. North Am. 45:245–260, 1998.

Barness, L. A. Nutrition update. Pediatr. Rev. 15:321–326, 1994.

Cutts, D. B., A. M. Pheley, and J. S. Geppert. Hunger in midwestern inner-city young children. Arch. Pediatr. Adolesc. Med. 152:489–493, 1998.

Dusdieker, L. B., and C. I. Dungy. Nitrates and babies: a dangerous combination. Contemp. Pediatr. 13:91–102, 1996.

Greer, F. R. Formulas for the healthy term infant. Pediatr. Rev. 16:107–112, 1995.

Hendricks, K. M., C. Duggan, L. Gallagher, et al. Malnutrition in hospitalized pediatric patients: current prevalence. Arch. Pediatr. Adolesc. Med. 149:1118–1122, 1995.

Klish, W. J. Childhood obesity. Pediatr. Rev. 19:312–315, 1998.

Kneepkens, C. M. F., and J. H. Hoeksra. Chronic nonspecific diarrhea of childhood: pathophysiology and management. Pediatr. Clin. North Am. 43:375–390, 1996.

Lawrence, R. A. The pediatrician's role in infant feeding decision making. Pediatr. Rev. 14:265–272, 1993.

Lawrence, R. A. Breastfeeding: A Guide for the Medical Profession, 4th ed. St. Louis, Mosby–Year Book, 1994.

Powers, N. G., and W. Slusser. Breastfeeding update 2: clinical lactation management. Pediatr. Rev. 18:147–161, 1997.

Slusser, W., and N. G. Powers. Breastfeeding update 1: immunology, nutrition, and advocacy. Pediatr. Rev. 18:111–119, 1997.

Smith, M. M., M. Davis, F. I. Chasalow, et al. Carbohydrate absorption from fruit juice in young children. Pediatrics 95:340–344, 1995.

CHAPTER 12

SLEEP: NORMAL PATTERNS AND COMMON DISORDERS

Geeta Grover, M.D.

H_x   During a routine 6-month health maintenance visit, a mother states that although her 6-month-old son falls asleep very easily at about 10 PM every night while breast-feeding, he wakes every 2–3 hours and cries until she nurses him back to sleep. A review of the dietary history reveals that the infant is breast-fed about every 3 hours and was begun on rice cereal 2 weeks ago. His immunizations are current; he should receive his third dose of DTaP/IPV/Hib today. The boy has no medical problems, and his physical examination is normal.

Questions

1. How old are most infants when they can begin to sleep through the night (at least 5 hours at a stretch) without a feeding?
2. What factors contribute to frequent nighttime wakings during infancy?
3. What advice can be given to parents to facilitate an infant's sleeping through the night?

Sleep disorders are common during infancy and childhood. Getting children to go to bed, fall asleep, stay asleep, and stay in bed can be no small challenge. Parents frequently ask pediatricians about sleep-related problems at routine health maintenance visits. Age-appropriate suggestions on how to help children sleep well are usually welcomed by parents.

EPIDEMIOLOGY

Bedtime struggles and frequent night wakings occur in 20–25% of children under 3 years of age. In preschool-age children, nighttime fears (e.g., fear of noises, fear of the dark) or separation anxiety often contribute to these problems. As children get older, nightmares and night terrors may contribute to difficulties with night wakings. About 5% of individuals experience nightmares, which usually begin before the age of 10 years and are seen more often in girls than in boys. Night terrors are a specific form of partial night waking from deep sleep that may begin during the preschool years. The incidence in children is reported to be 1–4%, with the greatest frequency between 5 and 7 years of age. Such terrors are more common in boys than in girls, and a familial tendency has been reported. Febrile illness and obstructive sleep apnea may be predisposing factors.

In most Western countries, children are expected to sleep in their own beds. However, in many cultures, it is not uncommon for infants and young children to sleep in their parents' bed (the "family bed"). **Co-sleeping** is not a problem in and of itself, and the decision to cosleep, like the decision to breast- or bottle-feed, is an entirely personal one. Parents who are interested in cosleeping should be cautioned that bed-sharing is not a solution to sleep problems, however; in the long term it may even contribute to them. Parents who share a bed with their children commonly have to lie down with them for 20–30 minutes to get them to fall asleep. Several studies have shown that cosleeping infants are two to three times more likely to have night awakenings than those who sleep alone. Furthermore, infants who are both breast-feeding and bed-sharing sleep the shortest periods prior to awakening.

PATHOPHYSIOLOGY

To understand the problems associated with sleep, the physiology of normal sleep and the development of normal sleep behavior in children must be understood.

Sleep States

Normal sleep has two distinct states, **rapid eye movement (REM)** and **non–rapid eye movement (NREM)** sleep. REM sleep develops at about 29 weeks' gestation and then persists throughout life. It is an active, lighter stage of sleep that occurs in association with rapid eye movements. Other features of REM sleep include suppression of muscle tone; rapid, irregular pulse and respiratory rate; and body twitches. Dreams occur during REM sleep. The EEG pattern of REM sleep is very similar to stage 1 NREM sleep.

NREM sleep begins at about 32–35 weeks' gestation. During NREM sleep, pulse and respiratory rates are slower and more regular, and body movements are minimal. Most of the restorative functions of sleep occur during this state. After the first several months of life, NREM sleep may be divided into four stages ranging from drowsiness to very deep sleep. Each stage represents a progressively deeper state of sleep and has a characteristic EEG tracing: stage 1 has low-voltage, fast activity; stage 2 is notable for the presence of sleep spindles and K complexes against a low-voltage background; and stages 3 and 4 are identified by varying amounts of high-amplitude, slow waves known as delta waves (Fig. 12–1).

The Sleep Cycle

REM and NREM sleep together make up the sleep cycle. Typically, the deepest sleep takes place during the first several hours of the night, with lighter stages of NREM sleep and REM sleep occurring during most of the rest of the night. Although sleep stages are the same in both infants and adults, several differences concerning the onset and duration of REM and NREM sleep between infants and adults exist. First, the sleep cycle is shorter in infants (50–60 minutes) than in adults (90–100 minutes), which means that infants have more periods of active REM sleep as compared to adults. Second, the total amount of time spent in REM sleep decreases with increasing age. Term newborns spend about 50% of their

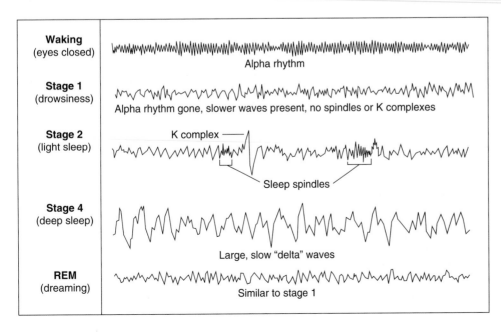

Waking (eyes closed)	Alpha rhythm
Stage 1 (drowsiness)	Alpha rhythm gone, slower waves present, no spindles or K complexes
Stage 2 (light sleep)	K complex — Sleep spindles
Stage 4 (deep sleep)	Large, slow "delta" waves
REM (dreaming)	Similar to stage 1

FIGURE 12–1. Brain wave patterns in waking and sleep. (Reproduced from Ferber, R. Solve Your Child's Sleep Problems. New York, Simon & Schuster, 1985, p. 24. Copyright 1985 by Richard Ferber, M.D. Reprinted by permission of Simon & Schuster, Inc.)

total sleep time in REM sleep (up to 80% in premature infants); this decreases to about 30% by 3 years of age and to 20% by adulthood. Third, infants may have very little REM latency, entering their first REM cycle very shortly after falling asleep. Adults, in comparison, generally enter their first REM period about 90 minutes after the onset of sleep.

Sleep-Wake Patterns

Sleep patterns follow a normal developmental sequence in children; the amount of sleep children need changes with maturation (Fig. 12–2). Healthy term newborns sleep 16–17 hours per day. Because they are unable to sleep for more than a few hours at a time, sleeping and waking periods are fairly evenly distributed throughout the day and night. Many infants are able to sleep through the night (at least 5 hours uninterrupted) by the age of 3 months; most infants are capable of this by 4 months. Brief arousals are a normal part of the sleep cycle at all ages, but children should be able to return to sleep on their own without requiring parents' attention. Children should definitely be able to fall asleep on their own by the age of 4–6 months. Otherwise, parental participation to fall asleep becomes required at every awakening throughout the night.

By 12 months of age, infants sleep about 14 hours per day, divided into two naps during the day and a period of about 10 hours at night. During the second year of life, most children stop napping in the morning. By 2 years of age, they require about 13 hours of sleep per day (1–2 hours in an afternoon nap and 11–12 hours at night). Most children take an afternoon nap until 3 years of age, and some children continue this until 5 years of age. The amount of nighttime sleep children need gradually continues to decline, decreasing from about 12 hours during the preschool years to about 8–9 hours during adolescence.

Sleep Abnormalities

The etiology of sleep disorders can be complex, involving the interaction of children's temperamental characteristics, psychosocial stressors in the home, parental childrearing philosophies, and the developmental nature of normal sleep states and sleep cycles.

DIFFERENTIAL DIAGNOSIS

The differential diagnosis of sleep disorders may be distinguished by problems associated with falling asleep or frequent night wakings (Table 12–1). Falling asleep may present two types of difficulties: problems associated with settling children to sleep and bedtime refusal.

In infants, **inappropriate sleep-onset associations** are the most common reason for difficulty settling to sleep. These infants require parental participation (e.g., holding, rocking, feeding) to fall asleep. They have not learned the critical skills of self-calming and initiating sleep on their own. Because these infants do not have

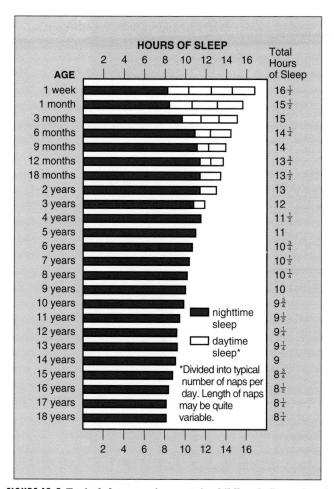

FIGURE 12–2. Typical sleep requirements in childhood. (Reproduced from Ferber, R. Solve Your Child's Sleep Problems. New York, Simon & Schuster, 1985, p. 19. Copyright 1985 by Richard Ferber, M.D. Reprinted by permission of Simon & Schuster, Inc.)

the self-soothing behaviors necessary to fall back asleep after normal nighttime arousals, they may also have nighttime wakings. Brief arousals are a normal component of sleep. Nighttime wakings are different, because parents' participation is needed to resettle children. The difficulty that the children experience falling back to sleep on their own, not the waking itself, is the problem.

An example of an inappropriate sleep-onset association is the child who needs to be nursed or fed to fall asleep. The term **"trained night feeder"** has been coined to describe children who need to be fed before going back to sleep after normal nighttime awakenings. Although they are developmentally old enough to receive all nutrition during the day, they have become conditioned to require nighttime feedings. These children are often nursed or bottle-fed until they fall asleep and only then placed in the crib. They are conditioned to require feeding to initiate sleep, and when they experience normal nighttime arousals, they require the breast or bottle to go back to sleep.

The term **"trained night crier"** refers to children who, like "trained night feeders," lack the self-comforting and self-initiating skills necessary to fall asleep on their own. Trained night criers awaken, cry, and want to be held,

---

TABLE 12–1. Practical Approach to the Differential Diagnosis of Sleep Disorders in Children

---

Difficulty Falling Asleep
Circadian and sleep schedule disturbances
Irregular sleep/wake patterns
Advanced sleep phase
Delayed sleep phase
Regular but inappropriate sleep schedules without phase shifts (e.g., late evening naps)
Habits, associations, and expectations
Inappropriate sleep-onset associations
Bedtime refusal/bedtime struggles
Poor or inconsistent limit setting
Overstimulation
Psychosocial
Separation anxiety
Nighttime fears (e.g., fears of the dark, monsters)
Family and social stresses
Medical
Acute illness
Underlying medical problems
Medications (e.g., antihistamines, stimulants, codeine, anticonvulsants)
Nighttime Waking
Normal variation (e.g., breast-fed infant)
Habits, associations, and expectations
Inappropriate sleep-onset associations: (e.g., age-inappropriate night wakings for feeding)
Psychosocial
Nighttime fears
Family and social stresses
Medical
Acute illness
Underlying medical problem
Medications
Nightmares
Arousal disorders (e.g., night terrors, sleep walking, and sleep talking)
Miscellaneous Sleep Disorders
Intrinsic sleep disorders
Narcolepsy
Sleep apnea (obstructive or central)
Sleep-wake transition disorders (e.g., head banging, rocking)

---

comforted, or entertained before they can go back to sleep.

Acute illness may also be a cause of sleep disturbances. Children with otitis media may awaken at night because of pain. They may continue to experience awakenings after the infection has resolved, however, and require comforting or some sort of attention to fall asleep again.

In children between the ages of 9 and 18 months, **separation** and **separation anxiety** may also affect sleep patterns. Children may cry when parents leave the room and have difficulty settling to sleep. Ability to climb out of the crib or bed can be associated with nighttime wakings in older toddlers. The transition from a crib to a bed is usually made between 2 and 3 years of age. Children who can climb out of their cribs or beds may come out of their rooms repeatedly for drinks of water, trips to the bathroom, or to sleep in the parents' bed. Such factors as nighttime fears of the dark influence sleep behaviors during the preschool years (3–5 years of age). Children's growing needs for autonomy and control over their environment may lead to bedtime refusals during both the toddler and preschool years.

Disorders of the sleep-wake cycle may contribute to sleep schedule irregularities. Circadian rhythms govern the regularity and degree of wakefulness and sleepiness. The circadian clock inherent in humans is not an exact 24-hour pattern but can be modified or entrained onto one by environmental cues. Regular and consistent structure needs to be provided by parents, because development of children's sleep-wake rhythms depend on an interaction of the child's inherent biologic rhythms with the environment. Entrainment requires predictable occurrence of time cues such as light and dark, mealtime, and bedtime. A consistent waking time in the morning is one of the most important of these cues.

Irregular sleep-wake cycles may be seen in children living in chaotic environments with irregular mealtimes and sleep-wake schedules. A delayed sleep phase and regular but inappropriate sleep-wake schedule are the most common forms of sleep rhythm disturbance. Children with **delayed sleep phase** have a resetting of their circadian rhythm; they are not sleepy at bedtime and have excessive morning sleepiness. This is a common problem, because the inherent circadian clock has a cycle closer to 25, not 24, hours. This clock has not been entrained to a 24-hour schedule in these children.

Examples of **regular but inappropriate sleep-wake schedules** include children who nap at the "wrong" time (e.g., a child who regularly naps at 7 PM for one hour and then has trouble going to bed at 9 PM) and infants who seem to have day and night confused. These children sleep most of the day and stay up most of the night.

Night terrors (pavor nocturnus), **sleepwalking** (somnambulism), and **sleeptalking** (somniloquy) are all forms of partial awakenings that occur during deep or stage 4 NREM sleep, most often during the transition from stage 4 NREM sleep to the first REM sleep period. Sleepwalking and sleeptalking usually occur during the school-age years, whereas night terrors begin during the preschool years.

Both nightmares and night terrors may begin during the preschool years and may continue throughout childhood. Night terrors are different from nightmares and occur during a different stage of the sleep cycle (Table 12–2). With night terrors, children usually sit up in bed and cry or scream inconsolably for up to 15 minutes. They may appear dazed and have signs of autonomic arousal such as tachycardia, tachypnea, and

---

TABLE 12–2. Nightmares Versus Night Terrors

Characteristic	Nightmare	Night Terror
Time of night	Late	Early, usually within 4 hours of bedtime
Sleep stage	REM sleep	Partial arousal from deep NREM sleep
State of child	Scared, but consolable	Disoriented, confused, and inconsolable
Memory of event	Clear recall of dream	Usually none
Return to sleep	Reluctant because of fear	Easily, unless fully awakened
Management	Reassure child	Reassure parents

sweating. These children cannot be consoled. When they finally go back to sleep, they do not remember the event in the morning. Because parents are often frightened by the experience, they may think the child is having a seizure or is suffering from an emotional disturbance and may seek medical advice. Although attacks may be precipitated by stressful events or fatiguing daytime activities, night terrors do not indicate excessive stress or emotional disturbance in children's lives unless they recur.

Nightmares usually occur during the last third of the night during REM sleep, whereas night terrors more often take place during the early part of the night. Nightmares are scary dreams that may awaken children, who can often remember them. Children can usually be consoled by parents but are reluctant to go back to sleep because of their fears.

Excessive daytime sleepiness can be a symptom of medical problems such as depression, sleep apnea, or illness. Viral illness is perhaps the most common medical cause of such sleepiness in children. Inadequate sleep at night may also be a potential cause of sleepiness during the day. Narcolepsy, a disorder of excessive sleepiness, is characterized by an overwhelming desire to sleep during the daytime despite adequate sleep at night. Its symptoms include excessive daytime sleepiness, cataplexy, sleep paralysis, and hypnagogic hallucinations. Cataplexy is an abrupt loss of muscle tone that is usually precipitated by an emotional reaction such as laughter or anger. Sleep paralysis is an inability to move or speak that occurs as patients fall asleep or awaken. Hypnagogic hallucinations, which can be visual or auditory, occur while falling asleep.

Narcolepsy affects about 0.05–0.1% of the general population. The prevalence increases to 50% when the family history is positive. The exact genetic basis of inheritance is unknown. The age of onset is usually between 10 and 20 years. The diagnosis is often delayed or missed for months to years in some cases because not all symptoms may be present initially. Diagnosis is important because pharmacologic therapy with CNS stimulants may provide some symptomatic relief.

EVALUATION

History

Evaluation of children with sleep difficulties begins with a thorough, detailed sleep history taken from both parents and children, if old enough (Questions Box).

Evaluation should also include an assessment of children's temperament and psychological well-being. Children's developmental status and level of function should also be evaluated.

Physical Examination

Physical examination is important to rule out organic causes of sleep difficulties. Acute illness (e.g., otitis media), obstructive sleep apnea resulting from adenoidal or tonsillar hypertrophy (most commonly), colic, gastroesophageal reflux, and any CNS disease or abnormality may all alter the sleep-wake cycle.

Questions: Sleep

- Does the child have regular nap times and bedtimes, or do these depend on changing parental schedules?
- What activities does the child participate in during the evening before going to bed?
- Where does the child sleep?
- Does the child sleep in his or her own room or in the parents' room in his or her own bed or crib?
- Does anyone else sleep in the room?
- Is the child able to fall asleep on his or her own, or does he or she require the parent's participation?
- Does the child require feeding or fluids at night?
- What typically happens when the child wakes at night? Which parent attends to the child? What does the parent do?
- Is there a family history of sleep disturbances?
- Is there any stress within the home due to marital or financial difficulties that may affect the home environment and cause the child to be anxious or stressed?
- Is the child taking any medications that may affect sleep patterns?
- How long has the child been having sleep disturbances?
- Does the child experience problems every night or only intermittently?

Laboratory Tests

Laboratory assessment is usually not necessary. An EEG may be useful if a central abnormality such as a seizure disorder is suspected. Polysomnography, the simultaneous monitoring of EEG, ECG, chin muscle tone, eye movements, and respirations during a night of sleep in a sleep laboratory may be very useful in certain children when significant sleep disturbances such as apnea are suspected.

MANAGEMENT

The goal of management is to help children develop a healthy pattern of sleeping, not simply eliminate the immediate problem. Healthy sleep associations include providing a consistent schedule of naps and bedtime, along with a pleasant bedtime routine. It is important to put infants in their cribs while they are relaxed and drowsy but not already asleep. This gives them the opportunity to develop skills to put themselves to sleep. If they become accustomed to being fed or rocked until they fall asleep, they will seek the same means of falling asleep every time they normally wake up during the night. In addition, overstimulation in the evening may make settling to sleep difficult for toddlers or young children. Instead, a routine such as a bath followed by a story in the child's bedroom with a clearly defined end point when the parent leaves the child in the crib or bed sleepy but awake may help facilitate sleep. Children must learn to fall asleep on their own.

Trained night feeders and trained night criers are infants who have not learned to fall asleep on their own. The basic treatment for these children is to put them in their cribs when they are sleepy but awake and ignore the subsequent crying. Their last memory before falling asleep should not be of their mothers holding or feeding them. If the crying persists, the contact with the infants should be brief and boring. Scheduled awakening is a technique in which infants are slightly aroused by the parent 15–60 minutes before an expected spontaneous awakening in an effort to prevent spontaneous awakening. Scheduled awakenings may be an effective treatment alternative for some trained night criers. If infants awaken for a feeding, parents should try to stretch the interval between waking and feeding so that children have an opportunity to practice self-calming techniques.

Specific sleep disorders can be addressed individually. Older toddlers and preschoolers who delay going to bed or refuse to stay in their room at night need clear, firm limits. It is important that these children have consistent bedtime routines and nighttime interventions for when they awaken. A gate may need to be installed in the bedroom doorway to prevent children who refuse to stay in their rooms at night from moving about the house and potentially hurting themselves or disturbing others. Parents of children who have night terrors may require reassurance that their children are not suffering from significant emotional problems or stressors. A night-light may help alleviate the anxieties of preschoolers who are unable to sleep at night because of their fears of darkness. Disturbances of the sleep-wake schedule can be corrected over time by gradually shifting children's schedules in the desired direction. For example, children with a delayed sleep phase who go to bed very late can have their morning wake-up time progressively advanced about 15 minutes per day; this is followed by a progressive advancement in their bedtime until the desired schedule is reached.

PROGNOSIS

Unfortunately, infants with sleep problems tend to grow into children with sleep problems. Researchers have found that about 40% of infants with sleep problems at the age of 8 months still had a problem at 3 years. It is to the parents' advantage to help their children develop healthy sleep habits rather than ignore the problems and hope that the children outgrow them.

Case Resolution

The 6-month-old infant described in the case history has disordered sleep associations. He has been conditioned to nighttime feedings, although he is old enough not to require them for nutrition. The physician suggests several things the mother can do to try to solve her son's sleep problem. She can begin by gradually lengthening the interval between daytime feedings to 4–5 hours. When he cries at night, she can wait progressively longer before feeding him and can then eventually eliminate the feedings altogether. He will learn to fall asleep on his own without requiring feeding.

Selected Readings

American Academy of Pediatrics: Sleep Problems. *In* Guidelines for Health Supervision III. Elk Grove Village, IL, American Academy of Pediatrics, 1997, pp. 207–210.

Blader, J. C., et al. Sleep problems of elementary school children. Arch. Pediatr. Adoles. Med. 151:473–480, 1997.

Blum, N. J., and W. B. Carey. Sleep problems among infants and young children. Pediatr. Rev. 17:87–93, 1996.

Ferber, R. Solve Your Child's Sleep Problems. New York, Simon & Schuster, 1985.

Kemper, K. J. Sleep Problems. *In* The Holistic Pediatrician. New York, HarperCollins, 1996, pp. 265–284.

McKenna, J. J., S. S. Mosko, and C. A. Richard. Bedsharing promotes breastfeeding. Pediatrics. 100:214–219, 1997.

Rickert, V. I., and C. M. Johnson. Reducing nocturnal awakening and crying episodes in infants and young children: A comparison between scheduled awakenings and systematic ignoring. Pediatrics. 81:203–211, 1988.

Schmitt, B. D. Sleep. *In* Your Child's Health, rev. ed. New York, Bantam Books, 1991, pp. 239–268.

Wise, M. S. Parasomnias in children. Pediatr. Ann. 26:427–433, 1997.

CHAPTER 13

DENTAL CARE

Geeta Grover, M.D.

Hx The parents of a 9-month-old girl bring her to the office because they are concerned that their daughter has no teeth yet. Growth and development have proceeded normally, and the physical examination is unremarkable.

Questions

1. What is the mean age and range for the eruption of the first tooth?
2. What is meant by the term "mixed dentition?"
3. At what age should fluoride supplementation begin?
4. When should oral hygiene using a toothbrush begin?

Pediatricians play an important role in the maintenance and evaluation of the oral health of children. Routine examination and screening of the oral cavity allow physicians to monitor normal development of teeth and screen for early signs of disease and abnormalities that involve the teeth or supporting structures. Parental counseling regarding preventive dental care and oral hygiene is also important.

NORMAL ANATOMY OF THE ORAL CAVITY

The oral cavity consists of teeth and supporting structures. Individual teeth have four major components (Fig. 13–1): the outer layer, or **enamel;** the inner layer, or **dentin,** which constitutes the bulk of the tooth; the **pulp,** which contains the neurovascular structures; and the **root,** which secures the tooth into its socket in the maxilla or mandible. The **supporting structures** consist of the **bones of the face** (maxilla and mandible) and the **periodontal tissues** (gingiva, alveolar bone, periodontal ligament, and cementum). The visible portion of an erupted tooth is called the **crown.**

GROWTH AND DEVELOPMENT OF TEETH

Unlike the other calcified tissues of the body, which are mesodermal, the teeth originate from both ectoderm (enamel) and mesoderm (dentin and pulp). Tooth development occurs both pre- and postnatally in four stages, which may be summarized as growth, calcification, eruption, and exfoliation. **Growth** begins at about 6 weeks of gestation with the establishment of the organic matrix of the primary teeth. **Calcification,** or hard tissue formation, which involves the deposition of enamel, first occurs at about 3–4 months' gestation; the permanent teeth also begin to develop at this time. Although the major part of enamel deposition of the primary teeth has occurred by birth, this process may continue until the age of 12–16 years in one or more of the permanent teeth. **Eruption** occurs when approximately two thirds of root development is complete, and the tooth protrudes through the gingiva. **Exfoliation** of the primary teeth may be referred to as the final stage of tooth development. Table 13–1 summarizes the chronology of tooth development for both the primary and permanent teeth.

Normal Dentition

There is a relationship between the pattern of tooth eruption and skeletal maturation ("poor man's bone age"). Knowledge of the chronology of dental development can help physicians monitor normal growth and development and identify specific disease.

Primary Dentition

The period of primary dentition begins with the eruption of the first tooth, usually at about 6 months of age (normal range, about 4–12 months). In the vast majority of infants, the first tooth to appear is the man-

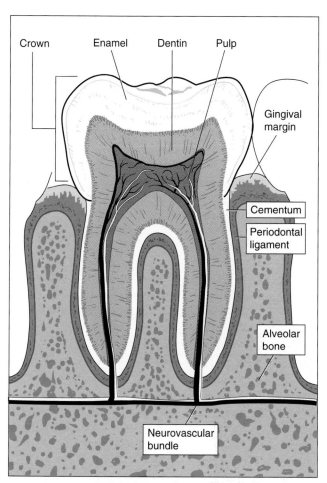

FIGURE 13–1. Tooth anatomy.

Crown   Enamel   Dentin   Pulp

Gingival margin

Cementum

Periodontal ligament

Alveolar bone

Neurovascular bundle

TABLE 13–1.   Chronology of Human Dentition

Primary or Deciduous Teeth

	Eruption		Shedding	
	Maxillary	Mandibular	Maxillary	Mandibular
Central incisors	6–8 mo	5–7 mo	7–8 yr	6–7 yr
Lateral incisors	8–11 mo	7–10 mo	8–9 yr	7–8 yr
Cuspids (canines)	16–20 mo	16–20 mo	11–12 yr	9–11 yr
First molars	10–16 mo	10–16 mo	10–11 yr	10–12 yr
Second molars	20–30 mo	20–30 mo	10–12 yr	11–13 yr

Secondary or Permanent Teeth

	Eruption	
	Maxillary	Mandibular
Central incisors	7–8 yr	6–7 yr
Lateral incisors	8–9 yr	7–8 yr
Cuspids (canines)	11–12 yr	9–11 yr
First premolars (bicuspids)	10–11 yr	10–12 yr
Second premolars (bicuspids)	10–12 yr	11–13 yr
First molars	6–7 yr	6–7 yr
Second molars	12–13 yr	12–13 yr
Third molars	17–22 yr	17–22 yr

Adapted, with permission, from Behrman, R.E. (ed.). Nelson Textbook of Pediatrics, 14th ed. Philadelphia, W.B. Saunders, 1992, p. 40.

dibular central incisor. The **incisors** (central and lateral) erupt first; these are followed by the **first molars,** the **cuspids,** and the **second molars.** The mnemonic device used to recall this sequence is "forward-forward-back-forward-back" (incisor-incisor-molar-cuspid-molar). Maxillary teeth generally erupt 1–2 months after their mandibular counterparts. The 20 primary teeth should all be in place by the age of 24–36 months. In general, it is more important to know that one tooth should appear per month once eruption has begun than it is to remember how many teeth should be present at a given age.

During the period of primary dentition, extra space between the teeth may be apparent. This space is actually normal and beneficial because it gives the larger permanent teeth more room. Crowding of the primary teeth may be an early indication of similar problems with the permanent teeth.

The time of eruption of primary teeth varies considerably. Late eruption is probably no cause for concern in children who are otherwise growing and developing normally. Significant delays in eruption, especially when associated with other developmental delays, however, may be associated with a variety of nutritional and systemic disturbances such as rickets, Down syndrome (trisomy 21), hypopituitarism, and hypothyroidism.

Teething, the eruption of the primary teeth, is a normal part of development that usually occurs uneventfully. However, many symptoms have been attributed to teething by parents, grandparents, and physicians. Low-grade fever; drooling; local, temporary discomfort at the site of tooth eruption; and increased fussiness are some of the symptoms more commonly ascribed to teething. Otitis media, upper respiratory infection, and diarrhea are all common conditions during infancy whose appearance may coincide with the eruption of primary teeth. High fever, irritability, or signs of systemic illness should not be attributed to teething alone; further evaluation is necessary.

An eruption hematoma, a bluish swelling of the overlying gum, may precede the eruption of a tooth. It usually ruptures when the tooth appears and requires no further treatment. Symptoms of teething may be treated with acetaminophen, infant teething rings, and infant teething gels (if used correctly). Several other teeth remedies that have been suggested include hard or frozen bagels, ice, or firm rubbing of the gums. Caution is warranted when preparations containing topical anesthetics are used, because cases of seizures secondary to excessive absorption of the anesthetic have been reported.

Mixed Dentition

Mixed dentition occurs during the transition from primary to permanent dentition. It begins at about 6 years of age with the exfoliation of the primary teeth, usually the central incisors, followed by the eruption of the first permanent molars. The early appearance of primary teeth may herald the early eruption of permanent teeth. This stage continues until the last primary tooth has been shed, at about 12 years of age.

Two common, normal variations may give the children an awkward appearance temporarily. Either the maxillary permanent incisors may erupt in a widely spaced, outwardly inclined position ("ugly-duckling" stage) or the mandibular incisors may erupt behind the primary incisors ("double teeth"). These variations generally self-correct as dental development continues.

Permanent Dentition

Permanent dentition begins with the exfoliation of the last primary tooth, usually the cuspid or second molar, at 10–12 years of age. The permanent teeth number 32 (Fig. 13–2). Each of the four quadrants of the mouth

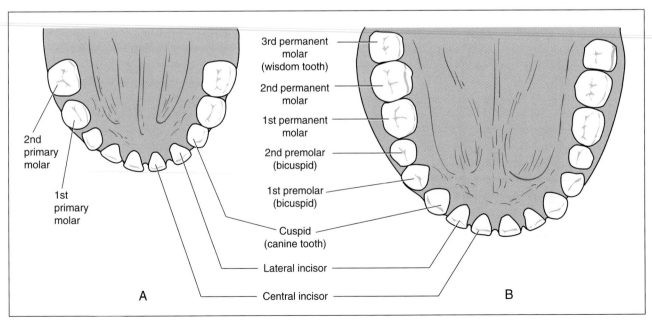

FIGURE 13–2. Primary dentition (A) and permanent dentition (B). (From Zitelli, B. J., and H. W. Davis [eds.]. Atlas of Pediatric Physical Diagnosis, 2nd ed. Philadelphia, J. B. Lippincott, 1992, with permission.)

contains two incisors, one cuspid, two premolars (bicuspids), and three molars (the third molar is the wisdom tooth).* The manner in which the teeth of the mandibular and maxillary arches fit together is referred to as **occlusion.** Normally, the maxillary incisors slightly overlap their mandibular counterparts. Occlusion is fully established on completion of the permanent dentition, but it may be altered during the pubertal growth spurt secondary to jaw growth.

PREVENTIVE DENTAL CARE

Pediatricians can begin preventive oral health counseling during routine health maintenance visits. The role of nutrition, oral hygiene, daily fluoride intake, and nonnutritive sucking can be discussed with parents and children at this time. The American Academy of Pediatric Dentistry recommends that all children have their first visit to the dentist for examination and oral health counseling by 12–18 months of age.

Nutrition

Proper nutrition is essential to the development of healthy teeth. **Vitamins A, C, and D** as well as **calcium** and **fluoride** are particularly important in the formation of teeth. Maintenance of a diet low in sugar to help prevent caries is also important. It is particularly critical that pediatricians inform parents about nursing bottle caries, because these caries may harm both the primary teeth and any unerupted permanent teeth (see Chapter 51, Common Oral Lesions).

Oral Hygiene

Counseling parents about oral hygiene should begin during their child's first year of life. During infancy, parents can **wipe children's teeth and gums** with a damp washcloth after feedings. A soft **toothbrush** moistened with **water** may be used after several teeth have appeared. **Toothpaste** may be introduced to children between the ages of 2 and 3 years. Parents should be warned that children of this age often swallow the toothpaste. A small, pea-sized amount should be used to minimize fluoride ingestion. **Flossing** should also be initiated when children are 2–3 years of age. It is usually not necessary before this age because tooth-to-tooth contact before this time is minimal.

Parents should continue to brush and floss their children's teeth at least once a day until the age of 6 years, when children should be encouraged to perform additional brushings themselves, with supervision. Although children usually begin to brush their teeth independently at age 6, they still require assistance with flossing. Not until the age of 8–10 years do children have the fine motor coordination necessary to brush and floss effectively.

Fluoride

Fluoride is one of the most effective prophylactic agents in the prevention of dental caries. Dramatic reductions in the rate of dental caries have been demonstrated when systemic fluoride therapy is begun during infancy. Fluoride may be provided both systemically and topically (e.g., fluoride-containing toothpaste and rinses or direct application in the dentist's office).

Systemic fluoride is incorporated into the enamel of the developing tooth, thus serving as an effective preeruptive cariostatic agent. Fluoride in the saliva provides a topical cariostatic effect by interfering with plaque-related microorganisms. For maximum protection against caries, **systemic fluoride** should be provided while teeth are developing; **topical fluoride** may be applied after teeth begin to erupt.

Because the incidence of fluorosis in children living in the United States correlates with early use of supplemental fluoride, it is now recommended that systemic fluoride therapy begin at 6 months of age. Fluoridation of drinking water is the most effective way of providing systemic fluoride. The optimal concentration of fluoride in the local water supply varies in accordance with the climate (climate determines the amount of water children drink); it ranges between 0.7 and 1.2 ppm. Fluoride supplements may be prescribed in the form of drops or tablets based on children's age and the amount of fluoride in the drinking water (Table 13–2). Infants who are breast-fed or drink premixed formula require full fluoride supplementation until they begin drinking fluoridated water. Ideally, supplementation should be continued until all of the permanent teeth, excluding the third molars, have erupted, which is usually between 12 and 14 years of age (see Table 13–1). The American Academy of Pediatrics recommends that supplementation continue until 16 years of age to ensure maximum benefit.

The recommended therapeutic fluoride dosage is 0.05–0.07 mg/kg/day. Children who consistently consume 0.1 mg/kg or more of fluoride per day are likely to develop dental fluorosis. Fluorosis is the result of disruption in enamel formation; therefore, it can only be caused by the preeruptive ingestion of systemic fluoride. Small white specks on the enamel surfaces of teeth are the only signs of mild fluorosis, whereas pitting and brown discoloration of teeth surfaces are associated with severe fluorosis.

TABLE 13–2. Fluoride Supplementation*			
Age	**Water Fluoride Content (ppm)**		
	<0.3	**0.3–0.6**	**>0.6**
Birth–6 mo	0	0	0
6 mo–3 yr	0.25	0	0
3–6 yr	0.50	0.25	0
6–16 yr	1.00	0.50	0

*Fluoride daily doses are given in milligrams.

Reproduced, with permission, from the Committee on Nutrition: Fluoride Supplementation for Children: Interim Policy Recommendations. Pediatrics 95:777, 1995.

*The widsom teeth generally erupt between the ages of 17 and 22 years. The timing of their eruption is highly variable, however.

Although acute fluoride toxicity is rare, ingestion of large amounts can be potentially fatal (e.g., 500 mg of fluoride is a lethal dose for a 3-year-old child). To avoid accidental overdoses, no more than 120 mg of supplemental fluoride should be prescribed at one time.

Nonnutritive Sucking

Nonnutritive sucking is a normal and essential activity for infants and young children. They may suck as a means of enjoyment, to cope with stress, or for comfort. Sucking is initially a reflex activity but later becomes an adaptive or learned behavior. The thumb, fingers, and pacifier are the most common objects used for sucking. An estimated 70% of children still practice some form of nonnutritive sucking at the age of 12 months. This decreases to 40% by the age of 24 months and to 1% by the age of 6 years. Most children discontinue the habit themselves by age 3. Generally, nonnutritive sucking has no long-term effects on permanent dentition if the habit ceases by the age of 4 or 5 years (see Chapter 32, Thumb-sucking and Other Habits). The most common dental problem associated with prolonged sucking is development of malocclusion.

Case Resolution

The parents of the infant in the case history should be reassured that the absence of teeth in their 9-month-old daughter is normal. Her first tooth may not appear until she is 12 months old. As long as she is growing and developing normally, there is no cause for concern.

Selected Readings

Griffen, A. L., and S. J. Goepferd. Preventive oral health care for the infant, child and adolescent. Pediatr. Clin. North Am. 38:1209–1226, 1991.

Jaber, L., I. J. Cohen, and A. Mor. Fever associated with teething. Arch. Dis. Child. 67:233–234, 1992.

Nazif, M. M., et al. Oral disorders. *In* Zitelli, B. J., and H. W. Davis. Atlas of Pediatric Physical Diagnosis, 3rd ed. St. Louis, Mosby-Wolfe, 1997, pp. 603–624.

Nowak, A. J. Promoting oral health in the school-age child. Contemp. Pediatr. 11:27–51, 1994.

Nowak, A. J. What pediatricians can do to promote oral health. Contemp. Pediatr. 10:90–106, 1993.

Schuman, A. J. How much fluoride is too much? The new guidelines. Contemp. Pediatr. 12:65–74, 1995.

Schusterman, S. Pediatric dental update. Pediatr. Rev. 15:211–218, 1994.

CHAPTER 14

NORMAL DEVELOPMENT AND DEVELOPMENTAL ASSESSMENT

Geeta Grover, M.D.

Hx The parents of a 12-month-old child are concerned that she is not walking yet. They report that she sat independently at 7 months and began crawling at 8 months. She can pull herself up to stand while holding on but is not cruising. Her birth and medical history are both unremarkable. The physical examination is within normal limits.

Questions

1. What are the major areas in which development is assessed?
2. What are the gross motor, fine motor, and personal/social milestones for a 12-month-old child?
3. What tests are useful for assessing child development?
4. How is developmental delay in children defined?

Development refers to the acquisition of functional skills during childhood. Monitoring the growth and development of children is an integral part of the assessment of pediatric patients. Recording the acquisition of developmental milestones provides a systematic approach by which to observe the progress of children over time. For ease of monitoring, these developmental milestones may be divided into five major domains or areas: gross motor, fine motor/adaptive, personal/social, language, and cognitive. This chapter discusses these major areas of development and the principles that govern them.

Four principles apply to all aspects of development. First, motor development is a continuous process that proceeds in the cephalocaudal direction and parallels neuronal myelination; therefore, developmental milestones reflect the maturation of the nervous system. Second, the sequence of development is the same in all children, but the rate of development may vary from child to child (e.g., all children must walk before they run, but the age at which children walk or run varies from child to child). Third, the rate of attainment of milestones in one area may not parallel that in another. Fourth, certain primitive reflexes must be lost before corresponding voluntary movements can be attained (e.g., the asymmetric tonic neck reflex must disappear before children can roll over).

PATHOPHYSIOLOGY

Development is influenced by both biological and environmental factors. Biological factors such as prematurity, exposure to drugs in utero, or the presence of chronic disease may place children at increased risk for developmental problems and delays. Environmental factors influencing development include parental attitudes and actions, sociodemographic factors, and cultural and societal influences. The quality of parental stimulation may influence the rate of acquisition of certain skills, especially cognitive and language abilities in preschool-age children. Poverty and other socioeconomic factors may make it difficult for parents to provide their child with an optimal environment for growth and development.

Development in Newborns and Infants

Normal, full-term newborns enter the world capable of responding to visual, auditory, olfactory, oral, and tactile stimuli. They can be quieted and can even soothe themselves. Newborns can signal needs (e.g., crying when hungry or wet), but they have a limited ability to respond to caregivers, primarily exhibiting disorganized and seemingly purposeless movements when stimulated. The newborn's reflexive generalized symmetric movements (e.g., arm waving and kicking) in response to environmental stimuli, are eventually replaced by cortically mediated voluntary actions in older infants and children. Additionally, in newborns, certain primitive reflexes can be elicited by appropriate peripheral stimuli. Eventually, primitive reflexes are replaced by reactions that allow children to maintain postural stability in response to a variety of sensory inputs (proprioceptive, visual, and vestibular).

Primitive reflexes are mediated by the brainstem; they are involuntary motor responses that are elicited by appropriate peripheral stimuli. They are present at birth and disappear during the first 6 months of life. Normal motor development appears to be related to the suppression of these reflexes (Fig. 14–1). Persistence or reappearance of these reflexes may indicate the presence of brain damage. **Postural reactions,** which are ultimately smoothly integrated into adult motor function (Fig. 14–1), appear between 2 and 9 months of age. These reactions help maintain the orientation of the body in space and the interrelationship of one body part to another. The three major

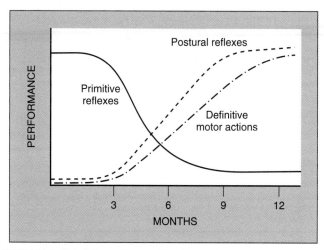

FIGURE 14–1. Primitive reflex profile. (Reproduced, with permission, from Capute, A. J., et al. Primitive Reflex Profile. Baltimore, University Park Press, 1978, p. 10.)

categories of postural reactions are righting, protection, and equilibrium.

The profile generated by combining primitive reflexes and postural reactions can be used to monitor the course of normal development and identify cases of problematic development. Persistence of primitive reflexes or failure of development of postural reactions can signal developmental problems. Authorities estimate that there are over 70 primitive reflexes and postural reactions. Researchers do not agree on which of these reflexes or reactions are the most useful in the monitoring of development. The seven most commonly used primitive reflexes are described in Table 14–1, and selected postural reactions are presented in Table 14–2.

TABLE 14–1.   Selected Primitive Reflexes

Moro Reflex
Allowing the infant's head to drop back suddenly results in abduction and upward movement of the arms followed by adduction and flexion. This reflex disappears by 4 months.

Rooting Reflex
Touching the corner of the infant's mouth results in lowering of the lower lip on the same side and movement of the tongue toward the stimulus.

Sucking Reflex
Placing an object in an infant's mouth causes vigorous sucking.

Grasp Reflex
Placing a finger in an infant's palm causes the infant to grasp it; the infant reinforces the grip as the finger is drawn upward. A similar response is seen in the foot grasp. Both these reflexes disappear by 2–3 months.

Placing Reflex
Stroking the anterior aspect of the tibia against the edge of a table results in the lifting of the infant's leg to step onto the table.

Stepping Reflex
Holding the infant upright and slightly leaning forward produces alternating flexion and extension movements of the legs that simulate walking. This reflex disappears by 5–6 weeks.

Asymmetrical Tonic Neck Reflex
With the infant lying supine, turning the head to one side results in extension of the extremities on that side and flexion of the opposite extremities ("fencer position"). This reflex disappears by 3–4 months.

TABLE 14–2.   Selected Postural Reactions

Righting Reactions

These allow the body to maintain normal postural relationships of the head, trunk, and extremities during all activities. The different reactions appear at different ages, beginning shortly after birth and ranging up to 12 months of age.

Protection and Equilibrium Reactions

Protective Equilibrium Response

When gently pushed toward one side while in a sitting position, infants increase trunk flexor tone toward that side to regain their center of gravity and extend the arm on the same side to protect against falling. This response usually emerges at about 4–6 months of age.

Parachute Reactions

When held in ventral suspension and suddenly lowered (downward parachute), infants extend their arms as if to protect themselves from a fall; similar reactions are seen with forward and backward stimulation. These reactions appear at 8–9 months.

Normal Development

A developmental assessment should include an evaluation of milestones in each of the five major areas. **Gross motor skills** are overall movements of large muscles (e.g., sitting, walking, running). **Fine motor-adaptive skills** involve use of the small muscles of the hands, the ability to manipulate small objects, problem-solving skills, and eye-hand coordination. **Language skills** include hearing, understanding, and use of language. **Personal-social skills** involve socialization and ability to care for personal needs. **Cognitive skills** involve the ability to use higher mental processes including comprehension, memory, and logical reasoning.

Table 14–3 outlines the normal pattern of development with regard to each of these skills. Although the table lists the average ages for the attainment of these skills, it is important to remember that there is a wide normal range. Development is an orderly and sequential process, and children must proceed through several stages before any given milestone is attained. Therefore, the physician should document not only *what* children can do but *how* they do it. For example, to sit without support, children first achieve head control. Several stages later they are able to sit in a "tripod" position with arms extended in front for support, and finally sit with the head steady and back straight without support (Fig. 14–2).

Gross Motor Skills

During the first year of life, the ultimate goal of gross motor development is walking. The first step toward this

TABLE 14–3.   Normal Pattern of Development

Gross Motor Skills		Personal-Social Skills	
Newborn	Reflex head turn; moves head side to side	Newborn	Regards face
1 mo	Lifts head when prone	6 wk	Spontaneous social smile
2 mo	Lifts shoulders up when prone	6 mo	Discriminates social smile
3 mo	Lifts up on elbows; head steady when upright	7 mo	Displays stranger anxiety; plays peek-a-boo (7–9 mo)
4 mo	Lifts up on hands; rolls from front to back; no head lag when pulled to sitting from supine position	12 mo	Drinks from a cup
5 mo	Rolls back to front	15–18 mo	Uses a spoon, spilling a little
6 mo	Sits alone 30 seconds or more	2 yr	Washes and dries hands
7–8 mo	Crawls/sits well	3 yr	Uses a spoon well; uses buttons
9–10 mo	Pulls to stand	4 yr	Washes and dries face; engages in cooperative play
10–11 mo	Cruises	5 yr	Dresses without assistance
12 mo	Walks	**Language Skills***	
15 mo	Walks backwards	Newborn	Alerts to bell
18 mo	Runs; kicks a ball	2 mo	Cooing; searches with eyes for sound
2 yr	Walks up and down stairs (taking one step at a time and holding on; stands on one foot [2.5 yr])	4 mo	Turns head to sound of voice or bell; laughs (3 mo)
3 yr	Walks up stairs alternating steps; rides a tricycle	6 mo	Babbles
4 yr	Walks down stairs alternating steps/hops on one foot	8 mo	Mama/dada nonspecific
5 yr	Skips	9 mo	Understands the word "no"
Fine Motor-Adaptive Skills		12 mo	Mama/dada specific; follows one-step command with gesture/3–5-word vocabulary
1 mo	Tracks horizontally to midline	14 mo	Follows one-step command without gesture
2 mo	Tracks past midline/tracks vertically	16 mo	Can point to several body parts
3 mo	Unfisted for >50% of the time; tracks 180 degrees; visual threat; discovers midline	2 yr	50-word vocalary; two-word sentences; uses pronouns indiscriminately
4 mo	Reaches for bright object; brings object to mouth	2.5 yr	Gives first and last names; uses plurals
5 mo	"Rakes" at bright object	3 yr	250-word vocabulary; three-word sentences; speech intelligible to strangers 75% of time; uses pronouns discriminately
6 mo	Transfers object from one hand to the other	**Cognitive Skills**	
7 mo	Three-finger pincer grasp	Newborn–2 yr	Sensorimotor
9 mo	Neat pincer grasp bangs cubes in midline	2–6 yrs	Preoperational
14 mo	Tower of two cubes; scribbles spontaneously	6–11 yrs	Concrete operational
18 mo	Tower of four cubes	>11 yrs	Formal operations
2 yr	Copies vertical and horizontal line; tower of six cubes	**Miscellaneous Cognitive Milestones**	
3 yr	Copies circle	24 mo	Concept of today
4 yr	Copies "+" (3.5 yr)	30 mo	Concept of tomorrow
5 yr	Copies square; draws person with three parts (4.5 yr)	36 mo	Concept of yesterday
6 yr	Copies triangle; draws person with six parts	7 yr	Concept of right and left

*Detailed milestones are presented in Chapter 15, Table 15–1.

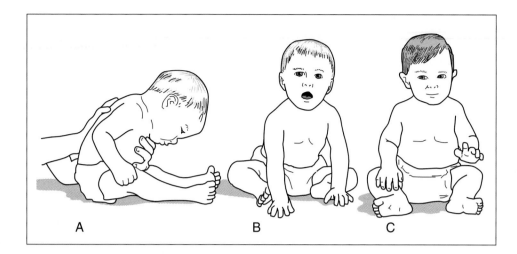

FIGURE 14–2. Stages in the development of sitting.
A. Head control.
B. "Tripod sitting."
C. Head steady and back straight without support.

goal is head control. By 6 months of age, children are able to sit without support for a few seconds. At 9–10 months children are able to pull themselves to a standing position, and by 12–14 months of age they are able to walk. Children then learn to run, negotiate stairs, hop on one foot, and skip—in that order.

Fine Motor Skills

Development of the two-finger pincer grasp is the major goal of fine motor development during the first year (Fig. 14–3). The hands primarily remain in a fisted position until 3 months of age. Infants also discover the midline at this age, and shortly thereafter they may play with the hands in the midline. Five-month-old children begin "raking" at desired objects; by 6 months of age they are able to transfer objects from one hand to the other. By 7 months they have a three-finger pincer grasp, and by 9–12 months they have developed the two-finger grasp, which allows them to manipulate small objects such as raisins and pencils. By 14 months they begin to

scribble, and by 3–5 years they are able to copy geometric shapes. Children with early preference for the use of one hand over another should be assessed for the presence of paresis or other neuromuscular problems. Handedness may develop by 3 years but often is not firmly established until the age of 4–5 years.

Language Skills

The development of normal speech and language skills is discussed in Chapter 15, Language Development.

Personal-Social Skills

These skills enable children to interact and respond to the surrounding world. The spontaneous social smile appears at 6 weeks of age followed by the discriminate social smile at 6 months. Stranger anxiety appears at 7 months, when games such as peek-a-boo become appealing.

FIGURE 14–3. Development of the pincer grasp.
A. Rake (4 months).
B. Inferior pincer grasp (7 months).
C. Fine pincer grasp (9–12 months).

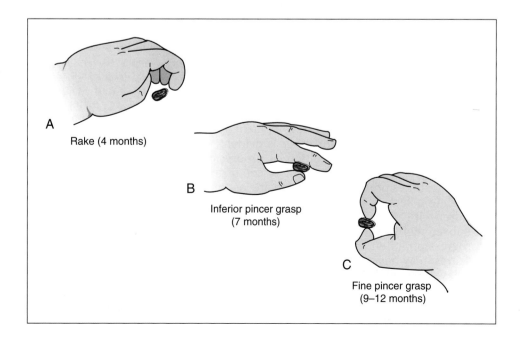

A
Rake (4 months)

B
Inferior pincer grasp (7 months)

C
Fine pincer grasp (9–12 months)

TABLE 14-4. Stages of Development of Piaget

Sensorimotor (birth-2 years)
Children approach the world through sensations and motor actions. They develop a sense of object permanence, spatial relationships, and causality.

Preoperational (2-6 years)
Children's mental processes are linked to their own perception of reality. They do not separate internal and external reality.

Concrete Operational (6-11 years)
Children can perform mental operations in their heads if they relate to real objects. They develop concepts of conservation of mass, volume, and number.

Formal Operations (>11 years)
Children develop the capacity for abstract thought.

Cognitive Skills

These abilities allow children to think, reason, problem-solve, and understand the surrounding environment. The concept of object permanence or object constancy, the realization that objects may exist even if they cannot be seen, develops at approximately 7–9 months of age. The understanding of time comes much later. Children develop the concept of "today" at 24 months of age, "tomorrow" at 30 months, and "yesterday" at 36 months. It is extremely important that health care providers realize that children's perception and understanding of pain, disease, and illness are guided by their stage of cognitive development. The psychologist Jean Piaget generated complex generalizations by observing what children did and how they did it; his theories are the cornerstone of knowledge in this area. Piaget's four stages of cognitive development are presented in Table 14–4.

Developmental Delay

Children are said to be developmentally delayed if they fail to reach developmental milestones at the expected age. This age ranges widely because of the wide variation among normal children. Individual children may be delayed in one area or several areas of development.

DIFFERENTIAL DIAGNOSIS

Three factors are involved in the differential diagnosis of children with developmental delays: (1) determination of the area or areas of development in which delay is apparent; (2) if motor delay is evident, determination of whether the condition is progressive or nonprogressive; and (3) assessment to see if developmental milestones previously achieved are lost or if age-appropriate milestones were achieved at all.

Children with an early history of normal development who subsequently experience a slowing of developmental progression, often associated with cognitive delays or seizures, may have a metabolic defect. Children who attain developmental milestones and subsequently lose them may have a neurodegenerative disease (e.g., multiple sclerosis, adrenoleukodystrophy) or a lesion of the spinal cord or brain. The presence of habitual rhythmic body movements (e.g., body rocking, head banging) may be a sign of a pervasive developmental disorder such as autism.

Cerebral palsy, the classic example of nonprogressive motor abnormality, is a form of static encephalopathy characterized by abnormal movement and posture. The type of cerebral palsy depends on which area of the brain is injured. Spastic cerebral palsy, seen most commonly, is secondary to upper motor neuron injury. The ataxic form of the disease is related to lesions of the cerebellum or its pathways. Dyskinetic cerebral palsy manifests as uncontrolled and purposeless movements that often result from a basal ganglia lesion (e.g., athetosis following bilirubin deposition in the basal ganglia [kernicterus]). The onset of symptoms is either in infancy or early childhood. The key factor in making the diagnosis is establishing that the motor deficits are static and nonprogressing.

EVALUATION

When evaluating children for possible delays in development, it is important to remember that there is a great deal of variation in the age of attainment of milestones. In addition, the rate of acquisition of milestones in one area of development may not parallel that in another. Routine and ongoing assessment of a child's level of development at all periodic health maintenance visits through observation, history, physical examination, and screening tests allows the physician to form a longitudinal view of the child. The physician is thus able to identify and differentiate true deficits and delays from temporary setbacks.

History

Evaluation of children for suspected delays in development includes a complete history (Questions Box). Family history is important, because other family members may have relatively delayed attainment of milestones. Perinatal factors that place children at high risk for developmental difficulties include a history of maternal drug or alcohol use during pregnancy, prematurity in the infant, and congenital infections. Other historical risk factors for developmental delay include history of seizures, sepsis or meningitis, exposure to lead or other toxins, and poor feeding or growth. Environmental factors such as stressful home conditions, history of abuse or neglect, and lack of stimulation may also contribute to delayed development.

Questions: Normal Development

- Has anyone in the child's family had developmental problems or delays?
- Did the mother use any drugs or alcohol during pregnancy?
- Was the child premature?
- Does the child have a history of seizures?
- Has the child had meningitis or sepsis?
- Does the child have any history of not feeding well or poor growth?
- Is the child's home environment characterized by any stresses (e.g., divorce, limited financial resources)?

Physical Examination

Both height and weight should be checked. Abnormal growth (i.e., height or weight less than the fifth percentile or head circumference either less than the fifth percentile or greater than the 90th percentile) may be a risk factor for developmental delay. The presence of congenital anomalies (e.g., cataracts, hypertelorism, spina bifida) or neurocutaneous lesions (e.g., café-au-lait spots) may be suggestive of chromosomal anomalies or other genetic diseases. Neuromuscular examination should emphasize age-appropriate milestones. Abnormalities in muscle tone (e.g., hypotonia, hypertonia) or bulk or strength may be clues to the presence of neuromuscular disease (e.g., muscular dystrophy), cerebral palsy, or Down syndrome.

Laboratory Tests

Age-appropriate assessment of the child's vision and hearing should be performed if signs of motor, cognitive, or language delays are apparent. Chromosomal studies may be conducted if dysmorphic features are noted on the physical examination. Evidence of cognitive or motor delays may warrant metabolic studies (e.g., organic and amino acids).

Imaging studies of the head such as MRI scans or EEGs may be necessary if the child has a history of seizures or an abnormal neurologic examination.

Developmental Testing

Developmental screening tests provide an objective assessment of children's performance on age-appropriate tasks in each area and allow for comparison with peers. Screening tests may be used regularly at routine well child care visits, most commonly the 9, 24, and 36 month visits, to help identify, in a timely manner, potential developmental problems and delays. Most pediatricians, however, use screening tests as a second stage evaluation when developmental delay is suspected based on routine developmental surveillance.

Although several screening tests for early development are available (Table 14–5), the Denver II (formerly, the Denver Developmental Screening Test–Revised) is probably the most widely used screening instrument for children from birth to 6 years of age. The test, divided into four areas (gross motor, fine motor-adaptive, personal-social, and language), consists of 125 tasks or items and takes 15–20 minutes to administer. It assesses the presence of developmental delays rather than simply giving each child an overall numerical score. Examiners should be trained in the administration of the Denver II prior to using it. Studies examining the accuracy of the Denver II in identifying children with developmental problems have shown that it has good sensitivity but limited specificity. Therefore, potentially normal children may be referred for additional evaluation.

When screening tests confirm suspicions of delay, children should be referred for more extensive developmental assessment and testing. Formal developmental testing should be performed by trained examiners.

TABLE 14–5.   Frequently Used Psychological Tests

Developmental Screening Tests
Bayley Infant Neurodevelopmental Screen
Denver-II

Developmental Tests
Gesell Developmental Schedules
Bayley Scales of Infant Development II

Intelligence Tests
Stanford-Binet Intelligence Scale, 4th edition
Kaufman Assessment Battery for Children
Wechsler Preschool and Primary Scale of Intelligence–Revised
Wechsler Intelligence Scale for Children–III

Achievement Tests
Wechsler Individual Achievement Test
Wide Range Achievement Test–III
Woodcock-Johnson Psycho-Educational Battery–Revised

Personality Tests
(projective and objective)
Draw-A-Person Test
Minnesota Multiphasic Personality Inventory–2
Rorschach Test
Thematic Apperception Test

Behavior Rating Scales
Connors Rating Scale
Achenbach Child Behavior Checklist
Vineland Adaptive Behavior Scale

Many infant/child assessment scales are currently used. The Gesell Developmental Schedules, first developed by Arnold Gesell and colleagues in 1925, are primarily of historical significance today. They emphasize the importance of maturation of the central nervous system and deemphasize the influence of the environment. The Bayley Scales of Infant Development II, first published in 1933 by Nancy Bayley, is one of the most commonly used scales today. It has three sections: mental, psychomotor, and a behavior rating scale. The Bayley II may be used for children 1–42 months of age. Developmental tests, like the Bayley II, (emphasizing sensorimotor-based skills), have a poor correlation with later measures of intelligence, (emphasizing language and abstract reasoning), especially before 24–30 months of age. As such, developmental tests are best used as measures of current developmental functioning, rather than as predictors of future functioning. Intelligence tests, achievement tests, personality tests or behavior rating scales may be used for preschool and school-age children having behavioral or emotional concerns, learning disabilities, or developmental disabilities (Table 14–5).

MANAGEMENT

Children with identified developmental delays in one or more areas should be referred to the appropriate specialist, agency, or state program for further testing and assessment. Detailed neurologic examination may be necessary if gross motor delays are identified. Language delays may warrant formal hearing and speech assessment by an audiologist or speech pathologist. Cognitive impairment requires formal psychometric assessment, which in some cases can be performed through the child's school.

PROGNOSIS

The goal of early identification and intervention is to allow individual children to reach their maximum potential. Identification and treatment of underlying disease (e.g., hypothyroidism or infection) prevents further damage. Removal of children from adverse home environments or placement of children from impoverished home environments in early intervention programs can greatly stimulate their developmental potential. The prognosis for children with mild developmental delays can sometimes be improved greatly from participation in such infant stimulation programs.

Case Resolution

The parents of the child described in the case history may be reassured that their child is developing normally for her age. Although the majority of children begin walking at about 12 months of age, commencement of walking anywhere up to the age of 17 months is considered to be within normal limits.

Selected Readings

Colson, E. R., and P. H. Dworkin. Toddler development. Pediatr. Rev. 18:255–259, 1997.

First, L. R., and J. S. Palfrey. The infant or young child with developmental delay. N. Engl. J. Med. 330:478–483, 1994.

Frankenburg, W. K., et al. Denver II Screening Test and Screening Manual. Denver, Denver Developmental Materials, Inc. 1990.

Gilbride, K. Developmental testing. Pediatr. Rev. 16:338–346, 1995.

Glascoe, F. P. Parents' concerns about children's development: Prescreening technique or screening test? Pediatrics 99:522–528, 1997.

Johnson, C. P., and P. A. Blasco. Infant growth and development. Pediatr. Rev. 18:224–242, 1997.

Olsen, R. D., W. J. Barbaresi, and G. P. Olsen. Development in the first year of life. Contemp. Pediatr. 15:81–117, 1998.

Sahler, O. J. Z., and B. I. Wood. Theories and concepts of development as they relate to pediatric practice. In Hoekelman, R. A. (ed.). Primary Pediatric Care, 3rd ed. St. Louis, Mosby-Year Book, 1997, pp. 581–601.

Stein, M. T. Preparing families for the toddler and preschool years. Contemp. Pediatr. 15:88–110, 1998.

CHAPTER 15

LANGUAGE DEVELOPMENT: SPEECH AND HEARING ASSESSMENT

Geeta Grover, M.D.

H$_x$ The parents of a 3-year-old girl bring her to see you. They are concerned because their daughter has only an 8- to 10-word vocabulary, and she does not put words together into phrases or sentences. They report that she seems to have no hearing problems; she responds to her name and follows directions well.

In general, she has been in good health. Her development, aside from delayed speech, is normal. During the physical examination, which is also normal, the girl does not speak.

Questions

1. What language skills should children have at 1, 2, and 3 years?
2. Approximately how many words should 3-year-olds have in their vocabulary?
3. By what age should children's speech be intelligible to strangers at least 75% of the time?
4. What factors may be associated with delayed speech development?
5. What tests are used to assess children's hearing, speech, and language development?

The ability to communicate through language is a uniquely human skill. Speech refers to the production of sounds, whereas language involves both comprehension and expression; it is the use of words, phrases, and gestures to convey intent. Normal hearing is essential for the development of speech and language.

The development of normal speech and language skills is an extremely important developmental milestone, that is eagerly awaited by parents. Normal patterns of language development should be as familiar to pediatricians as all other aspects of child development (see Chapter 14, Normal Development and Developmental Assessment). It is important that children with suspected language delays be referred to specialists as early as possible. Children with delayed speech or language development should be suspected of having a hearing deficit. Diminished hearing is an important cause of delayed language development.

EPIDEMIOLOGY

Sensorineural hearing loss is estimated to affect approximately 1/1000 live births in the United States. Many more infants are born with less severe hearing impairments, and still others develop hearing impairments during childhood. The prevalence of moderate to severe bilateral hearing loss is 1.5–2/1000 in children under 6 years of age. If less severe hearing losses and transient losses secondary to middle ear effusions are included, the prevalence increases significantly.

Language disorders may affect 5–10% of all children; they are one of the most common childhood disabilities. Although speech and hearing problems are common, they are often missed or minimized, and referral for evaluation and remediation is delayed significantly. Some researchers have estimated that the time from parents' first suspicion that their child may have a hearing loss to referral by the pediatrician to an audiologist for evaluation is as much as 12 months. On average, children with profound congenital hearing losses are not identified until they are approximately 2½–3 years of age, and children with less severe hearing losses may not be diagnosed until they are 4 years of age. These statistics are disturbing because the critical period for language development is within the first 3 years of life.

CLINICAL PRESENTATION

Lack of response to sound at any age, failure to achieve age-appropriate expressive language skills, and parental concern regarding a child's hearing are the most important signs of hearing or language impairment. Deaf infants coo normally and may even babble; therefore, an infant's vocalizing does not preclude a hearing loss.

PATHOPHYSIOLOGY

The left hemisphere of the brain is responsible for language skills in 94% of right-handed adults and approximately 75% of left-handed adults. Peripheral auditory stimuli are transmitted to the primary auditory areas in both temporal lobes. Sounds then undergo a series of analyses, primarily in three main areas in the left cerebral cortex: Wernicke's area (or auditory association area), which is responsible for the comprehension of language; Broca's area (or motor encoding area), which is responsible for the preliminary conversion of language into motor activity; and the primary motor cortex and supplementary motor cortex, which control the movements necessary for speech. This complex process is responsible for the comprehension and production of language.

Speech and language develop in a predictable, orderly sequence. Language skills can be either receptive or expressive. Early receptive milestones refer to ability to hear and respond to sound, whereas later milestones reflect ability to understand spoken words. Early expressive milestones relate to speech production; later, children use language to convey their intent to others. In the first year of life, receptive skills are more advanced than expressive skills.

Knowledge of normal receptive and expressive language skills (Table 15–1) is essential to recognition and identification of developmental delays. Table 15–2 lists "danger signals" that indicate possible delays and serves as a guide for referral to specialists. It is most important to remember that by the age of 3 years, 75% of children's speech should be intelligible to strangers.

DIFFERENTIAL DIAGNOSIS

The various causes of delayed language development include hearing loss, disorders of CNS processing, anatomic abnormalities, and environmental deprivation (Table 15–3). Although birth order (e.g., the belief that younger children speak later than first-born children because older siblings speak for them), laziness (e.g., "Don't give him what he wants when he points. Make him ask for it"), and bilingualism are commonly believed to lead to speech and language delay, their contributory role has never been proved.

Hearing loss, (see Chapter 53, Hearing Impairments) which may lead to language delays, is either congenital or acquired. The majority of cases of congenital deaf-

---

TABLE 15–1.   Receptive and Expressive Language Milestones (birth to three years)*

	Receptive Milestones
Newborn:	Alerts to sound (e.g., startling, widening eyes, crying)
4 mo:	Orients to sound (e.g., looks to where sound came from); responds to own name
9 mo:	Understands "no"
12 mo:	Follows one-step commands accompanied by gesture (e.g., "bring me the bottle")
14 mo:	Follows one-step commands without gesture
17 mo:	Can point to several body parts
24 mo:	Follows two-step commands (e.g., "come here and sit down")
36 mo:	Listens to stories
	Expressive Milestones
2 mo:	Cooing (vowel sounds)
4 mo:	Laughs, "ah-gooing"
6 mo:	Babbling (consonants added to vowel sounds)
8 mo:	Indiscriminate use of "mama" and "dada"
12 mo:	Discriminate use of "mama" and "dada"; three- to five–word vocabulary; one-word utterances; immature "jargoning" (e.g., essentially gibberish with intonation and inflection)
16 mo:	Mature jargoning (e.g., gibberish with occasional intelligible word)
24 mo:	50-word vocabulary; two-word sentences; indiscriminate use of pronouns
36 mo:	250-word vocabulary; three-word sentences; discriminate use of pronouns; 75% of speech intelligible to strangers

*The language skills appropriate for each age should be viewed as general guidelines.

TABLE 15–2. Danger Signals in Language Development

Inconsistent or lack of response to auditory stimuli at any age
No babbling by 9 months
No intelligible speech by 18 months
Inability to respond to simple directions or commands (e.g., "sit down," "come here") by 24 months
Speech predominantly unintelligible at 36 months
Dysfluency (stuttering) of speech noticeable after five years
Hypernasality, inappropriate vocal quality, pitch, or intensity at any age

ness are the result of genetic factors. The TORCHS infections (**t**oxoplasmosis, **r**ubella, **c**ytomegalovirus, **h**erpes simplex, **s**yphilis), especially CMV and rubella, are the most common nongenetic causes of hearing loss in the newborn period. Factors associated with high risk for infant hearing loss are outlined in Table 15–4. The leading cause of acquired hearing loss in older infants and children is meningitis.

On the basis of etiology, hearing loss can be divided into two categories: central (cortical hearing impairment) and peripheral. Peripheral causes are further subdivided into two broad groups: conductive (problems with transmission of sound through the external or middle ear) and sensorineural (inadequate transduction of sound waves into neural activity at the level of the inner ear or cranial nerve VIII).

Otitis media with effusion is the most common cause of conductive hearing loss in children (see Chapter 52, Otitis Media). Fluid in the middle ear can decrease sound conduction by an average of 25 decibels (dB). Other conditions that may result in conductive hearing loss include impaction of cerumen in the external ear canal, perforation of the tympanic membrane, atresia or stenosis of the ear canal, otosclerosis, abnormalities of the ossicles, and cholesteatoma. Injury to cranial nerve VIII or damage or maldevelopment of inner ear structures due to ototoxic agents, noise, cochlear agenesis, or perilymphatic fistula of the round or oval window membrane may lead to sensorineural hearing loss. Mixed hearing loss, a combination of conductive and sensorineural loss, may be seen in some children with developmental abnormalities.

Disorders of CNS processing include global developmental delay, mental retardation, autism, and developmental language problems. Developmental language disorders produce speech or language delays in children in the absence of hearing loss, anatomic abnormalities of the vocal tract, mental retardation, or global

TABLE 15–3. Causes of Delayed Language Development

Hearing impairment
Perinatal risk factors leading to hearing impairment
Disorders of central nervous system processing
   Global developmental delay
   Mental retardation
   Autism
   Developmental language disorders
Disorders of language production (disorders of articulation)
Presence of anatomic abnormalities (e.g., cleft lip, cleft palate)
Environmental deprivation

TABLE 15–4. Factors Associated With High Risk for Infant Hearing Loss

Neonatal Period (birth to 28 days)
Family history of hereditary childhood hearing loss
In utero infection (e.g., TORCHS infections [toxoplasmosis, rubella, cytomegalovirus, herpes simplex, syphilis])
Anatomical malformations of the head and neck region
Low birth weight (<1500 g)
Hyperbilirubinemia at a level requiring exchange transfusion
Exposure to ototoxic medications (e.g., aminoglycoside antibiotics)
Bacterial meningitis
Severe neonatal asphyxia or low Apgar score
Mechanical ventilation for 5 days or more
Stigmata of syndromes known to be associated with hearing loss

Infants and Children (28 days to 3 years of age)
Family history of hereditary hearing loss
Parental suspicion that the child does not hear
Bacterial meningitis or other infections associated with hearing loss
Severe head trauma (associated with loss of consciousness or skull fracture)
Stigmata of syndromes known to be associated with hearing loss
Exposure to ototoxic medications
Recurrent or persistent otitis media with effusion

Adapted, with permission, from the Joint Committee on Infant Hearing 1994 position statement. Pediatrics 95:152–156, 1995.

developmental delay. "Late talkers," or children who have normal comprehension but simply begin speaking late, have mild developmental language problems. Children who are completely nonverbal have more severe problems.

Anatomic abnormalities may also result in both speech and language delays. Cleft palate is the abnormality most commonly associated with difficulties in speech production. Children with cleft palate characteristically have hypernasal speech secondary to velopharyngeal incompetence (e.g., dysfunction of the soft palate). In addition, conductive hearing losses may result from chronic serous otitis media, which is common in these children. The presence of a submucous cleft palate, characterized by a bifid uvula, diastasis of the muscles in the midline of the soft palate with intact mucosa, and notching of the posterior border of the hard palate, should be considered in children without an overt cleft palate who have recurrent symptomatic serous otitis media and phonation difficulties.

Environmental deprivation is another cause of delayed language development, especially in families where children are not spoken or read to. Sometimes there is additional historical or physical evidence of deprivation (e.g., profound FTT, physical or sexual abuse) or emotional trauma (e.g., domestic violence).

EVALUATION

History

At present, an estimated 70% of children with acquired hearing loss are initially identified by their parents. Therefore, parental suspicion that their children do not hear should be sufficient reason to initiate a formal hearing evaluation. When evaluating children less than 3 years of age, pediatricians must rely primarily on parental reports of children's language capabilities (Questions Box). Children who are 3 years of age and older can usually be engaged in conversation during the visit, but younger children are more likely to be uncooperative or remain silent when confronted by strangers or new situations.

Historical factors such as a family history of childhood deafness, exposure to ototoxic agents (e.g., aminoglycoside antibiotics) neonatal asphyxia, hyperbilirubinemia, maternal cocaine abuse, or low birth weight provide valuable information in the identification of high-risk infants (see Tables 15–2 and 15–4).

Physical Examination

Examination should include a thorough assessment of the head and neck region. Microcephaly may indicate the presence of mental retardation or structural abnormalities. Abnormalities of the external ear (e.g., microtia) may be associated with sensorineural hearing loss. Otoscopic examination of the ear is essential. Presence of a middle ear effusion may be associated with a conductive hearing loss. The tympanic membrane should be examined for evidence of scarring or perforation, often secondary to recurrent otitis media. Pneumatic otoscopy provides subjective assessment of tympanic membrane mobility (compliance) when it is subjected to a pulse of air. Tympanometry (impedance audiometry) performed in the office can provide objective information regarding the mobility of the tympanic membrane and the presence of middle ear effusions (Fig. 15–1). Tympanometry is not a hearing test but rather an assessment of middle ear functioning that uses sound energy to determine the compliance of the tympanic membrane and pressure in the middle ear.

Physical stigmata of any syndromes that may be associated with deafness (Table 15–5) should be noted.

Laboratory Tests

The advantages of early identification of hearing loss cannot be overemphasized. The 1994 position statement of the Joint Committee on Infant Hearing has endorsed universal hearing evaluation of all infants prior to discharge from the newborn nursery and no later than 3 months of age. The use of high-risk criteria (see Table 15–4) to identify the population of infants to be screened is estimated to exclude approximately 50% of infants with hearing impairment. Until universal

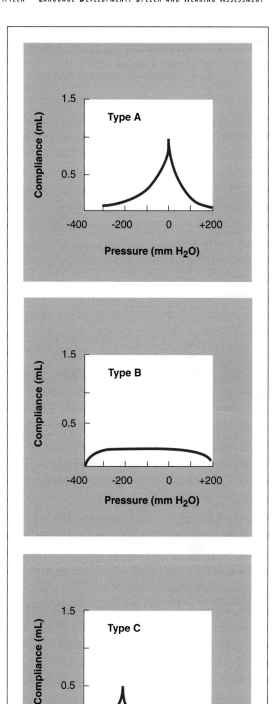

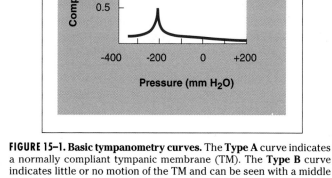

FIGURE 15–1. Basic tympanometry curves. The **Type A** curve indicates a normally compliant tympanic membrane (TM). The **Type B** curve indicates little or no motion of the TM and can be seen with a middle ear effusion, a perforation of the TM, or a patent eustachian (PE) tube. The **Type C** curve indicates negative middle ear pressure, and may be seen with a resolving middle ear effusion or eustachian tube dysfunction. Other variations can occur in these basic curves that are not illustrated here.

TABLE 15–5.   Syndromes Commonly Associated With Hearing Impairment

Autosomal Dominant Conditions

Brachio-otorenal syndrome
Goldenhar's syndrome (facioauriculovertebral dysplasia)
Stickler syndrome
Treacher Collins syndrome
Waardenburg's syndrome

Autosomal Recessive Conditions

Alport's syndrome
Jervell and Lange-Nielsen syndrome
Pendred's syndrome
Usher's syndrome

Chromosomal Disorders

Trisomy 13 syndrome
Trisomy 18q syndrome

Miscellaneous Disorders

CHARGE association (coloboma, congenital heart disease, choanal atresia, growth and mental retardation, genitourinary anomalies, ear anomalies and genital hypoplasia)
TORCHS syndrome

---

screening can be implemented, however, these factors should be used.

The evaluation of any child with delayed language development or suspected hearing loss begins with a hearing assessment. Various techniques are available, depending on the child's age and the degree of sophistication required. The brain stem auditory evoked response (BAER) may be used in children at any age, including newborns. This electrophysiologic measure, which does not require a child's cooperation, records brain waves as a function of sound stimuli (most commonly, clicks). The BAER provides an objective assessment of the integrity of auditory pathways. Behavioral audiometry, which involves rewarding children visually for turning their heads toward sounds can be used in infants over 6–8 months of age. Conventional pure tone audiometry with headphones can be used in children over the age of 3–4 years and allows for the evaluation of each ear independently. Within the frequency range of normal hearing (500–2000 hertz), a hearing threshold of 0–15 dB defines the normal range. A hearing threshold of 15–25 dB indicates minimal hearing loss; 25–40 dB, mild; 40–65 dB, moderate; 65–95 dB, severe; and 95 dB or greater, profound.

Language assessment may be aided by the use of screening tests such as the Denver II or the Early Language Milestone Scale (Coplan, J.; Austin, TX, PRO-ED, 1987). These tests are used to supplement the clinical history of a child's language abilities.

MANAGEMENT

The first 3 years of life are extremely important to language development. Hearing impairment is one of the most common causes of delayed language development

in young children. The history, physical examination, and initial screening can be used to suggest referral to various specialists (e.g., audiologists, speech pathologists, child psychologists, otolaryngologists) for further clarification of hearing, speech, or language deficits and treatment. Early identification of hearing impairment and its degree of severity allow for early intervention in the form of amplification of sound, special education for children, and counseling and support services for the families with affected children.

As soon as a diagnosis of significant hearing loss is made, **hearing aids** may be provided. **Cochlear implants** are experimental at present, but they may be useful in children with acquired hearing loss, such as toddlers with meningitis. With severe hearing loss, training in **sign language** and **lip reading,** which are most helpful for those children who already know a language, may be begun as early as possible. Special education is of prime importance in the management of children with language difficulties. The Education for All Handicapped Persons Act, federal legislation passed in 1975, requires that public schools provide an individualized and appropriate education for all children with disabilities. A knowledge of available community resources (e.g., special schools) can aid pediatricians in providing **support services** such as special community agencies and support groups for disabled children and their parents.

Case Resolution

The child described in the case history has delayed development of expressive language skills. At the age of 3 years, she should have a 250-word vocabulary and speak in three-word sentences; in addition, her speech should be primarily intelligible to strangers. Because of the delay, she should be referred immediately for a hearing assessment and speech and language evaluation. Hearing loss is an important diagnosis to rule out. Simply because her parents report no hearing problems does not mean she does not have a deficit. She may have learned to respond to nonverbal cues, or she may hear only some things.

Selected Readings

Bachmann, K. R., and J. C. Arvedson. Early identification and intervention for children who are hearing impaired. Pediatr. Rev. 19:155–165, 1998.

Coplan, J. Normal speech and language development: An overview. Pediatr. Rev. 16:91–100, 1995.

Joint Committee on Infant Hearing. Joint Committee on Infant Hearing 1994 position statement. Pediatrics 95:152–156, 1995.

Klein, S. K. Evaluation for suspected language disorders in preschool children. Pediatr. Clin. North Am. 38:1455–1467, 1991.

Montgomery, T. R. When "not talking" is the chief complaint. Contemp. Pediatr. 11:49–70, 1994.

Schuman, A. J. Universal newborn hearing screening: the time is right. Contemp. Pediatr. 15:49–60, 1998.

CHAPTER 16

GIFTED CHILDREN

Iris Wagman Borowsky, M.D., Ph.D.

H$_x$ A 3-year-old girl is brought to your office for well child care. Her parents believe that she may be gifted because she is much more advanced than her sister was when she was the same age. The parents report that their younger daughter walked at 11 months of age and was speaking in two-word sentences by 18 months. She is very "verbal," has a precocious vocabulary, and constantly asks difficult questions such as, "How do voices come over a radio?" The girl stays at home with her mother during the day but recently began going to a preschool program two mornings a week. She enjoys preschool and plays well with children her own age. She also likes to play with her sister's friends from school.

The girl is engaging and talkative. She asks questions about what you are doing during the examination and demonstrates impressive knowledge of anatomy. The physical examination is normal.

Questions

1. How are gifted children identified?
2. What characteristics are associated with giftedness?
3. What are the best approaches for dealing with the education of gifted children?
4. What is the role of the pediatrician in the management of gifted children?

Giftedness has been defined in several ways. The psychometric definition of giftedness is based on scores obtained on standardized intelligence tests. The two most frequently used cut-off points are two standard deviations above the mean (intelligence quotient [IQ] = 130–135) and three standard deviations above the mean (IQ = 145–150). Children with these scores are in the upper 2% and 0.1% of the IQ distribution, respectively. IQ, which is considered to be fairly stable after the age of 3 or 4 years, is the best single predictor of scholastic achievement at all levels, from elementary school to college.

A second definition of giftedness is based on real-life achievements or performance of exceptional skills rather than on test scores. Children with special talents (other than general intelligence) in areas such as music, mathematics, ice skating, chess, or drama fit this description. Other definitions of giftedness recognize motivation, commitment, perseverance, high self-esteem, and creativity as personality traits that allow children with above average ability to develop exceptional talents.

EPIDEMIOLOGY

The prevalence of giftedness depends on the somewhat arbitrary definitions of giftedness and the varied approaches for identification of gifted children. Traditional screening systems identify 3–5% of students for participation in gifted programs in schools. Some schools use an alternative system, where 10–15% of children are recognized as above average. In an effort to foster giftedness in these children, schools offer them enriched programs.

Intellectual giftedness in children has been associated with the social, economic, and educational background of their families. Factors that correlate with higher IQ scores in children are more years of parental education, higher IQ scores of mothers, increased family income, smaller family size, and longer intervals between siblings. Children from low-income and minority backgrounds are less likely to be identified as gifted than other children. African Americans, Hispanics, and Native Americans are underrepresented by 30–70% in gifted programs in the United States.

Larger head size at 1 year of age and greater height and weight at 4 years of age have also been reported in children with high IQs. Although researchers have found that academically gifted children, as a group, begin to walk, verbalize, and read earlier, such factors are not useful for predicting giftedness in individual children.

EVALUATION

One of the primary goals of child health promotion is **developmental monitoring.** The early identification of developmental delays, which allows for prompt intervention, is one of the primary purposes of such monitoring. Techniques for developmental assessment include **review of developmental milestones** with parents and discussion of parental concerns, **informal observation** of children in the office, and **formal screening with standardized tests** such as the Denver II.

Identification of Gifted Children

Although parents' first concern is usually to confirm that their child is developing normally, it is not uncommon for parents to ask if their child is gifted. Such questions are typically motivated by parents' desire to optimally encourage their child's development. Sharing information and observations with parents during de-

TABLE 16–1. Factors Used in the Identification of Giftedness in Children

Intelligence tests
Standardized achievement tests
Grades
Classroom observations
Parent and teacher rating scales
Evaluation of creative work in a specific field (e.g., poems, drawings, science projects)

velopmental monitoring may facilitate parent-child interaction and child development. In a competitive society, the pediatric provider should look for signs that above average abilities are the result of undue pressures placed on children, such as incessant teaching or overscheduling of time.

Infancy and early childhood may not be the best time to determine whether a child is gifted. Age of attainment of developmental milestones and performance on standardized tests (e.g., Bayley Scales of Infant Development) during the first 2 years of life are both unreliable predictors of intellectual giftedness. Reasons for this lack of reliability may include weaknesses in the tests and variable rates of child development that result in transient precocity or delay. Tests that focus on visual memory tasks in infants may be better predictors of later academic intelligence; this possibility requires more research. In addition, many special talents that comprise giftedness, such as creativity or artistic or musical ability, may not manifest themselves until children are older.

The determination of giftedness in older children may involve several factors (Table 16–1). The early identification of giftedness allows for the development of an appropriate educational program that is optimally matched to a particular child's ability to learn. Without early identification and intervention, intellectually gifted children may become disillusioned with school, lose interest in learning, fail to develop study skills because they are never challenged to think and work hard, and develop a pattern of underachievement that may be difficult to reverse by the middle grades.

Special Groups of Gifted Children

Giftedness is harder to identify in some children. In **physically disabled children,** giftedness is often obscured by their obvious physical disability, which demands attention. These children may participate in special programs where their physical needs are the major concern at the expense of their academic or artistic potential. In addition, poor self-esteem associated with the disability may prevent these children from realizing their potential. To identify giftedness in physically disabled children, parents and teachers must make a concerted effort to search for potential and encourage its development. Strengthening a child's capacities may involve training in the use of a wheelchair or computer or taking frequent breaks to prevent fatigue.

Giftedness also commonly goes unnoticed in **learning-disabled children.** It is quite possible for exceptional and poor abilities to coexist in a given child. In fact, an estimated 10% of gifted children have a reading problem, reading two or more years below grade level. Albert Einstein, Auguste Rodin, and John D. Rockefeller are famous examples of brilliant individuals who had reading and writing problems. An extreme example of the occurrence of both extraordinary and deficient abilities together in one individual is the "child savant." Affected children possess amazing abilities in one area (e.g., music, drawing, mathematics, memory), but they are retarded in other respects. In addition, they have behavioral problems that resemble autism, such as repetitive behavior, little use of language, and social withdrawal.

Learning disabilities may obscure children's talents, thus preventing awareness of their potential. Conversely, children's giftedness may mask their weaknesses, depriving them of needed help. Worst of all, gifted learning-disabled children may manage to barely "get by" in the regular classroom setting and fail to receive recognition for strengths or weaknesses. Large differences on intelligence and achievement tests between scores in different areas, such as language and spatial abilities, may indicate both giftedness and a learning disability. Attention should be given to both weaknesses and strengths. Research suggests that programs that focus on strengths, not deficits, however, enhance self-esteem in gifted learning-disabled children and can be extremely beneficial in their academic development.

The identification of giftedness is also difficult in **underachieving children.** Parents may approach the pediatrician with the following frustrating problem: their child is doing poorly at school, although they believe that the child is bright because of the child's abilities and participation in advanced activities at home. Underachievement may result from a learning disability; poor self-esteem; lack of motivation; or the absence of rewards, either at home or at school, for succeeding in academics.

As previously stated, giftedness is less likely to be recognized in children from low-income or ethnically diverse families. Many of the tests used to identify giftedness have been "normed" on white, English-speaking, middle-class children. In the absence of tests that are sensitive to socioeconomic differences, other means for identifying giftedness, such as assessment of creative work and teacher and student nominations, should be stressed. Schools with students from low-income or minority backgrounds tend to use their limited resources to help students who are doing poorly in school, not those students who are gifted. Research has shown that programs for gifted children from such backgrounds benefit all students by creating positive role models and promoting the school as a place for the cultivation of excellence.

MANAGEMENT

At Home

Loving, responsive, stimulating parenting should be encouraged for all children, including gifted children. Parents of gifted children may feel inadequate, fearing that their child is smarter than they are. The pediatrician can provide **parental reassurance** by telling parents, "You must have been doing something right for your child to have been identified as gifted." Children's librarians, periodicals written for parents and teachers of gifted children (e.g., *The Gifted Child Today*), and the local chapter of the National Association for Gifted Children are good resources for parents.

Parents are often overwhelmed with complex questions from their precocious preschool children about issues ranging from homelessness and world hunger to theology and the creation of the universe. The pediatrician should tell parents that they (1) should not be afraid to admit that they do not know all the answers and (2) should work together with their child to find the answers.

The pediatrician may need to warn parents about putting too much pressure on their gifted children. For example, enrolling children in multiple classes often leaves little free time for unstructured play. Play affords many opportunities for self-learning, interaction with peers, and development of creativity and initiative. Parents of infants, toddlers, and preschoolers should be encouraged to take cues from their children. If children have a rich environment with plenty of objects and books to explore, diverse experiences, and stimulating interactions, they will develop their own interests. Other educational materials and special instruction can then be provided in a particular area of interest.

Gifted children are often mistakenly considered to fit the stereotype of troubled, socially awkward "nerds." With the exception of children at the genius extreme (IQ> 180), gifted children are generally more sociable, well-liked, trustworthy, and emotionally stable than their peers, with lower rates of mental illness and delinquency. Nevertheless, they have the same emotional needs as do other children. Gifted children may prefer to play with older children whose interests and abilities are closer to their own. This should be allowed as long as these relationships are healthy.

Parents should be encouraged to treat gifted children the same way they do their other children. Siblings of gifted children may become resentful if attention is centered on their brother or sister. They may feel inferior, particularly if gifted children surpass them in school. Tensions may be magnified if gifted children become friends with their older sibling's friends. All tensions should be openly discussed within the family. To preserve a sense of self-worth and competence in siblings, the pediatrician should recommend to parents that they set aside special time to spend with each of their children. Parents should encourage other talents (e.g., musical or athletic abilities) in siblings. Older siblings should receive the special privileges and responsibilities that come with age, such as staying up later or doing different chores. Any tensions within the family should be openly addressed.

At School

Parents often seek advice from their pediatrician about educational planning for gifted children. A learning environment with the optimal degree of challenge—hard enough to require new learning and stave off boredom, but not so hard as to be discouraging—is the goal for all children. Parents of young children should look for preschools with flexible programs and capable teachers to accommodate children with precocious skills. Parents of school-age children must decide whether **acceleration** (starting school earlier or skipping grades) or **enrichment** (staying in the same grade but supplementing the regular curriculum) is more appropriate (Table 16–2). The choice depends on the particular child.

Parents and teachers of gifted children are usually concerned that children in accelerated programs may have problems with social adjustment if their classmates are older. Existing evidence suggests gifted children benefit socially from acceleration, however. Gifted children in accelerated programs participate in school activities (except contact sports) more often than gifted children placed with classmates of the same age. Even when gifted children are placed with children their own age, they tend to make friends with older children with whom they share more interests. Gifted children also make up any curricular content missed by grade-skipping. Because the process may be difficult to reverse, it may not be the best option when the decision is a borderline one.

Enrichment involves keeping gifted children with same-age classmates but supplementing the regular curriculum. Regular class placement with a teacher who is willing to offer extra work (e.g., special projects) in addition to grade-level assignments, part-time programs to supplement regular classwork (e.g., field trips, foreign language classes), "honors" classes that group bright children together for their basic curriculum, and independent study by the family at home are all examples of enrichment programs. These programs may work well for some gifted children, depending in large part on the resources and funding available and the experience, creativity, and enthusiasm of the teachers involved.

TABLE 16–2. Acceleration Versus Enrichment in Gifted Education

	Advantages	Disadvantages
Acceleration	May provide suitable academic challenge	Difficult to reverse
	May have social benefits	May have to skip more than one grade to be properly challenged
	Can be offered by all schools	
	Inexpensive	
Enrichment	Classmates are same age	May be expensive
	May expose children to subjects they would not otherwise learn	Inadequate for highly gifted children
	Appropriate for mildly gifted children	May isolate gifted from nongifted children and encourage "elite" label
		May lead to excessive homework if children have to make up work of regular class

Some enrichment programs may isolate gifted from nongifted children, however, and encourage labeling of the gifted students as "elite." If children are required to make up the regular class work that they miss when they are involved in the enrichment program, they may find themselves overloaded with homework.

Often a **combination of acceleration and enrichment** programs is the best option. Either acceleration or enrichment alone may not be enough for the brightest children. Acceleration may not be sufficient for markedly advanced children who would have to skip two or three grades to be appropriately challenged. The pediatrician should recommend that parents work closely with teachers to achieve the best learning environment for their children. Some factors that should be considered are age, physical size, motor coordination, emotional maturity, personality, and particular areas and degrees of giftedness of the child. Acceleration may be a better option for a large, outgoing child than for a small one. Gifted children should be asked what they would like to do.

When evaluating the suitability of an educational situation for their gifted child, parents should watch for some warning signs. Excessive homework should neither be expected nor tolerated, as it cuts into the child's time to play and develop socially. The emphasis in gifted education should be on broadening perspectives, not increasing busy work. If gifted children are developing a sense of elitism or peer animosity, the nature and philosophy of the program should be questioned. Boredom with schoolwork, the lack of a need to study, signs of depression, or symptoms suggestive of school phobia such as recurrent abdominal pain or headaches on school mornings should prompt investigation of the suitability of the child's program.

Case Resolution

In the case presented, the physician should reaffirm the parents' observations that their child is gifted. The parents should be encouraged to explore programs in which their daughter's talents may be fostered, but at the same time, they should understand that even gifted children need time for play and unstructured activities.

Selected Readings

Brody, L. E., and C. J. Mills. Gifted children with learning disabilities: A review of the issues. J. Learn. Disab. 30:282–296, 1997.

Ciba Foundation Symposium. The origins and development of high ability. 178:1–258, 1993. (Entire issue on giftedness.)

Colangelo, N., and G. A. Davis, eds. Handbook of Gifted Education, 2nd ed. Needham Heights, Mass. Allyn & Bacon, 1996.

Csikszentmihalyi, M., K. Rathunde, and S. Whalen. Talented Teenagers: The Roots of Success and Failure. Cambridge, UK. Cambridge University Press, 1993.

Freeman, J. Recent studies of giftedness in children. J. Child Psychol. Psychiatry 36:531–547, 1995.

Kranzler, J. H. Assessment of children and youth from culturally and linguistically diverse backgrounds with mental chronometric techniques. Perceptual & Motor Skills 86:321–322, 1998.

Pediatr. Ann. 14:691–768, 1985. (Entire issue on the gifted child.)

Robinson, A., and P. R. Clinkenbeard. Giftedness: An exceptionally examined. Ann. Rev. Psychol. 49:117–139, 1998.

Robinson, N. M., and P. M. Olszewski/Kubilius. Gifted and talented children: Issues for pediatricians. Ped. Rev. 17:427–434, 1996.

CHAPTER 17

IMMUNIZATIONS

Geeta Grover, M.D.

H_x An 8-month-old infant is evaluated in the emergency department for a history of fever for 2 days. The mother reports that her daughter has been pulling at her ears and is not sleeping well at night. The girl's past medical history is unremarkable. She is taking no medications except for acetaminophen for fever, and no family members are ill at home. Review of her immunization record reveals that she has received immunizations only at 2 and 4 months.

On examination, the girl's temperature is 101° F (38.3° C), but she is alert and appears nontoxic. Except for bilateral otitis media, the rest of the examination is within normal limits. Discharge orders for appropriate immunizations to be given today in addition to antibiotics and antipyretic medications are written. The nurse questions the orders to give immunizations to an ill infant.

Questions

1. According to the recommended schedule of immunizations, what immunizations should infants have received by the age of 8 months?
2. Can febrile infants with conditions such as otitis media be immunized?
3. What are the contraindications to immunizations?
4. What are some of the barriers that prevent children from being immunized?
5. How can physicians keep abreast of current recommendations regarding immunizations?

Immunizations are one of the simplest and most cost-effective preventive health care measures available today. They are an essential component of comprehensive well child care, and immunization coverage levels of infants and children are a measure of quality of preventive health services. The immediate goal of immunizations is to prevent disease in susceptible individuals, but the ultimate goal is to eradicate disease in populations. The global eradication of smallpox in 1980 is an example of disease eradication through immunizations and effective public health control measures. The incidence of vaccine-preventable diseases has declined tremendously in the United States as a result of immunizations. The reported number of cases of diphtheria, measles, mumps, pertussis, poliomyelitis, rubella, and tetanus have declined by 97% or more during this century.

Over 95% of school-age children in the United States are fully immunized by the time they are 5 or 6 years of age because of the enforcement of laws requiring adequate immunizations prior to school entry. However, according to a recent study by the CDC, only 76% of children aged 19–35 months are adequately immunized. This disparity between immunization levels at 5 years of age versus approximately 2 years of age is the **immunization dichotomy,** which states that although children are adequately immunized by the time of school entry, they are inadequately protected during the first few years of life. This is the period when they are most susceptible to the morbidity and mortality associated with vaccine-preventable diseases.

An example of the high cost of inadequate immunization is an increase in the occurrence of vaccine-preventable disease. This is currently best represented by the recent measles epidemic. In 1983, the United States had 1500 cases of measles, an all-time low. This number rose to about 25,000 at the peak of the epidemic in 1990, with case fatality rates as high as four deaths per 1000 cases in some areas. This increase in the incidence of measles infection may have been related to waning immunity or failure to immunize and has led to the current requirement of a second dose of MMR in all children.

TYPES OF IMMUNIZATION

Active immunity is the development of specific immunity within the host in response to contact with infectious organisms (e.g., bacteria, viruses). Natural active immunity is spontaneously obtained through community-acquired contact with the organism and protects the host against subsequent exposures to that organism (e.g., as in hepatitis A). When the morbidity and mortality associated with infections is significant (e.g., with measles or diphtheria), electively induced immunity, or immunoprophylaxis, is considered. Immunoprophylaxis may be accomplished by means of active immunization.

Vaccines may either contain live and attenuated or killed (inactivated) infectious agents. Although live vaccines are more likely to induce long-lasting or permanent immunity than killed vaccines, they carry the risk of causing vaccine-induced disease in recipients or spreading the vaccine strain to secondary hosts. Killed vaccines are noninfectious, but they can only induce immunity for relatively short periods. They therefore require booster injections to maintain immunity.

In **active immunization,** a vaccine that contains all or part of a microorganism or a modified product of that microorganism (e.g., toxoid, purified antigen, genetically engineered antigen) is administered to evoke an immunologic response without producing significant clinical illness. This immunologic response protects recipients from future exposures to the involved microorganism.

Passive immunization, in contrast to active immunization, involves providing preformed human or animal antibodies to individuals who have no active immunity against a particular infectious agent but have already been exposed or are at high risk for exposure. Indications for the use of passive immunizations include high risk of developing significant complications from certain disease exposure (e.g., immunocompromised children exposed to varicella or measles); insufficient time for adequate protection by active immunization alone (e.g., postexposure rabies); certain immunodeficiency states that result in deficient antibody synthesis; and preexposure prophylaxis with immune globulin against hepatitis A (e.g., for persons traveling to high-risk areas). Passive immunization provides immediate, relatively brief protection. In contrast, active immunization requires time to develop but provides prolonged or lifelong immunity.

CURRENT RECOMMENDED IMMUNIZATION SCHEDULE

Whether to immunize for a particular disease in a given region depends on the severity of the disease and the probability of exposure as compared to the cost and effectiveness of the vaccine. The earliest a vaccine may be administered is the youngest age at which children can mount a protective immunologic response to it. For example, measles, mumps, and rubella (MMR) vaccine is usually given at 12–15 months of age because transplacentally acquired maternal measles antibodies may persist up to 12 months of age.

In the United States, recommendations for childhood immunizations are made by three organizations: the Committee on Infectious Diseases of the AAP, the Advisory Committee on Immunization Practices (ACIP) of the Centers for Disease Control and Prevention (CDC), and the American Academy of Family Physicians. In developing countries, the Expanded Program on Immunization (EPI) of the World Health Organization (WHO) prepares guidelines for immunization practices.

Children are currently required to receive immunizations against 10 different diseases from birth until the time of school entry in the United States. Although many of these vaccines are provided in combination form, all except the varicella vaccine (Var) require more than one dose. The current recommended schedule of immunization for normal children includes the following vaccinations: hepatitis B virus vaccine (HBV); diphtheria, tetanus, and pertussis-containing vaccines (DTP or DTaP); poliovirus vaccines (OPV or IPV); *Haemophilus influenzae* type b vaccine (Hib); MMR; and Var. The

TABLE 17–1. Routine Childhood Vaccinations in the United States

Vaccine	Type	Route
DTP	Toxoids and inactivated bacteria	IM
DTaP	Toxoids and inactivated bacterial components	IM
HBV	Inactivated viral antigen	IM
Hib	Polysaccharide-protein conjugate	IM
MMR	Live viruses	SC
Poliovirus		
IPV	Inactivated virus (trivalent)	SC
OPV	Live virus (trivalent)	Oral
Var	Live virus	SC

Modified, with permission, from Committee on Infectious Diseases, American Academy of Pediatrics. Active and passive immunization. *In* 1997 Red Book: Report of the Committee on Infectious Diseases, 24th ed. Elk Grove Village, IL, American Academy of Pediatrics, 1997, p. 5.

Abbreviations: DTP, diphtheria, tetanus, and pertussis vaccine; DTaP, diphtheria, tetanus and acellular pertussis vaccine; HBV, hepatitis B virus vaccine; Hib, *Haemophilus influenzae* type b vaccine; MMR, measles, mumps and rubella vaccine; IPV, inactivated poliovirus vaccine; OPV, oral poliovirus vaccine; Var, varicella vaccine; IM, intramuscular; SC, subcutaneous.

composition and route of administration of each vaccine is provided in Table 17–1, and the recommended schedule of administration for the United States is summarized in Figure 17–1. Six visits are required prior to school entry to immunize children fully.

Hepatitis B Virus Vaccine

About 300 million people worldwide are infected with HBV. Although an effective vaccine to combat hepatitis B infection has been available for use in high-risk individuals since 1982, the incidence of the infection continued to increase through 1989. The recommendation for universal immunization of all children against hepatitis B came because of this failure of selective immunization to control the disease. Two types of vaccines have been licensed in the United States: an older vaccine that contained HBsAg purified from the plasma of chronic carriers of HBsAg, no longer in use, and a recombinant vaccine containing particles of hepatitis B surface antigen (HBsAg). Only the recombinant vaccine is currently available in the United States, however. The recommended three doses may be administered at birth, 2, and 6–18 months of age, or at 2, 4, and 6–18 months of age. Most states now require immunization against hepatitis B prior to entry into junior high school. Preteens who have not been previously vaccinated should be vaccinated at the 11- to 12-year-old visit.

Diphtheria, Tetanus, and Pertussis-Containing Vaccines

Diphtheria, tetanus, and pertussis can each produce very serious illness with high mortality rates, especially in young infants. DTP vaccine contains diphtheria and tetanus toxoids and whole-cell, killed *Bordetella pertussis*. The toxoids are obtained by formalin inactivation of the respective bacterial toxins. Unlike the whole-cell vaccine, acellular pertussis vaccines are prepared from one or more purified components of *B. pertussis* and then combined with diphtheria and tetanus toxoids

(DTaP). The DTaP vaccine has the advantage of lower rates of common systemic reactions, including vaccine-associated seizures, fever, and of local reactions, than the whole-cell preparation. For these reasons, DTaP is now the preferred vaccine for all doses in the vaccination series. Whole-cell DTP vaccine is an acceptable alternative during the transition period from use of DTP to DTaP. DTaP is administered at 2, 4, and 6 months of age; booster doses are given at 15–18 months and 4–6 years.

The dT vaccine contains about one-tenth the dose of diphtheria toxoid compared to the pediatric preparation of diphtheria and tetanus toxoids (DT); dT is administered to individuals over the age of 7 years. A routine dT booster is recommended at 11–12 years of age if at least 5 years have elapsed since the last dose of DTaP. Subsequent routine dT boosters are recommended every 10 years. At present, pertussis immunization of persons 7 years of age or older is not routinely indicated. Adults at high risk may receive acellular pertussis vaccine.

Poliovirus Vaccines

Poliovirus is an enterovirus that has a propensity for CNS invasion. Paralytic poliomyelitis occurs in approximately 1:250 infections and results in permanent paresis or paralysis of one or more of the extremities. Trivalent poliovirus vaccine used to immunize against polio is available either as a live-attenuated vaccine that is administered orally (OPV) or as an inactivated vaccine that is given parenterally (IPV). Both vaccines are highly immunogenic and effective in preventing poliomyelitis, but induction of intestinal immunity against poliovirus reinfection is better with OPV.

Polio is being eradicated. The Western hemisphere was certified as free of indigenous wild-type poliovirus in 1994. In the United States where there has been no reported disease secondary to wild-type poliovirus since 1979, an additional goal is to eliminate vaccine-associated paralytic poliomyelitis (VAPP). About 8–10 cases of VAPP are reported annually in the United States.

A sequential IPV-OPV schedule (IPV at 2 and 4 months and OPV at 12–18 months and 4–6 years of age) has been the recommended schedule for poliovirus vaccination in the United States. The sequential schedule is recommended to decrease the risk of VAPP (greatest risk with the first dose of vaccine) while inducing optimal intestinal immunity. Administration of OPV for the first two doses of the schedule is only acceptable in certain circumstances, such as imminent travel to a polio-endemic area or parental refusal of the recommended number of injections. Use of IPV for all doses is acceptable and is recommended for adults who need the polio vaccine, immunocompromised children, and for children living with immunocompromised individuals such as persons with cancer or HIV infection. Beginning January 1, 2000, all children will require a total of four doses of IPV: one dose at 2, 4, and 6–18 months, and another at 4–6 years. When administered orally, the live virus is excreted in the stool and may infect exposed individuals.

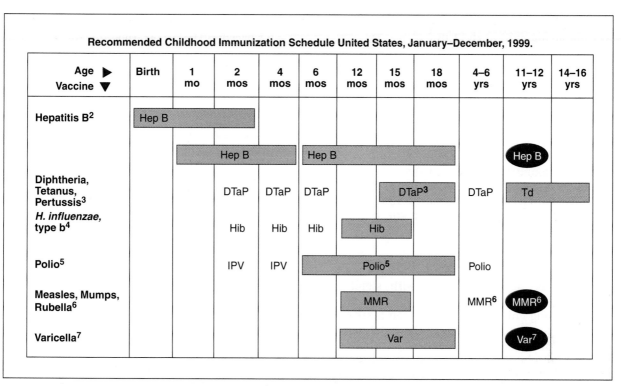

FIGURE 17-1. Recommended childhood immunization schedule—United States, January–December, 1999. Approved by the Advisory Committee on Immunization Practices (ACIP), the American Academy of Pediatrics (AAP), and the American Academy of Family Physicians (AAFP). Vaccines are listed under routinely recommended ages. Bars indicate range of recommended ages for immunizations. Any dose not given at the recommended age should be given as a "catch-up" immunization at any subsequent visit when indicated and feasible. Ovals indicate vaccines to be given if previously recommended doses were missed or given earlier than the recommended minimum age. (Reproduced, with permission, from Committee on Infectious Diseases, American Academy of Pediatrics. Recommended childhood immunization schedule—United States, January–December, 1999. Pediatrics 103:182, 1999.)

[1]This schedule indicates the recommended ages for routine administration of currently licensed childhood vaccines. Combination vaccines may be used whenever any components of the combination are indicated and its other components are not contraindicated. Providers should consult the manufacturers' package inserts for detailed recommendations.

[2]*Infants born to HBsAG-negative mothers* should receive the 2nd dose of hepatitis B vaccine at least 1 month after the 1st dose. The 3rd dose should be administered at least 4 months after the 1st dose and at least 2 months after the 2nd dose, but not before 6 months of age for infants.
Infants born to HBsAG-positive mothers should receive hepatitis B vaccine and 0.5 mL hepatitis B immune globulin (HBIG) within 12 hours of birth at separate sites. The 2nd dose is recommended at 1–2 months of age and the 3rd dose at 6 months of age.
Infants born to mothers whose HBsAG status is unknown should receive hepatitis B vaccine within 12 hours of birth. Maternal blood should be drawn at the time of delivery to determine the mother's HBsAG status; if the HBsAG test is positive, the infant should receive HBIG as soon as possible (no later than 1 week of age).
All children and adolescents (through 18 years of age) who have not been immunized against hepatitis B may begin the series during any visit. Special efforts should be made to immunize children who were born in or whose parents were born in areas of the world with moderate or high endemicity of HBV infection.

[3]DTaP (diphtheria and tetanus toxoids and acellular pertussis vaccine) is the preferred vaccine for all doses in the immunization series, including completion of the series in children who have received 1 or more doses of whole-cell DTP vaccine. Whole-cell DTP is an acceptable alternative to DTaP. The 4th dose (DTP or DTaP) may be administered as early as 12 months of age, provided 6 months have elapsed since the 3rd dose and if the child is unlikely to return at age 15–18 months. Td (tetanus and diphtheria toxoids) is recommended at 11–12 years of age if at least 5 years have elapsed since the last dose of DTP, DTaP, or DT. Subsequent routine Td boosters are recommended every 10 years.

[4]Three *H. influenzae* type b (Hib) conjugate vaccines are licensed for infant use. If PRP-OMP (PedvaxHIB and COMVAX [Merck]) is administered at 2 and 4 months of age, a dose at 6 months is not required. Because clinical studies in infants have demonstrated that using some combination products may induce a lower immune response to the Hib vaccine component, DTaP/Hib combination products should not be used for primary immunization in infants at 2, 4, or 6 months of age, unless FDA-approved for these ages.

[5]Two poliovirus vaccines currently are licensed in the United States: inactivated poliovirus vaccine (IPV) and oral poliovirus vaccine (OPV).
The ACIP, AAP, and AAFP had recommended that the first two doses of poliovirus vaccine should be IPV, followed by two doses of OPV at 12–18 months and 4–6 years. Use of IPV for all doses is recommended beginning January, 2000.

[6]The 2nd dose of measles, mumps, and rubella vaccine (MMR) is recommended routinely at 4–6 years of age but may be administered during any visit, provided at least 4 weeks have elapsed since receipt of the 1st dose and that both doses are administered beginning at or after 12 months of age. Those who have not previously received the second dose should complete the schedule by the 11- to 12-year-old visit.

[7]Varicella vaccine is recommended at any visit on or after the first birthday for susceptible children, i.e., those who lack a reliable history of chickenpox (as judged by a health care provider) and who have not been immunized. Susceptible persons 13 years of age or older should receive 2 doses, given at least 4 weeks apart.

Haemophilus Influenzae Type B Vaccines

Before the availability of the Hib vaccine, Hib was a major cause of such serious illnesses in young children as epiglottitis, meningitis, and septic arthritis. Since 1988 when Hib conjugate vaccines were introduced, the incidence of invasive Hib disease has declined by 95% in infants and young children. Several Hib conjugate vaccines are currently available in the United States. The Hib capsular polysaccharide is linked to various protein antigens such as diphtheria or tetanus toxoids to augment the immune response, particularly in young infants. Hib vaccine is administered either at 2, 4, and 6 months of age, with a booster dose at 12–15 months, or at 2, 4, and 12 months, depending on the particular vaccine conjugate used.

Measles, Mumps, and Rubella Vaccine

Measles can be a severe illness with significant mortality due to complications such as pneumonia, especially in young children. Orchitis, seen more commonly in adolescents and adults, is the most serious complication of mumps infection. Although rubella is a mild disease in childhood, infection of susceptible women during the first trimester of pregnancy can result in congenital rubella infection, a serious multisystem infection in neonates. To prevent development of measles, mumps, and rubella, MMR, a trivalent vaccine containing live attenuated viruses, was developed. This vaccine is administered at 12–15 months of age and again at 4–6 years. Children who have not previously received the second dose should complete the series no later than the 11–12 year visit.

Varicella Vaccine

Primary infection with varicella-zoster virus results in chickenpox, a generally innocuous infection that manifests as a generalized vesicular rash with fever and mild constitutional symptoms. Complications include bacterial superinfection, pneumonia, or meningitis. Even though most cases of varicella infection in healthy children are uncomplicated, the cost of the disease is high, secondary to parents' absence from work. Varicella vaccine is a live attenuated vaccine that may be given to susceptible children after 12 months of age.

SIDE EFFECTS AND CONTRAINDICATIONS

Common side effects following vaccination include local reactions such as erythema, swelling or tenderness at the site of the injection, and low-grade fever (temperature: 100.4° F [38° C]) especially following DTP immunization. Side effects are common, whereas adverse reactions, such as an anaphylactic reaction to a vaccine, are quite uncommon.

A guide to contraindications and precautions to vaccine administration is presented in Table 17–2. Low-grade fever, minor acute illness (e.g., otitis media), mild diarrheal illness in children who otherwise appear well, and current antimicrobial therapy are not contraindications to vaccine administration. Other common misconceptions about contraindications to vaccine adminis-

TABLE 17–2. General Contraindications and Precautions for Vaccines (DTP/DTaP, OPV, IPV, Hib, HBV, MMR, and Var)

True Contraindications and Precautions

Anaphylactic reaction to a vaccine (this contraindicates further doses of that vaccine)

Anaphylactic reaction to a vaccine constituent (this contraindicates the use of vaccines containing that substance)

Moderate or severe illness with or without a fever

Not True Contraindications (vaccines may be given)

Mild to moderate local reaction (e.g., soreness, redness, swelling) following a dose of an injectable antigen

Mild, acute illness with or without a low-grade fever

Current antimicrobial therapy

Convalescent phase of illness

Prematurity

Recent exposure to an infectious disease

History of penicillin or other nonspecific allergies or relatives with such allergies

Adapted from Committee on Infectious Diseases, American Academy of Pediatrics. 1997 Red Book: Report of the Committee on Infectious Diseases, 24th ed. Elk Grove Village, IL, American Academy of Pediatrics, 1997. (The reader is referred to this source for a more detailed discussion of immunization recommendations.)

tration include prematurity and a personal or family history of seizures. Generally, premature infants should be immunized at the same chronologic age as other infants; full, not reduced, vaccine doses should be used. A history of seizures usually is not a contraindication to whole-cell pertussis immunization unless the seizure followed a previous immunization for pertussis. The role of pertussis vaccine in causing epilepsy or permanent neurologic damage, if any, remains as yet unconfirmed. Children who have had seizures do have an increased risk of vaccine-associated seizures, which are usually febrile convulsions with no permanent sequelae.

True contraindications to vaccine administration are anaphylactic reactions to a vaccine or vaccine constituent (e.g., neomycin found in IPV, MMR, and Var); immunocompromise (live-virus vaccines); pregnancy (live-virus vaccines); moderate or severe febrile illness (e.g., pneumonia, meningitis, suspected bacteremia); and severe prior reaction to a particular vaccine. Specific contraindications include encephalopathy within 7 days of administration of a previous dose of DTP or DTaP and administration of OPV to immunologically normal children living in a home with an immunocompromised child. (MMR may be administered to such normal siblings because transmission of these viruses does not occur.) MMR vaccine (prepared in chick-embryo fibroblast-cell cultures) can be safely given to children with isolated anaphylactic allergies to eggs. Children with chronic illness, acquired or congenital immunodeficiency, malignancy, and those on chronic corticosteroid therapy should be individually evaluated regarding appropriate vaccinations.

Although live-virus vaccines usually are not given to immunocompromised children, exceptions to this guideline do exist. For example, it is recommended that children infected with HIV who are not severely immunocompromised, should receive MMR because of the severity of measles as compared to the potential risks of the vaccine. OPV is contraindicated because possible vaccine-associated poliomyelitis in these children may occur. These children can receive IPV instead.

OTHER CONSIDERATIONS

Informed Consent

Although the risk of serious adverse reactions following immunizations is small, informed consent has become an important issue in the last several years. The National Childhood Vaccine Injury Act of 1986 requires notification of patients or parents about vaccine risks and benefits. Distribution of standardized vaccine information pamphlets prior to vaccine administration and written informed consent is required for administration of all vaccines.

Simultaneous Administration of Multiple Vaccines

In general, immune responses to one vaccine do not interfere with those of other vaccines.* Simultaneous administration of routine immunizations is not contra-

*Simultaneous administration of the yellow fever and cholera vaccines limits their effectiveness.

indicated. Live virus vaccines not administered on the same day should be given at least 30 days apart because the immune responses to the live virus vaccines may interfere with each other. In addition, live vaccines (e.g., MMR) may have decreased efficacy when administered shortly before or within several months after the administration of immune globulin (IG). The duration of this effect depends on the dose of IG. Exceptions to the admonition against the simultaneous administration of IG and vaccines include OPV administration and simultaneous administration of hepatitis B IG, tetanus IG, and rabies IG given in conjunction with the corresponding inactivated vaccine or toxoid in postexposure situations.

Immunization of Children Not Immunized During Infancy

Children not immunized during the first year of life should be vaccinated according to the appropriate schedule (Table 17–3). Pertussis vaccination is not routinely recommended for children 7 years of age or older, and Hib vaccination is also unnecessary after 5 years of age.

TABLE 17–3.   Recommended Immunization Schedules for Children Not Immunized in the First Year of Life*

Recommended Time/Age	Immunization(s)[†‡§]	Comments
Younger Than 7 Years		
First visit	DTaP (or DTP), Hib,[‖] HBV, MMR, OPV[¶]	If indicated, tuberculin testing may be done at same visit. If child is 5 y of age or older, Hib is not indicated in most circumstances.
Interval after first visit		
1 mo (4 wk)	DTaP (or DTP), HBV, Var[#]	The second dose of OPV may be given if accelerated poliomyelitis vaccination is necessary, such as for travelers to areas where polio is endemic.
2 mo	DTaP (or DTP), Hib,[‖] OPV[¶]	Second dose of Hib is indicated only if the first dose was received when younger than 15 mo.
≥8 mo	DTaP (or DTP), HBV, OPV[¶]	OPV and HBV are not given if the third doses were given earlier.
Age 4–6 y (at or before school entry)	DTaP (or DTP), OPV,[¶] MMR**	DTaP (or DTP) is not necessary if the fourth dose was given after the fourth birthday; OPV is not necessary if the third dose was given after the fourth birthday.
7–12 Years		
First visit	HBV, MMR, Td, OPV[¶]	
Interval after first visit		
2 mo (8 wk)	HBV, MMR,** Var,[#] Td, OPV[¶]	OPV also may be given 1 mo after the first visit if accelerated poliomyelitis vaccination is necessary.
8–14 mo	HBV,[††] Td, OPV[¶]	OPV is not given if the third dose was given earlier.
Age 11–12 y	See Fig 1–1 in source	

Reproduced, with permission, from Committee on Infectious Diseases, American Academy of Pediatrics. 1997 Red Book: Report of the Committee on Infectious Diseases, 24th ed. Elk Grove Village, IL, American Academy of Pediatrics, 1997, p. 20.

*Table is not completely consistent with all package inserts. For products used, also consult manufacturer's package insert for instructions on storage, handling, dosage, and administration. Biologics prepared by different manufacturers may vary, and package inserts of the same manufacturer may change from time to time. Therefore, the physician should be aware of the contents of the current package insert.

Vaccine abbreviations: HBV indicates hepatitis B virus vaccine; Var, varicella vaccine; DTP, diphtheria and tetanus toxoids and pertussis vaccine; DTaP, diphtheria and tetanus toxoids and acellular pertussis vaccine; Hib, *Haemophilus influenzae* type b conjugate vaccine; OPV, oral poliovirus vaccine; IPV, inactivated poliovirus vaccine; MMR, live measles-mumps-rubella vaccine; Td, adult tetanus toxoid (full dose) and diphtheria toxoid (reduced dose), for children ≥7 years and adults.

†If all needed vaccines cannot be administered simultaneously, priority should be given to protecting the child against those diseases that pose the greatest immediate risk. In the United States, these diseases for children younger than 2 years usually are measles and *Haemophilus influenzae* type b infection; for children older than 7 years, they are measles, mumps, and rubella. Before 13 years of age, immunity against hepatitis B and varicella should be ensured.

‡DTaP, HBV, Hib, MMR, and Var can be given simultaneously at separate sites if failure of the patient to return for future immunizations is a concern.

§For further information on pertussis and poliomyelitis immunization, see Pertussis, and Poliovirus Infections in source.

‖See *Haemophilus influenzae* Infections, and Table 3–9 in source.

¶IPV is also acceptable. However, for infants and children starting vaccinations late (ie, after 6 months of age), OPV is preferred in order to complete an accelerated schedule with a minimum number of injections (see Poliovirus Infections in source). Effective January 1, 2000, all children will require a total of four doses of IPV: one at 2 months, 4 months, 6–18 months, and at 4–6 years of age.

#Varicella vaccine can be administered to susceptible children any time after 12 months of age. Unvaccinated children who lack a reliable history of chicken pox should be vaccinated before their 13th birthday.

**Minimal interval between doses of MMR is 1 month (4 weeks).

††HBV may be given earlier in a 0-, 2-, and 4-month schedule.

Interruptions in the Immunization Schedule

An interruption does not require restarting the entire immunization schedule. Immunizations should resume from the point of interruption, regardless of the time since the last dose.

Unknown or Undocumented Immunization Status

Children with unknown or undocumented immunization status should receive all appropriate vaccinations. No evidence indicates that immunization of already immune individuals with MMR, Hib, HBV, Var, IPV/OPV, or DTP/DTaP (dT for those age 7 years or more) is harmful.

SPECIAL VACCINES AND NEW VACCINES

Aside from the primary series of childhood immunizations that all children are required to receive, several other vaccines are available for use in specific circumstances. Rotavirus vaccine, a live attenuated vaccine, was licensed by the Food and Drug Administration (FDA) in August 1998, for oral administration to infants at 2, 4, and 6 months of age. Epidemiologic studies have estimated that rotavirus causes about 3 million cases of diarrhea and 20–40 deaths annually in the United States. Unfortunately, reports of a possible link between rotavirus vaccine and intussusception resulted in its removal from the market in August 1999. Annual influenza vaccination is recommended for children who are immunocompromised, or those who have chronic cardiovascular or pulmonary disease or any other underlying condition that may make them more susceptible to complications after influenza infection. Pneumococcal vaccine is recommended for children with sickle cell disease, anatomic or functional asplenia, nephrotic syndrome, and immunocompromise, but can only be given to children over 2 years of age. Hepatitis A vaccine is an inactivated whole virus vaccine that is recommended for persons ≥ 2 years of age at high risk of exposure (e.g., those living in communities with high rates of disease, or international travelers to regions of endemic disease) and patients with chronic liver disease. Several vaccinations, including vaccines for cholera, yellow fever, and tuberculosis, are available for persons traveling abroad. The requirements for different countries may be obtained from the Centers for Disease Control and Prevention.

Vaccine technology is increasing every day. Some combination vaccines are already available, and in the future it is likely that even more vaccines already in routine use will be combined. Vaccines against malaria, HIV, herpes simplex, RSV, group B streptococcus, and CMV are all investigational at the present time.

PUBLIC HEALTH PERSPECTIVE ON IMMUNIZATIONS

Worldwide Immunization Programs

Dramatic declines in the rates of vaccine-preventable diseases have occurred worldwide; these are largely a result of the efforts of the WHO through the EPI and the United Nations Children's Fund (UNICEF). At the time of the inception of the EPI in 1974, fewer than 5% of children in the developing world were immunized. The objectives of the EPI are to reduce the morbidity and mortality from diphtheria, pertussis, tetanus, measles, poliomyelitis, and tuberculosis by making immunizations against these diseases available to all the world's children. Today, 75–85% of the children in the developing world are protected by immunizations, and the rate continues to rise. The goal is the immunization of at least 85% of all 1-year-old children by the year 2000.

National Immunization Coverage Rates and Year 2000 Goals

Although the United States spends more money on health care than any other nation, it lags behind many other countries with regard to most aspects of child health, including immunizations. In 1992, the United States ranked 88th worldwide with regard to the percentage of 1-year-olds fully immunized against polio, and the ranking for DTP was 115th. Studies consistently show that nonwhite children and children from economically disadvantaged populations are far less likely to be adequately immunized than their peers.

In response to the current low levels of vaccine coverage of infants and young children in the United States, the U.S. Public Health Service has made immunization coverage of children one of its national year 2000 health goals. By the year 2000, 90% of 2-year-old children and 95% of school-age children should be appropriately immunized with the recommended immunizations.

Barriers to Immunization

Immunization coverage is a good example of the difference between the capacity to provide a service compared to availability, affordability, and ultimate utilization. Reasons for failure to immunize all children fully by 2 years of age may be classified into three main groups (Table 17–4): parental barriers, provider barriers, and systems barriers.

Parental barriers to immunizations may stem from false notions about the hazards of immunization, par-

---

TABLE 17–4. Barriers to Immunization

Parental Barriers
Financial (15% of children uninsured in the United States)
Lack of knowledge regarding value of immunizations
Concerns about adverse reactions

Provider Barriers: "Missed Opportunities to Vaccinate"
Using inappropriate contraindications (e.g., minor illness)
Failure to review the immunization record during all visits to the health care provider, including visits to emergency departments
Failure to administer all required immunizations at one visit

Systems Barriers
Economic
Limited clinic hours and locations
Administrative
Requiring appointments in advance for immunizations

ticularly involving certain vaccines. Sometimes these misconceptions are promoted by the media. In 1999, for instance, concern about a link between hepatitis B vaccine and demyelinating conditions such as multiple sclerosis was aired on a popular television show, in spite of the lack of medical evidence that such an association existed. Physicians must remain knowledgeable about vaccine recommendations and reputed adverse reactions so as to be able to address parental concerns. Updated information is available through the American Academy of Pediatrics and its website at www.aap.org.

Two other significant barriers involve economic factors (not just parental) and those known collectively as the "missed opportunities to vaccinate." One economic factor is cost. In 1980 the cost to completely immunize one child in the public sector was $6.69; in 1990, this value had risen to $91.20 (not taking into account the Hib or HBV immunizations), and this figure continues to increase today. A second economic factor is lack of health insurance coverage. At present, about 15% of children under the age of 18 have no health insurance coverage, which makes access to health care difficult. One of the easiest "missed opportunities" to remedy is the failure of health care providers to review immunization status at all health care visits. State-wide immunization registries, which exist in states such as Washington, may serve to make information about the immunization status of children available to all providers. Misinformation regarding contraindications to vaccination also means that many children are not immunized on schedule.

Possible solutions include such creative ideas as providing immunizations at federally funded programs such as Women, Infants, and Children (WIC) or on-site in child care settings. Such ideas acknowledge the busy and complex schedules of young families today and make access to preventive services easier. Decreasing administrative barriers, especially for economically disadvantaged families; improved, centralized tracking and monitoring systems; and continuing education for health care providers regarding appropriate contraindications are a few of the other solutions currently available. Universal access to health care, a system that eliminates all financial barriers to health care, will also help make health care more accessible and ensure children's immunization status.

Case Resolution

The infant described in the case history should be immunized today. She should receive DTaP, IPV, Hib, and HBV. Minor illness, including low-grade fever and otitis media, is not a contraindication to immunization.

Selected Readings

Bellanti, J. A. Basic immunologic principles underlying vaccination procedures. Pediatr. Clin. North Am. 37:513–530, 1990.

Centers for Disease Control and Prevention. National, state, and urban area vaccination coverage levels among children aged 19–35 months—United States, 1997. MMWR 47:547–554, 1998.

Committee on Infectious Diseases, American Academy of Pediatrics. Recommended childhood immunization schedule—United States, January–December, 1999. Pediatrics 103:182–185, 1999.

Committee on Infectious Diseases, American Academy of Pediatrics. Poliomyelitis prevention: Revised recommendations for the use of inactivated poliovirus vaccine and live oral poliovirus vaccine. Pediatrics 103:171–172, 1999.

Committee on Infectious Diseases, American Academy of Pediatrics. Prevention of rotavirus disease: Guidelines for use of rotavirus vaccine. Pediatrics 102:1483–1491, 1998.

Committee on Infectious Diseases, American Academy of Pediatrics. Active and Passive Immunization. *In* 1997 Red Book: Report of the Committee on Infectious Diseases, 24th ed. Elk Grove Village, IL, American Academy of Pediatrics, 1997, pp. 4–68.

Committee on Infectious Diseases, American Academy of Pediatrics. Immunization of adolescents: Recommendations of the Advisory Committee on Immunization Practices, the American Academy of Pediatrics, the American Academy of Family Physicians, and the American Medical Association. Pediatrics 99:479–488, 1997.

Harris, N., and K. Edwards. A progress report on hepatitis A vaccination. Contemp. Pediatr. 15:64–69, 1998.

James, J. M., et al. Safe administration of the measles vaccine to children allergic to eggs. N. Engl. J. Med. 332:1262–1265, 1995.

Johnson, C. E., et al. A long-term prospective study of varicella vaccine in healthy children. Pediatrics 100:761–766, 1997.

Lannon, C., et al. What mothers say about why poor children fall behind on immunizations. Arch. Pediatr. Adolesc. Med. 149:1070–1075, 1995.

Marwick, C. Rotavirus vaccine a boon to children. JAMA 279:489–490, 1998.

HEALTH MAINTENANCE IN OLDER CHILDREN AND ADOLESCENTS

Monica Sifuentes, M.D.

Hx Before a 13-year-old girl enters a new school, she is required to have a physical examination. She has not seen a physician in 5 years and has been healthy. Currently she has no medical complaints. Her examination is completely normal.

Questions

1. What are the important components of the history and physical examination in apparently healthy older children and adolescents?
2. What immunizations are recommended for older children and adolescents?
3. What laboratory tests should be performed at health maintenance visits? Why?
4. What are the results of screening tests likely to show?

Older children and adolescents are relatively healthy individuals who infrequently visit physicians. Visits are often for acute complaints such as pharyngitis or bronchitis and are therefore very problem-oriented. Statistics regarding health maintenance visits in this age group are not readily available, because patients go to several different sites for health care and often do not receive comprehensive care at any of these places. Older children and adolescents seek treatment for both acute and chronic conditions in private offices, public health clinics, public hospitals, and emergency departments. It is estimated that less than 15% of adolescents go to pediatricians for health care in general, and the same percentage probably applies to older children.

This all too common practice contributes to missed opportunities for adequate health screening for preventable conditions. Screening tests can also be used to identify treatable conditions such as hypertension, anemia, and tuberculosis. Ideally, older children and adolescents should receive recommended booster immunizations; counseling concerning sexual activity, contraception, and STDs, including HIV; guidelines for adequate nutrition; education about tobacco, drugs, and alcohol; and information about physical fitness and exercise.

Guidelines for preventive child and adolescent health care have been published by the Committee on Practice and Ambulatory Medicine of the AAP, the federal Child Health and Disability Prevention Program (CHDP), the section on adolescent health of the AAP, and the AMA (Table 18–1).

TABLE 18–1. Preventive Health Services by Age and Procedure

	Early				Middle			Late			
Procedure	11	12	13	14	15	16	17	18	19	20	21
Health Guidance											
Parenting*		•				•					
Development	•	•	•	•	•	•	•	•	•	•	•
Diet and fitness	•	•	•	•	•	•	•	•	•	•	•
Lifestyle†	•	•	•	•	•	•	•	•	•	•	•
Injury prevention	•	•	•	•	•	•	•	•	•	•	•
Screening											
History											
Eating disorders	•	•	•	•	•	•	•	•	•	•	•
Sexual activity‡	•	•	•	•	•	•	•	•	•	•	•
Alcohol and other drug use	•	•	•	•	•	•	•	•	•	•	•
Tobacco use	•	•	•	•	•	•	•	•	•	•	•
Abuse	•	•	•	•	•	•	•	•	•	•	•
School performance	•	•	•	•	•	•	•	•	•	•	•
Depression	•	•	•	•	•	•	•	•	•	•	•
Risk for suicide	•	•	•	•	•	•	•	•	•	•	•
Physical Assessment											
Blood pressure	•	•	•	•	•	•	•	•	•	•	•
Body Mass Index	•	•	•	•	•	•	•	•	•	•	•
Comprehensive exam			•			•			•		
Tests§											
Cholesterol	——1——				——1——			——1——			
TB	——2——				——2——			——2——			
GC, chlamydia, and HPV	——3——				——3——			——3——			
HIV and syphilis	——4——				——4——			——4——			
Pap smear	——5——				——5——			——5——			
Immunizations											
MMR		•									
Td						•					
HBV	——6——				——6——			——6——			
Varicella	——7——				——7——			——7——			

*A parent health-guidance visit is recommended during early and middle adolescence.
†Includes counseling regarding sexual behavior and avoidance of tobacco, alcohol, and other drugs.
‡Includes history of unintended pregnancy and STDs.
§1: Perform screening test once if family history is positive for early cardiovascular disease or hyperlipidemia. 2: Screen if positive for exposure to active tuberculosis or if patient lives or works in high-risk situation (e.g., homeless shelter, jail, health care facility). 3: Screen at least annually if sexually active. 4: Screen if high-risk for infection. 5: Screen annually if sexually active. 6: Vaccinate regardless of risk for hepatitis B infection. 7: Vaccinate if no reliable history of chicken pox.

Reproduced and modified, with permission, from Elster, A. (ed.). American Medical Association Guidelines for Adolescent Preventive Services (GAPS): Recommendations and Rationale. Baltimore, Williams & Wilkins, 1994, p. 179.

THE HEALTH MAINTENANCE VISIT

The purpose of the health maintenance visit is to assess the general health and well-being of the child or adolescent. Questions asked during this visit should initially be simple and focus on how the patient feels in general. More specific questions can then be formulated from the initial responses. In healthy patients, the medical history can be obtained using a questionnaire that parents and children complete in the waiting room. If this method is used, a separate form should be given to adolescents if they are accompanied by one or both parents. The information is then reviewed at the start of the interview. Chronic medical conditions also should be addressed at this time.

Medical History

Older children and adolescents should always be questioned directly about their medical history (Questions Box: Screening in Older Children and Adolescents). Parents should be encouraged to participate only after their children have responded to questions or if invited by children or adolescents themselves. The degree of parental participation is also influenced by the current cognitive as well as developmental stage of patients.

Questions: Screening in Older Children and Adolescents

Questions for both the patient and parent:
- How has the child or adolescent been lately? Does he or she have any complaints or concerns?
- How does the child or adolescent like school?
- What activities does the child or adolescent currently participate in? Does he or she have any hobbies?
- With whom does the child or adolescent live?
- Are there any significant illnesses in the immediate or extended family, such as hypertension, diabetes, or cancer?
- Does the child or adolescent take any medications (prescribed or over-the-counter) regularly?

Questions for the child or adolescent alone:
- Do you have any questions or concerns?
- How are things at home? Are there any problems with parents or siblings?
- Are you attending school?
  - Do you like school?
  - Have you ever been truant?
- Do you have friends?
- What do you do for fun?
- Do you or your friends use tobacco, drugs, or alcohol?
- Are you or your friends sexually active?
- Do you or any of your friends use contraception?
- Are you ever really sad?
  - Have you ever thought of, or tried to commit, suicide?
  - Do you have access to a gun?
- Do you or your friends diet?
- Are you using medications, exercise, or self-induced vomiting to control your weight?

Psychosocial History

The psychosocial component of the interview should be conducted with older children or adolescents alone as well as together with parents (Questions Box). General questions about school, outside activities or hobbies, and family are often less threatening than inquiries about friends and tobacco or drug use. More sensitive topics relating to sexuality and sexual activity should be addressed after parents have left the room. Subjects initially discussed with parents should also be reviewed in their absence.

A useful tool for conducting the psychosocial interview has been developed and refined by physicians who specialize in pediatrics and adolescent medicine. Known by the acronym **HEADSSS**, it reviews the essential components of the psychosocial history: **h**ome, **e**ducation or **e**mployment, **a**ctivities, **d**rugs, **s**exual activity, **s**uicide or depression, and **s**afety (see Chapter 4, Talking to Adolescents).

Dietary History

A general dietary history should be obtained, with particular focus on eating habits, level of physical activity, and body image. Daily calcium and iron intake also should be reviewed, especially in adolescent females.

Family History

Significant illnesses such as hypertension, hyperlipidemia, obesity, and diabetes in first- and second-degree family members should be reviewed. Family use of alcohol, tobacco, and illegal substances should also be determined. Age and cause of death in immediate family members should also be recorded.

Medications and Allergies

Prescription as well as nonprescription medications should be reviewed along with the indications and frequency of usage.

Physical Examination

The height and weight of patients should be plotted on a growth curve, with particular attention paid to the velocity of growth and the body mass index $(BMI = weight (kg) \div [height(m)]^2)$. The blood pressure should also be noted.

Aspects of the physical examination that are influenced by puberty should be emphasized. The skin should be carefully inspected for acne, and clinicians should offer treatment whether or not patients state that they have skin problems. The oropharynx should be examined for any evidence of gingivitis or other signs of poor hygiene or malocclusion. The neck should be palpated for adenopathy and the thyroid gland for hypertrophy or nodules, especially in adolescent females. The back should be examined for any evidence of scoliosis, which is important to diagnose during this time of rapid growth.

Assessment of the pubertal development of the breasts and pubic hair in preadolescent or adolescent females and the genitalia and pubic hair in adolescent males is essential. The Tanner stage can then be correlated with other signs of puberty, such as the appearance of acne and body odor. For example, the adolescent female with Tanner stage 4 breasts and immature pubic hair distribution may have a problem such as testicular feminization syndrome.

The abdomen should be palpated for organomegaly, the testicles for masses, and the external female genitalia for lesions. A speculum examination should be performed in sexually active females or in adolescents with a vaginal discharge or unexplained bleeding. (See Chapter 22, Reproductive Health, for additional indications for a pelvic examination.) A rectal examination is reserved for patients with chronic abdominal pain or a history of sexual activity.

Immunizations

Practitioners should verify that patients received the primary immunization series, and they should administer a second dose of MMR (if not given at 4–6 years of age) as well as a dT booster to adolescents ages 11–12 years or older. Although booster doses of dT are recommended at 10-year intervals, administration of the first dT booster at this age increases compliance and reduces the susceptibility of adolescents to tetanus and diphtheria. Routine vaccination against hepatitis B also is recommended, regardless of sexual activity, if it has not been administered previously. In addition, a Mantoux skin test for tuberculosis should be given, as well as the varicella vaccine, if the patient has not been vaccinated and does not have a reliable history of chicken pox. Other immunizations, such as influenza, pneumococcal, hepatitis A, and meningococcal vaccines, should be considered on an individual basis.

Laboratory Tests

A hemoglobin level should be obtained to check for anemia and a urinalysis performed, especially in sexually active adolescents, to assess for protein, blood, and pyuria. Other suggested screening tests include hearing and vision tests, and a cholesterol and lipid profile. Cholesterol screening remains controversial, but it is important to consider in patients who are morbidly obese or have a positive family history for hyperlipidemia or premature atherosclerotic heart disease.

In addition to the above laboratory tests, sexually active adolescents should be screened for STDs. A cervical culture for gonorrhea, a fluorescent antibody test for chlamydia, and a Pap smear should be performed on adolescent females. Males should be screened if they are symptomatic or have a history of multiple partners and unprotected intercourse. In addition, an RPR test for syphilis should be obtained, especially if another venereal disease is evident or suspected. HIV testing is not usually emergently indicated and should be offered in the clinically appropriate setting after patients have received pretest counseling.

Patient Education

At the conclusion of the health maintenance visit, positive as well as negative findings should be reviewed with patients and their parents. Depending on the nature of these findings and the age of patients, practitioners may initially choose to address these findings with patients alone. All recommended screening laboratory studies and immunizations should also be reviewed before administration, including the need for further follow-up with tests such as the Mantoux test. Subsequent vaccine doses must be outlined for patients or parents. The timing of the next visit and reasons for this visit should be discussed.

The remainder of the visit should then be spent addressing any specific concerns of patients and parents, highlighting health care problems (e.g., obesity, high blood pressure), and identifying any factors that may be related to high-risk behavior such as drug or alcohol use. Older children or adolescents who are not participating in any deleterious activities should be praised for their positive behavior as well as provided with information regarding injury prevention.

PREPARTICIPATION PHYSICAL EXAMINATION FOR SCHOOL-AGE AND ADOLESCENT ATHLETES

The preparticipation physical examination (PPE) is essentially the "sports physical" that many schools require for participation in organized athletic programs. The primary objective of the PPE is to assess the young athlete's readiness to compete safely and effectively in a given sport. Ideally, it should also identify athletes at risk for injury or sudden death as well as those with an underlying medical condition that may affect athletic participation.

Controversy exists about the appropriate location for performance of the PPE. Community physicians are often asked to perform limited en masse examinations at schools, or a group of clinicians is asked to perform the examinations in the gymnasium using "stations." Either way, the patient does not truly receive a complete physical examination or assessment, and neither approach lends itself to privacy. In addition, parents have a false sense of security and believe that their children have received adequate medical care. Ideally, primary care physicians should perform the PPE annually in their office during a scheduled visit at least 4–6 weeks before the beginning of the athletic season. Pediatricians can use this required visit as an opportunity to perform an annual comprehensive health maintenance examination on older children and adolescents, including the various screening tests.

History

The medical history for the PPE should primarily focus on previous athletic participation and any injuries that may have occurred (Questions Box: Preparticipation Physical Examination). A standard questionnaire developed by the AAP for this purpose may be used in the office setting. In addition, many practitioners record the results of the physical examination as well as their recommendations regarding the degree of athletic participation on this standard form (Table 18–2).

TABLE 18–2.   Sports Participation Health Record

This evaluation is only to determine readiness for sports participation. It should not be used as a substitute for regular health maintenance examinations.

NAME _____ AGE _____ (YRS) GRADE _____ DATE _____

ADDRESS _____ PHONE _____

SPORTS _____

The Health History (Part A) and Physical Examination (Part C) sections must both be completed, at least every 24 months, before sports participation. The Interim Health History section (Part B) needs to be completed at least annually.

PART A — HEALTH HISTORY:
To be completed by athlete and parent

1. Have you ever had an illness that: YES   NO
   a. required you to stay in the hospital?   ____ ____
   b. lasted longer than a week?   ____ ____
   c. caused you to miss 3 days of practice or a competition?   ____ ____
   d. is related to allergies (e.g., hay fever, hives, asthma, insect stings)?   ____ ____
   e. required an operation?   ____ ____
   f. is chronic (e.g., asthma, diabetes)?   ____ ____
2. Have you ever had an injury that:
   a. required you to go to an emergency room or see a doctor?   ____ ____
   b. required you to stay in the hospital?   ____ ____
   c. required x-rays?   ____ ____
   d. caused you to miss 3 days of practice or a competition?   ____ ____
   e. required an operation?   ____ ____
3. Do you take any medication or pills?   ____ ____
4. Have any members of your family under age 50 had a heart attack, heart problem, or died unexpectedly?   ____ ____
5. Have you ever:
   a. been dizzy or passed out during or after exercise?   ____ ____
   b. been unconscious or had a concussion?   ____ ____
6. Are you unable to run ½ mile (2 times around the track) without stopping?   ____ ____
7. Do you:
   a. wear glasses or contacts?   ____ ____
   b. wear dental bridges, plates, or braces?   ____ ____
8. Have you ever had a heart murmur, high blood pressure, or a heart abnormality?   ____ ____
9. Do you have any allergies to any medicine?   ____ ____
10. Are you missing a kidney?   ____ ____
11. When was your last tetanus booster? _____
12. For Women
    a. At what age did you experience your first menstrual period?_____
    b. In the last year, what is the longest time you have gone between periods?
    _____

EXPLAIN ANY "YES" ANSWERS _____
_____
_____

I hereby state that, to the best of my knowledge, my answers to the above questions are correct.

Date _____

Signature of athlete _____

Signature of parent_____

PART B — INTERIM HEALTH HISTORY:
This form should be used during the interval between preparticipation evaluations. Positive responses should prompt a medical evaluation.

1. Over the next 12 months, I wish to participate in the following sports:
   a. _____
   b. _____
   c. _____
   d. _____
2. Have you missed more than 3 consecutive days of participation in usual activities because of an injury this past year?
   Yes _____ No _____
   If yes, please indicate:
   a. Site of injury _____
   b. Type of injury _____
3. Have you missed more than 5 consecutive days of participation in usual activities because of an illness, or have you had a medical illness diagnosed that has not been resolved in this past year?
   Yes _____ No _____
   If yes, please indicate:
   a. Type of illness _____
4. Have you had a seizure, concussion or been unconscious for any reason in the last year?
   Yes _____ No _____
5. Have you had surgery or been hospitalized in this past year?
   Yes _____ No _____
   If yes, please indicate:
   a. Reason for hospitalization _____
   b. Type of surgery _____
6. List all medications you are presently taking and what condition the medication is for.
   a. _____
   b. _____
   c. _____
7. Are you worried about any problem or condition at this time?
   Yes _____ No _____
   If yes, please explain: _____
   _____
   _____

I heareby state that, to the best of my knowledge, my answers to the above questions are correct.

Date _____

Signature of athlete _____

Signature of parent_____

Table continued on following page

18–2.   **Sports Participation Health Record** *Continued*

PART C: PHYSICAL EXAMINATION RECORD

NAME _____ DATE _____ AGE _____ BIRTHDATE _____

Height _____   Vision: R _____/_____, corrected _____, uncorrected _____

Weight _____   L _____/_____, corrected _____, uncorrected _____

Pulse _____ Blood Pressure _____ Percent Body Fat (optional) _____

	Normal	Abnormal Findings	Initials
1. Eyes			
2. Ears, Nose, Throat			
3. Mouth and Teeth			
4. Neck			
5. Cardiovascular			
6. Chest and Lungs			
7. Abdomen			
8. Skin			
9. Genitalia—Hernia (male)			
10. Musculoskeletal: ROM, strength, etc.			
a. neck			
b. spine			
c. shoulders			
d. arms/hands			
e. hips			
f. thighs			
g. knees			
h. ankles			
i. feet			
11. Neuromuscular			
12. Physical Maturity (Tanner Stage)		1. 2. 3. 4. 5.	

Comments re: Abnormal Findings: _____

_____

_____

_____

PARTICIPATION RECOMMENDATIONS:

1. No participation in: _____

_____

2. Limited participation in: _____

3. Requires: _____

_____

4. Full participation in: _____

Physician Signature _____

Telephone Number _____ Address _____

Reproduced, with permission, from Sports Medicine: Health Care for Young Athletes, 2nd ed. Elk Grove Village, IL, American Academy of Pediatrics, 1991.

Questions: Preparticipation Physical Examination

- What sport(s) does the child or adolescent wish to participate in?
- Has the child or adolescent ever experienced a sports injury? If so, how much time did the athlete miss doing sports activities as a result of this injury?
- Has the athlete ever suffered a concussion?
- Does the child or adolescent have a significant underlying health problem?
- Is the child or adolescent taking any medications?
- Does the child or adolescent have any allergies?
- Has the child or adolescent ever had syncope, palpitations, or angina during exercise?
- Does the child or adolescent have a family history of sudden, early, nontraumatic deaths?

Physical Examination

A complete physical examination should be performed when possible. If circumstances preclude this, specific attention should be paid to the eyes, heart, abdomen, skin, and musculoskeletal system. Height, weight, blood pressure, and visual acuity also should be measured. Examination of the eyes is essential to document physiologic anisocoria. A thorough cardiac evaluation should be performed for murmurs, abnormal heart sounds, or arrhythmias. The abdomen should be palpated for an enlarged liver or spleen, especially in the adolescent with a recent viral illness that could suggest mononucleosis. In males, the genitalia should be examined for sexual maturity in addition to absence or atrophy of a testis. The skin should be inspected for lesions such as tinea corporis, impetigo, or herpes simplex infection.

The "two-minute orthopedic examination" consists of a head-to-toe assessment of all muscle groups and joints; any deformities, anomalies, or evidence of previous injuries should be noted (Table 18–3). Recent studies suggest expanding this examination to include a more detailed evaluation of high risk areas for injury such as the knee, ankle, and shoulder.

Laboratory Tests

Routine laboratory screening tests, except for those performed during the general health maintenance visit, are not recommended for the PPE. Screening young athletes for anemia or proteinuria has not been found to be particularly helpful. Such screening may be useful with highly competitive professional athletes, however.

Exclusion Criteria

Medical exclusion criteria for athletic participation are based on information obtained in the medical as well as family history. Findings discovered during the physical examination such as stature consistent with Marfan's syndrome, a cardiac arrhythmia, or the midsystolic click of mitral valve prolapse could preclude the adolescent from participation in a particular sport.

TABLE 18–3.   The Two-Minute Orthopedic Examination

Instructions	Points of Observation
Stand facing examiner	Acromioclavicular joints, general habitus
Look at ceiling, floor, over both shoulders; touch ears to shoulders	Cervical spinal motion
Shrug shoulders (examiner resists)	Trapezius strength
Abduct shoulders 90 degrees	Deltoid strength
Full external rotation of arms	Shoulder motion
Flex and extend elbows	Elbow motion
Arms at sides, elbows 90 degrees flexed; pronate and supinate wrists	Elbow and wrist motion
Spread fingers; make fist	Hand or finger motion and deformities
Tighten (contract) quadriceps; relax quadriceps	Symmetry and knee effusion; ankle effusion
"Duck walk" four steps (away from examiner with buttocks on heels)	Hip, knee, and ankle motion
Back to examiner	Shoulder symmetry, scoliosis
Knees straight, touch toes	Scoliosis, hip motion, hamstring tightness
Raise up on toes, raise heels	Calf symmetry, leg strength

Reproduced, with permission, from Sports Medicine: Health Care for Young Athletes, 2nd ed. Elk Grove Village, IL, American Academy of Pediatrics, 1991, p. 54.

Specific conditions, such as the athlete with one eye or one kidney, should be evaluated on an individual basis by a physician qualified to assess the safety of the particular sport for the athlete (contact/collision versus limited contact).

Significant historical clues include a family history of sudden, nontraumatic death; premature coronary artery disease in a first- or second-degree relative; a history of palpitations, angina, or syncope during exercise; and recent, documented infection with the Epstein-Barr virus (EBV). Controversy exists regarding when athletes can return to collision sports after infectious mononucleosis. The most common causes of unexpected death during athletics include cardiomyopathies, anomalous coronary arteries, heart valve defects, primary cardiac rhythm disorders, and pulmonary hypertension.

Special circumstances to consider during the PPE are menstrual disorders and the female athlete; exercise-induced bronchospasm; anabolic steroid use; and eating disorders that may be associated with certain activities such as gymnastics, ballet, and wrestling.

Case Resolution

The young adolescent described in the case history should first be interviewed with the parent and then alone. Her medical and psychosocial history should be reviewed. A complete physical examination should be performed as well as a pelvic examination if she is sexually active. General laboratory screening tests should be performed and the results reviewed with the patient. The remainder of the visit should be spent discussing issues such as nutrition, exercise, illicit substance abuse, sexuality and sexual activity, and safety. Results of the physical examination and screening tests should then be discussed with the parent who accompanied her to the office. If necessary, a follow-up visit should be scheduled. Otherwise, the adolescent should be seen annually.

Selected Readings

American Academy of Pediatrics, Committee on Nutrition. Cholesterol in Childhood. Pediatrics 101:141–147, 1998.

American Academy of Pediatrics, Committee on Sports Medicine and Fitness. Medical conditions affecting sports participation. Pediatrics 94:757–760, 1994.

Cavanaugh, R. M. Anticipatory guidance for the adolescent: Has it come of age? Pediatr. Rev. 15:485–489, 1994.

Centers for Disease Control. Immunization of Adolescents. M.M.W.R. 1996:45 (RR–13).

Cromer, B. A., C. S. McLean, and F. P. Heald. A critical review of comprehensive health screening in adolescents. J. Adolesc. Health 13:1S–65S, 1992.

Elster, A. (ed.). American Medical Association Guidelines for Adolescent Preventive Services (GAPS): Recommendations and Rationale. Baltimore, Williams & Wilkins, 1994.

Hergenroeder, A. C. The preparticipation sports examination. Pediatr. Clin. North Am. 44:1525–1540, 1997.

Igra, V., and S. G. Millstein. Current status and approaches to improving preventive services for adolescents. J.A.M.A. 269:1408–1412, 1993.

Jenkins, R. R., and S. B. Saxena. Keeping adolescents healthy. Contemp. Peds. 12:76–89, 1995.

Krowchuk, D. P. The preparticipation athletic examination: A closer look. Pediatr. Ann. 26:37–49, 1997.

Sports Medicine: Health Care for Young Athletes, 2nd ed. American Academy of Pediatrics, 1991.

CHAPTER 19

WELL CHILD CARE FOR CHILDREN WITH TRISOMY 21

Monica Sifuentes, M.D.

H$_x$ A 9-month-old girl with trisomy 21 whom you have known since birth is brought to your office for well child care. She and her parents have been doing well and report no intercurrent problems or illnesses since her last visit. Her past medical history is significant for a small ventricular septal defect, which has since closed spontaneously, and one episode of otitis media at 7 months of age. Her weight gain has been good—along the 25th percentile on the trisomy 21 growth chart. She now sleeps through the night and has a bowel movement once a day. She has received all of the recommended immunizations for her age without any problems. Except for an oral fluoride supplement, she takes no medications.

The infant can now roll from a supine to prone position but is still unable to sit unassisted. She grasps objects in both hands, however, and babbles appropriately with her siblings. Since she was 1-month-old, she has been enrolled in an early intervention program. An occupational therapist visits her at home twice a month.

On physical examination, she has typical facial features consistent with trisomy 21, a single palmar crease on each hand, and mild diffuse hypotonia.

Questions

1. What is the prevalence of trisomy 21 (Down syndrome) in the general population? What is the association of maternal age with trisomy 21?

2. What are the clinical manifestations of this syndrome?
3. What medical conditions are associated with trisomy 21 in the newborn period, during childhood, and in adolescence? When should screening tests for these conditions be performed?
4. What is the role of early intervention services for these patients and their families?
5. What specific psychosocial issues should be included in your anticipatory guidance and health education?
6. What is the prognosis for children with trisomy 21?

Trisomy 21, or Down syndrome, is one of the most common genetic disorders causing developmental delay. Infants and children with trisomy 21, like children with other developmental disabilities and chronic illnesses, need to be evaluated and monitored for associated conditions concurrently with their well child visits. The primary care provider is thus in the unique position to offer affected children routine health care maintenance and follow-up for intercurrent illnesses or chronic problems, as well as anticipatory guidance for families. In addition, the general pediatrician has the opportunity to develop a strong rapport with children and families given the frequency of well child visits. Such relationships are particularly important when considering the complex medical and social challenges associated with raising children with trisomy 21. An important goal of the well child visit is to provide children with trisomy 21 and their families with counseling about educational, social, and financial resources and support to ensure a healthy and productive transition into adulthood.

EPIDEMIOLOGY

The prevalence of trisomy 21 is approximately 1 in 800 to 1000 live births. Although the degree of mental retardation is variable, some authors claim it is responsible for up to one-third of all cases of moderate to severe mental retardation. Trisomy 21 occurs more commonly in males than in females, with a male-female ratio of 1.3:1.0.

The vast majority of cases of Down syndrome are caused by trisomy 21. This chromosomal nondisjunction occurs in the egg 95% of the time and in the sperm 5%, and it is strongly influenced by maternal age. For a 35–39-year-old woman, the risk of having a child with trisomy 21 is 6.5 times greater than for a 20–24-year-old woman. For the 40–44-year-old woman, the risk is 20.5 times greater. It is estimated that about one-half of embryos with trisomy 21 abort spontaneously.

The risk of recurrence in subsequent pregnancies is 1 in 100 until maternal age 35, after which the risk determined by age takes precedence. Other family members are not at increased risk of bearing children with this chromosomal abnormality.

CLINICAL PRESENTATION

Infants and children with trisomy 21 have a characteristic appearance (D_x Box). They may be microcephalic, with flattening of both the occiput and face. The eyes have an upward slant, with prominent epicanthal folds, the ears are low-set and small, the nasal bridge is flattened, and the tongue appears large. The feet, hands, and digits are small and stubby, and the fifth digit is slightly turned in (clinodactyly). A single palmar crease and a wide spacing between the first and second toes may be evident. After the newborn period, diffuse hypotonia and developmental delay are universally seen.

D_x Trisomy 21
• Microcephaly, with flattening of both occiput and face • Upward slant to the eyes with epicanthal folds • Brushfield spots in eyes • Small ears and mouth (therefore tongue appears large) • Low-set ears • Flat nasal bridge • Broad, stocky neck, with loose skin folds at the nape • Funnel-shaped or pigeon-breasted chest • Small, stubby feet, hands, and digits, with brachyclinodactyly of the fifth digits • Single transverse palmar crease on each hand • Wide space between first and second toes • Fair, mottled skin in newborns; dry skin in older children • Hypotonia

PATHOPHYSIOLOGY

All sources agree that in almost all cases (95%), Down syndrome is caused by nondisjunctional trisomy 21. The remaining cases are translocations (3–4%) and mosaics (1–2%). The translocations are unbalanced and usually occur with another acrocentric chromosome, usually 14/21 or 15/21. Approximately 75% of these are new mutations, and 25% are the result of a familial translocation. Therefore, if a child has a translocation, the parents must be evaluated for a balanced translocation. Mosaicism implies the presence of two cell lines: one normal and one with trisomy 21. As might be expected, children with Down syndrome as a result of mosaicism are affected less severely than those with nondisjunctional trisomy 21 or translocations.

EVALUATION

Routine health care maintenance for infants, children, or adolescents with trisomy 21 should cover the same issues in health education, prevention, and counseling that are discussed with other healthy patients and their families. In addition, specific medical as well as psychosocial issues pertinent to patients with trisomy 21 need to be addressed periodically.

Newborn Period

Verification of the diagnosis of trisomy 21 is perhaps the single most important focus of the initial family visit. Sometimes, the diagnosis has been made prenatally by chorionic villus sampling or amniocentesis, carried out because of maternal age or other risk factors, such as low maternal serum alpha-fetoprotein levels. If trisomy 21 was unsuspected prenatally, and the diagnosis is based on the physical examination performed shortly after birth, a karyotype must be sent from the nursery. The results can be reviewed with the family when they return to the office for the 1–2-week visit.

Several conditions that are associated with trisomy 21 are important to identify in the newborn period. They are congenital heart disease (risk: 30–50%), most commonly an endocardial cushion defect; GI malformations and obstructive disorders (risk: 12%) such as duodenal atresia, imperforate anus, tracheoesophageal fistula, pyloric stenosis, and Hirschsprung's disease; congenital hypothyroidism (risk: 1%); congenital ocular anomalies (risk: 60%), including cataracts, strabismus, and nystagmus; hip dysplasias; and leukemoid reactions that resemble leukemia but resolve during the first month of life. Leukemia is more common in individuals with trisomy 21 than in the general population, but it still occurs rarely (<1%).

History

Although associated conditions may not have been apparent in the newborn nursery, it is important to inquire about any symptoms that may indicate their current presence (Questions Box). In addition, the routine

Questions: Trisomy 21

- Is the infant or child having any feeding problems?
- Does the infant or child appear to be gaining weight?
- Does the infant or child appear to hear?
- Does the infant or child vocalize? What words does the young child know?
- Does the infant or child appear to see?
- Does one eye ever wander or appear "lazy" by the end of the day?
- Has the infant or child had many ear infections?
- Is the infant or child constipated? If so, is the hair coarse and the skin dry?

nutritional and developmental history should be documented. A detailed family and social history should also be obtained if this was not done in the hospital.

Physical Examination

All growth parameters (e.g., length, weight, head circumference) should be recorded and compared with those obtained at birth. Neonates with trisomy 21, like other term newborns, should regain birth weight by 2 weeks of life.

A complete physical examination must be performed on all neonates. In particular, the size of the fontanelles should be evaluated because of the increased incidence of congenital hypothyroidism. A bilateral red reflex and conjugate gaze should be documented to exclude congenital cataracts. A careful cardiac examination must be performed, noting any murmurs, irregular heart rates, abnormal heart sounds, or asymmetry of pulses. In addition to endocardial cushion defects, other associated cardiac malformations include ventricular septal defects, tetralogy of Fallot, and atrial septal defects. Cyanosis should also be evaluated. The abdomen should be palpated for organomegaly or any masses, and patency of the anus should be verified. An Ortolani test should also be performed for hip laxity. Finally, the neonate's tone should be evaluated; hypotonia is not an uncommon finding, although it may be less apparent in the newborn.

Laboratory Assessment

Prior to discharge from the nursery or when trisomy 21 is initially suspected based on clinical examination, a karyotype on peripheral lymphocytes should be performed to confirm the diagnosis although results may not be available for 1–2 weeks. In addition, an ECG and a chest x-ray should be obtained in the nursery or shortly thereafter. Some physicians advocate including an echocardiogram in the initial evaluation of all infants for congenital heart disease, regardless of the findings on physical examination, ECG, or chest x-ray. Other laboratory tests that should be performed include a thyroid screen to check for congenital hypothyroidism, which may have been missed on the state neonatal screen; a CBC to look for a leukemoid reaction or polycythemia; and a brain stem auditory evoked response (BAER) as a baseline study for hearing.

Anticipatory Guidance

Routine topics related to nutrition, growth, and development should be discussed in the newborn period. Other important issues to address include those pertaining to available resources for children and families such as early intervention programs and Down syndrome support groups in the community. Educational materials such as pamphlets and books may also be supplied at this time. Upcoming appointments with other physicians and allied health professionals should be reviewed. The schedule of health maintenance visits for infants and young children with trisomy 21 is essentially the same as that recommended by the AAP for other children (Table 19–1).

INFANCY AND EARLY CHILDHOOD

History

Some additional historical issues to address at this time include a detailed developmental assessment focusing on progress made since the last visit. Inquiries regarding the development of any new conditions associated with Down syndrome such as hearing deficits or hypothyroidism should be made. Oropharyngeal problems such as sleep apnea secondary to the underdevelopment of the nasopharynx and enlarged tonsils should also be reviewed.

Physical Examination

All growth parameters (height, weight, and head circumference) should be measured at each visit and plotted on growth charts for children with Down syndrome (Fig. 19–1 through 19–4). Children with trisomy 21 are

TABLE 19–1. Health Supervision for Children With Down Syndrome

	Newborn Period	Infancy and Early Childhood*	Older Childhood and Adolescence†
History	X	X	X
Developmental Assessment (by test or report)		X	X
Physical Examination (including measurements)	X	X	X
Visual testing	X	X	X
Hearing	X	X	X
Laboratory Assessment			
Karyotype	X		
Annual thyroid screen	X	X	X
Echocardiogram	X		
Neck radiographs		X	X
Consultation			
Genetics	X		
Cardiology	X	X	X
Ophthalmology	X	X	X
Ear-nose-throat	X	X	X
Dental		X	X

*Visits should be scheduled every 2–3 months.
†Visits should be scheduled every 1–2 years.

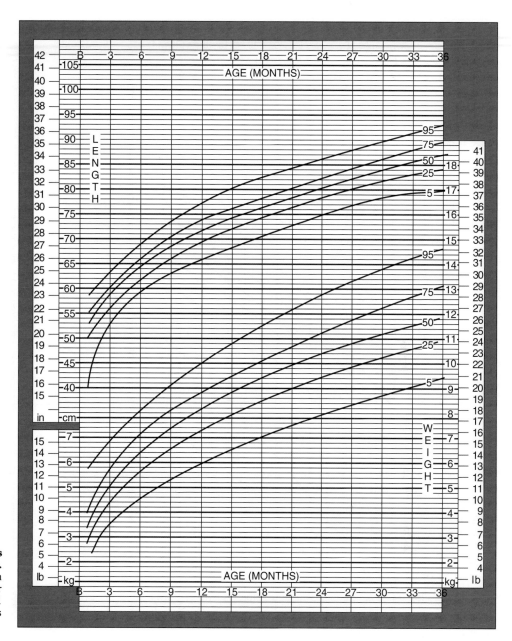

FIGURE 19–1. Growth chart for boys with Down syndrome: 1–36 months. (Reproduced, with permission, from Cronk, C., et al. Growth charts for children with Down syndrome: 1 month to 18 years of age. Pediatrics 81:102–110, 1988.)

shorter than other children and may have poor weight gain in their first year. Later in life, obesity unrelated to the syndrome may become a problem, however.

As with routine well child visits in other infants and children, a complete physical examination should be performed at each patient encounter. Noteworthy aspects of the examination in infants and children with trisomy 21 are given in Table 19–2.

Laboratory Assessment

Infants with trisomy 21 should have all routine screening tests and immunizations. In addition, they should have their hearing monitored during the first year of life. A BAER with a tympanogram should be performed by 8 months of age; hearing should be checked annually thereafter. Referral to an audiologist should be considered in any infants who appear to have a hearing deficit or significant speech delay. A history of

recurrent otitis media may also warrant referral to an otolaryngologist.

Developmentally appropriate gross visual screening should be performed in infants between 6 and 12 months of age at each visit. Positive findings on physical examination or indeterminate visual assessments warrant referral to an ophthalmologist. Children's vision should continue to be checked annually in the office until 5 years of age, because there is a 30–50% risk of refractive errors between 3 and 5 years. A formal ophthalmology consult should occur at about 4 years.

Thyroid screening tests should be performed early in infancy, if not in the neonatal period. Current AAP recommendations include repeating these studies at 4–6 months of age, at 12 months, and then annually.

Lateral cervical radiographs with flexion and extension views to detect atlantoaxial instability or subluxation are recommended once in early childhood. Much controversy exists regarding whether neck films are an

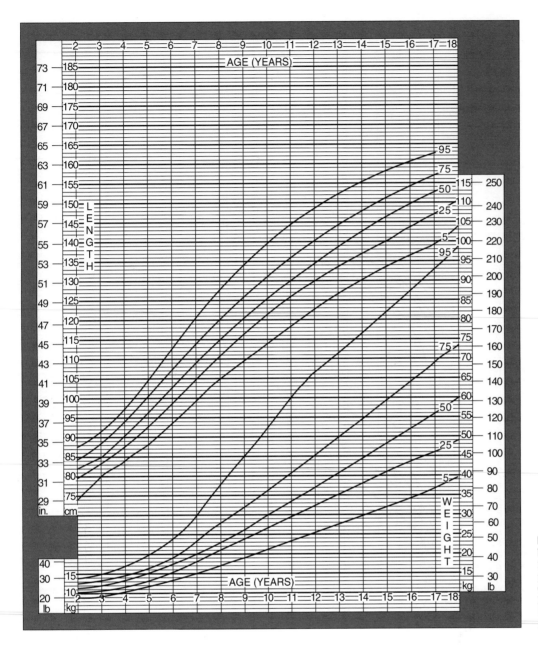

FIGURE 19–2. Growth chart for boys with Down syndrome: 2–18 years. (Reproduced, with permission, from Cronk, C., et al. Growth charts for children with Down syndrome: 1 month to 18 years of age. Pediatrics 81: 102–110, 1988.)

adequate screening tool for any potentially serious complication. Some authorities have suggested that these studies are more important in children who participate in contact sports or athletic activities (e.g., the Special Olympics) and in those who are symptomatic. Neck films should then be repeated at 3–4-year intervals. Regardless of radiographic findings, however, children with Down syndrome should be discouraged from activities that require acute flexion of the neck (tumbling, diving).

A cardiac evaluation should be made early in infancy if it was not performed in the newborn period. The primary care practitioner may prefer to have a pediatric cardiologist complete this examination (depending on the practitioner's experience and comfort level).

A dental referral should be made by the age of 4 years or earlier if the children have any dental problems.

Anticipatory Guidance

Growth and developmental progress should be reviewed with parents at the end of each visit, and any concerns or unmet expectations should be addressed at this time. Often the developmental delay associated with trisomy 21 is not apparent to families until infants are 4–6 months of age and not achieving the expected milestones of rolling over or sitting. The diagnosis and associated conditions should then be reviewed once again. It should also be emphasized to families that the degree of mental retardation in trisomy 21 is quite variable, ranging from mild to severe. Social function is not necessarily related to IQ. If the child is not already enrolled in an early intervention program, the positive role of such an experience should be addressed. The availability of support groups for parents and other family members should also be discussed.

In the early childhood years, plans for preschool attendance and future educational opportunities should be reviewed with families. The role of discipline and the presence of common behavioral problems such as temper tantrums and biting should be assessed in preparation for school entry and socialization. Developmentally appropriate safety issues such as toddler car seats and adult supervision while in the bathtub or pool should also be discussed. Some experts suggest that the advantages and disadvantages of reconstructive craniofacial surgery during early childhood to alter the characteristic features of Down syndrome should be reviewed.

OLDER CHILDHOOD AND ADOLESCENCE

History

Older, school-age children with Down syndrome should continue to visit their primary care physician at least annually. Although annual visits are not recommended in general, children with trisomy 21 require visits for screening for the development of common medical conditions and for assisting families with educational planning. Specific medical issues to address during the history pertain to possible signs or symptoms of visual or hearing deficits; evidence of hypothyroidism, such as a decrease in activity, coarse, dry hair, and constipation; and skin or dental problems such as eczema and caries, which are not uncommon in patients with Down syndrome. A careful nutritional history should also be taken because of the propensity for obesity.

Physical Examination

A complete physical examination should be performed. Growth parameters should continue to be plotted, although head circumference is probably now

FIGURE 19–3. Growth chart for girls with Down syndrome: 1–36 months. (Reproduced, with permission, from Cronk, C., et al. Growth charts for children with Down syndrome: 1 month to 18 years of age. Pediatrics 81:102–110, 1988.)

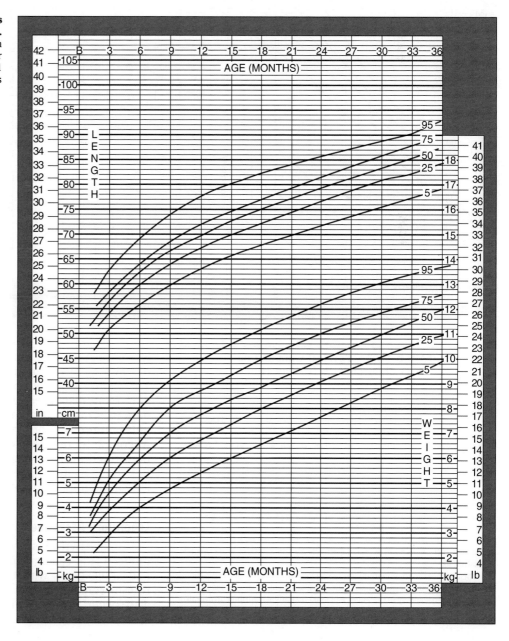

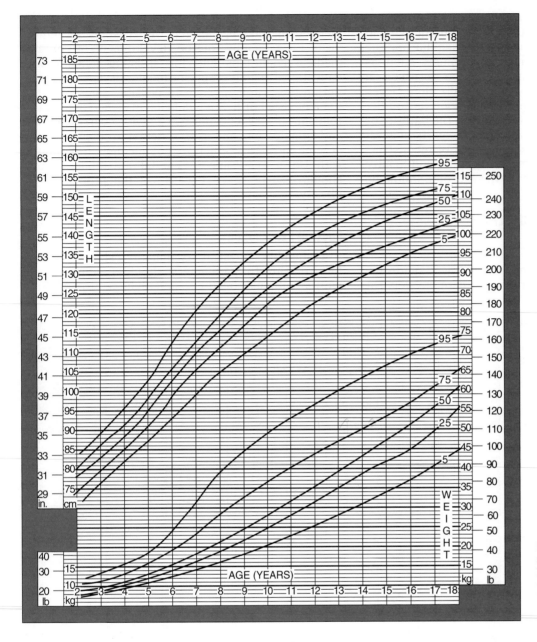

FIGURE 19–4. Growth chart for girls with Down syndrome: 2–18 years. (Reproduced, with permission, from Cronk, C., et al. Growth charts for children with Down syndrome: 1 month to 18 years of age. Pediatrics 81:102–110, 1988.

TABLE 19–2. Physical Examination of Children With Trisomy 21

Look for dry sensitive skin and alopecia, which develops in approximately 10% of children and resolves spontaneously.

Monitor the size of the anterior and posterior fontanelles, since delayed closure may indicate hypothyroidism.

Check for visual abnormalities, such as strabismus, nystagmus, cataracts, refractive errors, and blepharitis.

Document recurrent serous otitis media. It is estimated that 40–60% of children with trisomy 21 have significant conductive hearing loss, and 20–30% have some degree of neurosensory loss.

Examine the oropharynx carefully for delayed dentition, malocclusion, and caries.

Perform a thorough cardiac examination, and note any evidence of previously unrecognized congenital heart disease.

Palpate the abdomen for distention or organomegaly. Children with trisomy 21 have a slightly increased risk of developing acute nonlymphoblastic or acute lymphoblastic leukemia.

Perform a rectal examination in infants or children with a history of constipation.

Evaluate any musculoskeletal abnormalities such as overall hypotonia and joint laxity (most commonly in the knees and hips) that might contribute to overall gross motor delay.

---

less important. The skin should be examined closely for dryness or any evidence of acne during adolescence. The Tanner stage of both males and females should be noted and discussed with the parents. A pelvic examination is not indicated as a part of the routine visit unless there is concern about sexual abuse or an STD. A complete neurologic examination should also be performed in the patient participating in sports activities such as the Special Olympics to look for signs indicating impending atlantoaxial dislocation.

Laboratory Assessment

Annual thyroid screening (thyroid-stimulating hormone, T_4) is recommended for all school-age children and adolescents with trisomy 21, in addition to other routine screening tests. An audiologic evaluation should also occur at least once in older children and then annually thereafter. Because of the risk of keratoconus, an annual ophthalmology consultation should be arranged after the age of 10 years. In addition, children with trisomy 21 should be encouraged to continue annual dental visits because gingivitis, periodontal disease, and bruxism (teeth grinding) are common in these individuals.

Anticipatory Guidance

The major part of the visit with school-age and adolescent children should be spent on developmental, educational, and vocational anticipatory guidance. Educational placement and future goals should be both developmentally appropriate for the child and acceptable for the parent. Activities requiring socialization and the development of responsibility should continue to be encouraged; these can be very stressful for parents and other family members, however. Injury prevention should be highlighted as well, especially since older children are becoming more independent. In early adolescence, prevocational and vocational training within the school curriculum should be reviewed. In addition, brief discussions regarding independent living, group homes, and financial resources (e.g., community-supported employment for young adults) should begin during adolescence.

Puberty, fertility, and contraception are extremely important to address with adolescents and their parents. The patient's psychosocial development and physical sexual maturation should be discussed, including menstrual hygiene and any foreseeable problems with its management. Contraception and the potential for victimization must be addressed as well, particularly with female patients. Males with trisomy 21 are usually sterile.

MANAGEMENT

If a prenatal diagnosis of Down syndrome is made, and the general pediatrician is asked to participate in counseling the family, the points listed in Table 19–3 should be covered.

In addition to providing preventive health care during well child visits, the management of children with trisomy 21 is influenced by the presence of any associated conditions and the age at diagnosis. The primary goal should be to help affected infants and children reach their full potential. For example, if a newborn is found to have congenital heart disease and is clinically stable,

---

TABLE 19–3. Counseling the Family After a Prenatal Diagnosis of Down Syndrome

Review the data that established the diagnosis in the fetus.
Explain the mechanism of occurrence and risks for recurrence.
Review the manifestations of trisomy 21, commonly associated conditions, and the variable prognosis based on the presence of these conditions.
Discuss other modalities that confirm the presence of associated anomalies such as a fetal echocardiogram in the case of congenital heart disease.
Explore treatment options and interventions for associated conditions.
Offer resources to assist the family with decisions related to completing or terminating the pregnancy.
Refer the family to a clinical geneticist or genetics counselor.

---

then referral to a pediatric cardiologist is necessary but not emergent. However, suspected GI atresia or obstruction in a neonate is a medical emergency, and surgical consultation should be sought immediately.

Conditions such as congenital or acquired hypothyroidism should be treated aggressively with thyroxine and monitored closely during the first 2 years of life. Evaluation by a pediatric endocrinologist is warranted at the time of diagnosis and periodically thereafter. Other conditions associated with Down syndrome such as sensorineural hearing loss or refractive errors can be followed by the primary care practitioner in conjunction with the appropriate pediatric subspecialist.

PROGNOSIS

Individuals with trisomy 21 can be expected to live well into their sixties unless they are born with a congenital heart lesion, which may limit life expectancy. The major cause of morbidity and mortality is the development of symptomatic Alzheimer's disease, which occurs in approximately 15% of adults after the fourth decade. Fortunately, most adults with Down syndrome remain asymptomatic, despite histopathologic evidence of the disease.

Case Resolution

In the case described at the beginning of the chapter, the family should be encouraged by the healthy progress of their daughter. For this visit, anticipatory guidance should consist of a review of early intervention services, available resources, and general support services for the patient and her family. Medical screening should include vision and hearing, in addition to the routine hemoglobin or spun hematocrit that is performed in all healthy children. If the results are normal, the next visit should take place in 3 months.

Selected Readings

American Academy of Pediatrics, Committee on Children with Disabilities. General principles in the care of children and adolescents with genetic disorders and other chronic health conditions. Pediatrics 99:643–644, 1997.

American Academy of Pediatrics, Committee on Children with Disabilities. Sexuality education of children and adolescents with developmental disabilities. Pediatrics 97:275–278, 1996.

Carey, J. C. Health supervision and anticipatory guidance for children with genetic disorders (including specific recommendations for trisomy 21, trisomy 18, and neurofibromatosis I). Pediatr. Clin. North Am. 39:25–53, 1992.

Committee on Genetics, American Academy of Pediatrics. Health supervision for children with Down syndrome. Pediatrics 93:855–859, 1994.

Cronk, C., et al. Growth charts for children with Down syndrome: 1 month to 18 years of age. Pediatrics 81:102–110, 1988.

Hayes, A., and M. L. Batshaw. Down Syndrome. Pediatr. Clin. North Am. 40:523–535, 1993.

Levy, S. E., and S. L. Hyman. Pediatric assessment of the child with developmental delay. Pediatr. Clin. North Am. 40:465–477, 1993.

Toomey, K. E. Medical genetics for the pediatrician. Pediatr. Rev. 17:163–174, 1996.

CHAPTER 20

WELL CHILD CARE FOR PRETERM INFANTS

Monica Sifuentes, M.D.

H$_x$ A 2½-month-old infant girl was discharged from the neonatal intensive care unit 2 weeks ago, where she had been since birth. She was the product of a 29-week gestation born via spontaneous vaginal delivery to a 32-year-old primigravida. The perinatal course was complicated by premature rupture of membranes and maternal amnionitis. Several aspects of the neonatal course were significant, including respiratory distress that required surfactant therapy and 2 weeks of endotracheal intubation; a grade II intraventricular hemorrhage on head ultrasound at 1 week of life; group B streptococcal bacteremia; hyperbilirubinemia, which was treated with phototherapy; several episodes of apnea, presumably associated with the prematurity; and a history of poor oral intake with slow weight gain.

The infant's parents have a few questions about her feeding schedule and discontinuing the apnea monitor, but they feel relatively comfortable caring for their daughter at home. She is feeding well (2 oz of formula every 2–3 hours) and is becoming progressively more alert according to the family.

The infant's weight gain has averaged 25 g/day. The rest of the physical examination is normal, except for dolichocephaly and a left esotropia.

Questions

1. What constitutes well child care in preterm infants?
2. What are the nutritional requirements of preterm infants in the months following discharge from the hospital?
3. What information must be considered in the developmental screening of preterm infants?
4. What immunization schedule is appropriate for preterm infants? Do they require any special immunizations?
5. What specific conditions or illnesses are more likely to affect preterm infants than term infants?

Preterm, or premature, infants are born at less than 36 weeks' gestation and often weigh less than 2500 grams. Providing primary care for these infants is an important and challenging task for general pediatricians and other allied health practitioners. Well child care for preterm infants often requires coordination of medical, developmental, and social services for multiple chronic conditions. Because preterm infants are at increased risk for both developmental and neurologic sequelae as a result of their prematurity, routine well child care must also include formal developmental assessments as well as the usual screening tests. In addition, more frequent, longer visits may be necessary to evaluate preterm infants' nutritional and developmental progress and to assess how families have adjusted to caring for infants

at home. Primary care physicians must learn to manage these and many other complex issues while providing families with comprehensive anticipatory guidance.

EPIDEMIOLOGY

The number of preterm infants discharged from neonatal intensive care units (NICUs) has increased tremendously in the past 20 years. Improvement in both morbidity and mortality for infants weighing less than 1500 grams is quite impressive. For example, in the 1970s, less than 10% of extremely low-birth-weight infants (weight <750 g) survived. Today, 40–50% of such infants may live. Infants who weigh 750–1000 grams have also shown a marked decrease in mortality from approximately 70% in the 1970s to less than 30% in the late 1980s. Similarly, the survival rate of infants who weigh between 1000 and 1500 g is now 90%, a dramatic increase from 50% in the early 1970s.

Several factors have contributed to this improvement. Advances in technology, a better understanding of the physiology of preterm infants, important antenatal and perinatal interventions, and the development of specific medical treatments such as surfactant therapy are a few of these factors. In addition, these contributions have greatly affected the morbidity associated with prematurity, which may directly influence long-term outcome.

EVALUATION

The purpose of the health maintenance visit for preterm infants is the same as for other healthy children: to provide consistent preventive health care and education for patients and their parents. Prematurity, however, places the infants at risk for additional medical and neurodevelopmental conditions.

History

At the initial visit, it is imperative to review the entire past medical history and hospital course with the family. Ideally, the NICU should provide a discharge summary that includes the following information:

1. Birth weight and significant prenatal and perinatal information.
2. An overview of the hospital course, including significant illnesses, events, surgical procedures, and pertinent radiographic studies.
3. Nutrition information and present feeding regimen.
4. A list of current medications, including dosing intervals and, if appropriate, serum drug levels.

5. Immunizations given in the hospital or at the time of discharge.

6. Pertinent laboratory data, such as most recent hemoglobin, newborn screening results, and highest bilirubin.

7. Discharge physical exam including most recent height, weight, and head circumference.

8. Problems remaining at discharge.

9. Follow-up appointments.

Any significant complications or concerns should be discussed with the parents as soon as possible to assess their understanding of these issues as well as expectations for improvement.

Specifically, growth, nutrition, and developmental issues should be addressed at each visit (Questions Box). Adequate or desirable weight gain should be explained to the caregivers in terms of the infants' current weight versus the discharge weight. Infants under the age of 6 months should gain, on average, 20–40 g/day while at home. To ensure continued weight gain, many preterm infants are discharged from the NICU on a 24-hour feeding schedule, which requires that parents feed infants at least every 3 hours. The necessity for this practice should be reevaluated during the first few weeks following discharge after infants have demonstrated adequate weight gain.

The need for supplementation with iron, fluoride, and vitamins should also be addressed (see Management).

Probably the most important part of the preterm health maintenance visit is the developmental history. Parental expectations and observations should be noted and any developmental concerns should be evaluated. The adjusted developmental age should be calculated by subtracting the number of weeks the infant was born prematurely from the current chronologic age in weeks. The adjusted age should then be used for all formal and informal developmental assessments. The importance of correcting for prematurity until children are approximately 2½ years of age must be emphasized when discussing developmental progress and giving anticipatory guidance to parents.

Physical Examination

A complete physical examination should be performed at each visit to monitor the status of associated medical conditions. All growth parameters (weight, height, and head circumference) should be plotted on the growth chart and adjusted for prematurity. Because catch-up head growth generally precedes catch-up weight and length, preterm infants may appear to have disproportionally large heads. The onset of accelerated head growth may begin within a few weeks after birth (36 weeks post-conception) or as late as 8 months adjusted age. Average daily weight gain in grams/day should also be calculated. In addition, blood pressure must be recorded, especially if an umbilical catheter was used during the neonatal period.

Some findings of the physical examination are consistent with prematurity, whereas others are signs of complications of prematurity. The size and shape of the head must be evaluated, especially if the infant has a history of intraventricular or intracranial hemorrhage or hydrocephalus. An increase in head circumference of more than 2 cm per week should be cause for concern in these infants. In infants who have been treated neurosurgically for hydrocephalus, ventriculoperitoneal shunt and tubing may be palpated. Visual abnormalities such as strabismus must be carefully ruled out by examination as well as by history, because up to 20% of preterm infants may have an ophthalmologic problem (see Chapter 56, Strabismus). Oropharyngeal abnormalities such as a palatal groove, high arched palate, or abnormal tooth formation may occur as a result of prolonged endotracheal intubation. Discoloration of teeth may also result from exposure to high bilirubin levels. Baseline intercostal, substernal or subcostal retractions, wheezing, stridor and tachypnea in former premature babies with moderate-to-severe bronchopulmonary dysplasia (BPD) should be documented (see Chapter 118, Chronic Lung Disease).

Chest scars secondary to the placement of chest tubes should be noted. Adult female breasts may be affected if scarring occurs on or close to breast tissue. The umbilicus may appear hypoplastic as a result of umbilical catheter placement and suturing. Multiple scars on the heels from blood sampling or on the distal extremities from intravenous catheters and cutdowns may be evident.

The genitalia of both male and female preterm infants should be examined closely for inguinal hernias. The male scrotum should be examined for cryptorchidism. A careful evaluation for developmental dysplasia of the hip should be performed until children are ambulatory (see Chapter 79, Developmental Hip Dysplasia).

The most important part of the physical examination is probably the neuromuscular examination. Increased muscular tone, asymmetry, and decreased bulk should be noted along with the presence of any clonus or asymmetry of deep tendon reflexes. Inappropriate reflexes such as a persistent Moro or fisting beyond 4

Questions: Well Child Care for Preterm Infants

- How much did the infant weigh when discharged from the hospital?
- Is the infant breast-fed or bottle-fed? Is the infant on any special formula?
- How often and how much does the infant feed? How long do feedings take?
- Does the infant have any feeding problems (e.g., pain, vomiting, gastroesophageal reflux)?
- Does the infant take dietary supplementation of vitamins and minerals?
- Is the infant's development appropriate for the adjusted chronological age?
- What developmental milestones has the infant reached? Does the infant roll over? Smile? Sit up?
- Does the infant appear to hear and see?
- Who cares for the infant?
- Do the parents have any concerns regarding growth, development, or nutrition?
- Is the infant on an apnea monitor? Have there been any apneic episodes?

months of age should also be documented. Other abnormalities (e.g., scissoring or sustained clonus) in the neurologic examination may become more apparent as infants become older. The detection of subtle early findings is important, so appropriate intervention, such as physical therapy, can be instituted as soon as possible.

Laboratory Tests

In addition to the standard screening tests performed on all healthy infants and children during health maintenance visits, several laboratory studies are particularly important in preterm infants. Such tests include a CBC and reticulocyte count to check for anemia; electrolytes in infants with BPD on diuretics to detect hypokalemia or alkalosis; and serum calcium, phosphorus, and alkaline phosphatase levels in infants with documented rickets or an increased risk for rickets (birth weight <1000 g or prolonged history of total parenteral nutrition) to evaluate the need for specific vitamin and mineral replacement therapy. Therapeutic drug levels for commonly used medications such as phenobarbital, theophylline, or caffeine should also be measured if appropriate.

Results of screening tests for conditions such as phenylketonuria or hypothyroidism performed before discharge should also be reviewed and repeated as indicated. This applies to auditory evaluations and ophthalmologic examinations as well. EEGs and pneumograms should be reserved for preterm infants with a history of seizures or apnea and bradycardia of prematurity, respectively. Pulse oximetry is indicated for infants with severe BPD receiving supplemental oxygen who are going to be weaned gradually from therapy.

Imaging Studies

A head ultrasound should be repeated only if necessary. A baseline chest x-ray in infants with BPD is usually not warranted, because multiple films have already been taken in the NICU. A head CT scan may be considered in infants with a progressively abnormal neurologic examination and abnormal rate of head growth.

MANAGEMENT

Well child care in relatively healthy preterm infants has two components. One is the provision of routine health care maintenance for infants and appropriate developmental anticipatory guidance for parents, and the other involves the incorporation of treatment for chronic conditions into each visit. Health care maintenance should include nutrition counseling, developmental surveillance, immunizations, and assessment of vision and hearing, in addition to standard screening tests discussed above. Outside resources concerning developmental delay can be reviewed with parents (Table 20–1). Care related to chronic conditions includes adjusting medication doses such as diuretic therapy, weaning from supplemental oxygen, and discontinuing the apnea monitor.

TABLE 20–1. Physician Support and Education of Parents With Preterm Infants

Understand parental expectations
Legitimize parental fears
Be a source of support and encouragement
Provide consistent, honest information
Assume the role of the overall "coordinator of care"
Provide referrals to outside resources, including respite care

Nutrition

According to the Committee on Nutrition of the AAP, most healthy preterm infants require 110–130 kcal/kg/day to achieve adequate growth. Physicians must keep in mind, however, that caloric requirements vary with individual infants depending on associated chronic conditions such as BPD and malabsorption. In cases of inadequate weight gain, the number of calories in each feeding may be raised either by increasing the volume or concentrating the formula, thus raising its caloric density. The introduction of solid foods is appropriate once infants have developed acceptable oral motor skills for swallowing solids.

Preterm infants require vitamin and mineral supplements. Breast-fed preterm infants should receive multivitamins as well as iron. Although formulas for full-term infants supply most vitamins and minerals needed by preterm infants, daily multivitamins can also be given. Additional vitamin D, calcium, and phosphorus are necessary only in infants who have documented rickets or are at high risk (i.e., <1000 g birth weight) for the disease. Mature breast milk contains low levels of nutrients. A human milk fortifier alleviates the need for these supplements. Folate and vitamin E are usually no longer needed by the time infants weigh 2000–2500 g and are taking full feeds. Iron supplementation should be continued until infants are eating adequate iron-fortified solids. Daily fluoride should be prescribed at 6 months of age depending on the amount of fluoride contained in the drinking water and should be continued into adolescence.

Developmental Assessment

Both informal and formal developmental surveillance should include referral to an early intervention program, particularly in extremely low-birth-weight infants since routine screening tests are probably not sensitive enough to pick up subtle neurodevelopmental abnormalities (Table 20–2; see Chapter 14, Normal Development).

Immunizations

Routine immunization schedules recommended by the Committee on Immunization Practices of the AAP should be followed. The administration of any vaccine is determined by the chronologic or postnatal age, not the gestational age. Standard doses and intervals should also be used (see Chapter 17, Immunizations). Several studies have shown an adequate serologic response

TABLE 20–2. Guidelines for Developmental Surveillance

For pediatricians using developmental screening tests, the yielded score should be used to determine when to refer. For those who choose not to use standardized tests, the following guidelines are suggested. Be concerned if:

At 6 months adjusted age, the infant:
Is not sitting, even with support
Makes no effort to reach or bat at objects
Does not localize sound
Only momentarily grasps
Keeps hands fisted
Does not mouth objects

At 12 months adjusted age, the infant:
Is sitting but not crawling
Does not search for hidden objects
Does not vocalize consonant and vowel combinations
Does not attend to books
Does not respond to simple, familiar directions such as "pat-a-cake"

At 18 months adjusted age, the child:
Does not walk
Does not imitate sounds or motor actions
Cannot build a tower with blocks
Is most interested in putting toys in mouth at play
Knows fewer than eight words

At 24 months adjusted age, the child:
Does not put two words together in speech
Has play skills that remain primarily imitative
Has gross motor skills that are lacking in balance and control
Cannot complete a simple puzzle or shape sorter
Cannot identify basic body parts

At 36 months chronologic age, the child:
Does not follow simple commands, including "give me"
Does not use prepositions in speech
Cannot copy a circle
Has such poor articulation that it is impossble for others to understand
Does not jump with both feet off the ground

At 4 years, the child:
Still uses phrases instead of sentences
Does not know color names
Cannot give first and last name
Cannot pedal a tricycle

Modified and reproduced, with permission, from Bernbaum, J.C., and M. Hoffman-Williamson. Primary Care of the Preterm Infant. St. Louis, Mosby-Year Book, 1991, p. 71.

despite a history of prematurity. Absolute and relative contraindications to specific vaccine components or to live vaccines for preterm infants are identical to published guidelines for term infants and children. Physicians should note that in preterm infants greater than 6 months of age with chronic lung disease, administration of influenza vaccine is recommended during the winter.

Assessment of Vision and Hearing

Specialized follow-up visits for visual and auditory sequelae of prematurity must be arranged at the health maintenance visit. An initial ophthalmologic screening examination should have been performed between 5 and 7 weeks of age in infants less than 1500 g or less than 30 weeks' gestation, irrespective of oxygen exposure, and in infants between 1500 and 1800 g or between 30 and 35 weeks' gestation who have been exposed to oxygen. A repeat examination prior to discharge or 1 month later may also be required to detect the extent and progression of retinopathy of prematurity (ROP). Further follow-up is then dictated by the ophthalmolo-gist. Preterm infants are also at increased risk for the development of strabismus, myopia (independent of ROP), amblyopia and glaucoma.

A BAER or a behavioral audiogram should be performed by 3 months of age but no later than 6 months of age. Referral to an audiologist should be made if infants "fail" the initial screening or if parents or practitioners have any concerns.

Other Possible Problems

Preterm infants with chronic lung disease are at increased risk for respiratory illness, especially during the winter. Parents should be informed of this risk and counseled about symptoms such as tachypnea and wheezing associated with a simple URI. Practitioners should have a low threshold for considering a diagnosis of pneumonia in these infants in the appropriate clinical setting. Primary care providers should also keep in mind that preterm infants with BPD are at increased risk for SIDS.

Preterm survivors who were critically ill can be particularly at risk for developing the **vulnerable child syndrome,** because their parents often perceive them as fragile and vulnerable. Features of this syndrome include abnormal separation difficulties for both mother and child, sleep difficulties, parental overprotectiveness and overindulgence, lack of appropriate discipline, and excessive preoccupation with the infant's health. Serious behavioral problems may arise as a result of such parent-child interactions. Primary care providers must be cognizant of early signs of this syndrome and should try to prevent its occurrence by reassuring parents about the infant's well being. Every effort should be made to normalize the family's schedule once the infant is stable and to encourage parent-infant interactions unrelated to health care.

PROGNOSIS

No single risk factor successfully predicts the long-term prognosis for premature infants. Although some aspects of prognosis are indeed influenced by the complexity of the infant's hospital course, birth weight has been found to be one of the best predictors of mortality and morbidity. Large, comprehensive studies evaluating the morbidities associated with extremely low birth weight are only now being published, however. Thus most predictions made regarding the long-term outcome of premature infants, especially those who weigh less than 1000 grams, are incomplete. Research has shown that despite the decrease in respiratory distress syndrome in surfactant-treated infants, the incidence of other preterm complications such as intraventricular bleeds or ROP has not been reduced significantly. The implications of these findings on long-term development remain to be seen.

Prematurity does not seem to affect children's overall height significantly. Several studies have shown that preterm infants are smaller and thinner than their normal term peers in the first few years of life but often "catch up" by the time they reach middle childhood—about 7 or 8 years of age. Genetic factors continue to influence ultimate stature in these children.

Studies of developmental outcome are much more equivocal; the concept of "catch up" varies with each individual case. Vague definitions of developmental delay and what is appropriate for age make gathering data very difficult. In addition, reports about the incidence of moderate-to-severe disabilities are conflicting, especially in extremely low-birth-weight infants. Regardless, neurodevelopmental impairment is a concern for physicians who care for preterm infants.

Case Resolution

In the case presented at the beginning of the chapter, the infant's current feeding schedule should be continued because appropriate weight gain has occurred. Iron and multivitamin supplementation should be given. The apnea monitor can be discontinued after the infant reaches 40 weeks' gestation and has a normal pneumogram. The first set of immunizations should be administered at this visit, and any questions that the family has should be answered. A follow-up visit with the general pediatrician should be scheduled in 3–4 weeks. Vision, hearing, and formal developmental testing should be arranged in 1–2 months.

Selected Readings

American Academy of Pediatrics, Committee on Nutrition. Pediatric Nutrition Handbook. Evanston, IL, American Academy of Pediatrics, 1993.

Bernbaum, J. C., S. Friedman, and M. Hoffman-Williamson. Preterm infant care after hospital discharge. Pediatr. Rev. 10:195–206, 1989.

Bernbaum, J. C., and M. Hoffman-Williamson. Primary Care of the Preterm Infant. St. Louis, Mosby–Year Book, 1991.

Bernstein, S., et al. Approaching the management of the neonatal intensive care unit graduate through history and physical assessment. Pediatr. Clin. North Am. 45:79–105, 1998.

Bregman, J., and L. V. S. Kimberlin. Developmental outcome in extremely premature infants: Impact of surfactant. Pediatr. Clin. North Am. 40:937–953, 1993.

Gross, R. T. Day care for the child born prematurely. Pediatrics 91:189–192, 1993.

Hack, M., et al. School-age outcomes in children with birth weights under 750 g. N. Engl. J. Med. 331:753–759, 1994.

Hirata, T., and E. Bosque. When they grow up: The growth of extremely low birth weight (≤1000 gm) infants at adolescence. J. Pediatr. 132:1033–1035, 1998.

McCormick, M. C., et al. The health and developmental status of very low birth weight children at school age. J.A.M.A. 267:2204–2208, 1992.

O'Shea, M. T., et al. Survival and developmental disability in infants with birth weights of 501 to 800 grams, born between 1979 and 1994. Pediatrics 100:982–986, 1997.

Phelps, D. L. Retinopathy of prematurity. Pediatr. Rev. 16:50–56, 1995.

Piecuch, R. E., et al. Outcome of extremely low birth weight infants (500 to 999 grams) over a 12-year period. Pediatrics 100:633–639, 1997.

Siegel, M. D. Advances in neonatology: view from a practicing pediatrician. Pediatr. Clin. North Am. 40:1105–1114, 1993.

Toder, D. S., and J. T. McBride. Home care of children dependent on respiratory technology. Pediatr. Rev. 18:273–280, 1997.

CHAPTER 21

NEEDS OF CHILDREN WITH PHYSICAL AND SENSORY DISABILITIES

Monica Sifuentes, M.D.

Hx A 6-year-old physically disabled girl is brought to the office for a routine physical examination for school.

The girl was the full-term product of a normal pregnancy and delivery. The mother, who received regular prenatal care, was 25 years of age at the time. She used no illicit drugs, alcohol, or any other medications. At delivery, skin defects of the scalp, abdomen, and both knees were noted. The anterior fontanelle was enlarged. In addition, the infant had transverse, bilateral limb defects of both feet and fingers and short, dysplastic thumbs.

During the first year of life, the girl was admitted to the hospital several times for leakage of CSF from the calvarium defect. Although the skin defects have healed, a bony defect measuring 3 x 4 cm remains at the crown of the head.

The girl now attends special education classes and will be mainstreamed in the upcoming year. She uses prostheses for her legs and has undergone several procedures to give her better opposition in her primitive thumbs. She also wears a protective helmet at all times. Her growth and development are normal for age.

Questions

1. Why is early identification and intervention important for infants and children with disabilities?
2. What are the unique needs of infants and children with disabilities?
3. What role do primary care practitioners play in the care of children with disabilities?
4. What are the appropriate referrals and resources for families of children with disabilities?
5. What specific psychosocial issues should be addressed whenever children with disabilities visit their primary care practitioners?

Disabilities range from mild to moderate, depending on the nature and extent of the condition. For unprepared parents, however, the diagnosis of any disability can be overwhelming and disappointing. Early identification of a disabling condition by physicians leads to appropriate, definitive treatment for certain disabilities. Even when such treatment is not available, prompt identification improves children's long-term outcome and allows families to obtain appropriate resources for their children. Through early intervention, infants and children with irreversible conditions can be introduced to medical, educational, and psychosocial services available in the community. These services are crucial if children with disabilities are to reach their full potential.

EPIDEMIOLOGY

The prevalence of children in the United States with disabilities is difficult to assess. Recent studies report that approximately 17% of children under the age of 17 years have at least one disability, including deafness or trouble hearing, blindness, cerebral palsy, epilepsy, speech impediments, and other learning and behavioral problems. In addition, an estimated 30% of these children have more than one disability. A single sensory disability such as deafness affects approximately 3.5% of children, and blindness occurs in 1% of children.

The presence of any disabling condition has a profound impact on the health and education of affected children. Studies show that children with disabilities have 1.5 times more doctor visits and spend 3.5 more days in the hospital than children without these conditions. Children with disabilities miss twice the number of school days and are twice as likely to repeat a grade compared to children without disabilities.

In addition, numerous associated conditions occur more commonly in children with disabilities. These include mental retardation, growth failure, nutrition problems, and behavioral and emotional disorders. Problems with dentition, respiratory infections, and bowel and bladder continence may also develop.

CLINICAL PRESENTATION

Children with disabilities can present in a variety of ways depending on their age. They may be seen for a routine health maintenance visit, and delayed development is apparent on examination. Children can also present with specific complaints, such as poor vision or hearing, or with more general concerns, such as growth failure (Dx Box). Behavioral problems or difficulties in school may be the reason for the initial visit.

PATHOPHYSIOLOGY

Disabilities include a variety of childhood conditions that are manifested as physical, sensory, psychological, or cognitive impairments. They may be acquired or congenital and static or progressive. Etiologies are often multifactorial.

Cerebral palsy, for example, is a collection of non-progressive disorders resulting from a CNS insult early in brain development. It is characterized by abnormal motor movements and posturing and may be accompanied by other disabilities. Causes of cerebral palsy include prematurity (i.e., low birth weight), asphyxia, prenatal abnormalities (e.g., placental insufficiency), congenital infections (e.g., toxoplasmosis, CMV), and biochemical abnormalities (e.g., severe hyperbilirubinemia). Other rarer causes are environmental toxins (e.g., alcohol [maternal alcoholism]) and genetic disorders (e.g., inborn errors of metabolism). Severe postnatal injuries or infections can also lead to cerebral palsy; classic examples are shaken baby syndrome and meningitis. An estimated 25%–50% of cases of cerebral palsy have no discernible cause, however.

DIFFERENTIAL DIAGNOSIS

Multiple conditions can lead to physical or sensory disabilities, the most common being cerebral palsy. Other etiologies include prematurity complicated by intraventricular hemorrhage, exposure to ototoxic drugs such as aminoglycosides, refractory seizures, congenital infections such as toxoplasmosis, and endocrine disorders such as poorly treated congenital hypothyroidism.

EVALUATION

History

When initially evaluating children with newly diagnosed disabilities, practitioners should first assess any

---

D$_x$ Children With Physical and Sensory Disabilities*

- Growth failure
- Microcephaly
- Abnormal neurologic examination, including hypertonicity, spastic diplegia or quadriplegia, and brisk deep tendon reflexes
- Developmental delay
- Speech or hearing deficit
- Visual deficit

* May not be present in all children.

primary parental concerns. A complete medical history should then be obtained, including information about the pregnancy and birth. General screening questions about development are also important to ask (Questions Box) so that children's developmental progress can be assessed. Specific questioning is warranted if parents are concerned about delayed development or if any of their answers indicate that their children are not attaining age-appropriate developmental milestones.

In cases of children with known sensory or physical disabilities, families should be asked directly at each visit about daily activities. Because many children with disabilities are also on daily medication for either seizures or other chronic conditions, it is also important to ask about any potential side effects of drugs.

In addition, an overall assessment of family dynamics should be made. It is important to inquire about the relationships between children with disabilities and their siblings, as well as the impact of these children on the parents' marriage.

Physical Examination

In general, a complete physical examination, including a neurologic assessment, should be performed at each visit. The height, weight, and head circumference should be plotted on the growth chart and compared to previous measurements. A failure of adequate growth as measured by any of these parameters should be examined closely. For example, microcephaly, nutritional problems, and growth failure are not uncommon in children with cerebral palsy. Depending on the disability, the main part of the examination should then focus on physical findings associated with the particular condition. For children with physical disabilities such as

congenital or acquired amputations, for instance, assessment of the skin that comes in contact with prosthetic devices is a pertinent aspect of the physical examination. In children with sensory disabilities such as unilateral hearing loss, the evaluation of a middle ear effusion or infection in the unaffected ear should be a priority.

Overall, for most children with disabilities, the neurologic examination is extremely important. The following questions should be addressed: Are normal primitive reflexes such as the Moro and rooting reflexes present in neonates? Have all primitive reflexes been extinguished in older children? Do infants appear to visualize and track objects appropriately? Are there any abnormal movements of the trunk or extremities at rest? Is the muscle tone normal? Is any hyper- or hypotonicity evident? Is any asymmetry of the upper and lower extremities apparent? Are the deep tendon reflexes normal and symmetric? Is the gait appropriate for age?

Laboratory Tests

The laboratory evaluation of infants or children with physical or sensory disabilities depends on the specific condition. Not all patients need a costly array of diagnostic procedures. A ***chromosomal*** **karyotype** using peripheral blood is helpful in children with suspected genetic disorders (e.g., abnormal facies or a major anomaly and developmental delay). Routine testing for Fragile X syndrome in all mentally retarded boys remains controversial.

Metabolic screening for inborn errors should be performed on children with mental retardation and any of the following symptoms: intermittent vomiting or lethargy, loss of developmental milestones, or seizures. Such screening is not needed in the routine evaluation of children with developmental delay and no other symptoms.

A screening test for visual acuity (Snellen test) and hearing (audiogram) should be performed in all children suspected of having sensory deficits, even mild ones. For infants or toddlers, a BAER (brain stem auditory evoked response) or behavioral audiogram is a more appropriate screening test for hearing. A visual evoked response (VER) can be performed to test vision.

Psychometric testing may be helpful in certain school-age children to assess intellectual function.

Imaging Studies

An EEG is indicated in all patients who have a history of seizures or seizurelike episodes. Other brain imaging studies, such as CT or MRI scans of the head, can be performed when intrauterine infection, intraventricular hemorrhage, or genetic disorders with associated developmental delays are suspected. An EMG can be used to differentiate cerebral palsy from a congenital myopathy.

MANAGEMENT

Caring for children with a single disability or multiple disabilities can be both a rewarding and challenging task

---

Questions: Children With Physical and Sensory Disabilities

- Were there any perinatal complications, such as premature rupture of membranes or fetal distress?
- Was the infant born prematurely? If so, how long did the infant remain in the hospital and for what reasons?
- Was the infant exposed to any toxins in utero?
- Is there any history of infection during the perinatal period or infancy?
- What developmental milestones has the infant or child mastered?
- Is the child attending school or some type of early intervention program?
  - How does the child get there?
  - What does the child do upon returning from school?
- Who feeds and bathes the child?
- Can the older child use the toilet without assistance?
- How is the child sleeping? Does the child take naps at school and at home?
- Has respite care been arranged for the family?
- Does the caregiver appear overwhelmed or excessively tired, especially one who is caring for a child with multiple disabilities?
- Do other family members help care for the child?
- Is the extended family available to help with the siblings?
- Are there any other disabled people in the family?
- Does the family receive any financial assistance for care of the child?

for primary pediatricians. Although all cases should be handled individually, general guidelines have been developed for the provision of pediatric services for infants and children with special health care needs. They include recommendations for medical services, suggestions for parental involvement, assistance from community agencies, and fulfillment of specific federal requirements for educational opportunities for children with disabilities. Pediatricians who care for children with disabling conditions should be familiar with these principles of care, which are published by the American Academy of Pediatrics, and should incorporate them into the overall treatment plan.

General Considerations

The major role of primary pediatricians who care for children with disabilities is threefold: (1) to make therapeutic decisions for patients and families, (2) to serve as an advocate and overall coordinator of care, and (3) to inform families of available community resources. The most difficult part of providing care for children with disabilities is initially establishing the diagnosis. Whether the diagnosis is blatantly apparent or completely unsuspected, physicians are placed in the challenging position of breaking the news to families. Parents should be informed of the diagnosis as soon as possible, but care should be taken to refrain from discussing the prognosis, especially if it is still unknown. The cause of the disability and the possible complications of the condition should also be reviewed. *The primary goal is to help children with disabilities reach their full potential.*

Health care providers are in a unique position to establish a treatment plan with families that includes medical, psychosocial, and educational services. A multidisciplinary team that includes the pediatrician, a member of the school system, a social worker, and a representative of an early intervention program should be identified. Federally funded, nonprofit, regional centers can provide an organized treatment plan and entry into an early intervention program to some children with disabilities. To qualify, children must be diagnosed with certain disorders such as cerebral palsy, epilepsy, autism, or global developmental delay. In addition, infants considered "at risk" for developing disabilities qualify for assistance (e.g., premature infants with bronchopulmonary dysplasia and intraventricular hemorrhage). For children who do not qualify, similar services can be coordinated on an individual basis by the physician's office or the school district.

Children with severe physical and sensory disabilities are often cared for by many medical subspecialists in addition to primary care pediatricians. Pediatric orthopedic surgeons, plastic surgeons, geneticists, ophthalmologists, otolaryngologists, child neurologists, and psychologists or psychiatrists may be necessary. In addition, speech and language therapists, occupational therapists, and physical therapists are often an integral part of the medical team. Initial and ongoing therapeutic services provided by each of these individuals must be monitored periodically to assess the progress and overall effectiveness of the treatment plan. Ideally, services should be coordinated so that children as well as parents miss a minimum number of school and work days (e.g., Saturday and after-school appointments, visits to several providers on one day).

All information from diagnostic studies and initial evaluations should be shared among each of the health care providers to determine the eligibility of individual children for special services such as Supplemental Social Security (SSI). The case worker can then assist families to apply for the appropriate services.

Specific Medical Conditions

A number of medical conditions commonly occur in children with moderate to severe disabilities. While providing children with comprehensive well child care, general pediatricians can also address and treat these conditions.

Problems with adequate nutrition, which usually result from insufficient caloric intake, are manifested by growth failure. Depending on the degree of disability and amount of oropharyngeal dysfunction, the placement of a nasogastric or gastrostomy tube may be necessary. Caloric needs are 10–50% higher than normal basal needs to ensure growth.

Respiratory illness is not uncommon among these children. Close observation and conservative treatment of viral illnesses are often necessary. Aspiration pneumonia is likely to occur, especially in children with severe developmental delay, because of poor handling of oral secretions or severe malnutrition. To help minimize respiratory infections, influenza vaccine should also be administered during the winter months.

Maintaining good oral hygiene is another challenge, because some children with disabilities do not clear secretions well and retain food in their mouths, predisposing to cavity development. In addition, many children are treated with anticonvulsants and antibiotics that can cause gingival and enamel dysplasias. Abnormal oromotor coordination, tone, and posturing also contribute to the development of oropharyngeal deformities such as high, arched palate and overcrowded teeth. As with other children, fluoride supplementation and consistent preventive dental care are recommended.

Bowel and bladder continence is important to attain for several reasons. It allows children to function in a socially acceptable fashion, provides independence, and prevents the development of complications such as recurrent UTIs, diaper dermatitis, and decubitus ulcers. Behavior modification techniques coupled with positive reinforcement are associated with complete or partial success for bowel training.

Community Resources

Optimal care for children with developmental disabilities depends on maximum utilization of community agencies and resources. An assessment of parental and patient needs should first be performed and prioritized.

The appropriate resources should then be identified for individual children. Primary care physicians may need to help determine the appropriateness of specific services for patients and families. Emphasis should be placed on integrating each child into support services used by all patients and their families to avoid any feelings of isolation. Support groups for siblings as well as parents, respite care, and in-home health service programs should also be investigated. Physicians should act as liaisons between all agencies. Case conferences are occasionally necessary to review the progress of individual children with each member of the health care team.

Education

Every effort should be made to enroll children with disabilities in conventional schools and to provide opportunities for socialization at an early age. Although this may be difficult for families to accept initially, it is important to introduce the concept of structured independence and mainstreaming, the placement of disabled children in classes with nondisabled children.

Until mainstreaming is achieved, several different educational possibilities can be considered, and each case should be evaluated on an individual basis. Choices include special education classes in separate schools (full- or part-time), special education classes in regular schools (full- or part-time), or part-time special education classes and part-time regular classes. The decision can be facilitated through the development of an Individual Education Plan (IEP) by a multidisciplinary team at the school. Parents and primary physicians are encouraged to participate in this evaluation.

PROGNOSIS

The prognosis for children with physical and sensory disabilities depends on the underlying etiology, the severity and extent of the disability, and early participation in an intervention program that includes services such as physical and occupational therapy. The major-

ity of affected children are able to lead productive, independent lives when they receive adequate early intervention and education.

Case Resolution

Although the girl's medical condition appears stable, the physician should inquire about any ongoing problems or concerns. A complete examination should be performed; head growth, skin healing, and callus formation as a result of prosthetic devices should be assessed. Routine screening laboratory tests required for school entry should be obtained. Integration into the regular classroom should be addressed with both the child and the mother at this visit, and a follow-up phone call to the school should also be made.

Selected Readings

American Academy of Pediatrics, Committee on Children with Disabilities. Managed care and children with special health care needs: A subject review. Pediatrics 102:657–660, 1998.

American Academy of Pediatrics, Committee on Children with Disabilities. Pediatric services for infants and children with special health care needs. Pediatrics 92:163–165, 1993.

American Academy of Pediatrics, Committee on Children with Disabilities. Screening infants and young children for developmental disabilities. Pediatrics 93:863–865, 1994.

American Academy of Pediatrics, Committee on Children with Disabilities and Committee on Adolescence. Transition care provided for adolescents with special health care needs. Pediatrics 98:1203–1206, 1996.

Boyle, C. A., P. Decoufle, and M. Yeargin-Allsopp. Prevalence and impact of developmental disabilities in U.S. children. Pediatrics 93:399–403, 1994.

Eicher, P. S., and M. L. Batshaw. Cerebral palsy. Pediatr. Clin. North Am. 40:537–551, 1993.

Fewell, R. R. Child care for children with special needs. Pediatrics 91:193–198, 1993.

Liptak, G. S. The pediatrician's role in caring for the developmentally disabled child. Pediatr. Rev. 17:203–210, 1996.

McPherson M., et al. A new definition of children with special health care needs. Pediatrics 102:137–140, 1998.

Menacker, S. J. Visual function in children with developmental disabilities. Pediatr. Clin. North Am. 40:659–674, 1993.

Taft, L. T. Cerebral palsy. Pediatr. Rev. 16:411–418, 1995.

REPRODUCTIVE HEALTH*

Monica Sifuentes, M.D.

H$_x$ An 18-year-old female college student in good health comes in for a routine health care visit during her spring break. She is unaccompanied by her parents and has no complaints, stating that she just needs a checkup. She likes college, passed all of her fall and winter classes, and has some new friends. She denies tobacco use but says most of her friends smoke. She occasionally drinks alcohol and has tried marijuana once. Although she is not sexually active, she is interested in discussing oral contraception. Her last menstrual period (LMP), which occurred 2 weeks ago, was normal. She is taking no medications. Her physical examination is entirely normal.

Questions

1. What issues are important to discuss with adolescents at reproductive health maintenance examinations?
2. What are the indications for a complete pelvic examination?
3. Which patients should have Pap smears? How often should this procedure be performed?
4. What methods of contraception are most successful in adolescent patients? What factors regarding each method should be considered?
5. What are the legal issues involved in prescribing contraception to minors in the absence of parents?

Adolescent visits to primary care physicians are relatively few and infrequent by the time teenagers reach puberty. At most, healthy adolescent patients are seen once or twice during high school for preparticipation sports physicals. If adolescents are not athletic or if their schools do not require such assessments, these teenagers will probably never visit their health care providers again while in school. Therefore, it is extremely important to use any interactions with adolescents as opportunities for anticipatory guidance and health education, particularly reproductive health education.

Reproductive health can be defined as sexuality-related services, screening, and counseling. Such services should be included as a part of the routine health maintenance examination of both male and female adolescents, for several reasons. The current rise of sexually transmitted disease (STDs) in teenagers, the risk of AIDS, and the reality of unplanned pregnancy make reproductive health issues increasingly important. In addition, adolescents rarely schedule appointments with health care providers prior to the initiation of coitus. Experimentation with drugs and alcohol also contributes to early, unplanned sexual experiences (Box 22–1).

Aside from issues of sexual activity, adolescents may also have questions about their progression through puberty. Normal variants in body habitus or certain physical characteristics can be a source of unnecessary anxiety for uninformed teenagers. Health education to alleviate these fears is ideal. Adolescents who come for physical examinations should be allotted extra time so that topics such as puberty, abstinence, sexual activity, STDs, and contraception can be discussed. In addition, during more acute, problem-oriented visits, adolescents should be encouraged to voice any other problems or concerns they may have. Depending on the nature of these issues, follow-up appointments can be scheduled.

NORMAL PHYSICAL DEVELOPMENT

Puberty begins during early adolescence with the development of secondary sexual characteristics. A sexual maturity rating scale or Tanner staging is used to describe breast and pubic hair development in females and genital development and pubic hair growth in males (Fig. 22–1, 22–2, and 22–3). The average age of menarche in the United States is 12.5 years and menarche usually occurs between Tanner stages 4 and 5. On average, male ejaculation or "wet dreams" occur at 13 years of age; they are unrelated to pubic hair development. Full fertility is achieved by age 15 years, or midadolescence, in most boys and girls.

EVALUATION

History

The history obtained at a reproductive health visit should include two parts: the medical history, which focuses primarily on the gynecologic history in females, and the psychosocial interview. Regardless of the type of visit scheduled, practitioners should take a few moments at the beginning of the interview to address routine health maintenance issues with adolescents (Questions Box: Reproductive Health). Physicians should find out whether female adolescents have ever

---

*This chapter is largely devoted to a discussion of the reproductive health of adolescent females. However, "Evaluation" is divided into two sections—one for females and one for males. The reader is referred to Chapter 76, Sexually Transmitted Diseases, for more information regarding male reproductive health.

BOX 22–1. Reproductive Health: Sexual Activity

Statistics regarding sexual activity among adolescents in the United States are startling. One in four females and one in three males have had sexual intercourse by 15 years of age. Among adolescents from 15–19 years of age, more than half are sexually active, and only one-third of these teenagers use contraception. As a result, nearly one million adolescent females under 20 years of age, or one out of every ten, become pregnant each year. A large majority of these pregnancies are unintended and occur premaritally, especially among certain racial and ethnic minority groups. The outcome of these pregnancies in 15–19-year-olds varies. An estimated 40–50% of these pregnancies result in live births, 30–40% end in abortion, and 10% are miscarried or stillborn.

Unprotected sexual activity among adolescents has several adverse health consequences, the most obvious being teenage pregnancy. Of the adolescents who continue their pregnancies, prematurity (< 37 weeks' gestation) and low birth weight < 2500 g) are two of the most frequently reported neonatal complications. Long-term maternal psychosocial sequelae of adolescent pregnancy include undereducation/school failure, limited vocational training and skills, economic dependency on public assistance, subsequent unwanted births, social isolation, depression, and high rates of separation and divorce among teenaged couples.

In addition to unintended pregnancy, the risk of contracting an STD such as chlamydia, human papillomavirus (HPV), herpes, and HIV is increased. In cases of pelvic inflammatory disease (PID) from either gonorrhea or chlamydia, future problems with fertility and an increased risk of ectopic pregnancy may occur. HPV, which has been associated with the development of cervical cancer, has a prevalence of up to 40% in adolescents. Other STDs are also on the rise. More alarming, however, is the relationship between acquired immunodeficiency syndrome in young adults aged 20–29 and probable exposure to HIV during adolescence.

Many factors have been associated with the initiation of early coitus in adolescents. They include male gender; race/ethnicity; poverty; a large, single-parent family; previous teen pregnancy in the household (either mother or sibling); poor academic achievement; discrepancy between the onset of physical puberty and cognitive development; peer group encouragement; and problem behaviors such as drug use. In addition, religious affiliation and cultural norms probably influence this decision. The role of hormonal changes during puberty and their influence on behavior has yet to be determined.

An estimated 6% of adolescents have limited normal functioning because of a chronic illness. However, a majority of these adolescents experience normal pubertal development and fertility because of advances in medical treatment for conditions such as diabetes and sickle cell disease. Like their healthy peers, many of these adolescents begin sexual intercourse at an early age. Pregnancy and childbirth can exacerbate some illnesses and increase risks significantly for both adolescents and fetuses. The genetic implications and specific patterns of inheritance of certain chronic conditions must also be considered. For this reason, attention to sexual issues is essential for adolescents with chronic medical illness.

had a pelvic examination. The gynecologic history should also be reviewed with these patients.

In addition, current methods of contraceptive use, if any, should be reviewed (Questions Box: Contraceptive Use). If adolescent females take oral contraceptives, a review of the more emergent danger signs of birth control pills is warranted, especially at an initial visit. **ACHES** (**a**bdominal pain, **c**hest pain, **h**eadaches, **e**ye problems, **s**evere leg pain) is a useful acronym (Table 22–1).

The rest of the psychosocial history, otherwise known as the **HEADSSS** interview (**h**ome, **e**mployment and education, **a**ctivities, **d**rugs, **s**exual activity/sexuality, **s**uicide and depression, **s**afety), should be completed whether or not adolescents are currently sexually active (see Chapter 4, Talking to Adolescents). Risk factors for

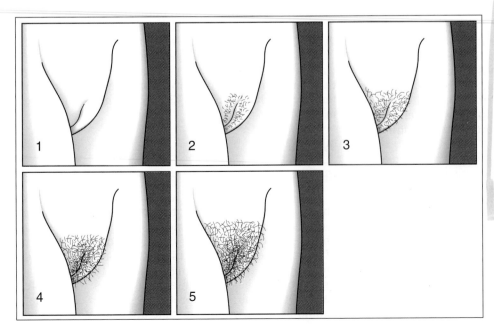

FIGURE 22–1. Female pubic hair development. Sex maturity rating 1: prepubertal, no pubic hair; sex maturity rating 2: straight hair is extending along the labia and between ratings 2 and 3, begins on the symphysis pubis; sex maturity rating 3: pubic hair is increased in quantity, is darker, coarser and curlier, and is present in the typical female triangle; sex maturity rating 4: pubic hair is more dense, curled, and adult in distribution but is less abundant; sex maturity rating 5: abundant, adult-type pattern; hair may extend on the medial aspect of the thighs.

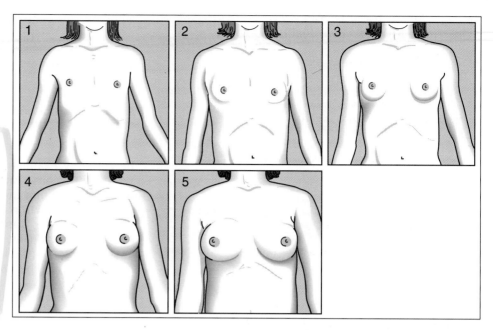

FIGURE 22–2. Female breast development. Sex maturity rating 1: prepubertal, elevations of papilla only; sex maturity rating 2: breast buds appear, areola is slightly widened and projects as small mound; sex maturity rating 3: enlargement of the entire breast with no protrusion of the papilla or of the nipple; sex maturity rating 4: enlargement of the breast and projection of areola and papilla as a secondary mound; sex maturity rating 5: adult configuration of the breast with protrusion of the nipple, areola no longer projects separately from remainder of breast.

teenage pregnancy or multiple exposures to STDs should be kept in mind when formulating health care plans with adolescents.

Physical Examination

A complete physical examination should be performed on all adolescents, with particular attention paid to their Tanner stage, also termed Sexual Maturity Rating (SMR).

Males

The genitalia should be examined closely for penile and testicular size, distribution of pubic hair, and pres-

ence of any ulcerative, vesicular, or wartlike lesions. Any urethral erythema or discharge should also be noted. Clinicians can use this opportunity to teach male adolescents how to perform a testicular self-examination.

Females

Prior to performing the physical examination, the physician should determine whether a full speculum examination is indicated (Table 22–2). Each decision should be made on an individual basis. Proper preparation of adolescents is imperative. This should include an explanation of the procedure and the physical sensations felt while the Pap smear and cervical cultures are being obtained, choice of who should be

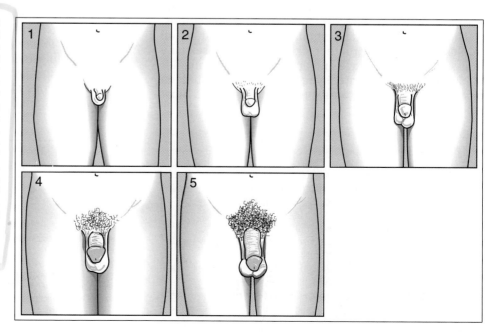

FIGURE 22–3. Male genital and pubic hair development. Sex maturity rating 1: prepubertal, no pubic hair, genitalia unchanged from early childhood; sex maturity rating 2: light, downy hair develops laterally and later becomes dark, penis and testes may be slightly larger, scrotum becomes more textured; sex maturity rating 3: pubic hair is extended across pubis, testes and scrotum are further enlarged, penis is larger, especially in length; sex maturity rating 4: more abundant pubic hair with curling, genitalia resemble those of an adult, glans has become darker; sex maturity rating 5: adult quantity and pattern of pubic hair, with hair present along the inner borders of the thighs. The testes and scrotum are adult in size.

Questions: Reproductive Health

For males and females:

- How is the adolescent feeling overall?
- Has the adolescent had any recent illnesses or conditions that the health care provider should know about?
- When was the last physical examination performed?
- Is the adolescent sexually active?
  - If so, when was the last episode of sexual intercourse?
  - Was the last episode of sexual intercourse protected or unprotected intercourse?
  - How old was the adolescent when he or she initiated coitus? Was it consensual?
  - How many sexual partners does the patient have? What gender are they (all contacts may not be heterosexual)?
- Is there any history of physical or sexual abuse?
- Has the adolescent or any of his or her partners ever been treated for an STD or tested for HIV?

For females only:

- What was the age at menarche?
- What was the date of the LMP and the duration and amount of flow?
- Are any symptoms such as cramping, bloating, or vomiting associated with menses?
  - Are any of these symptoms incapacitating? Do they cause the adolescent to miss school or work?
  - Do the mother or siblings have similar problems? If so, what do they do to manage them, if anything?

---

present during the examination (e.g., parent or friend who may have accompanied the patient), and a discussion of the desired positioning (i.e., supine versus semisitting). In addition, speculums and other equipment should be shown to adolescents. The goal is to minimize the adolescent's fears, anxieties, misconceptions, and discomfort regarding the examination.

A breast examination should be performed on female adolescents, and any breast tenderness, nodularity, or masses should be noted. Again, this portion of the examination can be used to educate patients about the purpose and importance of breast self-examinations.

The external genitalia should be examined in all adolescent females whether or not they are sexually active. The Tanner stage and any congenital anomalies such as an imperforate hymen should be noted. In sexually active adolescents, the external genitalia must

Questions: Contraceptive Use

- What percentage of the time are condoms used?
- Is any other method, such as spermicidal foam or jelly, also used?
- Is the adolescent female currently using oral contraceptives?
  - If so, what particular type is she taking, and how long has she been using this method of contraception?
  - How often does she forget to take the pill? *or* What does she do when she forgets to take the pill?
  - Does she experience common minor side effects such as breakthrough bleeding, nausea, weight gain, or acne?
  - Is the adolescent female using a long-acting progestin, such as Depo-Provera? If so, has she experienced irregular bleeding, weight gain, hair loss, headache, or acne?

TABLE 22–1.   Danger Signs Associated With Oral Contraceptive Use

A	Abdominal pain (severe)
C	Chest pain (severe), shortness of breath
H	Headaches
E	Eye problems (visual loss or blur)
S	Severe leg pain (calf/thigh)

---

be carefully examined for venereal warts, ulcers, and vesicular lesions. Any urethral erythema, edema, or discharge that may indicate an otherwise asymptomatic chlamydial infection should be noted. A vaginal discharge may be appreciated prior to inserting the speculum, but ideally, the cervix should be examined for cervical ectopy, friability, and any lesions or discharge from the os. The vaginal mucosa should also be inspected as the speculum is withdrawn.

During the bimanual examination, the cervix should be palpated for any cervical motion tenderness. Uterine size and position should be appreciated, and adnexal tenderness or masses should be noted. Because normal ovaries are approximately the size of almonds, they are often not palpated by the inexperienced clinician. A rectovaginal examination is necessary to rule out fistulas, especially in postpartum adolescents. If the practitioner is unable to perform a vaginal bimanual examination, a rectoabdominal examination can be done to assess uterine size and position and the presence of adnexal masses.

Laboratory Tests

A gonorrhea culture and a chlamydia rapid assay should be obtained in sexually active adolescents who have had unprotected intercourse or vaginal discharge or who have cervical friability noted on speculum examination. A saline and KOH wet mount should also be collected in symptomatic patients. A Pap smear should be performed in females who are sexually active or who have external genital warts, persistent vaginal discharge, or *in utero* exposure to DES. The Pap smear can also help detect *Trichomonas vaginalis* or the cytologic changes associated with human papillomavirus (HPV). Herpes simplex cultures should be done if painful vesicles are noted on examination.

TABLE 22–2.   Indications for a Complete Pelvic Examination

Contraceptive management
Pregnancy
Request by adolescent
Sexual activity
Partner with sexually transmitted disease (STD)
Previous history of STD
History of hepatitis B
Unexplained lower abdominal pain
Abnormal vaginal discharge
Unexplained vaginal bleeding
External venereal warts
Urinary symptoms

Other laboratory tests include an RPR test for syphilis and an HIV test (after appropriate pretest counseling). Baseline CBC, liver function tests, cholesterol, and fasting glucose may be indicated before starting oral contraceptives but are not mandatory. A pregnancy test is warranted only in sexually active females if the practitioner chooses to begin oral contraceptives midcycle.

MANAGEMENT

Reproductive Health Education

All management plans during reproductive health visits should include a frank **discussion of puberty, sexuality, and STDs** regardless of sexual activity. The adolescent should be counseled about abstinence as an acceptable choice. Ideally, preventive health care measures such as **breast and testicular self-examinations** have been reviewed during the physical examination. It is hoped that by encouraging adolescents' familiarity with these self-examinations, they will continue to perform them throughout their adult lives. The use of posters, plastic models, and written materials to support the discussion is greatly encouraged. The goal of education should be to assist adolescents in identifying and communicating their thoughts and feelings about sexual abstinence as well as sexual activity and to aid in the prevention of unintended pregnancies, parenthood, and STDs. Prevention programs offered by schools must be supplemented by open parental communication in the home about sexuality.

Legal Issues

The issue of **confidentiality** is important to consider when providing reproductive health care for adolescents. Parental involvement should be strongly encouraged, but health care practitioners are not required to disclose any information to parents except in cases of suicide or harmful intent to others. Contraceptive services can be provided to adolescents of any age without parental knowledge or consent. The complex issue of abortion varies from state to state.

Papanicolaou Smear

A Pap smear should be performed annually in all sexually active adolescent females. Although this is a conservative recommendation, it seems justified given adolescents' high rate of exposure to HPV and the association of certain types of HPV with the progression of cervical dysplasia. The general recommendation of the American Cancer Society and the American College of Obstetricians and Gynecologists is an annual Pap smear with the onset of sexual activity or at the age of 18 years (whichever comes first) until three or more consecutive smears are documented as normal. The Pap smear should be performed at least every 2–3 years thereafter. Because of the increased rate of abnormal cervical cytology in recent years in younger women, there may be a need for more frequent examinations.

Management following an abnormal Pap smear depends on the presence of atypia versus low-grade or high-grade squamous intraepithelial lesions. Further evaluation with colposcopy and cervical biopsy may be warranted. This decision should be made in consultation with the cytopathologist who reviewed the specimen and a gynecologist familiar with the management of cervical dysplasia in young women.

Contraceptive Methods

The appropriate method of contraception should be individualized. Barrier methods include condoms (male and female), diaphragms, and cervical caps. Vaginal spermicides such as nonoxynol 9 are available in a variety of forms (foams, gels, creams, and suppositories) and can be used alone or can provide extra protection if used with a barrier method. Hormonal methods include oral contraceptives and long-acting progestin agents. Intrauterine devices are not used in teenagers because of the prevalence of STDs and risk of pelvic inflammatory disease (PID). The withdrawal method, or coitus interruptus, and natural family planning are ineffective methods for adolescents for protection against pregnancy.

Hormonal Contraception

Combined low-dose oral contraceptives are an effective means of birth control for adolescents. Monophasic pills contain a fixed dose of estrogen and progestin throughout the 21-day pill cycle. Biphasic preparations contain a lower dose of the progestin component during the first 10 days of the cycle. In the newest type of oral contraceptive, triphasic pills, the doses of both estrogen and progestin or the progestin component alone is varied. This contraceptive was created to decrease the overall progestin-related side effects such as hypertension, acne, and lipid abnormalities. Clear benefits associated with oral contraceptive use include prevention of pregnancy, protection against ovarian and endometrial cancers, decreased risk of functional ovarian cysts, and decreased menstrual symptoms such as dysmenorrhea. The potential risks, which include thromboembolic phenomena, hypertension, and changes in the lipid profile, are minimal compared to the morbidity and mortality associated with teenage pregnancy and childbirth.

The long-acting progestins, medroxyprogesterone acetate (Depo-Provera) and levonorgestrel (Norplant), have been approved for use in the United States. Depo-Provera, which is given intramuscularly every 3 months, inhibits ovulation for at least 14 weeks. Norplant provides continuous contraception for 5 years via six subdermal plastic rods inserted through a small incision in the upper, inner arm. Common side effects are irregular bleeding, especially in the first few months, and eventual amenorrhea with prolonged use of either method.

Emergency Postcoital Contraception

Postcoital contraception, or the "morning-after pill," can be an effective way to prevent unintended pregnancy in adolescents. It requires, however, that the physician educate teens about its availability and usage

82and

that teens feel comfortable contacting their health care provider within 72 hours of unprotected intercourse. Although not meant to be used repeatedly as the sole method of contraception, emergency contraception is useful for the "unplanned" sexual encounter, which is often the case with adolescents. The "morning-after pill" contains a high dose of hormone that is thought to alter the endometrium, making it unsuitable for implantation. It may also interfere with fertilization itself.

The most common regimen is a combination of estrogen and progestin. The recommended dose is 100 µg ethinyl estradiol and 1.0 mg norgestrel taken initially, then repeated 12 hours later. This can be provided by prescribing 2 tablets of Ovral or 4 tablets of Lo/Ovral, (120 µg ethinyl estradiol/1.2 mg norgestrel) per dose. The most common side effect is nausea and vomiting, which occurs in about 25%–30% of patients. If this occurs after the first dose, an antiemetic can be taken 30 minutes before the second dose. Other side effects include transient headache, dizziness, and breast tenderness, which usually resolve within 24 hours. Emergency contraception does not produce withdrawal bleeding and usually does not alter the timing of the next menses.

The patient should be given a follow-up appointment 3 weeks after using emergency contraception for a pregnancy test to identify any treatment failures and to discuss the importance of ongoing contraception.

Nonhormonal Contraception

Numerous studies and clinical experience have shown that nonhormonal methods are less effective in adolescents. However, condoms in conjunction with a spermicide have become crucial as a method of contraception since the emergence of AIDS. They help prevent transmission of other STDs as well as HIV. A few moments, therefore, should be taken during the visit to explain and demonstrate proper use of condoms. Risks of condom use are minimal, except for allergic reactions to the spermicide, latex, or lubricants. The female condom, the most recent development in barrier contraception, has been heralded as a possible answer to teenage pregnancy and STDs because it is controlled by the female partner. Other nonhormonal methods should be reviewed with adolescents as needed.

Sexually Transmitted Diseases

All STDs should be treated according to specific guidelines published by the Centers for Disease Control and Prevention (CDC) based on current epidemiology. Readers should see Chapter 76, Sexually Transmitted Diseases, for details regarding the diagnosis and management of STDs in adolescents.

Case Resolution

In the case scenario presented at the beginning of the chapter, a more detailed history should be obtained regarding the adolescent's menstrual history and daily activities (e.g., Who does she spend most of her time with?, What does she do in her spare time?). In addition, the indications for a pelvic examination should be reviewed. If they do not apply, the pelvic examination can be deferred until the next visit or until she becomes sexually active. A discussion should then follow regarding both barrier and hormonal methods of contraception and their role in the prevention of pregnancy and STDs.

Selected Readings

Beach, B. K. Contraception for adolescents: Part 2. Adol. Health Update 7:1–8, 1995.

Blum, R. W. Sexual health contraceptive needs of adolescents with chronic conditions. Arch. Pediatr. Adolesc. Med. 151:290–297, 1997.

Brown, R. T., and B. A. Cromer. The pediatrician and the sexually active adolescent. Pediatr. Clin. North Am. 44:1379–1390, 1997.

Centers for Disease Control and Prevention. Trends in sexual risk behaviors among high school students—United States, 1991–1997. M.M.W.R. 47:749–752, 1998.

Centers for Disease Control and Prevention. Youth risk behavior surveillance—United States, 1997. M.M.W.R. 47:1–89, 1998.

Gold, M. A., A. Schein, and S. M. Coupey. Emergency contraception: A national survey of adolescent health experts. Fam. Plann. Perspect. 29:15–19, 1997.

McAnarney, E. R., and W. R. Handee. Adolescent pregnancy and its consequences. J.A.M.A. 262:74–77, 1989.

Nelson, A. L. Adolescent contraception. West. J. Med. 165:374–376, 1996.

Rauh, J. L. The pediatrician's role in assisting teenagers to avoid the consequences of adolescent pregnancy. Pediatr. Ann. 22:90–98, 1993.

Rosenfeld, W. D., and J. B. Swedler. Role of hormonal contraceptives in prevention of pregnancy and sexually transmitted diseases. Adol. Med. State Art Rev. 3:207–222, 1992.

Sikand, A., and M. Fisher. The role of barrier contraceptives in prevention of pregnancy and disease in adolescents. Adol. Med. State Art Rev. 3:223–240, 1992.

Stevens-Simon, C. Providing effective reproductive health care and prescribing contraceptives for adolescents. Pediatr. Rev. 19:409–417, 1998.

Task Force on Pediatric AIDS. Adolescent and human immunodeficiency virus infection. The role of the pediatrician in prevention and intervention. Pediatrics 92:626–629, 1993.

INJURY PREVENTION

Iris Wagman Borowsky, M.D., Ph.D.

H$_x$ A 3-year-old girl was brought to the emergency department with a BB in her right eye. The girl's 10-year-old brother inadvertently fired his BB gun, and a BB lodged in her right eye. The BB was surgically removed, but as a result of the injury, the girl is legally blind in that eye.

Questions

1. How extensive is the injury problem in children?
2. What are the different methods for injury prevention? How could this particular injury have been prevented?
3. What injury prevention program has been developed by the AAP?
4. What are some general guidelines for effective injury prevention counseling?

Traditionally, unintentional injuries have been called accidents. The problem with the term "accident," however, is that it implies unpredictability, carrying with it connotations of chance, fate, and unexpectedness. The perception that injuries are random, chance occurrences that cannot be predicted or prevented has been a major barrier to progress in injury prevention and the study and control of injury as a scientific discipline. According to the modern view of injury, "accidents" must be anticipated in order to be prevented. Specialists in injury prevention have tried to replace the word "accident" with "injury" and have developed the idea of "reducing injury risk." Thus, injuries are not random events at all; rather, they occur in predictable patterns determined by identifiable risk factors. For example, if a 10-year-old boy plays unsupervised with a "toy" BB gun, which is capable of expelling projectiles at velocities much greater than those required to penetrate the eye, the resulting injury can hardly be called an accident. On the contrary, the injury is entirely predictable.

EPIDEMIOLOGY

Injuries are the leading health problem among children and adolescents in the United States. Over 20,000 children and adolescents under the age of 20 die from injuries each year. Injuries are the leading cause of death in individuals from the ages of 1–34 years. The leading cause of injury deaths is motor vehicle crashes. Intentional injuries, homicide and suicide, rank second and third, respectively, as causes of injury deaths in young people aged 10–34. After motor vehicle crashes, drowning and burns are the leading causes of unintentional injury deaths in children. Falls, poisoning, aspiration, suffocation, and firearms account for most of the remaining unintentional injury deaths in children.

Several epidemiologic factors are associated with higher death rates from unintentional injuries. These include male sex, low income, family stressors (e.g., death in the family, new residence, birth of a sibling), and residence in a rural area or a southern or mountain state. Injuries vary by race; Native Americans have the highest death rate from unintentional injuries and Asian Americans the lowest. The incidence of injuries varies seasonally, with July being the peak month.

Deaths from injury are only part of the problem. For every injury-related death, many more children are admitted to hospitals for the treatment of injury; for every injured child admitted, many more are treated in emergency departments. Injury is a major cause of permanent disability and is associated with much unmeasurable grief and suffering. Overall, one of every five children in the United States receives medical attention for an injury each year.

STRATEGIES FOR INJURY PREVENTION

During this century, efforts to prevent injuries have shifted from changing the behavior of individuals to modifying the environments in which injuries occur. William Haddon, a medical epidemiologist, devised two useful frameworks for developing injury prevention strategies.

Haddon Matrix

This matrix relates three factors (host, vector, and environment) to the three phases of an injury-producing event (preevent, event, and postevent). The host, vector, and environment are viewed as elements that interact over time to produce injury. Table 23–1 shows a Haddon matrix of motor vehicle crash injuries. The precrash phase describes elements that determine whether a crash will occur; the crash phase, the variables that influence the nature and severity of the resultant injury; and the postcrash phase, the factors that determine the degree to which the injury is limited and repaired after the crash occurs. By describing the "anatomy" of an injury, the Haddon matrix illustrates the numerous characteristics that determine an injury and the many corresponding strategies for interfering with the production of an injury.

Haddon also developed a list of **10 countermeasures to prevent injuries** or reduce the severity of their effects. These 10 general strategies are:

TABLE 23–1. The Haddon Matrix

Phase	Host (human)	Vector (vehicle)	Environment
Precrash	Driver vision Alcohol consumption	Brakes Tires Speed	Speed limit Road curvature Road signs
Crash	Use of safety belts Osteoporosis	Vehicle size	Median barriers Laws about use of safety belts
Postcrash	Age Physical condition	Fuel system integrity	EMS personnel training

Adapted and reproduced, with permission, from Haddon, W. Advances in the epidemiology of injuries as a basis for public policy. Public Health Rep. 95:411–421, 1980. Originally adapted from Baker, O'Neill, and Karpf. The Injury Fact Book. Lexington, MA, 1989, and Haddon, W. Options for the prevention of motor vehicle crash injury. Isr. J. Med. 16:45–68, 1980.

Abbreviations: EMS, emergency medical service.

1. Prevent creation of the hazard (e.g., stop producing poisons, toys with small parts, and nonpowder firearms; do not participate in dangerous sports).

2. Reduce the amount of the hazard (e.g., package drugs in smaller, nonlethal amounts; reduce speed limits).

3. Prevent the release of the hazard (e.g., use child-resistant caps for medications, toilet locks, and safety latches on cabinets and drawers).

4. Modify the rate or spatial distribution of release of the hazard (e.g., require air bags in cars, use child safety seats and seat belts, make poisons taste bad).

5. Separate people from the hazard in space or time (e.g., make sidewalks for pedestrians, bikeways for bicyclists, and recreation areas separated from vehicles).

6. Separate people from hazards with material barriers (e.g., use bicycle helmets and protective equipment for athletes; install fences around swimming pools; build window guards).

7. Modify relevant basic qualities of the hazard (e.g., place padded carpets under cribs, require guns to have safety locks).

8. Increase resistance to damage from the hazard (e.g., train and condition athletes, make structures more earthquake-proof, use flame-retardant sleepwear).

9. Limit the damage that has already begun (e.g., use syrup of ipecac or fire extinguisher; begin cardiopulmonary resuscitation).

10. Stabilize, repair, and rehabilitate injured individuals (e.g., develop pediatric trauma centers and physical rehabilitation programs).

Haddon's work served as a practical guide for thinking about ways to prevent injury. It emphasized the importance of considering injuries as a result of a sequence of events, with many opportunities for prevention. The shift of emphasis away from changing human behavior to prevent injury is particularly appropriate with regard to injuries in children, since inhibiting children's curiosity is impractical as well as undesirable.

Passive and Active Interventions

Interventions to prevent injuries can also be categorized as passive or active. **Passive or automatic strate-** gies protect whenever they are needed **without the action of parents or children.** An example is the automobile air bag. In a crash, the air bag automatically inflates to cushion the occupants. Other examples of strategies that work automatically are lowered water heater temperatures, not having guns in the home, and energy-absorbing surfaces under playground equipment. In contrast, **active interventions require action to become effective.** For example, nonautomatic safety belts are active strategies; every time protection is needed, individuals must "buckle up." Watching children continuously is another example of an injury prevention strategy that requires constant activity.

Some strategies are partially automatic, requiring some action by individuals. Smoke detectors are one example. Functional smoke detectors can be very effective in preventing injury and death in house fires. Roughly one-third of smoke detectors, however, do not have working batteries. Batteries should be changed once a year, and, ideally, tested once a month. As might be expected, the greater the effort required for children to be protected, the smaller the chance that protection occurs. Therefore, whenever possible, passive measures are preferable because they are the most effective.

Several approaches have been used successfully to prevent childhood injuries, including education, legislation, enforcement, and engineering. Often these approaches can be effectively combined, as with child safety seats. Between 1977 and 1985 every state in the United States passed child restraint laws to protect infants and children by requiring that they be in an approved safety seat when riding in a motor vehicle. The car seat, an engineering intervention, is extremely effective when used correctly. Unfortunately, studies indicate that between one-third and two-thirds of car seats are used incorrectly. Education, an important factor in the passage of the child restraint laws, as well as strict enforcement of child safety seat laws, is essential to compliance. Parents must be urged to obtain and use the seats properly. Multifaceted efforts must continue because problems still exist. For example, there are illogical loop-holes in the laws, including exemptions when feeding, changing, or rocking a child to sleep; when an automobile has an out-of-state registration; or when an automobile is driven by someone other than a parent or legal guardian. Such exemptions reinforce parental misconceptions, particularly that the lap of an occupant (the "child crusher" position) is a safe position.

COUNSELING BY PEDIATRICIANS

Although the existence of significant gaps in parental knowledge about injury prevention has been clearly established, studies have shown that pediatricians spend surprisingly little time counseling parents about childhood safety. One study found that physicians spent an average of 12.4 seconds counseling parents of 6–11-month-old infants about injury prevention; the time was even less for children in other age groups. Some of the reasons for this limited discussion of safety issues may include lack of emphasis on preventive medical care in medical schools and pediatric training programs, as well as absence of solid evidence showing that anticipatory guidance works. Recent research, however, suggests that educational efforts by pediatricians can make a difference in preventing injuries, particularly if they are combined with other prevention strategies. Parents report that they would listen to physicians much more than any other group regarding child safety.

The injury prevention program (TIPP) developed by the AAP is widely used for office safety counseling. The aim of TIPP is to firmly establish injury prevention as a standard of care for pediatricians. The AAP suggests that pediatric providers focus their safety counseling on a few topics; other topics should be discussed depending on the injury risk factors that apply to each child (e.g., age, sex, location, season of the year, socioeconomic status of family). In its 1994 policy statement on injury prevention, the AAP recommends that pediatricians advise parents of all infants and preschool children about (1) traffic safety (e.g., car seats for child, seat belts for parents), (2) burn prevention (e.g., smoke detectors, safe hot water temperatures), (3) fall prevention (e.g., window and stairway guards/gates, avoiding use of infant walkers), and (4) poison prevention (e.g., use of syrup of ipecac). For all elementary school-age children, the AAP recommends that pediatric practitioners advise all patients and their parents about (1) traffic safety (e.g., seat belts, bicycle helmets, pedestrian safety), (2) water safety (swimming or boating), (3) sports safety (e.g., safety equipment, physical condition), and (4) firearm safety. Specific areas of injury prevention guidance recommended for adolescents include (1) traffic safety (e.g., seat belts, alcohol use, motorcycle and bicycle helmets, (2) water safety (e.g., alcohol use and diving injuries), (3) sports safety, and (4) firearm safety.

Injury prevention has been likened to immunizations. Because all children are at risk for injury, they all need a standard package of injury prevention counseling, just as all children need the standard immunizations to protect against infectious diseases. In addition, just as extra immunizations are given to certain high-risk children (e.g., pneumococcal and meningococcal vaccines for children with sickle cell disease), children who are at high risk for injuries need more injury prevention counseling, which should focus on the injuries that are most likely to occur.

Table 23–2 shows the age-specific counseling schedule of TIPP, which indicates the minimum topics to cover at each visit. Topics are scheduled for discussion before children reach a particular developmental milestone. For example, a discussion of falls is scheduled for the 2- or 4-week visit before infants normally begin to roll over, and a discussion of choking is scheduled for 4 months, before they can grasp and put things in their mouths. Specific preventive measures should also be reinforced at each visit. Other relevant topics include toy safety, safety around animals, poisonous plants, and adolescent injury prevention topics.

Some guidelines for health care professionals to keep in mind when counseling about injury prevention in children include involving parents and patients in educational efforts (e.g., have a bicycle helmet in the

TABLE 23–2. The Injury Prevention Program (TIPP) Safety Counseling Schedule for Early and Middle Childhood

Visit	Introduce	Reinforce
Prenatal/newborn	Infant car seat, smoke detector, crib safety	
2 day–4 wk	Falls	Car seat
2 mo	Burns—hot liquids	Car seats, falls
4 mo	Choking/suffocation	Car seat, falls, burns
6 mo	Poisonings, burns—hot surfaces	Falls, burns, choking
9 mo	Water/pool safety, toddler car seat	Poisonings, falls, burns
1 yr	Firearm hazards, auto—pedestrian	Water/pool safety, falls, burns
15 mo		Auto—pedestrian, poisonings, falls, burns
18 mo	Auto—pedestrian	Poisonings, falls, burns, firearm hazards
2 yr	Falls—play equipment, tricycles	Auto—restraints, water/pool safety, burns, firearm hazards
3 yr		Auto—restraints, pedestrian safety, falls, burns, firearm hazards
4 yr	Car seat, booster seat, or seat belt	Pedestrian safety, falls—play equipment, firearm hazards
5 yr	Water/pool safety, bicycle safety	Pedestrian and auto safety
6 yr	Fire safety	Bicycle, pedestrian, and auto safety
8 yr	Sports safety	Bicycle and auto safety
10 yr	Firearm hazards	Sports, bicycle and auto safety

Adapted and reproduced, with permission, from the American Academy of Pediatrics. Committee and Section on Injury and Poison Prevention. TIPP: The Injury Prevention Program, Implementing Safety Counseling in Office Practice. Elk Grove Village, IL, American Academy of Pediatrics, 1994.

office for children to try on). Parents and children should be given simple, practical advice rather than general information (e.g., write the poison control number on the phone, buy a bottle of syrup of ipecac, never leave children unattended in a bathtub, wear a bicycle helmet). Objectives should be well defined and finite. Safety counseling probably will not be especially effective if parents are given a long list of hazards; most people have a limited attention span and memory. Two or three topics should be discussed per visit. Whenever possible, pediatricians should coordinate their educational efforts with current injury prevention efforts (e.g., bicycle helmet campaigns, handgun regulation) in the community.

PEDIATRICIANS AS ADVOCATES

Pediatricians can play a major role in injury prevention outside of the clinical setting. As advocates for child safety, health care professionals can contribute to community efforts in injury prevention either by starting a program or by providing support to ongoing programs.

Supporting legislation and regulatory intervention in injury prevention is another powerful advocacy role for pediatricians and other health care professionals. Dramatic reductions in injuries often follow safety legislation. After the Poison Prevention Packaging Act of 1970, deaths from ingestion of aspirin decreased by 65%. The Flammable Fabrics Act of 1967, the law mandating flame-resistant children's sleepwear, and child passenger safety legislation are other examples. Pediatric practitioners can heighten awareness among policy makers of the magnitude of the injury problem in children (e.g., telephoning or writing letters to legislators, testifying about the benefits of specific safety legislation). They can initiate injury prevention legislation individually or collectively (e.g., through the AAP). Pediatricians can also direct attention to hazardous products on the market; they can help initiate changes in the design of products and enact appropriate regulations (e.g., federal crib standards of 1974 mandating close spacing of vertical slats to reduce the risk of entrapment).

Case Resolution

Some of the factors that influenced the injury suffered by the girl in the case history are the ease with which BB guns are purchased, the marketing of BB guns as toys, the design of the guns, the recreational activities available to children in the community, and the availability of emergency ophthalmologic services. Health care professionals have the opportunity to teach injury prevention to children and their parents as well as to influence the individuals who manufacture the products and pass the laws that affect children's risk of injury.

Selected Readings

American Academy of Pediatrics. Committee on Injury and Poison Prevention. Office-based counseling for injury prevention. Pediatrics 94:566–567, 1994.

American Academy of Pediatrics. Committee and Section on Injury and Poison Prevention. TIPP: The Injury Prevention Program, Implementing Safety Counseling in Office Practice. Elk Grove Village, IL, American Academy of Pediatrics, 1994.

Baker, S. P., et al. The Injury Fact Book. New York, Oxford University Press, 1992.

Bass J. L., K. K. Christoffel, M. Widome, et al. Childhood injury prevention counseling in primary care settings: A critical review of the literature. Pediatrics 92:544–550, 1993.

Childhood injuries. Am. J. Dis. Child. 144:625–731, 1991. (Entire issue.)

Rivara F. P., D. C. Grossman, and P. Cummings. Injury prevention. (2 parts). N. Eng. J. Med. 337:543–548, 613–618, 1997.

Widome, M. Pediatric injury prevention for the practitioner. Curr. Probl. Pediatr. 21:428–468, 1991.

Wilson, M. H., et al. Saving Children: A Guide to Injury Prevention. New York, Oxford University Press, 1991.

CHAPTER 24

FOSTERING SELF-ESTEEM

Monica Sifuentes, M.D.

H$_x$ A 4-year-old girl is brought to the office for a physical examination for preschool. Except for an episode of bronchiolitis at 8 months of age, she has been healthy. Her mother expresses concern that her daughter is shy and does not always play well with other children. She has never participated in a day-care program; she spends most of her time with her mother, grandmother, and 7-year-old sister, with whom she gets along fairly well. Both parents work outside the home, her father full-time and her mother part-time.

The girl's medical history is unremarkable. She has reached all of her developmental milestones at appropriate ages, currently speaks well in sentences, is able to dress herself without supervision, and can balance on one foot with no difficulty.

The physical examination is entirely normal. However, numerous times during the visit, the mother tells her daughter to "sit up straight," "stop fidgeting," and "act your age."

Questions

1. What is self-esteem?
2. How do parents or other caregivers affect the development of their children's self-esteem both positively and negatively?
3. What observable warning signs in parent-child relationships negatively affect normal development of self-esteem?
4. What role does discipline play in the development of self-esteem?
5. What suggestions can primary practitioners give parents and other caregivers to help foster positive self-esteem in children?

Self-esteem can be defined as how one feels about oneself. According to educator Dorothy Briggs, the development of self-respect incorporates two basic concepts: "I am lovable" and "I am worthwhile." To children, "I am lovable" implies that they are valued and deserve to be loved. "I am worthwhile" means that children have something to offer others. Self-esteem is essential to children's health and well-being and influences the development of relationships during both childhood and adulthood.

As children develop into articulate and more social human beings, their interactions with others reflect their feelings of self-worth and security. This self-image is a product of several factors: individual personality, developmental stage, familial environment, degree of parental discipline, sibling and peer interactions, and school experiences. All parents hope that their children will develop a positive self-identity that will aid them throughout their lives. Primary care practitioners should offer parents useful suggestions to ensure this outcome. What parents and other adults can do to foster children's self-esteem is an important part of anticipatory guidance that is often not considered a critical part of the health care maintenance visit. Unfortunately, discussions related to self-esteem are usually held only as a result of a crisis or an observation noted by worried parents or teachers.

Parents should understand the difference between encouragement and pressure and should be introduced to the concept of positive communication. They should also understand the complex relationship between discipline and self-esteem. Pediatricians and other allied health professionals are in a unique position to offer specific recommendations for fostering self-esteem that may have a major impact on their patients' lives. Practitioners may also act as role models for parents by fostering children's self-esteem during health maintenance visits.

SELF-ESTEEM AND GROWTH AND DEVELOPMENT

Although some experts contend that self-esteem necessitates the development of certain cognitive functions, many professionals believe that parents and other caregivers can influence children early on in infancy. Crying newborns quickly adapt to the calming influence of a maternal figure. Infants who are 3–4 months of age often smile at all individuals for social interaction and protest being left alone. Once infants become more verbal and develop more advanced motor skills, they begin to respond consistently to both verbal and nonverbal cues from parents (e.g., laugh with parents, follow simple commands, are taken aback by a stern voice). If parental figures are warm and loving as well as supportive and consistent, infants learn to trust and enjoy these interactions.

By the time children are toddlers, they have developed a specific relationship with their caregivers and the rest of their environment. Presumably they have learned the meaning of "no" and have been reprimanded for going beyond the limits set by caregivers in their attempts at exploration. All children, regardless of

temperament, exhibit negative behaviors such as temper tantrums and selfish behavior, which elicit some type of response from parents.

Preschool children become much more independent, and they spend more time away from primary caregivers. Despite this newly acquired independence, however, they still require attention from parents and often look to them for approval. They also enjoy playing alongside other children, although not necessarily in cooperative play (e.g., helping each other in addition to playing together).

Thus, from a very early age, children's concept of self-worth and competence is established and reinforced by those around them, especially their primary caregivers. This continues into the school years, with peers and teachers eventually assuming a more influential role in the continued development and reinforcement of self-esteem.

ENCOURAGEMENT VERSUS PRESSURE

To build positive self-esteem, children need encouragement at all levels of their development (Table 24–1). This can be in the form of verbal as well as nonverbal communication and should be distinguished from overt pressure. For example, infants should be allowed to explore new surroundings at their own pace rather than being overstimulated and forced to interact in an unfamiliar environment. They should be allowed to develop at their own rate and not be coaxed into activities before they are ready.

Inadvertent pressure can also be detrimental to toddlers who are not yet ready to complete certain tasks. For instance, if parents wait to begin toilet training until toddlers are ready, the likelihood of success, and therefore a positive experience, is greater. Pressuring young children to give up pacifiers or another security object before they are emotionally ready may be quite anxiety-provoking.

Well-intentioned pressure may be equally harmful later in childhood. Forcing children to participate in rigid, structured play does not foster individual creativity or independence; children are merely doing what parents have arranged. Ideally, children should be encouraged to explore and occasionally take risks. Mistakes should be acceptable and even expected under these circumstances. They should be considered learning rather than humiliating experiences. Pressuring children to do things "right" or "perfectly" discourages normal, healthy, risk-taking behavior. In addition, it interferes with future efforts by children to participate in activities unless they are certain they can succeed.

TABLE 24–1. Encouraging Self-Esteem

Don't's	Do's
Have negative expectations	Show confidence in children's abilities
Focus on mistakes	Build on children's strengths
Expect perfection	Value children as they are
Overly protect children	Stimulate independence

COMMUNICATION THAT BUILDS SELF-ESTEEM

Specific ways to communicate that build self-esteem include active listening, use of positive language, discarding "labels," use of encouragement rather than pressure, and the use of the "I" method of communication (Table 24–2). The purpose of active listening is to hear the child's message and understand its meaning. Parents must be attentive, stop what they are doing, and look directly at children. Nonverbal cues such as body posture and facial expression should be appreciated. If children are having trouble understanding their feelings, the parent should repeat what they hear them saying ("It sounds like . . . ").

A nonjudgmental response is warranted if children have a question or concern. The basic message should be simple, clear, and directed specifically at the child. Words should be easily understood and spoken in a moderate tone, especially when discipline is necessary. Facial expression and body language should also be consistent with the message parents or caregivers are trying to convey.

Positive language should be used at all times, even when disciplining children. For instance, when children are playing kick ball in the house, most parents initially reprimand children by yelling, "Don't play ball in the house!" or "Haven't I told you before? No ball playing inside!" Instead of prefacing each sentence with "don't" or "no," parents or other adults should tell children what they can do, what the limits are, and the reason for these rules. For example, caregivers should say: "You may kick the ball outside in the backyard. If you kick it inside, you may break a window or hurt yourself or someone else." Communicating in this manner prevents normally active children from feeling as if they are always being reprimanded.

"Labels" such as "good" or "bad" should be avoided. If children repeatedly hear themselves referred to as "dumb-dumb" or "turkey," they begin to believe these phrases, no matter how innocuous they may initially seem to parents. Seemingly complimentary labels such as "smart" or "bright" may also create undue anxiety for children who then try to live up to these expectations continuously.

Parents should praise their children for successes and achievements. Failures should be minimized whenever possible, although the acknowledgment of mistakes can be important. For example, correcting a child's homework assignment for errors should be done in a nonthreatening manner. Parents should involve the child in the review process rather than simply marking up the paper with a red pen and telling the child to redo the assignment.

TABLE 24–2. Communication That Builds Self-Esteem

Active listening
Use of positive language
Discarding "labels"
Use of encouragement
Use of the "I" method of communication

In addition, talents and abilities should be recognized and highlighted. Children should know that parents have confidence in their abilities and that any display of effort is appreciated. Small successes should be valued as much as large ones, no matter how seemingly insignificant they may be at the time. Parents and other caregivers should keep in mind that although extra positive reinforcement is never detrimental to children's self-esteem, lack of encouragement can hurt their self-image.

Many parenting courses teach primary caregivers to use the "I" method of communication, which requires that parents explain their feelings to children rather than blame them for their actions. This approach is believed to be less threatening and demeaning for children, especially in situations requiring discipline. The "I" method has four recommended steps:

1. Statement of behavior or situation to be addressed (e.g., "When you . . . ").
2. Statement in specific terms how one feels about the effect of the situation on oneself (e.g., "I feel . . . ").
3. Statement of reason (e.g., "because . . . ").
4. Statement of expectations (e.g., "I would like . . . " or "I want . . . ").

Using this approach, a parent's statement might be: "When you bite me, I feel pain because it hurts a lot. I would like you to please tell me what makes you angry instead of biting me."

VULNERABLE TIMES IN A CHILD'S LIFE

There are certain instances when a child's self-esteem can be particularly vulnerable, and the primary care provider should be especially cognizant of these specific circumstances. Problems with self-esteem may be found in overweight children and in those with conditions such as enuresis or encopresis. Negative experiences in school and at home can predispose the child to feelings of shame and worthlessness. Other circumstances that may negatively influence the self-esteem of children are marital conflict and divorce. Children may believe they are responsible for the problem. In order to minimize the lasting effects on self-esteem, parents must communicate honestly and openly with their children and make an extra effort to provide additional support for them during these difficult times (see Chapter 111, Divorce).

DISCIPLINE AND SELF-ESTEEM

Ideally, parents or other adults should feel good about disciplining their children. Two general principles of discipline are to teach by example and to state expectations. Several different approaches to discipline have been adapted by various ethnic, cultural, religious, and socioeconomic groups. A discussion of each of these methods is beyond the scope of this chapter (see Chapter 28, Discipline). Parents and other caregivers should remember that certain methods of discipline can be very destructive to children's self-esteem. For instance, making an enuretic child "wear" the wet bedsheets or reprimanding a child with physical punishment (e.g., spanking) in public places can be demeaning.

temperament when considering involvement in multiple school activities.

Case Resolution

In the case history, the health maintenance visit is a good opportunity for fostering the child's self-esteem. The health care provider can begin by reassuring the girl and her mother that the child's overall health and development are normal. The shy child should be approached by inviting her to tell you some things about herself (e.g., "What do you like to do for fun?," "What is your favorite color?") and giving her some sincere general compliments (e.g., "What a pretty dress you are wearing!," "You have very pretty eyes"). The hope is that this approach will be repeated by the parent at home. In addition, the practitioner should offer concrete suggestions to the parent for positive communication, such as avoiding "don't" and "no" phrases. Parents should be encouraged to think about the child's

Selected Readings

American Academy of Pediatrics. Committee on Psychosocial Aspects of Child and Family Health. Guidance for effective discipline. Pediatrics 101:723–728, 1998.

Berman, B. D., et al. After-school child care and self-esteem in school-age children. Pediatrics 89:654–659, 1992.

Briggs, D. C. Your Child's Self-Esteem. New York, Doubleday, 1970.

Brooks, R. B. Self-esteem during the school years: Its normal development and hazardous decline. Pediatr. Clin. North Am. 39:537–550, 1992.

Coleman, W. L., and R. L. Lindsay. Making friends: Helping children develop interpersonal skills. Contemp. Pediatr. 15:111–129, 1998.

Howard, B. J. Discipline in early childhood. Pediatr. Clin. North Am. 38:1351–1369, 1991.

Sieving, R. E., and S. T. Zirbel-Donish. Development and enhancement of self-esteem in children. J. Pediatr. Health Care 4:290–296, 1990.

CHAPTER 25

SIBLING RIVALRY

Carol D. Berkowitz, M.D.

H$_x$ An 8-year-old boy is brought to the office for an annual checkup. During the course of the evaluation, his mother complains that her son and his 6-year-old sister are always fighting. She says her son hits his sister and pulls her hair, and nothing she does prevents them from fighting. The boy is a B+ student and has no behavior problems in school. The past medical history and the physical examination are completely normal.

Questions

1. What is sibling rivalry?
2. What is the physician's role in counseling a family about sibling rivalry?
3. What is the role of anticipatory guidance in preparing older children for the birth of a new sister or brother?

Sibling rivalry refers to the rivalry between siblings based on the need for parental love and esteem. Historical examples of sibling rivalry include relationships between the biblical figures Cain and Abel, Joseph and his brothers, and Jacob and Esau. Sibling rivalry is also noteworthy in pairs of celebrities, such as actresses Joan Fontaine and Olivia de Havilland.

Sibling rivalry, a universal phenomenon, results from the fear of displacement, dethronement, and loss of love that occurs with the birth of a new brother or sister. Older children fear they are not good enough and need to be replaced. Such feelings lead to a fear of abandonment. Jealousy also plays a role, and older children may be angry at younger siblings for displacing them within the family.

Sibling rivalry frequently has a negative effect on parents because it is hard for them to see one of their children hurt, even if it is by a sister or a brother. The challenge for parents is to know when, and when not, to intervene and what strategies to use to minimize conflicts. Physicians can help by offering anticipatory guidance to all parents and specific recommendations to parents who are experiencing such individual problems.

EPIDEMIOLOGY

Sibling rivalry is a universal phenomenon, and a number of factors influence its development. Time interval between children affects the degree of rivalry. Close spacing results in more problems, particularly when the children are less than 2 years apart. In such situations, older children still have dependency needs, often feel less secure, and experience a need for maternal attention. They stay closer to mothers, are less playful, and more tense. Closely spaced children engage in less spontaneous play, appear more angry, and issue sterner commands to their playmates.

Position in the family also influences sibling rivalry. Middle children experience what is referred to as "middle child syndrome;" they lack the prestige of older children or the privileges of younger ones. These children are often least secure and strive hardest to gain affection. Special difficulties may develop if middle children are the same sex as older ones. Middle children grow up to be flexible, adaptable, and good negotiators. In myths and folklore, youngest children are "favorites." They are often the ones defended by parents when there are bouts of fighting.

Twins rarely present a problem of sibling rivalry; instead they have a problem maintaining their individuality. However, sets of twins create problems for older siblings because they are not as unique as the pair of twins.

Step siblings also present a unique problem in sibling rivalry. Children of divorce frequently feel abandoned by one parent and in competition for the time and love of the custodial parent (see Chapter 111, Divorce). Competition with step siblings is especially difficult if the step siblings are in the same home.

CLINICAL PRESENTATION

Parental complaints related to sibling rivalry consist of fighting between siblings, including physical violence and verbal abuse; bickering; and regression to immature behavioral patterns. Although such immature behavior occurs most often following the birth of a new baby, it may also be apparent if one sibling is receiving more attention, such as during an illness or after a major accomplishment. Regressive behavior includes bedwetting, drinking from a bottle, and wanting to be carried to bed. Substitution behavior, such as nail biting, in place of biting the new sibling, may occur after the birth of a new baby.

Before the birth of a new baby, parents may complain that their children exhibit temper tantrums, irritability, and solemnness. They may mimic the pregnancy by eating a lot and putting a pillow under their clothes. In addition, children may have psychosomatic complaints such as stomachaches or headaches. Risk factors for maladjustment following the addition of a sibling include family discord, physical or emotional exhaustion in parents, and housing insecurity. Conversely, a good marital relationship and family support facilitates the adjustment to new siblings.

DIFFERENTIAL DIAGNOSIS

Dilemmas concerning the correct diagnosis of sibling rivalry most often relate to the appearance of behavioral changes such as regressive or aggressive patterns after the birth of a new sibling. For example, a child who was previously toilet-trained may become incontinent of urine. Although UTI may be considered in the diagnosis, a careful history concerning the birth of the sibling reveals the correct etiology.

EVALUATION

The evaluation of children with suspected sibling rivalry involves a history of the problem and parental strategies for dealing with the difficulties. The parent should be particularly queried about one-on-one opportunities between parents and individual children. The physical examination and laboratory assessment are noncontributory.

MANAGEMENT

The focus of management is to allow the parents to recognize the normalcy of sibling rivalry while helping them define the behaviors that are acceptable and not acceptable within the family context. Parents may not appreciate their child's fear of loss of parental love. They should be told that many children think, "If I am so good, why do I have to be replaced?" Physicians can also help parents deal with sibling rivalry by having them consider their treatment of children in terms of uniformity versus uniqueness and quality versus inequality.

Birth of New Siblings

Parents may notice the behavioral changes in their children before the birth of the new sibling. These changes depend on the age of the children and the presence of other siblings. Children should be told about the upcoming birth. The timing depends on the children's age; younger children do not need much lead time. Some studies have evaluated the inclusion of older children in the birthing process. The results of these studies vary, but they suggest that children under the age of 4 need their mother for emotional support and are concerned about her physical exertion during the birthing process. Some older children may also want to distance themselves from the actual events.

Physicians should suggest that older children be involved in planning for the arrival of the new baby as a means of minimizing their feelings of exclusion. For example, they can help purchase clothes or prepare the baby's room. Physicians should also suggest that parents purchase a gift for older children that represents a present from the new baby. In addition, older siblings may be given a doll to serve as a baby they can care for. Parents should point out the advantages of being older with comments such as, "You can stay up later" or "You can walk and play with all these toys." Frequently, the birth of a new baby is met with regressive behavior in older siblings. Regressive behavior should be handled with tolerance and a realization that symptoms resolve with time.

Once the mother goes to the hospital, she should be advised to maintain contact with older children by writing or telephoning. At present, hospital stays are so brief that this period of separation is much shorter than previously. Household changes that may be necessitated by the birth of the new baby, such as room changes, the substitution of a bed for a crib, and entrance into nursery school, should be made before the arrival of the new baby.

Rivalry Between Older Children

Physicians need to consider individual parenting techniques when counseling parents of older children. Parents who compare one child to the other may foster contentious behavior, and those who strive to treat all children equally may inadvertently perpetuate rivalry. Children need to feel that they are unique rather than ordinary. For example, parents who buy both children the same presents may think they are preventing rivalry from developing, but they are actually depriving each child of a sense of uniqueness. The harder parents try to be uniform, the more vigilantly the children may look for inequality. Each child needs a parent's undivided attention, time alone together. The more agreeable a parent-child relationship, the more agreeable a sibling-sibling relationship, because each child has good self-esteem. Practitioners should recommend uniqueness and quality in each parent-child relationship.

Parents sometimes have to deal with sibling rivalry between older children. Physicians should reassure parents that these older children should be allowed to vent their negative feelings toward each other. For example, if a girl refers to her brother by saying "I hate him," the parents should respond by validating these emotions and saying something like, "It sounds as if he's done something to really annoy you." Parents should also be advised not to take sides. They should examine how they usually respond to squabbling between siblings. Is one child's name always called first during a fight? Do they perpetuate sibling rivalry by using certain nicknames (e.g., "turkey brain") or other derogatory terms? Parents should assume that both parties are at least partially guilty and should not allow themselves to be drawn into the fight as referees. Parents can respond to a request for arbitration with a statement such as, "I wasn't here when things started, so I don't know who is right or wrong." The parents should also advise siblings that they do not have to be friends with one another, but they should not hurt each other's feelings.

Anticipatory guidance helps parents anticipate conflictual situations such as who sits where during long car rides. Children should be allowed to work out a solution by themselves, with the stipulation that the parents will solve the problem if the children do not reach an agreement. Table 25–1 lists suggestions for parents who are seeking advice about fighting between children.

TABLE 25–1. Coping With Rivalry Between Siblings: Physician's Advise to Parents

Do's	Don'ts
Allow children to vent negative feelings	Take sides
Encourage children to develop solutions	Serve as a referee
Anticipate problem situations	Foster rivalry
Foster individuality in each child	Use derogatory names
Spend time with children individually	Permit physical or verbal abuse between siblings
Compliment children when they are playing together	
Tell children about the conflicts you had with your siblings when you were children	
Define acceptable and unacceptable behavior	

PROGNOSIS

Although sibling rivalry may last for years, most siblings become good friends as adults.

Case Resolution

In the case history presented at the beginning of the chapter, the mother should be advised not to serve as a referee. She should learn how to validate each child's feelings about the other. The physician can help her by talking to her son about his feelings. She should be advised to have a discussion with her children during which each child has the opportunity to define areas of conflict and the means to resolve them. The mother has the right and responsibility to prohibit physical fighting and encourage verbal dialogue.

Selected Readings

Dunn, J. Annotation: sibling influences on childhood development. J. Child. Psychol. Psychiatry 29:119–127, 1988.

Hass, E., and P. Light. Talking about the new baby. Parents Magazine 58:68–70, October 1983.

Leung, A. K., and W. L. Robson. Sibling rivalry. Clin. Pediatr. 30:314, 1991.

Pakula, L. C. Sibling rivalry. Pediatr. Rev. 13:72–73, 1992.

Samalin, N., and P. McCormick. How to cure sibling fights. Parents Magazine 68:147–150, May 1993.

Schmitt, B. D. Sibling rivalry toward a new baby. Contemp. Pediatr. 7:111–112, 1990.

Schmitt, B. D. When siblings quarrel. Contemp. Pediatr. 8:73–74, 1991.

CHAPTER 26

TOILET TRAINING

Carol D. Berkowitz, M.D.

Hx A 2-year-old boy is brought to the office for a well child visit. His mother, who is about to begin toilet training her son, asks your advice. The mother says that by the time her daughter was two, she was already toilet trained, and she wants to know if training her son will be any different. The boy was the product of a full-term pregnancy and a normal delivery. He has been in good health, and his immunizations are up to date. He is developmentally normal, has a 30-word vocabulary, and has been walking since the age of 13 months. His physical examination is normal.

Questions

1. When should physicians begin discussing toilet training with parents?
2. What factors help determine children's readiness to begin toilet training?
3. Is toilet training in boys different from toilet training in girls?
4. What are some of the methods used to toilet train children?

The age at which toilet training is carried out is culturally determined. Some cultures train children at a very early age. For example, in the East African Digo culture, some children between 2–3 months of age are conditioned to urinate or defecate when placed in certain positions. Similar conditioning practices are carried out in China. Chinese children are kept without diapers, and when caregivers who are holding them sense a change in their bodies in response to a need to eliminate, they place their children in an appropriate position. In addition, children are dressed in clothing that facilitates toileting. "Split pants," with the back and bottom portion missing, are used so that children can squat and eliminate without removing complicated clothing.

American culture has emphasized the learning aspects of toilet training as opposed to the conditioning aspects. This training focuses on the cognitive development of children and children's readiness to learn the complexity of the task. It has been demonstrated that infants as young as 6 months can be trained to signal the need to urinate or defecate, and suppress emptying for brief periods of time.

Toilet training is potentially both a rewarding and frustrating experience for children and parents. Parents may have unrealistic expectations of children's capability or may be very intolerant of normal accidents that occur in the training process. It is important for

physicians to introduce the topic of toilet training early on to prevent these unrealistic expectations. Children's refusal to toilet train is the second most common precipitant of fatal child abuse. It is recommended that the issue of toilet training be introduced and anticipatory guidance provided by the age of 9 months.

EPIDEMIOLOGY

The age at which children are toilet trained varies depending on social considerations and social pressures. Prior to the 1920s, the American approach to toilet training was permissive. This attitude then changed, and the methods became more rigorous, requiring that children be trained at an earlier age. In 1947, only 5% of children were not trained by 33 months of age, but by 1975, this figure had increased to 42%. There has been a renewed interest in earlier toilet training in the United States. This has been attributed to three societal factors: requirement that toddlers attending preschool are toilet trained, concerns about contagious illnesses such as hepatitis and infectious diarrhea in daycare facilities where diapers are changed, and the adverse environmental effects of nonbiodegradable disposable diapers.

As a general rule, girls are trained a bit earlier than boys, but only by a matter of a few months. The large majority of children (80%) are trained simultaneously for bladder and bowel control. Approximately 12% are trained first for bowel control and about 8% for bladder control. Girls achieve nighttime continence at a younger age than boys.

PATHOPHYSIOLOGY

Toilet training involves the ability both to inhibit a normal reflex release action and then relax the inhibition of the involved muscles. For the process to be successful, a certain degree of neurologic and biologic development is essential. Myelinization of the pyramidal tracts and conditioned reflex sphincter control are necessary. Voluntary control is evidenced by myelinization of the pyramidal tracts by the age of 12–18 months. Conditioned reflex sphincter control occurs by 9 months of age and voluntary cooperation between 12–15 months. In assessing the neurologic development of children, walking is viewed as one of the milestones that indicate motor readiness for toilet training.

Toilet training depends on both physiologic and psychological readiness. Cognitive development is assessed by children's ability to follow certain instructions.

Two years of age has been suggested as the appropriate age to initiate toilet training. As a rule, parents of clinic patients expect that their children will learn at an earlier age. Toilet training usually takes 2 weeks to 2 months to learn, although training may occur in less time using more intense conditioning methods.

DIFFERENTIAL DIAGNOSIS

The differential diagnosis focuses on factors that contribute to a delay in acquisition of skills. Physicians should look for associated symptoms, such as dysuria, a weak urinary stream, constantly wet underwear, or fecal soiling, when assessing children who continue to manifest signs of either urinary or stool incontinence. In addition, it is important to determine if children are essentially toilet trained but are having intermittent accidents.

The most common cause of isolated daytime wetting in previously trained children is **UTI** (see Chapter 33, Enuresis). **Chemical urethritis** may also be associated with urinary incontinence. **Stress incontinence,** which has also been called giggle incontinence, may result in wetting. **Urgency incontinence** occurs when children delay going to the bathroom and then are unable to hold urine any longer. Some children have ectopic ureters, which can empty into the lower portion of the bladder, vagina, or urethra and cause a constant dribble of urine. **Labial fusion** may also be associated with daytime wetting. Urine pools behind the fused labia during voiding, and when children stand up, the urine exits. Children with **neurogenic bladders** may also have symptoms of daytime wetting.

Stooling accidents may be associated with chronic constipation and overflow incontinence or with Hirschsprung's disease. (See Chapter 34, Encopresis.)

EVALUATION

History, Behavioral Assessment, and Physical Examination

Toddlers who appear normal should be assessed for both their physiologic and psychological readiness to undertake this task. Physicians should provide anticipatory guidance to parents about toileting readiness. Affirmative answers should be obtained to the following three questions:

1. Do children exhibit bladder control as evidenced by (1) periods of dryness that last up to 2 hours and (2) facial expressions that show their physiologic response to the elimination process?
2. Do children have the motor skills necessary to get around? This essentially involves the children's ability to walk and remove their clothing.
3. Do children have the cognitive ability to understand the task at hand?

Cognitive ability can be assessed by giving children ten tasks to carry out and seeing if they are able to carry out at least eight of the ten tasks (Table 26–1).

TABLE 26–1. Requests or Imperatives Used to Help Assess Toilet Training Readiness

Bring me the ball
Go to the door
Sit on the chair
Pick up the doll
Open the door
Give the pen to your Mom
Put the ball on the table
Put the doll on the floor
Take off your shoes
Open the book

Stress in the home may negatively affect a toddler's ability to master the task of toilet training. The physician might counsel a family to delay toilet training if the family has moved recently, the birth of a new baby is expected, or there has been a major family crisis such as a death or serious illness.

Children who have had difficulties with toilet training need to undergo a similar assessment. In addition, a physical examination to rule out underlying problems such as spina bifida occulta, which may be associated with a neurogenic bladder, should be performed. A careful examination of the genitalia is important in children who are having urinary incontinence to determine if conditions such as labial fusion are evident. In children who are having stooling problems, physicians should check for an abdomen with feces-filled intestines, a sign of obstipation. In addition, a rectal examination should be performed to determine the presence of hard or impacted stools or any other abnormalities in the anal area.

Laboratory Tests

Although a laboratory assessment is not indicated in normal toddlers who are being toilet trained, diagnostic studies may be appropriate in children who are having problems with training. In older children, urinalysis may show evidence of a UTI.

MANAGEMENT

Physicians should help parents understand the appropriate approach to the toilet training process. Unfortunately, most parents do not obtain the necessary advice from physicians. In one report, no parents attending a clinic and only 7% of patients in a private practice received advice about toilet training from their physicians. Therefore, it is important for physicians to initiate the discussion early enough to prevent the development of any problems. Emphasis on the use of **rewards,** not punishments, is essential.

When toilet training children, parents should be advised to take the following approach:

1. Teach children the **appropriate vocabulary** related to the toilet training process. This could include words such as "pee," "poop," "dry," "wet," "clean," "messy," and "potty."

2. Tell children what the **purpose of the potty** is. Adapter rings fit directly onto the toilet and do not require emptying as do separate potty chairs. They require that the toddler climb up on the toilet, and they need to be removed for others to use the toilet. In general, a child potty chair should be purchased. The potty chair has a number of advantages over the toilet. Children can sit on the potty and have their feet on the floor, which is more physiologically sound and gives them a greater sense of security.

Parents can encourage children to decorate the potty and put their names on it. The potty should be kept in a place where children spend a lot of time, such as the kitchen. Children should be allowed to sit on the potty with their clothes on for about a week before the process of toilet training begins. Then children should sit on the potty without their clothes on, but no attempt to catch either stool or urine should be made.

3. Encourage cleanliness and dryness by **changing children frequently.** Parents should ask their children whether they need to be changed using the appropriate vocabulary. This phase is important to continue as the toilet training process proceeds. Some parents mistakenly do not change their soiled children as a means of punishing them for having accidents. This gives children a confusing message about the need for cleanliness.

4. Explain the **connection between dry pants and going to the potty** to children. Children should understand that dry pants feel good and that they can keep their pants dry by going to the potty.

5. Help children understand the **physiologic signals** for using the toilet. Parents can facilitate this by observing children's behavior around the time of elimination and making comments such as, "When you jump up and down like that, Mommy knows you have to go to the bathroom."

6. Children must have the physiologic ability to postpone the "urge to go." This usually occurs when children have the ability to delay voiding for at least 2 hours. Parents then can initiate toilet training by taking children to the bathroom at 2-hour intervals. In addition, children should sit on the toilet immediately after naps and 20 minutes after meals. Children should not be left on the toilet for more than 5 minutes and should be permitted to get up if they want. While sitting on the potty, they can be entertained with reading a story or playing games.

Additional suggestions involve allowing children to have their clothes off and keeping the potty chair near them during play. This facilitates using the potty and is reminiscent of the practice of using split pants in China.

Children who use the potty successfully should be rewarded. Rewards can be in the form of verbal comments such as "Mommy is so proud of you," hand clapping, or the use of candy, cookies, or star charts. Children can be consulted about what rewards they like. Punishment should not be used, particularly physical punishment. One report indicates that 15% of parents of clinic patients believe that spanking their children for accidents is acceptable. Parental disapproval of accidents can be articulated; however, parents should understand that accidents may continue to occur for months.

If children are trained on a potty chair, they can generally begin using a toilet between 2½–3½ years of age. Children can also use training pants, which are thickened underwear, or pull-ups, which are diaperlike underwear, rather than diapers. Regular underwear are promoted as advantageous because they feel different from diapers and encourage the use of the potty. Using a bigger size or snipping the waistband facilitates children's ability to remove their underpants and can be recommended.

If children demonstrate resistance to toilet training, the process should be delayed for 1–2 months. Children who learn how to withhold need additional time to learn how to relax their sphincter when sitting on a potty. It is important for parents to avoid an aggressiveness-resistance struggle, because this then may become the source of future bowel problems, including constipation. Children who are regular, particularly those who have a bowel movement at the same time every day, are more easily toilet trained. Some children appear fearful of certain aspects of the toilet training process. These include fear of falling into the toilet (this is circumvented with the use of a potty) or fear of the loud noise of the flush. Allowing the child to flush the toilet without using it may dispel the fear. Some children become fascinated with flushing or rolling toilet paper, and parents have to prevent children from wasting water or paper. Children who prefer to stand in a corner to defecate should be commended for recognizing their physiologic urge. Parents should suggest that children stand fully clothed in the bathroom as an initial step in encouraging their use of a potty.

One of the major components of toilet training children is **modeling.** Children should be allowed to enter the bathroom with the parents and even sit on the potty as one or the other parent sits on the toilet. Some children are very strong willed and independent. Strong-willed children, coupled with perfectionist parents, may have problems with toilet training.

Special considerations have to be made for children attending day care. Their teachers should be advised about the toilet training. Children should have "open bathroom privileges," which means that they should be permitted to leave the room to go to the bathroom without raising their hands or other reminders.

Medications have a limited role in toilet training. Some physicians recommend the use of drugs to increase bladder capacity. Although oxybutynin (Ditropan) increases bladder capacity and decreases the frequency of bladder contraction, it should not be used because it does not actually assist children with the toilet training process. However, children who are constipated may require stool softeners such as mineral oil or the addition of fiber bulk to their diet to facilitate the stooling process. Physicians should see children who appear to have toilet training problems on a weekly or biweekly basis until they show improvement.

Parents can also be referred to the many books on toilet training, particularly if problems develop. Many books are geared for children, to help them understand their body and the elimination process. Videotapes are also available to help children with toilet training. Children may also have the opportunity to practice with dolls designed to wet or poop after being fed.

PROGNOSIS

All normal children are eventually toilet trained. The age when this occurs varies and is significant only if it restricts children from participating in school.

Case Resolution

The mother in the case history should be advised that this is a good time to initiate the toilet training process. She should be told that boys, as a group, are successfully toilet trained at a later age than girls. Her son can be assessed to see if he can follow at least eight out of ten instructions (see Table 26–1). If he can, the mother should be given the stepwise approach to initiating the toilet training process.

Selected Readings

Physicians

Azrin, N. H., and R. M. Foxx. Toilet Training in Less Than a Day. New York, Simon & Schuster, 1974.

Berk, L., and P. Friman. Epidemiologic aspects of toilet training. Clin. Pediatr. 29:278–282, 1990.

Christophersen, E. R. Toileting problems in children. Pediatr. Ann. 20:240–244, 1991.

Howe, A. C., and C. E. Walker. Behavioral management of toilet training, enuresis, and encopresis. Pediatr. Clin. North Am. 39:413–432, 1992.

Luxem, M., and E. Christophersen. Behavioral toilet training in early childhood: Research, practice and implications. J. Dev. Behav. Pediatr. 15:370–378, 1994.

Neifert, M. It's potty time. Parenting 66–72, August, 1996.

Robson, W. and A. Leung. Advising parents on toilet training. Amer. Fam. Phys. 44:1263–1268, 1991.

Schmitt, B. D. Toilet training refusal: avoid the battle and win the war. Contemp. Pediatr. 3:32–50, 1987.

Schmitt, B. D. Toilet training without tears. Contemp. Pediatr. 8:47–49, 1992.

Van Pelt, K. Potty Training Your Baby. Garden City Park, NY, Avery, 1988.

Parents and Children

Brooks, Joae Graham. I'm a Big Kid Now. Neenah, WI. Kimberly-Clark Corporation, 1990.

Frankel, Alona. Once Upon a Potty. Hauppauge, New York, Barron's Educational Series, Inc. 1980.

Mack, Alison. Toilet Learning: The Picture Book Technique for Children and Parents. Boston, Little, Brown and Company, 1978.

Miller, Virginia. On Your Potty. Cambridge, Massachusetts, Candlewick Press, 1994.

Rogers, Fred. Going to the Potty. New York, Penguin Putnam Books for Young Readers, 1986.

CHAPTER 27

CRYING AND COLIC

Geeta Grover, M.D.

H$_x$ The parents of a 2-week-old infant bring their son to the emergency department because he has been crying persistently for the past 4 hours. He has no history of fever, vomiting, diarrhea, upper respiratory tract infection, or change in feeding. The infant is breast-fed.

On physical examination, the infant appears well developed and well nourished. His weight is 7 lb, 7 oz—seven ounces more than when he was born. Although he is fussy and crying, he is afebrile with normal vital signs. The remainder of the physical examination is within normal limits.

Questions

1. What is the normal crying pattern in young infants?
2. What is colic?
3. What conditions are associated with prolonged crying in young infants?
4. What are key factors in the history of crying infants?
5. What laboratory tests are indicated in crying infants?
6. List a few of the management strategies that can be used by parents to soothe their crying or colicky infants.

Crying, an important method of communication between infants and caregivers, is nonspecific, and many stimuli can produce the same response (e.g., hunger, fatigue, pain). Parents report that they can discriminate among various types of cries in their infants. Crying can be divided into three categories: (1) normal or physiologic crying, (2) excessive crying secondary to distress (e.g., hunger) or disease, and (3) excessive crying without an apparent cause.

The difference between normal and excessive crying may be more qualitative than quantitative. Deciding whether crying is excessive varies with parents' expectations and thresholds. Expressed parental concern about extreme crying or fussiness requires attention. If parents complain that infants cry inconsolably or continuously as well as excessively, the crying may have an underlying organic etiology.

Colic, a poorly understood, benign, self-limited condition, falls into the third category. It manifests as unexplained crying or fussing in infants that usually occurs in the late afternoon or evening. During an episode of colic, infants cry and may either draw the knees up to the chest or rigidly stiffen the legs, flex the elbows, clench the fists, and turn red (Fig. 27–1). Although infants may appear to be totally miserable during an episode of colic, they are otherwise healthy, eat well, and demonstrate good weight gain.

EPIDEMIOLOGY

Qualitatively, **excessive crying** is any amount of crying that concerns or worries parents. Quantitatively, definitions of excessive crying have been based on the results of Brazelton's study of normal infants. This study found that the median daily crying time at 2 weeks of age is 1¾ hours; this time increases to a peak of 2¾ hours at 6 weeks of age and then decreases to less than 1 hour by 12 weeks. Apparently, more crying occurs during the evening hours, especially between the ages of 3 and 6 weeks.

Colic affects 10–20% of infants less than 3 months of age. There is no seasonal variation in its occurrence, and breast-fed and formula-fed infants are affected equally.

Colic usually begins at 2–3 weeks, peaks at 6–8 weeks, and resolves by 3–4 months of age. Colicky infants cry for at least 3 hours per day for at least 3 days per week, usually around 3 PM ("rule of threes").

CLINICAL PRESENTATION

Colicky infants are otherwise healthy infants under three months of age who cry or fuss inconsolably for extended periods of time, usually during the afternoon or evening. The crying usually resolves within a few hours.

PATHOPHYSIOLOGY

Crying is a complex vocalization that changes during the first year of life as infants develop. In the first few weeks of life, crying is a signal that infants are experiencing a disturbance in homeostatic regulation (e.g., hunger, discomfort). As infants mature and begin to differentiate internal from external stimuli, crying may also be an indication of too little or too much environmental stimulation. During the second half of the first year, as infants mature neurologically and gain voluntary control over vocalizations, crying can be an expression of different affects (e.g., frustration, fear).

A variety of explanations for the etiology of **colic** have been proposed. Some authorities believe that colic may not be a pathologic entity but simply an extreme variant of normal crying. The condition may result from an allergy, cow's milk intolerance, abnormal intestinal peristalsis, or increased intestinal gas, which are some of the more frequently associated factors. Others have proposed that colic is caused by problems in the interaction between infants and their environment, specifically their parents. This interactional theory requires not only excessive crying on the part of the infant, but also an inability of the parents to soothe the crying infant. Whether maternal anxiety has any role in colic remains a controversial issue. More than one of these factors may contribute to the pathogenesis of colic.

DIFFERENTIAL DIAGNOSIS

An acute episode of excessive crying may be secondary to disease (e.g., fever, otitis media). An organic etiology should be suspected in infants who present with inconsolable crying of acute onset. Table 27–1 lists the most common causes. Some conditions occur in a more chronic or recurrent pattern, particularly if the condition is not treated.

The differential diagnosis of infants who experience recurrent episodes of excessive crying focuses more on behavior and temperament. Colic, persistent night awakening, difficult infant temperament (e.g., extreme fussiness, neonatal drug withdrawal) may cause recurrent crying. Persistent night awakening and difficult infant temperament are discussed in Chapter 12, Sleep, and Chapter 29, Temper Tantrums, respectively.

EVALUATION

A thorough history and physical examination usually provide clues to the diagnosis in instances of acute onset of crying.

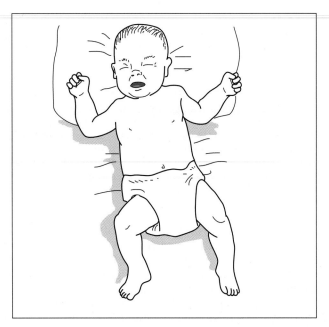

FIGURE 27–1. Colicky infant.

TABLE 27–1. **Most Common Causes of Acute Unexplained, Excessive Crying in Infants**

Idiopathic*
Colic*
Infectious
    Otitis media
    Urinary tract infection (UTI)
    Stomatitis
    Meningitis
Gastrointestinal*
    Constipation
    Anal fissure
    Gaseous distention
    Peristalsis problems
    Reflux
    Intussusception
Trauma
    Corneal abrasion
    Foreign body in the eye
    Hair tourniquet syndrome
Behavioral*
    Overstimulation
    Persistent night awakening
Drug Reactions
    Immunization reactions (most common: diphtheria-tetanus-pertussis vaccine)
    Neonatal drug withdrawal (narcotics)
Child Abuse
    Long bone fractures
    Retinal hemorrhage
    Intracranial hemorrhage
Hematologic*
    Sickle cell crisis
Cardiovascular
    Arrhythmia (supraventricular tachycardia)
    Congestive heart failure
    Anomalous left coronary artery

*May present as acute or recurrent episodes of excessive crying.

History

The focus of the history should be on determining the presence of any associated symptoms. In addition, the circumstances surrounding the crying (e.g., occurrence during day or night) should be ascertained (Questions Box).

Physical Examination

A thorough physical examination is required for accurate diagnosis. Particular attention should be given to the following aspects of the examination:

1. Careful inspection of the skin after all clothing has been removed to look for any suspicious bruises or marks.
2. Palpation of all long bones to detect fractures.

Questions: Crying and Colic

- Is this the first time the infant has cried inconsolably or does this happen on a recurring basis?
- Has the infant had a fever?
- Does the infant have any cold symptoms, vomiting, or diarrhea?
- Is the infant having any difficulty feeding? Is the infant formula- or breast-fed?
- Has the infant had a recent fall or accident?

3. Examination of all digits and the penis to check for "hair tourniquets" (single strands of hair wrapped around digits or the penis).
4. Examination of the retina to look for retinal hemorrhages (a sign of intracranial hemorrhage).
5. Eversion of the eyelids to check for foreign bodies.
6. Fluorescein staining of the cornea to look for corneal abrasion.

Laboratory Tests

Except for urinalysis, most screening laboratory tests are probably not useful. Test selection can be guided by the history and physical examination (e.g., infants with fever without an apparent cause should have a septic workup, with an examination of blood, urine, and CSF). Urinalysis, which may provide clues to an underlying metabolic deficiency, is sometimes helpful. Even when the initial history and physical examination are nondiagnostic, infants who persist in crying inconsolably should be suspected of having a serious underlying condition (e.g., intracranial hemorrhage, drug ingestion). Such infants may warrant an extended period of observation or a more extensive workup that includes laboratory assessment.

Imaging Studies

Roentgenographic studies such as long bone x-rays may be necessary in some situations (e.g., infants with long bone pain on palpation, suspicion of child abuse). Infants with retinal hemorrhages should have a CT scan.

MANAGEMENT

Management and treatment depends on identification of the cause of the crying. Underlying organic conditions (e.g., UTI, fractures) should be treated. Management of colic depends on presumptions regarding its etiology. It is important for practitioners to **reassure** parents regarding the benign nature of colic and its resolution over time. Physicians should provide a caring and supportive environment in which the parents may express their concerns and frustrations. Reassurance along with practical suggestions regarding infant feeding and handling techniques (e.g., cuddling, swaddling, or rocking) may often suffice.

Management suggestions for colic should be customized for infants and families. The more common management techniques are listed in Table 27–2.

TABLE 27–2. **Management of Colic**

Parental reassurance
Alteration in techniques of infant feeding and handling
Alteration of sensory input to infant
Prevention of swallowed air from passing through pylorus
Dietary alterations
Medication
Folk remedies
Increase carrying
Respond quickly to crying

Changes in sensory input (e.g., soothing sounds or motions) may resolve crying and soothe colicky infants.

Prophylactic measures to prevent the passage of swallowed air through the pylorus can also be useful. Such techniques include feeding in an upright position and limiting the period of sucking at the breast or bottle to about 10 minutes (after this time, greater amounts of air are swallowed relative to the amount of milk ingested). Some infants eat very fast and swallow a lot of air. Burping these infants every 5–10 minutes during feeds may help alleviate discomfort due to excessive air swallowing (aerophagia).

Methods to decrease intestinal spasm (e.g., abdominal massage, warm baths, avoidance of overfeeding) may be helpful. The use of suppositories or rectal thermometers to break up rectal spasm and thereby release retained gas should be discouraged.

Formula changes to eliminate possible allergens should be reserved for those infants with additional symptoms of allergy (e.g., wheezing, rash) or intolerance (e.g., vomiting, diarrhea, hematochezia, or weight loss).

Various drugs, including anticholinergics, motility-enhancing agents, barbiturates, laxatives, and antiflatulents, have limited success and are best avoided. Currently, antiflatulents (e.g., simethicone) are prescribed most commonly. Despite lack of scientific evidence to support their efficacy, parents indicate that they are effective.

As long as no adverse effects are evident, limited amounts (e.g., 1–2 oz/d) of **folk remedies** (e.g., chamomile tea) can be supported if parents report satisfaction. Over-the-counter homeopathic preparations are also innocuous but may be advocated as efficacious by some parents.

Finally, the pratitioner should encourage parents to respond to the infants' cries quickly and carry their infants as much as possible (e.g., at least 3–4 hours daily). Parents should be advised that they cannot "spoil" young infants under 4 months of age and that they might actually improve behavior by their own increased responsiveness.

PROGNOSIS

Fortunately, the natural history of persistent crying during infancy is resolution over time. To date, no long-term sequelae of infantile colic have been identified except for a possible relationship with irritable bowel syndrome in childhood.

Case Resolution

The infant described in the case history is experiencing an acute episode of unexplained crying. Despite a normal physical examination, he was observed for 1 hour in the emergency department because his crying persisted. Subsequently a septic workup was initiated, which revealed that a UTI was the source of the irritability.

Selected Readings

Barr, R. G. The normal crying curve: what do we really know? Dev. Med. Child Neurol. 32:356–362, 1990.

Brazelton, T. B. Crying in infancy. Pediatrics 29:579–588, 1962.

Fleisher, D. R. Coping with colic. Contemp. Pediatr. 15:144–156, 1998.

Kemper, K. J. Colic. In The Holistic Pediatrician. New York, Harper Collins, 1996.

Markestad, T. Use of sucrose as a treatment for infant colic. Arch. Dis. Child. 76:356–358, 1997.

Metcalf, T. J., et al. Simethicone in the treatment of infant colic: a randomized, placebo-controlled, multicenter trial. Pediatrics 94:29–34, 1994.

Parkin, P. C., C. J. Schwartz, and B. A. Manuel. Randomized, controlled trial of three interventions in the management of persistent crying of infancy. Pediatrics 92:197–201, 1993.

Poole, S. R. The infant with acute, unexplained excessive crying. Pediatrics 88:450–455, 1992.

Sferra, T. J., and L. A. Heitlinger. Gastrointestinal gas formation and infantile colic. Pediatr. Clin. North Am. 43:489–507, 1996.

CHAPTER 28

DISCIPLINE

Carol D. Berkowitz, M.D.

Hx A 3-year-old boy is being threatened with expulsion from preschool because he is biting the other children. His mother states that he is very active and aggressive toward other children. In addition, his language development is delayed. She is at her wits end about what to do. The birth history is normal, and the mother denies the use of drugs or cigarettes, but she drank socially before she realized she was pregnant. The past medical and family histories are noncontributory, and the physical examination is normal.

Questions

1. What is the definition of discipline?
2. What strategies can parents use to discipline children?
3. What are the guidelines for using "time-out"?
4. What is the relationship between corporal punishment and child abuse?

Discipline can be defined as an educational process in which children learn how to behave in a socially acceptable manner. It involves a complex set of interactions of attitudes, models, instructions, rewards, and punishments. Discipline is not synonymous with corporal punishment. The goal is to help children gain self-control and respect for others and to learn behavior that is appropriate for given situations. Proactive discipline is action taken by parents to encourage good behavior, and reactive discipline is parental action following misbehavior.

PHYSICIAN-PARENT INTERACTIONS CONCERNING DISCIPLINE

Practitioners can assist parents by giving them guidelines for appropriate childhood discipline related to both routine and problem development. The age and temperament of the child are important factors to consider. In addition, pediatricians can discourage corporal punishment as the major method of discipline. It is important to encourage parents to establish a positive interactive environment with verbal communication, monitoring children's behavior and commending desirable behavior, ignoring trivial problems, and consistently applying predetermined consequences for misbehavior. Frequently physicians fail to inquire about children's behavior. Unless the topic is brought up by parents, it is not discussed during the physician visit. On average, physicians spend only 90 seconds per visit on anticipatory guidance and counseling. However, one survey of mothers in a physician waiting room showed that up to 90% were concerned about one aspect of behavior. Sixty percent of mothers surveyed found physician intervention quite helpful. The American Academy of Pediatrics recommends anticipatory guidance about discipline at each health maintenance visit between 9 months and 5 years. Such counseling is especially important to help parents understand the value of appropriate discipline in shaping their children's self-esteem. Information about discipline in the media may be confusing, contradictory, and support the unfounded approaches of nonprofessionals.

Early in the physician-parent relationship, physicians may express their interest in behavioral problems by saying, "I am interested not only in your child's physical well being, but also in his (or her) growth and development and how he (or she) gets along with friends and family." They may then question parents about how children spend their days. During subsequent visits, pediatricians may say, "Parents of children of (child's name)'s age frequently worry about discipline. I wonder if you have any concerns." In making these inquiries, the physician may establish what factors such as religious or ethnic beliefs, or family influences are shaping parents' decisions about discipline.

PROBLEM BEHAVIORS

Behavioral problems can be placed in five major categories.

1. **Problems of daily routine.** Such problems refer to the refusal of children to go about their daily activities, such as eating, going to bed, awakening at a certain time, and toilet training.
2. **Aggressive resistance behavior.** This behavior is characterized by negativism and includes temper tantrums and aggressive responses to siblings and peers.
3. **Overdependent or withdrawal behavior.** Such behavior is typical of children who are very attached to their mothers. These clingy children find separation difficult, especially in a preschool setting.
4. **Hyperactivity or excessive restlessness.**
5. **Undesirable habits,** which include thumb sucking, nail biting, throat clearing, and playing with genitals.

Some of the behaviors listed above are age-appropriate, and physicians can help parents by counseling them about stage-related behavior, such as oppositional behavior in a 2-year-old and independence-dependence problems in a 3–5-year-old. Parents may be more tolerant of a particular behavior if they understand what is normal at a given age. Just because something is normal, however, does not mean that it should be tolerated. Physicians can suggest to the parents ways of dealing with age-appropriate behavior (e.g., placing breakable objects out of reach of toddlers).

Certain behavioral problems reflect differences in childhood temperaments. Temperament is the biological predisposition to style of behavior. Carey has compiled a series of temperament scales to assess children and adolescents of different ages. For example, some children are shy and have a hard time adjusting to new situations. If parents anticipate such problems, they are often less angry when difficulties arise. Parental expectations can vary with a child's gender. Boys may be permitted to act a certain way ("He's all boy!") that would be disapproved of in girls. Physicians can discuss such expectations at health maintenance visits.

Physicians can also be particularly helpful in detecting and advising parents about disparities in the achievement of different developmental skills. Some children acquire motor skills before verbal skills, yet parents expect their children to be equally versatile in speech and movement.

PSYCHOPHYSIOLOGY

All behaviors are modified by the responses and reactions of other individuals. The basic premise of discipline is to discourage unwanted behavior and to encourage desired behavior. This is accomplished by using techniques that are based on conditioning modalities.

Several factors contribute to an increased incidence of behavioral problems in children. Ten to fifteen percent of all preschool children are raised in grossly disturbed family situations. These homes are torn by divorce, death, separation, parental substance abuse, mental illness, or extreme poverty. Parental insecurity may also be a factor. In addition, families may have fewer social contacts than they once did because of greater mobility within society. As a result, they face greater social isolation.

DIFFERENTIAL DIAGNOSIS

In addition to providing anticipatory guidance about discipline, physicians must make two diagnostic decisions. First, they must determine whether a specific behavioral problem represents normal childhood behavior or an abnormality in behavior that warrants more specific intervention. Between 8 and 18% of behavioral disturbances may deserve physician intervention. More intensive management may be necessary for problems related to aggressive-resistant behavior and hyperactivity. Hyperactive behavior, which may exist as part of ADHD, may be a sign of a significant underlying problem that warrants one-on-one intervention or the use of neuropharmacologic agents (see Chapter 103, Attention Deficit/Hyperactivity Disorder).

Second, physicians must differentiate between acceptable corporal punishment and child abuse. Some individuals feel that any form of corporal punishment is unacceptable. The use of physical punishment is widely accepted in our society, however, and it is legally condoned in the home setting. Fractures and bruises are not acceptable, and physical abuse should be suspected in children who present with such injuries.

EVALUATION

History

The key component in the evaluation process is the assessment of the means parents use to discipline children (Questions Box). To obtain this information, physicians may simply ask parents, "How do you get your child to mind you?" This question is designed to lead to a discussion of how parents interact with their children. If parents have specific complaints, such as oppositional behavior, they should be questioned about the strategies they have used in their effort to discipline their children.

Physical Examination

Children's behavior should be assessed during the office visit. A general physical examination is useful to check for any signs of physical abuse as well as to evaluate children's well being. A developmental assessment is also helpful because it may delineate disparities in the achievement of certain skills. Some hyperactive children may warrant a more extensive psychodevelopmental assessment to look for findings consistent with ADHD. Behavioral checklists may be used to evaluate children's temperament.

Laboratory Tests

No specific laboratory or imaging studies are indicated for children with discipline problems.

MANAGEMENT

Physicians should assist parents in establishing appropriate guidelines for disciplining their children and reinforce the role of parents as the source of authority (Table 28-1). It is important for parents to realize that total freedom results in uncontrollable anxiety.

Children mimic behavior, and **parents should act as role models.** If parents have temper tantrums when they are frustrated, their children may act in a similar manner. **Consistency** is also important. A system with a limited number of enforced rules is better than one with many different rules. In families where both parents are working, especially if they have overlapping time schedules, consistency is sometimes difficult to attain.

Physicians should emphasize to parents that it is best to **avoid power struggles.** Children engaged in a struggle often win because they have final control (e.g., refusing to eat). Children should always be given the opportunity to graciously back out of a situation and save face. It is easier to avoid situations that lead to head-on confrontations than to get out of them once the confrontation has occurred. Parents should be the source of information for physicians. This helps strengthen parents' egos and validates their ability to handle their children appropriately.

In the past, specific methods of dealing with children with discipline problems concerned the issues of permissiveness versus overpermissiveness and accommodation versus strict punishment. Overpermissiveness refers to the allowing of undesirable acts and may exacerbate anxiety and increase demands for privilege.

Questions: Discipline

- What does the child do that the parents wish he or she would not do?
- What do the parents do to stop unwanted behavior?
- Does the child usually obey the parents?
- Where does most of the unwanted behavior occur?
- Which parent is responsible for disciplining the child?

TABLE 28–1.   Advice for Parents about Discipline

Set limits
Define consequences
Be consistent
Ignore trivial problems
Compliment desirable behavior
Take time-out when angry

Physicians should remind parents that preventing many behavioral disorders is easier than treating them. Discipline should not only discourage bad behavior but also reinforce good behavior.

The five types of reactive discipline described below are used today.

Redirection

Redirection is a simple and effective method in which the parent removes the problem and distracts the child with an alternative. This technique is frequently used to remove some object (such as a valued knic-knac) from the hands of an infant and replacing it with a toy. Parental patience, ingenuity, and enthusiasm facilitates this approach.

Spanking

Spanking involves inflicting physical pain, which is usually successful in bringing about the immediate cessation or a decrease in problem behavior. Spanking tends to clear the air and get the punishment over with rather than producing a lingering guilt. To be truly effective, however, physical punishment must immediately follow the act. The "wait until Daddy comes home" approach is less effective because of the lack of temporal association. In addition, spanking tends to become situation-specific so that children associate a particular action with being spanked. This learning does not generalize to other situations. Spanking can teach children to be afraid of adults rather than to respect them.

Spanking may actually be damaging to the parent-child relationship. Differentiation of physical punishment from child abuse is often difficult. In general, punishment with the hands is acceptable, but punishment with objects and spanking on parts of the body other than the buttocks or thighs is unacceptable. Spanking may be an early precursor of later physical violence and subsequent abuse. Again, parents act as role models. Children should never be allowed to hit their parents. This makes children feel extremely insecure.

Scolding

Scolding involves the excess use of reasoning and explanations and is used by most parents as part of the discipline process. In families where communication or interaction is minimal, scolding may result in an initial increase in inappropriate behavior because this is the only way children receive any attention. Scolding, because of its negative focus, can be damaging to children's self-esteem.

Ignoring

Ignoring represents the opposite of explaining and reasoning. This form of discipline is difficult to use successfully because parents must totally ignore children's behavior. If even the least flicker of recognition occurs, then activity increases. A brief initial increase in unwanted behavior, a so-called response burst, may occur with ignoring. This disciplinary method works better in younger children.

Time-Out

"Time-out," the most recommended form of discipline, refers to time out from positive reinforcement. In sports, teams call a "time-out" to rethink what they are doing and to replan their strategies. Children are placed in a neutral or boring environment whenever they engage in inappropriate behavior. The time out technique can be used to discourage undesired habits. For example, parents may say, "You can suck your thumb, but you may only do it in such and such a room." This type of discipline is better than ignoring, especially if "ignored" children are receiving attention from siblings and peers. Children should understand the rules ahead of time and why the behavior is unacceptable. Once this is accomplished, time out may occur without any warning.

A timer should be used, and children should stay in the time-out area for 1 minute per 1 year of age. An appropriate area must be selected. This area should be fairly boring, so children's rooms are often not appropriate. A laundry room, a corner, or specific chair may be better. If children act unacceptably during the time out, the timer should be reset. If children have to go to the bathroom during time out, they are allowed one trip. After they return from the bathroom, the timer is reset.

The use of the time-out method is sometimes difficult. If the inappropriate behavior occurs in the morning when children are getting ready for school, time out just encourages children's desire to delay. "Beat the buzzer" is another idea that may be used in such situations. With "beat the buzzer," the timer is set. If children are dressed before the timer goes off, they may be rewarded for the behavior by being allowed to go to bed one half hour later. If the buzzer "beats" them, then they have to go to bed one half hour earlier.

Inappropriate behavior away from home presents the greatest difficulty. These situations can be dealt with in numerous ways, particularly if the behavior problem involves temper tantrums. When children are crying or screaming uncontrollably, it is best to remove them from the embarrassment of the situation. This "manual guidance" often occurs in a supermarket, where children select something that parents do not wish to buy. Parents can often circumvent this problem easily by walking into the supermarket and saying, "If you are a good boy (or girl) during the whole trip, then I will get you something at the checkout counter." If children still have temper tantrums, then they should be removed from the area and brought to a neutral place such as the automobile or a restroom and allowed to finish their crying and screaming. It has been said that a glass of cold water splashed in a child's face is sometimes very therapeutic. If the inappropriate behavior does not develop into a temper tantrum, then "marking" time out is helpful. This consists of putting a mark on the child's hand every time he or she engages in an inappropriate behavior. When the child returns home, the marks are totaled, and the time-out method is used.

Parents who complain about inappropriate behavior should be asked to keep a record of children's behavior for 1–2 weeks. This helps determine if the behavior is really inappropriate and what is motivating it. Parents should be encouraged to talk to their children in a reasonable manner and to verbalize what they think children are feeling. They might say something like this, "It's terrible to be three years old and get so upset. You feel that you can't get the things you want, but some day you will grow up and then you will be in charge. I am really sorry it is so hard for you right now." Physicians should tell parents that it is important to set limits for children and to avoid threatening, judging, and constantly criticizing children. Parents should ask themselves, "If someone said this to me, how would I feel?" Many parents have themselves been disciplined only with spanking and know no other means, and the advice that physicians offer is valuable.

PROGNOSIS

Children raised in a supportive environment that teaches respect for others and self-control grow up as caring adults. Children who have been exposed to excessive corporal punishment show aggressive behavior later.

Case Resolution

In the case presented at the beginning of the chapter, further history should be elicited about the mother's disciplining techniques. It is also significant that the child is speech-delayed. The boy's ability to articulate his feelings may be limited, and a formal speech and hearing assessment is warranted. The preschool should be advised that the evaluation is underway. A report from the preschool concerning the boy's behavior would be appreciated.

Selected Readings

Barkley, R. A. Defiant Children: A Clinician's Manual for Assessment and Parent Training, 2nd ed. New York, The Guilford Press, 1997.

Carey, W. B. Pediatric assessment of behavioral adjustment and behavioral style. In Levine, M.D., W.B. Carey, and A.C. Crocker (eds.). Developmental-Behavioral Pediatrics, 2nd ed. Philadelphia, W. B. Saunders, 1992, pp. 609–612.

Carey, W. B. Temperament issues in the school-aged child. Pediatr. Clin. North Am. 39:564–584, 1992.

Christophersen, E. R. Discipline. Pediatr. Clin. North Am. 39:395–411, 1992.

Christophersen, E. R. Oppositional behavior in children. Pediatr. Ann. 20:267–273, 1991.

Corwin, D. G. The fine art of the time-out. Parenting 171–172, November, 1996.

Howard, B. J. Discipline in early childhood. Pediatr. Clin. North Am. 38:1351–1369, 1991.

Schmitt, B. D. Discipline: rules and consequences. Contemp. Pediatr. 8:65–69, 1991.

Schmitt, B. D. Time-out: intervention of choice for the irrational years. Contemp. Pediatr. 10:64–71, 1993.

Schmitt, B. D. When a child hurts other children. Contemp. Pediatr. 7:81–82, 1990.

Socolar, R. R. S., et al. Research on discipline: The state of the art, deficits, and implications. Arch. Pediatr. Adolesc. Med. 151:758–760, 1997.

Socolar, R. R. S., and R. E. K. Stein. Maternal discipline of young children: Context, belief, and practice. J. Dev. Behav. Pediatr. 17:1–8, 1996.

Socolar, R. R. S., and R. E. K. Stein. Spanking infants and toddlers: maternal belief and practice. Pediatrics 95:105–111, 1995.

Smith, J. R., and J. Brooks-Gunn. Correlates and consequences of harsh discipline for young children. Arch. Pediatr. Adolesc. Med. 151:777–786, 1997.

Straus, M. A., D. B. Sugarman, and J. Giles-Sims. Spanking by parents and subsequent antisocial behavior of children. Arch. Pediatr. Adolesc. Med. 151:761–767, 1997.

Wissow, L. S., and D. Roter. Toward effective discussion of discipline and corporal punishment during primary care visits: findings from studies of doctor-patient interaction. Pediatrics 94:587–593, 1994.

CHAPTER 29

TEMPER TANTRUMS

Geeta Grover, M.D.

H$_x$ During a routine office visit, the parents of a 3-year-old boy express concern about his recent behavior. They report that whenever he is asked to do something he does not want to do, he throws a "fit." He cries fiercely, falls to the floor, bangs his hands, and kicks his feet until his parents give in. He often displays such behavior at bedtime or mealtime if he is asked to turn off the television or eat foods that he does not want. He has two to three such episodes per week. The parents state that their home life has not changed, and the boy's teacher reports that he displays no such behaviors at preschool.

Questions

1. At what age are temper tantrums common in children?
2. How do parents' reactions encourage or discourage temper tantrums?
3. What appropriate management strategies may help control such oppositional behavior?
4. What factors or aspects of such oppositional behavior indicate underlying pathology?

Temper tantrums are common, normal, age-related behaviors in young children. To a certain degree, oppositional behaviors such as negativism, defiance, and tantrums are part of the normal progression toward self-reliance and independence. Toddlers need to assert their freedom and explore their environment, which often puts them at odds with the limitations imposed by society and well-meaning parents. Young children cannot appreciate that rules and limitations have been established in the interest of their own safety and well being. They see only that their own desires have been thwarted, and they may react to this disappointment with intense emotions. Children are not simply upset because they cannot have their way. They are angry and frustrated, and they lose control over their emotions. During tantrums children cry and scream uncontrollably. They may fall to the floor, bang their heads, kick their feet, pound their hands, and thrash about wildly. Some children may throw things, try to hit one another, or destroy property.

Such intense displays of anger may be a terrifying experience for both children and parents. Some children use tantrums to gain attention, whereas others use them to achieve something or to avoid doing something. Recurrent temper tantrums may strain relationships among parents, children, and other family members.

EPIDEMIOLOGY

Temper tantrums are noted most often in children who are 2–3 years of age, but they may occur any time between the ages of 12 months and 5 years. Parental surveys reveal that about 20% of 2-year-olds, 18% of 3-year-olds, and 10% of 4-year-olds have at least one tantrum per day. Boys and girls are affected equally. Although temper tantrums are unusual in school-age children, they often reappear in the form of verbal tantrums during adolescence when autonomy and independence once again become developmental issues.

BEHAVIORAL PATHOPHYSIOLOGY

Appreciation of children's level of maturity and the developmental tasks normally associated with the toddler and preschool years, when temper tantrums occur most often, facilitates an understanding of tan-

trum behavior. Young children who are exploring the world and developing a sense of autonomy think primarily in egocentric terms. They view reality from their own perspective and are unable to appreciate the perspective of other individuals. Only as they mature and enter school do they learn to recognize the position of others and begin to develop a sense of morality, of right and wrong. Toddlers may become frustrated or angry because of their lack of control over the world, inability to communicate, or limitations of their cognitive and motor abilities, which do not allow them to accomplish desired tasks. Unlike adults who have the ability to verbalize frustrations or simply walk away from unpleasant situations, young children have neither the sophisticated ability to articulate their feelings nor the freedom to walk away. Therefore, they may react to disappointments with temper tantrums.

Temper tantrums may be classified as normal or problematic based on their cause, frequency, and characteristics. Normal tantrums can simply be demands for attention or signs of frustration, anger, or protest. In the interval between tantrums, the child's disposition and mood are normal. The well-behaved 3-year-old boy who has an occasional tantrum following the birth of a sibling, the 2½-year-old girl who throws a tantrum to express frustration because no one understands what she is trying to say, and the 2-year-old boy who cries uncontrollably because he cannot complete the puzzle he has started or run fast enough to keep up with his 4-year-old brother are all examples of normal tantrums. A typical reason for an avoidance-type tantrum is not wanting to go to bed at bedtime. All types of tantrums are more common when children are tired, ill, or hungry, because their ability to cope with disappointment and frustration is limited under these circumstances.

Frequent tantrums (>5 per day) or tantrums that result in destruction of property or physical harm to the child or others are signs of problematic tantrums (Table 29–1). These tantrums result from factors that are beyond the child's control such as parental problems, school difficulties, or health-related conditions (Table 29–2). For example, the child with unrecognized hearing loss may be performing poorly at school and resort to tantrum behavior in frustration. Marital discord or domestic violence may create anxiety for a child, which may manifest as frequent or destructive tantrums.

EVALUATION

Thorough history taking is essential (Questions Box). The frequency of the temper tantrums, circumstances

---

TABLE 29–1.   Features of Problematic Tantrums

Tantrums that persist or get worse beyond 5 years of age
Frequent tantrums (> 5 per day)
Persistent negative mood or behavior in intervals between tantrums
Recurrent tantrums at school
Destruction of property during tantrums
Harm to self or others during tantrums
Other behavioral problems (e.g., sleep disorders, aggressive behaviors, enuresis)

TABLE 29–2. Underlying Causes of Problematic Tantrums

Parent-Related Factors

Marital discord
Abusive behavior toward children
Domestic violence
Substance abuse
Depression
Inappropriate parental expectations

Child-Related Factors

Health problems
    Chronic or recurrent illnesses
    Unrecognized illnesses (e.g., otitis media, sinusitis)
Disabilities
    Hearing loss
    Speech and language difficulties
    Learning disabilities
Emotional problems (e.g., low self-esteem, depression)
Attention-deficit/hyperactivity disorder (ADHD)
Temperament

Data from Needlman, R., B. Howard, and B. Zuckerman. Temper tantrums: when to worry. Contemp. Pediatr. 6:12–34, 1989.

that provoke them, a description of actual tantrums, and parental reaction must be ascertained. In some instances, this reaction may provide insight as to why the tantrums recur. In addition, parental expectations should be assessed. Expectations that are inappropriate for children's age and developmental maturity may create unnecessary tensions between parents and children and lead to tantrum behavior. Factors associated with problematic tantrums should also be assessed (see Table 29–2).

Tantrums that are frequent (>5 per day), severe, or persist after the age of 5 years may be a sign of underlying conditions such as depression or low self-esteem. Frequent tantrums may also be associated with attention-deficit hyperactivity disorder (ADHD). Children with a history of impulsivity, hyperactivity, and inattention that are inappropriate for age should be evaluated for ADHD. Children who hurt themselves or others or destroy property during tantrums may have significant emotional problems. Peer pressure may inhibit tantrum behavior; if tantrums occur frequently at school, the presence of learning disabilities or speech and hearing deficits should be considered.

Questions: Temper Tantrums

- How often does the child have temper tantrums?
- What circumstances provoke the tantrums?
- How does the child behave during the tantrums? What does the child do?
- How does the child behave in the interval between tantrums?
- How do the parents react to the child during the tantrums? What do they do or say?
- Are parental expectations consistent with the child's developmental stage?
- Have there been any changes at home or school (e.g., birth of a sibling, new school)?
- Is the child having any other behavioral problems (e.g., enuresis, sleep difficulties)?

It is important to remember that physicians usually see children whose tantrums are frequent, severe, or cannot be controlled by parents. First, pediatricians must determine whether any underlying pathology may be contributing to the behavior and, if so, what parental or child factors may be provoking it. Second, they must differentiate between normal tantrums and problematic tantrums. Identification and remediation of the cause of problematic tantrums are the first steps toward cure. Children with suspected underlying conditions such as ADHD or mood disturbances should be referred to the appropriate specialist for further evaluation.

MANAGEMENT

Punishment is not the solution to temper tantrums (see Chapter 28, Discipline). Health maintenance visits are an ideal time to provide **anticipatory guidance** regarding tantrums and discuss strategies to prevent or minimize this behavior. Parents typically report that their children become defiant and difficult to manage during the "terrible twos." At the 12- and 15-month visits, physicians should alert parents that this period is approaching and remind them that it is a normal part of development. Preventive strategies such as **child proofing** the home to minimize unnecessary conflicts should be discussed. In addition, parents can give young children **frequent opportunities to make choices** (e.g., which color shirt to wear or which of two foods to have for lunch). These opportunities allow children to exercise independence and autonomy in a positive rather than a negative manner. Physicians can provide **reassurance** that this unpleasant stage will pass; children will eventually become more cooperative and agreeable.

Parents should be told that helping children learn self-control and how to handle anger are keys to management. To expect that children will never get angry is unrealistic. Children should be taught how to **vent their anger and frustration in an acceptable manner** (e.g., articulating their feelings, or hitting a designated punching bag or pillow). As children mature, their ability to verbalize their feelings increases, but even young toddlers can say "me angry."

Physicians should emphasize that it is **important for parents to remain calm** during children's temper tantrums. Shouting and spanking indicate to children that parents are also out of control. Children feel more secure if the adults around them are calm and in control.

Different types of temper tantrums may require specific treatment and management strategies. Parents should **be supportive** of children who are having tantrums resulting from frustration or fatigue by letting the children know that they understand. Children's energy should be redirected into activities they can do well. Parents should be encouraged to **praise positive behavior** (e.g., completing tasks properly, handling anger in an acceptable fashion). They should **ignore some tantrums,** such as those for purposes of attention seeking or wanting something. If children have no audience, they have no need to perform. **Time-outs** may also be used in such situations (see Chapter 28, Discipline). Parents should not give in to children's wishes; this may reinforce tantrum behavior. **Physical movement** of children to where they belong may be necessary if they are refusing to do something (e.g., bed for the child who is refusing to go to sleep at bedtime) or in danger of hurting themselves. **Holding children** who are raging may give them a sense of security and help calm them. If temper tantrums occur outside the home, it may be necessary to accompany children to a **quiet, private place** such as an automobile until they calm down.

Case Resolution

The child in the case scenario appears to be having normal, age-appropriate tantrums. The boy's tantrums oc-cur when he is asked to do something that he does not want to do. In these situations the parents should try to ignore the tantrums as much as possible and not give in to the child's wishes.

Selected Readings

Christophersen, E. R. Oppositional behavior in children. Pediatr. Ann. 20:267–273, 1991.

Cruikshank, B. M., and L. J. Cooper. Common behavior problems. *In* Greydanus, D. E., and M. L. Wolraich (eds.). Behavioral Pediatrics. New York, Springer-Verlag, 1992.

McIntosh, B. J. Spoiled child syndrome. Pediatrics 83:108–114, 1989.

Needlman, R., B. Howard, and B. Zuckerman. Temper tantrums: when to worry. Contemp. Pediatr. 6:12–34, 1989.

Schmitt, B. D. Temper tantrums. *In* Your Child's Health, rev. ed. New York, Bantam Books, 1991.

C H A P T E R 3 0

BREATH-HOLDING SPELLS

Geeta Grover, M.D.

H_x A 15-month-old girl is brought to the office because of parental concern about seizures. In the last month she has passed out momentarily three times. Each episode seems to be precipitated by anger or frustration on her part. Typically she cries, holds her breath, turns blue, and passes out. Each time she awakens within a few seconds and seems fine. The medical history and family history are unremarkable, and the physical examination is entirely within normal limits.

Questions

1. What are breath-holding spells (BHS)?
2. What is the differential diagnosis of BHS?
3. What, if any, laboratory studies are indicated in the evaluation of BHS?
4. What measures can be taken to prevent BHS? Are anticonvulsants necessary?
5. What, if any, are the long-term sequelae of BHS?

Breath-holding spells (BHS) are a benign, recurring condition of childhood in which anger or pain produce crying that culminates in noiseless expiration and apnea. The frequency of BHS, an involuntary phenomenon, is variable and ranges from several episodes a day to only several episodes per year. Although the spells are innocuous, they usually provoke parental fear and anxiety, because children often turn blue and become limp. The diagnosis can usually be made on the basis of a characteristic history and description of the episode, but the possibility of seizures should be considered.

EPIDEMIOLOGY

BHS occur in about 5% of all children between the ages of 6 months and 6 years, but they are most common in children between 12 and 18 months of age. The vast majority of children have experienced their first episode by 18 months and virtually all by 2 years of age. Although BHS have been described in children under 6 months of age, occurrence in such young infants is uncommon. Boys and girls are affected equally. A positive family history is found in about 25% of cases.

CLINICAL PRESENTATION

The typical clinical sequence of the two major types of BHS is described later in the chapter (see Pathophysiology and D_x Box). After the spells, children may experience a short period of drowsiness.

PATHOPHYSIOLOGY

BHS may be classified as one of the nonepileptic paroxysmal disorders of childhood. These recurrent

---

D_x Breath-Holding Spells

- Identifiable precipitating event or emotion
- Brief duration
- Color change, if present, prior to loss of consciousness and rhythmic jerking of extremities
- Rapid restoration of full activity
- Normal neurologic examination

---

conditions, which have a sudden onset and no epileptiform focus, resolve spontaneously. Other disorders in this heterogeneous group include syncope, migraine, cyclic vomiting, benign paroxysmal vertigo, paroxysmal torticollis, sleep disorders (narcolepsy, night terrors, somnambulism), and shudder attacks.

Types of Breath-Holding Spells

The two major types of BHS are **cyanotic** and **pallid**. The cyanotic type is more common. Approximately 60% of children with BHS have cyanotic spells, 20% have pallid spells, and 20% of affected children have both types. Most commonly, affected children experience several spells per week. Approximately 15% of children with breath-holding spells have complicated features. Complicated breath-holding spells are defined as typical breath-holding spells followed by seizure-like activity or rigid posturing of the body.

Cyanotic episodes are more often provoked by an upsetting event, anger, frustration, or scolding rather than by injury or fear. Children usually cry or scream loudly. The cries becomes noiseless as children open their mouths and hold their breath in expiration. After approximately 30 seconds of apnea, a color change is apparent as children become cyanotic. The spell may terminate at this point, or children may proceed to lose consciousness and become limp. Rarely, loss of consciousness may be followed by a few seconds of rhythmic clonic jerking of the extremities, mimicking seizure-like activity, or rigid opisthotonic posturing of the body. The entire attack lasts less than one minute. Children generally resume full activity within a few minutes. Unlike the postictal period of epileptic seizures, prolonged periods of lethargy or drowsiness following spells are uncommon.

Pallid spells are similar to cyanotic BHS with some exceptions. Pallid episodes are more commonly provoked by minor injury, pain, or fear rather than frustration or anger; the initial cry is minimal prior to apnea and loss of consciousness; and children become pale rather than cyanotic. In pallid BHS, children often lose consciousness or tone after only a single gasp or cry, whereas in the cyanotic form, the period of apnea prior to loss of consciousness is much longer.

Etiology

Although the spells are triggered by identifiable stimuli, they are involuntary phenomena. It is believed that loss of consciousness in both the cyanotic and pallid forms is caused by cerebral anoxia. The actual mechanisms of the two types of BHS are different. The processes involved in cyanotic BHS are not clear. Proposed mechanisms include centrally mediated inhibition of respiratory effort and altered lung mechanics, which may inappropriately stimulate pulmonary reflexes, thus resulting in apnea and hypoxia. In the pallid form, the pale coloration and loss of tone are thought to result from vagally mediated severe bradycardia or asystole. Pallid spells have been spontaneously induced in the EEG laboratory using ocular compression to trigger the oculocardiac reflex. Vagally mediated bradycardia or asystole lasting more than 2 seconds has been produced by this maneuver.

An association between iron-deficiency anemia and breath-holding spells has been recognized for many years, but is poorly understood. It may be related to iron's importance in the function of various enzymes and neurotransmitters in the central nervous system.

DIFFERENTIAL DIAGNOSIS

The differential diagnosis primarily includes seizures and syncope secondary to cardiac arrhythmia or a vasovagal episode. Although vasovagal syncope, like BHS, may be provoked by fear or pain, it is uncommon in children under 12 years of age. Three factors may help differentiate BHS from true epileptic seizure activity. First, spells are usually provoked by some upsetting event or emotion, unlike seizures, which generally do not have a recognizable precipitating event. Second, episodes are brief in duration and followed by rapid restoration of full activity. Third, color change precedes loss of consciousness and rhythmic jerking of the extremities, whereas in the typical epileptic seizure, convulsive activity and loss of muscular tone usually precede change in color. See Table 30–1 for the differential diagnosis of BHS.

EVALUATION

History

The history alone may be diagnostic (Questions Box). A family history of BHS should be obtained. It is essential to record a detailed history of the suspected breath-holding episode. The sequence in which the

---

TABLE 30–1. Differential Diagnosis of Breath-Holding Spells

Epileptic seizures
Syncope
    Cardiac arrhythmia
    Vasovagal
    Orthostatic
Benign paroxysmal vertigo
Cataplexy (transient loss of muscle tone associated with narcolepsy; rare before adolescence)
Occult or overt brainstem lesions (causing dysfunction within the pontomedullary area)
Central or obstructive apnea

Questions: Breath-Holding Spells

- What happened before the episode?
- Was the child crying?
- What was the child's color before and during the episode?
- Was the child lethargic after the episode?
- Does the family have a history of breath-holding spells?

events occurred may help differentiate BHS from epileptic seizures.

Physical Examination

Children should have a complete physical examination, including a thorough neurologic evaluation. Focal neurologic signs or evidence of structural lesions such as meningomyelocele or hydrocephalus may lead the physician away from a diagnosis of BHS.

Laboratory Tests

If the history is consistent with BHS and the physical examination is normal, laboratory evaluation is usually unnecessary. Because of the association of BHS with iron-deficiency anemia in some children, it is appropriate to determine a hemoglobin level. An EEG may be performed if the physician is concerned about the possibility of epileptic seizures. In both forms of BHS, the EEG shows generalized slowing followed by flattening (a pattern characteristic of cerebral anoxia) during attacks, although it is unusual to record the EEG during BHS. Simultaneous EEG and video recordings can be very useful in helping to distinguish breath-holding spells from seizures, especially in children having frequent episodes. The interictal EEG is normal in children with BHS, whereas it may often be abnormal in children with epilepsy. An ECG may be obtained if there is any question about cardiac arrhythmia (e.g., prolonged QT syndrome).

MANAGEMENT

Management of BHS includes **parental support and reassurance.** BHS may be extremely frightening for parents to witness, especially if the episodes are routinely associated with loss of consciousness or seizure-like activity. Parents should be told about the involuntary nature of the attacks and be cautioned against reinforcing the spells by giving in to the child's wishes. They should be advised to avoid unnecessary discipline. Similarly, it is impossible to ensure that the child will never be frustrated or injured. Instead, they should be encouraged to handle the episodes in a "matter-of-fact" manner and continue age-appropriate discipline. They should be reassured that the long-term prognosis is excellent.

Pharmacologic therapy is usually not necessary, but atropine sulfate may be considered in the management of children with frequent pallid BHS because of atropine's anticholinergic action. Anticonvulsants are not effective. A recent clinical trial showed that iron therapy was effective in the treatment of both cyanotic and pallid breath-holding spells, especially in children who were iron deficient. Referral to a neurologist or psychiatrist may be considered at the family's request if the episodes are frequent and associated with loss of consciousness or if there is uncertainty regarding the diagnosis or management.

PROGNOSIS

BHS resolve spontaneously in the vast majority of children by 5–6 years of age. About 50% of cases resolve by the age of 4 years. Neither pallid nor cyanotic BHS are associated with an increased risk of development of epilepsy, although children with pallid BHS do have an increased incidence of developing syncopal attacks during adulthood.

Case Resolution

The child presented in the opening case scenario has a history and physical examination suggestive of BHS. The girl's episodes are consistent with cyanotic BHS. The episodes are preceded by an identifiable emotion, are brief in duration, and are followed by a rapid recovery of normal consciousness and activity. Assessment of the hemoglobin level revealed mild iron-deficiency anemia. The child received iron therapy, and the parents were reassured about the benign nature of BHS.

Selected Readings

Daoud, A. S., et al. Effectiveness of iron therapy on breath-holding spells. J. Pediatr. 130:547–550, 1997.

DiMario, F. J. Breath-holding spells in childhood. Am. J. Dis. Child. 146:125–131, 1992.

Evans, O. B. Breath-holding spells. Pediatr. Ann. 26:410–414, 1997.

Golden, G. S. Nonepileptic paroxysmal events in childhood. Pediatr. Clin. North Am. 39:715–725, 1992.

Lombroso, C. T., and P. Lerman. Breath-holding spells (cyanotic and pallid infantile syncope). Pediatrics 39:563–581, 1967.

Nathanson, L. W. Breath-holding spells. *In* The Portable Pediatrician for Parents. New York, Harper Collins, 1994.

CHAPTER 31

FEARS AND PHOBIAS

Carol D. Berkowitz, M.D.

H$_x$ A 5-year-old girl is brought into the office by her mother, who complains that her daughter has been frightened of sleeping alone since the occurrence of an earthquake. The house did not sustain any significant damage, but the entire family was awakened. The mother says that the girl has become more timid. As nighttime approaches, she becomes particularly fearful. She will not stay in her bed, and she is comforted only by sleeping with her parents. In addition, the girl has had some bed-wetting accidents since the earthquake, and the mother wonders whether she should put her daughter in diapers. The physical examination, including the vital signs, is normal, except for the observation that the child is very clingy and whiny.

Questions

1. What are normal childhood fears?
2. When do these fears commonly occur?
3. What strategies are used to deal with these fears?
4. What are simple phobias? What are social phobias?
5. What is school phobia and how is it best handled?

Fears are normal feelings that cause emotional, behavioral, and physiologic changes that are essential for survival. Fears are associated with psychological discomforts such as a negative, unpleasant feeling. Children may develop fears in response to actual events (e.g., earthquakes) or as a result of the temporal association of two events (e.g., seeing a scary movie on a rainy day and then becoming afraid of rain). Some fears appear to be innate, and others seem to be developmental. Children fear different things at different ages. For example, school phobia is sometimes particularly problematic in young, school-age children.

Phobias are overwhelming, intense, highly specific, and often irrational fears. Social phobias are specific to social situations that arouse intense concerns about humiliation or embarrassment. Fear of speaking in public may represent a social phobia. When these fears are combined with avoidance behavior, they may be incapacitating. Anxiety refers to fear without a definable source. It is a vague feeling of uneasiness, apprehension, and foreboding of impending doom.

Different strategies are useful for dealing with different fears. It is important for parents not to trivialize these fears, nor to reinforce them, but to empower children to deal with them.

It is also important to realize that parents sometimes foster fears by using threats with children such as "the doctor will give you a shot unless you eat your spinach" or "the boogie man will get you." By fostering fears, the parents are also fostering dependency. Parents lack the imagination that children have and find it difficult to understand the degree of fear that children experience.

FEARS CHARACTERISTIC OF CHILDREN OF VARIOUS AGES

Fears follow a developmental pattern. Neonates are believed to have no fear, although young infants whose faces are covered with a blanket struggle to toss off the blanket. Infants who are 6 months of age exhibit what is known as **stranger anxiety** in response to unfamiliar persons, places, or objects. To combat this anxiety, infants seek refuge with a parent. Stranger anxiety becomes equated with separation anxiety and reaches a peak at 2 years of age. Children between 6 months and 2 years of age are also frightened by loud noises and falling or quickly moving objects.

Children between the ages of 2 and 5 years are in what is termed the **"age of anxiety."** They fear many things, including animals, abandonment, loud noises, and darkness. Children in this age group are particularly fearful of physicians, hospitals, and getting hurt. Young children are afraid of the physically disabled, who represent bodily injury, and monsters and scary movies. They sometimes displace their anger onto monsters and witches and attribute to these imaginary characters the bad feelings they are experiencing. Children in this age group have strong imaginations, which makes it difficult for them to differentiate fantasy from reality.

School-age children between 6 years of age and adolescence tend to have more abstract thoughts, and their fears are less relevant to physical immediacy. These children are afraid of the death of their parents or the burning of their home. They also fear war, growing up (expressed as "How will I know what to do?"), going into the next grade, being alone or being kidnapped, and the divorce of their parents. Children in this age group are often reluctant to bother their parents with their fears, and they can easily misinterpret parental concerns when they overhear parental conversation.

Separation anxiety, which may appear as school phobia, may also be evident in school-age children. It is defined as developmentally inappropriate, excessive anxiety precipitated by actual or anticipated separation from home or family. Affected children develop physical complaints (e.g., stomachaches) on school days. The mother-child relationship is often disturbed, and the child is fearful of leaving the parent alone. The prevalence of school phobia is reported to be less than 5%. Childhood school phobia and parental history of panic attacks and agoraphobia may be associated.

Fears during adolescence relate to social functioning such as public speaking or talking to members of the opposite sex. Older children are also concerned about school failure and physical injury. They have many of the same fears expressed by younger school-age children, although phobias are uncommon. Phobias, which occur in less than 1.7% of the general population, are reported in 13% of disturbed children.

Panic disorders are rare in childhood, but more common during adolescence. They involve the sudden onset of intense fear or discomfort associated with physiologic symptoms such as palpitations and shortness of breath. Fear about a panic attack may lead to agoraphobia, the avoidance of going away from home.

PATHOPHYSIOLOGY

Fear has its basis in a series of psychophysiologic reactions, which are mediated through a series of neurotransmitters. Elevated levels of certain transmitters such as γ-aminobutyric acid and norepinephrine are associated with feelings of anxiety. Excess serotonin has also been related to anxiety disorders. Patients with panic attacks and anxiety disorders have disturbances in neurotransmitter regulation.

DIFFERENTIAL DIAGNOSIS

The challenge for physicians is to assess the etiology of the fear and to differentiate normal fears from those which may be signs of unusual stresses or signs of psychopathology. Appropriate fears represent a real reaction to a real danger. As a rule, children are more resilient than adults and recover more rapidly from traumatic events. On the other hand, children are prone to inappropriate fears, which may develop for a number of reasons.

Inappropriate fears may occur because of operant conditioning, in which a conditioned stimulus becomes associated with another object. Fear for the other object becomes reinforced through this association. Inappropriate fears may also develop in a child whose parent has the fear (modeling) or through witnessing a fearful event in the media (informational). True phobias represent neuroses and may occur in more than one family member.

School phobia, also called school refusal, may occur under three distinct conditions. Not uncommonly, young children who are entering school for the first time are frightened. This fear is a normal component of separation anxiety, which usually resolves within a few days of starting school. In contrast, older children may experience school phobia because they are truly afraid of a school situation. They may fear a teacher, violence, or a bully. To avoid the problem, children may actually request to change classrooms or schools. It is important to talk to children to find out what is behind their fear of school.

On the other hand, some children who appear fearful of school are actually concerned about parental separation (i.e., separation anxiety). Frequently these children enjoy school and miss attending it. Absences occur when feelings of separation from parents are so intense that they do not allow children to function well in school settings. This separation anxiety may result from parental illness or parents' fostering dependency in children. Children then see parents as vulnerable and are uncomfortable about leaving them alone.

School refusal is the third leading cause of school absenteeism after transient illness and truancy. Fifty percent of children with school refusal have other problems, including depression (28%), tantrums (18%), sleep disturbances (17%), obsessive-compulsive behavior (11%), other fears (10%), enuresis (3%), and learning disabilities (3%). Overall, school refusal has a good prognosis, although adolescents do not do as well as younger children, and individuals with a higher IQ have a poorer outcome. Twenty percent of parents of children with school refusal have a diagnosable psychiatric disorder. Issues of mother-child dependency are often a concern.

Another type of childhood fear concerns physicians and hospitals. Children have many concerns about what happens to them at the doctor's office. They are particularly fearful of needles. To children, needles represent possible mutilation. When asked to represent needles in drawings, children often portray needles as larger than themselves and very pointed. They comment that needles are sharp (e.g., "needles can make you pop, just like a balloon"; "needles can also take out all your blood until you die"). In addition, children are preoccupied with what happens to their blood. One youngster commented, "They check out your blood to see if it's good or bad, and if your blood is bad, then it means that you need to have more tests."

Hospitalization raises other issues concerning parental separation as well as painful procedures. As children adjust to hospitalization, they progress through three stages: protest, during which they complain about the hospital and cry; despair, during which they have given up hope that their parents will return; and detachment, during which they seem to be adjusting but actually have distanced themselves from their parents.

EVALUATION

Physicians should explore the area of childhood fears and phobias at routine health maintenance visits, even if parents do not have specific concerns. Sometimes parents are embarrassed by children's fears (e.g., the fear of an older child to sleep without a night light). Parents may not report children's fears unless these fears seem to be unusually intense. Practitioners may ask children, "What is the scariest thing you can think of?" If children are having difficulty providing details, physicians may ask them to name things that other children fear or to complete the sentence, "I feel afraid when _____ ." Alternatively, practitioners may suggest things that other children may fear: "Do the kids you know seem to be worried about kidnapping?"

History

The evaluation of children with specific fears demands a careful history that provides information about situations in which children are fearful (Questions Box). Physicians should consider fears within a developmental context, because many childhood fears are normal and experienced by all children. It is also important to look at changes in the family situation. Children sometimes develop what appear to be fears but in fact are behaviors designed to manipulate other family members. For instance, young children who sense marital discord may insist on sleeping with their parents as a way of ensuring that the parents are together rather than separate.

Physical Examination

A routine examination is warranted, but findings are usually normal.

Laboratory Tests

As a rule, laboratory tests are not required.

MANAGEMENT

The management of the fear or phobia is determined by the degree to which children are incapacitated. As a general rule, **children should be empowered to conquer their fears.** Children's books that address the issues of certain fears can help achieve this empowerment. Books such as *The Berenstain Bears in the Dark* (Random House, 1982) discuss specific worries such as fear of lightning and thunder. These books often explain the basis of such natural phenomena in easy-to-understand terms. The books also normalize particular fears and show how one character is fearful. Parents can also re-create some of the sounds that children fear. For example, children who are afraid of the noise the wind makes are shown a teakettle where the hot steam blows through the whistle, creating the same noise as the wind. For fears about nuclear war, empowering children to become active, such as joining a nuclear protest group, may be useful.

Parents may feel helpless because they do not know how to deal with children's fears. Physicians should give them the necessary information. Children's fears should not be trivialized. Even if the **fears** are unfounded, they should be validated. In general, children should be questioned about whether they are fearful about a situation. The following two examples illustrate the proper handling of fears in children.

If children are visiting the dentist for the first time, it is appropriate for parents to ask, "Are you afraid?" If children reply, "Yes, a little bit," parents can say, "Almost everybody is afraid. Tell me what it is you're afraid of. Fear is a normal emotion, and I'm glad you told me about it."

Parents of children who express fear of imaginary characters can reassure children that they do not exist. In addition, parents can tell children what the parents would do if such characters did exist. For instance, the father of a little girl who was afraid of witches told her, "There are no such things as witches. But if there were, and they came into your room, I would punch them in the nose and punch them in the stomach and beat them up, and then there would be no more witches to hurt you." By doing this, parents establish the reality of the situation and then also create a plan to deal with the problem should it actually happen.

Parents can also help to limit or reduce children's fears by **minimizing** their **exposure to fear-provoking situations** such as television shows or scary movies. These programs can be particularly frightening for some children, who should not watch them without adult supervision.

When dealing with children who have school phobia because of problems in school, it is important to determine if a change in school would be appropriate to facilitate their school attendance. This may be particularly appropriate in children whose schools are plagued with violence.

If, on the other hand, children's refusal to attend school is linked to separation anxiety, then a program of **desensitization** is recommended. Desensitization may involve the participation of mothers in the classroom for a period of time. When children acclimate and can tolerate some separation, mothers move to another area in the school such as the principal's office. Next they go outside the school grounds. As children reestablish a sense of well-being in spite of the separation, the mothers gradually move farther and farther away. This solution is somewhat problematic for mothers who work outside the home. Children with significant school refusal may need the assistance of child psychologists or psychiatrists.

Phobias may be treated using the concept of **flooding,** which consists of rapid, prolonged exposure to the feared item. For example, a child who is afraid of dogs is exposed to a friendly, docile, small dog while in the company of his or her parents. Alternatively, systematic desensitization, during which children are exposed to the feared objects over a series of weeks, coupled with relaxation techniques, is also utilized. Phobias usually require the help of mental health specialists. The routine use of **medications** such as benzodiazepines to control anxiety or propranolol to lessen the peripheral autonomic nervous system symptoms of social phobias is not usually recommended. Medications are, however, useful in the treatment of panic disorder.

Children who must undergo hospitalization benefit from a prehospital visit, when possible. This visit familiarizes the child with the facilities and explains proposed procedures. Many hospitals have child life specialists who ease the adjustment of children as well as their parents to the hospital stay.

PROGNOSIS

Most childhood fears resolve with time, nurturing, and reassurance. Most fears last only several weeks, and then new fears develop. As a rule, specific fears should not last longer than 2 years, and the younger the child, the shorter the duration of the fear.

Prognosis is good for children with true phobias, with 100% resolution of monosymptomatic phobias.

Case Resolution

In the case scenario, the girl's fear of sleeping in her bed was triggered by a significant environmental event. Although earthquakes are uncontrollable, the girl can be empowered to deal with manageable aspects of an earthquake as much as possible. She should be assured that in the same situation, many adults probably would also fear sleeping alone. The parents should stock a box with shoes, flashlight, radio, and water and place the box under the child's bed. In addition, they may also have their daughter get into her bed and then shake it, simulating the jiggling that she would experience during an earthquake. The girl should also practice getting out of bed and standing in the doorway. To combat the child's fear of separation during times of natural disaster, the parents should reassure their daughter that they will all be together.

Selected Readings

Physicians

American Psychiatric Association. Diagnostic and Statistical Manual of Mental Disorders, 4th rev. ed. Washington, DC, American Psychiatric Association, 1994.

Emotions and moods. *In* Wolraich, M. L. (ed.). The Classification of Child and Adolescent Mental Diagnoses in Primary Care. Elk Grove Village, IL, American Academy of Pediatrics, 1996. pp. 145–149.

Jellinek, M. S., and M. E. Kearns. Separation anxiety. Pediatr. Rev. 16:57–61, 1995.

Klein, R. G., H. S. Koplewicz, and A. Kanner. Imipramine treatment of children with separation anxiety disorder. J. Am. Acad. Child Adolesc. Psychiatry 31:21, 1992.

Klein, R. G., and C. G. Last. Anxiety Disorders in Children. Newbury Park, CA, Sage Publications, 1989.

McMenamy, C., and R. C. Katz. Brief parent-assisted treatment for children's nighttime fears. J. Dev. Behav. Pediatr. 10:145–148, 1989.

Sarafino, E. P. The Fears of Childhood. New York, Human Sciences Press, 1986.

Scholwalter, J. E. Fears and phobias. Pediatr. Rev. 15:384–388, 1994.

Parents and Children

Berenstain, S., and J. Berenstain. The Berenstain Bears and the Bully. New York, Random House, 1993.

Berenstain, S., and J. Berenstain. The Berenstain Bears in the Dark. New York, Random House, 1982.

Berenstain, S., and J. Berenstain. The Berenstain Bears Visit the Dentist. New York, Random House, 1981.

Ziefert, H. Nicky's Noisy Night. New York, Penguin Books, 1986.

CHAPTER 32

THUMB SUCKING AND OTHER HABITS

Carol D. Berkowitz, M.D.

H$_x$ A 5-year-old boy is brought to the office because of thumb sucking. His mother claims that she has tried nearly everything, including tying his hands at night and using aversive treatments on his thumbs, but nothing has worked. She reports that her son has been teased at school and has few friends. He is in good general health, and his immunizations are up to date.

His growth parameters are at the 50th percentile. Except for a callus on the right thumb, the physical examination is normal.

Questions

1. What are common habits in children?
2. What is the significance of transitional objects?
3. What are the consequences of the common habits in children?
4. What are strategies used to break children of habits?

Habits are defined as somewhat complicated, repetitive behaviors. They are different from tics, which are rapid, repetitive muscle twitches involving the head, face, or shoulders. Tics are also referred to as habit spasms (see Chapter 96, Tics). Children have many socially unacceptable habits, including thumb sucking, nail biting, hair pulling (trichotillomania), rocking, biting other children, and teeth grinding (bruxism). Some habits, such as pica, are potentially harmful. Children engage in most of these habits because of their soothing potential.

One third of children use transitional objects for comfort. Blankets or favorite toys are traditional transitional objects that represent an age-appropriate coping mechanism. Most transitional objects are strokable, and the stroking often occurs in association with thumb sucking. Transitional objects sometimes present a problem because children experience distress if these objects are lost, misplaced, or need cleaning.

EPIDEMIOLOGY

Thumb sucking probably represents the most common habit of children. A reported 50–87% of children engage in this habit. The median age for the onset of hand sucking is 54 minutes of life, and 90% of newborns show hand sucking behavior by the age of 2 hours. Forty percent of children between the ages of 1 and 3 years, 33% of children between the ages of 3 and 5, and 25% of children at the age of 5 still suck their thumbs. Some children suck their fingers rather than thumbs.

Other oral behavior may involve lip sucking, lip biting, and toe sucking. Lip sucking and biting begin at about 5–6 months of age and occur in about 90% of infants. It is unusual for these actions to persist as habits. Toe sucking is noted in infants who are 6–7 months of age, and it is reported in 80% of normal infants.

Trichotillomania is a disorder once believed to be uncommon but now thought to affect eight million Americans (about five per thousand). The term, first coined in 1889, refers to alopecia from compulsive hair pulling. Hair pulling may involve hair from the head, eyebrows, eyelashes, or pubic area. Although trichotillomania appears to peak during early childhood and adolescence, the disorder is reported from infancy to adolescence. In young children, boys and girls are equally affected, but in older children and adolescents, females outnumber males.

Rhythmic habits are stereotypic, repetitive behaviors that usually occur in infants under the age of 1 year. These habits are reported in 15–20% of the population. Rhythmic habits include rocking (about 19% of infants), when infants rock back and forth; jouncing (5–10%), when they move up-and-down on their hands and knees so that the whole crib rocks; head rolling (8%); and head banging (5%). Rhythmic habits are seen more commonly in boys; the male-female ratio is 3:1. These habits usually occur with a frequency of 60 to 80 movements per minute, often when infants are tired, and last for less than 15 minutes before they fall sleep.

Rhythmic movements have been equated with **sleep tics.** These tics are reported in 20% of children, most often between the ages of 6 and 10 years. As a rule, tics are three times more common in boys than in girls. They tend to be noted with increased frequency in children who are shy, overly self-conscious, or have obsessive-compulsive tendencies. Tics usually occur when children are under stress.

Biting, an aggressive habit noted in toddlers, may be related to teething. It occurs more often in children with slow verbal skills.

Nail biting (onychophagia) is usually believed to be a sign of internal tension. The disorder affects 10–40% of children. Nail biting begins between the ages of 3 and 6, and the peak age is 13 years. One third of adolescents bite their nails, but 50% of these adolescents break the habit by the time they reach adulthood. Nail biting in adults is regarded as a sign of emotional and social immaturity and regression. The family history for nail biting is often positive. Identical twins are concordant for the condition in 66% of cases. In contrast, the incidence in dizygotic twins is 34%.

Pica, which is not a normal behavior, is defined as the ingestion of nonfood products. The peak incidence of pica is between the ages of 1 and 3 years. The incidence is increased in children from lower socioeconomic levels, and the behavior occurs in 10% of children who present with lead poisoning.

Teeth grinding (bruxism) is reported in 5–15% of children. Boys are more commonly affected than girls, and the disorder appears to regress later in life. It is reported with increased incidence among mentally retarded children. The cause is unknown, although it may be associated with malocclusion in some children.

CLINICAL PRESENTATION

Children with common habits, such as thumb sucking or rhythmic movements, may be brought to the physician with these particular complaints because the parent wants advice about stopping the behavior. Other children may present with consequences of habits, such as alopecia (trichotillomania), paronychia (nail biting), or lead intoxication (pica) (D$_x$ Box).

PSYCHOPHYSIOLOGY

Children engage in habits to reduce stress and provide comfort. Thumb sucking is related to nonnutritive sucking. Although the initial purpose of sucking is nutritional, the pleasure associated with sucking reinforces the behavior. Infants who are served from a cup from birth develop no interest in sucking. Humans and other primates spend more time in nonnutritive than in nutritive sucking. Monkeys use a five-point hold, with two hands, two feet, and mouth (holding on to their mother's nipple) for attachment. Universal thumb sucking is noted even in orphan monkeys, and sucking is thought to be an important aspect of environmental adaptation. Nonnutritive sucking occurs even in the

---

D$_x$ Childhood Habits

- History of a habit
- Callus on thumb or fingers
- Short, chewed nails
- Alopecia
- Lead intoxication
- Iron deficiency anemia

absence of fatigue, hunger, or discomfort, and has a purpose in itself—to provide comfort and be self-soothing. The maximum intensity of sucking occurs at 7 months.

In bottle-fed infants, thumb sucking appears to commence when feeding stops. Some infants, described as "type A," seem to be satisfied only when their thumb is in their mouth. As infants spend more time engaged in motor activity, they spend less time thumb sucking. Placid infants who cry less also do less sucking. Some studies have shown that thumb sucking is less common in breast-fed infants, and that thumb suckers as a group feed less frequently (every 4 hours rather than 3 and for 10 minutes rather than 20).

Nail biting is related to thumb sucking, a form of oral gratification, and children may progress from thumb sucking to nail biting. The pattern of nail biting usually involves placement of the hand in the vicinity of the mouth, tapping of the fingers along the teeth, quick spasmodic bites with the fingers around the central incisors, and the removal and inspection of the hands. Other oral habits, such as pencil gnawing, gum chewing, lip biting, and nail picking are related activities, as is nose picking. The cause of teeth grinding is unclear.

Rocking habits are believed to be kinesthetically pleasing and soothing and a means of autostimulation. The etiology of hair pulling is less apparent. In recent years, investigators have linked trichotillomania to disorders of serotonin reuptake and placed it in the category of obsessive-compulsive behavior. Some individuals who engage in trichotillomania have abnormal head positron emission tomography. Pica, which is also considered abnormal, may be associated with mental retardation, environmental deprivation, or inadequate nutrition, particularly iron deficiency.

DIFFERENTIAL DIAGNOSIS

The differential diagnosis of most habits is not difficult. Tics or habit spasms should be differentiated from Tourette's syndrome. This syndrome, which is reported in 1 in 3000 children, is a neurologic disorder characterized by severe, frequent, and multiple tics. These tics are also often vocal and consist of sounds such as hissing, barking, grunting, or coprolalia (repeating profanities). Some of the rhythmic habits may be mistaken for seizures but can be easily distinguished because of the stereotypic, repetitive nature of the behavior.

Trichotillomania usually has a classic physical appearance that has been referred to as the "tonsure Friar Tuck" pattern baldness, with baldness around the vertex of the head. Unilateral temporal baldness is also a consequence of trichotillomania. The differential diagnosis of trichotillomania includes alopecia areata, tinea capitis, syphilitic alopecia, and androgenic alopecia (see Chapter 98, Disorders of the Hair and Scalp). Alopecia secondary to trichotillomania is usually characterized by broken hairs of variable length. Other disorders in the differential diagnosis include traction alopecia, related to tight braids or hair brushing; atopic eczema; seborrheic dermatitis; hypothyroidism; systemic lupus erythematosus (SLE); and dermatomyositis.

EVALUATION

Habits must be evaluated in the context of the child's developmental level and home situation. Children who present with thumb sucking, nail biting, and teeth grinding usually do not require an assessment other than a routine health maintenance history and physical examination. The physical examination may reveal thumb calluses, candidal infection of the nails, or evidence of malocclusion with an overbite (Fig. 32-1). Children who present with movements that resemble tics should be carefully questioned about the frequency and duration of the tics, the effect of the tics on their behavior, and whether coughing is associated with the tics (sign of Tourette's syndrome). The occurrence of obsessive-compulsive mannerisms should also be noted. A careful neurologic examination should be performed in children with tics.

Children with trichotillomania should be evaluated for the disorders listed above. An easy evaluation process for trichotillomania involves shaving the hair in the middle of the area of baldness. The growth of these small hairs is uniform because children are unable to pull them out. Disorders such as syphilis and collagen vascular diseases can be ruled out using appropriate laboratory studies. Fungal infections can be differentiated by the use of appropriate cultures. A Wood's lamp examination may reveal fluorescence noted with certain fungal infections.

Children who present with pica should be evaluated for the presence of iron deficiency anemia and lead poisoning.

MANAGEMENT

The management of childhood habits should be directed at the specific symptoms. The issue of thumb sucking versus the use of pacifiers can be addressed by anticipatory guidance. **Pacifiers,** which were initially

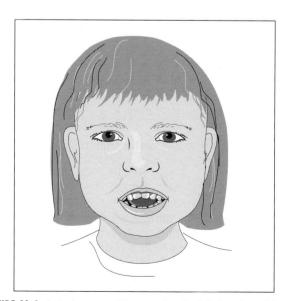

FIGURE 32-1. Anterior open bite associated with thumb sucking.

discouraged, are now believed to have some advantages over thumb sucking. With pacifiers, the risk for dental disturbances is lower, because the pacifiers are softer and are accompanied by a plastic shield that puts counter pressure on the teeth. Pacifiers are also detachable and cleanable.

Pacifiers can be lost, however. Parents should be advised not to attach a pacifier to the child's shirt with a string because of risk of strangulation. For children who are pacifier-dependent and are unable to go back to sleep if they lose their pacifier at night, multiple pacifiers can be placed in the crib to make finding one easier. For infants who desire pacifiers because they complete their feeding in under 20 minutes, a nipple with a smaller hole can be used or the cap can be screwed on the bottle more tightly to prolong the time spent in nutritive sucking. Dental problems may develop when pacifiers are used upside down, all day long, or after the eruption of permanent dentition.

It is suggested that parents do not try to stop thumb sucking behavior until children have reached the age of four years. Dental problems in late thumb suckers include anterior open bite, increased overjet (protruding upper incisors), intruded and flared upper incisors, lingually flipped lower incisors, and warped alveolar ridge. When thumb sucking persists to school age, tongue-thrust is noted, as are articulation problems, specifically with consonants s, t, d, n, z, l, and r. The physician should reassure parents that children who stop sucking their thumb prior to the onset of the secondary dentition are not at risk for poor dentition.

Numerous devices have been proposed to help with the cessation of thumb sucking, but reported success has been variable. The use of arm restraints, particularly at night, is not recommended and may result in rumination. Bitter paints such as Stop Zit seek to reduce thumb sucking by subjecting children to a bitter, aversive taste. This medication consists of 49% toluene, 19% isopropyl alcohol, 18% butyl acetate, 11% ethylcellulose, and 0.3% denatonium benzoate. A ¾-ounce bottle is toxic if ingested in its entirety. The principle of retraining, where thumb sucking becomes a duty and children are required to suck all ten fingers, one at a time, has also been recommended. Some recommend that elastic bandages be put on the hand of nocturnal thumb suckers. Problems associated with thumb sucking include sore thumbs, calluses and candidal infections. Dentists may fashion a reminder appliance, called a palatal crib, making it difficult for children to suck their thumbs.

Encouragement works better than nagging, as a rule, and a **reward system** is particularly useful in children who are 5–6 years of age. Parents may be referred to books such as *Danny and His Thumb* (K.F. Ernst; Prentice-Hall, Englewood Cliffs, NJ, 1973) and encouraged to talk to their children about how good it feels not to suck their thumb. A star chart and diary are also useful. Sometimes telling children something like, "Mommy would be so proud of you if you didn't suck your thumb now that you're such a big girl or a big boy" is effective. In addition, the pressure to stop thumb sucking becomes greater during the school years.

Children who suck their thumbs are regarded by their peers in first grade as less intelligent, less happy, less likable, and less desirable as friends.

In children who suck their thumbs and twirl their hair at the same time, the hair twirling stops once the thumb sucking ends. Hair pulling in young children seems to often resolve spontaneously but is more problematic in adolescents and adults. In children, behavior modification, including putting socks on the hands and the use of time out for hair pulling, in addition to extra attention for not pulling the hair, is recommended. In older individuals, hair pulling may be related to obsessive-compulsive disorders. Trichotillomania may lead to the presence of bezoars (hairballs) from swallowed hair. The results of treatment with agents such as isocarboxazid, amitriptyline, clomipramine, fluoxetine, and clonazepam are more successful in adults than in children.

Nail biting also often responds to behavior modification. Olive oil may be put on the nails to make them soft so there are fewer jagged edges to bite.

Rhythmic habits are less easy to modify. For the most part, reassurance is all that is available. The use of metronomelike devices has had no demonstrable effect. Children over the age of 3 years who disturb the family's sleep with their rhythmic habits may be given mild sedatives such as diphenhydramine. Medications to reduce head banging include transdermal clonidine and thioridazine (Mellaril). Other maneuvers involve placing the crib or bed on carpeting to decrease the amount of noise from movement.

Children who engage in biting behavior should be managed with behavior modification, including praising of good behavior and time out for inappropriate behavior.

Iron deficiency resulting from pica requires iron supplementation. Lead intoxication should be managed with chelation and environmental manipulation.

PROGNOSIS

Most habits are not harmful to children's health. The major problem is social acceptability. Parents should be encouraged to stop a habit before it becomes ingrained. This can often be done by praising good behavior and encouraging activities during which the unwanted behavior does not appear. Habits that do not respond to parental influence often resolve spontaneously under peer pressure.

Case Resolution

In the case history presented at the beginning of the chapter, it is important for the physician and the mother to empower the boy to stop thumb sucking before he finds himself ridiculed by his classmates. He might be allowed to suck his thumb at certain times and in certain places (e.g., "You can suck in your room after school for fifteen minutes"). Books geared at children and parents to help stop the thumb sucking are recommended, and the boy is rewarded for times when he is not sucking his thumb.

Selected Readings

Blum, N. J., V. J. Barone, and P. C. Friman. A simplified behavioral treatment for trichotillomania: report of two cases. Pediatrics 91:993–995, 1993.

Brazelton, T. B. Sucking in infancy. Pediatrics 17:400–404, 1956.

Dimino-Emme, L., and C. Camisa. Trichotillomania associated with the "Friar Tuck sign" and nail biting. Cutis 47:107–110, 1991.

Friman, P. C., and B. Schmitt. Thumb sucking in childhood: guidelines for the pediatrician. Clin. Pediatr. 28:438–440, 1989.

Friman, P. C., et al. Influence of thumb sucking on peer social acceptance in first-grade children. Pediatrics 91:784–786, 1993.

Johnson, E. and B. Larson. Thumb-sucking: Literature review. J. A.S.D.C. Dent. Child. 60:385–391, 1993.

Peterson, J. E., and P. E. Schneider. Oral habits: a behavioral approach. Pediatr. Clin. North Am. 38:1289–1307, 1991.

Repetitive behavioral patterns. In Wolraich, M. L. (ed.). The Classification of Child and Adolescent Mental Diagnoses in Primary Care. Elk Grove Village, IL, American Academy of Pediatrics, 1996, pp. 269–275.

Rosenberg, M. D. Thumbsucking. Pediatr. Rev. 16:73–74, 1995.

Schmitt, B. Helping the child with tics (twitches). Contemp. Pediatr. 8:31–32, 1991.

CHAPTER 33

ENURESIS

Carol D. Berkowitz, M.D.

H$_x$ A 9-year-old boy who is in good general health is evaluated for a history of bed-wetting. He is the product of a normal pregnancy and delivery and achieved his developmental milestones at the appropriate time. The boy was toilet trained by the age of 3 years, but he has never been dry at night for more than several days at a time. Enuresis occurs at least three to four times a week even if he is fluid-restricted after 6 PM. The boy never wets himself during the day, has normal stools, and is an average student. His father had enuresis that resolved by the time he was 12 years old.

The boy's physical examination is entirely normal.

Questions

1. What conditions account for the symptoms of enuresis?
2. What is the appropriate evaluation of children with enuresis?
3. What is the relationship between enuresis and emotional stresses or psychosocial disorders?
4. What management plans are available for enuresis?
5. How do physicians decide which management technique is appropriate for which patients?

Enuresis is defined as involuntary or intentional urination in children whose age and development suggest achievement of bladder control. Voiding into the bed or clothing occurs repeatedly (at least twice a week for at least 3 consecutive months). Urinary continence is reached earlier in girls than in boys, and the diagnosis of enuresis is reserved for girls over the age of 5 years and boys over the age of 6. Diurnal enuresis is wetting that occurs during the day. Nocturnal or sleep enuresis refers to involuntary urination that occurs during the night. The term **primary enuresis** is used when children have never achieved sustained dryness, and **secondary enuresis** is used when urinary incontinence recurs after 3–6 months of dryness. Monosymptomatic nocturnal enuresis means that nighttime wetting is the only complaint. Children who experience urgency, frequency, dribbling, or other symptoms have polysymptomatic enuresis.

Physicians can be particularly helpful by routinely questioning parents about bed-wetting during health maintenance visits. Many families are otherwise reluctant to bring up this embarrassing complaint, because enuresis is viewed as socially unacceptable. It poses particular difficulties if children wish to sleep away from home. In addition, enuresis may be a marker for other behavioral problems.

EPIDEMIOLOGY

Enuresis affects 5–7 million patients in the United States. It is one of the most common conditions of childhood, affecting 10–20% of first-grade boys and 8–17% of first-grade girls. By age 10 years, 5–10% of boys have enuresis (1% of army recruits are enuretic). Seventy-four percent of affected children have nocturnal enuresis, 10% diurnal enuresis, and 16% both. Primary enuresis affects the large majority (75–80%) of children with enuresis. Although the overall incidence of secondary enuresis is lower (20–25%), it increases with age; secondary enuresis makes up 50% of cases of enuresis in children 12 years of age.

Several epidemiologic factors have been associated with enuresis, including low socioeconomic level, large

D_x	**Enuresis**

- Bed-wetting
- Old enough to be toilet trained
- Precipitating problem such as diabetes or UTI
- Encopresis
- ADHD
- Family history of enuresis

family size, single-parent family, low birth weight, short height at 11–15 years of age, immature behavior, relatively low IQ, poor speech and coordination, and encopresis (fecal incontinence; 5–15% of cases). Enuresis occurs more often in institutionalized children. Enuresis has a familial basis, and as many as 77% of children are enuretic if both parents were similarly affected. Concordance for enuresis is reported in 68% of monozygotic twins and 48% of dizygotic twins.

CLINICAL PRESENTATION

A history of enuresis may be obtained as a presenting complaint or elicited by physicians during a health maintenance visit. Medical complaints such as encopresis or ADHD may be associated with the enuresis (D_x Box). The physical examination is usually normal.

PATHOPHYSIOLOGY

Delayed control of micturition has several possible causes (Table 33–1).

1. **Faulty toilet training.** Faulty toilet training may perpetuate both diurnal and nocturnal enuresis but is not expected to selectively perpetuate the latter. Parental expectations are believed to play a role in the toilet training experience. Parents who allow children to sleep in diapers may be delaying the achievement of nighttime dryness, but it is unlikely that the use of diapers causes nocturnal enuresis. Poor toilet habits, particularly infrequent voiding or constipation, may be associated with UTIs.

2. **Maturational delay.** The development of the inhibitory reflex of voiding may be delayed in some children, which may contribute to enuresis until the age of 5 years. It is unlikely that maturational delay persists as

a cause of enuresis beyond this age. Experts believe that maturational delay is not a reasonable explanation if children can achieve dryness in the daytime but not at night.

3. **Small bladder capacity.** Evidence suggests that some children with enuresis have smaller bladder capacities. Bladder capacity in ounces is estimated as the age in years plus two. For example, five-year-old children have a bladder capacity of 7 ounces (210 mL). Adult bladder capacity is 12–16 ounces (360–480 mL). Small bladder capacity is associated with diurnal frequency or incontinence.

4. **Sleep disorder/impaired arousal.** It has been suggested that children with enuresis are in "deep sleep" and do not sense a full bladder. However, studies have shown that enuresis occurs during all stages of sleep, particularly in the first one third of sleep and in transition from non-REM stage 4 to REM sleep. During this period body tone, respiratory rate, and heart rate increase, and erection and micturition occur. Children with enuresis do not appear to sleep more deeply than other children. However, enuretic children may have dimished arousal during sleep. In one study, 40% of enuretic children, compared to only 8.5% of nonenuretic children, failed to awaken to an 80 db noise.

5. **Allergens.** No evidence confirms the notion that exposure to certain foods (e.g., food additives, sugar) contributes to enuresis. However, some parents believe that bed-wetting is decreased if certain foods such as sodas and sweets are eliminated from the diet. The ingestion of caffeine-containing beverages may exacerbate nocturnal enuresis.

6. **Nocturnal polyuria/relative vasopressin deficiency.** Research has shown that although nonenuretic children exhibit a diurnal variation in vasopressin secretion, this rhythm is disturbed in some children with enuresis, resulting in nocturnal polyuria.

7. **Dysfunctional bladder contraction.** In cases of diurnal enuresis, contractile disturbances of the bladder affect normal voiding. Children with an "uninhibited bladder" have not learned to inhibit bladder contraction. They may assume a certain posture, called Vincent's curtsy, in an effort to prevent micturition. Some children exhibit discoordinated, incomplete voiding and the urine exits the urethra in a staccato stream. Trabeculations or bladder wall thickening may be noted on imaging studies.

DIFFERENTIAL DIAGNOSIS

Primary nocturnal enuresis is usually related to the conditions discussed in Pathophysiology. An organic problem is rarely the cause. However, secondary enuresis frequently results from an organic problem, such as UTI, diabetes mellitus, diabetes insipidus, nocturnal seizures, genitourinary anomalies (e.g., ectopic ureter), sickle cell anemia, medication (e.g., diuretics, theophylline), or emotional stress. When primary enuresis is both diurnal and nocturnal, some of these conditions should also be considered. Additional diagnoses include neurogenic bladder, which may occur in association with cerebral palsy, sacral agenesis, or myelomeningocoele.

TABLE 33–1. Causes of Enuresis

Primary Enuresis	Secondary Enuresis
Faulty toilet training	Urinary tract infection
Maturational delay	Diabetes mellitus
Small bladder capacity	Diabetes insipidus
Sleep disorder/impaired arousal	Nocturnal seizures
Allergens	Genitourinary anomalies
Nocturnal polyuria/relative vasopressin deficiency	Sickle cell anemia
	Medication use
	Emotional stress

EVALUATION

History

A thorough history should be obtained when evaluating children with enuresis (Questions Box).

Physical Examination

A general physical examination should be performed, with particular attention to certain areas. The pattern of growth should be plotted. Blood pressure should be obtained. The abdomen should be assessed for evidence of organomegaly, bladder size, and fecal impaction. A rectal examination should be performed to evaluate rectal tone.

If possible, physicians should watch children void. Practitioners should determine whether children can start and stop micturition and whether the stream is forceful. Dribbling in girls may indicate an ectopic ureter. The appearance of the genitalia should be assessed. A rash in the genital area may be secondary to wetness from urinary incontinence. Labial fusion in girls may trap urine, allow reflux into the vagina, and lead to dribbling. Meatal stenosis, epispadias, hypospadias, or cryptorchidism may be present in boys. Any of these conditions suggests a possible underlying genitourinary anomaly.

The neuromuscular integrity of the lower extremities should be evaluated. This may provide a clue to a disorder such as spina bifida occulta. The presence of some anomaly in the sacral area, such as a sacral dimple or a tuft of hair, may also be a sign of this condition.

Laboratory Tests

Only a minimal laboratory evaluation is indicated in most children with primary enuresis. Urinalysis, including specific gravity is usually indicated. A CBC, hemoglobin electrophoresis, serum electrolytes, and BUN should also be considered. Studies such as urine culture and blood glucose are more often indicated in cases of secondary enuresis.

Diagnostic Studies

In cases in which the urinalysis is abnormal, the culture is positive, or genitourinary anomalies are apparent on physical examination, a renal ultrasound and vesicoureterogram may be warranted. Vertebral x-rays or MRI are appropriate in the diagnosis of spina bifida. An EEG is indicated if nocturnal epilepsy is suspected. Urodynamic studies to evaluate bladder contractility are controversial but are recommended by some urologists.

MANAGEMENT

Primary Enuresis

Family counseling about enuresis should be part of all management plans. Issues related to psychosocial stress should be explored, particularly in cases of secondary enuresis. Families should be advised that the wetting is not intentional and that punishing children for accidents is inappropriate. However, children may take some responsibility for the consequences of their actions, such as removing soiled bedding or helping with the laundry. They should be rewarded for "dry" nights. Star charts, in which a sticker or gold star is applied to a calendar for each dry night, have traditionally been used. The exclusive use of these charts without other interventions has limited success, however, and suggests that the enuresis may have a volitional component. Star charts should be used in conjunction with other management strategies.

Two treatment modalities are acceptable for managing enuresis. Most studies do not support the use of fluid restriction as a reliable isolated means of controlling enuresis.

Conditioning therapy involves the use of an alarm that is triggered when children void during the night. Children are awakened by the sounding of the alarm, and further urination is inhibited. Eventually bladder distention is associated with inhibition of the urge to urinate. When conditioning therapy is used for 4–6 months, it is associated with a success rate of 70%. If the alarm is used for 4 more weeks with sustained dryness, relapses are uncommon.

Because patient cooperation is needed with the alarm system, its use is reserved for children over the age of 7 years. A newer system is a transistorized version of the original device that contains a small sensor in the underwear and an alarm on the wrist or collar.

Overall, conditioning devices have a cure rate of 70–85%, and a relapse rate of 10–15%. They incur a one-time cost of $45–60. Conditioning without the use of auxilliary alarms may also be undertaken. One proposed method involves instituting a self-awakening program. Older school age children practice lying in bed during the daytime and simulating the experience of awakening, sensing a full bladder and going to the toilet. Another dry bed training program involves parents' awakening their children first hourly, and then at longer intervals over the period of about 1 week. Children eventually learn to self-awaken. A 92% success rate with a relapse rate of 20% is reported with this program.

Pharmacologic agents include tricyclic antidepressants (TCAs) and desmopressin. TCAs, especially imipramine, have been successfully used to treat nocturnal enuresis, although the mechanism of action is uncertain. The antidepressant action of the drug, its effect on sleep and arousal, and its anticholinergic properties may all play a role. The bladder capacity of individuals with enuresis may be increased by 34%, which indicates that the anticholinergic effects of the drug may be the most significant.

Imipramine should not be prescribed for children under the age of 6 or 7 years because of potential adverse effects. The recommended dosage is 0.9–1.5 mg/kg/d. In general, children under the age of 8 years are given 25 mg 1–2 hours before bedtime, and older children are given 50–75 mg. Beneficial results usually occur within the first few weeks of therapy. Medication is usually continued for 3–6 months to prevent relapses, which are reported in up to 75% of cases. The drug should be tapered by reducing the dose or using an alternate-night regimen. Side effects are rare and include insomnia, nightmares, and personality changes. Acute overdoses are potentially fatal secondary to cardiac complications. The initial cure rate is 10–60% with a relapse rate of 90%. The monthly cost of imipramine is about $5.

Desmopressin (DDAVP), an analog of vasopressin, the antidiuretic hormone, is another pharmacologic agent used for enuresis. DDAVP probably works to decrease nocturnal urine production. Most patients respond rapidly to DDAVP and become dry within 1–2 weeks of the initiation of therapy. The medication is sprayed into the nostril although an oral preparation is being evaluated. The initial dose, which can be doubled if patients fail to respond, is one puff (10 mg) in each nostril. Complications, such as epistaxis, nasal pain, congestion, and headache, may occur at higher doses. Severe hyponatremia has also been reported with DDAVP in the face of high fluid intake. If patients achieve a 2-week period of dryness, the dose can be tapered at 2-week intervals. The cure rate is 40–50% with a relapse rate of 90% off medication. Intranasal DDAVP is expensive, with an average monthly cost of $90–180.

Oxybutynin is an antispasmodic, anticholinergic agent used in the management of diurnal or polysymp-tomatic nocturnal enuresis. The dosage is 5 mg hs for children 6–12 years and 10 mg hs over the age of 12. The response rate is 33%, and the major side effects include drowsiness, flushing, dry mouth, constipation, and hyperthermia. Hyoscyamine sulfate and flavoxate hydrochloride are two other medications used for diurnal enuresis.

Treatment of enuresis in children with small bladder capacities includes bladder retention training. Such children are fluid loaded and asked to delay voiding for 5–10 minutes. This strategy is generally reserved for children with diurnal enuresis.

Secondary Enuresis

The management of secondary enuresis should focus on the treatment of the causal disorder, such as a UTI or diabetes mellitus.

PROGNOSIS

The prognosis for children with enuresis is good. The spontaneous cure rate is 15% per year. Medical management results in a reduction in symptoms in over 70% of affected children.

Case Resolution

The boy in the case scenario has primary nocturnal enuresis. The history of childhood enuresis in the father is significant. Two management options, behavior modification and treatment with DDAVP or imipramine, can be discussed with the family. The child's symptoms will probably spontaneously improve over time.

Selected Readings

Belman, A. B., and H. G. Rushton. Voiding dysfunction and enuresis. Washington, DC, Children's National Medical Center, 1995.

Moffat, M. E., et al. Desmopressin acetate and nocturnal enuresis: how much do we know? Pediatrics 92:420–425, 1993.

Rappaport, L. The treatment of nocturnal enuresis–where are we now? Pediatrics 92: 465–466, 1993.

Robson, W. L. Diurnal enuresis. Pediatr. Rev. 18:407–412, 1997.

Schmitt, B. D. Nocturnal enuresis. Pediatr. Rev. 18:183–191, 1997.

Treatment of childhood enuresis. Clin. Pediatr. 32: 1993. (Entire issue.)

Wan, J., and S. Greenfield. Enuresis and common voiding abnormalities. Pediatr. Clin. North Am. 44:1117–1131, 1997.

Warady, B. A., U. Alon, and S. Hellerstein. Primary nocturnal enuresis: current concepts about an old problem. Pediatr. Ann. 20:246–255, 1991.

CHAPTER 34

ENCOPRESIS

Carol D. Berkowitz, M.D.

H$_x$ A 7-year-old boy presents with the complaint of soiling his underpants. His mother states that he has never been completely toilet trained, and that stooling accidents occur at least 2–3 times a week, mainly during the day. The boy rarely has a spontaneous bowel movement without assistance. He sits on the toilet for just a few minutes and has small pelletlike stools. His mother has never sought medical care before for this problem.

The boy is very fidgety during the physical examination. The vital signs are normal and the child's height and weight are at the 25th percentile. His abdomen is soft but distended, with palpable loops of stool-filled bowel. A small amount of stool is present around the anus and in the boy's underpants. Digital examination of the rectum reveals hard stool. The rectal tone is normal as is the rest of the physical examination.

Questions

1. What is the definition of encopresis?
2. What is the difference between retentive and nonretentive encopresis?
3. What are some physiologic conditions that contribute to encopresis?
4. What conditions may be mistaken for encopresis?

Encopresis is the repeated passage of stool into inappropriate places (e.g., clothing) either voluntary or involuntary, in children who should be toilet trained on the basis of age and developmental level and who have no primary organic pathology. One such encopretic event occurs each month for at least 3 months. The term "encopresis," which was originally used for children with psychogenic soiling, is similar to enuresis. Now encopresis is used in a broader sense to refer to all types of fecal incontinence.

Retentive encopresis occurs in the face of constipation (obstipation) in which chronic rectal distention leads to the seepage of liquid stool around hard, retained feces. Sometimes this is called overflow soiling. The onset of symptoms is usually about 4 years of age. Approximately 95% of cases of encopresis are retentive. **Nonretentive encopresis** is characterized by the passage of soft stool without colonic distention or retention of stool. Primary encopresis occurs when children have never been completely toilet trained. Secondary encopresis occurs in children who have had a period of complete continence of stool. The majority of encopretic children have secondary encopresis.

EPIDEMIOLOGY

Encopresis is reported in approximately 2% of 8-year-old boys and about 0.7% of 8-year-old girls, making the condition three times more prevalent in boys than in girls. This sex ratio reverses in the elderly, in which the prevalence of encopresis is twice as high in females as in males. An association between encopresis, enuresis, and ADHD is sometimes present. About 15% of children with enuresis also have encopresis. Family history for encopresis may also be positive; 16% of affected children have one affected parent, usually the father. An association between encopresis and child sexual abuse has been reported in a small number of children.

CLINICAL PRESENTATION

Children with encopresis have a history of staining of the underpants, which may be hidden in drawers or under beds by embarrassed children. Occasionally parents are unaware of the problem. Stooling accidents occur more frequently at home than in school. Some children have a history of constipation (D$_x$ Box).

PATHOPHYSIOLOGY

A history of constipation, often with painful defecation, is associated with retentive encopresis. With time, the colon distends and liquid feces seep around impacted stool (Fig. 34–1). In 30–50% of children, anal spasm, referred to as animus, occurs and contraction rather than relaxation occurs during evacuation of feces. In another 40%, rectal hyposensitivity is apparent so that the children are unaware of the presence of the stool. Some children have an evacuation release disorder, in which the presence of the stool does not result in relaxation and stool evacuation. In such cases, the rectum is chronically distended by stool. Water is

D$_x$ Encopresis

- Incontinence of stool
- Constipation
- Hyperactivity
- Distended abdomen
- Stool-filled loops of bowel
- Lax rectal tone
- Soiled clothing or bedding

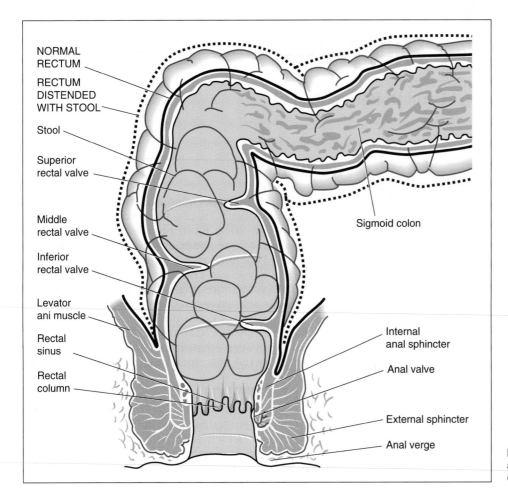

NORMAL
RECTUM

RECTUM
DISTENDED
WITH STOOL

Stool

Superior
rectal valve

Middle
rectal valve

Inferior
rectal valve

Levator
ani muscle

Rectal
sinus

Rectal
column

Sigmoid colon

Internal
anal sphincter

Anal valve

External sphincter

Anal verge

FIGURE 34–1. Diagram of the rectum, anal canal, and sigmoid colon distended with stool.

absorbed and the stool becomes harder and drier. The distended rectum fails to sense the presence of the stool. When evacuation is attempted, the process is painful, leading to further retention (see Chapter 90, Constipation).

Encopresis has been associated with a short attention span and a high level of motor activity. Affected children are unable to sit on a toilet for more than a few minutes and do not adequately attend to the task of stool evacuation. As a result, they get off the toilet after the incomplete evacuation of only small amounts of stool. In some toddlers, constipation is related to the struggle of toilet training and an unwillingness to sit on the toilet (see Chapter 26, Toilet Training).

The pathophysiology of nonretentive encopresis appears to be psychogenic. Some children who have been chronically sexually abused have lax anal tone, which may contribute to the fecal incontinence.

DIFFERENTIAL DIAGNOSIS

The differential diagnosis of encopresis focuses on organic conditions associated with chronic constipation. These conditions include Hirschsprung's disease, disorders of intestinal motility (e.g., pseudo-obstruction), disorders of anal tone and anal anatomy (e.g., imperforate anus with fistula), disorders of the lumbosacral spine (e.g., meningomyelocele), and previous surgeries (e.g., repair of imperforate anus). Neuro-

fibromatosis, lead poisoning, and hypothyroidism are also associated with constipation. Congenital anorectal anomalies, which are reported in 1 in 5000 live births, are rare.

Most of these conditions can be ruled out on the basis of a careful history and physical examination. In some cases, specific testing such as anal manometry or rectal biopsy may be necessary to exclude a particular disorder.

EVALUATION

History

The age of onset of the problem, as well as the age of initiation of toilet training, should be determined. In general, affected children are 4 years of age and older. A detailed history of the stooling pattern should be obtained (Questions Box). The frequency and consistency of stools as well as quantity of stools should also be noted. In addition, the presence of nocturnal episodes of encopresis should be determined. In cases of secondary encopresis, the duration of fecal continence and the occurrence of any events such as the birth of a sibling or the start of school that may have precipitated the episodes of encopresis should be noted. Some children experience the onset of encopresis when they start school. Because of "toilet phobia," they are unwilling to use the public toilet in the school setting.

Physical Examination

The next step involves the performance of a comprehensive physical examination, paying particular attention to the abdomen to check for the presence of distended, stool-filled loops of bowel. The rectal area should be assessed for rectal tone, an anal wink, and the presence of hard stool. Children with retentive encopresis have normal or tight anal tone on rectal examination because they are frequently contracting their external anal sphincter to prevent the seepage of the liquid stool.

Dysmorphic features should be noted and may suggest a syndrome in which constipation is a feature. Abnormalities around the anus such as fistulas should also be noted. Fistulas are found in Crohn's disease. The underpants should be evaluated for the presence of stool, mucus, or pus. A sensory and motor examination of the lower extremities helps determine if any signs of spinal cord dysfunction are evident. An evaluation of the skin over the spinal area may reveal abnormalities such as sacral dimples or tufts of hair.

Children who do not exhibit abdominal distention may have soft stool on rectal examination, which indicates nonretentive encopresis. If patulous anal tone is noted, spinal cord abnormalities or prior child sexual abuse should be suspected.

Diagnostic Tests

Most children with encopresis require few laboratory studies. Urinalysis and urine culture are recommended in children with fecal impactions to exclude urinary tract infection. Anorectal manometry, which may be used to measure the pressure generated by the anal sphincter, may also reveal abnormalities of anal tone or evidence of aganglionosis. The Child Behavioral Checklist is useful to determine if certain behavior problems exist. Such problems may either potentiate the encopresis or result from it.

Imaging Studies

In most encopretic children, imaging studies are not necessary. If x-rays of the abdomen are taken in children with retentive encopresis, distended, stool-filled bowel may be noted. A barium enema is useful if Hirschsprung's disease is to be ruled out. Strictures, which may occur following necrotizing enterocolitis, will also be detected. EMG to determine whether the innervation of the external anal sphincter is intact is recommended for children with encopresis who fail to respond to routine treatment.

MANAGEMENT

The management of encopresis focuses on complete rectal evacuation, and patient and parent education and counseling.

Rectal evacuation requires **pharmacologic management** to ensure an adequate cleanout of retained stools. The decision about which laxatives to use depends on the degree of constipation. If the degree of fecal retention is mild, a high-fiber diet and stool-bulking agents or oral laxatives such as senna derivatives or bisacodyl may be used in association with stool softeners or lubricants such as mineral oil. The amount of mineral oil may be titrated up to ensure success. Some practitioners recommend that mineral oil be given until it oozes from the rectum. The amount may then be titrated back to a lower level.

If the degree of retention is more severe, suppositories or enemas may be needed. Occasionally, children have to be disimpacted manually. Alternative methods to manual disimpaction include two to three sodium phosphate enemas over 1–2 days or 8 ounces of mineral oil a day for 4 days. "Pulsed irrigation-enhanced evacuation" involves the insertion of a rectal tube and the installation of pulses of warm irrigating solution, simultaneously draining rectal contents. If the above modalities are not successful, children may need to be admitted to the hospital for oral lavage using polyethylene glycol-electrolyte solution at 30–40 mL/kg/hr until successful evacuation has occurred. This procedure often requires insertion of a nasogastric tube and 6–8 hours of treatment. Once the fecal accumulation has been relieved, every effort should be made to keep children regular. This can be accomplished with the combined use of toilet retraining, stool softeners or laxatives, and enemas or suppositories. Prokinetic agents such as cisapride or metaclopramide may also be used.

Dietary manipulation is important to assure sustained regular stooling. Parents should be told that children require a high-fiber diet with decreased milk (≤16 oz/d) and fruit juices such as pear or peach. It has been suggested that a "team and coach" approach is the most successful route, and that bowel training be likened to fitness training.

The toilet retraining process requires that children sit on the toilet at least two or three times a day, usually after meals, for about 10 minutes or until they have had a bowel movement. Some practitioners recommend the use of an egg timer to ensure that children spend the appropriate amount of time on the toilet. Children should be requested to maintain a diary of their evacuation, which may take the form of a star chart. Stars or other rewards are given for successful bowel movements in the toilet.

If children skip a day between bowel movements, they may be treated with a suppository, such as a glycerin or a bisacodyl suppository. If they still have not succeeded in having a bowel movement, then an enema may be appropriate. This sequence should be maintained until children are having bowel movements in the toilet and not soiling for at least 1 month. In general, stool softeners are required for at least 3–6 months. The regimen may have to be modified, particularly in younger children.

Behavior modification and biofeedback are two other modalities that can be used to help manage encopresis. Consultation with specialists such as pediatric gastroenterologists may be required.

Thirty percent of children with encopresis may need psychological consultation. Children with evidence of child sexual abuse or nonretentive encopresis should be referred to a psychologist early in the course of therapy. The underlying psychosocial problems of children with nonretentive encopresis must be adequately addressed before their condition can improve.

PROGNOSIS

The prognosis for children with retentive encopresis is reportedly good with appropriate intervention. In one study, children who were able to defecate a rectal balloon filled with 100 mL of water within 5 minutes were twice as likely to recover from constipation and encopresis. It is estimated that about two thirds of affected children experience long-lasting remission within 6 months of the initiation of medical management, and another 30% are considerably improved.

The prognosis for children with nonretentive encopresis is less predictable and highly dependent on the underlying psychopathology.

Case Resolution

In the case scenario, the boy exhibits typical manifestations of retentive encopresis. His condition should be managed with the use of laxatives, stool softeners, and toilet retraining with a star chart. The possible ADHD should be addressed separately but may be contributing to his inability to attend to the task of toileting.

Selected Readings

Abi-Hanna, A., and A. M. Lake. Constipation and encopresis in childhood. Pediatr. Rev. 19:23–31, 1998.

Howe, A. C., and C. E. Walker. Behavioral management of toilet training, enuresis, and encopresis. Pediatr. Clin. North Am. 39:413–432, 1992.

Loenig-Baucke, V. Balloon defecation as a predictor of outcome in children with functional constipation and encopresis. J. Pediatr. 128:336–340, 1997.

Madoff, R. D., J. G. Williams, and P. F. Caushaj. Fecal incontinence. N. Engl. J. Med. 326:1002–1007, 1992.

Nolan, T., and F. Oberklaid. New concepts in the management of encopresis. Pediatr. Rev. 14:447–451, 1993.

Partin, J. C., et al. Painful defecation and fecal soiling in children. Pediatrics 89:1007–1009, 1992.

Schmitt, B. D. Soiling with constipation in the school-age child. Contemp. Pediatr. 9:75–78, 1992.

Schmitt, B. D. Soiling without constipation. Contemp. Pediatr. 9:69–70, 1992.

Schmitt, B. D., and R. D. Mauro. Twenty common errors in treating encopresis. Contemp. Pediatr. 9:47–65, May 1992.

Young, M. H., L. C. Brennen, R. D. Baker, and S. S. Baker. Functional encopresis: Symptom reduction and behavioral improvement. J. Develop. Behav. Pediatr. 16:226–232, 1996.

ACUTE AND EMERGENT PROBLEMS

C H A P T E R   3 5

FEVER AND BACTEREMIA

Geeta Grover, M.D.

H_x An 8-month-old girl is brought to the emergency department with a 2-day history of fever and increased fussiness. She is irritable but consolable by parents. On examination, she has a rectal temperature of 103.1° F (39.5° C). The rest of the physical examination is within normal limits, and no source for the fever is apparent.

Questions

1. How do the height of fever and the age of the patient influence the evaluation and management of infants and young children with fever?
2. What, if any, laboratory studies are required in the evaluation of infants with fever?
3. What are the management options for children with fever of unknown source? How does clinical appearance affect management?

Normothermia, which is equivalent to a body temperature of 98.6° F (37.0° C), is the result of the delicate balance of heat gain and heat loss that allows the body to maintain a constant core temperature. Mean body temperature exhibits a diurnal variation, with a peak in the early evening (approximately 6 PM) and a nadir in the early morning (approximately 6 AM). With fever, the central thermostat of the body increases to a new "set point," and heat loss and heat gain are again balanced at this higher temperature. Fever is not a disease but a nonspecific symptom of some underlying condition or process that involves inflammation. Although there is no consensus regarding the exact temperature that denotes fever, it is generally accepted that a rectal temperature of at least 100.4° F (38.0° C) represents a fever in children.

Bacteremia is the presence of bacteria in the blood. **Occult bacteremia** is bacteremia in children with a benign clinical appearance and no apparent source of serious infections (e.g., pneumonia, UTI). **Septicemia** is the presence of microorganisms in the blood with localized or systemic disease in an ill-appearing child.

EPIDEMIOLOGY

Children in the first 2–3 years of life have approximately six to ten infectious illnesses each year. Thus fever is one of the most common presenting complaints seen in children. Up to one third of outpatient visits by children to both emergency departments and private practitioners are for fever. By some estimates, 20–30% of after-hours calls to pediatricians concern fever.

The risk of serious bacterial illness (SBI) in infants under 3 months of age with fever is generally believed to be higher than in older infants with fever. For the purposes of this discussion, SBIs include meningitis, bacteremia, UTI, osteomyelitis, septic arthritis, pneumonia, bacterial gastroenteritis, and serious skin and soft tissue infections (e.g., cellulitis, adenitis). In febrile infants (rectal temperature ≥100.4° F [38.0° C]) under 3 months of age, the prevalence of SBI is approximately 5–9%, whereas the prevalence of occult bacteremia is about 3–4%. Historical, physical, and laboratory criteria may help to identify infants at low risk for SBI (Table 35–1). The organisms commonly implicated in SBI in this age group are presented in Table 35–2. Although group B streptococci and *Escherichia coli* account for the vast majority of infections, other pathogens such as *Salmonella* species are important after the first month of life.

The risk of occult bacteremia in children 3–36 months of age with fever without localizing signs (FWLS) is approximately 3–5%. Recent data suggest that the universal immunization of children with *Haemophilus influenzae* vaccine has reduced the risk of occult bacteremia in these children to about 2%. Children 7–18 months of age are at the highest risk for bacteremia. Occult bacteremia is more common in children with FWLS and in children with fever who are the same age and have common childhood infections that are usually treated on an outpatient basis (e.g., otitis media, pharyngitis). Factors increasing the risk of bacteremia are high fever, and high WBC count. Authorities estimate that approximately 8–15% of children with temperatures over 102.2° F (39.0° C), WBC counts over 15,000/μL, and no focus of infection have bacteremia. Hyperpyrexia (temperature >106.0° F [41.1° C]) has been associated

TABLE 35–1. The Rochester Criteria for Evaluation of Febrile Infants Aged 60 Days or Less*

Low Risk Factors for SBI

Infant appears generally well
Infant has been previously healthy
    Born at term (≥37 weeks' gestation)
    Did not receive perinatal antimicrobial therapy
    Was not treated for unexplained hyperbilirubinemia
    Had not received and was not receiving antimicrobial agents
    Had not been previously hospitalized
    Had no chronic or underlying illness
    Was not hospitalized longer than mother
No evidence of skin, soft tissue, bone, joint, or ear infection
Laboratory values
    Peripheral WBC count: 5000–15,000/μL
    Absolute band count: ≤1500/μL
    Urinalysis WBC count: ≤10/hpf on microscopic examination of a spun urine sediment
    Stool WBC count: ≤5/hpf on microscopic examination of a stool smear (only for infants with diarrhea)

*Rectal temperature ≥100.4° F (38.0° C).

Abbreviations: SBI, serious bacterial infection; hpf, high-power field; WBC, white blood cell.

Reproduced, with permission, from Jaskiewicz, J.A., et al. Febrile infants at low risk for serious bacterial infection—an appraisal of the Rochester Criteria and implications for management. Pediatrics 94:390–396, 1994.

D$_x$ Serious Bacterial Illness

- Lethargy, irritability, or change in mental status
- Tachycardia disproportionate to the degree of temperature elevation
- Tachypnea or labored respirations
- Bulging or depressed anterior fontanelle
- Nuchal rigidity
- Petechiae
- Localized erythema, pain, or swelling
- Abdominal or flank pain
- Fever

---

with an increased incidence of bacteremia and meningitis.

The routine use of Hib conjugate vaccines has virtually eliminated *H. influenzae* type b disease in the United States. It is estimated that *Streptococcus pneumoniae* now accounts for about 90% of cases of occult bacteremia in children 3–36 months of age. Less common causes include *Neisseria meningitidis*, *Salmonella* species, *Staphylococcus aureus*, or *H. influenzae* (unvaccinated children) (see Table 35–2).

CLINICAL PRESENTATION

In some febrile children fever may be the only complaint, and these children otherwise look fine and behave normally. Other children with fever may appear less interactive, quieter, and less energetic than children of the same age without fever. Appetite decreases, and children may become more fussy. Because young children, especially infants under 3 months of age, have fewer and more subtle behavioral signs when febrile,

---

physicians must maintain a high index of suspicion for SBI even in the absence of localizing signs. Physical findings associated with fever include flushed cheeks; hot, dry skin; shivering (uncommon in young infants); cool distal extremities; tachycardia; and tachypnea (D$_x$ Box). Occult bacteremia, by definition, has no additional abnormal physical manifestations.

PATHOPHYSIOLOGY

Fever is an elevation in the thermoregulatory set point of the body. The thermoregulatory center is located in the preoptic region of the anterior hypothalamus, and an elevation in the hypothalamic set point above the normal body temperature initiates the physiologic changes that lead to fever. Exogenous pyrogens (e.g., bacteria, viruses, antigen-antibody complexes) stimulate host inflammatory cells (e.g., macrophages, polymorphonuclear cells) to produce endogenous pyrogens (EPs). Interleukin-1 is currently regarded as the prototypical EP. EPs cause the hypothalamic endothelium to increase intermediary substances such as prostaglandins and neurotransmitters, which then act on the preoptic neurons of the anterior hypothalamus to produce an elevated set point. The body uses physiologic mechanisms (e.g., peripheral vasoconstriction, shivering) and behavioral actions (e.g., bundling up, drinking hot tea) to increase body temperature to reach and maintain this higher set point, thus producing fever (Fig. 35–1).

In contrast, the thermoregulatory set point of the body is normal in hyperthermia. Due to abnormal physiologic processes, heat gain exceeds heat loss, and the body temperature rises in spite of efforts to return to the control set point.

DIFFERENTIAL DIAGNOSIS

In the vast majority of cases, the duration of fever in children is short, and signs and symptoms are localized. FWLS is an acute episode of fever that lasts 1 week or less in children in whom history, physical examination, and preliminary laboratory tests fail to find a source. The majority of children with FWLS are eventually found to have acute, generally self-limited, infectious illnesses. Occult bacteremia is a major concern in young children

---

TABLE 35–2. Organisms Implicated in Serious Bacterial Infection/Occult Bacteremia in Children

Infants Less Than 3 Months of Age
Group B *Streptococcus*
Escherichia coli
Listeria monocytogenes
Salmonella species (infants >1 mo)
Haemophilus influenzae type b* (infants >1 mo)
Children Between 3 and 36 Months of Age
Streptococcus pneumoniae
Neisseria meningitidis
Salmonella species
Staphylococcus aureus
H. influenzae type b (Hib)*

*Hib disease has been virtually eliminated with the routine use of Hib conjugate vaccines.

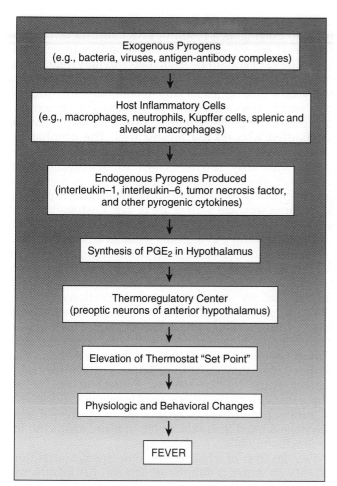

FIGURE 35–1. Pathophysiology of fever production. Antipyretics work by blocking the synthesis of PGE_2.

with FWLS, primarily in infants less than 36 months of age. High-risk factors for occult bacteremia are presented in Table 35–3. Fever of unknown origin (FUO) is fever of at least 8 days' duration in infants or children in whom routine history, physical examination, and laboratory assessment fail to reveal a source.

The differential diagnosis of children with an acute febrile illness is primarily infectious (Table 35–4), including both benign, generally self-limited illness such as URI, and less common, more serious illness such as meningitis and osteomyelitis. Occasionally, a child with FWLS turns out to have a noninfectious illness such as a collagen vascular disease or neoplasia. By comparison, the differential diagnosis of children with FUO is quite broad (Table 35–5) and contains both infectious and noninfectious disorders.

TABLE 35–3.   Risk Factors for Occult Bacteremia

Age ≤ 36 mo
Temperature ≥ 103.1° F (39.5° C)
White blood cells ≥ 15,000/μL or ≤ 5000/μL
Total band cells ≥ 500/μL
Erythrocyte sedimentation rate ≥ 30 mm/hr
Underlying chronic disease (malignancy, immunodeficiency, sickle cell disease, malnutrition)
Clinical appearance (irritability, lethargy, toxic appearance)

TABLE 35–4.   Common Infectious Causes of an Acute Episode of Fever in Children

Upper Respiratory Tract
Upper respiratory infection (common cold)
Otitis media
Sinusitis
Pulmonary
Bronchiolitis
Pneumonia
Oral Cavity
Gingivostomatitis
Pharyngitis
Dental abscess
Gastrointestinal Tract
Acute gastroenteritis (bacterial or viral)
Appendicitis
Genitourinary Tract
Urinary tract infection
Pyelonephritis
Musculoskeletal
Septic arthritis
Osteomyelitis
Central Nervous System
Meningitis
Miscellaneous (including noninfectious causes)
Bacteremia
Immunization reaction
Viral exanthems (e.g., chickenpox, measles)
Neoplasia
Collagen vascular disease

TABLE 35–5.   Common Causes of Fever of Unknown Origin (FUO) in Children*

Infectious Diseases
Bacterial
   Localized infection: mastoiditis, sinusitis, pneumonia, osteomyelitis, pyelonephritis, abscess (e.g., abdominal, pelvic)
   Systemic disease: tuberculosis, brucellosis, salmonellosis, leptospirosis, tularemia
Viral
   Hepatitis viruses
   Cytomegalovirus
   Epstein-Barr virus (infectious mononucleosis)
   Human immunodeficiency virus
Fungal
   Disseminated coccidioidomycosis
   Disseminated histoplasmosis
Miscellaneous
   Malaria
   Rocky Mountain spotted fever
   Syphilis
   Lyme disease
Neoplasia
Leukemia
Lymphoma
Hodgkin's disease
Neuroblastoma
Collagen Vascular Diseases
Juvenile rheumatoid arthritis
Systemic lupus erythematosus
Rheumatic fever
Miscellaneous
Inflammatory bowel diseases
Kawasaki disease
Thyroiditis
Drugs
Factitious fever

*For a complete discussion of FUO, the reader is referred to Lorin, M.I., and R.D. Feigin. Fever without localizing signs and fever of unknown origin. *In* Feigin, R.D., and J.D. Cherry (eds.). Textbook of Pediatric Infectious Diseases, 4th ed. Philadelphia, W.B. Saunders, 1998, pp. 820–830.

EVALUATION

History

The medical history can provide a great deal of valuable information in the evaluation of children with fever (Questions Box). The history should focus on the duration and severity of the fever. The presence of associated symptoms that may be signs of specific organ system involvement should also be noted.

Physical Examination

Vital signs provide important diagnostic clues. The effect of fever on the heart and respiratory rates should be noted. The heart rate increases by 10 beats per minute for each degree Fahrenheit of temperature elevation above normal (98.6° F). Tachycardia disproportionate to the degree of temperature elevation may suggest dehydration or sepsis. Tachypnea, which is often the only sign of a respiratory infection, may also be seen in response to metabolic acidosis (most commonly secondary to sepsis or shock). These changes may be clues to an occult focus.

Observation of the overall hydration and well-being of children is extremely important. An attempt should be made to determine whether children are behaving and responding in an age-appropriate fashion. Physicians should look for spontaneous movements, negative responses to adverse stimuli, and positive responses to pleasant stimuli.

In addition, all febrile children should receive a complete physical examination. This is important even when the history may suggest involvement of one organ system. For example, in young children, vomiting and fever may often be the only signs of a UTI, and the problem is not necessarily gastroenteritis, as suggested by the history. The condition may go undiagnosed unless a thorough examination, including evaluation of the urine, is performed.

Growth parameters should be measured. Weight loss, although nonspecific, can be an important finding.

The anterior fontanelle should be palpated. It may be normal, bulging as a result of CNS infection or congestive heart failure, or depressed secondary to dehydration. The ears should be examined carefully; pneumatic otoscopy should be used. Careful inspection may reveal the source of fever, especially in children under the age of 3 years. The occurrence of otitis media should not preclude further workup for invasive bacterial disease in children who do not appear well. The oropharynx should also be examined. Dry or "tacky" mucous membranes may provide clues to dehydration. Enlarged, inflamed, or exudative tonsils often signal the presence of a group A streptococcal infection, especially in children who are 5–10 years of age. Epstein-Barr and adenoviral infections should also be considered in such cases. Respiratory symptoms such as labored respirations, retractions, nasal flaring, stridor, rales, rhonchi, or wheezing may all be clues to respiratory tract infections. Enanthems on the buccal mucosa, or exanthems on the skin, are often signs of viral infections.

The presence of petechiae in association with fever may indicate serious underlying infection. Children with such conditions should receive a comprehensive evaluation. Localized areas of pain, erythema, swelling, or all of these signs may point to cellulitis, septic arthritis, or osteomyelitis. Nuchal rigidity, if present, can be an important clue to the presence of meningitis. Because it is rarely present in infants under 2 years of age, physicians must maintain a high index of suspicion for meningitis in children of this age.

Two groups of children require special attention: (1) infants under 3 months of age and (2) infants and young children 3–36 months of age with FWLS. Determining the cause of fever in young infants can be diagnostically challenging. Nonspecific signs and symptoms such as irritability, increased fussiness, feeding intolerance, or mild respiratory distress may be the only clues to the presence of SBI. Elevated rectal temperatures in children in this age group should not be attributed to overbundling.

The evaluation of children 3–36 months of age with FWLS should be guided by clinical appearance and the criteria for occult bacteremia (see Table 35–3). Neither the infants' response to antipyretics nor improvement in clinical status after defervescence helps in predicting bacteremia.

Thorough and repeat physical examinations are important in the evaluation of children with FUO. For these reasons, children with FUO are often hospitalized for workup. Significant weight loss may be suggestive of a chronic illness such as inflammatory bowel disease. Joint pain or rashes may be signs of collagen vascular disease. A rectal examination should be performed to look for tenderness, which may be indicative of an abdominal or pelvic abscess or fissures suggestive of inflammatory bowel disease.

Laboratory Tests

Infants less than 3 months of age with fever should receive a thorough laboratory assessment, including a CBC, blood culture, urinalysis and urine culture, and lumbar puncture. If bacterial gastroenteritis is suspected, a stool smear should be examined for the presence of WBCs. At present, no single laboratory test can accurately predict the likelihood of bacteremia in febrile children.

Older infants and children may be classified as either low or high risk for SBI or occult bacteremia based on overall clinical impression, history, and physical examination. Routine laboratory assessment may not be required for low-risk children, but high-risk children should at least have a CBC and blood culture. The CBC provides additional information that can aid in the decision of whether or not to obtain further laboratory or imaging studies.

A focus of infection in an ill-appearing child should not prevent further workup. In addition, the laboratory assessment of ill-appearing children with fever and petechiae should be aggressive, because the incidence of invasive bacterial disease is 8–20% and the incidence of meningococcal meningitis or sepsis is 7–10%. Data from a recent prospective study finds an overall 2% rate (8 of 411 patients) of bacteremia or sepsis in children 3–36 months of age with fever and petechiae. Eleven percent (6 of 53 patients) of ill-appearing children had serious invasive bacteremia, while no well-appearing children had serious invasive bacteremia, although two did have *S. pneumoniae* occult bacteremia.

All children with FUO should have a CBC. Other appropriate initial screening laboratory studies include tuberculin skin testing, blood and urine cultures, chest radiograph, ESR, or C-reactive protein and liver enzymes.

Imaging Studies

Routine imaging studies, except for chest radiography, are not usually necessary. Chest radiographs should be performed in febrile infants under 3 months of age with respiratory symptoms. In older infants and children, chest radiographs should be obtained if lower respiratory tract signs (e.g., wheezing, rales) of pulmonary disease are present. Other imaging studies, such as bone or gallium scans, may be performed if indicated.

MANAGEMENT

Management of children with fever includes both controlling the fever and treating the underlying process causing the fever. There is no evidence that fever itself is harmful. To the contrary, animal studies have suggested that fever may have some survival advantage.

Despite the possible beneficial effects of fever, febrile children may still feel uncomfortable. Fever should be reduced to relieve the associated discomfort and malaise. **Antipyretics** such as acetaminophen and ibuprofen can be used. Aspirin should be avoided in children because of the association with Reye's syndrome and viral illnesses. **Sponging** or **bathing** with tepid water and **unbundling** children aid in fever reduction. Ice water or alcohol baths should be avoided.

Some authorities have argued that fever should be reduced in an effort to prevent febrile seizures. However, the occurrence of such seizures may be related more to the rapidity of rise in temperature than the height of the temperature itself. In addition, febrile seizures usually occur at the onset of a febrile illness before the need for antipyretics is even realized (see Chapter 36, Febrile Seizures).

Any focal bacterial infection should be treated with appropriate antimicrobial therapy. In the absence of a focal infection, management of febrile children depends on age. Infants under 1 month should be hospitalized for observation and administered **intravenous antibiotics** pending culture results. Infants between 1 and 3 months can be managed safely at home if they satisfy the following criteria: (1) they do not have symptoms of serious infection, (2) results of their laboratory tests are within normal limits, and (3) reliable follow-up is assured.

Ill-appearing children between 3 and 36 months of age with FWLS who are suspected of having an SBI should be hospitalized for repeat assessments and intravenous antibiotics (e.g., cefotaxime or ceftriaxone). Because of the increasing prevalence of drug-resistant *S. pneumoniae*, current initial therapy for children suspected of having bacterial meningitis is to begin vancomycin with either cefotaxime or ceftriaxone. If children appear well but have a risk for SBI based on high-risk factors (see Table 35–3), empiric outpatient **ceftriaxone** therapy (50 mg/kg intramuscularly) can be considered. Individual assessment of risk for bacteremia is necessary. Such therapy is not an alternative to hospitalization for children who appear clinically ill. Before administering ceftriaxone, a minimal laboratory workup, including CBC, blood culture, and urinalysis and urine culture should be performed. A lumbar puncture is highly recommended, especially in infants under 1 year of age. A chest radiograph may be performed if clinically appropriate. The widespread use of ceftriaxone is discouraged by some who cite cost and emergence of drug-resistant organisms as negative effects of such therapy.

In febrile children over the age of 36 months, expectant antibiotics are generally not indicated. Children of any age who are at high risk for SBI include those with fever and petechiae, immunocompromised children (e.g., children with HIV, malignancy, sickle cell disease) and children with some types of congenital heart disease (e.g., cyanotic lesions). These children require an intensive evaluation and often the institution of expectant antibiotic therapy before a pathogen is isolated.

PROGNOSIS

Occult bacteremia may resolve without therapy and have no sequelae, but it may persist or produce localized infections such as meningitis or septic arthritis. In bacteremic children who do not receive antimicrobial therapy, the risk of persistent bacteremia is approximately 20% and the risk of meningitis is about 5–10%. These risks vary depending on which organism is isolated from the blood. In general, the risk of developing serious sequelae is greater with bacteremia caused by *H. influenzae* than by *S. pneumoniae* (25% vs. 5%).

Case Resolution

The infant presented in the case history is irritable and has a high fever of unknown source. She should receive a thorough history and physical examination in addition to a complete laboratory assessment, including a lumbar puncture. Management should be based on reassessment after all laboratory data are available. If laboratory assessment reveals a focus of infection such as a UTI, she should be managed with antibiotics. If laboratory assessment fails to reveal a source for the fever, and her WBC is greater than 15,000/mm^3, she can receive an intramuscular injection of ceftriaxone as expectant management for occult bacteremia and be reevaluated in 24 hours or be managed without antibiotics.

Selected Readings

Avner, J. R. Occult bacteremia: How great the risk? Contemp. Pediatr. 14:53–65, 1997.

Baraff, L. J., et al. Practice guidelines for the management of infants and children 0 to 36 months of age with fever without source. Pediatrics 92:1–12, 1993.

Bonadio, W. A. The history and physical assessments of the febrile infant. Pediatr. Clin. North Am. 45:65–77, 1998.

Grover, G., et al. The effects of bundling on infant temperature. Pediatrics 94:669–673, 1994.

Jaskeiwicz, J. A., et al. Febrile infants at low risk for serious bacterial infection—an appraisal of the Rochester Criteria and implications for management. Pediatrics 94:390–396, 1994.

Kluger, M. J. Fever revisited. Pediatrics 90:846–850, 1992.

Lee, G. M., and M. B. Harper. Risk of bacteremia for febrile young children in the post-*Haemophilus influenzae* Type b era. Arch. Pediatr. Adolesc. Med. 152:624–628, 1998.

Lorin, M. I., and R. D. Feigin. Fever of unknown origin. *In* Feigin, R. D., and J. D. Cherry (eds.). Textbook of Pediatric Infectious Diseases, 3rd ed. Philadelphia, W. B. Saunders, 1992, pp. 1012–1022.

Mandl, K. D., A. M. Stack, and G. R. Fleisher. Incidence of bacteremia in infants and children with fever and petechiae. J. Pediatr. 131:398–404, 1997.

McCarthy, P. L. Fever. Pediatr. Rev. 19:401–407, 1998.

Steinhoff, M. C. Resistant pneumococcus: The challenge for pediatrics. Contemp. Pediatr. Supp: 4–11, 1998.

Willoughby, R. E., and F. S. Polack. Meningitis: What's new in diagnosis and management. Contemp. Pediatr. 15:49–70, 1998.

CHAPTER 36

FEBRILE SEIZURES

Kenneth R. Huff, M.D.

H$_x$ A 12-month-old girl is brought to the emergency department by paramedics because she is having a seizure. She is unresponsive and hypertonic, with arched trunk and extended arms and legs that are jerking rhythmically. Her eyes are open, but her gaze is directed upward. She has bubbles of saliva around her lips as well as circumoral cyanosis. Her vital signs are a respiratory rate of 60/min, heart rate of 125 beats/min, blood pressure of 130/78, and temperature of 105.8° F (41.0° C). An assessment of her respiratory status discloses that she is moving air in all lung fields, and there is no evidence of upper airway obstruction.

The paramedics inform you that the girl has been convulsing for approximately 6 minutes. Glucometer testing reveals a normal serum glucose. Blood samples for other tests are sent to the laboratory, and urine is collected. An intravenous line is started, and the girl is given lorazepam by intravenous push. Within 2 minutes, the movements cease, and her respirations become slow and even. Her physical examination shows no signs of trauma. Her only abnormality other than her unresponsive mental status is an inflamed and bulging right tympanic membrane.

The girl's parents tell you that she has had a mildly stuffy nose for 2 days but has been afebrile and has seemed to be her usual self. While she was playing, she became cranky, and her parents put her in her crib for her nap. Thirty minutes later they heard grunting noises, found her in the midst of a seizure, and called the paramedics. The girl has never had a seizure before. Her father recalls that his mother once told him that he had several "fever seizures" as an infant.

Questions

1. What are the characteristics of simple febrile seizures?
2. What is the appropriate evaluation of children with febrile seizures, whether it is the first one or a recurrence?
3. What is the recurrence risk for febrile seizures and the risk of developing unprovoked seizures following a febrile seizure?
4. What are the treatment options for children with febrile seizures?

Febrile seizures are easily recognized, dramatic, generalized convulsions. These seizures are defined by the presence of a fever (often sudden) from a source outside the nervous system; age of less than or equal to 5 years; and absence of chronic brain pathology, including developmental delay; and the absence of acute or chronic chemical or structural aberrations of the brain. Frequently, familial predisposition to similar seizures plays a role. Despite the relatively uniform presentation of the seizure, individual clinical variables and social factors may affect the treatment and prognosis.

EPIDEMIOLOGY

Febrile seizures occur in children between the ages of 6 months and 5 years but are more common in those who are less than 3 years of age. Some studies indicate that as many as 5% of all children experience at least one febrile seizure. The recurrence rate is 30–50% in children less than 1 year of age, but drops to 25% between 1 and 3 years, and is only 12% after 3 years. Seizures usually occur with the increase in temperature and often so suddenly that the febrile illness is not recognized by the family prior to the seizure. Frequently, the febrile illness is eventually diagnosed as a URI or influenza infection. Febrile seizures are seen more often in children who have a first-degree relative who experienced the problem at the same age.

CLINICAL PRESENTATION

Febrile seizures are characterized by generalized, symmetric, tonic posturing and clonic movements of a few minutes' duration that occur suddenly in children whose developmental progress is generally normal. Fever is present, although it may not have been recognized before the seizure, and its source is outside the nervous system. A short time after the seizure (approximately 1 hour), children become neurologically well again (D$_x$ Box).

PATHOPHYSIOLOGY

The susceptibility of young children to febrile seizures may be related to an increased incidence of sudden high fevers in this age group, a developmental genetic factor that may lower the seizure threshold, or both. A sudden increase in temperature to a sufficiently high level can provoke seizures regardless of age. Seizures occur more frequently with fever in many seizure-prone patients who have seizures of different etiologies, including epilepsy. Perhaps circulating pyrogens interact with a brain cellular circuitry mechanism, causing hypersynchronous depolarization and a seizure. The multigenerational familial history that is often seen suggests an autosomal dominent form of genetic transmission. Both the definition of the genetic marker and the mechanism of generalized seizures are not yet fully understood.

DIFFERENTIAL DIAGNOSIS

When a young child presents with a fever and a seizure, the possibility that the seizure is symptomatic of meningitis, encephalitis, or brain abscess must be considered. Signs of meningeal irritation may not be reliable in children less than 18 months old, and these and other signs of the illness may be obscured in the postictal period. If there is a history of lethargy or persistent vomiting, or the seizure was focal in onset, prolonged, or multiple, an examination of the CSF must be done. The fever may be coincidental to a seizure of different etiology such as trauma, toxic ingestion, metabolic derangement, degenerative or neurocutaneous disorder, or stroke.

A useful concept for the physician caring for children with seizures with fever is the differentiation of "simple febrile seizures" from "complex febrile seizures" (Table 36–1). A question that has prognostic implications is whether children in the appropriate age range have had a true "febrile seizure" or a "seizure with fever," which may be an early fever-provoked episode of a nonfebrile seizure disorder. The factors defining a complex febrile seizure also predict an increased likelihood of later unprovoked nonfebrile seizures. The length of a complex febrile seizure is greater than 15 minutes. Most febrile seizures last less than 90 seconds, although a significant number present in status epilepticus. More than one febrile seizure during the same infectious illness or 24-hour period makes these recurrent seizures complex febrile seizures. The history of a focal or partial onset or the presence of postictal focal neurologic signs makes the febrile seizure complex. The presence of an abnormal neurodevelopmental history prior to the febrile seizure or abnormal neurologic examination or brain imaging study before or after the seizure also increases the likelihood of later unprovoked seizures.

D$_x$ Febrile Seizures

- Sudden unresponsiveness, tonic posturing, and generalized rhythmic jerking
- Fever source outside nervous system
- Age 6 months to 5 years
- Normal neurodevelopmental history

TABLE 36–1.   Simple Versus Complex Febrile Seizures

Feature	Simple	Complex
Onset of clonic movements	Generalized	Focal
Length	<15 minutes (usually <90 seconds)	>15 minutes
Number of seizures/ 24 h febrile illness	1	Recurrent
Neurodevelopmental history	Normal	Abnormal
Parent-sibling history of a febrile seizure	Negative	Positive

EVALUATION

History

After the seizure has been controlled and the child has been stabilized, a more detailed history relating to the circumstances of the seizure; the child's state leading up to the seizure; prenatal, birth, and developmental histories; and family seizure history should be obtained (Questions Box).

Physical Examination

Children should be examined completely after stabilization, noting the possibility that the fever may be coincidental. Physicians should look for bruises, fractures, retinal hemorrhages, or other signs of trauma. The presence of dysmorphic features, enlarged organs, or bony changes should be noted. The skin should be examined for abnormal, pigmented or textured spots. Lateralized signs of tone or strength should be assessed. An appropriate evaluation to determine the etiology of the fever should be performed (see Chapter 35, Fever and Bacteremia).

Laboratory Tests

If the seizure is prolonged, focal, or multiple; if there is a history of lethargy, stupor, or persistent vomiting before the seizure; or if the patient still appears ill after the postictal period, cultures should be obtained and metabolic and toxicologic blood and urine studies sent. A spinal tap for CSF examination should be done unless there are signs of increased intracranial pressure or a lateralized neurologic examination, in which case antibiotics should be given and an imaging study obtained prior to the spinal tap.

If the seizure is a simple febrile seizure, an EEG has limited usefulness. There is a high rate of abnormality that is nonspecific and many believe nonpredictive of either future simple febrile seizures or unprovoked seizures. If the patient does not fully recover after the postictal period, the EEG may be useful to help define the nature of the encephalopathy.

Imaging Studies

CT and MRI scans have a low yield of abnormal results in children with simple febrile seizures. Children who have had an abnormal neurodevelopmental history or who have had a focal or partial onset to their seizure should have an imaging study to detect a structural lesion that may be the source of the seizure provoked by the fever or serve as a nidus for future seizures provoked or unprovoked by fever.

MANAGEMENT

If children are still convulsing on presentation and have been for at least 5 minutes, they should be managed as for status epilepticus (see Chapter 122, Seizures and Epilepsy). The airway must be secure, blood tests drawn and sent to the laboratory, an intravenous line started, and lorazepam administered in the appropriate dose to stop the seizure.

If children are not in status epilepticus, management decisions are made on a more long term basis (Table 36–2). Whether to recommend **anticonvulsant prophylaxis** for children who have experienced febrile seizures is **controversial**. Factors that must be considered include (1) the benign, age-limited nature of the condition; (2) the morbidity of the anticonvulsant treatment; (3) the chance of recurrence of febrile or nonfebrile seizures; (4) the risk of overmedication during an acute recurrence; and (5) the family's reaction and social disruption caused by the seizures.

Daily doses of phenobarbital or valproic acid are effective prophylactic anticonvulsants. The most commonly used regimen is daily phenobarbital, but its potential side effects include hyperactive behavior disorder and depressed cognition. Valproic acid can produce thrombocytopenia and may have the potential of provoking acute liver dysfunction in the patient younger than 2 years who is taking other medications. Fever control measures should be instituted to make the patient more comfortable but have not been found effective as prevention for seizures. Intermittent anticonvulsant therapy has the advantage of reducing side effects but relies on recognizing the fever prior to the seizure and mandates greater vigilance for compliance during each fever. Diazepam administered intermittently is effective within this sometimes considerable limitation.

Recommendations for prophylactic anticonvulsant treatment are often individualized. Anticonvulsants are usually not recommended unless the child has presented in status epilepticus, has experienced marked respiratory compromise (perhaps needing ventilatory support) during the seizure, or has had complex febrile seizures. There is no definitive evidence yet that anticonvulsant prophylaxis for simple febrile seizures pre-

TABLE 36–2. Treatment Options for Febrile Seizures

Cooling measures during febrile illness (antipyretics or bathing in tepid water)
Family reassurance and education
Diazepam, 0.3 mg/kg PO or 5–10 mg rectal gel (Diastat) PR q8h (during febrile illness only)
Phenobarbital, 3–5 mg/kg PO daily, for prophylaxis
Valproic acid, 30 mg/kg PO divided twice daily, for prophylaxis

vents the development of unprovoked seizures. Children who have had frequently recurring seizures that are extremely disruptive for the family and deleterious to parent-child interactions despite educational efforts by the medical caretakers may also be candidates for prophylactic anticonvulsant treatment.

PROGNOSIS

Febrile seizures are a common age-limited problem. The prognosis for children with simple febrile seizures is generally good; the incidence of seizure episodes later in life is 3–6 times higher than in the general population at the same age but is still low: 2–3%. Those who have a complex presentation have a higher likelihood of developing a nonfebrile seizure disorder, but at only 6% if two of the first three factors (Table 36–1) are present or 17% if they are neurodevelopmentally abnormal. Overall, one-third of children with febrile seizures experience a recurrence. The risk of febrile seizure recurrence is most dependent on age: 50% of infants less than 1 year old at the time of their first seizure will have a recurrence, but only 20% of children over 3 years will have a recurrence. Other factors that have a lesser influence on the recurrence risk include family history of seizures, temperature at the initial seizure, time since the previous seizure, and history of previous recurrences.

Case Resolution

In the case history presented at the beginning of this chapter, the girl had a somewhat prolonged simple febrile seizure, a diagnosis supported by a family history positive for febrile seizures. Her family is educated about treatment options. They became comfortable with a decision to use intermittent therapy with diazepam for her subsequent febrile illnesses, realizing that a fever may not be recognized before the seizure.

Selected Readings

Al-Eissa, Y. A. Lumbar puncture in the clinical evaluation of children with seizures associated with fever. Pediatr. Emerg. Care 11:347–350, 1995.
Duchowny, M. Febrile seizures in childhood. In Wyllie, E. (ed.). The Treatment of Epilepsy: Principles and Practice. 1st ed. Philadelphia, Lea & Febiger, 1993, pp. 647–653.
Nelson, K. B., and J. H. Ellenberg. Febrile Seizures. New York, Raven Press, 1981.
Offringa, M. Seizures associated with fever: Current management controversies. Semin. Pediatr. Neurol. 1:90–101, 1994.
Rosman, N. P. A controlled trial of diazepam administered during febrile illnesses to prevent recurrence of febrile seizures. N. Engl. J. Med. 329:79–84, 1993.
Practice parameter: The neurodiagnostic evaluation of the child with a first simple febrile seizure. Pediatrics 97:769–772, 1996.
Technical Report: The neurodiagnostic evaluation of the child with a first simple febrile seizure. Pediatrics 97:773–775, 1996.

CHAPTER 37

RESPIRATORY DISTRESS

James S. Seidel, M.D., Ph.D.

Hx A 6-month-old boy has been coughing and breathing fast for the past day. This morning he refused his bottle and has been irritable. On examination, the infant is fussy. He has a respiratory rate of 60 breaths/min, a pulse of 140/min, and a normal blood pressure and temperature. In addition, he has nasal flaring, intercostal and supraclavicular retractions, and occasional grunting.

Questions

1. What are the causes of respiratory distress in infants and children?
2. What are the signs and symptoms of respiratory distress in infants and children?
3. What are the signs and symptoms of impending respiratory failure in infants and children?
4. What are the critical interventions for infants and children in respiratory distress?

Respiratory distress and respiratory failure may cause significant morbidity and mortality in infants and children. The signs and symptoms of respiratory compromise may be subtle, particularly in small infants. Decompensation may occur rapidly if ventilation or oxygenation is inadequate. Respiratory distress is defined as increased work of breathing, and it usually precedes respiratory failure. Respiratory failure occurs when ventilation or oxygenation is not sufficient to meet the metabolic demands of the tissues. Thus oxygenation of the blood is inadequate or carbon dioxide is not eliminated.

TABLE 37-1.   Causes of Respiratory Distress in Infants and Children

Infection
   Bronchiolitis
   Pneumonia
   Croup
   Epiglottitis
Congenital anomalies
Foreign body aspiration
Reactive airway disease (asthma)
Submersion injuries
Pneumothorax
Smoke inhalation
Toxin exposure
Cardiac disease
Metabolic disease
Neuromuscular disease

This may be caused by diseases of the airway or poor respiratory effort (Table 37–1).

EPIDEMIOLOGY

Primary care physicians frequently care for children in respiratory distress in both offices and emergency departments. In 1990 there were 701,000 hospital admissions for respiratory disease, many of which were in young infants with infections. Other admissions were for reactive airway disease (asthma).

CLINICAL PRESENTATION

Increases in respiratory rate and work of breathing are the most common signs of respiratory disease. Tachycardia is often present, although bradycardia may be a sign of impending cardiopulmonary failure. Signs of poor oxygenation include alterations in mental status, head bobbing, and change in skin color. Cyanosis is often a late sign; it occurs when the amount of unsaturated hemoglobin is at least 5 g/dL. Children may first appear dusky or pale. If children are anemic, cyanosis may not be evident, although the oxygen saturation is low (D$_x$ Box).

D$_x$ Respiratory Distress

- Increased respiratory rate
- Changes in tidal volume or minute ventilation
- Presence of retractions: intercostal, substernal, diaphragmatic, or supraclavicular
- Nasal flaring
- Decreased or absent breath sounds
- Changes in inspiratory-expiratory ratio
- Production of sounds with respiration (e.g., gurgling, stridor, rhonchi, grunting)
- Alterations in mental status
- Inability to speak in sentences
- Presence of pale or cyanotic skin
- Presence of central cyanosis

BOX 37-1.   Comparison of Respiratory Systems in Children and Adults

- The head in children is proportionally larger and has less muscular support.
- The tongue in children is larger in relation to the mouth and can cause airway obstruction.
- The airway diameter is smaller in children. Reductions in size due to secretions or inflammation cause greater resistance to air flow.
- The larynx is higher and more anterior in children, which makes visualization of the vocal cords more difficult.
- The narrowest part of the airway in children is at the cricoid ring, unlike in adults, where the narrowest point is at the vocal cords.
- The trachea in children is short. In newborns it is 4 cm long, and in 18-month-old infants, 7 cm. In adults, it is 12 cm.
- The major muscle of respiration in children is the diaphragm. Any interference with diaphragmatic motion in young children impedes respiratory function. Intercostal muscles are immature in children.
- Children have less pulmonary reserve volume.
- Normal respiratory rates are higher in children and vary by age.

PATHOPHYSIOLOGY

The adequacy of respiration depends on effective gas exchange and the ability to move an adequate volume of gas in and out of the airways. Infants and children generally breathe with minimal effort. In very young children, the diaphragm and abdominal musculature are used for respiration, and the tidal volume is approximately 6–8 mL/kg. If the tidal volume is decreased because of obstruction, children compensate by increasing the respiratory rate, thus attempting to maintain an adequate minute ventilation (minute ventilation = respiratory rate × tidal volume). If the minute ventilation is still insufficient for adequate gas exchange, or children can no longer sustain the increased work of breathing, then respiratory failure ensues. Respiratory failure may progress to cardiopulmonary arrest.

Infants and children are more prone than adults to respiratory distress because of the differences between their respiratory systems (Box 37–1).

EVALUATION

History

A brief history should be taken (Questions Box).

Questions: Respiratory Distress

- For how long has this problem been occurring? Has a similar problem ever occurred before?
- Did the problem begin while the child was eating?
- Has the child had any recent infections?
- Are any members of the household ill?
- Is the child taking any medications?

Physical Examination

Before a complete assessment can proceed, critical interventions that may change children's clinical status should be made. Children should be placed in a position of comfort, and oxygen should be applied. Both ventilation and oxygenation should be assessed.

Respiratory and heart rates should be determined for a period of at least 30 seconds. In infants, abdominal excursions should be counted, and in older children, chest excursions should be counted. Respiratory rates in children are higher than in adults; infants may breathe 40 times per minute, 1-year-olds 25 times per minute, and 10-year-olds 18 times per minute (Table 37–2). These rates vary with age and changes of activity, emotion, and illness. Abnormal respiratory rates are defined as being faster than normal (tachypnea), slower than normal (bradypnea), or absent (apnea). Neonates may exhibit periodic breathing, with periods of regular respirations alternating with irregular breathing. This is a normal variant for age. True apnea (cessation of respiration) is accompanied by change in skin color or altered level of consciousness.

The depth of respiration should be noted. Whether breaths are deep, gasping, or shallow should be determined. Rapid, shallow respirations may not provide enough inspiratory time for adequate gas exchange. The heart rate may also reflect respiratory compromise.

Breath sounds should first be listened to in the axillae and then at the bases and apices. The absence of breath sounds may be an ominous sign. Children's breath sounds are usually well transmitted across the thorax because of the thin chest wall. It is not uncommon to hear upper airway noises when auscultating the lungs.

Abnormal sounds are caused by turbulent air passing through a narrowed airway. Resistance to flow through a hollow tube increases exponentially. Thus the smaller the airway, the greater the resistance to flow generated by even small changes in the radius (e.g., as with edema, secretions, or foreign bodies). The nature of the sounds produced depends on the location of the narrowing in the airway. Gurgling and stridor come from the upper airway, and rhonchi and wheezing from the lower airway. If no abnormal sounds are evident, and breath sounds are absent or decreased, the airways may be totally obstructed. Grunting is caused by turbulent air coming in contact with a partially closed glottis. Children who grunt are generating their own Valsalva maneuver, which results in the partial obstruction of the upper airway and the production of positive end-expiratory pressure.

The physician should also observe the effort children expend in breathing. Increased work of breathing occurs when intercostal, subcostal, or supraclavicular retractions are present, the accessory muscles of respiration are used, breathing is abnormally noisy, or nasal flaring is seen.

In addition, the physician should observe the inspiratory-expiratory ratio while assessing the work of breathing. The ratio is approximately 1:1 in most patients. Prolonged expirations are most often seen with reactive airway disease.

Laboratory Tests

Although the physical examination is the most important tool for assessing children in respiratory distress, laboratory tests such as complete and differential blood counts, ESRs, and blood cultures may help in the diagnosis of infection. It should be remembered that meningitis and metabolic derangement may present with tachypnea not associated with increased work of breathing. Arterial blood gases should be reserved for patients in impending respiratory failure.

Peak expiratory flow or forced expiratory volume in one second (FEV_1) determinations can be helpful in assessing children with reactive airway disease.

Imaging Studies

Chest radiographs can aid in assessing children in respiratory distress but should not be routinely performed in patients with known reactive airway disease unless children have a fever or are in status asthmaticus.

MANAGEMENT

All infants or children in respiratory distress should be managed emergently. In such situations, assessment and intervention often occur simultaneously. All children in respiratory distress should be assessed frequently. The highest possible oxygen concentration should be delivered. Children should never be forced to use an airway adjunct, because this may cause increased anxiety and distress. Patients with clear airways can be maintained with simple interventions such as oxygen blown by the face or given by mask or nasal prongs. More advanced airway management (bag-valve-mask ventilation or endotracheal intubation) may be necessary for children who need assisted ventilation, airway protection, or hyperventilation.

Position

Children in respiratory distress who are alert and breathing spontaneously should be allowed to choose a position of comfort. Small infants who are incapable of positioning themselves are best placed upright

TABLE 37–2. Vital Signs by Age			
Age	Respiration (breaths/min)	Pulse (beats/min)	Systolic Blood Pressure (mm Hg)
Newborn	30–60	100–160	50–70
1–6 wk	30–60	100–160	70–95
6 mo	25–40	90–120	80–100
1 yr	20–30	90–120	80–100
3 yr	20–30	80–120	80–110
6 yr	18–25	70–110	80–110
10 yr	15–20	60–90	90–120

with care taken not to flex or extend the neck. Children and their caregivers should be kept together to reduce anxiety.

The proper position for unconscious children is the "sniffing position," with the neck slightly flexed and the head extended to open the airway. This can be facilitated by placing a towel under the occiput of the head. If simple positioning does not relieve an obstruction, then the airway should be opened using the chin lift or jaw thrust. If spinal trauma is a possibility, only the jaw thrust should be used.

Monitoring

All infants and children in respiratory distress should be carefully monitored. Pulse oximetry will assist the clinician in determining degree of oxygen saturation and, if available, a cardiac and respiratory monitor will provide constant readings of respirations and heart rate. Frequent assessments of the patient are critical to assure a good outcome.

Oxygen Administration

Oxygen should be delivered by any method tolerated by children.

Nasal Prongs. Nasal prongs have two advantages; they are noninvasive and allow maintenance of a constant gas flow even when talking and eating. The concentration of oxygen delivered is limited, however, and irritation and drying of the mucous membranes may result.

Oxygen Masks. Masks deliver a higher concentration of humidified oxygen. Disadvantages include obstruction of children's visual field, potential for carbon dioxide retention, and anxiety because the face is covered. Various types of masks can be used.

The **simple mask** can deliver 35–65% oxygen concentration at flow rates of 6–10 L/min. Room air is drawn into the mask through the exhalation ports in the side of the mask.

A **partial rebreathing mask** is desirable when higher concentrations of oxygen (50–60%) are required. During exhalation, oxygen flows into the reservoir bag along with one third of the exhaled gas. Entrapment of room air is minimized when patients breathe oxygen from the reservoir bag.

A **nonrebreathing mask** has valves that allow only oxygen (85–95%) to flow from the reservoir bag to the patient on inhalation and additional valves on the exhalation ports of the mask that prevent entrapment of room air (Fig. 37–1).

The **face tent** is a soft plastic bucket shaped to the chin that is well tolerated by children. The face tent allows high-flow oxygen to be delivered, and it has the advantage of allowing access to the face and mouth (Fig. 37–2).

A **Venturi mask** is rarely used in children but has the advantage of precisely titrating the oxygen concentration to be delivered from 24–60%.

Assisted Ventilation. Children with potential respiratory failure require assisted ventilation with bag-valve-

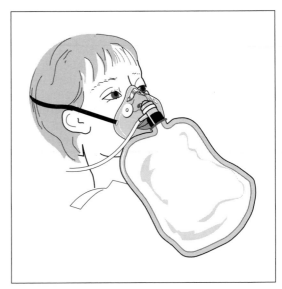

FIGURE 37-1. A non-breathing mask can deliver a high concentration of oxygen to a patient in respiratory distress.

mask devices or endotracheal intubation. Masks of the proper size should be used. The upper edge of the mask should fit snugly over the bridge of the nose without touching the eyes. The lower edge should rest directly on or just above the mandible. An oropharyngeal airway should be inserted in unconscious children to prevent the tongue from obstructing the upper airway. If a bag-valve mask is not available, assisted ventilation can be given with a pocket mask with a one-way valve. Oxygen can be attached to the mask at the side port (Fig. 37–3). Endotracheal intubation is indicated in those children who require control of the airway, who need airway protection, or who require hyperventilation.

PROGNOSIS

Respiratory failure and resulting cardiopulmonary arrest are preventable in most infants and children if their condition is carefully assessed and appropriate

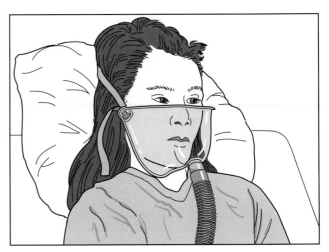

FIGURE 37-2. Use of a face tent.

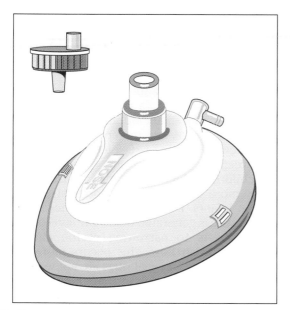

FIGURE 37–3. A pocket mask with a one-way valve and side oxygen port that can be used for assisted ventilation in the office setting.

critical interventions are made. Careful attention to ventilation and oxygenation of patients usually results in a good outcome.

Case Resolution

The fussy infant discussed in the case history has obvious signs of respiratory distress, including tachypnea, tachycardia, grunting, nasal flaring, and retractions. The differential diagnosis includes foreign body, infection, and reactive airway disease. It is important to place the infant in a position of comfort and provide supplemental oxygen before any diagnostic studies, such as chest x-ray, are performed. Pulse oximetry should be monitored. The clinical status of the infant should be reassessed periodically to prevent further deterioration.

Selected Readings

American Heart Association. Guidelines for cardiopulmonary resuscitation and emergency cardiac care: pediatric basic life support. J.A.M.A. 268:2251–2261, 1992.

Chameides, L., and M. F. Hazinski (eds.). Textbook of Pediatric Advanced Life Support. Dallas, American Heart Association, 1994.

Downes, J. J., Fulgencio, and R. C. Raphaely. Acute respiratory failure in infants and children. Pediatr. Clin. North Am. 19:423–445, 1972.

Seidel, J. S. Respiratory emergencies and cardiopulmonary arrest. *In* Barkin, R. (ed.). Pediatric Emergency Medicine: Concepts and Clinical Practice. St. Louis, Mosby–Year Book, 1992, pp. 73–83.

CHAPTER 38

STRIDOR AND CROUP

James S. Seidel, M.D., Ph.D.

H$_x$ A 2-year-old boy has been breathing noisily for 1 day. For the past week he has had a "cold," with a runny nose, fever (temperature: up to 100.4° F [38° C]), and a slight cough. The cough has gradually become worse and now has a barking quality.

On examination, the child is sitting up, has a respiratory rate of 48 breaths/min with marked inspiratory stridor, and an occasional barking cough. His other vital signs include heart rate, 100 beats/min, and temperature of 101.1° F (38.4° C). He has intercostal retractions, his breath sounds are slightly decreased bilaterally, and his skin is pale. The remainder of the examination is normal.

Questions

1. What are the common causes of stridor?
2. What is the pathophysiology of viral croup?
3. How are children with stridor managed?

Noisy breathing is a common symptom that often accompanies respiratory infections in children. The presence of **stridor,** a crowing sound, often concerns children's caregivers. Some parents try home remedies to alleviate the symptoms, whereas others immediately seek help in the office or emergency department setting. **Croup,** a type of noisy breathing, is an inflammation of the larynx, trachea, and upper bronchioles (laryngotracheobronchitis). It is one of the most common causes of barking cough in children.

EPIDEMIOLOGY

Croup most commonly affects children between 6 months and 3 years of age, generally in the fall or early winter. Children less than 1 year of age make up 26% of cases. The condition is more common in boys than girls; two-thirds of all hospitalized children with croup are boys.

Noisy respiration, which may be indicative of croup, may also be a sign of epiglottitis. The incidence of epiglottitis in children has been dramatically reduced in the past 10 years because of immunization against *Haemophilus influenzae*. Many young children are incompletely immunized, however, and epiglottitis should be considered in toxic-appearing children with rapid onset of symptoms of upper airway obstruction. Prior to *H. influenzae* type b immunization, the ratio of cases of epiglottitis to croup was 1:100.

PATHOPHYSIOLOGY

Stridor

Stridor is generally caused by obstruction of the airway between the nose and the larger bronchi. Obstruction at the level of the nose or pharynx may produce snoring or gurgling sounds. The level of the obstruction determines the quality of the sounds produced by turbulence of airflow across a narrowed airway. Turbulence of airflow in the laryngeal area or upper trachea causes the crowing sound characteristic of stridor. Edema and inflammation at the cords and subglottic areas result in inspiratory stridor, whereas obstruction below the cricoid cartilage may lead to both inspiratory and expiratory stridor.

Some of the more common causes of stridor are listed in Table 38–1. The sounds produced at various levels of obstruction can give the primary care provider clues as to the etiology of the problem. The most

---

TABLE 38–1. Causes of Stridor

Congenital Anomalies
Tracheomalacia
Laryngomalacia
Choanal atresia
Laryngeal web
Laryngocele
Subglottic stenosis
Vascular ring
Macroglossia (Beckwith's syndrome)
Tracheal web or cyst
Inflammatory Lesions
Viral croup
Epiglottitis
Abscess (retropharyngeal, peritonsillar, parapharyngeal)
Tracheitis
Bronchitis
Severe tonsillitis
Angioneurotic edema
Infectious mononucleosis
Diphtheria
Trauma
Direct trauma to the upper airway
Postintubation subglottic stenosis
Neurogenic
Laryngeal paralysis
Poor pharyngeal muscle tone
Caustic or Thermal Injury
Lye or caustic ingestion
Hot liquid
Foreign Body
Neoplasm

---

common cause of stridor that begins shortly after birth is tracheomalacia, a condition secondary to the immaturity of the cartilage of the trachea. Laryngomalacia, which is caused by floppy supraglottic structures, resolves after several months.

The upper airway of infants and children is more susceptible to obstruction as a result of anatomic differences between children and adults. The tongue of children is relatively large, and the epiglottis is floppy and shaped somewhat like the Greek letter omega (Ω). The angle between the epiglottis and the glottis is more acute in children, which makes direct visualization of the airway more difficult. Cartilaginous structures are less rigid in infants. During inspiration, negative intraluminal pressure is generated below the level of obstruction, which leads to narrowing of the airway and turbulence of the air flow. This occurs more often in children because the tracheal rings are not well formed. In addition, the smaller size of the airway in children makes resistance to air flow greater when obstruction is present.

The smaller the airway, the greater the resistance to flow (resistance increases exponentially). Alterations in the diameter of the airway are most often caused by edema and inflammation from a variety of conditions, including congenital anomalies, infection, allergic and anaphylactic reactions, cysts, tumors, and trauma. Even localized areas of airway narrowing in infants and children can lead to respiratory distress because the airway is so small, particularly at the cricoid ring, which is the narrowest portion of the airway in children.

Croup

Croup is most often caused by an infection with parainfluenza virus (type I or II), respiratory syncytial virus, or influenza virus. Particularly severe disease may be associated with influenza A infection. Infection occurs via droplets spread from other infected individuals.

The virus first attacks the nasopharynx and subsequently spreads to the larynx and upper trachea. The infection causes inflammation and edema of the airway that often involves the vocal cords, producing the typical barking cough, hoarseness, and inspiratory stridor. In severe cases the lower airways also may be involved, leading to impaired alveolar ventilation. In some children, bacterial infection may occur with bacterial tracheitis or extension of infection to the lower airway. Airways of infants are small and particularly susceptible to obstruction because of the narrow subglottic region and the laxity of the cartilaginous structures.

Spasmodic croup, which occurs at night, may be recurrent. It is characterized by the sudden onset of hoarseness, barking cough, and stridor. This condition may resolve when children are exposed to humid air. The etiology is unknown but is probably either a reaction to a viral infection or an allergic phenomenon. There may be a family history of recurrent stridor in children with spasmodic croup.

TABLE 38–2. Differential Diagnosis of Stridor

Data	Viral Croup	Spasmodic Croup	Epiglottitis	Foreign Body
Age	3–36 mo	3–36 mo	1–8 yr	All ages
Prodrome	URI symptoms; onset over 2–5 d	None; sudden onset at night	Usually none; rapid onset over several hours	None; sudden onset
Fever	Low-grade	None	Usually above 39° C	None
Cough	Barking	Barking	None or dry	May or may not be present
Respiratory distress	Present	Present	Present	Usually present
White blood cell count	Normal or slightly elevated	Normal	Elevated	Normal
Blood culture	No growth	No growth	H. influenzae	No growth
Radiograph	Subglottic narrowing; steeple sign	Subglottic narrowing (±)	Swollen epiglottis	Air trapping; may show a foreign body

DIFFERENTIAL DIAGNOSIS

The differential diagnosis of stridor is presented in Table 38–2.

EVALUATION

History

A complete history should be obtained (Questions Box).

Physical Examination

It is important to assess the degree of respiratory distress and to place children in a position of comfort; monitor heart rate, ventilation, and oxygenation; and deliver oxygen (see Chapter 37, Respiratory Distress). The stridorous sounds produced are usually inspiratory but may be inspiratory and expiratory if the disease progresses to the lower airway. The presence of stridor at rest or with sleep should be assessed. Breath sounds may be decreased bilaterally, and severe tachypnea, with respiratory rates from 40–80 breaths/min, may occur. The peripheral or central cyanosis associated with severe disease should be noted. Assessment of the croup score may be helpful (Table 38–3).

Laboratory Tests

Laboratory tests such as a CBC and blood culture are rarely helpful unless the physician is concerned about bacterial infection. The WBC count may be normal or mildly elevated, and the differential count may show a predominance of polymorphonuclear cells. If epiglottitis is being considered, no blood should be drawn until the airway has been visualized and secured.

Imaging Studies

Radiographs of the soft tissues of the upper airway are often helpful. In children with croup, lateral neck films may reveal ballooning of the hypopharynx, a normal epiglottis, and narrowing of the subglottic area (Fig. 38–1). The frontal view shows the classic "steeple sign" of the subglottic area where the airway narrows like a steeple or pencil tip. Radiographic studies should not delay the management of children with suspected epiglottis. Widening of the epiglottis (thumb-shaped rather than pinky-shaped) may be seen on lateral neck films in such patients if radiographs are obtained.

Other imaging studies, such as a barium swallow or CT scan of the thorax, are helpful in diagnosing congenital anomalies (e.g., vascular ring).

MANAGEMENT

Most children with croup and stridor can be managed as outpatients. Caregivers should be given careful instructions so that they understand the course of the illness, know what to expect, and realize when emergency care is needed. Children with a prolonged history of stridor may require consultation with a head and neck specialist. If a specific cause of stridor, such as a foreign body, is identified, appropriate management should be instituted.

Children with croup should be treated with gentleness and should not be upset. Agitation and crying increase respiratory distress and oxygen demand. Procedures should be kept to a minimum.

Cool mist should be provided by "blow by" or mask. Airway adjuncts that cause increased agitation should not be used. **Humidified oxygen or air,** which decreases the viscosity of secretions and reduces the edema of the airway, is the most important therapy for croup. Management of spasmodic croup requires only humidified air, and symptoms usually resolve within 6 hours of the onset.

The heart rate, respiratory status, and oxygen saturation should be monitored. Pulse oximetry should be used.

Questions: Stridor and Croup

- Did the child have an antecedent respiratory infection?
- Does the child have a fever? If so, how high is the temperature?
- Was the onset of stridor abrupt?
- Does the child have any ill contacts?
- Does the child have any associated symptoms such as vomiting, diarrhea, or rash?
- Is the child feeding normally?
- Is the child drooling?

TABLE 38–3. Croup Score 0–4

	0	1	2	3
Stridor	None	Only with agitation	Mild at rest	Severe at rest
Retraction	None	Mild	Moderate	Severe
Air entry	Normal	Mild decrease	Moderate decrease	Marked decrease
Color	Normal	Normal	Normal	Cyanotic
Level of consciousness	Normal	Restless when disturbed	Restless when undisturbed	Leghargic

Disease Category by Score

Score	Degree	Management
≤4	Mild	Outpatient—mist therapy
5–6	Mild to moderate	Outpatient dexamethasone 0.6 mg/kg PO, if child improves in ED after mist, is older than 6 months, and has a reliable family
7–8	Moderate	Dexamethasone 0.6 mg/kg PO or IM, consider admission—racemic epinephrine
≥9	Severe	Admit—racemic epinephrine, oxygen, intensive care unit

Modified, with permission, from Taussig, L. M., et al. Treatment of laryngotracheobronchitis (croup). Use of intermittent positive-pressure breathing and racemic epinephrine. Am. J. Dis. Child 129:790, 1975.

Treatment of croup with **corticosteroids** has been controversial; however, a number of studies have demonstrated that dexamethasone given as a single dose of 0.6 mg/kg is effective in shortening the course of the illness if given in the first 3 days. It may be given orally or as an intramuscular injection for children who are unable to take oral medication. Use of the tablet preparation ground up in apple sauce is recommended as the liquid preparation does not taste good and is not well tolerated. Recent studies using nebulized budes-onide also demonstrate some efficacy in reducing respiratory distress and lowering of the croup score. The combined use of oral dexamethasone and nebulized budesonide has also been shown to improve the clinical croup score. Continuous or long-term therapy with steroids does not seem to alter the clinical course of the disease or the period of hospitalization. Treatment with antibiotics is not indicated unless infection with bacteria is evident.

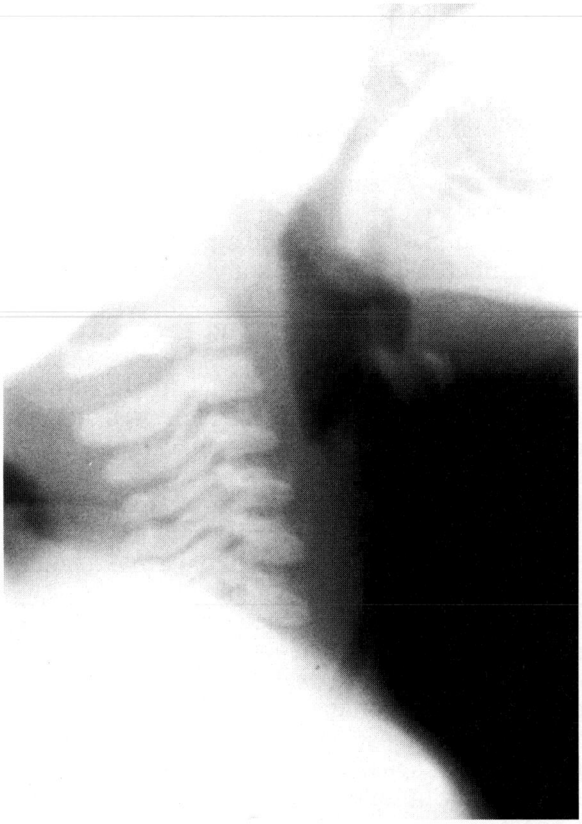

Use of racemic epinephrine is also controversial. Several studies have shown that there was no difference in the long-term outcome between those children who were treated with epinephrine and those who received a placebo. Other studies have clearly demonstrated an acute effect of the drug when given via nebulizer. "Rebound" respiratory distress after the drug effects have worn off has been reported in the literature. Racemic epinephrine may be used on patients who are going to be discharged if they can be observed for 3–4 hours after treatment.

Hospitalization should be considered for children in severe respiratory distress, those who are unable to eat, and those whose parents are unable to cope with the tasks required to manage children at home. It is always indicated for children with a bacterial infection such as epiglottitis or tracheitis.

About 10% of infants and children with croup may need **controlled ventilation with endotracheal intubation.** The indications for intubation include severe respiratory distress, hypoxia, and hypercapnia. A major complication of endotracheal intubation in children with croup is subglottic stenosis, which develops because the endotracheal tube may traumatize the inflamed airway, leading to permanent damage. Patients should be extubated as soon as possible.

Direct laryngoscopy may be necessary in some children where the etiology of the stridor is not clear. This procedure should be done by a practitioner who is experienced in managing the airway.

PROGNOSIS

Stridor is a serious sign, which is indicative of upper airway obstruction and potential respiratory compro-

FIGURE 38–1. Lateral neck radiograph of viral croup. Note the ballooning of the hypopharynx and the narrowing in the subglottic area. (Courtesy of Dr. J. S. Seidel, Division of General and Emergency Pediatrics, Harbor-UCLA Medical Center.)

mise. Although it has many causes, the prognosis is usually determined by the rapidity of diagnosis and the institution of appropriate therapeutic measures, particularly stabilizing the patient and ensuring patency of the airway. Certain conditions such as croup often resolve spontaneously within a few days, although some children require hospitalization and, rarely, assisted ventilation. Other conditions, such as foreign bodies or tumors, necessitate aggressive intervention to prevent death from airway obstruction.

Case Resolution

In the case history at the beginning of this chapter, the 2-year-old with the antecedent infection and stridor has the classic signs of croup and a croup score of 6. First, adequate ventilation and oxygenation should be ensured. As soon as the assessment and management of airway, breathing, and circulation are completed, other diagnostic studies and specific therapy, such as dexamethasone or racemic epinephrine, or both, can be considered.

Selected Readings

Cherry, J. D. Croup, laryngitis, laryngotracheitis, spasmodic croup, laryngotracheobronchitis, bacterial tracheitis, and laryngotracheobronchopneuomonitis. *In* Feigin R. D., and J. D. Cherry. Pediatric Infectious Diseases, 4th ed. Philadelphia, W. B. Saunders, 1998, pp. 237–241.

Johnson, D. W., S. Jacobson, P. C. Edney, et al. A comparison of nebulized budesonide, intramuscular dexamethasone, and placebo for moderately severe croup. N. Engl. J. Med. 339:498–503, 1998.

Kaditis, A. G., and E. R. Wald. Viral croup: Current diagnosis and treatment. Pediatr. Infect. Dis. J. 17:827–834, 1998.

Klassen, T. P., W. R. Craig, D. Moher, M. H. Osmond, et al. Nebulized budesonide and oral dexamethasone for the treatment of croup: a randomized controlled trial. J.A.M.A. 279:1629–1632, 1998.

Kunkel, N. C., and M. D. Baker. Use of racemic epinephrine, dexamethasone, and mist in the outpatient management of croup. Peds. Emerg. Care. 12:156–159, 1996.

Ledwith, C. A., L. M. Shae, and E. D. Mauro. Safety and efficacy of nebulized racemic epinephrine in conjunction with oral dexamethasone and mist in the outpatient treatment of croup. Ann. Emerg. Med. 25:331–337, 1995.

Super, D. M., et al. A prospective double-blind study to evaluate the effect of dexamethasone in acute laryngotracheitis. J. Pediatr. 115:323–329, 1989.

CHAPTER 39

SIDS AND ALTE

Carol D. Berkowitz, M.D.

Hx A 4-month-old male infant is brought to the emergency department by paramedics after being found blue and not breathing by his mother. He had previously been well except for a mild upper respiratory infection. His mother fed her son at 2:00 AM, and when she checked on him at 6:00 AM, she found him blue and lifeless. Although the mother smoked cigarettes during pregnancy, the pregnancy and delivery were otherwise normal. The infant received the appropriate immunizations at 2 months of age.

Questions

1. What factors are associated with SIDS?
2. How are SIDS and ALTE related?
3. What is the appropriate evaluation of infants who present with an ALTE?
4. What services are available to families who have lost infants to SIDS?

Sudden infant death syndrome (SIDS), also referred to as crib death, is defined as the sudden, unexplained death of an apparently well infant that is not adequately explained by a comprehensive medical history of the infant and family, a thorough postmortem examination, or a death scene examination. The term SIDS was officially designated in 1963 to describe the syndrome of sudden, unexpected death of infants less than 1 year of age in whom no pathologic etiology could be determined after a careful autopsy. The syndrome has been known since biblical times; parents were advised not to lie with their children for fear of suffocating them. SIDS is the second leading cause of death of infants between the ages of 1 month and 1 year, second only to congenital anomalies. Most of the recent SIDS research has sought to determine the etiology of the disorder, define the relationship between SIDS and apnea, and determine patient and environmental risk factors.

SIDS-like events associated with successful resuscitation were once described as near-miss SIDS or aborted crib death. The term that is now used is apparent life-threatening event (ALTE). ALTE episodes are characterized by some combination of apnea, color change, marked change in muscle tone, and choking or gagging. Infants who experience ALTEs may appear to have died, which makes the events frightening to observers. The relationship between ALTE and subsequently succumbing to SIDS is controversial.

EPIDEMIOLOGY

SIDS had accounted for 5000 to 10,000 deaths per year in the United States, with an overall incidence of slightly under 2 per 1000. These figures have been dramatically reduced by the campaign of the American Academy of Pediatrics (AAP) to place babies in the supine position for sleep. Following the institution of the "Back to Sleep" program, the annual death rate from SIDS dropped to 3000 with an incidence of 0.8 per 1000. SIDS affects boys more commonly than girls and occurs more often in the winter months. This seasonality may be related to infection with respiratory syncytial virus. Infants are usually 2–3 months of age. The frequency of SIDS differs in different populations in both the United States and other countries. The disorder is reported less frequently in Asian Americans, with an incidence of 0.51 per 1000, and more often in Native Americans, with an incidence of 5.93 per 1000. In recent years, ethnic variation in compliance with supine sleeping position may account for some of these differences.

Numerous epidemiologic, maternal, and infant factors have been associated with SIDS, including prematurity and intrauterine growth retardation (Table 39–1). Recent studies have not confirmed initial reports of a higher incidence of SIDS among premature infants with bronchopulmonary dysplasia. A disproportionate number of infants with SIDS come from lower socioeconomic groups, although this is true for infants dying from all causes. Mothers of children with SIDS are frequently young and unwed; smoke cigarettes or use drugs, such as heroin, methadone, or cocaine; and have had fewer doctor visits during the prenatal and postpartum periods.

CLINICAL PRESENTATION

Victims of SIDS present in cardiopulmonary arrest, with a history of previous good health or antecedent URI. They often present in the early morning hours, having succumbed during sleep. Infants who have experienced an ALTE may appear pale, cyanotic, hypotonic, lethargic, and have bradycardia. They often present during the day between the hours of 8 AM and 8 PM (D$_x$ Box). If resuscitation is successful, infants may look normal and be fully alert.

TABLE 39–1. Risk Factors for Sudden Infant Death Syndrome

Lower socioeconomic class
Maternal youth
Unmarried mother
Maternal smoking
Maternal substance abuse
Prematurity
Poor prenatal care
Sleeping in prone position

D$_x$ SIDS and ALTE

- Apnea
- Bradycardia
- Hypotonia
- Cyanosis
- Pallor
- Altered level of consciousness

PATHOPHYSIOLOGY

The exact cause of SIDS is unclear. More than 70 different theories have been proposed. The relationship between SIDS and apnea engendered a great deal of interest in the 1970s and 1980s. Studies assessed ventilatory response of infants with ALTE to different conditions (e.g., hypoxia) as well as the appearance of postmortem tissue from SIDS victims. The postmortem tissue has often shown evidence of long-standing hypoxia such as brainstem gliosis. Markedly increased neuronal apoptosis in the brain stem and hippocampus of SIDS victims supports the role of hypoxia. Other changes initially observed on autopsy such as thickening of smooth muscle and small blood vessels in the lungs, hypertrophy of the right ventricle, and hematopoiesis in the liver have not been borne out by subsequent studies.

Research concerning the relationship between ALTE and control of ventilation suggests that three separate components are associated with respiratory abnormalities in some infants who have experienced ALTEs. First, central apnea, which may be associated with immaturity, infection, or congenital anomalies, results from primary failure of the respiratory control center. Affected infants fail to respond appropriately to hypercarbia and hypoxia. Second, airway obstruction may be associated with apnea. Obstructive apnea is noted in infants with craniofacial anomalies and Down syndrome. Obstructive apnea contributes to ALTE an estimated 5% of the time. Infants with obstructive apnea demonstrate increased chest wall movement in the face of decreasing heart rate and decreasing oxygen levels (pO$_2$). Third, expiratory apnea may play a role. Infants with expiratory apnea experience sudden atelectasis, ventilation perfusion inequalities, hypoxia, and marked cyanosis, which occurs in 5–10 seconds. Expiratory apnea is often associated with sudden death. Cardiac arrhythmias or anomalies do not appear to be causative in SIDS.

As noted above, recent studies have implicated sleeping in the prone position with an increased incidence of SIDS. Researchers have examined the relationship between the worldwide incidence of SIDS and infant sleep positions. No association between aspiration and sleeping in the supine position in normal infants apparently exists. A number of mechanisms have been postulated linking SIDS to sleeping in the prone position. Sleeping in the prone position may be associated with upper airway obstruction, rebreathing of expired air, or hyperthermia. Because of the link between sleeping in a prone position and apnea, the American Academy of Pediatrics recommends a supine or side sleeping position for normal infants.

The association between SIDS and fatal child abuse has also received attention. The evaluation of the home environment of SIDS victims, referred to as death scene investigations, may reveal accidental causes of death for some of these children. Alternatively, such investigations may reveal that children died from inflicted injuries. A comprehensive autopsy should include an assessment for long bone fractures as well as intracranial hemorrhage, which establish inflicted trauma as the cause of the sudden death. In some municipalities, child fatality boards review each case of reputed SIDS to determine whether an etiology other than SIDS is present. Infants with Munchausen's syndrome by proxy (MSBP) may present with SIDS or ALTE. Such infants are suffocated by the parents until they become apneic or die. The use of in-hospital covert videosurveillance has facilitated the recognition of apnea secondary to MSBP.

DIFFERENTIAL DIAGNOSIS

The major challenge for physicians who care for children with SIDS or ALTE is to determine if any underlying condition may have caused the symptomatology (Table 39–2). Sepsis, respiratory infections, seizures, gastroesophageal reflux, inborn errors of metabolism, infantile botulism, cardiac anomalies, and child abuse should all be considered. The circumstances surrounding ALTEs suggest which of these conditions is suspect. A sepsis evaluation is particularly warranted in children who have symptoms such as fever, vomiting, or diarrhea. Infants with respiratory symptoms such as tachypnea and wheezing may have respiratory syncitial virus (RSV) infection, which is associated with apneic episodes, particularly during the first week of illness in infants under 3 months of age who had been premature and experienced apnea of prematurity. Young infants with pertussis do not exhibit the classic cough with whoop and may present with respiratory distress and apnea. Infants with abnormal movements or ALTEs when awake may be experiencing seizures. The apnea may represent the seizure or a postictal event. Infantile botulism causes decreased

muscle tone and weakness. Apnea may also accompany gastroesophageal reflux. In general, affected infants have a history of eating, regurgitating, and then developing apnea. As previously noted, child abuse, particularly with intracranial hemorrhage, or MSBP may result in apnea or SIDS.

Inborn errors of metabolism are reported in 4–8% of cases of ALTE. Most commonly, there is abnormal fat oxidation. Medium chain acyl-CoA dehydrogenase deficiency is the most common disorder. Inborn errors of metabolism should be considered in infants with other symptoms, such as vomiting or failure to thrive, or in the context of a positive family history. Symptoms may first appear when a previously well infant is metabolically stressed as by an acute infectious illness. Rarely, cardiac arrhythmias, most notably long QT interval or Wolff-Parkinson-White syndrome, are associated with apnea or sudden episodes of bradycardia.

EVALUATION

History

The history may provide the clue to the etiology of SIDS or ALTE (Questions Box).

Physical Examination

A complete examination should be conducted. If infants are floppy and have poor color or have required either mouth-to-mouth resuscitation or vigorous stimulation, significant events are likely. Physicians should check for the presence of bruises, dysmorphic features, growth impairment, abnormal neurologic or developmental findings, which may suggest an alternative etiology. The presence of tachypnea, retractions, wheezing, or cough is consistent with a respiratory infection such as RSV or pertussis.

Laboratory Tests

In general, the laboratory workup is guided by the findings of the history and physical examination (Table

---

TABLE 39–2. Differential Diagnosis of Sudden Infant Death Syndrome (SIDS)/Apparent Life-Threatening Event (ALTE)

ALTE
Sepsis
Pertussis
Respiratory syncitial virus
Infantile botulism
Seizures
Cardiac arrhythmias/anomalies
Gastroesophageal reflux
Inborn errors of metabolism
Child abuse
Intracranial hemorrhage

Questions: SIDS and ALTE

- What were the events leading up to the episode?
  - Was the child awake and eating, indicating that gastroesophageal reflux should be considered?
  - Was the child awake and did the eyes roll back or the body stiffen or jerk, suggesting that a seizure may have occurred?
- How serious was the event? Did breathing resume spontaneously or did cardiopulmonary resuscitation have to be initiated?
- Have similar events occurred in the past?
- Is the infant basically well? Has the infant been ill recently?
- Has the child had respiratory symptoms such as wheezing or cough?
- Do the siblings have a history of SIDS or ALTE that would suggest the presence of a familial disorder or child abuse?
- Were there any problems with the pregnancy or delivery?
- Is there a history of maternal drug use during pregnancy?
- Is there a history of maternal pre- or post-natal smoking?
- Does the infant sleep in a supine, prone, or side down position?

TABLE 39–3. Laboratory Studies to Consider in Evaluating Infants with Apparent Life-Threatening Event (ALTE)

Often Indicated
Complete blood count
Blood culture
Lumbar puncture
Urine culture
Chest x-ray
Serum electrolytes
Blood sugar
Serum ammonia
Sometimes Indicated
Electroencephalogram
Computed tomographic scan
Barium swallow

39–3). A sepsis evaluation, including a CBC, blood culture, lumbar puncture, and urine culture, is appropriate to rule out sepsis in toxic-appearing infants. Serum electrolytes and glucose are important to check because they may indicate an inborn error of metabolism or other abnormalities (e.g., hypoglycemia), which may be associated with apnea with or without the presence of a seizure. When a metabolic etiology is suspected, a test for serum ammonia level should be performed. Hypotonic infants should be evaluated for infantile botulism by sending a stool specimen for testing. All infants with a history of apnea or ALTE should be admitted to the hospital for observation, workup, and monitoring.

Imaging Studies

A chest x-ray should be performed to rule out pneumonia if sepsis is suspected. If the history and physical examination suggest other etiologies, CT, and barium swallow may also be ordered.

Diagnostic Studies

An EEG should be obtained if a seizure disorder is suspected. In-hospital covert videosurveillance is a complex procedure that may be undertaken if MSBP is suspected. Pneumograms detect apnea and associated bradycardia, and document such episodes. Polysomnography assesses for upper airway obstruction, but is usually available only in tertiary care centers.

MANAGEMENT

In addition to the diagnostic workup, other evaluation to determine if infants are at risk for repeated episodes of apnea, bradycardia, or upper airway obstruction is warranted. Infants who have not been fully resuscitated in the field should be resuscitated, stabilized, and admitted. Any identifiable conditions such as sepsis or seizures should be appropriately managed. In most cases, no etiology for the apneic episodes can be determined. Only 5–10% of children who succumb to SIDS have had a previous ALTE.

The administration of **xanthine derivatives** such as caffeine, 5–7.5 mg/kg/day, or theophylline, 6–9 mg/kg/day to a serum level of 5–15 mg/dL, may be used to manage infants who have experienced ALTEs. These medications stimulate the respiratory center and prevent central apnea. The efficacy of xanthine derivatives in the management of apnea other than that associated with prematurity has not been established, however.

A second treatment method involves **home apnea monitoring.** A 1986 consensus statement of the National Institutes of Health described three groups of infants who should be candidates for home monitoring: term infants who have unexplained apnea of infancy, which is usually manifested by an ALTE or an abnormal pneumogram; preterm infants who have experienced apnea of infancy beyond 40 weeks postconception; and subsequent siblings of two or more SIDS victims. Apnea monitoring involves an apparatus that measures both chest wall movement and heart rate. Parents must be instructed in equipment maintenance, alarm interpretation, and cardiopulmonary resuscitation. In general, monitoring equipment is distributed by companies who provide 24-hour service to ensure that the equipment is functioning. The cost of evaluating infants with ALTE is $3000–$5000, and the monthly rental and maintenance costs of monitoring devices are $150–$300. Whether monitoring has made any difference in the incidence of SIDS in infants who have experienced an ALTE is unclear. Poor parental compliance may be a factor in monitor failure. Frequent false alarms may dissuade parents from use of the home monitor. Monitoring may be discontinued if infants have had no periods of apnea that require stimulation or resuscitation for a minimum of 2–3 months. Underlying neurologic problems should be adequately addressed and corrected before monitoring is discontinued.

In addition to managing infants with ALTE, physicians must provide care to families whose infants have succumbed to SIDS. In most jurisdictions, cases of SIDS must be reported to the coroner's office. Some coroners maintain a Child Death Review Board that further investigates each case, sometimes initiating a death scene investigation. The diagnosis of SIDS can only be reached following a full autopsy, a complete history of the infant and family, and a death scene investigation. It is important for physicians to tell families when they think the cause of death is SIDS even before definitive autopsy results are available. Parents of children who have succumbed to SIDS should be referred to support groups and agencies to help them deal with the loss of their children. Information about these organizations can be obtained from the SIDS Alliance, 10500 Little Patuxent Parkway, Suite 420, Columbia, MD 21044, 800-221-SIDS.

PROGNOSIS

Prevention of SIDS has become a focus of public health measures. Improving maternal risk factors involves drug and smoking cessation, access to prenatal care, and implementing breast-feeding. Mothers must be instructed to avoid soft bedding for their infants and place their infants in the supine position for sleep.

The prognosis for children who have experienced an ALTE varies and depends on predisposing conditions. Abnormal neurodevelopmental conditions are generally associated with a poor prognosis.

Case Resolution

The infant presented in the case history succumbed to SIDS. In spite of resuscitative efforts by the paramedics, he could not be revived. The mother is advised of the diagnosis of suspected SIDS and referred to the appropriate agency. The coroner is notified about the case and the presence of any associated physical findings such as bruises.

Selected Readings

American Academy of Pediatrics, Task Force on Infant Sleeping Position and SIDS. Infant sleep position and sudden infant death syndrome (SIDS) in the United States: Joint Commentary from the American Academy of Pediatrics and selected agencies of the federal government. Pediatrics 93:820, 1994.

Assessment of infant sleeping position–selected states, 1996. M.M.W.R. 47:873–874, 1998.

Bass, M., R. E. Kravath, and L. Golass. Death-scene investigation in sudden infant death. N. Engl. J. Med. 315:100–105, 1986.

Boles, R. G., et al. Retrospective biochemical screening of fatty acid oxidation disorders in postmortem livers of 418 cases of sudden death in the first year of life. J. Pediatr. 132:924–933, 1998.

Brooks, J: (guest editor) SIDS. Pediatric Annals 1995; 24(7). Entire issue.

Carroll, J. L., and G. M. Loughlin. Sudden infant death syndrome. Pediatr. Rev. 14:83, 1993.

Chiodini, B. A., and B. T. Thatch. Impaired ventilation in infants sleeping face down: potential significance for sudden infant death syndrome. J. Pediatr. 123:686–692, 1993.

Emery, J. L. Child abuse, sudden infant death syndrome, and unexpected infant death. Am. J. Dis. Child. 147:1097–1100, 1993.

Goyco, P. G., and R. C. Beckerman. Sudden infant death syndrome. Curr. Probl. Pediatr. 20:229–346, 1990.

Gray, P. H., and Y. Rogers. Are infants with bronchopulmonary dysplasia at risk for sudden infant death syndrome? Pediatrics 93:774–777, 1994.

Haas, J. E., et al. Relationship between epidemiologic risk factors and clinicopathologic findings in the sudden infant death syndrome. Pediatrics 91:106–112, 1993.

Taylor, J. A., and M. Sanderson. A reexamination of the risk factors for the sudden infant death syndrome. J. Pediatr. 126:887–891, 1995.

Willinger, M., E. Hoffman, and R. B. Hartford. Infant sleep position and risk for sudden infant death syndrome: Report of meeting held January 13 and 14, 1994, National Institutes of Health, Bethesda, MD. Pediatrics 93:814–819, 1994.

C H A P T E R   4 0

SYNCOPE

Elizabeth A. Edgerton, M.D., M.P.H.

H$_x$ The school nurse refers a 14-year-old adolescent female to your office. The patient states that she fainted during marching band tryouts that afternoon. This is the first time she has ever fainted. She reports that after standing in formation for an hour she suddenly felt light-headed and nauseous, and that the next thing she knew she was on the ground. Witnesses said that she was unconscious for less than a minute and did not have any unusual movements. She denies taking any medication or using any illicit drugs. There is no family history of sudden death, seizures, breath-holding spells, or pallid spells. The patient does admit to not eating anything during the day because she has been busy practicing for the tryouts. Her mother is concerned because she read that fainting might be associated with sudden death. The mother wants to know whether her daughter should still participate in physical activities.

Her physical examination reveals no unusual findings, and her vital signs are within normal limits. A serum glucose test is normal, and a urine pregnancy test is found to be negative. Her ECG shows normal rate, rhythm, and axis. No arrhythmias or prolonged QT intervals are detected.

Questions

1. What are the causes of syncope?
2. What type of workup is done primarily to evaluate for syncope?
3. Which pediatric subspecialists assist in the evaluation of syncope?
4. When are referrals to subspecialists indicated?
5. Which patients who present with syncope are at greatest risk for sudden death?

Pediatricians are often called upon to evaluate children and adolescents with syncopal events. An episode of syncope, commonly referred to as fainting, frequently leads to much anxiety among family members. Although sudden cardiac death is a rare complication, it is usually of foremost concern to the patient, family members, and health professionals. The workup of syncope can easily result in costly evaluations that provide little in the way of new information beyond that obtained by the history and physical. The dilemma for the pediatrician is knowing the type of and extent of the evaluation, which patients are at risk for sudden death, and when a referral to a subspecialist is indicated. In a time of managed care, being able to develop a cost-effective and medically sound approach to the assessment is imperative. A step-wise approach, based on key findings in the history and physical examination, is often effective.

EPIDEMIOLOGY

Syncope is defined as a sudden loss of consciousness, usually associated with a rapid recovery. Syncope results from a decrease in cerebral perfusion that can occur through many different mechanisms. It is estimated that syncope occurs in up to 50% of children by the time they reach adolescence and that it accounts for approximately 1–3% of all emergency department visits. Since many syncopal events resolve quickly, the care of a physician is never sought. These numbers may therefore actually underestimate the true prevalence of syncope among children.

CLINICAL PRESENTATION

The clinical presentation of syncope varies with the etiology. In the vasovagal form of syncope, there can be a prodrome of symptoms, which include lightheadedness, visual disturbances, nausea, pallor, and diaphoresis. The patient has usually been in the upright position for a long period of time or has suddenly changed from a sitting position to standing one. Dehydration, fatigue, hunger, or illness can precipitate a syncopal event. If the patient experiences a syncopal event, the length of unconsciousness is usually less than a minute and there are typically no residual sequelae. Syncope of a cardiac etiology may lack the prodrome of the vasovagal form. Patients may complain of palpitations, angina, or tightness in the chest. This type of syncope often occurs during physical activity. Syncope can be accompanied by abnormal movements or a complete loss of body tone. Syncope related to seizures is marked by a longer recovery time often associated with a postictal phase; also these episodes may occur when the patient is recumbent rather than upright.

PATHOPHYSIOLOGY

The mechanisms leading to syncope can be multiple, but three broad categories are used to explain the pathophysiology: **autonomic, cardiac,** and **noncardiac.** Many of these mechanisms overlap, and these categories serve only to provide a broad framework for understanding, assisting in history taking, and diagnosing the cause.

Autonomic

In this category, the most common type of syncope is **vasovagal,** accounting for more than 50% of patients presenting with syncope. It begins with a sudden loss of vasovagal tone followed by hypotension (vasodepressor spells) that can be associated with bradycardia or asystole (cardioinhibitory spells). Patients may present with hypotension only or with both hypotension and paradoxical bradycardia. The vasovagal type of syncope usually occurs while the patient is in an upright position, a situation that leads to decreased venous return. The patient's heart then responds with either an increased sensitivity or excessive response to the decreased venous return. This then elicits a central vagal reflex causing a sympathetic withdrawal, resulting in hypotension and bradycardia. A similar mechanism is seen in adolescents and athletes who have excessive vagal tone. In situational syncope or reflex syncope, the performance of an activity (e.g., coughing, micturition, defecation, and hair grooming) causes an increase in vagal tone. In the younger child, pallid breath-holding spells can lead to syncope. The child usually suffers a painful event, followed by crying, pallor, then loss of consciousness. In orthostatic syncope, the patient is intravascularly volume depleted secondary to dehydration or blood loss that leads to tachycardia and hypotension when changing to the upright position. This form of syncope is considered a variant of the vasovagal form.

Cardiac

Cardiac mechanisms of syncope can be due to structural or functional abnormalities. Structural lesions are usually obstructive lesions and lead to decreased ventricular outflow, which results in diminished cerebral perfusion and syncope. Functional abnormalities primarily include arrhythmias, which affect the cardiac output, thus decreasing cerebral perfusion. Cardiac causes of syncope are more likely to be associated with sudden death, so it is particularly important to identify and treat these abnormalities.

Among patients with obstructive outflow lesions, aortic stenosis and hypertrophic cardiomyopathy are the most common. Less common cardiac lesions include pulmonic stenosis, mitral stenosis, atrial myxoma, cardiac tamponade, and primary pulmonary hypertension. Syncope often occurs during exertion owing to the heart's inability to provide the increased cardiac output needed with physical activity. Another proposed mechanism for cardiac-related syncope is decreased perfusion to the myocardium, leading to ischemia, dyskinesia, or an arrhythmia that ultimately leads to decreased ventricular output. When arrhythmias occur in patients who have an underlying structural heart disease, the risk of syncopal events is greater and arrhythmias should be the presumed cause of syncope until proven otherwise. Different structural abnormalities produce different types of arrhythmias. Patients who have undergone correction of atrial defects can have supraventricular tachycardia (SVT), atrial flutter or fibrillation, or bradycardia. Patients with repaired ventricular lesions are more prone to ventricular tachycardia (VT), and those with repaired AV canal defects are prone to heart block.

For patients with syncope but no underlying cardiac disease, arrhythmias are much less common but can occur in all forms (SVT, VT, heart block). When they do occur, the most common type of arrhythmia is SVT, which is associated with Wolff-Parkinson-White (WPW) syndrome. It is characterized by a short PR interval and an abnormal QRS complex with a delta wave in the initial phase. Ventricular tachycardia can be brought on by infection, dilated cardiomyopathy, drugs (cocaine, amphetamines), drug interactions (nonsedating antihistamines in combination with erythromycin or ketoconazole), and long QT syndrome. Patients with long QT syndrome have a prolonged refractory period, which can place them at risk for **torsades de pointes,** a malignant form of ventricular tachycardia. Two forms of congenital long QT syndrome exist: the autosomal dominant Romano-Ward syndrome and the autosomal recessive Jervell and Lange-Nielsen syndrome, which is associated with congenital deafness. The congenital form of long QT syndrome is due to mutations in either the cardiac potassium channel or the sodium channel gene, with higher mortality being associated with mutations on the potassium channel gene. The acquired form of long QT syndrome can be a result of electrolyte imbalance, increased intracranial pressure, and use of some medications, particularly tricyclic antidepressants and nonsedating antihistamines. In the patient without underlying structural abnormalities, heart block or slowed rhythms can be seen with neonatal lupus syndrome and Lyme carditis.

Noncardiac

Noncardiac causes of syncope include neurologic etiologies (seizures, migraines), metabolic disturbances (hypoglycemia), hyperventilation (panic attacks or self-induced), and hysteria. Seizures may be difficult to distinguish from vasovagal events because both can have tonic-clonic movements. Unlike vasovagal or cardiac syncope, seizures result in unconsciousness secondary to neurologic dysfunction. Syncope associated with hypoglycemia is due to insufficient substrate being delivered to the brain. Cerebral vasoconstriction secondary to arterial hypocapnia produces syncope with hyperventilation, which may be secondary to panic attacks or may be self-induced. Hysterical syncope lacks a true prodrome, and patients usually suffer no injury when they fall. This form of syncope is thought to be related to Munchausen syndrome.

DIFFERENTIAL DIAGNOSIS

The differential diagnosis of syncope is presented in Table 40–1. Events that precede and follow the syncopal event are key in determining the etiology of syncope.

EVALUATION

History

A thorough history should be obtained from the family and patient focusing on the patient's symptoms, the situation surrounding the event, and the family history (Questions Box). A primary goal of the history is to identify any underlying cardiac problems because these patients are at the greatest risk for sudden death.

TABLE 40–1. Differential Diagnosis of Syncope

Autonomic

Vasovagal	Excessive vagal tone
Pallid spells	Orthostatic hypotension
Situational	
Coughing	
Micturition	
Defecation	
Hair combing	
Swallowing	

Cardiac

Structural (outflow obstruction)	Functional (arrhythmias)
Aortic stenosis	Structurally normal heart
Hypertrophic cardiomyopathy	Wolff-Parkinson-White syndrome
Pulmonic stenosis	Long QT syndrome
Mitral stenosis	Acquired
Myxoma	Electrolyte imbalance
Cardiac tamponade	CNS abnormalities
Pulmonary hypertension	Infection
Coronary arterial abnormalities	Drugs
	Congenital
	Romano-Ward syndrome
	Jervell and Lange-Nielsen syndrome
	Structurally abnormal heart
	Supraventricular tachycardia
	Ventricular tachycardia
	Bradycardia/heart block

Noncardiac

Neurologic	Metabolic
Seizures	Hypoglycemia
Migraines	Hyperventilation
Transient ischemic attacks	Panic attacks
	Self induced
	Hysterical

Physical Examination

A complete physical examination is necessary for all patients. Vital signs should include blood pressure to screen for hypotension and hypovolemia. The cardiac examination should include palpation of the chest for the point of maximal intensity (PMI), thrills, and lifts and auscultation for assessment of heart sounds and murmurs. Upper and lower extremity pulses should be palpated for their presence and quality. The remainder of the examination should focus on identifying any abnormal neurologic findings.

Questions: Syncope

- What was the patient doing when the episode occurred?
- What was the position of the patient?
- Did the patient have any symptoms before the syncopal event?
- Did the patient have any chest pain or palpitations during the event?
- How long did it take the patient to recover from the syncopal event?
- Were any residual symptoms present after the syncopal event?
- When did the patient eat with reference to the syncopal event?
- Has the patient recently been ill, dehydrated, or fatigued?
- Does the patient have a history of underlying cardiac disease?
- Is the patient taking any type of medication (prescribed, over-the-counter, or illicit)?
- Does the patient have a history of breath holding or pallid spells?
- Is there a family history of sudden death, seizures, deafness, or cardiac abnormalities?

Laboratory Tests

The history and physical should guide which laboratory tests are necessary. In general, few tests are needed. Serum glucose shortly after the syncopal event may reveal hypoglycemia. Fasting glucose or glucose tolerance tests are usually normal, and such testing usually is not indicated. In pubertal females, a pregnancy test should be considered.

Diagnostic Tests

All patients who experience syncope should have an ECG to detect cardiac disease. The ECG may reveal WPW or long QT syndrome, which otherwise are not diagnosed by history and physical alone. The ECG can also identify underlying structural abnormalities such as RVH (right ventricular hypertrophy) secondary to pulmonary hypertension, LVH (left ventricular hypertrophy) seondary to hypertrophied cardiomyopathy, or Q waves associated with anomalous origin of the coronary arteries. For patients with findings consistent with cardiac disease (positive history, physical findings, or abnormal ECG), a referral to a pediatric cardiologist for further cardiac workup is indicated. The cardiac workup usually includes either a Holter monitor or an event monitor. Usually worn for only 24 hours, the Holter monitor catches arrhythmias only 13% of the time during this interval. Event monitors are worn for a longer time period and can retain the rhythm before and after the patient's identified symptom. When a patient becomes symptomatic, the event monitor can be activated. It records the cardiac rhythm prior to, during, and following the event, thus providing the clinician with more information than the Holter monitor does. Stress tests are often used to assess the patient's response to exertion and allow for replication of symptoms in a monitored setting. For patients with heart disease and arrhythmias, intracardiac electrophysiologic studies may be indicated.

For patients without evidence of cardiac disease (no family history of sudden death, no symptoms on exertion, and no angina), the workup should focus on noncardiac or autonomic causes of syncope. Patients with prolonged recovery or persistent neurologic symptoms after the event should have an EEG to rule out a seizure.

The tilt test is often used to diagnose vasovagal syncope. The patient is placed on a table that is tilted to simulate standing in the upright position, a condition that may be associated with vasovagal syncope. Unfortunately, there is great variability in the tilt test. Factors that influence the results include the time of day, whether the patient has fasted, duration in the supine position, whether invasive monitoring is used, and whether the test is augmented with isoproterenol. Concerning reproducibility of the tilt test, among those patients with a positive test, 36–80% will have a second positive test, and among those with a negative test, 85–100% will have a second negative test. Thus, very few false negatives occur, but 15% or more may have a false positive. Current recommendations suggest using the tilt test primarily for recurrent and unexplained syncope.

MANAGEMENT

Key to the initial management of syncope is determining its cause. For recurrent vasovagal syncope, various treatments are used. The most common in the pediatric population is **fludrocortisone.** It works via mineralocorticoid effects and is frequently used with salt. Other treatments include **beta-blockers** (propranolol), **vagolytic drugs** (disopyramide), and **centrally acting drugs** (imipramine, fluoxetine). These medications have varied benefits. One study reports a 90% success rate with the use of fludrocortisone, while in a placebo-controlled study using beta-blockers no significant difference was found between placebo and control (70% of the treated and 67% of the placebo group improved). Less information is available about the vagolytic and centrally acting agents.

Patients with neurologic syncope secondary to seizures should be treated with anticonvulsants. Patients with hyperventilation, hysteria, or hypoglycemia are most amenable to behavioral interventions. Patients with syncope secondary to a cardiac etiology should be referred to a cardiologist for further evaluation and correction of the underlying problem. These types of syncopal episodes may require more aggressive management, such as surgery or cardiac pacing, because they are more likely to result in sudden death.

PROGNOSIS

Overall, the prognosis for the autonomic and noncardiac syncope is good. Often patients with vasovagal syncope will have only a single event. Those with recurrent events can be treated with medication. One subgroup to be aware of is children with pallid breath-holding spells (see Chapter 30, Breath-Holding Spells); while a majority will have resolution of these spells by 5 years of age, up to 17% will continue to have syncope in adulthood. Patients with a cardiac etiology have the greatest risk for sudden death, and it is only by identification and treatment of these cardiac abnormalities that sudden death may be prevented.

Case Resolution

In the case presented at the beginning of the chapter, the adolescent describes symptoms consistent with a vasovagal form of syncope. Her family history, physical, and ECG do not indicate underlying cardiac disease. The patient and her family should be informed that certain factors, such as dehydration, fatigue, and hunger, can precipitate syncope, and behavioral changes such as eating breakfast should be implemented to prevent these. Management with medication is not indicated at this time, since this is the first syncopal event.

Selected Readings

Braden, D. S., and G. H. Gaymes. The diagnosis and management of syncope in children and adolescents. Pediatr. Ann. 26:422–426, 1997.

Benson, D. W., and G. Muller. Ambulatory electrocardiography. *In* Moss and Adams' Heart Disease in Infants, Children, and Adolescents,

Including the Fetus and Young Adult, 5th ed. Baltimore, Williams & Wilkins, 1995, pp. 165–172.

Corrado, D., C. Basso, M. Schiavon, et al. Screening for hypertrophic cardiomyopathy in young athletes. N. Engl. J. Med. 339:364–369, 1998.

Feit, L. R. Syncope in the pediatric patient: diagnosis, pathophysiology, and treatment. Adv. Pediatr. 43:469–496, 1996.

Hannon, D. W., and T. K. Knilans. Syncope in children and adolescents. Curr. Probl. Pediatr. 23:358–384, 1993.

Linzer, M., E. H. Yang, M. Estes, et al. Diagnosing syncope. 1. Value of history, physical examination and electrocardiography. 2. Unexplained syncope. Ann. Intern. Med. 126:989–996; 127:76–86, 1997.

Ross, B. A. Syncope and hypotension. In Burg, F. D., et al. Gellis & Kagan's Current Pediatric Therapy 15. Philadelphia, W. B. Saunders, 1996, pp. 205–207.

Scott, W. A. Assessment of the autonomic nervous system. In Moss and Adams' Heart Disease in Infant, Children, and Adolescents, Including the Fetus and Young Adult, 5th ed. Baltimore, Williams & Wilkins, 1995, pp. 172–179.

Zareba, W., A. J. Moss, P. J. Schwartz, et al. Influence of the genotype on the clinical course of the long QT syndrome. N. Engl. J. Med. 339:960–965, 1998.

CHAPTER 41

SHOCK

Kelly D. Young, M.D.

H$_x$ A 7-month-old infant boy is brought in by his parents with a history of vomiting and diarrhea for 2 days. He also has had a low-grade fever and, according to his parents, has become progressively more listless. Vital signs show a heart rate of 200 beats/min, respiratory rate of 30 breaths/min, and blood pressure of 72/35 mm Hg. The infant is lethargic and mottled. Capillary refill time is 3 seconds. His anterior fontanelle is sunken, and his mucous membranes are dry. The abdomen is flat and nontender and displays hyperactive bowel sounds.

Questions

1. What is shock, and what clinical signs can help in the recognition and assessment of shock?
2. What are the stages of shock?
3. What different types of shock are there, and what are the possible causes for each type?
4. What are the management priorities in treating shock?

Shock is defined as a state of circulatory dysfunction resulting in insufficient delivery of oxygen and other metabolic substrates to the tissues. Shock is not a disease but rather an abnormal physiologic state that may result from many disease processes. Early recognition and prompt therapy of shock are critical to avoid permanent end-organ damage or death.

EPIDEMIOLOGY

The most common type of shock is hypovolemic shock, and the most common causes are dehydration from gastrointestinal infections that cause vomiting and diarrhea, and hemorrhage from traumatic injury. Overwhelming sepsis is another common cause of shock.

Shock may be seen in any age group, but it is more difficult to recognize the early stages in young children because early clinical signs of shock in children are subjective and may be attributed to other causes. By the time children have developed more typical signs such as thready pulses and hypotension, they are in the late stages of shock.

CLINICAL PRESENTATION

Early signs of shock include tachycardia; cool, clammy, pale, or mottled skin; and delayed capillary refill time. There may be a history of decreased urine output. In this early stage, perfusion to vital organs such as the brain and heart is maintained by compensatory physiologic processes. As the shock state progresses, it becomes uncompensated, resulting in impairment of vital organ perfusion. Signs of uncompensated shock include hypotension; altered mental status; weak, thready, or absent pulses; and severely mottled or cyanotic skin. (D$_x$ Box). Irreversible shock occurs when multiple organs fail and death occurs.

PATHOPHYSIOLOGY

Shock occurs when oxygen delivery to tissues is impaired. Adequate oxygen delivery depends on sufficient blood oxygen content and adequate circulatory blood flow (Fig. 41–1). The oxygen content in blood depends primarily on the concentration of hemoglobin and the amount of oxygen bound to hemoglobin.

Blood flow, or cardiac output, is determined by heart rate and stroke volume. Stroke volume depends on preload, contractility, and afterload. Preload refers to the amount of blood entering the heart from the systemic vasculature. Increasing preload, for example, via administration of intravenous fluid boluses, will

D_x Shock

Compensated
Tachycardia
Normal blood pressure
Normal or bounding pulses
Normal or cool, clammy skin
Pale or mottled skin color
Alert, anxious mental state
Mildly delayed capillary refill time
Decreased urine output

Uncompensated
Tachycardia or bradycardia
Hypotension
Weak, thready, or absent pulses
Cool, clammy skin
Severely mottled or cyanotic skin color
Altered mental state, lethargic
Delayed capillary refill time
Decreased or absent urine output

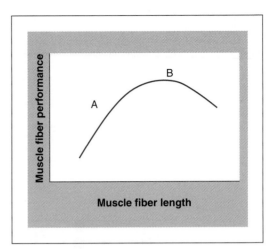

FIGURE 41–2. Starling curve of cardiac output. A. As muscle fiber length increases, performance increases. **B.** Muscle fiber reaches its optimal length, after which performance declines.

increase cardiac output until a point of optimal heart muscle fiber length is reached. The Starling curve demonstrates that increased stretching of a muscle fiber results in improved performance of that muscle fiber (i.e., improved stroke volume and cardiac output); but after the point of optimal stretching is reached, there is decreased performance (Fig. 41–2).

Contractility, or inotropy, is the heart's intrinsic ability to contract and pump blood to the body. Afterload refers to the systemic vascular resistance impeding ejection of blood from the ventricles. Optimal cardiac output depends on sufficient preload, unimpaired cardiac contractility, and the ability of the heart to overcome any afterload. During states of decreased cardiac output leading to decreased tissue perfusion, adults compensate primarily by increasing cardiac contractility, whereas children compensate primarily by increasing their heart rate.

DIFFERENTIAL DIAGNOSIS

There are several types of shock depending on the underlying pathophysiology (Table 41–1). **Hypovolemic shock** is the most common type seen in children and usually results from dehydration or traumatic hemorrhage. Hypovolemia results in inadequate preload, which leads to impaired cardiac output and impaired perfusion. Other causes of hypovolemic shock include diabetic ketoacidosis (dehydration due to osmotic diuresis) and peritonitis and burns leading to third-spacing of fluids (shifting from intravascular to extravascular sites) with resultant intravascular hypovolemia.

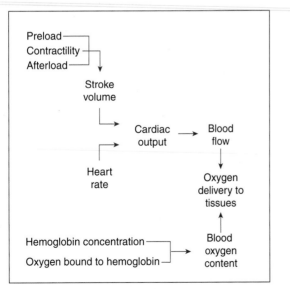

FIGURE 41–1. Pathophysiology of shock. Factors affecting oxygen delivery to tissue.

TABLE 41–1. Types of Shock

Type of Shock	Pathophysiologic Mechanism	Common Causes
Hypovolemic	Decreased preload	Dehydration Traumatic hemorrhage Diabetic ketoacidosis Peritonitis Burns
Distributive	Relative hypovolemia due to vasodilation	Sepsis Anaphylaxis Neurogenic Toxin-mediated
Cardiogenic	Decreased contractility	Congestive heart failure from congenital lesions Myocarditis Tachydysrhythmias Ductal-dependent cardiac lesions
Obstructive	Impaired cardiac filling	Pulmonary embolus Pericardial tamponade Tension pneumothorax
Dissociative	Abnormal hemoglobin— inadequate oxygen bound	Carbon monoxide poisoning Methemoglobinemia

Distributive shock is a relative hypovolemia; vasodilation results in inadequate circulating blood volume relative to the vasodilation (i.e., the "tank" has been made larger by vasodilation, and now there is insufficient fluid to fill the tank). Causes include anaphylaxis and sepsis, which result in the release of vasoactive mediators that cause vasodilation. Spinal cord injury **(neurogenic shock)** may result in loss of sympathetic nerve–mediated vascular tone and subsequent vasodilation. Finally, certain intoxications such as iron, barbiturate, and tricyclic antidepressant can cause vasodilation and distributive shock.

Cardiogenic shock is an uncommon but important cause of shock in children. Congestive heart failure from a congenital heart lesion, myocarditis, or cardiomyopathy result in impaired cardiac contractility and decreased cardiac output. Tachydysrhythmias, such as supraventricular tachycardia, do not allow sufficient time for the ventricles to fill with blood, resulting in decreased stroke volume. Closure of the ductus arteriosus in a neonate with a duct-dependent congenital heart lesion is another cause of insufficient cardiac output and cardiogenic shock.

Rare causes of shock in pediatric patients include obstructive and dissociative types. In **obstructive shock,** there is obstruction to cardiac filling due to pulmonary embolus, cardiac tamponade, or tension pneumothorax. In **dissociative shock** an abnormal hemoglobin such as methemoglobin or carboxyhemoglobin from carbon monoxide poisoning results in decreased oxygen bound to hemoglobin and decreased oxygen delivered to tissues.

Septic shock combines elements of distributive, hypovolemic, and cardiogenic shock. Vasoactive mediators lead to vasodilation and a relative hypovolemia. Third-spacing of fluid leads to a true intravascular hypovolemia as well. In addition, mediators of sepsis cause impaired cardiac function.

EVALUATION

Early recognition and prompt treatment of shock is the goal. A rapid, focused history and physical examination should be performed to identify patients in shock, and then early therapy should be instituted before returning for a more complete evaluation. Recognition of shock depends on physical examination alone; therapy should never be withheld while awaiting results of diagnostic tests.

History

A history of vomiting with or without diarrhea, decreased oral intake, and decreased urine output, especially in infants, should alert the clinician to possible hypovolemic shock. Children presenting with major trauma should be evaluated for hemorrhagic shock. A history of fever, lethargy or irritability, and sometimes a rash may point toward septic shock. Patients with asplenia, sickle cell disease, or indwelling catheters and those who are immunocompromised (e.g., young infants or children on chemotherapy) are at increased risk for sepsis. Children in cardiogenic shock may have a history of a murmur, poor feeding, sweating with feeds, cyanosis, tachypnea and dyspnea, and, in the older child, palpitations.

Physical Examination

A brief examination to identify shock focuses on mental status, vital signs, pulses, and skin signs. Impaired level of consciousness, such as lethargy or lack of recognition of parents, occurs late in shock. Earlier, children are anxious or fussy but alert. Tachycardia occurs early in shock but must be interpreted in the context of other signs of shock, since tachycardia may also result from fever, pain, or simply the child's fear of the examination process. Bradycardia is a late, ominous sign in shock and often results from hypoxemia. Hypotension is also a late sign in shock. It is important to remember that normal values for heart rate and blood pressure vary by age. The lower limit of acceptable systolic blood pressure in a neonate from birth to 1 month is 60 mm Hg; in an infant from 1 month to 1 year is 70 mm Hg. For a child 1 year or older, the lower limit can be estimated using the formula $70 + (2 \times \text{age in years})$ mm Hg.

Presence and quality of pulses should be checked. Weak, thready, or absent peripheral pulses are indicative of shock. Skin color, moisture, and temperature give valuable clues to diagnosis. Children in shock may have pale, cyanotic, or mottled skin. Early in shock, however, skin color may be normal. Some infants may also have mottled skin normally. As with tachycardia, isolated signs must be correlated with the bigger clinical picture to diagnose shock. Decreased perfusion in shock leads to cool and clammy skin. This is often best appreciated in the hands and feet initially.

Capillary refill is tested by compressing the capillary bed of a fingertip, palm, or dorsal foot with gentle pressure until it blanches. Upon release, color should return in 2 seconds or less; a capillary refill time of 3 seconds or more is abnormal and indicative of shock. Capillary refill should be tested with the extremity elevated above the heart so that arterial, not venous, perfusion is tested. Also, cool ambient temperatures can falsely delay capillary refill times.

In hypovolemic shock due to dehydration, look for signs of dehydration such as dry mucous membranes, lack of tears, sunken eyes, sunken anterior fontanelle in infants, and tenting of the skin. The degree of dehydration can often be estimated clinically (see Chapter 46, Fluid and Electrolyte Disturbances).

Children with congestive heart failure and cardiogenic shock may demonstrate dyspnea on exertion, tachypnea, orthopnea, rales, hepatomegaly, gallop rhythm, and a heart murmur. Jugular venous distention and peripheral edema are appreciated less often in children compared with adults.

Laboratory Tests

The suspected cause of the shock will determine which laboratory tests are performed. In hypovolemic shock secondary to dehydration, a chemistry panel should be obtained for electrolyte abnormalities and acidosis. Serial hematocrit determinations and a type and crossmatch are important studies in traumatic hemorrhage. In septic shock, a complete blood count and blood cultures should be obtained. Coagulation studies including panels to rule out disseminated intravascular coagulopathy, and electrolyte studies including calcium and magnesium levels, are frequently abnormal in sepsis. Hypoglycemia is a common finding in any type of shock, and a rapid bedside glucose determination should be performed. Arterial blood gases can demonstrate adequacy of oxygenation and degree of acidosis.

Diagnostic Studies

Invasive monitoring with arterial lines for systemic arterial blood pressure and central venous lines for central venous pressure or pulmonary artery wedge pressure may be helpful in the ongoing management of shock. Chest radiography, electrocardiogram, and echocardiogram may be obtained in cardiogenic shock to further elucidate the etiology. Workup of stabilized trauma patients may include radiographs or CT scans.

MANAGEMENT

The first management priority in the treatment of any critically ill child is attention to airway patency and ventilation. If there is significant respiratory compromise, bag-valve-mask ventilation followed by endotracheal intubation is performed. Usually, however, patients in compensated shock do not require immediate attention to airway management. Instead, the immediate priorities are administration of **oxygen** and initiation of **cardiorespiratory monitoring.** Elective, rather than emergent, endotracheal intubation should be considered to reduce metabolic demands caused by increased work of breathing.

Almost concurrently with the above, the next priority is achieving **intravascular access** and, in most cases, administering fluids. Peripheral intravenous access should be attempted. If this is unsuccessful after three attempts or 90 seconds, an intraosseous line may be placed in younger children, or intravenous access may be obtained by placement of a central venous catheter or by cut-down technique. Decreased preload and hypovolemia (actual or relative) are present in the most common causes of shock. Only cardiogenic shock may not benefit from increasing preload via a fluid bolus. Generally, an **initial fluid bolus of 20 mL/kg isotonic crystalloid fluid,** such as normal saline or lactated Ringer's, should be rapidly infused. The patient should be assessed for improvement in mentation, vital signs, peripheral pulses, and skin signs after each fluid bolus. Repeat fluid boluses of 20 mL/kg to a total of 80 mL/kg may be necessary to restore intravascular volume. Colloid fluid (e.g., albumin) theoretically has the advantage of staying intravascular longer, but this has not been proved to result in a measurable benefit. Crystalloid fluid is recommended because it is less expensive

and more readily available. If a patient with traumatic hemorrhage is still hemodynamically unstable after two crystalloid fluid boluses, packed red blood cells at 10 mL/kg may be required.

Further management depends on the specific etiology. Patients in septic shock should receive empiric broad-spectrum antibiotic coverage. A surgeon must assist in identifying the source of hemorrhage and controlling the bleeding in patients with traumatic hemorrhage. Spinal cord injury is treated with supportive care and high-dose methylprednisolone in consultation with a neurosurgeon. Anaphylactic shock is treated with intravenous epinephrine, diphenhydramine, glucocorticoids, and nebulized albuterol. Pericardial tamponade is relieved by pericardiocentesis, tension pneumothorax by needle thoracotomy or tube thoracostomy, and pulmonary embolus with supportive care and thrombolytics. Carbon monoxide poisoning is treated with 100% oxygen and, if severe, hyperbaric oxygen. Patients with methemoglobinemia appear cyanotic even while receiving 100% oxygen and may be treated with methylene blue. Supraventricular tachycardia should be treated with adenosine if the patient is stable and with synchronized cardioversion if the patient is hemodynamically unstable.

Patients with cardiogenic shock require **inotropic agents** to increase cardiac contractility and improve tissue perfusion. Patients in the later stages of other forms of shock (hypovolemic, distributive, septic) may suffer cardiac dysfunction. In such patients, only after adequate fluid resuscitation has been performed and there are still signs of shock or hypotension should inotropic agents be started. Central venous pressure monitoring may be needed to determine whether fluid resuscitation is adequate.

Dopamine or epinephrine is often the first-line inotropic agent. At low doses (2–5 µg/kg/min), dopamine improves renal blood flow and enhances urine output. At midrange doses (5–10 µg/kg/min), dopamine exerts primarily a β-adrenergic effect, improving contractility and increasing heart rate. At higher doses (10–20 µg/kg/min), dopamine's α-adrenergic effects cause peripheral vasoconstriction to improve hypotension. **Epinephrine** has predominantly β-adrenergic effects at lower doses (0.05–0.1 µg/kg/min) and α-adrenergic effects at higher doses. **Dobutamine** may be the most useful drug for cardiogenic shock because it is selective for β-adrenergic effects, increasing cardiac contractility. However, if hypotension is present, dobutamine-mediated peripheral vasodilation may be detrimental. Dobutamine is typically used in a range of 10–20 µg/kg/min. Combinations of inotropic agents may be beneficial to maximize improvements in cardiac contractility and cardiac output without compromising renal perfusion or worsening hypotension.

Patients in cardiogenic shock may also benefit from afterload reduction using systemic vasodilators such as nitroprusside (0.5–5 µg/kg/min). If these are used, blood pressure should be continuously monitored, typically in the setting of the intensive care unit. Neonates with duct-dependent lesions typically present with a sudden onset of shock and cyanosis in the second half of the first week of life. Common lesions include hypoplastic left heart syndrome, aortic coarctation, and tricuspid atresia. Prostaglandin E_1 (0.1 μg/kg/min, titrated to effect), which acts to keep the ductus arteriosus open, should be immediately infused if a duct-dependent lesion is suspected as the cause of shock.

Vasoactive infusions may be mixed using the **rule of 6 and 0.6.** For dopamine, dobutamine, and nitroprusside, mix 6 mg/kg of drug with enough D5W to produce a final volume of 100 mL. Infusion at 1 mL/h provides a dose of 1 μg/kg/min). For epinephrine and prostaglandin E_1 mix 0.6 mg/kg of drug with enough D5W to produce a final volume of 100 mL. Infusion of 1 mL/h provides a dose of 0.1 μg/kg/min.

Treatment of patients in shock must include attention to conditions that increase metabolic demand. Acidosis should be assessed and, if severe, treatment with bicarbonate considered. Temperature should be kept neutral with heating lamps for hypothermia and antipyretics for fever as needed. Electrolyte abnormalities and hypoglycemia must be assessed and corrected.

PROGNOSIS

Children in shock are critically ill and at risk for progression to multiorgan failure and death. Prognosis depends on how early shock is recognized and treated and on the underlying etiology. Prompt, appropriate therapy has a significant impact on morbidity and mortality.

Case Resolution

The boy in the case history is in barely compensated (he is not hypotensive) hypovolemic shock due to diarrhea, vomiting, and dehydration. He should receive oxygen and cardiorespiratory monitoring, and intravenous access should be rapidly established. Isotonic fluid boluses of 20 mL/kg should be given with reassessment between each bolus. As much as 80 mL/kg may be needed before improvements in mentation, vital signs, pulses, and skin signs are seen.

Selected Readings

Chameides, L., and M. F. Hazinski (eds.). Textbook of Pediatric Advanced Life Support. Dallas, American Heart Association, 1994.
Core Lecture: Shock. *In* Gausche, M. (ed.). APLS: The Pediatric Emergency Medicine Course Instructor Manual. Elk Grove Village, IL, American Academy of Pediatrics, 1998, pp. 62–74.
Hazinski, M. F., and R. M. Barkin. Shock. *In* Barkin, R. M. (ed.). Pediatric Emergency Medicine: Concepts and Clinical Practice. St. Louis, Mosby-Year Book, 1992, pp. 118–146.
Shock. *In* Strange, G. R. (ed.). APLS: The Pediatric Emergency Medicine Course. Elk Grove Village, IL, American Academy of Pediatrics, 1998, pp. 29–39.

CHAPTER 42

APPROACH TO THE TRAUMATIZED CHILD

Jill M. Baren, M.D.

H_x A 6-year-old boy is brought to the emergency department after being struck by an automobile while crossing the street. He was found unconscious at the scene. Initial evaluation shows that the boy has an altered level of consciousness; shallow respirations; ecchymosis across the upper abdomen; and a deformed, swollen left thigh. The pediatric emergency physician is called on to discuss an initial assessment and management plan for the injured child with the trauma surgeon.

Questions

1. What are the most common mechanisms of injury responsible for trauma in children?
2. What are some of the physiologic differences between adults and children that make children more susceptible to certain types of injuries?
3. Which areas of the body are most likely to be injured in a typical automobile-versus-pedestrian crash?
4. What are the components of a primary survey in pediatric trauma patients?
5. What radiographic and laboratory studies should be performed in children with multiple injuries?

Trauma is often referred to as the neglected disease of modern society. Childhood trauma, in particular, is poorly understood. Death from trauma is higher in pediatric patients than in adults. Mechanisms of injury may be similar in adults and children, but children have particular physiologic and psychologic responses to injury. Health care professionals should realize that children have unique anatomic and physiologic features

(Box 42–1); they are not just small adults. Evaluation and management of traumatized children may require specialized equipment. Recognition of such facts, coupled with expertise in the performance of emergency procedures, should improve the outcome of children who sustain major injuries.

EPIDEMIOLOGY

More than 50% of the deaths of children who are 1–14 years with the peak at 8 years of age are caused by traumatic injuries. Approximately 1.5 million pediatric injuries result in 500,000 hospitalizations, and 15,000 to 25,000 deaths (1.5%) occur each year. This figure may be an underestimation, as most childhood injury fatalities occur in the field prior to arrival at a health care facility. The magnitude of the problem becomes even more evident when morbidity is considered. Between 50,000 and 100,000 children per year become permanently disabled as a result of their injuries. Such disabilities have an enormous impact on society; they result in financial and emotional losses for families and many years of lost productivity for individuals.

Blunt trauma, which is more common than penetrating injury in children, represents about 87% of all childhood injuries. In certain age groups (e.g., 13–18-year age group), however, penetrating injury accounts for a higher percentage of the total, especially among minority populations in urban areas. Causes of non-penetrating trauma, listed in order of frequency, are motor vehicle crashes (>40%), falls (25–30%), drownings (10–15%), and burns (5–10%). Included in the remainder are bicycle crashes and automobile-versus-pedestrian injuries which predominates among school-aged children. Male children are injured twice as often as females. Different mechanisms of injury predominate in different age groups; the figures given above refer to overall causes of trauma.

CLINICAL PRESENTATION

Children who sustain severe trauma present with multiple organ system injury manifested by shock, respiratory failure, or altered mental status (singly or in combination). Those with mild to moderate injury may present in this way or simply with localized signs and symptoms in the injured area.

PATHOPHYSIOLOGY

Patterns of injury are important to identify to develop strategies for injury prevention. One common pattern in the United States is the triad of injuries that results from an automobile-versus-pedestrian crash (Waddell's triad) (Fig. 42–1). Multisystem injury is the rule rather than the exception in children. Internal injury should not be ruled out, even if no evidence suggestive of external trauma is apparent. Because children are anatomically and physiologically different from adults, they are more susceptible to different types of injury (see Box 42–1). The most striking physiologic differences between adults and children concern responses to acute blood loss.

Hypovolemic shock secondary to acute blood loss is the most common cause of shock in pediatric trauma patients. In general, hemorrhagic shock is a clinical state where the cardiac output is unable to meet the metabolic demands of the tissues for oxygen and nutrients; it is not defined by any absolute blood pressure value.

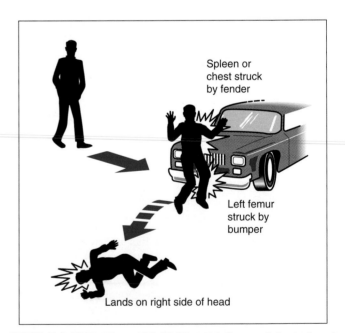

Spleen or chest struck by fender

Left femur struck by bumper

Lands on right side of head

FIGURE 42–1. Illustration of Waddell's triad. Femur, abdominal, and contralateral head injuries (Waddell's triad) should be expected to result from automobile-versus-pedestrian crashes in the United States. A child crossing the street is struck on the left side of the body by an automobile traveling on the right side of the road. The left femur is likely to be injured by the bumper, and the abdomen or chest strikes the grille as the child is lifted into the air and lands on the opposite side of the head, sustaining blunt head trauma. Waddell's triad illustrates the necessity of having a high degree of suspicion for a complex of injuries based on a well-known mechanism.

Acute blood loss stimulates peripheral and central receptors and results in an increased production of catecholamines and adrenocorticoids. The body responds by increasing peripheral vascular resistance, stroke volume, and heart rate. Children are able to tolerate increases in heart rate and peripheral vascular resistance very well at first, and they exhibit normal blood pressure in the presence of hypovolemic shock. By the time their blood pressure falls, they have probably already lost 20–25% of their circulating blood volume. In adults, blood pressure tends to decline after a less significant blood loss and therefore may be recognized sooner (Fig. 42–2). Another obstacle to the recognition of shock in children is the lack of knowledge on the part of many health professionals of age-appropriate vital signs, particularly blood pressure. Table 42–1 gives the normal blood pressure ranges for children of different ages.

Three stages of shock correspond to the progression of volume loss. In the first stage, **compensated shock,** mechanisms for preserving blood pressure are still effective. Decreased capillary refill, diminished pulses, cool extremities, and tachypnea may be apparent, and blood pressure is normal and accompanied by tachycardia. Unrecognized, untreated compensated shock rapidly progresses to **uncompensated shock.** Examination reveals decreased level of consciousness, pallor, reduced urine output, and lower blood pressure with weak, thready pulses and tachycardia. Despite therapy, uncompensated shock becomes **irreversible shock,** resulting in irreparable organ damage. (See Chapter 41, Shock, for a more extensive discussion.)

Shock has several causes, and it is important to emphasize that shock should never be attributed solely to head trauma. The pathways resulting in decreased blood pressure in patients with head trauma are present only at the terminal stages. Therefore, the possibility of blood loss from internal organs should be pursued promptly. Children with spinal cord injuries may have

TABLE 42–1. Normal Vital Signs for Children of Different Ages

Age	Respiration (breaths/min)	Pulse (beats/min)	Blood Pressure (systolic)
Newborn	30–60	100–160	50–70
1–6 wk	30–60	100–160	70–95
6 mo	25–40	90–120	80–100
1 yr	20–30	90–120	80–100
3 yr	20–30	80–120	80–110
6 yr	18–25	60–110	80–110
10 yr	15–20	50–80	90–120

spinal shock, but this tends to be a rare occurrence. Spinal shock may be distinguished from hypovolemic shock by its manifestation of decreased blood pressure with a lack of concommitant rise in heart rate secondary to decreased sympathetic tone.

EVALUATION AND MANAGEMENT

Because of the high potential for serious morbidity and mortality in trauma patients, evaluation and management are performed simultaneously. This care is best handled using an organized, multidisciplinary team approach, with preestablished criteria for activation of the trauma team. History of the event provides important information when implementing these criteria. For example, the entire team responds for all falls greater than 10 feet. The types of subspecialists that make up a trauma team are decided by individual institutions.*

Several approaches to the assessment of trauma patients have been developed by professional organizations. The Advanced Trauma Life Support (ATLS) course of the American College of Surgeons and the Basic Trauma Life Support (BTLS) course of the American College of Emergency Physicians are two such approaches. Both the ATLS and the BTLS methods stress the importance of a primary evaluation, or primary survey, to identify and treat life-threatening injuries and a more detailed regional examination, or secondary survey, after stabilization. In addition, they both adhere to the principles of serial examination and reassessment after each intervention. The primary survey and initial resuscitation efforts must occur simultaneously and within the first 5–10 minutes of the evaluation. The secondary survey is meant to enhance the primary survey. Vital signs should be repeated every 5 minutes during the primary survey and every 15 minutes during the secondary survey until the trauma team feels the patient has been adequately stabilized. The reader should understand the rationale for the trauma examination and its parts. (See Selected Readings for articles that explain the rationales for trauma examination and provide detailed descriptions of evaluation and management techniques.)

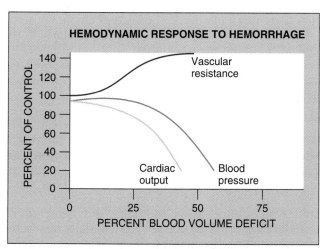

HEMODYNAMIC RESPONSE TO HEMORRHAGE

Vascular resistance

Cardiac output

Blood pressure

PERCENT OF CONTROL

PERCENT BLOOD VOLUME DEFICIT

FIGURE 42–2. Graph showing cardiovascular response to hypovolemia in children. Blood pressure does not begin to decline until the volume deficit is more than 25% because of the compensatory increase in vascular resistance. Cardiac output drops earlier and is manifested clinically as skin signs (delayed capillary refill; cool, clammy skin), tachycardia, and so on.

*Most institutions have trauma teams composed of pediatric emergency and critical care specialists, anesthesiologists, trauma surgeons, neurosurgeons, emergency nurses, respiratory therapists, and x-ray technicians.

Physical Examination

The **primary survey** begins with an assessment of level of consciousness, patency of the airway, and quality of breathing. When evaluating injured patients, physicians should always assume that the cervical spine has been injured and should use in-line immobilization to secure it. Basic airway maneuvers for positioning should be performed. The safest method is the jaw thrust or chin lift to avoid moving the cervical spine (Fig. 42–3). The oral cavity should be examined for foreign bodies, blood, or secretions; the most common form of airway obstruction in children is a posteriorly displaced tongue, which is relieved by good airway positioning. Advanced airway maneuvers (bag-valve-mask ventilation or endotracheal tube intubation) are performed in the primary survey if children have apnea, significant respiratory distress or head trauma, or an airway that cannot be maintained with basic techniques. All trauma patients are given supplemental oxygen by mask or nasal cannula at a concentration of 100%.

After adequate ventilation has been secured, circulatory status is assessed. All pediatric trauma patients require placement of the largest bore intravenous catheter obtainable for that patient; two of these should be placed, if possible. In life-threatening situations, peripheral vascular access is attempted either three times or for 90 seconds, whichever comes first. If peripheral attempts fail, then intraosseous infusion or central venous access should be used. A bolus of 20 mL/kg of an isotonic fluid (normal saline or Ringer's lactate) should be given. This may be repeated, if necessary, to treat hypovolemic shock. After 80 mL/kg, administration of blood or other crystalloid products should be considered, and the likelihood of surgical exploration is high. Acutely exsanguinating wounds are treated using direct pressure bandages.

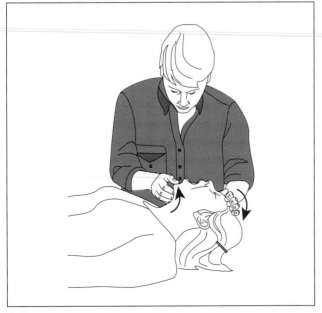

FIGURE 42–3. Correct method for positioning the head with chin lift or jaw thrust.

TABLE 42–2. AMPLE History
A Allergies
M Medications
P Past history/Hospitalizations/Surgeries
L Last meal
E Events preceding trauma

A brief neurologic assessment to assess patient disability is also performed during the primary survey. One rapid assessment technique is the AVPU system: **A** (alert), **V** (responds to verbal stimuli), **P** (responds to painful stimuli), and **U** (is unresponsive). Subsequently, a Glasgow Coma Scale score or Children's Coma Scale score may be calculated.

Once life-threatening conditions are stabilized, more information can be collected. The **secondary survey** involves a head-to-toe examination of children, fully exposed, to identify additional injuries, while taking great care to maintain normothermia. It also includes an **AMPLE** history (allergies, medications, past history/hospitalizations/surgeries, last meal, events preceding trauma) (Table 42–2). A detailed history of events preceding trauma should ensure that injuries are consistent with the causal mechanism. Health care professionals should be prepared to consider abuse when specific diagnoses do not correlate with either the history given by the care giver or the developmental ability of the child. Measurement of vital signs should occur as previously described, and other devices such as Foley catheters, nasogastric tubes, and pulse oximetry should be used at this time. Every time an intervention is performed, repeat assessments that incorporate the elements of the primary survey are made.

Laboratory Tests

Most institutions have a standardized trauma panel (CBC with differential, electrolytes, BUN, creatinine, glucose, amylase, PT, PTT, and blood typing and cross-matching). In addition, drug and alcohol screens may provide important information, particularly in the child with altered mental status.

Imaging Studies

When major trauma is suspected, radiographs of at least the chest, pelvis/abdomen, and cervical spine should be obtained. This prevents missing injuries in children who may be unconscious or who need life-saving procedures during resuscitation, which obscure an area of injury from examination. Additional radiographs, for example, of the extremities, may be indicated when other areas of injury are detected on secondary survey. Children are often initially distracted from one injury because of the presence of a more painful one.

More sophisticated imaging techniques such as CT scans and ultrasound are a usual part of the evaluation of the seriously injured pediatric trauma patient. The choice of test depends on the experience of the trauma team and the individual characteristics of the patient.

PROGNOSIS

The highest survival rates for seriously injured children have been found among those who are brought to the operating room for treatment within 1 hour of the injury. Definitive care for trauma takes place in the operating room, and initial stabilization takes place in the emergency department. An organized, preestablished, multidisciplinary approach to care is therefore essential. Studies have shown that the single most important element for any hospital treating injured children is the committment on the part of the institution and its surgeons. Regional pediatric trauma centers have increased resources for dealing with severely injured patients that include long-term care and rehabilitation. Other nondesignated hospitals may do an excellent job in the initial stabilization phase of care. Indications for transfer to a specialty center include: inability to provide definitive surgical intervention, inability to provide an appropriate intensive care environment, the presence of multisystem injuries or injuries requiring extensive orthopedic or plastic surgery procedures, or major burns. Health care professionals who treat children should not only become adept at the recognition and initial stabilization of injuries, but should also serve as advocates for injury prevention and coordinated prehospital care services in the community.

Case Resolution

The 6-year-old boy in the case history sustained multiple trauma from an automobile-versus-pedestrian crash. He presents with altered level of consciousness; respiratory failure (shallow respirations); potential internal organ injury, which may lead to shock; and probable fracture of the left femur, which may also contribute to the development of shock. These injuries are identified by performance of a primary and secondary survey. Proper management includes stabilization of the cervical spine, airway management, aggressive early shock treatment with fluid replacement, and a vigilant search for additional injuries. Continued reassessment is also an integral part of emergency department stabilization. Due to the presence of multisystem injuries, after initial stabilization, the patient should be transferred to a regional pediatric trauma center for extended care.

Selected Readings

Cantor, R. M., and J. M. Leaming. Evaluation and management of pediatric major trauma. Emerg. Med. Clin. North Am. 16:229–256, 1998.

Chameides, L., and M. F. Hazinski (eds.). Textbook of Pediatric Advanced Life Support. Dallas, American Heart Association, 1994.

Fitzmaurice, L. S. Approach to multiple trauma. *In* Barkin, R. M. (ed.). Pediatric Emergency Medicine Concepts and Clinical Practice. St. Louis, Mosby-Year Book, pp. 223–235, 1997.

Maksoud, J. G., M. L. Moront, and M. R. Eichelberger. Resuscitation of the injured child. Sem. Ped. Surg. 4:93–99, 1995.

Polhgeers, A., and R. M. Ruddy. An update on pediatric trauma. Emerg. Med. Clin. North Am. 13:267–289, 1995.

Ruddy, R. M., and G. R. Fleisher. An approach to the injured child. *In* Fleisher, G. R., and S. Ludwig (eds.). Textbook of Pediatric Emergency Medicine, 3rd ed. Baltimore, Williams & Wilkins, 1993.

Ziegler, M. M., and J. M. Templeton. Major trauma. *In* Fleisher, G.R., and S. Ludwig (eds.). Textbook of Pediatric Emergency Medicine, 3rd ed. Baltimore, Williams & Wilkins, 1993.

CHAPTER 43

ABDOMINAL TRAUMA

Jill M. Baren, M.D.

H$_x$ An 8-year-old boy who is riding a bicycle at a speed of 20 miles per hour accidentally crashes into a tree. On arrival at the trauma center, the paramedics report that the bike handlebars rammed into the child's stomach, "knocking the wind out of him." The boy complains of dizziness and vomits several times. Initial vital signs show a heart rate of 135 beats/min and a respiratory rate of 24 breaths/min. The abdomen is flat but tender to palpation in the midepigastric region and left upper quadrant.

Questions

1. What are the most frequent types of intra-abdominal trauma in children?
2. What are the diagnostic studies used to evaluate abdominal trauma?
3. What are the basic components of the treatment of shock that occurs following abdominal trauma?
4. What is a simple rule for establishing the lower limit of normal blood pressure in children?

D$_x$ Abdominal Trauma

- Pain
- Tenderness
- Distention
- Peritoneal signs (absent or diminished bowel sounds, rebound tenderness)
- Ecchymoses
- Tire tracks
- Seat belt marks
- Urine, stool, or nasogastric aspirate positive for blood
- Unexplained hypotension or other signs of hypovolemic shock

---

Abdominal trauma is the leading unrecognized cause of fatal injury, specifically because early shock is not recognized. Death results when the extent and nature of abdominal injuries are neither appreciated nor appropriately managed, fluid replacement is inadequate, and airway maintenance is not implemented soon enough. Abdominal trauma is the third leading cause of traumatic death, following death due to head and thoracic injury. Clinicians should be knowledgeable about mechanisms of injury that result in abdominal trauma, the early manifestations of shock, and the methods for aggressive treatment of hemorrhagic shock.

EPIDEMIOLOGY

Twenty-five percent of children who sustain multisystem trauma have significant abdominal injury. When both head and abdominal injury occur simultaneously, the risk of death is higher than when either occurs alone. Blunt force mechanisms are responsible for almost 85% of abdominal injuries; the remainder are a result of penetrating force. Examples of blunt force, presented in order of frequency, are motor vehicle crashes, pedestrian versus automobile collisions, falls, sports injuries, and direct blows from both abuse and assault. Injuries to the liver and spleen predominate; injuries to the kidney, bowel, and pancreas occur less often. In multiple injuries, the incidence of trauma involving pelvic organs (bladder, ureter, iliac vessels) is also high, especially when pelvic fractures occur. A straddle injury (e.g., fall that occurs when climbing over a fence) can also result in abdominal and pelvic trauma.

CLINICAL PRESENTATION

Pain, distention, and ecchymoses tend to be more reliable signs of pathology, whereas the absence of bowel sounds is less consistent as a marker for injury. (See D$_x$ Box for signs and symptoms suggestive of abdominal trauma.) No particular sign, however, is completely reliable.

PATHOPHYSIOLOGY

Blunt trauma largely involves injury to solid, not hollow, intraabdominal organs (i.e., liver and spleen rather than small bowel) for a variety of reasons. First, the rib cage is flexible in children. Therefore, rib fractures are less likely to occur, reducing the potential for penetration of abdominal organs by broken ribs. Second, children have less well developed abdominal musculature and less adipose tissue than adults, and thus blunt force is transmitted to abdominal organs more easily. Third, because the diaphragm is oriented more horizontally in children than in adults, the liver and spleen lie more anteriorly and caudally within the abdomen.

It is important to emphasize that abdominal injury may lead to excessive blood loss. The pathophysiology of hemorrhagic shock is discussed in detail in Chapter 42, Approach to the Traumatized Child and Chapter 41, Shock. The liver and spleen are highly vascularized organs that bleed profusely when lacerated. Even the accumulation of subcapsular hematomas without rupture may cause a profound drop in hematocrit. Because intraabdominal organs are not directly visible when a patient is examined, signs and symptoms of injury are not always obvious. Therefore, hemorrhagic shock should always be suspected with abdominal trauma. Likewise, large volumes of blood can accumulate in the pelvis, and because of its proximity to the abdomen, the pelvis should always be considered as a reservoir for hemorrhage in abdominal as well as pelvic trauma.

DIFFERENTIAL DIAGNOSIS

Physicians should be familiar with the most common patterns of abdominal injury, and they should consider the possibility of specific injuries. Any abdominal organ can be injured by any mechanism, either blunt or penetrating. The spleen is the most common intraabdominal organ injured by a blunt force. **Hepatic injuries** are the most common fatal abdominal injuries, although they are less frequent than splenic injuries. The right lobe of the liver is injured more frequently than the left lobe.

Injuries to hollow viscera such as the stomach and intestines, which represent only about 5–15% of injuries from blunt forces, are difficult to diagnose. Three mechanisms lead to injuries of hollow structures: (1) "crush" between the anterior wall of the abdomen and the vertebral column; (2) deceleration, which causes shearing of the bowel from its mesenteric attachments; and (3) "burst," which occurs when an air-filled or fluid-filled loop of bowel is closed at both ends at the time of impact. Peritonitis may develop in 6–48 hours secondary to fecal spillage (soiling) or devascularization as a consequence of any of these mechanisms. Occasionally, a diagnosis of hollow viscera injury is made incidentally or may be delayed more than 48 hours, highlighting the need for serial examinations. Duodenal and pancreatic injuries are examples of potentially delayed diagnoses that can have grave consequences. Leakage of bile and enzymes may activate autodigestion of the pancreas and result in sepsis.

EVALUATION

Determining which organ or organs may be injured from abdominal trauma is difficult. Physicians tend to focus on injuries to the extremities, pelvis, face, or chest that are painful and distracting to children and more clinically obvious to the examiner. Initial clinical impressions may be incorrect, causing delay in diagnosis or unnecessary surgical exploration.

History

The history should focus on the mechanism of injury and the physiologic response of the child, especially in the prehospital setting (e.g., initial hypotension, tachycardia, cyanosis) (Questions Box). A poor history concerning the circumstances of the injury may contribute to a delayed diagnosis.

Physical Examination

An abnormal physical examination may not always be indicative of pathology. Clinicians should avoid relying on physical examination alone as a predictor of abdominal injury. Studies have demonstrated that patients with and without proven injuries often showed no significant differences with respect to physical findings.

Vital signs should be monitored. In children, the range for normal heart rate, respiratory rate, and blood pressure is age dependent. A simple rule for calculating the lower limit of normal systolic blood pressure is 70 + (2 × age in years). Physicians should always remember that a drop in blood pressure is a late sign in the development of shock (see Chapter 42, Approach to the Traumatized Child and Chapter 41, Shock).

Serial abdominal examinations increase the likelihood of detecting a previously missed condition. Inspection of the abdomen to look for ecchymosis, distention, tire

---

> **Questions: Abdominal Trauma**
>
> - How was the child injured?
> - How long ago did the injury occur?
> - What parts of the body were injured?
> - Has the child received any treatment prior to coming to the hospital?

---

tracks, penetrations, or paradoxical motion should occur first. Auscultation for bowel sounds follows this inspection, and palpation should come last. Palpation should be done in all four quadrants to elicit tenderness, rebound, and guarding. If a hepatic or splenic injury is initially suspected, palpation should be minimized to avoid further hemorrhaging.

Laboratory Tests

Laboratory evaluation should be guided by the history and physical examination. A urinalysis to look for hematuria and check for associated genitourinary injuries is helpful. Elevated serum transaminases, amylase, and alkaline phosphatase may be indicative of injury, but normal values do not exclude pathology. A comprehensive trauma panel should be carried out for all patients with serious or multiple injuries (see Chapter 42, Approach to the Traumatized Child).

Diagnostic/Imaging Studies

Multiple imaging modalities are available to assess the pediatric trauma patient with suspected abdominal injuries. The time to perform an imaging study is after the patient is responding appropriately to resuscitation (i.e., fluid therapy). Unstable patients will require surgical exploration for definitive treatment of abdominal or pelvic injury.

In the United States, CT scanning is the standard of care for imaging the injured abdomen of a pediatric trauma patient. CT scans have a greater than 97% accuracy in identifying abdominal injury, are noninvasive, and provide detailed specific information regarding injuries. The images can also be extended to include the pelvis, if necessary. Disadvantages of CT scanning include the lack of proximity to the trauma suite, which may not be ideal for unstable patients; the length of time it takes to perform the procedure; and the need for oral and IV contrast, which has inherent risks such as allergic reactions and aspiration.

In other countries, particularly European countries and Japan, the use of ultrasonography has become very popular, with encouraging results for the identification of abdominal injury. Ultrasound can rapidly and noninvasively document the presence of intraperitoneal and pelvic fluid (blood). Studies so far show that it is probably at least as effective as CT scanning for documenting the **presence of injury** but does not provide as much specific information about the **nature** of the injury. Ultrasound has a few additional advantages: it is relatively inexpensive; does not require contrast or radiation exposure; can be performed in 5–10 minutes in the trauma room, thus minimizing the risk to an unstable patient; and can be used many times for serial assessments.

Over the last several decades, diagnostic peritoneal lavage (DPL) has been a dependable method of detecting intra-abdominal hemorrhage. However, its use may be limited in the pediatric population since many children with blunt trauma to the abdomen are now managed nonoperatively.

MANAGEMENT

Management of abdominal trauma in children occurs simultaneously with evaluation. The stabilization of children with abdominal trauma, especially in the context of multiple trauma, requires a multidisciplinary team approach that includes surgeons, pediatricians, and emergency physicians. A discussion on the approach to trauma management can be found in Chapter 42, Approach to the Traumatized Child.

Hypovolemic shock, if present, is the primary complication of abdominal trauma on which to focus, because the leading unrecognized cause of death in affected children is profound blood loss. **Airway problems** and **breathing difficulties** should be addressed initially, followed by **vascular access** and **fluid replacement.** No more than three attempts at peripheral vascular access should be made (in 90 seconds or less) before moving on to more invasive procedures.

The intraosseous route should be used for the next vascular access attempt in children who are less than 6 years of age. The flat, medial portion of the proximal tibia is most commonly used for the procedure, which is performed with an intraosseous, bone marrow, or spinal needle (Fig. 43–1). Fluids and medications, delivered into the marrow cavity, then flow into the venous circulation. Intraosseous cannulation is rapid, simple, and may be life saving. It is limited by low flow rates (approximately 30 mL/minute), which can be augmented either by using pressure on the intravenous bag or by pushing fluid by hand through a syringe. Complications associated with intraosseous line placement are rare. All physicians who care for pediatric trauma patients should be familiar with this technique.

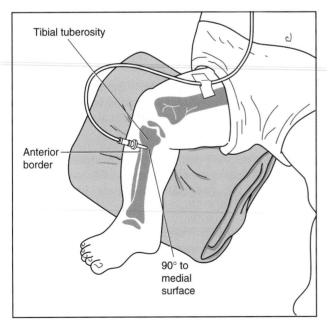

FIGURE 43–1. Intraosseous cannulation technique. (Adapted, with permission, from Chameides, L., and M. F. Hazinski [eds.]. Textbook of Pediatric Advanced Life Support. Dallas, American Heart Association, 1994.)

Labels on figure:
- Tibial tuberosity
- Anterior border
- 90° to medial surface

TABLE 43–1. Signs and Symptoms of Hemorrhagic Shock in Children

Tachycardia
Increased capillary refill (>2 sec)
Cool and mottled skin, pallor
Respiratory distress
Anxiety, irritability, decreased responsiveness
Thirst
Orthostatic fall in blood pressure, supine hypotension (late sign)

A variety of central venous access sites, such as femoral, subclavian, and internal jugular, may be used in older children. Upper and lower saphenous vein cutdowns are also possible access sites. The Seldinger technique, with insertion of a large-bore catheter over a guidewire, is often used. A description of these procedures is beyond the scope of this book but may be found in many other texts, including the *Textbook of Pediatric Advanced Life Support* published by the American Heart Association (see Selected Readings).

Fluid replacement begins with a 20–40-mL/kg bolus of crystalloid solution, either warmed normal saline or Ringer's lactate. If no improvement in circulation occurs, additional 10–20-mL/kg boluses may be given, and type-specific blood should be considered. In most scenarios, type-specific blood is given after 80 ml/kg of crystalloid has failed to improve circulatory parameters. Frequent hematocrits or hemoglobins should be determined to monitor ongoing blood loss. Vital signs should be repeated frequently. Serial examinations, which detect the signs and symptoms of shock (Table 43–1), are the most important gauge of hemodynamic recovery and stability. All children require close hospital observation, preferably in a pediatric trauma center and intensive care unit.

If hemodynamic stabilization is not achieved after appropriate vascular access and fluid resuscitation, the trauma surgeon will most likely perform an exploratory laparotomy. If children have been stabilized with initial airway and circulatory support, diagnostic procedures such as CT scans can be performed as part of the emergency department evaluation. Once identified, specific organ injury can be managed.

Other specific management concerns for pediatric patients with abdominal injury are early decompression of the stomach with a nasogastric or orogastric tube to prevent respiratory compromise, and urinary catheter insertion to decompress the bladder. Before inserting a urinary catheter, the trauma team should evaluate for possible urethral trauma and check for the present of blood in the urine, which may indicate other genitourinary trauma.

PROGNOSIS

Morbidity and mortality related to abdominal trauma depend on the specific organ injury and the style of management. More than 40% of patients with major liver injuries die in the prehospital setting. However, a large number of minor liver injuries can be managed nonoperatively. Currently, an increasing number of injuries to the spleen and liver are managed with observation in the pediatric intensive care unit. Surgical exploration and repair is performed only if patients become hemodynamically unstable. Reduction in anesthetic-related mortality, postsplenectomy sepsis, and a decrease in other postoperative complications have resulted from this shift in practice style. Without surgical intervention, however, an injury such as complete splenic rupture has a 90–100% mortality rate.

Case Resolution

The boy in the case scenario sustained isolated abdominal trauma. Initial presenting signs and symptoms are consistent with internal organ injury, specifically splenic hematoma, pancreatic injury, internal hemorrhage, and compensated shock (e.g., tachycardia, tachypnea). The child should undergo initial resuscitation with attention to the airway, breathing, and circulation, especially fluid

repletion. Serial hemodynamic measurement and hematocrits, if stable, permit diagnosis of specific injuries by CT scanning. Surgical consultation with expectant observation is the likely management choice. If the child deteriorates, surgical intervention would ensue. Trauma to the small intestine, particularly a duodenal hematoma, must also be suspected because of the mechanism of injury.

Selected Readings

Bennett, M. K., and D. Jehle. Ultrasonography in blunt abdominal trauma. Emerg. Med. Clin. North Am. 15:763–784, 1997.

Cantor, R. M., and J. M. Leaming. Evaluation and management of pediatric major trauma. Emerg. Med. Clin. North Am. 16:229–256, 1998.

Chameides, L. (ed.). Textbook of Pediatric Advanced Life Support. Dallas, American Heart Association, 1994.

Foltin, G. L., and A. Cooper. Abdominal trauma. *In* Barkin, R. M. (ed.). Pediatric Emergency Medicine Concepts and Clinical Practice. St. Louis, Mosby-Year Book, 1997, pp. 335–354.

Haller, J. A. Blunt trauma to the abdomen. Pediatr. Rev. 17:29–31, 1996.

CHAPTER 44

HEAD TRAUMA

Jill M. Baren, M.D.

H$_x$ A 2-year-old girl is playing on a window ledge unsupervised. She pushes the screen out and falls onto the concrete sidewalk below, striking her head. A neighbor reports that she is unconscious for 10 minutes. When paramedics arrive, the girl is awake but lethargic. She is transported to the emergency department. Her vital signs are normal. A scalp hematoma is present, and a depressed area of cranial bone is palpated.

Questions

1. What are the priorities in the initial stabilization and management of pediatric head trauma?
2. What is the difference between primary and secondary brain injury?
3. What are the common structural injuries sustained by children with head trauma?
4. What are the various modalities available for treatment of increased intracranial pressure (ICP)?
5. Name and briefly describe the scoring systems used in the evaluation of mental status in children with head trauma.

Although the vast majority of childhood head injuries are minor and can be treated on an outpatient basis, it is important for clinicians to become adept at recognizing and managing more severe forms of head injury. The various clinical presentations of pediatric head trauma range from simple scalp lacerations to intracranial hematomas. Familiarity with techniques for assessment of mental status and control of ICP can help reduce morbidity from traumatic brain injury. Furthermore, health care providers can help lower mortality from head trauma by actively promoting injury prevention to patients and communities.

EPIDEMIOLOGY

Head injury is the leading cause of morbidity and mortality in pediatric trauma patients. About 250,000 children per year sustain head trauma; 150,000 suffer injury to the brain tissue itself, and 20% of these injuries result in permanent neurologic sequelae. Overall mortality from isolated head trauma is believed to be 6–35%

but increases in the presence of other injuries. In children with trauma to multiple parts of the body, 70% of the deaths that occur within 48 hours of hospitalization are the result of trauma to the head. Major causes of head trauma in children include falls, motor vehicle crashes, and recreational activities. Falls are the most likely reason a child or adolescent will visit an emergency department. The severity of the head trauma sustained in a fall is usually related to the height from which the child fell. Falls from heights less than 10 feet usually do not result in severe injury to toddlers and older children. In infants under the age of 2 months, significant head injury rarely results from a fall of less than 4 feet. Therefore, this raises concern about nonaccidental trauma, and warrants further investigation.

Motor vehicle crashes are responsible for 25% of childhood head injury. Between the ages of 5–9 years, head injury is predominently the result of pedestrian injuries and secondarily of bicycle injuries. Adolescents are increasingly more likely to sustain head injury as motor vehicle occupants.

Sports-related trauma causes about 21% of head injury in children and adolescents, and roughly half of these involve bicycles. Child abuse (assaults) must be recognized as another important cause of head injury in children, particularly among children under the age of 2 years. Physical findings such as retinal hemorrhages support this diagnosis.

CLINICAL PRESENTATION

Children who have sustained head trauma may present with a history of an antecedent event (e.g., fall or collision with another child) or signs and symptoms related to the injury. These include external bruises or lacerations; alterations in the level of consciousness (LOC); and neurologic findings, including seizures. Vital signs may be altered; in particular, deep or irregular respiration, hypertension, or bradycardia may be apparent (D_x Box). These changes are indicative of elevated ICP.

D_x Head Trauma*

- LOC
- Somnolence
- Pallor
- Emesis/nausea/anorexia
- Irritability
- Lethargy
- Seizure
- Ataxia
- Weakness
- Pain
- Parasthesias
- Amnesia
- Headache
- Visual changes
- Confusion/altered mental status

*All these symptoms may not be present in head trauma.

PATHOPHYSIOLOGY

Compared to adults, children have a higher center of gravity, an increased head-to-body ratio, and weaker neck muscles that predispose the head to injury. Children also have other anatomic disadvantages such as thinner cranial bones and less myelinated brain tissue, which increases the risk of injury to brain parenchyma.

Normally, blood flow to the brain is maintained at a constant rate, a process known as autoregulation. With severe brain injury, autoregulation is lost and blood flow to the brain is equal to cerebral perfusion pressure (CPP). CPP is the difference between mean arterial pressure (MAP) and ICP. A CPP that is either too high or too low can be detrimental.

Control of CPP after head injury in children is challenging. Focal hematomas, which are seen more often in adults, can be evacuated surgically to relieve pressure. In contrast, children tend to develop diffuse cerebral edema that requires complex management. However, children have a greater capacity for recovery despite these initial difficulties. This is especially true in very young children, whose open sutures and fontanelles permit expansion of the skull from edema and blood.

It is important to understand the difference between primary and secondary brain injury. Primary injury is the structural damage that occurs to the cranium and its contents at the time of the injury. Secondary injury is damage to the brain tissue after the initial event. Such damage may result from hypoxia, hypoperfusion, hypercarbia, hyperthermia, and altered glucose or sodium metabolism. It is imperative that the overall goal of management involve the prevention of secondary brain injury; primary brain injury can be prevented only through education and safety.

DIFFERENTIAL DIAGNOSIS

Head trauma can result in a wide variety of clinical syndromes with different degrees of severity. Often the signs and symptoms of one type of injury overlap with another. Figure 44–1 illustrates the anatomic location of various head injuries.

Scalp lacerations, which are extremely common presentations of head trauma, may be either superficial or deep to the galea. They are caused by both blunt and penetrating mechanisms. Penetration of the skull table by a lacerating object (e.g., knife, bullet) is associated with a vast potential for damage and a poor outcome. Soft tissue injuries include abrasions, scalp hematomas, subgaleal hematomas, and cephalhematomas. These injuries are readily managed in the emergency department.

The majority of skull fractures are simple and linear. When fractures cross the path of a blood vessel or venous sinus, the potential for complications is increased. Other fracture types are compound, diastatic, base-of-skull, and depressed. Base-of-skull fractures usually present with **hemotympanum, blood** or **CSF in the ear canal, Battle's sign** (postauricular ecchymosis), **raccoon eyes** (periorbital ecchymosis), or **cranial nerve palsies.** Depressed skull fractures often require

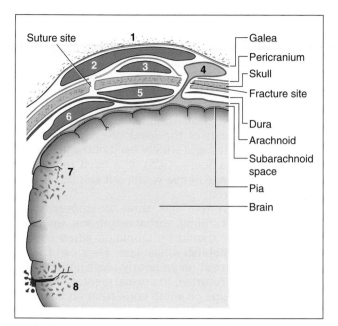

FIGURE 44–1. Functional anatomy of brain and surrounding structures with sites of pathology. 1, caput succedaneum; 2, subgaleal hematoma; 3, cephalhematoma; 4, porencephalic cyst or leptomeningeal cyst; 5, epidural hematoma; 6, subdural hematoma; 7, cerebral contusion; 8, cerebral laceration. (Redrawn, with permission, from Tecklenburg, F.W., and M.S. Wright. Minor head trauma in the pediatric patient. Pediatr. Emerg. Care 7:40–47, 1991.)

operative management to lift the depressed fragment away from the underlying brain.

Head injury may result in a concussion or concussive syndrome, which is defined as a transient LOC with amnesia with no abnormality detected on CT scan of the brain. Neurologic examination is usually normal, but patients may experience headache, vomiting, and other minor symptoms. Concussions can also have minor and subtle neurologic sequelae, such as dizziness or headache, for months following the injury (postconcussive syndrome). Concussions have a characteristic triangular appearance on MRI scan.

A cerebral contusion occurs with a more severe injury such as a high-speed motor vehicle crash. A coup-contrecoup injury may be produced when the brain strikes the skull, anteriorly bruising the frontal lobe and then posteriorly bruising the occipital lobe. Clinical manifestations depend on the location of the contusion but often include altered mental status, excessive sleepiness, confusion, and even combativeness. Bleeding and swelling of surrounding tissue are major concerns in the acute setting.

Epidural hematomas are collections of blood that accumulate between the skull bone and the tough outer covering of the brain (dura). They are often the result of tears in the middle meningeal artery caused by skull fractures. Classically, patients have initial LOC followed by a lucid interval and then rapid deterioration secondary to brain compression. On CT scan an epidural hematoma appears as a large collection of blood with convex borders next to the skull (Fig. 44–2A). Surgical evacuation is required in the majority of cases.

Subdural hematomas, which are five to ten times more common than epidural hematomas, accumulate between the dura and the underlying brain tissue. They are associated with both skull fractures and contusions. On CT scan they appear to have crescent-shaped borders (Fig. 44–2B). Large subdural hematomas usually require surgery for evacuation.

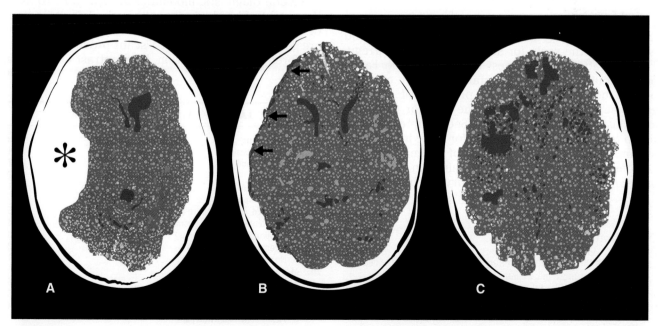

FIGURE 44–2.
A. Epidural hematoma, marked by the asterisk. Note convex borders and midline shift.
B. Subdural hematoma. Note crescent shape.
C. Diffuse axonal injury. Note ground-glass appearance and tightly compressed ventricles.
(Reproduced, with permission, from Harris, J. H., Jr., W. H. Harris, and R. A. Norelline. The Radiology of Emergency Medicine, 3rd ed. Baltimore, Williams & Wilkins, 1993. pp. 15, 16, 17.)

The initial force that results in severe head trauma may produce a shearing or tearing effect on the axonal white matter of the brain known as diffuse axonal injury (DAI) (Fig. 44–2C). As a result of DAI, cerebral edema and elevated ICP occur, maximally within 24–48 hours postinjury. It is difficult to predict which patients will recover from this diffuse damage. Children have a better prognosis than adults, although in many instances, even a long neurorehabilitation process may not correct severe neurologic disability.

EVALUATION

In children with acute head injuries, especially when other organ system trauma is present, assessment and management occur simultaneously. A primary survey is performed with attention to airway, breathing, circulation (ABC), and cervical spine immobilization as well as a rapid, gross neurologic assessment of responsiveness and pupillary size and reactivity (see Chapter 42, Approach to the Traumatized Child, for more information about treating trauma patients). Cervical spinal injuries are less common in children than head injuries. However, all children with altered LOC; painful, distracting injuries; inability to communicate; focal neurologic deficits; or localized pain, swelling, or ecchymosis of the cervical spine require careful evaluation of their spine.

History

Historical data are obtained during the secondary survey or reassessment phase of evaluation. Prehospital health care providers or witnesses to the injury should be asked about details of the event (Questions Box).

Physical Examination

Secondary survey actions include palpation and inspection of the scalp for soft tissue swelling, irregularity, lacerations, and fullness of the fontanelle. Facial bones should be tested for stability. Other clues to possible head trauma include presence of a septal hematoma, draining fluid from the nose or ears, and malocclusion of the mandible. (See Chapter 42, Approach to the Traumatized Child, for more information on primary and secondary survey of trauma patients.)

A comprehensive neurologic examination is the most important part of the secondary survey. This examina-

tion should include mental status, cranial nerves, deep tendon reflexes, muscle tone, muscle strength, sensation, cerebellar function, and funduscopic evaluation if possible. When describing mental status, imprecise terms such as "altered," "lethargic," and "obtunded" should be avoided. Several widely used scoring systems are available for mental status assessment of children who have suffered head trauma. A number of scales exist for assessment of the level of coma. The most universally accepted and widely used of these scales is the Glasgow Coma Score (GCS). It is used routinely in children over the age of five years, but can be modified for younger children.

Each scoring system has three components: eye opening to various stimuli, verbal responses, and motor responses. Scores should be tabulated when children first present to establish a baseline. They can then be used for reassessment on an hourly basis until patients have stabilized or returned to normal mental status. Use of these scores helps promote consistent and accurate communication among health care providers. Tables 44–1 and 44–2 show how to calculate the GCS and modified GCS scores. Classification of mild, moderate, or severe head trauma, based on the GCS score, is illustrated in Table 44–3.

Laboratory Tests

The most useful laboratory tests are a CBC, serum electrolytes, serum glucose, and possibly a toxicologic screen, if appropriate. These tests do not help establish a diagnosis but help guide management.

Imaging Studies

Several diagnostic modalities are available to assess the extent of head injuries. Although plain radiographs of the skull may be useful for identifying fractures, they are generally not justified. CT scans provide much more comprehensive information. Noncontrast CT scans are

---

Questions: Head Trauma

- What was the mechanism of injury (motor vehicle crash, ejection from motor vehicle, fall, assault)?
- What was the shape of the object(s) striking the head?
- What was the velocity of object(s) striking the head?
- What was the height of the fall?
- What was the type of impact surface?
- What was the child's immediate status after injury?
- What changes in status occurred before arrival at the hospital?
- Did the child lose consciousness? If so, for how long?

TABLE 44–1. Glasgow Coma Scale

	Points
I. Eye opening	
a. Spontaneous	4
b. To command	3
c. With pain	2
d. No response	1
II. Verbal response*	
a. Oriented, communicative (oriented)	5
b. Disoriented, confused (words)	4
c. Inappropriate (vocal sounds)	3
d. Incomprehensible (cries)	2
e. No response (no response)	1
III. Motor response	
a. Obeys commands	6
b. Localizes pain	5
c. Flexes with pain	4
d. Flexes abnormally with pain	3
e. Extensor response	2
f. None	1
Maximum score	**15**

*Assessment of verbal response is modified in children.

TABLE 44-2.   Modified GCS for Younger Children

	Points
I. **Eye opening**	
a. Spontaneous	4
b. To command	3
c. With pain	2
d. No response	1
II. **Verbal response**	
a. Coos and babbles	5
b. Irritable cry	4
c. Cries to pain	3
d. Moans to pain	2
e. None	1
III. **Motor response**	
a. Normal spontaneous movement	6
b. Withdraws to touch	5
c. Withdraws to pain	4
d. Abnormal flexion	3
e. Abnormal extension	2
f. None	1
Maximum score	15

adequate in the setting of acute trauma and detect skull fractures, soft tissue swelling, cerebral contusions, intracranial hematomas, diffuse cerebral edema, compression, midline shift of brain structures, and ventricular enlargement or compression.

All patients classified as having moderate to severe head trauma (GCS <14) should have a head CT scan performed on arrival at the emergency department. For minor head trauma (GCS = 14–15) with varying degrees of LOC, the decision to perform a CT scan is based on historical data, physical findings, physician experience, and the psychosocial situation of patients and their families. A list of suggested criteria for obtaining a CT scan for mildly injured patients can be found in Table 44–4.

Although MRI may be superior to CT for identifying diffuse axonal injury and certain types of hemorrhage, MRI has limited use for severely injured patients in the acute phase of injury. In general, MRI takes longer (30–60 minutes) to complete, and the scanners are often not in the vicinity of the emergency department. However, as MRI scanners become more widely available and efficient, they may be used more frequently in the assessment of acute head trauma.

MANAGEMENT

The ABCs are the initial management priorities for children with head injuries, as they are in other trauma

TABLE 44-3.   Definitions of Head Injuries in Children Secondary to Initial Glasgow Coma Scale (GCS) Score

Head Injury	Initial GCS		Duration of LOC
Mild	13–15	and	<20 min
Moderate	9–12*		
Severe	≤8	or	Coma ≥ 6 hr

*Denotes no deterioration below that range.
Adapted, with permission, from Goldstein, B., and K.S. Powers. Head trauma in children. Pediatr. Rev. 15:213, 1994.

TABLE 44-4.   Indications for CT Scans in Children with Head Trauma

Alteration in level of consciousness, waxing and waning or deteriorating mental status
Glasgow Coma score <14
Focal neurologic deficits on examination
Palpation of a depressed skull fracture
Posttraumatic seizures
Persistent vomiting, headache, lethargy
Trauma to multiple areas of the body
Associated facial or neck trauma
Age less than 2 yr

patients. The primary goal of management of acute head trauma is the prevention of all possible mechanisms of secondary brain injury. Prompt neurosurgical consultation should be obtained for all children with head trauma except those with very minor injuries.

Obtaining control over the airway is of paramount importance in patients with head trauma. Hyperventilation is one way to reduce ICP. Hyperventilation lowers arterial carbon dioxide (pCO_2), leading to cerebral vasoconstriction and decreased cerebral blood flow. The bag-valve-mask technique should be used initially, followed by rapid sequence intubation to minimize hypoxic and hypercarbic insult. Rapid sequence intubation often involves agents such as lidocaine and thiopental that either reduce ICP or blunt the rise in ICP that occurs during intubation. Care must be taken not to lower the pCO_2 too much, because this may deprive the brain of needed blood flow; the target range for pCO_2 is 27–32 mm Hg.

Circulation and MAP should be aggressively supported with fluids to prevent hypoperfusion to the brain. Hypovolemia or hypotension should never be assumed to result from head trauma alone. Children should be examined carefully for evidence of internal organ injury (see Chapters 42, Approach to the Traumatized Child, and 43, Abdominal Trauma).

Because CPP is determined by both MAP and ICP, increases in ICP may impede blood flow to the brain and exacerbate ischemic injury. Administration of diuretics and osmotic agents such as mannitol and elevation of the head of the bed to 30 degrees to promote venous drainage are examples of methods used to reduce ICP. Paralytic agents and sedatives may be needed to prevent agitation, which also leads to increased ICP. To assist in monitoring for sudden increases in ICP and to provide drainage of excess CSF, intraventricular pressure catheters can be placed.

Hyperthermia should be avoided, and alterations in serum electrolytes should be minimized. Patients with head injuries should be monitored closely for the development of diabetes insipidus or syndrome of inappropriate secretion of antidiuretic hormone. Prophylaxis with anticonvulsants is still controversial, but any seizure activity must be rapidly recognized and treated.

Children with minor head injuries (GCS = 14–15) with no LOC or a brief witnessed period of LOC, no focal deficits on neurologic examination, no high-risk skull fractures, and no persistent vomiting, who demonstrate improvement and normal mental status (GCS = 15) after 4–6 hours of observation can be discharged with written instructions if they have adequate transportation back to the hospital, a telephone, and a reliable parent or guardian. Children should be admitted if these criteria cannot be reliably fulfilled. Younger children (<4 years of age) are more difficult to assess accurately and consistently; therefore, admission should be strongly considered if their mental status is not completely normal or at baseline. Physicians should be wary of discharging children whose conditions have not improved to baseline following minor injuries even if their CT scans are normal.

More moderate head injuries (initial GCS = 9–12) necessitate a longer period of evaluation, probably in a monitored setting with neurosurgical consultation. Severe head injuries (GCS <8) require aggressive stabilization in the emergency department with the measures described above and admission to a pediatric intensive care unit.

PROGNOSIS

Age is the most important prognostic factor in outcome. Younger children tend to do better than older children. It is still difficult to predict the outcome of any individual patient, however. Scalp lacerations, most skull fractures, and concussions are low-risk injuries. Intracranial hemorrhage, specific skull fractures, head injury secondary to child abuse, and trauma accompanied by diffuse cerebral edema are high-risk injuries.

If untreated, severe head injury may lead to death from herniation. Herniation results when cranial contents are too large for the space inside the skull, and the brain is compressed down through openings of the skull. Herniation can occur at several locations, such as through the foramen magnum or by compression against the cerebellar tentorium. Depending on the area being stretched or compressed, different clinical syndromes are produced.

Other complications from severe head trauma are posttraumatic seizures, requiring lifelong treatment with anticonvulsants; hydrocephalus, necessitating a ventriculoperitoneal shunt catheter; and persistent vegetative or severely impaired mental states. Sequelae such as postconcussive syndrome may result from less severe head trauma. Some of the characteristics of this syndrome include dizziness, headache, irritability, memory deficits, impaired behavior, and impaired cognitive development. These may persist for months after the head injury.

PREVENTION

Despite advancing medical knowledge and excellent critical care available to children with head trauma, little can be done to reduce the severity of primary brain injury once it has occurred. Therefore, pediatric health care providers should make every attempt to educate patients and families about prevention strategies.

Some of the most successful prevention strategies involve the required use of restraint devices such as seatbelts, and of proper safety gear such as bicycle helmets. Educational efforts aimed at reducing the use of baby walkers, putting up gates in homes, and reducing teen use of alcohol are more complex, but also worthwhile. Finally, communities can contribute to injury prevention by providing playground resurfacing, reducing the height of playground equipment, and by changing traffic laws. It is only through a combination of these prevention strategies that morbidity and mortality of pediatric head trauma will be truly reduced.

Case Resolution

The case scenario involves a young child with a significant mechanism of injury; brief LOC; and a depressed, altered mental status. Initial physical findings prompt suspicion of a depressed skull fracture and overlying soft tissue injury. Appropriate diagnostic tools after evaluation of the ABCs are a cranial CT scan followed by admission for observation, monitoring, and serial neurologic examination. Operative repair of the skull fracture may be necessary.

Selected Readings

Bruce, D. A. Head trauma. *In* Fleisher, G. R., and S. Ludwig (eds.). Textbook of Pediatric Emergency Medicine, 3rd ed. Baltimore, Williams & Wilkins, 1993.

Goldstein, B., and K. S. Powers. Head trauma in children. Pediatr. Rev. 15:213–219, June 1994.

Michaud, L. J. , A. Duhaime, and M. L. Batshaw. Traumatic brain injury in children. Pediatr. Clin. North Am. 40:553–565, 1993.

Rivara, F. P. Epidemiology and prevention of pediatric traumatic brain injury. Pediatr. Ann. 23:12–17, 1994.

Tecklenburg, F. W., and M. S. Wright. Minor head trauma in the pediatric patient. Pediatr. Emerg. Care 7:40–47, February 1991.

Zuckerman, G. B., and E. E. Conway. Accidental head injury. Pediatr. Ann. 26:621–632, 1997.

INCREASED INTRACRANIAL PRESSURE

Kenneth R. Huff, M.D.

H_x   A 7-year-old boy has a 2-week history of recurrent vomiting. No fever, abdominal pain, or diarrhea has accompanied the vomiting, the vomiting has no particular relationship to meals, and the boy's appetite has decreased only slightly. The vomiting, has gradually increased in frequency and is occurring every night. Yesterday, there were four episodes. The boy's parents have noticed that their son is generally less active; he spends more time playing on the floor of his room and does not want to ride his bicycle or play with neighborhood friends. Some unsteadiness in the boy's gait has developed in the last few days. His parents attribute this to weakness from the vomiting.

The child's vital signs are normal except for a blood pressure of 130/80. Although the boy is somewhat pale and uncomfortable, he does not appear to be in acute distress. His abdominal examination is unremarkable. His speech is grammatically correct but sparse and hesitant, and he seems inattentive. On lateral and upgaze the boy has coarse nystagmus, and upgaze is somewhat limited. Some diplopia on left gaze is apparent, with slight failure of left eye abduction. The left eye does not blink as much as the right eye. Fundal examination discloses elevated disks with indistinct margins. No upper extremity weakness is evident. The right foot is slightly weaker than the left, ankle tone is bilaterally increased, and three to four beats of clonus on the right and bilateral, positive Babinski reflexes are present. Some tremor occurs in both arms with finger-to-nose testing. The boy walks with shuffling, small steps; his gait has a slight lurching character, and he veers to the right.

Questions

1. What clinical situations are associated with increased intracranial pressure (ICP)?
2. What is the pathophysiologic process leading to ICP?
3. What studies are used to evaluate children with ICP?
4. What measures are used to treat children with ICP?

The signs and symptoms of increased intracranial pressure (ICP) are often a signal of a serious intracranial process that may require surgical or intensive care intervention depending on the underlying cause. Because the process is frequently critical and dynamic, it has proven useful to quantitate intracranial pressure for management purposes, although values in children are not as well correlated with pathophysiology as in adults. Normal intracranial pressure levels are somewhat lower in the neonatal period, but in older children pressures are abnormal above 13 mm Hg (180 mm H_2O) and may become symptomatic above 20 mm Hg. Although it is possible to have normal mental function up to 40 mm Hg, the ICP becomes clinically significant when the perfusion pressure is compromised, which perhaps is when the ICP is 70–90 mm Hg below the mean arterial pressure, and it becomes dangerous as the ICP approaches 40–50 mm Hg below the mean arterial pressure. Decreased perfusion produces swollen damaged tissue, which further exacerbates the pressure-volume problem in a "snowballing" fashion.

Although only a relatively small number of effective treatments for increased ICP are available, greater understanding is accumulating about when to initiate them. It is important to recognize signs and symptoms early and determine the underlying cause; treatment of the cause may resolve the increased ICP, particularly if used early in the course. In other cases, however, increased ICP is a potentially life-threatening critical care issue whose management along with that of the underlying cause is key for survival.

EPIDEMIOLOGY

Head trauma is a leading cause of increased ICP. Infants may be victims of nonaccidental trauma; older children may be stricken pedestrians or bicycle riders, occupants of motor vehicles, or victims of falls; and adolescents may be victims of penetrating trauma such as gunshots. Such trauma is a major source of morbidity in children and requires careful monitoring and management of ICP.

Brain tumors are the most common solid neoplasms in children and frequently lead to increased ICP either by direct mass effect or blockage of CSF flow. Ischemic brain damage resulting from a difficult delivery at birth, a submersion incident, or a major cerebral vessel thrombosis is also a cause of increased ICP. Cytotoxic causes of brain swelling, such as lead intoxication and liver failure in Reye's syndrome, are less common etiologies.

Benign intracranial hypertension or pseudotumor cerebri may also lead to increased ICP. This condition is seen most frequently in obese adolescent females, with thrombosis of a lateral venous sinus following complicated otitis media, with therapy with high doses of vitamin A or tetracycline, and with withdrawal of steroid therapy.

CLINICAL PRESENTATION

Children with increased ICP may present with a history of recurrent vomiting, lethargy, and headaches of increasing frequency or severity or that awaken them

---

Dx   Increased ICP

- Loss of appetite, nausea, vomiting, headache, or lethargy
- Inattention, decreased arousability
- Papilledema, upgaze paresis
- Increased tone, positive Babinski reflex
- Focal signs and history compatible with an intracranial mass
- Mass lesion, cerebral edema, or enlarged ventricles in an imaging study

---

from sleep. A prior history of trauma, ischemia, or intoxication/metabolic aberration may also raise suspicions of increased ICP in the child with compatible examination findings. Physical findings may include elevated optic disk, failure of upward gaze, hypertonicity of the extremities, and depressed alertness or inattention. Localized findings on neurologic examination may point to a lesion indicative of a space-occupying intracranial mass, which contributes to increased ICP (Dx Box).

PATHOPHYSIOLOGY

The problem of increased ICP can be understood in terms of the Monro-Kellie doctrine, which applies to the theoretically rigid cranial compartment and pressure-volume relationships of the contents. Intracranial volume has three main components: brain parenchyma, cerebrospinal fluid (CSF), and blood. Except in the first 2 years of life before most of the cranial sutures are fused, the skull and dura form a relatively rigid compartment; any increase in one of the three intracranial volume components must occur at the expense of one or both of the other two. Decreased volume leads to increased pressure in a nonlinear relationship related to compliance of the skull, sutures, and dura. As compliance decreases, pressure rises rapidly. Irreversible damage to brain tissue occurs primarily as a result of pressure of the other components overtaking the arterial blood pressure and not allowing adequate tissue perfusion. In younger children, nonfused sutures allow more compliance if volume increases are relatively slow, but this factor is not true for acute volume increases. In addition, pressure gradients exist across compartments, sites of CSF flow obstruction, or even around lesions within brain parenchyma, which may lead to more focal disorders than can be explained by global intracranial pressure or perfusion changes.

Changes in any of the three components making up the intracranial volume may result in increased ICP in several ways. First, the brain parenchyma component may be directly increased by mass lesions such as neoplasms, abscesses, or hemorrhages. Edema may increase the brain parenchyma volume. Fluid may accumulate because of vascular leakage due to cytokines. Brain edema may also result from cytotoxic damage, cell death, and necrosis. Cytotoxic processes include swelling of intact cells, cell rupture producing increased interstitial oncotic pressure from released proteins and ions, and cellular inflammatory and repair processes. Cytotoxic brain edema may be caused by various cellular insults including hypoxemia; ischemia; toxins, including neuronal excitotoxins; and depletion of energy substrates. These cellular insults may be a consequence of a diversity of local or diffuse brain problems including major vessel thrombosis, trauma (e.g., local contusion or diffuse axonal injury), anoxia from cardiac arrest, hypertension, encephalitic infection, or metabolic poisoning.

Second, the pressure of the CSF volume component (ventricles or subarachnoid spaces) may increase in hydrocephalus. Hydrocephalus can result in two ways: (1) from a discrepancy in the rate of formation of CSF relative to absorption, and (2) from an obstruction between the point of formation in the lateral ventricles and the site of absorption at the arachnoid granulations. An obstruction can occur with a congenital malformation; parenchymal or CSF mass such as a cyst or neoplasm; CSF inflammatory cells from meningitis, ventriculitis, or hemorrhage; brain parenchyma; or arachnoid border. The small passageways connecting the ventricular system, the foramina of Monro and the aqueduct of Sylvius; the exits of the ventricular system, the foramina of Magendie and Luschka; and the cisterns surrounding the brain stem are particularly vulnerable points of obstruction.

Third, ICP may rise because the intravascular volume component may increase.

One process that leads to this increase is venous outflow obstruction such as occurs with a lateral sinus thrombosis, a cause of pseudotumor cerebri. Other processes that raise jugular venous pressure may also increase ICP. In addition, the intracranial arterial vascular volume is affected by carbon dioxide partial pressure. It not only increases with hypercarbia but also decreases with hypocarbia, which allows for iatrogenic lowering of ICP by hyperventilation.

As ICP increases, brain perfusion pressure may be maintained up to a point by a spontaneous increase in mean arterial pressure, a response referred to as Cushing's phenomenon. Although the relationship may not be direct and universally reliable, the rise in systemic pressure can be a useful clinical sign of increased ICP.

Acute or subacute changes in pressure in an intracranial compartment may produce a pressure gradient that may precipitate a brain herniation syndrome (Fig. 45–1). An ominous heralding sign of transtentorial herniation of the uncus of the temporal lobe is loss of the pupillary light reflex caused by entrapment of the third cranial nerve. This herniation often leads to irreversible brain stem damage as well as infarcts and additional secondary edema. Focally increased posterior fossa pressure may result in a pressure cone downward through the foramen magnum compressing medullary centers leading to apnea and death. A marginally compensated system could be decompensated by an ill-advised lumbar puncture when the spinal compartment pressure is acutely lowered and the pressure gradient from the posterior fossa is thereby increased.

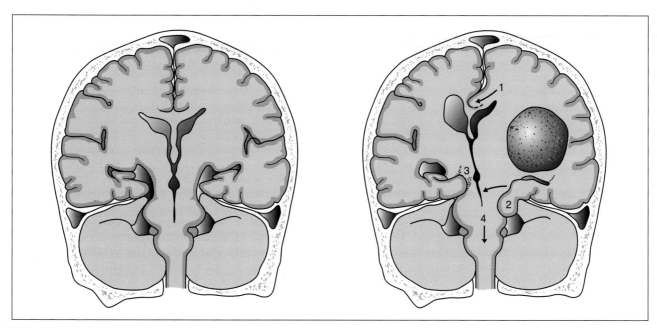

FIGURE 45–1. Depiction of the anatomy of several potential herniation syndromes caused by intracranial compartment pressure gradients related to a mass (hematoma, neoplasm, or acutely necrotic brain tissue) in a cerebral hemisphere. 1, trans-falxine herniation; 2, uncal herniation; 3, contralateral tentorial-midbrain damage; 4, central herniation and foramen magnum pressure cone. These syndromes often lead to further brain ischemia and additional increases in ICP. The drawing on the left depicts a normal brain.

DIFFERENTIAL DIAGNOSIS

Seizures, metabolic derangements, and complicated migraine sometimes have a clinical presentation similar to increased ICP. In children who are only partially responsive, distinguishing an ictal or postictal state from a condition that may be producing increased ICP is sometimes difficult. Findings that suggest a seizure include rhythmic, clonic movements or lightning, myoclonic jerks; rapid or variable changes of tone or posturing that are different from decerebrate posturing; and abrupt, fluctuating changes of autonomic function (e.g., heart rate, blood pressure, pupillary size); saliva production without swallowing; and history of prior seizures. Sometimes, however, only direct EEG monitoring and ICP monitoring are able to distinguish ongoing seizure activity from increased ICP as the cause of the change in level of responsiveness.

In some cases, diffuse brain dysfunction from a toxic or metabolic etiology mimics increased ICP. Such toxic/metabolic causes include medication toxicity, electrolyte or blood chemistry imbalances, and systemic infections. With toxic/metabolic disorders, inattention is often accompanied by a confusional state with disorientation, incoherency, and sometimes agitation. In contrast, with increased ICP, inattention is frequently accompanied by slowness of thought, perseveration, decreased mental activity, and impaired gait, although these differences are not universal.

The symptoms and signs of complicated migraine sometimes also mimic those of increased ICP. At the initial headache presentation or when only a short headache history is present, the complicated migraine diagnosis may be one of exclusion however. If children display focal neurologic signs along with some symp-toms of increased ICP, imaging studies to rule out space-occupying lesions and then laboratory confirmation of normal pressure by lumbar puncture manometry may need to be performed.

EVALUATION

History

A thorough neurologic history should be taken (Questions Box). Headache, nausea and vomiting, drowsiness, and changes in visual acuity are important historical factors.

Physical Examination

Vital signs and head circumference should be noted. A careful neurologic examination is warranted whenever increased ICP is suspected. Particular attention should be paid to the mental status and level of responsiveness of patients. The presence of papilledema and cranial nerve function should be assessed. Specific muscle tone and strength as well as gait should be evaluated in coop-

---

Questions: Increased ICP

- How long has the child been vomiting?
- When does the vomiting occur?
- Is the vomiting related to meals?
- Do the headaches awaken the child?
- Has there been a progressive decline in activity level or loss of developmental skills?
- Does the child display weakness or change in gait?
- Does the child have a recent history of trauma or lack of oxygen?

erative children. Posturing responses and the breathing pattern should be noted in comatose children to help ascertain brain stem localization of the lesion. In such children, findings should be reassessed at frequent intervals to follow a potentially rapid process such as impending tentorial or brain stem herniation, which necessitates immediate intervention.

Useful quick assessment instruments for initial, rapid evaluation and subsequent monitoring are the Glasgow and Children's (ages 4 years and below) Coma Scales (see Tables 44–1 and 44–2 in Chapter 44, Head Trauma). However, these scales do not contain adequate information for all clinical decisions related to patients with increased ICP.

In infants, a unique collection of signs—bulging, raised fontanelle, frontal bone bossing with prominent venous distention, "sunset sign" (inability to elevate the eyes and lid retraction from midbrain tectal pressure), hypertonicity, and hyperreflexia—may be secondary to increased ICP from hydrocephalus. Papilledema is not present, perhaps related to greater compliance of the infant skull.

Laboratory Tests

If mental status changes are suggestive of a toxic or metabolic aberration, appropriate laboratory screens should be performed. These may include electrolytes, toxicologic screen, liver function and kidney function tests, and CSF examination if signs of meningeal irritation or infection are present without lateralized signs of altered tone or strength or imaging study evidence of an intercompartmental pressure gradient that could lead to herniation after lumbar puncture.

Imaging Studies

A CT or MRI scan should be performed whenever children's signs or symptoms indicate the possibility of increased ICP. Intravenous contrast should be given if disruption in the blood-brain barrier (e.g., infection, inflammation, neoplasia) is suspected and children are not hypersensitive and have adequate kidney function.

MANAGEMENT

When diagnostic imaging studies reveal an etiology for the increased ICP, management is emergently directed at the cause if it is a rapidly enlarging surgically accessible lesion such as an epidural hematoma. In such cases, immediate **neurosurgical craniotomy** may be necessary. Other focal space-occupying lesions seen on scans may not require immediate craniotomy; neoplastic lesions may require diagnostic biopsy or excisional biopsy within a few days if surgically accessible. **Mineralocorticoids** are useful in situations in which the pressure is produced by a component of vasogenic edema, such as that surrounding neoplasms. If acute danger of herniation due to a pressure gradient produced by CSF flow blockage is present, then a temporary ventriculostomy may be indicated to relieve the CSF pressure. If an infectious process is present, including focal lesions, abscess, cerebritis, or encephalitis, **antibiotics** and/or **antiviral** agents are indicated after appropriate cultures, serology, and molecular diagnostic tests have been done. Following directed specific treatment of the underlying lesion, increased intracranial pressure may resolve spontaneously. If hydrocephalus is still present after initial therapy due to CSF flow obstruction, **ventriculoperitoneal shunting of CSF** may be necessary.

Children whose intracranial pressure is markedly elevated or likely to rise rapidly require treatment in an intensive care unit. Interventional measures are directed toward preventing eventual loss of brain perfusion. Intracranial pressure can be monitored on an ongoing basis with commonly used neurosurgically placed devices including the fiberoptic microtransducer and intraventricular catheter or ventriculostomy. The former device can measure pressure in brain parenchyma as well as in fluid-filled spaces. An advantage of the latter device is that it also allows for therapeutic CSF drainage to relieve pressure. It carries a slight risk of infection and may be difficult to place if ventricles are small or shifted. Intracranial pressure monitoring with neurosurgically placed devices has not been helpful in many cases of ischemic damage, infection, or poisoning.

Children with a decreased or fluctuating level of responsiveness may require EEG monitoring or cerebral electrical activity. The EEG helps diagnose the abnormal responsiveness as seizure activity that may fluctuate and occur even in the presence of increased ICP. Anticonvulsant therapy is indicated if evidence of seizures is present. In addition, the EEG may be used to monitor barbiturate-induced coma therapy, which is used for severely increased intracranial pressure.

Airway patency and ventilation are important in children with increased ICP, since hypoxia and hypercarbia can contribute to vasodilation and increased pressure. If acute lowering of pressure is necessary, hyperventilation to reduce the intracranial arterial blood volume is most effective, but care must be taken to avoid decreasing brain cell perfusion to the point of producing ischemic damage and exacerbating the problem. It is recommended that pCO_2 be kept at 30–35 mm Hg. Elevating the head to about 30 degrees and avoiding flexion or excessive turning of the neck to prevent jugular kinking are also effective in reducing ICP. Because the goal is to assure perfusion while lowering ICP, maintaining and even elevating mean arterial pressure by appropriate use of fluid therapy and pressor agents is key. Central venous pressure monitoring may also be helpful.

Diuretic agents such as mannitol (osmotherapy) may also be useful in reducing brain volume by removing water and changing the rheologic characteristics of blood and producing reflex vasoconstriction, but caution is advised. Mannitol, as a chronic infusion, can eventually cross the blood-brain barrier and draw more fluid into the brain. It is most effective where the blood-brain barrier is intact. Serum osmolarity greater than 320 mOsm/kg can lead to renal failure. By giving diuretic agents at intervals as a bolus and titrating up to the ICP-lowering dose, such effects can generally be

TABLE 45–1. Management Interventions in Increased ICP

Maintain serum osmols at 300–320 mOsm
Keep head elevated to 30 degrees
Maintain normal blood pressure
Controlled hyperventilation to $PaCO_2$ at 30–35 mm Hg
Supplemental O_2 and PEEP as needed to keep PaO_2 > 90 mm Hg and FiO_2 < 50%
If ICP progressively rises, pressure waves higher than 20 mm Hg last longer than 5 minutes, or any pressure in first 24 hours is higher than 30 mm Hg, then give mannitol, 250–1000 mg/kg IV
If mannitol needs repeating in less than 4 hours or osmolality is greater than 320 mOsm:
    Give pentobarbital, 5 mg/kg IV, then 2 mg/kg/hr IV monitoring to blood level of 25–35 μg/mL, burst-suppression pattern with 10 seconds between bursts on EEG, and cardiac index greater than 2.7 L/min/m²
    or
    Give midazolam by titrating the dose starting at 0.1 mg/kg/hr IV to the same EEG criteria and limited by the same cardiac index criteria

avoided. Sometimes these agents are used to counter intracranial pressure plateau waves or increased pressure with endotracheal suctioning or other procedures.

In children with severe refractory increased ICP, especially if secondary to an acute focal process, barbiturates such as pentobarbital or the benzodiazepine midazolam can be given as a continuous intravenous infusion with appropriate monitoring of brain electrical activity, serum levels, and systemic and brain perfusion pressures (Table 45–1). These agents may serve to reduce brain metabolism without impairing vascular autoregulation significantly. Their risk is in reducing cardiac output and with associated infections, particularly pneumonia.

PROGNOSIS

Children may recover fully from increased ICP if brain perfusion pressure is adequately maintained and the underlying brain lesion generating the increased pressure can be resolved. Ultimately the prognosis depends on the nature of the lesion; its propensity to generate ICP that may be refractory to treatment, leading to brain tissue damage or death; and its permanence or potential for recurrence.

Case Resolution

The boy in the case history has focal signs and symptoms referable to the brain in the posterior fossa of the intracranial cavity as well as symptoms of increased ICP. An emergent CT scan shows subacute hydrocephalus due to obstruction of CSF flow produced by a large mass in the cerebellum and brain stem on the left side. He begins taking dexamethasone. Two days later the mass is surgically excised and is found to be a medulloblastoma. Because the ICP remains high, a ventriculoperitoneal shunt is subsequently required for the hydrocephalus. The boy's recovery is otherwise uneventful, and he begins evaluation for further brain tumor therapy.

Selected Readings

American Academy of Pediatrics, Committee on Child Abuse and Neglect. Shaken baby syndrome: Inflicted cerebral trauma. Pediatrics 92:872–875, 1993.

Brown, J., and R. Minns. Non-accidental head injury, with particular reference to whiplash shaking injury and medico-legal aspects. Dev. Med. Child. Neurol. 35:849–869, 1993.

Fishman, R. A. Cerebrospinal Fluid in Diseases of the Nervous System, 2nd ed. Philadelphia, W. B. Saunders, 1992.

Hymel, K., et al. Coagulopathy in pediatric abusive head trauma. Pediatrics 99:371–375, 1997.

Johnson, D., et al. Accidental head trauma and retinal hemorrhage. Neurosurgery 33:231–235, 1993.

Klonoff, H., et al. Long-term outcome of head injuries: A 23-year follow-up study of children with head injuries. J. Neurol. Neurosurg. Psychiatry 56:410–415, 1993.

Luerssen, T. Intracranial pressure: Current status in monitoring and management. Semin. Pediatr. Neurol. 4:146–155, 1997.

Plum, F., and J. Posner. Diagnosis of Stupor and Coma, 3rd ed., Philadelphia, F. A. Davis, 1982.

Rekate, H. Recent advances in the understanding and treatment of hydrocephalus. Semin. Pediatr. Neurol. 4:167–178, 1997.

CHAPTER 46

FLUID AND ELECTROLYTE DISTURBANCES

Charlotte W. Lewis, M.D., R.D. and Sudhir K. Anand, M.D.

Hx A 2-year-old boy presents to your office after 2 days of vomiting and diarrhea. His siblings were both ill a few days ago with similar symptoms. Two weeks ago his weight was 12 kg at a well-child visit. Today his weight is 10.8 kg. He has a pulse of 130/min, respiratory rate of 28/min, blood pressure of 85/55. He is alert and responsive but appears tired. He has dry mucous membranes, no tears with crying, and slightly sunken appearing eyeballs. His capillary refill is 2 seconds. He urinated a small amount about 6 hours ago. Despite his mother's best efforts in your office, the patient has vomited all of the oral rehydration therapy (ORT) given to him. You draw serum electrolytes, BUN, and creatinine and initiate IV rehydration.

Questions

1. How does one assess the magnitude of dehydration in children?
2. What are the different types of dehydration?
3. How does one determine the type and amount of fluid that a dehydrated child requires?
4. How does one assess renal status in a dehydrated child?
5. What is the role of electrolyte and acid-base laboratory studies in the evaluation of the dehydrated child?

Pediatrics is unique among fields in medicine in its focus on the growing and developing individual. Within the scope of pediatric practice, patients may range in size and weight from the less than 1 kg preterm infant to the greater than 100 kg adolescent. Young children, like adults, maintain fluid and electrolyte balance under a variety of physiologic conditions; however, during illness their homeostatic adjustments may be less efficient than those of adult patients. Clinicians caring for children must feel comfortable in determining fluid and electrolyte needs for healthy children as they grow from infants into adults and understand how fluid and electrolyte needs are altered in dehydration and other illnesses.

EPIDEMIOLOGY

Dehydration is one of the most common medical problems encountered in pediatrics. In the United States, dehydration, usually as the result of common childhood illnesses, is responsible for approximately 10% of all pediatric hospital admissions. Worldwide, over 3 million children under 5 years die of diarrheal disease, mainly from dehydration, which usually is preventable with oral rehydration therapy (ORT).

Maintenance Fluid and Electrolyte Requirements

The body has a **maintenance fluid requirement** to replace daily normal losses that occur through the kidney, intestines, skin, and respiratory tract. Of the various methods available for the determination of fluid needs, the most physiologic is the **caloric method,** which is based on the linear relationship between metabolic rate and fluid needs. For every 100 calories expended in metabolism, a child requires about 100 mL of water. Metabolic rate in children is a function of body surface area. Infants, with higher relative surface areas per unit of body weight, have higher metabolic rates and therefore higher fluid requirements per unit weight. As children grow, their relative surface area decreases, as

TABLE 46–1.   Caloric Method of Determining Maintenance Fluid Requirements in Healthy Children

Weight of child	Maintenance Fluid Requirement for 24 Hours
3*–10 kg	100 mL/kg/d†
11–20 kg	50 mL/kg/d for each kg above 10 kg + 1000 mL (fluid requirement for first 10 kg)
>20 kg	20 mL/kg/d for each kg above 20 kg + 1500 mL (fluid requirement for first 20 kg)

*Children weighing less than 3 kg may have altered fluid requirements owing to prematurity or other conditions.
†During the first 2–3 days of life, normal term infants require less fluid (approximately 80 mL/kg), since they mobilize excess extracellular fluid.

does their metabolic rate and fluid requirement per unit weight. Using this relationship, maintenance fluid needs can be calculated for the healthy child using the method outlined in Table 46–1. These calculations of fluid needs are often used to determine the amount of intravenous (IV) fluids to provide a hospitalized child (Box 46–1), but this formula can also be used to calculate the usual amount of fluid a healthy child requires by mouth to maintain hydration.

This method makes no allowance for extra fluid needed for growth, activity, or pathophysiologic states that increase fluid needs (such as fever). The fluid requirement derived from the caloric method is valid to determine the daily needs for an essentially healthy child. Thriving infants normally drink more fluid than this method provides. On average, growing infants may take 150–200 mL/kg/d of milk on an ad lib basis to

---

BOX 46–1.   Example of Fluid Calculations

Part A
Case: A 22-kg boy is NPO in preparation for an elective abdominal surgery. How much IV fluid per hour should he receive as he awaits the surgery?

For first 10 kg: 100 mL/kg/d × 10 kg = 1000 mL
For next 10 kg (to get to 20 kg): 50 mL/kg/d × 10 kg = 500 mL
For next 2 kg (to get to 22 kg): 20 mL/kg/d × 2 kg = 40 mL

1000 mL + 500 mL + 40 mL = 1540 mL/24 h
IV rate per hour = 64.2 mL/h (with a healthy child, round off to 65 mL/h for ease of administration)

Part B
Question: How much sodium and potassium should this patient receive in his IV fluids?
Answer: 3 mEq Na$^+$/100 mL (1 dL) of fluid = 3 mEq × 15.4 dL = 46.2 mEq Na$^+$/d in 1540 mL of water or 30 mEq NaCl/L
2.5 mEq K$^+$/100 mL (1 dL) of fluid = 2.5 × 15.4 = 38.5 mEq K$^+$/d in 1540 mL of water or 25 mEq KCl/L

One possible way to write an IV order for this patient:
D5 0.2NS with 25 mEq KCl/L to run at 65 mL/h.

Note: D5 = 5% dextrose water; normal saline (NS) contains 154 mEq NaCl/L and 0.2NS contains 34 mEq NaCl. This solution is a widely available, pre-made IV solution that provides the approximate daily sodium requirement of the patient.

support the average weight gain of 30 g/d usually observed in the first few months of life.

Replacement of normal daily losses of electrolytes are considered when a child is not able to take adequate nutritional intake by mouth (as in the example in Box 46–1, where the child is NPO for surgery). These requirements are usually expressed as milliequivalent (mEq) amount per 100 mL fluid required. The usually recommended **sodium** (Na^+) requirement for a healthy child is 3.0 mEq/100 mL fluid required, and the **potassium** (K^+) requirement is 2.5 mEq/100 mL fluid (see Box 46–1, part B, for sample calculation and IV order). As discussed in more detail below, potassium should only be given to a patient after assurance of adequate renal function. These estimations of sodium and potassium requirements are meant to replace normal losses and would not be adequate in the face of increased electrolyte losses that can occur in a number of pathophysiologic conditions (such as diarrhea). Healthy, well-nourished children receiving IV fluids for a brief period of time (1 to 2 days) while hospitalized do not routinely require supplementation with other electrolytes such as calcium (Ca) and magnesium (Mg). However, one must realize that IV fluids containing only dextrose, NaCl, and KCl provide only minimal caloric needs and do not adequately support weight gain or provide other necessary nutrients. Children who require prolonged IV therapy because of inadequate gastrointestinal tract function should receive total parenteral nutrition (TPN) to better meet their caloric and nutritional needs.

Pathophysiologic Alterations in Fluid and Electrolyte Needs

A number of pathophysiologic conditions alter fluid requirements. Conditions that increase a patient's metabolic rate will also increase their fluid requirement, e.g., fever. A child's metabolic rate is increased 12% for each one degree celsius temperature elevation above normal. Most healthy children with free access to fluids will increase their own fluid intake to account for these increased needs during an episode of fever. Other less common hypermetabolic conditions, such as thyrotoxicosis or salicylate poisoning, may have an even more dramatic effect, perhaps increasing metabolic rate and fluid needs by 25–50% over maintenance. In these cases and for very young children who are dependent on others to provide their fluids, clinicians must be aware of the magnitude of increased need and provide supplemental fluids to avoid dehydration.

Other conditions may decrease a child's fluid requirement. In hypometabolic states such as hypothyroidism, metabolic rate and fluid needs are decreased by 10–25%. Fluid requirements are decreased by 10–25% in high environmental humidity unless the ambient temperature is also high and results in visible sweating. In these situations, a healthy child with normal renal function given extra fluid beyond what is needed can, within limits, effectively excrete any excessive intake. Children with renal failure, however, pose a special challenge for the clinician in the management of fluid and electrolytes. When a child is unable to adequately excrete excessive fluid intake, this fluid can accumulate and lead to complications such as congestive heart failure and pulmonary edema. Without functioning kidneys, only **insensible fluid losses** need to be replaced. Insensible losses occur primarily through the skin and respiratory tract; they account for approximately 40% of maintenance fluid needs. However, fluid needs for patients with renal failure are usually estimated at 25–30% of the maintenance requirement, with additional fluids provided if needed. This is to avoid giving excessive fluids that may require dialysis for removal.

PATHOPHYSIOLOGY AND DEHYDRATION

Dehydration is one of the most common pathophysiologic alterations in fluid balance encountered in pediatrics. The term dehydration, when rigorously defined, implies a deficit of water only; however, most children with dehydration have a deficit of both water and electrolytes. Dehydration can occur as a result of (1) diminished intake, (2) excessive losses through the gastrointestinal tract (e.g., diarrhea or vomiting), (3) excessive losses from the kidney or skin (e.g., polyuria due to osmotic diuresis in uncontrolled diabetes), or (4) a combination of these factors.

Children are at increased risk for episodes of dehydration for a number of reasons. Young children have 3–4 times the body surface area per unit body weight compared with adults, and this is associated with relatively higher fluid needs. It is therefore much easier for children to become dehydrated in the face of the decreased intake or increased losses that often accompany common childhood illnesses. For example, acute gastroenteritis, which is common in young children, often leads to anorexia as well as recurrent vomiting and frequent, large-volume stools with proportionately more severe fluid loss than in older children and adults. In addition, infants and young children are dependent beings who are unable to increase their own fluid intake in response to thirst and must rely on others to provide their fluid needs. If these fluid needs are not met or are underestimated, children can easily become dehydrated.

Dehydration is classified as **isotonic, hypotonic,** or **hypertonic.** When considering acute dehydration, these terms are often used interchangeably with **isonatremic, hyponatremic,** and **hypernatremic** dehydration, respectively, since it is the sodium content of the extracellular fluid (ECF) that largely determines the osmolality in otherwise healthy dehydrated children. In acute **isotonic** *or* **isonatremic dehydration** (serum sodium 130–150 mEq/L), the most common type of dehydration, there is net loss of isotonic fluid containing both sodium and potassium (Figure 46–1A). Sodium, the primary ECF cation, is lost not only to the environment but some also shifts to the intracellular fluid (ICF), to balance the loss of potassium because potassium losses from cells are generally not accompanied by anionic losses. The sodium that has shifted into the ICF will return to the ECF compartment with rehydration. There

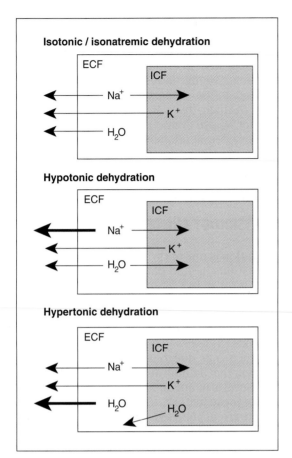

FIGURE 46–1. Pathophysiology of various types of dehydration. ECF, extracellular fluids; ICF, intracellular fluid.

is no net loss of fluid from the ICF in this process; the total water deficit in dehydration comes primarily from the ECF. (Some other authors suggest that two-thirds of the losses come from ECF and one-third from ICF.)

In **hypotonic** or **hyponatremic dehydration** (serum sodium <130 mEq/L), net solute loss exceeds that of water (Figure 46–1B). This may result from excessive sodium wasting in the stool or urine. However, most often it is due to a parent giving oral replacement with water or very low sodium beverages such as apple juice or tea. In hypotonic dehydration, the ECF osmolarity is reduced and fluid shifts from the ECF to the ICF until the osmolality between the two compartments is the same. In these circumstances, the ECF volume is compromised to a greater degree than in isotonic dehydration, resulting in more severe signs of dehydration.

Hypertonic or **hypernatremic dehydration** (serum sodium >150 mEq/L) occurs when net loss of water exceeds that of solute loss (Figure 46–1C). It is usually seen in clinical conditions where there is rapid loss of hypotonic fluid in stools, vomitus, or urine accompanied by failure of adequate water intake due to anorexia or vomiting. Fever or hyperventilation, if present, may intensify the disproportionate loss of water. Occasionally, hypernatremic dehydration may be due to excessive solute intake. The urinary excretion of the excess solute obligates loss of large volumes of water, resulting

in dehydration. The history may reveal that the child was accidentally fed a high sodium solution or concentrated formula. In hypernatremic dehydration, there is shift of fluid from the ICF to the ECF to attain osmotic balance. As such, the ECF volume is somewhat spared at the expense of the ICF and signs of dehydration may be delayed. However, fluid loss from the ICF results in intracellular dehydration, the most serious effect of which can occur in the brain. If hypernatremia occurs rapidly, there is not only a decrease in brain size but also a fall in CSF pressure owing to diffusion of water from CSF to the blood. As the brain shrinks, the bridging veins within the skull may stretch and even tear, resulting in subdural hemorrhage or other complication. If the hypernatremic state develops more slowly, the brain cell size may initially shrink but will gradually return to normal size even in the face of continued hypernatremia. The preservation of the brain cell volume despite hypernatremia is thought to be due to the generation of "idiogenic" osmoles (myoinositol, trimethylamines, taurine, and other amino acids) that attract water back into the cell and maintain cell volume. Rehydration of the patient with hypernatremia must occur slowly and cautiously to avoid brain cell swelling, which can occur if the hypernatremic state is corrected too rapidly (Figure 46–2).

EVALUATION OF THE DEHYDRATED CHILD

History

In addition to signs and symptoms of the current illness, the history should focus on the cause of dehydration. Parents should be questioned on the type and amount of oral intake; the duration, quality, and frequency of the vomitus and/or diarrhea; whether blood is present in the stool; the presence or absence of fever; frequency of urination; and whether a recent pre-illness weight is known for the child (Questions Box).

Physical Examination

The most accurate way to assess the degree of dehydration is to compare current weight to a recent pre-illness weight. In acute dehydration, the loss of weight is primarily due to fluid loss. The difference between pre-illness and current weight can be used to determine the degree of the fluid deficit. However, recent weights frequently are not available and clinicians must rely on vital signs and clinical signs and symptoms to assess the degree of dehydration (Table 46–2). Estimation of the magnitude of dehydration based on clinical findings is imprecise and subjective; any single indicator is likely to lack sensitivity. A recent study found that a subset of four factors—delayed capillary refill, absent tears, dry mucous membranes, and general ill appearance—predicted dehydration as well as all of the clinical parameters combined and that the presence of two or more of these four factors was correlated with a greater than 5% fluid deficit. In infants and young children (<5 years), the estimated fluid loss for mild dehydration is 5% deficit of body water;

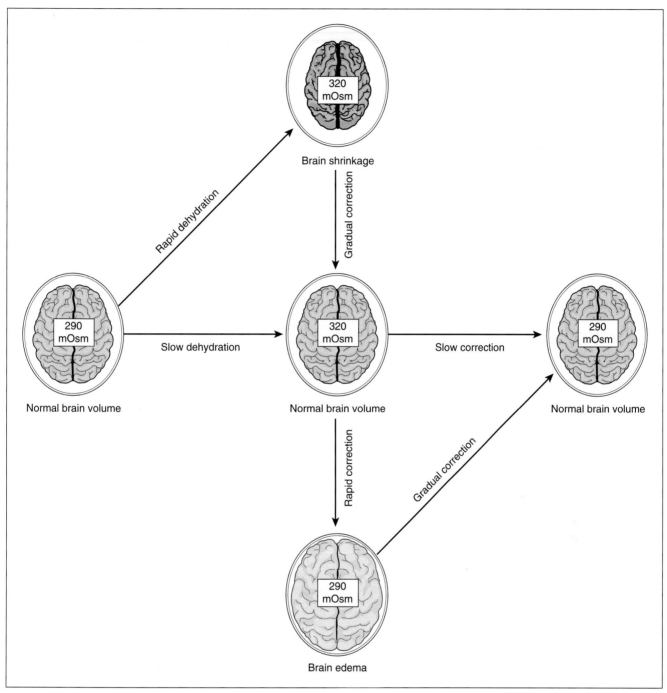

FIGURE 46–2. Hypernatremic dehydration. Effects upon brain volume of rapid versus slow development of hypernatremia and results of rapid versus slow correction of hypernatremia. Solid line = outline of skull; dotted line = outline of brain.

Questions: Dehydration

- Has the child had vomiting or diarrhea?
- Has the child had fever?
- What has the child been eating or drinking?
- Has the child been urinating? How many wet diapers did the child have?
- How much did the child weigh at the last visit to the physician?

moderate dehydration, 10%; and severe dehydration, 15%. The corresponding numbers for estimated fluid loss in older children are 3%, 6%, and 9%, respectively.

During the initial evaluation, it is important that the clinician recognize whether **shock** is present, since this is a life-threatening condition that requires emergent treatment. Accurate and rapid assessment of vital signs and physical examination is essential to this process (see Chapter 41, Shock).

TABLE 46–2. Clinical Assessment of Magnitude of Dehydration

Clinical Signs	Mild Dehydration	Moderate Dehydration	Severe Dehydration
Loss of body weight			
Infant/young child	5%	10%	15%
Older child/adult	3%	6%	9%
Skin turgor	Normal to slightly reduced	Decreased	Markedly decreased (tenting)
Skin color and temperature	Pale or normal	Ashen, cool	Mottled, cool
Dry mucous membranes	±	+	++
Absent tears	±	+	++
Sunken eyeballs	±	+	++
Increased pulse	±	+	++ (may be thready)
Blood pressure	Normal	Normal	Reduced (in late shock)
		Postural decrease ±	
Urine output	Normal or reduced*	Oliguria*	Oliguria/anuria
BUN	Normal†	Normal or mild increase	Usually >30 mg/dL

*Usually resumes with restoration of intravascular volume.
†Usually not necessary to check in mild dehydration.

Laboratory Studies

Laboratory studies are not indicated in children who present with mild dehydration or even most children with moderate dehydration unless they are unable to tolerate oral fluids and require IV therapy. Previously healthy children with mild or moderate dehydration who have urinated within the last 6 hours prior to presentation are unlikely to have significant renal impairment or electrolyte abnormalities as a result of their dehydration. The vast majority of children with dehydration have isonatremic or isotonic dehydration and can be treated without need for laboratory studies. Serial serum electrolytes, BUN, and creatinine should be assessed in children with (1) shock, (2) severe dehydration, (3) decreased urine output that does not improve after initial restoration of intravascular volume, or (4) history and clinical findings inconsistent with straightforward isotonic dehydration. If hyponatremic or hypernatremic dehydration is suspected, based on history or clinical findings, laboratory studies should be conducted, since these conditions can have serious complications and treatment requires special considerations. Hemolytic uremic syndrome, although uncommon, should be considered in any child with a history of gastroenteritis who also has decreased urine output.

Very ill children may require an arterial blood gas measurement to more accurately assess their acid-base status; in others, serum electrolytes are sufficient. The usual acid-base derangement in the moderately dehydrated child is a non–anion gap acidosis (with hyperchloremia) due to bicarbonate losses in the stool. Severely dehydrated children may have an anion gap acidosis due to lactic acid and/or ketone accumulation in the peripheral tissues secondary to the decreased perfusion that accompanies hypovolemia. An interesting exception is seen in infants with pyloric stenosis, who typically manifest a hypokalemic, hypochloremic metabolic alkalosis.

MANAGEMENT OF THE DEHYDRATED CHILD

The management of the dehydrated child involves consideration of three components (1) normal maintenance fluid and electrolyte requirement, (2) fluid and electrolyte **deficit** incurred during the present illness, and (3) **ongoing fluid and electrolyte losses.** Most commonly, ongoing losses result from continued vomiting and diarrhea. Losses from diarrhea are estimated at 10 mL/kg/stool and from vomit at 5 mL/kg/vomitus. Other forms of ongoing losses that occasionally must be considered and replaced include those associated with gastric secretions suctioned via nasogastric tube, burns, hyperventilation, prolonged fever, and intestinal stoma contents. The estimation of children's fluid and electrolytes needs and losses is only an approximation; the clinician must reassess and readjust as needed throughout the treatment.

Fluid given to dehydrated children may be provided either enterally or parenterally. **Oral rehydration therapy** (ORT) is preferred for children with mild dehydration and most children with moderate dehydration. **Parenteral fluid therapy** should be used in children with severe dehydration, when oral therapy has failed despite an *adequate* trial (e.g., due to intractable vomiting or lethargy), in children in shock or impending shock, or when an anatomic defect such as pyloric stenosis or ileus is suspected.

Parenteral Fluid Therapy

The parenteral management of moderate or severe dehydration can be divided into two phases: an **initial phase** (first 1–2 hours) and the **main phase** of rehydration. The aim of the initial phase is to restore intravascular volume, thus improving perfusion and renal function and reversing tissue hypoxia and acidosis. Regardless of the type of dehydration (iso-, hypo-, or hypernatremic), normal saline (0.9% sodium chloride) with 5% dextrose at 10 mL/kg/h provides the most rapid and effective means to expand the intravascular volume.

If **shock** is present or imminent, the treatment is more aggressive (see Chapter 41 Shock). The child should immediately receive a 20 mL/kg IV bolus of normal saline (NS) given over 20–30 minutes. After the first bolus, the child should be reassessed, and if signs and symptoms of intravascular depletion persist, a second IV bolus of 20 mL/kg of NS should be given over 20–30 minutes. If evidence of circulatory compromise continues after two boluses, the child should be admitted to a pediatric intensive care unit and reassessed for other causes of shock, e.g., sepsis.

During the main phase of IV rehydration, the remaining fluid and electrolyte deficits are replaced based upon the magnitude of their losses. This replacement is in addition to the daily maintenance requirements as well as any abnormal ongoing losses discussed above. Different schemes to restore deficits have been developed. Differences lie in the composition of the treatment fluid and the rate at which it is administered. Regardless of which scheme is used, the condition of most patients improves. Owing to well-functioning kidneys and the safeguards built into each scheme, most patients do not develop complications of therapy.

Some clinicians prefer to administer half the total fluid needs over the first 8 hours and the remainder over the next 16 hours; others replace the fluid at the same rate throughout the rehydration period. The latter method is presented in the case resolution at the end of this chapter. Usually, the fluid deficit is replaced within 24 hours. There are noteworthy exceptions, however. **Hypernatremic dehydration** is corrected more slowly, over 48–72 hours, to allow a decrease of serum sodium of about 12–15 mEq/L/24 h in order to avoid serious complications such as cerebral edema and herniation. The correction of profound **hyponatremia** (serum sodium <115 mEq/L) must also proceed slowly, with the aim to increase the serum sodium about 12–15 mEq/L/24 h, to avoid the potential complication of pontine demyelination.

Sodium replacement in the dehydrated child depends on the type of dehydration. In **isotonic dehydration**, some authors elect to replace the entire fluid deficit with normal saline, others with solution containing sodium 110 mEq/L, and still others with 0.5 normal saline. We prefer to calculate replacement of isotonic losses at 110 mEq sodium/1000 mL of fluid deficit (see the case resolution for an example). This is somewhat less than 154 mEq sodium/1000 mL in isotonic fluids because some of the sodium lost from the ECF during isotonic dehydration is shifted intracellularly to balance potassium losses and will return to the ECF during rehydration.

The management of **hyponatremic dehydration** is similar to that of isotonic dehydration except that an additional sodium deficit must be replaced. The amount of sodium required to correct the serum sodium into a normal range is calculated using the following formula:

$$\text{Additional sodium in mEq} = \text{patient's weight (in kg)} \times 0.6 \times (135 - X)$$

where 0.6 denotes sodium space, 135 desired and X actual sodium concentration

This amount of sodium is in addition to the patient's other fluid and electrolyte needs. The use of **hypertonic saline** (3% saline) is limited to children with symptomatic hyponatremia (e.g., seizing). Hypertonic saline is administered as 3.0 mL/kg of 3% saline given intravenously over 30 minutes; this amount will raise the serum sodium by approximately 5.0 mEq/L, which is usually sufficient to alleviate serious symptoms and improve CNS function. In general, hyponatremia that results from acute dehydration of the otherwise healthy child can be corrected over a 24-hour period. However, caution should be taken in the patient with profound hyponatremia or chronic hyponatremia or in patients suspected of SIADH (syndrome of inappropriate antidiuretic hormone secretion). Treatment of SIADH usually involves fluid restriction.

In **hypernatremic dehydration,** the patient is considered to have a relative free water deficit but usually has lost not only body water but also some sodium. The amount of free water a patient requires is calculated as follows: Patient weight (in kg) × [actual serum sodium − 145 mEq/L (desired serum sodium)] × 4 mL/kg = amount of free water to lower serum sodium to 145 mEq/L. (For serum sodium >170 mEq/L, the formula is changed to 3 mL/kg of free water for each mEq desired decrease in serum sodium.) This amount of fluid usually constitutes only a portion of the patient's total needs. The remainder of the fluid deficit is considered to have arisen from isotonic losses. Because hypernatremic dehydration must be corrected slowly and carefully in order to avoid cerebral edema or seizures, many clinicians will provide IV fluids with higher sodium concentrations than determined in the calculations.

Potassium Replacement

Potassium deficits are more difficult to determine, and there is no easy method to calculate the exact amount of potassium that a dehydrated child requires. Additionally, as the acidosis that commonly accompanies moderate and severe dehydration corrects, potassium shifts intracellularly. What initially appears to be a normal serum potassium may fall into the hypokalemic zone. Frequent reassessment of serum potassium and adjustment of potassium content of the IV fluids may be necessary. In general, once adequate urine output has been established, potassium may be added to the IV fluids to provide 3–4 mEq/kg/24 h. Children who have decreased urine output or other indicators of renal impairment *should not* receive potassium until normal urine output has been restored. Hyperkalemia, a serious and life-threatening condition, may occur if a child is unable to excrete excess potassium via the kidney because of renal impairment.

Oral Rehydration

Oral rehydration therapy (ORT) refers to specially prepared, balanced preparations of carbohydrates and electrolytes meant for oral consumption. Clinical trials have repeatedly shown that ORT is as efficacious as IV therapy in the treatment of the child with mild or moderate dehydration. Additional advantages of ORT over IV therapy are that it is less expensive, nonin-

TABLE 46–3. Composition of Various ORT Solutions

Solution	CHO (g/dL)	Na (mEq/L)	K (mEq/L)	Base (mmol/L)	Osmo-lality
Infalyte	3.0*	50	20	30	200
KaoLectrolyte†	2.0	50	20	30	N/A
Pedialyte	2.5	45	20	30	250
WHO/ UNICEF ORS‡	2.0	90	20	30	310

*Contains 3% rice syrup solids.
†Available as a powder that is reconstituted with water.
‡WHO Oral rehydration salt (ORS) available from Jianas Brothers Co., 2533 Southwest Blvd., Kansas City, MO 64108; 816–421–2880.

TABLE 46–4. Composition of Some Clear Liquids Not Appropriate for Rehydration

Liquid	CHO (g/dL)	Na (mEq/L)	K (mEq/L)	Base (mmol/L)	Osmo-lality
Cola	11.0	2	0	13	750
Apple juice	12.0	3	32	0	730
Chicken broth	0	250	8	0	500
Sport beverage	4.0	20	3	3	330

vasive, and low-technology. ORT has been credited with the dramatic reduction in death associated with diarrhea in the developing world. Previously, the treatment of dehydration with ORT was divided into two phases using two preparations. A higher sodium solution was given for initial rehydration and a lower sodium solution for the main rehydration phase. However, the ORT solutions commercially available in the United States (e.g., Infalyte, Pedialyte, KaoLectrolyte) are effective for both phases of rehydration in mildly and moderately dehydrated children. Flavored solutions and ice-pop versions of these solutions are available and often preferred by older children over the unflavored variety. It is not necessary to change to ORT in a breast-fed child who is tolerating breast milk; these children can continue to receive breast milk for rehydration, though they may require shorter, more frequent feedings.

The composition of various ORT solutions is presented in Table 46–3. The cost of commercially available ORT solution may be prohibitive for some families. Homemade ORT, using the recipes in Box 46–2, can be effective as long as families have and know how to use measuring spoons and cups and have a clean source of water. Some solutions such as fruit juices or teas do not contain the proper balance of sodium and carbohydrate to effectively rehydrate a dehydrated individual, may have detrimental effects, and are not appropriate for rehydration (Table 46–4).

The amount of ORT fluid needed can be calculated using the method described above for parenteral replacement. However, most children with mild dehydration can be rehydrated relatively quickly and then are likely to request the amount of fluid they need in response to their thirst. Therefore, a simplified method of determining ORT fluid requirements has been developed (Table 46–5). It is not necessary to determine children's exact electrolyte needs if they are taking ORT; they will receive adequate amounts of electrolytes in the food and ORT to meet maintenance needs and replace losses.

Parents must be given specific guidelines about the volume (converted into common household measures), the frequency, and the duration of home ORT. Small volumes of about 5–15 mL administered with a syringe or teaspoon every 2–5 minutes are much more likely to be retained by children who vomit larger volumes. Although this technique is labor intensive, it can be done by the parent and will deliver 150–300 mL/h. As dehydration is corrected, vomiting decreases and the child is able to tolerate larger volumes. With ORT the frequency and amount of stooling often increases during the initial period of treatment. Parents should be made aware that the primary purpose of ORT is to rehydrate and not to stop diarrhea, which will gradually decrease spontaneously. Once vomiting has resolved and rehydration has been achieved, early refeeding with a return to the usual formula or milk is recommended.

PROGNOSIS

Children with mild or moderate dehydration as a consequence of a self-limited childhood illness are likely to recover completely when given timely and appropriate rehydration therapy. It is more difficult to predict the prognosis of children with severe dehydration or significant aberrations in electrolyte balance. Most of these children if managed appropriately also completely recover; however, some, despite closely monitored care, may have permanent sequelae or poor outcomes.

BOX 46–2. Recipes for Two Homemade Oral Rehydration Solutions*

Starch-based solution
1 quart *clean* water (4 cups, or 32 oz)
½ teaspoon salt
1 cup dry baby rice cereal (about 2 oz in weight)

Sugar-based solution
1 quart *clean* water (4 cups, or 32 oz)
½ teaspoon salt
6 teaspoons sugar

One teaspoon of flavored gelatin powder may be added to either recipe to improve palatability.

---

*The proportion of ingredients in these recipes is important. These recipes should only be given to families who have and know how to use measuring spoons and cups. (Courtesy of Kathi Kemper, M.D.)

TABLE 46-5.   Treatment with ORT

Degree of Dehydration	ORT (>4 h)	Replacement of Losses	Dietary Therapy
Mild (5%) (older children = 3%)	50 mL/kg of oral rehydration solution (ORT)	10 mL/kg for each diarrheal stool 5 mL/kg for each vomitus	Return to formula or milk as soon as vomiting resolves. Children who eat solid food can continue their regular diet.
Moderate (10%) (older children = 6%)	100 mL/kg of ORT	10 mL/kg for each diarrheal stool 5 mL/kg for each vomitus	Return to formula or milk as soon as vomiting resolves. Children who eat solid food can continue their regular diet.

Case Resolution

The opening vignette describes a child who is moderately dehydrated. Based on clinical assessment and weight change since his last clinic visit, he is approximately 10% dehydrated. He does not show evidence of shock. His laboratory studies show a serum sodium of 138 mEq/L, potassium of 3.7 mEq/L, chloride of 108 mEq/L, bicarbonate of 14 mEq/L, BUN of 13 mg/dL, and creatinine 0.4 of mg/dL. His renal status is likely to be adequate because he is urinating and BUN as well as creatinine are normal for patient age. The child's serum sodium is 138 mEq/L, which is in the isonatremic range. The serum potassium is 3.7 mEq/L, which is within normal range; however, this may not accurately reflect this patient's total body potassium status. This level may decrease substantially as he is rehydrated and acidosis is corrected, indicating total body potassium depletion. His serum bicarbonate is 14 mEq/L, and his anion gap is 16 [138 − (108 + 14)] which is mildly increased and probably related to ketosis or mild lactic acidosis.

A calculation of this child's fluid and electrolyte needs follows:

His pre-illness weight was 12 kg.

Maintenance
   Fluid needs: 1000 mL for first 10 kg + 100 mL for next 2 kg = 1100 mL.
   Sodium needs: 33 mEq Na^+ (3 mEq/100 mL of maintenance fluid requirement).

Deficit
   Fluid: 10% of child's weight has been lost during this episode of dehydration = 1200 mL deficit.
   Sodium: 132 mEq Na^+ (110 mEq/1000 mL of isotonic losses): $^{110}/_{1000} \times 1200 = 132$ mEq.

Ongoing losses
   Fluid: Estimate this child's ongoing losses at 10 mL/kg for each stool. He had one loose stool while in the office, so add 120 mL of additional fluid.
   Sodium: The sodium content of diarrhea is variable; however, it is usually replaced with 0.5 NS or about 75 mEq/1000/mL. We estimate about 9 mEq of sodium in his one loose stool.

Total fluid needs: 1100 mL (maintenance) + 1200 mL (deficit) + 120 mL (ongoing losses) = 2420 mL/24 h.

Electrolyte needs
   Sodium: 33 mEq (maintenance) + 132 mEq (deficit) + 9 mEq (ongoing losses) = 174 mEq sodium/24 h.
   Potassium: Estimate his maintenance and replacement needs to be 20 mEq potassium/1000 mL fluid provided.

Treatment: In the initial phase of therapy, provide 10 mL/kg/h normal saline with 5% dextrose for about 2 hours. During this period, his heart rate normalizes and he urinates. The initial parenteral phase provides 240 mL fluid and 37 mEq sodium. This amount of fluid and sodium is subtracted from the patient's total fluid needs. The remaining amount to be provided is 2180 mL fluid and 137 mEq Na^+, or about 65 mEq Na^+/1000 mL fluid. It is not necessary to prepare a special IV solution; 0.5 normal saline (77 mEq NaCl/L) with 5% dextrose ordered as **D5 0.5 NS with 20 mEq KCl/L to run at 90 mL/h** is appropriate. As his gastrointestinal symptoms improve, IV therapy is discontinued and ORT instituted. The patient tolerates the ORT well and is discharged home.

Selected Readings

American Academy of Pediatrics. Practice parameter: The management of acute gastroenteritis in young children. Pediatrics 97(3): 424–435, 1996.

Gorelick, M. H., et al. Validity and reliability of clinical signs in the diagnosis of dehydration in children. Pediatrics 99(5): e6. 1997.

Halperin, M. L., and M. B. Goldstein. Fluid, Electrolytes and Acid-Base Physiology. Philadelphia. W. B. Saunders, 1999.

Jospe, N., and G. Forbes. Fluids and electrolytes—clinical aspects. Pediatr. Rev. 17:395–403, 1996.

Watkins, S. L. The basics of fluid and electrolyte therapy. Pediatr. Ann. 24:16–22, 1995.

Winters, R. W. (ed.). The Body Fluids in Pediatrics. Boston, Little Brown, 1973.

ACUTE RENAL FAILURE

Sudhir K. Anand, M.D.

H_x A 10-month-old girl has a 2-day history of fever, vomiting, and watery diarrhea. The child has previously been healthy. Her diet has consisted of Similac with iron, baby food, and some table food. Since the onset of her illness, she has not been drinking or eating well, and she has thrown up most of what she has eaten. Her mother has tried to give her Pedialyte and apple juice on several occasions but has had limited success. The child has had 8–10 watery stools without blood or mucus each day. Her temperature has varied between 98.6 and 101.8° F (37.0 and 38.8° C); her mother has given her daughter acetaminophen, which she has vomited. The girl's 4-year-old brother and her parents are doing well and have no vomiting or diarrhea.

The physical examination reveals a severely dehydrated (15%), listless infant. Her weight is 9.4 kg, her height is 74 cm, her temperature is 101.1° F (38.4° C), her heart rate is 168 beats/min, her respiratory rate is 30/min, and her blood pressure is 72/40 with an appropriately sized cuff. Capillary refill is 2–3 seconds. The skin appears dry, but no rash is present. Head and neck, chest, heart, and abdominal examinations are normal. Until the results of routine blood studies are available, an intravenous fluid bolus of 180 mL D5 normal saline (20 mL/kg) over 1 hour is administered. The girl is catheterized to obtain urine and determine the flow rate over the next several hours. Urinalysis is performed.

Questions

1. What are the three categories of acute renal failure?
2. What is the etiology of acute renal failure in children?
3. What tests distinguish the three types of acute renal failure?
4. What is the appropriate management for children with acute renal failure? What are the indications for dialysis?

Acute renal failure (ARF) is the sudden decrease in kidney function with accumulation of nitrogenous waste products (e.g., creatinine, BUN). Most children with ARF have oliguria (urine volume <400 mL/m^2/day or <25% of daily recommended fluid intake for age). In some children, however, urine output may remain normal (nonoliguric ARF). Unlike many other organ failures, ARF in children is usually completely reversible. Although ARF is still associated with considerable morbidity, with appropriate management, including use of dialysis, mortality due to renal failure itself is now minimal in children.

EPIDEMIOLOGY

ARF may occur in children with a wide variety of medical or surgical conditions, especially in children who are critically ill. The exact incidence of ARF in children is not known, but ARF is often observed in pediatric intensive care units (ICUs). The incidence of ARF is about 10–20% in neonatal ICUs.

CLINICAL PRESENTATION

Most children with ARF initially present with the clinical findings of the primary condition that led to the renal problem. Other findings, such as decreased urine output, edema, and heart failure (with administration of excessive fluids), result from ARF (D$_x$ Box). Hyperkalemia with cardiac arrhythmia, hyperventilation due to acidosis, and nausea and vomiting due to uremia may occur as renal failure progresses.

ETIOLOGY AND PATHOPHYSIOLOGY

The causes of ARF are usually grouped into three categories: prerenal, intrinsic renal, and postrenal disorders (Table 47–1). This classification helps with diagnosis and formulation of the initial treatment plan.

Prerenal Disorders

In these disorders, decreased total or "effective" circulating blood volume caused by such conditions as dehydration, heart failure, or third spacing leads to decreased renal perfusion. The resulting decrease in the glomerular filtration rate (GFR) in early stages can be easily reversed by improving renal perfusion. If hypoperfusion is prolonged, however, ischemic damage to the kidney occurs and intrinsic renal failure develops (see below).

Postrenal Disorders

Urinary obstruction due to posterior urethral valves or other lesions occasionally leads to ARF, especially during infancy.

D$_x$ Acute Renal Failure

- Decreased urine output
- Hematuria
- Edema
- Elevated serum creatinine
- Elevated BUN
- Elevated fractional excretion of sodium

TABLE 47–1. Etiology of Acute Renal Failure in Children

Prerenal Causes

Decreased plasma volume
> Dehydration, hemorrhage, third spacing of plasma volume in burns, sepsis, bowel obstruction

Other causes of renal hypoperfusion
> Shock, hypoxia, congestive heart failure, hepatorenal syndrome, bilateral renal artery stenosis, cardiac surgery

Postrenal Causes

Bilateral obstruction
> Posterior urethral valves, trauma to urethra, neurogenic bladder, bilateral ureteropelvic obstruction

Obstruction of only functioning kidney
> Ureteropelvic obstruction, stone

Intrinsic Renal Causes

Vascular
> Renal artery or vein thrombosis, disseminated intravascular coagulation

Glomerular
> Severe (rapidly progressive) glomerulonephritis from any etiology, hemolytic-uremic syndrome

Interstitial
> Interstitial nephritis due to allergic reaction to drugs (e.g., methicillin), sepsis

Tubular (acute tubular necrosis [ATN])
> Ischemia due to prolonged hypoperfusion: all causes listed in prerenal category; if sufficiently prolonged, it will lead to ATN
> Nephrotoxins: aminoglycoside antibiotics, indomethacin, radiocontrast agents, ethylene glycol, methanol, heavy metals
> Pigments: myoglobinuria, hemoglobinuria
> Uric acid: hyperuricemia, tumor lysis syndrome

Congenital renal anomalies (especially in newborns and young infants)
> Bilateral cystic dysplastic kidneys, reflux nephropathy, polycystic kidneys, oligomeganephronia

Intrinsic Disorders

Intrinsic renal failure occurs because of injury to the vascular, glomerular, interstitial, or tubular components of the kidney (see Table 47–1). ARF resulting from renal tubular lesions is called acute tubular necrosis (ATN), although in many patients with ATN, necrosis of tubular cells visible by light microscopy is minimal. Certain histologic changes that characterize ATN include loss of brush border microvilli in tubular cells, detachment of epithelial cells from basement membrane, and cast formation from cellular debris and protein.

Children with prolonged shock due to trauma (hemorrhage), sepsis, or dehydration often develop ATN. This is the most frequent type of intrinsic ARF observed in children. Hemolytic-uremic syndrome (HUS) is another common cause of ARF in young children. In newborns and young infants, ARF may result from or be superimposed on a preexisting congenital renal disorder.

The pathogenesis of ATN in humans is controversial, and no single mechanism completely explains the sequence of events that lead to ATN. Ischemic and toxic ATN result from a complex interplay of hemodynamic, nephronal, and cellular changes. These include hypoperfusion in glomerular and tubular capillaries, resulting in reduced GFR; injury to cortical and medullary tubules with their cellular debris, leading to tubular obstruction; and "back leak" of solute and water from the lumen to the interstitium with further decrease in GFR. Increased production of endothelin and reduced production of nitrous oxide in the capillaries lead to increased vasoconstriction and reduced vasodilation, perpetuating the renal injury. Renal tubular cells respond to the injury in many different ways including no or minimal damage, sublethal injury, apoptosis, or necrosis. At the renal cellular level, when the damage is severe, there is decreased production of adenosine triphosphate (ATP), damage to cell membranes and cell cytoskeletons, alterations in cell polarity, and entry of increased amounts of calcium and intracellular free radicals. These changes lead to altered function and cellular swelling and eventually result in cell necrosis. It is hoped that with better understanding of the pathophysiology of ARF, innovative, improved ways to both prevent and treat the disease will be developed.

DIFFERENTIAL DIAGNOSIS

The diagnosis of ARF is established by the demonstration of sudden increase in serum creatinine or BUN. Presence of decreased urine output is also helpful. Identification of the clinical disorder that led to ARF is often obvious, but at other times, extensive evaluation to discover the etiology of the primary disorder may be necessary. It should also be determined whether children have chronic renal failure or superimposition of ARF on a preexisting renal condition.

EVALUATION

Laboratory and radiologic tests are often more helpful diagnostically than history and physical examination.

History

Possible development of ARF should be anticipated in all critically ill children. A history of decrease in urinary volume, hematuria, dysuria, and nausea and vomiting should be sought in all such patients. The presence of previous urinary disorders and delayed growth may point to preexisting kidney conditions (Questions Box).

Physical Examination

Evaluation of physical growth, presence or absence of hypotension or hypertension, arrhythmia, dehydration, or edema should be made. Examination of the flank

---

Questions: Acute Renal Failure

- How frequently is the child passing urine?
- Is the amount of daily urine decreased, increased, or unchanged?
- Does the child have hematuria or dysuria?
- Does the child have nausea or vomiting?
- Has the child had any previous urinary problems?
- (Older children) Does the child have a history of enuresis or nocturia?
- Is the child's physical development normal or delayed?
- Does the child have a history consistent with the primary condition that may have led to the ARF?

area for renal enlargement or tenderness and of the bladder for distention is necessary to help determine the etiology of ARF.

Laboratory Tests

The following laboratory tests are recommended in all children with ARF: CBC, with red blood cell morphology and platelet count; serum sodium, potassium, and bicarbonate; BUN; creatinine, uric acid, calcium, and phosphorus; glucose; total protein and albumin serum concentration; urinalysis and urine culture (if indicated); and spot urinary sodium and creatinine concentration and osmolality. If children are not voiding frequently, catheterization of the bladder is advisable temporarily (4–6 hours) to obtain urine for analysis. Residual volume should also be assessed, and the urinary flow rate (especially the response to initial fluid therapy) and presence of an outflow obstruction should be determined. All children with ARF should have an ECG.

The diagnosis of ARF can easily be established by laboratory tests and determination of urinary output over a specific time. Oliguria is defined as urine output less than 400 mL/m^2/day or less than 1 mL/kg/hour in infants less than 1 year of age, less than 0.75 mL/kg/hour in children 2–6 years of age, and less than 0.5 mL/kg/hour in children more than 6 years of age. Urinalysis, urine specific gravity or osmolality, urine creatinine: plasma creatinine ratio, urinary sodium concentration, and fractional excretion of sodium help differentiate prerenal from intrinsic ARF (Table 47–2).

Tubular epithelial cells and brown pigmented casts are often seen in patients with ATN. Evidence of hematuria or proteinuria signifies glomerular disease, especially glomerulonephritis or HUS. Presence of blood on dipstick but absence of RBCs on sediment examination suggests hemoglobinuria or myoglobinuria as the basis of ATN.

Although urinary indices are helpful in differentiating prerenal from intrinsic ARF, a simple clinical method to distinguish between the two can be used. A therapeutic trial of volume expansion with 20 mL/kg of D5 normal saline is administered intravenously over 1 hour (after the possibilities of congestive heart failure and urinary obstruction are excluded). If oliguria persists at the end of 1 hour, furosemide, 2 mg/kg, is given. If urinary output does not increase following furosemide administration, intrinsic ARF should be suspected and fluid administration reduced. Some physicians believe that by increasing urinary output, furosemide may help prevent imminent ARF or may transform oliguric into nonoliguric ARF; its effectiveness has not been established, however. Once intrinsic ARF has developed, repeated administration of high-dose furosemide has few benefits and can cause toxicity, especially hearing loss.

Imaging Studies

All infants and children with ARF should have a chest x-ray. Renal ultrasonography is the most useful test for differentiating between intrinsic ARF and postrenal ARF or identifying congenital anomalies. Renal ultrasound can detect the presence or absence of kidneys, enlarged kidneys, dilated pelvocalyceal system, or a distended bladder. Other investigative tests such as voiding cystourethrography, renal scans, angiography, CT, MRI, or renal biopsy may occasionally be necessary but are generally not indicated in children with ARF.

MANAGEMENT

Currently, no treatment leads to recovery of renal function in humans with established intrinsic ARF. Certain drugs, such as ATP-MgCl$_2$, thyroxine, atrial natriuretic hormone, and insulin-like growth factors (IGF-1) have been used experimentally in animal and some human trials with variable results. The goal of therapeutic management of intrinsic ARF is maintenance of normal body homeostasis while awaiting spontaneous improvement.

After dehydration is corrected, **daily fluid intake** is limited to replacement of insensible water loss (about 30% of daily recommended fluid intake for age), urinary losses, and fluid losses from nonrenal sources (e.g., nasogastric drainage). Overhydration should be avoided in patients with ARF because it can cause edema, congestive heart failure, hypertension, hyponatremia, encephalopathy, and seizures.

Patients with complete anuria require no sodium intake. **Sodium** losses should be replaced daily in patients with urinary output, however. Preferably, the amount of sodium required should be determined by measuring daily urinary sodium losses.

Once ARF is suspected, **potassium** intake from all sources should be restricted. Severe hyperkalemia can often be avoided early in the course of the disease with strict adherence to potassium restriction. The level of serum potassium as well as ECG changes should be closely monitored. Patients with mild hyperkalemia may be treated with ion exchange resins; sodium polystyrene sulfonate (Kayexalate) may be given orally every 4–6 hours or by retention enema every 1–2 hours. Dialysis is more effective for treating hyperkalemia and may be

TABLE 47–2. Diagnostic Indices in Acute Renal Failure*

Test	Prerenal	Intrinsic Renal
Urinalysis	Normal, occasional granular casts	Renal epithelial cells; pigment casts
Urine osmolality (mOsm/kg H$_2$O)	> 600	< 400
Urine specific gravity	> 1.020	<1.015
Urine sodium (mEq/L)	< 15	> 40
U/P creatinine†	> 40	< 20
Fractional excretion of sodium (FENa)‡	< 1%	> 2%

*Values in patients with nonoligouric acute renal failure often overlap and fall between prerenal and renal values. In addition, values in newborn infants differ from those in children beyond 1 year of age (see Anand reference in Selected Readings for values in newborns).

†U/P creatinine = urinary-plasma creatinine ratio (mg/mg)

$$\ddagger FENa = \frac{UNa}{UCr} \times \frac{PCr}{PNa} \times 100$$

UNa = urine sodium (mEq/L)
UCr = urine creatinine (mg/dL)
PCr = plasma creatinine (mg/dL)
PNa = plasma sodium (mEq/L)

warranted if serum potassium has been rising slowly over several days. Dialysis is also indicated for other reasons (see below).

Hypocalcemia and hyperphosphatemia are common in ARF, and small alterations in levels of **calcium** and **phosphorus** require no treatment. For serum phosphate greater than 8 mg/dL, phosphate binders such as calcium carbonate may be used. If serum calcium is less than 8 mg/dL, intravenous or oral calcium should be given to prevent tetany.

Mild metabolic acidosis is common in ARF and requires no treatment. If blood pH is less than 7.2 or serum bicarbonate is less than 12 mEq/L, sodium **bicarbonate** may be administered.

Adequate nutrition is important in ARF because it prevents excessive tissue breakdown. If renal failure is expected to be short in duration (3–4 days), most calories may be provided as carbohydrates. If ARF is expected to last longer, adequate calories in the form of carbohydrates along with daily protein intake of 1 g/kg should be provided.

Many children with ARF can be managed by the conservative measures described above. If renal failure lasts more than 7 days or if complications develop, however, **dialysis** should be performed. The usual indications for dialysis include uncontrollable hyperkalemia or acidosis, volume overload with potential for pulmonary edema or congestive heart failure, and progressive uremia with BUN greater than 120 mg/dL or creatinine greater than 6 mg/dL. In children, peritoneal dialysis is usually preferred over hemodialysis. If peritoneal dialysis is contraindicated, continuous hemodiafiltration is another option.

ARF can often be prevented by anticipating its possible occurrence in children with high-risk conditions, such as dehydration, trauma, sepsis, and shock, or after cardiac surgery. Prompt recognition of prerenal failure and its aggressive management with volume expanders, inotropic agents, or judicious use of diuretics may prevent the development of intrinsic ARF. Nephrotoxic agents such as gentamicin should be avoided in high-risk patients if possible. When these drugs are used, they should be monitored meticulously, with frequent measurement of blood levels.

PROGNOSIS

The duration of oliguria in ARF may be short (1–2 days) or long (a few weeks). Recovery is usually first indicated by an increase in urinary output. BUN and creatinine may rise during the first few days of diuresis before beginning to return to normal. During diuresis, large quantities of sodium and potassium may be lost in the urine. Serum electrolytes should be closely monitored, and adequate replacements should be made to prevent hyponatremia or hypokalemia.

In children with ARF, outcome largely depends on the primary condition, the severity of damage to other organs, and physician expertise in managing ARF. Nonoliguric ARF is consistently associated with a shorter clinical course and better prognosis than oliguric ARF. Most children with ATN recover completely. However, children with more severe kidney involvement (cortical necrosis) may have residual renal impairment or chronic renal failure.

Case Resolution

In the case scenario, a series of diagnostic studies are performed. The laboratory results are: hemoglobin, 13.8 g/dL; hematocrit, 41%; WBC count, 12,400/μL; neutrophils, 58%; band forms, 6%; lymphocytes, 32%; monocytes, 3%; and eosinophils, 1%. The platelet count is 277,500/μL. Serum sodium is 136 mEq/L; potassium, 5.1 mEq/L; chloride, 110 mEq/L; bicarbonate, 10 mEq/L; BUN, 84 mg/dL; creatinine, 2.8 mg/dL; and glucose, 68 mg/dL. The specific gravity is 1.015, the specimen is protein trace, blood, WBC and nitrite negative, and the sediment has many epithelial cells, one to two RBCs, and many granular and pigmented casts. Spot urinary sodium is 65 mEq/L, creatinine is 39 mg/dL, and the fractional excretion of sodium is 3.4%.

These results are most consistent with the diagnosis of intrinsic renal failure because the fractional excretion of sodium is increased. Recovery may take a few days to a few weeks.

Selected Readings

Anand, S. K. Acute renal failure (in the newborn infant). *In* Taeusch, W., R. Ballard, and M. E. Avery (eds.). Diseases of the Newborn, 6th ed. Philadelphia, W. B. Saunders, 1991, pp. 892–897.

Anderson, R. J. Prevention and management of acute renal failure. Hosp. Pract. 28:61–75, 1993.

Gaudio, K. M., et al. Acute renal failure: clinical aspects. *In* Holliday, M. A., T. M. Barratt, and E. D. Avner (eds.). Pediatric Nephrology, 3rd ed. Baltimore, Williams & Wilkins, 1994, pp. 1186–1203.

Lieberthal, W. Biology of acute renal failure: Therapeutic implications. Kidney Int. 52:1102–1115, 1997.

Sehic, A., and R. W. Chesney. Acute renal failure: diagnosis and therapy. Pediatr. Rev. 16:101–106 and 137–141, 1995.

Thadani, R. et al. Acute renal failure. N. Engl. J. Med. 334:1448–1460, 1996.

INGESTIONS: DIAGNOSIS AND MANAGEMENT

Kelly D. Young, M.D.

H$_x$ A 2-year-old girl is found by her mother with an open bottle of pills and pill fragments in her hands and mouth. She is rushed into the emergency department. She is sleepy but arousable. The vital signs are temperature of 98.8° F (37.1° C), heart rate of 120 beats/min, respiratory rate of 12 breaths/min, and blood pressure of 85/42 mm Hg. Pupils are 2 mm and reactive. Skin color, temperature, and moisture are normal. She has no other medical problems.

Questions

1. What history questions should be asked to help identify the substance ingested?
2. What physical examination findings can give clues to the substance ingested and the seriousness of the ingestion?
3. What other diagnostic tests might be helpful in managing ingestion patients?
4. What are the management priorities?

Ingestions are a common problem faced by pediatric practitioners. Two scenarios frequently encountered are accidental ingestions by pre-school-age children and intentional suicide attempts by adolescents. This chapter discusses the general approach to the child who has ingested a potentially poisonous substance; ingestions of specific substances or groups of substances (sometimes referred to as "toxidromes") are beyond the scope of this chapter, as is toxicity occurring by dermal, ophthalmologic, or inhalational routes. However, the general approach to history, physical examination, laboratory tests and diagnostic studies, and management, especially decontamination, is useful for all ingestions.

EPIDEMIOLOGY

The majority of calls made to poison centers involve children under 18 years of age. Accidental ingestions by curious preschoolers and intentional ingestions by adolescents predominate. The most common substance ingested overall is acetaminophen. The most common fatal ingestion in young children is iron; in adolescents, tricyclic antidepressants. Fatalities are uncommon overall and are more likely to be seen in intentional ingestions by older children. Young children tend to ingest either nontoxic substances or small quantities of toxic substances. There has been a decline in pediatric fatalities due to poisoning over the last few decades, possibly owing to improved child-resistant packaging of

medications, increased education of parents and caretakers, and better supportive care.

CLINICAL PRESENTATION

The clinical presentation varies considerably depending on the substance ingested. Some patients may not present with a clear history of an ingestion. The clinician must maintain a high index of suspicion for poisoning as the cause of symptoms such as altered behavior, depressed level of consciousness, cardiac dysrhythmias, vomiting, seizures, and autonomic changes.

PATHOPHYSIOLOGY

The pathophysiologic picture depends on the substance. Some toxins act on a particular organ system (e.g., acetaminophen on the liver, ethanol on the central nervous system), while others act diffusely at the cellular level (e.g., cyanide). Generally, drugs are absorbed, distributed within the body, metabolized, then excreted. Drug levels obtained prior to completion of absorption and distribution may not reflect the peak level. Interventions focus on preventing absorption, sometimes on preventing metabolism into a more toxic by-product, and on enhancing excretion. Toxicity may be prolonged when an extended release form of a drug has been ingested.

EVALUATION

A detailed history of what and how much the patient ingested is key to the evaluation. Physical examination should focus on identifying symptoms and serious complications. Patients should be monitored and reassessed frequently. Laboratory and other diagnostic studies can be tailored to the specific ingestion.

History

The most important questions address the ingestion (Questions Box): What did the patient ingest, what is the maximum possible amount that was ingested, when did the ingestion occur, and what symptoms are occurring? History regarding previous medical conditions is also important, either to identify increased susceptibility to a particular toxin (e.g., seizure disorder with ingestion of a substance that causes seizures), or to assess for factors that may have precipitated the ingestion, such as depression.

Parents should be encouraged to bring in the container and any remains of the substance ingested. The practitioner should try to obtain the exact formulation, since generic and brand name drugs may differ. One must be aware also of possible combination products. Sleuthing methods such as calling or sending a family member to the home to identify the product, calling the pharmacy on a prescription label, or identifying a pill by comparing its picture and imprint to those in a pharmaceutics reference may be necessary. Parents should be questioned regarding all available drugs or other toxic substances in the household. The practitioner must ask about medications used by recent visitors, e.g., grandparents. It is important not to overlook the possibility of herbal preparations, vitamins, alternative medications, household products (including cleaning and personal care products), gardening products, chemicals used in hobbies or work, and alcohol or drugs of abuse belonging to an adult. One must maintain a high index of suspicion for unreported coingestants, especially in adolescent suicide attempts.

Although often difficult, it is important to attempt to determine the quantity of drug that was available to the patient and how much is currently missing. One may need to count pills or measure liquid to determine this. For estimating liquids, the approximate volume of a swallow is 0.3 mL/kg. The practitioner should always assume the "worst case," i.e., the patient took all of the drug that is missing. History concerning the amount ingested may be inaccurate, especially when taken from adolescents with intentional ingestion.

The practitioner should try to determine approximately what time the ingestion occurred. Symptoms are usually expected within a defined time range. Recommended observation periods before discharge usually take into account expected symptoms based on the length of time since the ingestion. Timing may also be important in determining expected toxicity. For example, ingestion of mushrooms that cause a self-limited illness usually causes gastrointestinal upset within 4–6 hours, whereas *Amanita* mushrooms that may ultimately cause hepatic failure typically present with gastrointestinal upset in 6–12 hours.

The practitioner should ask about current symptoms and when they started relative to the time of the ingestion. In a patient without a definite history of an ingestion, certain combinations of symptoms may point toward a specific substance. Whether the patient is symptomatic and what symptoms are present may guide the workup for an unknown ingestion, determine whether the patient needs to be hospitalized, or dictate therapy.

Physical Examination

If the substance ingested is known, the physical examination should be directed toward identifying expected symptoms of toxicity. A general physical examination should always be performed, however, since co-ingestion of another undisclosed substance must be considered. Particular attention should be paid to vital signs including temperature, pupillary size and reaction, breathing (e.g., Kussmaul's respiration seen in acidosis), mental status, distinctive breath odors, and skin color, temperature, and moisture. The patient's weight should be measured because toxicity is often estimated based on mg of drug ingested/kg of body weight. Since symptoms may develop or worsen if peak levels of the toxic substance have not been reached at the time of initial evaluation, continual reassessment and cardiorespiratory monitoring are imperative. A recognizable set of symptoms suggestive of a certain class of medications or toxins is called a toxidrome. If a symptomatic patient is noted to have a typical toxidrome, therapy may be initiated based on the toxidrome without confirmation of the exact substance ingested. Some common toxidromes and their treatments are listed in Table 48–1.

Laboratory Tests (Box 48–1)

Qualitative drug screens (reporting only presence or absence of the drug) of urine or blood are often used when poisoning is part of a broader differential for symptoms such as altered mental status or acute behavioral changes. Such drug screens are rarely helpful acutely in the poisoned patient because results are typically not rapidly reported, testing can only be done for a limited number of substances, and false positives and negatives may occur.

On the other hand, quantitative drug levels for specific drugs can be helpful to estimate severity of expected symptoms or to rule out ingestion of that drug.

TABLE 48–1.   Toxidromes

Toxin	Symptoms	Treatment
Narcotic	Respiratory depression, miosis, altered mental status or coma.	Naloxone
Organophosphate, cholinergic	SLUDGE mnemonic: *s*alivation, *l*acrimation, *u*rination, *d*iarrhea, *g*astrointestinal cramping, *e*mesis. Also bronchorrhea, bronchospasm.	Atropine 2-PAM (pralidoxime)
Tricyclic antidepressant	Seizures, prolonged QRS complex, altered level of consciousness, dysrhythmias.	Sodium bicarbonate
Anticholinergic	Flushing ("red as a beet"), dry skin and mucous membranes ("dry as a bone"), hyperthermia ("hot as a hare"), delirium ("mad as a hatter"). Also, mydriasis, tachycardia, urinary retention.	Supportive care
Sympathomimetic	Mydriasis, anxiety, tachycardia, hypertension, hyperthermia, diaphoresis.	Quiet environment and benzodiazepines

---

BOX 48–1. Laboratory Tests and Diagnostic Studies to Consider

- Specific drug levels as indicated
- Acetaminophen level, ethanol level
- Serum chemistries, calculated anion gap
- Serum osmolarity, calculated osmolar gap
- Arterial blood gas
- Rapid bedside glucose test
- Urinalysis
- Urine pregnancy test
- Pulse oximetry
- Electrocardiography
- Chest x-ray
- Abdominal film for radiopaque tablets

Examples are acetaminophen, salicylate, ethanol, methanol, ethylene glycol, iron, theophylline, lithium, and anticonvulsants and levels of carboxyhemoglobin or methemoglobin by blood gas analysis. Such levels should only be measured when suggested by history or physical examination, with the exception of acetaminophen and ethanol. Many experts in toxicology feel that because acetaminophen overdose produces few acute symptoms, may lead to fulminating hepatic failure, and is readily treatable with an antidote, all patients with history of an ingestion should have an acetaminophen level determined. In adolescents and adults, ethanol is a common co-ingestant, and ethanol levels are often routinely measured.

Serum chemistries and osmolarity may offer clues in ingestion of an unknown substance. The **anion gap** is calculated as $[Na] - ([Cl] + [HCO_3])$ and is normally 8–12 mEq/L. An elevated anion gap indicates presence of metabolic acidosis and is seen in ingestions and conditions identified by the **MUDPILES** mnemonic: **m**ethanol, **u**remia, **d**iabetic ketoacidosis, **p**araldehyde and **p**henformin, **i**ron and **i**soniazid, **l**actic acidosis, **e**thylene glycol and **e**thanol, **s**alicylates and **s**olvents (e.g., toluene). The **osmolar gap** is the difference between the measured serum osmolarity and the calculated osmolarity (given by the formula $2[Na] + [glucose]/18 + [BUN]/2.8$). The normal osmolar gap is less than 10 mOsm. An elevated osmolar gap is seen with ingestion of alcohols such as ethanol, methanol, ethylene glycol, and isopropanol.

Depending on suspicion for acidosis, hypoxemia, or abnormal hemoglobins (carboxyhemoglobin and methemoglobin), arterial blood gas analysis may be indicated. Because hypoglycemia may be seen with some ingestions and is easily treated, a rapid bedside glucose test should be done on all patients. Urinalysis may be performed to look for signs of rhabdomyolysis if the patient is deemed at risk. All females of child-bearing age should have a urine pregnancy test.

Diagnostic Studies

Pulse oximetry and cardiorespiratory monitoring should be instituted for all serious ingestions. An electrocardiogram may be indicated if cardiac toxicity is expected. Other studies are tailored to the specific ingestion, such as endoscopy after ingestion of caustic acids or alkalis.

Imaging Studies

Specific imaging studies may be indicated for certain ingestions, such as chest radiography in hydrocarbon ingestion to look for signs of aspiration. An abdominal film may be helpful in identifying ingestion of radiopaque substances and monitoring the effectiveness of gastrointestinal decontamination procedures for such substances. The mnemonic **CHIPS** can be used for radiopaque medications: **c**hloral hydrate, **h**eavy metals, **i**ron, **p**henothiazines, and **s**low-release (enteric-coated) medications. In practice, abdominal radiography is primarily used in iron ingestion.

MANAGEMENT

Management strategies are specific for the substance ingested. The regional poison center should be consulted for advice regarding management and length of time to observe asymptomatic patients. In general, the approach to management includes attention to the basic ABC's (*a*irway, *b*reathing, *c*irculation) or resuscitation, decontamination methods, specific antidotes when available, and meticulous supportive care, often in an intensive care unit.

Decontamination

Decontamination techniques are strategies used to prevent or minimize absorption of the toxic substance and to enhance its elimination. They are a critical part of the management of acutely poisoned patients and should be used whenever a significant ingestion is suspected (Table 48–2).

Syrup of ipecac has commonly been recommended for home use to induce vomiting in the event of an accidental ingestion. **Gastric lavage**, in which a large nasogastric tube is placed and the stomach is washed with normal saline, is the hospital counterpart to syrup of ipecac. Both techniques theoretically remove toxic substance from the stomach, thus preventing absorption. However, only a third of gastric contents are removed by these methods. In addition, these techniques may interfere with the use of activated charcoal, usually a more effective therapy. Gastric lavage is technically difficult to perform in young children owing to the need to pass a large-bore tube. Gastric lavage also has a high rate of complications such as aspiration and esophageal trauma. Many experts in toxicology no longer recommend syrup of ipecac or gastric lavage. Others recommend syrup of ipecac only for use at home if given within 30 minutes of ingestion of liquid products or 1 hour for solids. Those who recommend gastric lavage do so for use in the hospital only if it can be done within 1 hour of the ingestion.

Activated charcoal is the mainstay in treatment of ingestion. Charcoal binds toxins, and because it is not absorbed in the gastrointestinal tract, the charcoal-

TABLE 48–2. **Summary of Gastric Decontamination Techniques**

Technique	Dose	Contraindications
Syrup of ipecac	6 months–1 year: 10 mL (use with caution). 1–12 years: 15 mL. >12 years: 30 mL. Follow with 8 oz. water.	Altered level of consciousness (ALOC). Caustics: acids and alkalis. Hydrocarbons. Expected ALOC (e.g., tricyclic antidepressants).
Gastric lavage	15 mL/kg aliquots normal saline to maximum of 400 mL until lavage fluid is clear (may be several liters).	Altered level of consciousness (ALOC) with unprotected airway. Caustics: acids and alkalis. Hydrocarbons. Expected ALOC >1 h since ingestion.
Activated charcoal	1–2 g/kg or <6 years: 25–50 g >6 years: 50–100 g	Altered level of consciousness (ALOC) with unprotected airway. Absent bowel sounds or bowel obstruction. Substance not bound by charcoal.
Cathartics	Magnesium citrate 4 mL/kg. 70% sorbitol 1 g/kg.	Repeated doses can cause dehydration or electrolyte imbalances.
Whole-bowel irrigation	Toddler and preschool age: 500 mL/h. Adolescent and adult: 1–2 L/h. Continue until rectal effluent is clear.	Bowel obstruction, ileus, perforation, or hemorrhage. Altered level of consciousness (ALOC) with unprotected airway.

toxin complex passes through and is eliminated. The optimal dose of charcoal is 10 times the amount of substance ingested. Because the exact amount of toxin ingested is often unknown, activated charcoal is usually dosed at 1–2 g/kg. The amount of charcoal given is limited only by what the child is able to tolerate. Only a few substances are not absorbed by activated charcoal. The mnemonic **PHAILS** can be used to remember them: **p**esticides, **h**ydrocarbons, **a**cids, **a**lkalis and **a**lcohols, **i**ron, **l**ithium, and **s**olvents. The main complication of charcoal administration is aspiration pneumonitis, primarily seen in patients with altered level of consciousness and an unprotected airway. If charcoal is not voluntarily taken by the child, it may be administered via nasogastric tube. Endotracheal intubation to protect the airway may be necessary in the patient with altered mental status. It is imperative that nasogastric tube placement in the gastrointestinal tract (as opposed to the respiratory tract) be confirmed prior to charcoal administration.

Cathartics have been used to decrease transit time and improve elimination of the toxin through the gastrointestinal tract and to counteract activated charcoal-induced constipation. The cathartic is often mixed with the activated charcoal and may serve to improve the palatability of the charcoal. A significant benefit from cathartic use has never been demonstrated, however, and there is a risk of dehydration and electrolyte disturbances, particularly in young children. Many experts in toxicology no longer recommend routine use of cathartics. Under no circumstances should repeated doses of cathartics be given.

Multiple-dose charcoal may remove drug from the bloodstream by promoting diffusion back into the gastrointestinal tract and subsequent binding to charcoal. It has been called the "GI dialysis." Activated charcoal at the same dose previously used is repeated approximately every 4 hours. Cathartics should **not** be mixed with the charcoal for repeat doses. Multiple-dose charcoal is useful for a small number of drugs, such as phenobarbital, theophylline, and carbamazepine. It should not be used for drugs that can cause an ileus, e.g., tricyclic antidepressants.

Whole-bowel irrigation involves infusion of a solution usually used for cleansing of the bowel prior to gastrointestinal surgery (e.g., GoLYTELY). It is especially useful for slow-release medications, for tablets that dissolve slowly and may cause concretions (e.g., iron), and in ingestions where charcoal is not likely to be effective. A nasogastric tube is used to infuse the solution at a rate of 500 mL/h in young children, and 1–2 L/h in older children and adolescents. Clear rectal effluent is the endpoint; a bedpan may be necessary. Whole-bowel irrigation should not be used when there is bowel obstruction, ileus, perforation, or hemorrhage or altered mental status with an unprotected airway.

Hemodialysis may be used for serious ingestions of ethylene glycol, methanol, phenobarbital, lithium, salicylate, or theophylline. Charcoal hemoperfusion, in which blood goes through a charcoal cartridge instead of a dialysis machine, is used rarely for severe theophylline poisoning. Urinary alkalinization (by administration of sodium bicarbonate) can increase elimination of weak acids by keeping the drug in its ionic state, thus preventing reabsorption in the renal tubule. It is primarily used for significant salicylate and phenobarbital poisonings.

Antidotes

Antidotes or medications that counteract the pathophysiologic mechanisms of the toxin are available for only a few ingestions (Table 48–3). Important antidotes are N-acetylcysteine for acetaminophen, naloxone for narcotics, oxygen for carbon monoxide poisoning, bicarbonate for tricyclic antidepressant cardiotoxicity, Digibind for digoxin, and deferoxamine for iron.

ANTICIPATORY GUIDANCE AND PREVENTION

Most ingestions are nontoxic and require only observation for a few hours. They do, however, provide an excellent opportunity to discuss poisoning prevention with parents and caretakers. Possible toxins, including prescription and over-the-counter medications, cleaning and household products, toxic plants, gardening and hobby chemicals, and kitchen items such as alcohol should be kept out of reach of children. Visitors to the household should also be cautioned to keep medications out of reach of children. Substances should never be stored in unmarked containers, particularly in containers that typically hold beverages such as old soda bottles or cups. Medications should not be referred to as "candy" to entice youngsters to take them. Parents should have telephone numbers for the

TABLE 48–3. Antidotes

Toxin	Antidote
Acetaminophen	N-Acetylcysteine
Anticoagulants (coumadin-like)	Vitamin K
Anticholinergic	Physostigmine
Benzodiazepine	Flumazenil
Beta-blocker	Glucagon
Calcium channel blocker	Calcium, glucagon
Carbamate pesticide	Atropine
Carbon monoxide	Oxygen
Cyanide	Cyanide antidote kit
Digoxin	Digibind
Ethylene glycol	Ethanol
Iron	Deferoxamine
Isoniazid	Pyridoxine
Lead	BAL, EDTA, DMSA
Mercury	BAL, DMSA
Methanol	Ethanol, fomepizole
Methemoglobinemia	Methylene blue
Narcotics	Naloxone
Organophosphate pesticide	Atropine, 2-PAM (pralidoxime)
Tricyclic antidepressant	Sodium bicarbonate

regional poison center and local emergency department readily available.

PROGNOSIS

Prognosis depends on the toxicity of the substance ingested. For a few substances, a small amount can be fatal (e.g., oil of wintergreen), whereas for others, even large ingestions are generally benign (e.g., ibuprofen). Prognosis is generally excellent; fatalities are rare. Prognosis is worse for intentional ingestions, often because patients delay or fail to reveal that they attempted overdose.

Case Resolution

Because the respiratory rate of this 2-year-old is slow and there are symptoms of miosis and altered level of consciousness, narcotic ingestion is suspected and naloxone is administered. The child becomes more alert and respiratory rate increases to 24 breaths per minute. The father is instructed to retrieve the bottle, and it turns out to be a prescription narcotic analgesic left in the house by a recent visitor. The child is given activated charcoal, observed overnight in the hospital, and discharged on the following day without sequelae.

Selected Readings

American Academy of Pediatrics, Committee on Injury and Poison Prevention. Handbook of Common Poisonings in Children, 3rd ed. Elk Grove Village, IL. American Academy of Pediatrics, 1994.

Mack, R. B. (ed.). Poisoning. Pediatr. Ann. 25:19–29, 1996.

Tenenbein, M. General management principles for poisoning. In Barkin, R. M. (ed.). Pediatric Emergency Medicine: Concepts and Clinical Practice. St. Louis, Mosby–Year Book, 1997, pp. 527–534.

Tenenbein, M., S. Cohen, and D. S. Sitar. Efficacy of ipecac-induced emesis, orogastric lavage and activated charcoal for acute drug overdose. Ann. Emerg. Med. 16:838–841, 1987.

Toxicology: Ingestions, inhalation injuries, envenomations. In Strange, G. R. (ed.). APLS: The Pediatric Emergency Medicine Course. Elk Grove Village, IL. American Academy of Pediatrics, 1998, pp. 113–125.

HEAD, NECK, AND RESPIRATORY SYSTEM

C H A P T E R   4 9

APPROACH TO THE DYSMORPHIC CHILD

Julie E. Noble, M.D.

H*x*   A 12-year-old male presents to the office for the first time for an evaluation after moving to the area. Parents note that he has unexplained mental retardation and has had problems with hyperactivity in school. The pregnancy was uncomplicated and the mother, who was a 32-year-old gravida 1, para 1, at the time of the child's birth, denies alcohol or drug use or exposure to any teratogens during pregnancy. Delivery was by cesarean section secondary to cephalopelvic disproportion, but Apgar scores were 8 at 1 minute and 9 at 5 minutes. The infant was noted to have macrocephaly and to be large for gestational age. He did well in the newborn period and had no feeding problems. Subsequently, he had no significant medical illnesses including no seizures, but at 1 year of age was noted to be developmentally delayed. This delay continued, and he has been in special education classes throughout his school career. Family history is negative for any family members with retardation.

On physical examination, the boy is greater than 90th percentile for height and weight. He is mildly prognathic with large ears. He has hyperextensible fingers. A complete examination reveals that his testicles appear large (6 cm) and his Tanner stage is 2. The rest of the examination is normal.

Questions
1. What history is important to elicit in evaluating a child with dysmorphic features?
2. What are the possible causes of errors in morphogenesis?
3. What clues on physical examination can aid in establishing a specific diagnosis?
4. What laboratory tests can confirm a diagnosis?
5. When is it appropriate to obtain a genetics consultation or refer a patient for genetic counseling?
6. What are the benefits of establishing a specific diagnosis?

Evaluation for structural anomalies is an essential part of all pediatric examinations. Visible errors in morphogenesis give the physician valuable information in evaluating a patient with abnormal symptoms, such as seizures. Additionally, major malformations frequently require treatment, and the presence of one anomaly suggests that others may also exist.

The study of these congenital defects was termed dysmorphology by David Smith in 1966. The anomalies fall into two categories: minor and major. Minor malformations are those of "no medical or cosmetic consequence to the patient." An example would be a supernumerary nipple that appears as a hyperpigmented papule along the nipple line. Identification of minor malformations is important because they may indicate the presence of a more generalized pattern of malformation. Major malformations are those that have "an adverse effect on either the function or social acceptability of the individual." A cleft lip and palate is a major malformation that has functional as well as cosmetic relevance to the patient's health.

EPIDEMIOLOGY

Structural anomalies are common in the general population. The majority are minor. In the first comprehensive analysis of minor structural anomalies, Marden in 1964 identified 7–14% of newborn infants with at least one minor anomaly on surface examination. Other studies identify up to 40% of newborns with one anomaly. Three or more minor malformations have predictive value in identifying a major malformation. In newborns, 0.8% have two minor malformations, and 11% of these patients will have a major malformation. Three or more minor malformations occur in 0.5% of newborns, and 90% of these will have a major malformation. Data from the National Collaborative Perinatal Program revealed that 44.78% of these anomalies were craniofacial and 45.3% were skin. Males are affected with minor malformations more often than females. Autopsies of dead fetuses reveal an increased incidence of both minor and major malformations. Frequencies of both minor and major malformations vary along racial lines, depending on the specific malformations. For example, postaxial polydactyly is seen in 16 of 10,000 births in the white population and 140 of 10,000 births in the African American population. Hemangiomas are seen in 350 of 10,000 births in whites and only 100 of 10,000 African Americans.

Three percent of all pregnancies produce a child with a significant genetic disease or a birth defect. These malformations account for a great proportion of morbidity and mortality in the pediatric population. Of all pediatric hospital admissions, one-third to one-half involve a child with a disease with a genetic component.

CLINICAL PRESENTATION

With the advent of more prenatal tests and diagnostic modalities (see Chapter 8, Screening in Newborns), the detection of anomalies may first occur in the prenatal period. Routine prenatal screening tests that are abnormal raise the possibility that the infant will have an anomaly. For instance, an elevated maternal α-fetoprotein indicates the possibility of a spinal cord defect. Amniocentesis or chorionic villus biopsy may reveal abnormal chromosomes with associated structural defects. Prenatal ultrasound now demonstrates structural defects that can be diagnosed *in utero*.

Most structural anomalies develop during the first trimester of gestation and, if not detected prenatally, are noted at birth in the delivery room or the newborn nursery. Many major congenital defects are obvious on a thorough physical examination. Some major defects such as a tracheoesophageal fistula will not be manifest on surface examination but will be readily apparent as the infant adapts to extra-uterine life and experiences symptoms when feeding begins.

Minor anomalies may be overlooked on an infant's initial examination. However, if that infant manifests developmental delay at 6 months of age, the physician may be more inclined to evaluate for minor anomalies that may aid in identifying the cause of the developmental delay.

Sometimes dysmorphic features are not present at birth but become apparent later in life as the child grows and develops. These types of features are associated with dysplasias, defects in cellular metabolism that become manifest after birth. An example is a skeletal dysplasia that becomes more apparent as the bones grow.

PATHOPHYSIOLOGY

The pathophysiology of structural defects can be separated into four different types of errors in morphogenesis: malformations, deformations, disruptions, and dysplasias (Table 49–1).

TABLE 49–1. Pathophysiology

Malformation
Chromosomal abnormality
Single gene disorder
Deformation
Disruption
Vascular compromise
Viral infection
Mechanical—amniotic bands
Teratogens—alcohol, drugs, irradiation
Dysplasia
Metabolic disorder

Previously, the term **malformation** was used descriptively to denote an anomaly; but it is also used to denote a specific pathogenic mechanism. Malformations are permanent defects in a structure caused by an intrinsic abnormality in the development of that structure. An example of a malformation is an endocardial cushion defect in a patient with Down syndrome. Malformations frequently are caused by chromosomal abnormalities and single-gene disorders that program for abnormal structure.

Deformations occur in an infant when external forces exert a mechanical pressure on the developing fetus. There is no intrinsic defect of the fetus. These deformations can be caused by uterine constraint, an abnormally shaped uterus, or multiparous pregnancy. A flexible clubfoot is a deformation caused by uterine constraint.

Disruptions occur when an agent outside a fetus causes cell death and a permanent defect in development. These disruptive events result in tissue destruction. Disruptions can occur during development when there is tissue ischemia secondary to vascular compromise; when a viral infection disrupts development at a critical gestational age; or when a mechanical disruption interferes with normal development. An amniotic band is an example of a mechanical disruptive agent that can cause an amputation of a limb by constricting the extremity during development. Teratogens can also function as disruptive agents by interfering during a critical period in embryogenesis, causing dysgenesis of fetal organs. Alcohol, drugs, and irradiation are all teratogens. Fewer than 30 drugs have been proved to be teratogenic.

Dysplasias, often caused by a single-gene defect, are structural abnormalities that develop from abnormal cellular metabolism and organization. Mucopolysaccharidosis is a dysplasia that develops secondary to the absence of the lysosomal hydrolase of α-L-iduronidase. As a result, mucopolysaccharides accumulate in parenchymal and mesenchymal tissues. As affected children grow, they develop coarse facies, enlarged tongue, misshapen bones, and hepatosplenomegaly among other features.

DIFFERENTIAL DIAGNOSIS

In generating an appropriate differential diagnosis for a dysmorphic child, it is essential to identify all minor and major malformations. The differential will vary depending on the specific findings. A thorough history and physical examination will help greatly to establish the list of conditions to consider. If there are multiple anomalies, identifying the most specific and rarest anomaly can direct the practitioner to a narrower list of possible diagnoses. For example, nail hypoplasia, which is seen in fetal hydantoin syndrome, is much rarer than congenital cardiac disease, which is seen in multiple syndromes. A practitioner should be familiar with the prominent features of the more common syndromes but also should have readily available reference texts such as *Smith's Recognizable Patterns of Human Malformation* to aid in establishing differential lists as well as finalizing diagnoses.

In evaluating an infant with congenital anomalies, the practitioner should attempt to separate the findings into one of five categories: an isolated defect, a developmental field defect, a birth defect association, a sequence pattern, or a dysmorphic syndrome (Table 49–2). The first step is to determine whether the anomaly is **isolated.** If so, does it represent a failure in development in one location, such as a cleft lip? Most isolated anomalies are believed to have a multifactorial inheritance, representing the interaction between multiple genes and unknown external influences. They usually have a recurrence risk of 2–5%.

A **developmental field defect** is a pattern of anomalies that develop in structures that are together during embryologic development. These defects involve one limited region and are secondary to a disruptive event such as vascular compromise. They therefore have a low recurrence risk. An example would be hemifacial microsomia, where the defects are secondary to disruption in vascular flow to the first and second branchial arches. This disruption results in hypoplasia of the malar, maxillary, and mandibular region on one side with associated microtia and vertebral defects.

Birth defect associations are diagnosed when the combination of anomalies occurs together commonly but the pattern does not fit a known field defect or syndrome. The etiology of association defects is unknown at this time, and the recurrence risk is low. One of the more common associations is the VACTERRL association, where the acronym stands for *v*ertebral anomalies, *a*nal atresia, *c*ardiac defects, *t*racheoesophageal fistula, *r*adial defects, and *r*enal and *l*imb defects.

A **sequence pattern** of anomalies occurs when one malformation leads to multiple dysmorphic features. Potter's oligohydramnios sequence results from renal agenesis. The renal malformation causes oligohydramnios with resultant fetal contractures, pulmonary hypoplasia, and a flattened face.

A **syndrome** is a pattern of anomalies that are pathologically related. Chromosomal abnormalities such as Down syndrome (trisomy 21), single-gene disorders, and teratogens fall into this category. Alcohol is the most common teratogen to which fetuses are exposed. Alcohol causes growth failure, developmental delay, microcephaly, a short nose, and small distal phalanges. Children with developmental delay and anomalies have a higher likelihood of having a syndrome and should undergo a chromosome analysis.

EVALUATION

History

A complete history is essential (Questions Box). The history begins prenatally with information from the

---

TABLE 49–2.   Categories of Anomalies

Isolated defect
Developmental field defect
Birth defect association
Sequence pattern
Dysmorphic syndrome

Questions: The Dysmorphic Child

- How long was the pregnancy?
- Did the mother take any medications, smoke cigarettes, or use alcohol or any illicit drug?
- What was the fetal activity?
- Were there any complications of pregnancy?
- What was the type of delivery and presentation of the baby?
- What was the infant's size at birth?
- How did the infant feed?
- What is the subsequent medical and developmental history?
- Are the parents related?
- What are the parents' ages?
- Is there a history of fetal or infant deaths?
- Is there a history of birth defects in the family?
- Are any family members retarded?

mother on duration of pregnancy, possible teratogen exposure, fetal activity, diagnostic test results, and any complications of pregnancy. The delivery history should include type of delivery, infant presentation, and size at birth, including growth percentiles. Neonatal adaption and feeding patterns are important parameters to assess. The subsequent medical history should be obtained.

A thorough family history is equally important, and a pedigree should be outlined. Specifically, the family should be questioned for parental age, possible consanguinity, and history of fetal loss or early infant deaths. Family history of birth defects or retardation should be documented.

Physical Examination

The physical examination should be extremely thorough with all morphologic findings noted. Objective measurements should be obtained when possible. Normal grids are available for evaluating inner canthus distance, palpebral fissure length, ear length, etc. Hair whorl patterns and dermatoglyphics should be evaluated. Physical data, including height, weight, and head circumference, should be plotted and the growth percentiles noted. A complete ophthalmologic evaluation may be indicated to detect abnormalities such as cataracts or cherry-red spots.

Laboratory Tests

In assessments of dysmorphic-appearing children, the physical examination is the most important part. Findings on physical examination direct which further studies will be of benefit. Additional studies may give added or confirmatory information regarding a suspected diagnosis. Skeletal x-rays may be helpful in detecting skeletal anomalies. As mentioned, prenatal screening tests may be used to detect a fetal abnormality. Specific prenatal tests are available to assess a fetus at risk for a given disease. Chromosomal analysis is essential in evaluating a child with a suspected syndrome and also in evaluating a child with malformations and developmental delay. Small chromosomal aberrations can be detected by FISH analysis (fluorescent *in situ* hybridization), in which labeled probes are applied to chromosomal preparations. These probes are specific for given disorders and should be used to confirm a suspected clinical syndrome. Prader-Willi and DiGeorge syndromes may be diagnosed by FISH analysis. Molecular testing is available for many single-gene disorders.

Imaging Studies

Imaging studies are extremely useful in deriving information on internal malformations. Echocardiogram, ultrasound, CT scan, and MRI studies can all be utilized when appropriate.

MANAGEMENT

When children present with dysmorphic features, they should be evaluated to determine a specific diagnosis. Knowing the diagnosis can direct subsequent testing for associated abnormalities. Treatment options may be available for the condition. With a specific diagnosis, a prognosis can be established. Defining the developmental prognosis for children is very important. If developmental delay is not associated with the diagnosis, such as with cleft lip and palate, the parents should be reassured. Parents also need to know the recurrence risk for themselves and for their children. Occasionally, further testing of the parents may be necessary to determine the accurate recurrence risk. If one of the parents is a translocation carrier, the risk of subsequent children having the abnormality is increased.

If the diagnosis is in question, a genetic consultation should be obtained. Consultation with a geneticist can help the practitioner in establishing the correct diagnosis and provide the practitioner with the latest information regarding evaluation and possible treatment. New information in the field of genetic disease appears daily, and it is difficult for a primary care practitioner to stay abreast. A genetic consultation should also be obtained in most patients with major malformations to confirm the diagnosis and to help counsel parents.

Health supervision strategies have been established for specific disorders. For instance, published guidelines recommend hearing, ophthalmologic, and thyroid screening, among other tests, for patients with Down syndrome. A geneticist can give guidance regarding revised recommendations.

If support groups are available for specific conditions, parents should be referred to these groups. Such groups can be invaluable in helping parents understand as well as adjust to the disorder. They can also advise parents about community and educational resources available for their child's care and help parents advocate for their child's unique needs.

A referral to a genetics counselor can provide parents with education about prenatal testing, recurrence risk, and alternatives for dealing with this recurrence risk. Counseling is extremely useful to help parents understand the inheritance pattern.

PROGNOSIS

As for management, defining an accurate prognosis depends on recognition of the specific condition. Some conditions such as trisomy 13 are lethal, while other conditions allow for a normal life span.

Malformations are permanent defects that generally have a recurrence risk. They may be correctable with surgery or treatment but frequently leave a residual disability.

Deformations usually resolve with treatment and have no recurrence risk unless the deformation is secondary to a uterine abnormality such as a bicornuate uterus.

A disruption may be treated with surgery or therapy to improve function but, as in malformations, a residual disability frequently remains. When the disruption is due to tissue ischemia or a mechanical agent, there is no recurrence risk. If it is due to a teratogen, the disruption will recur with the same teratogenic exposure.

Dysplasias tend to persist or worsen with time unless a specific treatment is available. Only a limited number of diseases have specific treatments available. Generally, there is a recurrence risk.

Case Resolution

The child in the case scenario has features that suggest a dysmorphic syndrome. The most specific finding on examination is macro-orchidism. This finding is associated with fragile X syndrome. Specific DNA-based molecular analysis is performed and is positive for a fragile site on the X chromosome at Xq27.3.

Parents are counseled that this condition has an X-linked inheritance pattern. The child will have a normal life span but may need early intervention services and later a special education program and may not be capable of independent living as an adult. Parents are encouraged to attend a parents' support group and consult with experts to learn how their child's full potential may be realized.

Selected Readings

Aase, J. M. Dysmorphologic diagnosis for the pediatric practitioner. Pediatr. Clin. North Am. 39:135–156, 1992.

Frias, J. L., and J. C. Carey. Mild errors of morphogenesis. Adv. Pediatr. 43:27–75, 1996.

Friedman, J. M. A practical approach to dysmorphology. Pediatr. Ann. 19:95–101, 1990.

Jones, K. L. Smith's Recognizable Patterns of Human Malformation, 5th ed. Philadelphia, W. B. Saunders, 1997.

Koren, G., A. Pastuszak, and S. Ito. Drugs in pregnancy. N. Engl. J. Med. 338:1128–1136, 1998.

Toomay, K. E. Medical genetics for the practitioner. Pediatr. Rev. 17:163–174, 1996.

CHAPTER 50

CRANIOFACIAL ANOMALIES

Carol D. Berkowitz, M.D.

H$_x$ A 3500-gram boy is born by normal spontaneous vaginal delivery to a 28-year-old gravida III para III mother after an uncomplicated full-term gestation. The Apgar scores are 9 and 10. On physical examination, the infant is well but has an incomplete, left-sided unilateral cleft of the lip as well as of the palate.

No other family members have such a deformity, but the mother and father are distantly related. The mother had prenatal care. During the pregnancy she had no illnesses, took vitamins but no other medications, and did not smoke, drink alcohol, or use illicit drugs.

The mother is planning to feed the infant with formula and wonders if she should do anything special. She is also wondering if her son's lip deformity can be repaired before she takes him home from the hospital. Except for the cleft, the physical examination is normal.

Questions

1. What craniofacial anomalies are common in children?
2. What are feeding considerations in infants with cleft lip or palate?
3. What is the appropriate timing of surgery for the more common craniofacial anomalies?
4. What are the major medical problems that children with craniofacial anomalies, particularly clefts of the lip or palate, experience?

The most frequently seen major craniofacial anomalies in children are cleft lip and cleft palate. Other common craniofacial problems include microtia, craniosynostosis, and facial asymmetry.

EPIDEMIOLOGY

The overall incidence of cleft lip with or without cleft palate is 1 in 1000, and that of isolated cleft palate is 1 in 2500. There is racial, ethnic, and geographic variation in the incidence of clefts. For example, the incidence of clefts in parts of the Philippines is 1 in 200. The sex distribution varies with the type of cleft. Isolated clefts of the palate occur twice as frequently in girls, but clefts of the lip with or without clefts of the palate appear twice as often in boys.

The type of cleft, the sex of the child, and whether parents or other siblings are similarly affected influence the risk for recurrence of clefts in subsequent offspring. In general, the risk for recurrence of clefts is 4–7% for cleft lip with or without cleft palate and 3% for isolated cleft palate.

Clefts may occur either as isolated findings or as part of syndromes such as Pierre Robin sequence, where they are associated with micrognathia and glossoptosis. In Van der Woude's syndrome, clefts of the lip or palate are associated with lip pits. This condition is inherited in an autosomal dominant manner. There are now over 250 disorders associated with clefts, although only 20% of children with clefts fit a syndrome.

True craniosynostosis occurs in about 1 in 2–3000 births and this incidence is the same in all ethnic groups. There is gender variation among the different types of craniosynostosis. Microtia is less common and occurs in 1 in 6–8,000 births.

CLINICAL PRESENTATION

Most craniofacial anomalies are readily apparent (see D$_x$ Box). Some anomalies, such as cleft lips or microtia, are noted immediately in the delivery room. Other anomalies, such as craniosynostosis, develop over time. Because the onset of craniosynostosis may be gradual, parents may fail to recognize the condition, which usually appears as asymmetry of the face or skull.

Children with craniofacial anomalies may also have medical problems that occur secondary to the deformity. Infants with cleft palate may present with FTT (failure to thrive) because of difficulty feeding. Older infants and children may experience recurrent otitis media, speech impairments, or psychosocial stress. Nasal regurgitation of liquids may occur in children with obvious palatal clefts or more subtle deformities, such as submucous clefts of the soft palate.

PATHOPHYSIOLOGY

Clefts of the lip and palate (Fig. 50–1) are believed to develop as a result of an interruption in the merging of the middle and lateral portions of the face during the sixth to seventh week of gestation. The palate normally closes with an anterior to posterior progression. Any interference with this progression (e.g., tumor or encephalocele in the roof of the mouth) leads to a cleft. A

D$_x$ Craniofacial Anomalies

- Cleft of the lip or palate
- Small, atretic, or malformed ear
- Asymmetry of the face
- Misshapen skull
- Recurrent otitis media
- Speech impairment

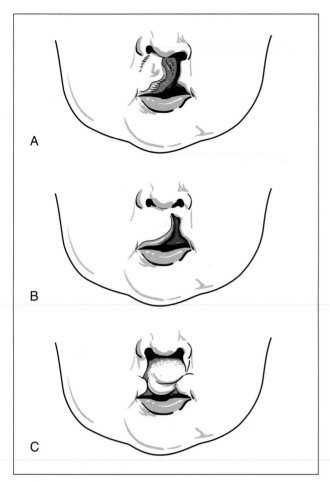

FIGURE 50-1. Cleft lips.
A. Unilateral, complete cleft lip.
B. Unilateral, incomplete cleft lip.
C. Bilateral, complete cleft lip.

vascular disruption may also result in ischemia in the involved areas. Although the etiology of clefts is not fully determined, it is felt to be multifactorial. New studies establish a link between clefting and transforming growth factor alpha (TGFα). The locus for TGFα is on the short arm of human chromosome 2 at band p 13. Infants with the A2 form of the TGFα gene are 8 times more likely to have facial clefts if their mothers smoke.

The presence of a cleft palate affects normal oropharyngeal functioning, including sucking and speech. Children may exhibit hypernasal speech due to the escape of air through the nose and have articulation problems. Recurrent otitis media appears to be related to dysfunction of the eustachian tube.

Microtia, a small atretic pinna of the ear, results from failure of development of the pinna and portions of the external auditory canal. It is most likely caused by a vascular accident during the twelfth week of gestation. Similar anomalies have been created in laboratory animals by ligature of the stapedius artery. Microtia is considered in the spectrum of branchial arch defects.

Craniosynostosis refers to the premature closure of the sutures, which should remain open until 2–3 years of age. What initiates this pathologic ossification is unclear. There is some evidence to suggest that skull compression, such as occurs *in utero* with breech presentation or twins, contributes to the process. When there are other associated anomalies, such as syndactyly, embryologic disturbances in fibrocartilaginous development are suspected. Abnormalities in one region of chromosome 10 are implicated in syndrome synostosis. Any or all of the sutures can be affected, and the closure may result in asymmetry of the skull or microcephaly. Single suture synostosis is classified as simple; multiple synostosis is classified as compound. When closure is related to pathology at the suture, the condition is primary. When there is underlying brain pathology, the disorder is secondary. Premature closure of all sutures is often associated with diseases of the central nervous system with failure of the brain to grow.

Microcephaly may result from premature closure of some or all of the sutures as a primary event or from impairment of the brain and its growth related to some other problem, such as hypoxic encephalopathy or congenital infection.

Fusion of individual sutures prevents growth of the skull perpendicular to the suture, and skull expansion proceeds in an axis parallel to that of the suture (Fig. 50–2). If the sagittal suture fuses prematurely, the head is long and narrow, a condition referred to as **scaphocephaly** (boat head). This is the most common type of craniosynostosis, occurring in about 54–58%. If the coronal sutures fuse too soon, the head is flattened; this condition is called **brachycephaly** and occurs in 18–29% of cases of craniosynostosis. The incidence is 1 in 10,000 live births. Premature closure of the metopic suture results in the triangular-shaped head characteristic of **trigonocephaly,** reported in 4–10%. Familial cases have been reported, as well as abnormalities of chromosomes 3, 9, and 11.

Premature closure of the lambdoidal sutures leads to **plagiocephaly** (oblique head) (Fig. 50–3). Plagiocephaly may also result from malpositioning in utero or after birth, a condition referred to as nonsynostotic or positional plagiocephaly. Malar and contralateral occipital flattening related to preferential positioning by infants are characteristically seen in affected infants. The skull has been likened to a parallelogram in appearance. Torticollis, often related to injury to the sternocleidomastoid muscle at birth (see Chapter 85, Musculoskeletal Disorders of the Neck and Back) and abnormal positioning after birth, may cause plagiocephaly. Plagiocephaly-torticollis sequence occurs in 1 in 300 live births. Some affected babies also have hip dislocation or positional club foot from *in utero* constraint. Current data suggest an increase in the incidence of positional plagiocephaly, which may be related to supine sleeping in infants.

DIFFERENTIAL DIAGNOSIS

In general, the differential diagnosis of clefts of the lip and palate presents few problems. However, submucous clefts may be more difficult to diagnose. Children with such clefts may present with recurrent otitis media or

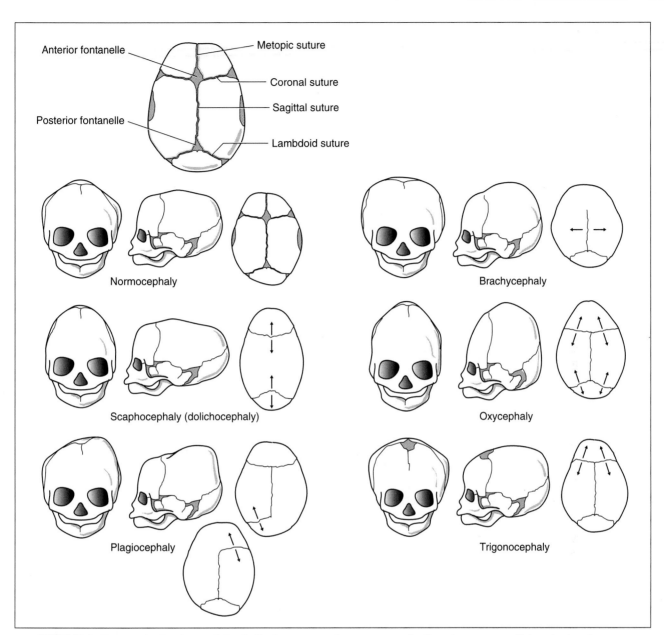

FIGURE 50–2. Changes in the shape of the skull when sutures fuse prematurely. Growth occurs parallel to the fused suture.

hypernasal speech. Physical examination may reveal a bifid uvula and occasionally a notch at the junction of the hard and soft palates.

Determining whether any physical finding represents an isolated anomaly or is part of a genetic syndrome may be challenging. Any associated anomalies (e.g., syndactyly or atrial septal defect) suggest the possibility of a genetic problem (Tables 50–1 and 50–2).

Microtia does not present a diagnostic dilemma. The anomaly usually appears sporadically as an isolated condition, although, like a cleft, it may be part of some other syndrome. Microtia is associated with midfacial hypoplasia and antimongoloid slant to the eyes in Treacher Collins syndrome. Microtia may also occur in Goldenhar's syndrome, which is characterized by several associated findings, including hemifacial microsomia (one side of the face smaller than the other),

epibulbar dermoids, hemivertebrae, microphthalmia, and renal and cardiac anomalies.

Craniosynostosis may also be an isolated finding or associated with a condition such as Apert's syndrome, in which clefts of the palate are also seen (Table 50–3). A careful neurodevelopmental assessment helps determine the cause of microcephaly. Plagiocephaly may present a diagnostic dilemma: Is the condition related to unilateral craniosynostosis or to torticollis and malpositioning after birth? A careful assessment of the neck for masses frequently helps differentiate between these two possibilities.

EVALUATION

Care must be taken to assess children and determine if the anomalies are isolated findings or components of

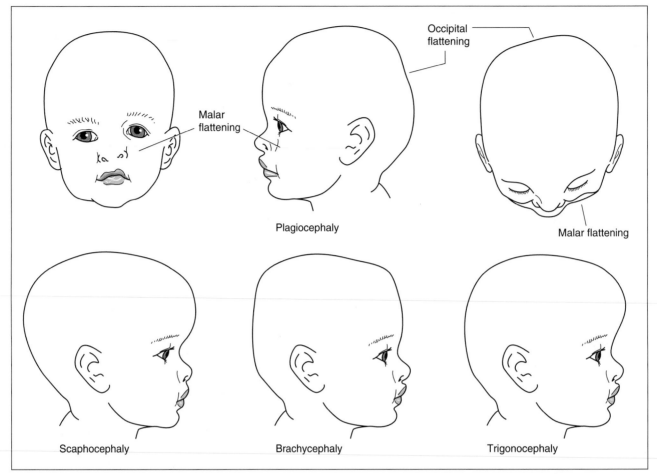

FIGURE 50-3. Classic appearance of an infant with facial asymmetry secondary to plagiocephaly (top row); classic appearance of infants with craniosynostosis (bottom row).

a syndrome. This information is important both in terms of patient care and genetic counseling for parents regarding the likelihood of having future offspring with similar anomalies.

History

A medical, family, and psychosocial history should be obtained (Questions Box). Whether the condition appeared at birth or some time later is particularly significant in lesions affecting the skull, such as craniosynostosis. Maternal use of certain medications, such as diazepam, phenytoin, and isotretinoin (Accutane), and alcohol is associated with an increased incidence of

clefts of the lip and palate. Maternal smoking also increases the risk of clefting, especially in a genetically vulnerable population. Maternal smoking and high altitude are associated with an increased occurrence of craniosynostosis.

Physical Examination

Height, weight, and head circumference should be measured and plotted at each visit. Head circumference is especially important in children with craniosynostosis or facial asymmetry. The skull should be palpated to detect perisutural ridging. Inner canthal distance may

---

TABLE 50-1. Genetic Syndromes Associated with Clefts

Apert's
Ectodactyly-ectodermal dysplasia-clefting
Goldenhar's
Meckel's
Optiz
Popliteal pterygium
Stickler's disease
Treacher Collins
Van der Woude's

TABLE 50-2. Anomalies Associated with Cleft Lips and Palates

Nasal glioma or meningoencephalocele	Aniridia
Persistent buccopharyngeal membrane	Cleft larynx
Congenital neuroblastoma	Polydactyly
Congenital heart disease	Anencephaly
Thoracopagus twins	Foot deformities
Congenital oral teratoma	Oral duplication
Forearm bone aplasia	Spina bifida
Lateral proboscis	Aplasia of trochlea
Sacral agenesis	Laryngeal web

TABLE 50–3.   **Genetic Disorders with Craniosynostosis**

Apert's syndrome
Crouzon's disease
Jackson-Weiss syndrome
Pfeiffer's syndrome

reveal hypotelorism, a finding seen in trigonocephaly. The neck should be palpated for masses, and the range of neck motion assessed. The growth of children with craniofacial anomalies must be carefully monitored. Problems with adequate weight gain are frequently experienced by infants with clefts.

The physical examination should focus on defining the extent of the anomaly and determining if associated abnormalities are present. Such abnormalities may involve the face or other parts of the body, including the skeleton. In children with microtia, the position of the ear should be noted. When the ear is displaced to the cheek, the condition is called auricular dystopia. Cardiac murmurs may be noted in children with clefts, and these murmurs should be carefully evaluated.

Children with clefts should be carefully assessed for the presence of otitis media at each visit. Periodic hearing assessments should be carried out in children with clefts or microtia. Speech and development should also be evaluated.

Laboratory Tests

Routine laboratory tests are not indicated in most children with craniofacial anomalies. Chromosomal studies are indicated if a genetic disorder is suspected.

Imaging Studies

X-rays and imaging studies may be indicated in children with facial asymmetry, micro- and macroceph-

Questions: Craniofacial Anomalies

- Did the child suffer any injuries at birth?
- Was the child born in an abnormal position?
- Have the findings been present since birth, or did they appear later?
- Has the anomaly led to any changes in the child's health, such as recurrent ear infections or speech difficulties?
- Does the child have any family history of craniofacial anomalies?
- Does the mother have a history of illness during pregnancy?
- Was the mother exposed to any medications, particularly teratogenic agents, during pregnancy?
- Did the mother use alcohol during pregnancy?
- Did the mother smoke during pregnancy?
- Is the child experiencing difficulties in school (e.g., teasing)?
- How is the child performing in school?
- Is development progressing normally? What are the child's milestones?
- Is the child's speech understandable?
- Does the child have any trouble with eating or drinking? Are fluids expelled through the child's nose with swallowing?

aly, and craniosynostosis. A three-dimensional CT scan of the skull is particularly helpful in defining which sutures are fused. Renal ultrasound may be necessary in children with microtia because of the association between ear and renal anomalies.

MANAGEMENT

The management of children with craniofacial anomalies usually requires the expertise of a multidisciplinary team, including a pediatrician, plastic surgeon, ear-nose-throat specialist, speech pathologist, social worker, psychologist, orthodontist, and prosthodontist. Primary care physicians who are not part of the team can receive information regarding appropriate patient care and follow-up. It is important for primary care physicians to be familiar with the appropriate nomenclature to be able to communicate with consultants. In brief, clefts of the lip are unilateral or bilateral and complete or incomplete. A complete cleft extends into the nares (see Fig. 50–1). Clefts of the palate may involve the entire palate or be confined to the secondary or soft palate.

Routine **well child care,** including monitoring of growth and administration of immunizations, is most important in the management of children with craniofacial anomalies. Some infants with clefts are slow feeders. Mothers should be told that although breastfeeding can be carried out, it is often slow and difficult. Some formula-fed infants require the use of special adaptive nipples or feeders. A specific cleft palate feeder, which consists of a plastic bottle that allows for compression of the unit during feeding, is available. A soft, premature-type nipple can also be obtained. Long nipples, such as lamb's nipples, which are used to feed infant lambs, are not routinely recommended because they cause infants to gag. Infants who gain weight slowly may need to be given concentrated formulas (see Chapter 106, Failure to Thrive).

Hearing and speech should be monitored. Chronic prophylactic **antibiotics** or the insertion of **pressure equalization tubes** may be needed to manage recurrent otitis media (see Chapter 52, Otitis Media). Speech problems require the expertise of a speech pathologist and placement of children in **speech therapy** in either the community or school.

Surgical correction is indicated for many anomalies. Clefts are usually repaired as staged procedures during the first 2 years of life. Repair of the cleft lip, the first procedure, is traditionally scheduled when infants weigh 10 pounds, are 10 weeks of age, and when their hemoglobin is 10 (rule of tens). Appropriate weight gain is therefore critical to ensure timely surgery. If skilled anesthesiologists and nurses are available, cleft lip repair can be carried out within the first 2 weeks of life. Early repair is recommended at some centers. Repair of the cleft palate, the second procedure, is usually undertaken when infants are between 12 and 18 months of age. Better speech develops with earlier palatal repair. Surgical correction of clefts does not alter children's propensity to otitis media. This condition improves as children get older, however. Refinement of the cosmetic results, including rhinoplasty, occurs throughout childhood. Orthodontia is frequently a key component to achieve a cosmetically acceptable result and appropriate occlusion of the dentition for speech and chewing.

Children with isolated unilateral microtia often hear, and surgery is recommended for cosmetic purposes. Surgical correction of microtia is usually initiated when children are 5 years of age, before they start school. At this time the ear has achieved 90% of its growth, and children are spared the potential embarrassment of their deformity in the school setting. Surgical reconstruction usually involves three procedures and implantation of the costal cartilage. If there are other facial anomalies, more extensive reconstructive surgery is indicated.

Craniosynostosis can be corrected surgically, although the procedure is major and has significant risks. The age of the infant and the site of the synostosis influence the complexity of the procedure. A controversy about whether neurodevelopmental problems are related to craniosynostosis or whether they represent a preexisting condition has arisen. In developmentally normal children with evidence of closure of all the sutures, surgical repair is believed to be warranted. In other cases, the procedure is thought to be reconstructive because it normalizes the appearance of children with a deformation.

In children with plagiocephaly, where the deformation is believed to be related to torticollis, **passive stretching of the neck** 5–6 times a day (with each diaper change) is used to manage the condition. In addition, it is recommended that bright objects such as mobiles be placed over children's cribs to encourage head turning. Children who do not improve with stretching, or who have a deformity at 6 months of age may be fitted with a specially designed helmet referred to as a dynamic orthotic cranioplasty (DOC) device that reshapes the skull. The device is generally worn for 4 months. In an effort to reverse the trend of increasing positional plagiocephaly related to supine sleeping, the AAP has recommended that parents rotate their infant's position when they are awake. Positional plagiocephaly secondary to supine sleeping usually resolves without surgical intervention.

Psychologic counseling should be available to affected children and their families to help them adjust to the anomalies and the reactions of society. Parents may be referred to community agencies such as the Cleft Palate Guild to help them cope with the potential stress related to giving birth to children with this anomaly and to advise them about the medical and surgical interventions that are available. FACES, the National Association for the Craniofacially Handicapped (PO Box 11082,

Chattanooga, TN 37401 (800) 332-2373) is a referral source for parents.

PROGNOSIS

Most anomalies can be surgically corrected, leaving little residual evidence of the deformity. School success and psychological well-being may be more resistant to remediation, and are highly dependent on the supportiveness of the family and their emotional resources. Children who grow up in settings where the deformity is thought to be embarrassing have long-term problems with low self-esteem.

Case Resolution

The infant in the case history has a cleft of the lip and palate. The mother is advised that the infant can be given formula, and she is given a supply of special feeders. She should have the opportunity either to meet other parents of children with similar anomalies or to view pictures of children who have undergone a repair.

The mother should also be advised about the timing of surgery. She should be told that the surgery is scheduled when the infant is approximately 10 weeks old. A follow-up appointment in about 2 weeks should be arranged. Weight gain can be monitored, and the adjustment between the mother and the infant should be assessed.

Selected Readings

Balasubrahmanyam, G., N. J. Schere, J. A. Martin, and M. L. Michal. Cleft lip and palate: Keys to successful management. Contemp. Pediatr. 15:133–153, 1998.

Berera, G. Index of suspicion: submucous cleft palate. Pediatr. Rev. 14:191–192, 1993.

Denk, M. J. Topics in pediatric plastic surgery. Pediatr. Clin. North Am. 45:1479–1506, 1998.

Fields, H. W. Craniofacial growth from infancy through adulthood. Pediatr. Clin. North Am. 38:1053–1125, 1991.

Kane, A. A., L. E. Mitchell, K. P. Craven, and J. L. Marsh. Observations on a recent increase in plagiocephaly without synostosis. Pediatrics 97:877–885, 1996.

Kaufman, F. L. Managing the cleft lip and palate patient. Pediatr. Clin. North Am. 38:1127–1147, 1991.

Keating, R. F. Craniosynostosis: Diagnosis and management in the new millennium. Pediatr. Ann. 26:600–612, 1997.

Liptak, G. S., and J. M. Serletti. Pediatric approach to craniosynostosis. Pediatr. Rev. 19:352–358, 1998.

Marion, R. W. Craniosynostosis. Pediatr. Rev. 16:115–116, 1995.

Nagata, S. A new method of total reconstruction of the auricle for microtia. Plast. Reconstr. Surg. 92:187–201, 1993.

Ripley, C. E., et al. Treatment of positional plagiocephaly with dynamic orthotic cranioplasty. J. Craniofac. Surg. 5:150–159, 1994.

Rohan, A. J., S. G. Golombek, and A. D. Rosenthal. Infants with misshapen skulls: When to worry. Contemp. Pediatr. 16:47–70, 1999.

Throkelsson, T., F. Mimouni, and W. S. Ball, Jr. Sagittal and lambdoidal craniosynostosis. Am. J. Dis. Child. 146:1311–1312, 1992.

COMMON ORAL LESIONS

Geeta Grover, M.D.

H$_x$ A 7-year old girl is brought to the office for evaluation of a swelling on the inside of her lower lip of 4–6 weeks' duration. Her mother reports that it increases and decreases in size. The girl says that the swelling is not painful, and she cannot remember hurting her lower lip. On examination, a raised, bluish, nontender, 1 x 1 cm swelling is apparent along the mucosa of the lower lip.

Questions

1. What is the differential diagnosis of lip masses?
2. What laboratory or radiographic tests are useful in the evaluation of oral lesions?
3. What management strategies are used to treat cystlike oral lesions?
4. When should children with oral lesions be referred to subspecialists?

Primary care physicians are often required to evaluate lesions in the oral cavity. Knowledge of common congenital, developmental, infectious, and neoplastic conditions that affect the mouth and its structures can help physicians recognize and manage these lesions appropriately. Although many lesions are benign and regress spontaneously, others may require drainage, administration of medications, or surgical excision. Evaluation and management of some oral conditions may necessitate interaction among the pediatrician, dentist, and oral surgeon.

EPIDEMIOLOGY

Oral pathology is common. Benign oral lesions, such as gingival cysts, occur in about 75% of newborns. The reported incidence of natal teeth (teeth present at birth) is about 1 in every 3000 live births; the incidence increases in infants with cleft lip or palate. Developmental abnormalities such as geographic tongue and hyper- or hypodontia are evident in 1–2% and 4–7% of individuals, respectively. The incidence of hypodontia in the permanent dentition is about 7% (less than 1% in the primary dentition). The teeth most commonly missing are the third molars, maxillary lateral incisors, and mandibular second premolars. The incidence of supernumerary permanent teeth is 3–4%, occurring most often in the area of the maxillary central incisors.

Infections of the mouth are even more common. Although the rate of dental caries in the United States has significantly declined in the past 10–20 years, largely because of the use of systemic fluoride, approximately 50% of school children either have dental caries or a history of gingivitis.

CLINICAL PRESENTATION

Little or no discomfort is associated with even extensive dental caries. Untreated caries may result in destruction of most of the tooth. When infection extends to the dental pulp (pulpitis), significant pain may occur. Dental abscesses may present with fever, severe facial pain, and swelling. Aphthous ulcers are characteristically extremely painful. Even small lesions can produce a disproportionate amount of discomfort.

Children with gingivitis present with red, swollen mucosa that may bleed with toothbrushing. Children with primary herpetic gingivostomatitis present with fever, often as high as 103–104° F (39.4–40.0° C); irritability; anorexia due to pain on chewing and swallowing; and scattered vesicular lesions on the mucous membranes of the lips, tongue, and gingivae, which may also be erythematous and swollen. Herpangina, like herpetic gingivostomatitis, may be associated with fever (frequently high), irritability, and anorexia. The vesicular lesions are usually confined to the oropharynx (e.g., pharynx, tonsils, soft palate), sparing the gingiva and anterior oral cavity.

Candidiasis, or thrush, typically appears as small, white plaques on the buccal mucosa or tongue. Children are usually asymptomatic.

PATHOPHYSIOLOGY

Neonatal Abnormalities

Gingival cysts in newborns are due to entrapment of tissues during embryologic development. Histologically, **congenital epulis** consists of sheets of granular cells in the connective tissue underlying the epithelium. **Melanotic neuroectodermal tumor of infancy** is characterized by clusters of small, neuroblast-type cells lying within the alveolar spaces lined with endothelial-type, melanin-containing cells.

Developmental Abnormalities

The etiology of **geographic tongue,** or benign migratory glossitis, is unknown, but this chronic, often recurring condition has been associated with stress. **Mucoceles** are usually due to trauma to one of the minor salivary glands. **Enamel abnormalities** may be due to local or systemic infections, excessive fluoride ingestion, or nutritional deficiencies.

Tooth Discoloration

Extrinsic staining is due to material adhering to the surfaces of the teeth. **Intrinsic staining** results from the incorporation of excessive levels of endogenous substances, including normal pigments, such as hemoglobin or bilirubin, or exogenous substances, such as tetracycline or fluoride, into the developing enamel.

Oral Infections

The process of the formation of **dental caries** requires the interaction of dietary carbohydrates, particularly sucrose, and dental plaque. Dental plaque is a dense material composed of salivary products, food debris, and bacteria that forms along the margins of the teeth and gums. The bacteria in plaque, most commonly *Streptococcus mutans*, produce organic acids that demineralize the outer surfaces of the teeth through the fermentation of carbohydrates. Left untreated, caries can progress, and eventually lead to necrosis of the pulp and cavitation of the tooth. The frequency of carbohydrate consumption and duration of contact with the tooth (relative stickiness of the substance) are more important than the total amount of carbohydrates consumed.

Nursing bottle caries are caused by the pooling of carbohydrate-containing liquids around the teeth. These caries are seen most often in infants who sleep with a bottle in their mouth, and they affect the maxillary central incisors.

Primary herpetic gingivostomatitis is caused by herpes simplex virus, usually type 1.

The etiology of **aphthous ulcers** is unknown, but stress and local trauma are believed to be predisposing factors.

DIFFERENTIAL DIAGNOSIS

Oral pathology may be divided into several categories: neonatal abnormalities, developmental abnormalities, tooth discoloration, and oral infections (Table 51–1).

Neonatal Abnormalities

Natal teeth are present in the oral cavity at the time of birth, whereas **neonatal teeth** erupt during the first month of life. Most natal teeth are primary teeth that have erupted early, not supernumerary teeth. The most commonly affected teeth are the mandibular central incisors. These teeth are often loose due to immature root development. The two most common associated problems involve difficulty with breast-feeding (biting the mother) and potential aspiration of teeth.

Benign gingival cysts are commonly seen in newborns. **Epstein's pearls** are most common. They are small, white, keratin-filled lesions located along the midline of the palate. **Bohn's nodules** appear as multiple, firm, grayish-white lesions located along the gums and only occasionally on the palate. Unlike Epstein's pearls, these contain remnants of mucous gland structures as well as keratin. **Dental lamina cysts** are

remnants of dental lamina epithelium that appear as small, cystic lesions along the crests of the mandibular and maxillary mucosa.

Two benign tumors that are seen during infancy are congenital epulis and melanotic neuroectodermal tumor of infancy. **Congenital epulis** is a rare, benign soft tissue tumor usually located on the anterior portion of the maxillary (most likely) or mandibular mucosa at birth. Over 90% of cases occur in girls. Solitary lesions are most common, but about 10% are multiple. **Melanotic neuroectodermal tumor of infancy** is a benign but locally aggressive tumor that presents during the first year of life. It usually appears as a grayish-blue, firm mass along the anterior aspect of the maxillary mucosa.

Developmental Abnormalities

Common soft tissue abnormalities include generalized gingival hyperplasia, geographic tongue, mucoceles, and ranulas. **Generalized gingival hyperplasia** may be idiopathic, secondary to drugs such as phenytoin and cyclosporine, genetically transmitted (fibromatosis gingivae), or transiently associated with tooth eruption. A nonspecific pathologic entity, it is characterized by gingival overgrowth that may secondarily become inflamed or edematous. **Geographic tongue** is characterized by painless, irregularly shaped, red patches with

---

TABLE 51–1. Common Oral Lesions in Children

Neonatal Abnormalities
Natal teeth
Benign gingival cysts
    Epstein's pearls
    Bohn's nodules
    Dental lamina cysts
Congenital epulis
Melanotic neuroectodermal tumor of infancy
Developmental Abnormalities
Soft tissues
    Generalized gingival hyperplasia
    Benign migratory glossitis (geographic tongue)
    Mucoceles and ranulas
Hard tissues (teeth)
    Variations in tooth number (hyper- and hypodontia)
    Variations in size and shape of teeth
    Defective enamel formation (hypoplasia or hypocalcification)
Tooth Discoloration
Extrinsic staining
    Poor oral hygiene
    Smoking
    Food or drink
    Medication
Intrinsic staining
    Endogenous (e.g., hemoglobin, bilirubin)
    Exogenous (e.g., tetracycline, fluoride)
Oral Infections
Bacterial
    Dental caries
    Nursing bottle caries
    Dental abscesses
    Gingivitis
Viral
    Primary herpetic gingivostomatitis
    Herpangina
    Aphthous ulcers
Fungal
    Candidiasis (thrush)

white borders located on the dorsum and lateral borders of the tongue. Affected areas are devoid of filiform papillae. Lesions regress and reappear spontaneously over a period of weeks to months, producing a migratory appearance.

Mucoceles and ranulas are benign soft tissue tumors of the oral cavity. **Mucoceles** are painless, smooth, fluid-filled translucent or bluish lesions that are most often found on the mucosa of the lower lip. They may increase and decrease in size. Ranulas are mucoceles located in the floor of the mouth.

Hard tissue abnormalities include variations in tooth number (hyperdontia and hypodontia), size and shape, and hypoplasia or hypocalcification of teeth. **Hypodontia** occurs when tooth buds fail to form. Hypodontia may be associated with ectodermal dysplasia syndromes. **Hyperdontia** is the occurrence of supernumerary teeth. **Variations in size and shape of teeth** result from disturbances during tooth development. These changes are clinically significant only if they cause problems with crowding or alignment of the other teeth. Defective enamel formation may present as **hypoplasia** (pitting or thinning of the enamel) or **hypocalcification** (chalky or white lesions on the surfaces of the teeth).

Tooth Discoloration

Discoloration may be extrinsic or intrinsic. **Extrinsic stains** are usually due to poor oral hygiene, smoking, foods or drinks and medications (e.g., children taking liquid iron supplements may develop brownish-black stains on their teeth). **Intrinsic stains** may be secondary to endogenous or exogenous substances. Infants with erythroblastosis fetalis or severe neonatal jaundice are at risk for staining secondary to high plasma levels of hemoglobin or bilirubin. Tetracycline is incorporated into calcifying teeth and produces a yellow to brown to dark gray discoloration.

Oral Infections
Bacterial Infections

Dental caries, a multifactorial disease, causes progressive destruction of teeth. Lesions initially appear as opaque or yellowish-brown defects on the surface of the enamel. Severe involvement can present as complete destruction of the involved teeth. Caries may affect the smooth surfaces of the teeth, especially those between adjacent teeth, but they occur more commonly in the pits and fissures of the chewing surfaces of the teeth.

Nursing bottle caries, or baby bottle tooth decay, is a specific form of caries that occurs typically in children 12–24 months of age. The most commonly affected teeth are the maxillary incisors, followed by the cuspids and the first molars. The lower incisors are usually spared because of the protective barrier provided by the tongue. Opaque or chalky discolorations of the teeth begin on the palatal, or backside, of the teeth first and are the earliest sign of decay. These areas become darkly eroded, and eventually tooth loss results.

Dental abscesses are most often the result of untreated dental caries. Once tooth necrosis occurs, bacteria may invade the alveolar bone and produce dental abscesses. Associated complications include sepsis and facial cellulitis.

Gingivitis is an infection of the gingiva that produces inflammatory changes. It is usually secondary to poor oral hygiene, resulting in accumulation of dental plaque around the apices of the teeth at the gingival margin (gum line). This condition may also be seen in children with diabetes mellitus, neutropenia, thrombocytopenia, and leukemia.

Viral Infections

Viral infections of the mouth are quite common in children. Gingivostomatitis is an infection of the gingiva and other parts of the oral mucosa. **Primary herpetic gingivostomatitis** primarily affects children 1–3 years of age. The associated vesicles are painful, and when these vesicles rupture, shallow ulcers form. **Herpangina,** a form of stomatitis, is an infection of the oral mucosa that spares the gingiva. Caused by the coxsackie A group of viruses, it is usually characterized by painful vesicles on the mucosa of the soft palate and posterior pharynx. Although herpangina most commonly affects children under 5 years of age, older children may also be afflicted. **Aphthous ulcers,** or canker sores, are of unclear etiology, but may be related to trauma or viruses. These shallow, 3–4-mm ulcers, with an erythematous ring, occur singly or multiply, most often on the floor of the mouth or the mucous membranes of the lips. The painful lesions usually begin during adolescence or young adulthood and often recur.

Fungal Infections

Candidiasis, or thrush, is caused by *Candida albicans*. This condition is seen mostly in infants, but it also occurs in children who are receiving antibiotic therapy or who are immunosuppressed. Creamy white plaques on the buccal mucosa or tongue that are difficult to remove and may cause bleeding when scraped are characteristic of candidiasis. Candidal diaper rash may be associated with oral thrush.

EVALUATION

History

Any parental concerns regarding disruptions in the child's daily activities (e.g., decreased appetite, irritability) due to the lesion in question should be noted. The length of time the lesion has been present, whether it is painful, and whether the child has recently taken or is currently taking any medications are important to determine (Questions Box).

Physical Examination

Physical examination begins with an inspection of all structures in the mouth (e.g., lips, gums, teeth, mucosal surfaces) and an assessment of oral hygiene. Gingival swelling, erythema, and friability should be noted. The number of teeth should be counted, and any unusual shapes or stains should be described. Any obvious lesions within the oral cavity should be assessed in terms of location, color, size, shape, and tenderness.

Laboratory Tests

A CBC and blood culture may be obtained if systemic symptoms (e.g., fever) are associated with a dental abscess. Ulcers can be scraped for viral isolation or microscopic examination (Tzanck smear), looking for the multinuclear giant cells characteristic of herpetic infection. The diagnosis of thrush can be made by scraping the lesion, mixing the material with KOH, and viewing the characteristic hyphae on microscopic examination. This is rarely necessary, however, because the diagnosis can usually be made on clinical appearance.

Imaging Studies

Dental x-rays may be required in the evaluation of natal teeth, dental caries, or dental abscesses. Such x-rays may also be used to differentiate supernumerary teeth from natal teeth that are prematurely erupted primary teeth. Early radiographic identification of supernumerary teeth is important because they may interfere with eruption and alignment of future teeth.

MANAGEMENT

Neonatal Abnormalities

The vast majority of natal teeth are true primary teeth. Premature extraction may lead to overcrowding of the permanent teeth because the space once occupied by the extracted tooth may become occupied by the adjacent primary teeth. Only loose teeth that pose a danger of aspiration, are supernumerary, or cause discomfort to the mother or child should be removed. All gingival cysts are benign and resolve within a few weeks. Both congenital epulis and melanotic neuroectodermal tumors respond to surgical excision with infrequent recurrence.

Developmental Abnormalities

Meticulous oral hygiene should be stressed for children on phenytoin therapy. Phenytoin-induced gingival hyperplasia may require surgical excision of the excessive tissue. However, recurrence is common. Both mucoceles and ranulas require surgical excision of the lesion and the associated minor salivary gland to prevent recurrence. Children with hard tissue abnormalities should be referred to a pediatric dentist for further evaluation.

Tooth Discoloration

Tetracycline should not be given to pregnant women or children under the age of 8–10 years because it produces intrinsic staining of the teeth. Because tetracycline crosses the placenta and affects developing teeth in the fetus, it should not be prescribed to pregnant women. Green staining may result from algal growth on the teeth. Such extrinsic stains can be removed with cleaning.

Oral Infections

Most dental caries can be prevented through **good oral hygiene, proper diet,** and **preventive dental care.** The best method for prevention of smooth surface caries involves the **regular use of systemic fluorides.** Initiation of caries on chewing surfaces may be prevented by the application of **dental sealants** to these surfaces. **Prevention** is the best treatment for nursing bottle caries. Parents should be counseled never to nurse their children to sleep or put them to bed with a bottle containing anything but water.

Gingivitis in its early forms responds to improved oral hygiene and daily plaque removal with toothbrushing. Professional dental care may be required for more extensive disease. In both primary herpetic gingivostomatitis and herpangina, lesions heal spontaneously in 1–2 weeks. Treatment is supportive. Acetaminophen may be used for fever and pain control, and fluids, including cold liquids and Popsicles, should be encouraged because they may be soothing to inflamed tissues. Rinsing with or topically applying a solution of equal parts diphenhydramine hydrochloride elixir and Maalox liquid may provide temporary pain relief for children with severe disease. Application of topical anesthetics such as viscous lidocaine should be discouraged because of the risk of absorption and seizures. Systemic acyclovir therapy may be considered for moderate to severe disease, especially in immunocompromised children. Controversy exists about the efficacy of topical acyclovir for less severe acute cases or cases of recurrent herpes labialis.

Aphthous ulcers (canker sores) heal spontaneously. Treatment is supportive and aimed at minimizing pain and shortening the duration of the lesions. Rinsing the mouth with a **topical antibiotic** (e.g., 250-mg capsule of tetracycline dissolved in 15 mL of water) may help reduce pain and prevent the overgrowth of opportunistic microorganisms. Mouthwashes containing hydrogen peroxide promote oral hygiene as well and should be used frequently. Topical steroid ointment (e.g., 0.1% triamcinolone dental paste) and systemic steroid therapy (in adults with extensive lesions) are other therapeutic options. Omeprazole has also been used for extensive, chronic aphthous ulcers, particularly in immunodeficient patients.

Treatment of candidiasis involves administration of **nystatin** suspension four times a day until the lesions resolve (generally 1–2 weeks). An alternative treatment is direct application to the lesions of a 1% gentian violet solution several times a day. Because it stains the skin and mucous membranes a bluish-purple color, it may not be well-accepted. Recurrent or refractory infection may warrant evaluation of the immune system.

Case Resolution

The child described in the case history at the beginning of this chapter appears to have a mucocele. She should be referred to either an oral or head and neck surgeon for surgical excision of the lesion.

Selected Readings

Acs, G. Oral manifestations of systemic disease. Pediatr. Basics 82:2–10, 1998.

Dunlap, C. L., B. F. Barker, and J. W. Lowe. Ten oral lesions you should know. Contemp. Pediatr. 8:16–28, 1991.

Mueller, W. A. When baby teeth decay. Contemp. Pediatr. 10:75–83, 1993.

Nazif, M. M., et al. Oral disorders. *In* Zitelli, B. J., and H. W. Davis. Atlas of Pediatric Physical Diagnosis, 3rd ed. St. Louis, Mosby-Wolfe, 1997.

Peter, J. R., and H. M. Haney. Infections on the oral cavity. Pediatr. Ann. 25:572–576, 1996.

CHAPTER 52

OTITIS MEDIA

Monica Sifuentes, M.D.

H$_x$ An 18-month-old male infant is brought to your office with a 2-day history of fever and decreased intake of feedings. He has had symptoms of an upper respiratory infection (URI) for the past 4 days but no vomiting or diarrhea. Otherwise he is healthy.

The infant appears tired but not toxic. On physical examination the vital signs are normal except for a temperature of 101° F (38.8° C). The left tympanic membrane (TM) is erythematous and injected, with yellow pus behind the membrane. The light reflex is splayed, and mobility is decreased. The right tympanic membrane is gray and mobile, with a sharp light reflex. The neck is supple with shotty anterior cervical adenopathy, and the lungs are clear.

This is the infant's fourth documented ear infection in 6 months. He has a 10- to 15-word vocabulary, and no one smokes in the household.

Questions

1. What are the differences between acute, persistent, and recurrent otitis media (OM)?
2. What factors predispose to the development of ear infections?
3. What are the most common presenting signs and symptoms of an ear infection in infants, older children, and adolescents?
4. How do the treatment considerations differ between acute, persistent, and recurrent ear infections?
5. What are the complications of OM?

Otitis media (OM) is the second most common reason after well child care for a visit to the pediatrician. It is estimated that approximately 30 million office visits per year involve the evaluation and treatment of OM and that billions of dollars are spent annually for OM care. Moreover, more than a quarter of all prescriptions written each year for oral antibiotics are for the treatment of middle ear infections. In addition, many surgical procedures such as myringotomy with tympanostomy tube placement or adenoidectomy are performed on children for treatment of recurrent disease. Therefore, the primary care physician must have a good understanding of this pediatric condition.

OM can be classified into the following four categories: acute OM, OM with effusion, recurrent acute OM, and chronic OM with effusion. It is important to distinguish between each of these entities because their presentation and management differ.

Acute OM (acute suppurative or purulent OM) is the sudden onset of inflammation of the middle ear, which is often accompanied by fever and ear pain. **OM with effusion** is the presence of middle ear fluid after antimicrobial treatment. Resolution of acute inflammatory signs has occurred, with persistence of a more serous, nonpurulent effusion. Although the fluid may persist for 2–3 months, it resolves within 3–4 weeks in 60% of cases. **Recurrent OM** is defined as frequent episodes of acute OM with complete clearing between each case. A more specific definition is three new episodes of acute OM requiring antibiotic treatment within a 6-month period, or four documented infections in 1 year. This condition affects approximately 20% of children who are "otitis prone"; such children are usually infants who have their first infection at less than a year of age. **Chronic OM with effusion** (serous OM, secretory OM, or nonsuppurative OM) is a chronic condition characterized by persistence of fluid in the middle ear for 3 months or longer. The TM is retracted or concave with impaired mobility and shows no signs of acute inflammation, and affected children may be asymptomatic. These individuals are at greatest risk for developing hearing deficits and speech delay.

EPIDEMIOLOGY

The overall prevalence of OM is 15–20%, with the highest peak at 6–36 months of age. An additional smaller peak occurs at about 4–6 years. OM is relatively uncommon in older children and adolescents. The condition is more common in boys than girls, and the prevalence is greater in Alaskan natives and Native Americans than in Caucasians.

Several epidemiologic risk factors for OM have been identified, including familial predisposition; presence of siblings in the household; low socioeconomic status; altered host defenses (acquired or congenital immuno-deficiencies); environmental factors, such as day care attendance and passive smoke exposure; and the presence of an underlying condition such as a cleft palate or other craniofacial anomaly. Children with Down, Goldenhar's, and Treacher Collins syndromes also have an increased risk of OM as well. As one might expect, the highest rate of OM occurs during the winter months and in early spring, coinciding with peaks in the incidence of URIs.

Breast-feeding, which provides infants with immunologic protection against URIs, other viral and bacterial infections, and allergies, is thought to have a preventive effect. It has also been hypothesized that facial musculature develops differently in breast-fed infants, thus influencing eustachian tube function and preventing aspiration of fluid into the middle ear. Positioning during breast-feeding also has been hypothesized to have some protective effect, although this may not be as important as the role of an immune factor in breast milk.

CLINICAL PRESENTATION

Children with acute OM often have a history of fever and ear pain. Associated symptoms include URI, cough, diarrhea, and nonspecific complaints such as decreased appetite, waking at night, or irritability in infants. Purulent otorrhea with minimal ear pain and hearing loss may also occur (D_x Box).

PATHOPHYSIOLOGY

The most important factor in the pathogenesis of OM is abnormal function of the eustachian tube (Fig. 52–1). Reflux, aspiration, or insufflation of nasopharyngeal bacteria into the middle ear via the dysfunctional

---

D_x Otitis Media

- Ear pain or otorrhea
- Possibly fever
- Abnormal TM:
  - Erythema or injection of TM
  - Pus or air-fluid level behind TM
  - Bulging appearance
  - Distorted or absent light reflex
  - Decreased mobility via pneumatic otoscopy

---

eustachian tube may lead to infection. Hematogenous spread of microorganisms is another cause of infection. Less often, primary mucosal disease of the middle ear from allergies or abnormal cilia may lead to OM.

The causative microorganisms for OM are *Streptococcus pneumoniae* (30–50% of cases), *Haemophilus influenzae* (20–30% of cases, a majority being nontypeable strains), and *Moraxella catarrhalis* (7–25% of cases). Group A streptococcus, *Staphylococcus aureus,* α-hemolytic *Streptococcus, Pseudomonas aeruginosa,* and anaerobic bacteria are other less common causes. Respiratory viruses such as RSV, adenovirus, rhinovirus, parainfluenza, coronavirus and influenza A also play a role. Gram-negative enteric bacteria are common etiologic agents in the neonate, occurring in approximately 20% of cases, but are rare in older patients.

Eustachian tube dysfunction occurs primarily for two reasons: abnormal patency and obstruction. Obstruction is either functional (secondary to collapse of the eustachian tube), mechanical (from intrinsic or extrinsic causes), or both. Functional obstruction or collapse of the eustachian tube occurs commonly in infants and young children because the tube is less cartilaginous and therefore less stiff than in adults. In addition, the tensor veli palatini muscle is less efficient in this age group. Intrinsic mechanical obstruction of the eustachian tube occurs as the result of inflammation secondary to a URI or allergy in patients beyond 5 years of age. Extrinsic causes of mechanical obstruction include masses such as tumors or adenoidal enlargement.

DIFFERENTIAL DIAGNOSIS

The most common cause of otalgia, or ear pain, is acute OM. Other causes include mastoiditis, which is almost always accompanied by OM; otitis externa; and referred pain from the oropharynx, teeth, adenoids, or posterior auricular lymph nodes. A foreign body in the canal can produce similiar symptoms. In children with ear pain, a search for any of these other conditions must be undertaken if the TM appears completely normal.

EVALUATION

History

It is important in the history to differentiate nonspecific symptoms of otitis media from those indicating

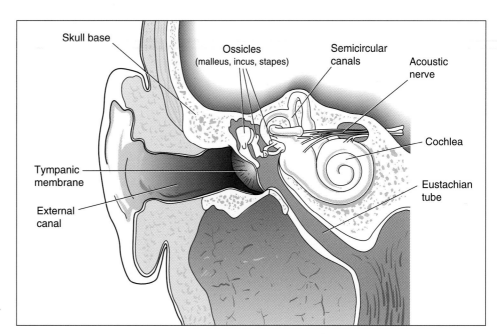

FIGURE 52–1. Relationship of middle ear to external and inner ears.

a more serious condition such as meningitis (Questions Box).

For infants or children with a history of persistent or recurrent OM, it is important to find out when they had their last documented infection and what treatment they received.

Physical Examination

To diagnose OM, the TM must be visualized. Occasionally this may be difficult because of otorrhea, and the diagnosis is then made clinically. In all other cases, the position, color, degree of translucency, and mobility of the TM must be evaluated. Classically, in acute OM the TM is full or bulging, hyperemic, opaque, and has limited or no mobility. In addition, the light reflex is usually distorted or absent. In the case of a persistent or chronic OM, signs of inflammation are usually absent and the TM may be retracted, with limited or no mobility.

Associated physical findings with an uncomplicated middle ear infection may include posterior auricular and cervical adenopathy. Other significant findings on physical examination are pain on movement of the pinna, anterior ear displacement, posterior auricular pain, and, rarely, evidence of peripheral facial nerve (cranial nerve VII) paralysis. The presence of these findings suggests other diagnoses such as an associated otitis externa or mastoiditis.

Positioning of infants or young children for examination of the ear can be difficult. Several methods have been described, including allowing parents to hold the child in their arms or on their laps or restraining the child on the examination table with or without a papoose board (Fig. 52–2). In addition, it may be difficult to visualize the TM in infants because the external auditory canal is slightly angulated. Lateral retraction of the pinna may help correct this problem.

Laboratory Tests

Although the diagnosis of OM is suspected on the basis of the history and then verified on physical examination, tympanometry may be helpful in distinguishing the normal ear from one with an effusion. In acute cases, audiometry is of limited diagnostic value, but it is helpful in evaluating the effects of a persistent, recurrent, or chronic middle ear effusion on hearing.

Tympanocentesis is the most definitive method of verifying the presence of middle ear fluid and of recovering the organism responsible for the infection. Indications for tympanocentesis or myringotomy are listed in Table 52–1. Nasopharyngeal cultures are not helpful because they do not seem to correlate highly with middle ear fluid cultures.

MANAGEMENT

Oral antibiotics continue to be the mainstay of medical treatment for acute OM (Table 52–2). Although some investigators recommend withholding antimicro-

---

Questions: Otitis Media

- Does the infant or child have fever, ear pain, hearing loss, or otorrhea?
- Is the infant or child inconsolable or lethargic?
- Has the infant or child had a previous ear infection? If so, when?
- Did the child complete the course of prescribed antibiotics?
- How many ear infections has the child had in the past year?
- Is the child taking any medication to prevent recurrent OM?
- Does the child attend day care?
- Is the child exposed to passive smoke?
- Is the infant breast-fed?
- Does the child appear to hear?
- Is the child's speech development normal?

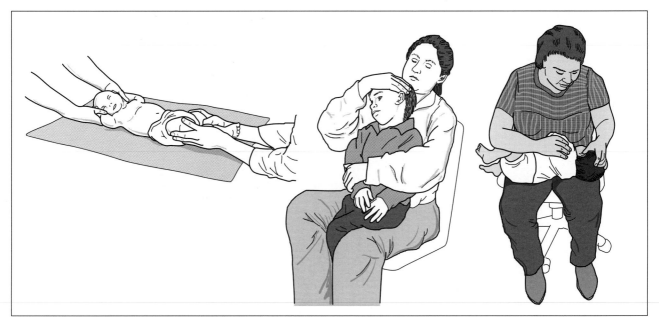

FIGURE 52–2. Three ways to position the infant or child for examination of the ear.

bial treatment since studies have shown the spontaneous resolution of acute OM without them, most health care providers continue to advocate their use. Several studies have been conducted to evaluate second- and third-generation cephalosporins as well as other newer antibiotics such as the macrolides. Amoxicillin remains the first-line drug of choice. It is effective in treating 80–85% of cases of acute OM, is well tolerated by children, has few adverse side effects, and is inexpensive. More important, amoxicillin is active both in vitro and in vivo against *S. pneumoniae* and nontypeable *H. influenzae,* the most common organisms that cause acute OM. The emergence of penicillin-resistant pneumococci has created a debate regarding the dose of amoxicillin required to treat acute infections of the middle ear. Most experts recommend 40–50 mg/kg/d. However, some advocate higher doses of amoxicillin (75–90 mg/kg/d) to cover highly resistant strains of pneumococci, although no data currently support this practice.

Trimethoprim-sulfamethoxazole (TMP-SMZ, Bactrim, Septra) and erythromycin-sulfisoxazole (Pediazole) are usually considered second-line therapy or can be used in penicillin-allergic individuals. They are both effective against β-lactamase-producing bacteria (10–30% of *H. influenzae* and most *M. catarrhalis*). TMP-SMZ, however, is not effective against group A streptococcus.

Factors to consider when prescribing these drugs are dosing intervals and side effects. Compliance may be an issue with Pediazole because it is taken four times a day. TMP-SMZ is taken twice daily. The erythromycin in Pediazole may also cause undesirable vomiting and abdominal pain. In addition, both of these medications contain a sulfonamide, so the risk of serious reactions such as Stevens-Johnson syndrome is not negligible.

Amoxicillin-clavulanic acid (Augmentin) and cefixime (Suprax) can be used in cases of resistant organisms. The main disadvantage of these medications is cost; in the case of Augmentin, side effects such as diarrhea, which occurs in some patients, may also be a problem. An attractive advantage of Suprax is the once-a-day dosing. Some clinicians have advocated cefaclor (Ceclor) as another treatment option; cost, inadequate antimicrobial coverage, and adverse reactions such as serum sickness make it less popular, however.

Although most practitioners prescribe these antibiotics for 10 days, they may be given for up to 14 days. After beginning correct medical therapy, children should be afebrile and subjectively feeling better in 48–72 hours. They should remain afebrile throughout the remainder of the antibiotic course. For those who fail initial antibiotic therapy, a second antimicrobial should be prescribed. Failure of the second antibiotic should alert the practitioner to the possibility of

---

TABLE 52–1. Indications for Tympanocentesis or Myringotomy in Children with Otitis Media

Otitis media (OM) in patients with severe ear pain, serious illness or appearance of toxicity

Onset of OM in children receiving appropriate and adequate antimicrobial therapy

OM associated with confirmed or potential suppurative complications, such as facial paralysis, mastoiditis or meningitis

OM in newborns, sick neonates, or immunodeficient patients, in each of whom an unusual organism may be present

---

TABLE 52–2. Considerations in Antimicrobial Drug Selection

Age
Associated illnesses
History of otitis media
Drug hypersensitivity
Cost and coverage
Compliance issues

highly resistant pneumococci, noncompliance, or misdiagnosis.

Adjunctive medications such as topical analgesics and antipyretics are important therapeutic options and should be prescribed for children with significant pain or fever. Antihistamines, decongestants, or steroids play no documented role in the treatment of OM with effusion.

Most resolving middle ear effusions seen after an acute OM in otherwise healthy children do not need to be treated, and the "wait-and-watch" approach can be taken. In the symptomatic patient (recurrent fever, pain, or hearing loss), second-line antibiotic treatment is in order. Children should then be reexamined in 1 month.

Environmental manipulation may help reduce recurrent OM in some children. Parents who smoke should be advised about the adverse effects of smoking on ear infections. They should be encouraged to stop smoking or to confine their smoking to outside of the home.

Chemoprophylaxis is indicated in "otitis prone" children as a means of protecting them from the serious consequences of recurrent OM such as language impairment and permanent hearing loss. Children who have three or more documented ear infections in 6 months or four episodes in 12 months and those with a positive family history of otitis are candidates for prophylaxis. In addition, infants who are plagued with ear infections beginning at less than 1 year of age should be considered for preventive therapy. Before the initiation of chemoprophylaxis, however, children must be free of all signs and symptoms of an acute infection.

Amoxicillin and sulfisoxazole are safe and effective drugs for daily prophylaxis. Half the therapeutic dose given once daily is appropriate. To increase compliance, the dosage should probably be given at the same time each day. Dosages are: Amoxicillin, 20 mg/kg/d, and sulfisoxazole, 75 mg/kg/d. Although TMP-SMZ is also effective and is used by some clinicians, it is currently not recommended for prophylaxis.

Current recommendations are to continue the chemoprophylaxis for 3–6 months or during the winter and spring seasons when the incidence of respiratory illnesses is highest. Children should then be reexamined at 1–2-month intervals to ensure the resolution of any residual effusions. Any acute infections should be treated accordingly with full dosages of an alternative regimen.

Frequent bouts of OM also require a further search for respiratory allergies, sinusitis, immunologic deficiencies, and anatomic abnormalities such as a submucosal cleft palate or nasopharyngeal tumor. Any suspicion of a hearing deficit requires that a BAER (brainstem auditory evoked response) or audiogram be performed, depending on the age of the child.

Failure of prophylactic medication and chronic effusions warrant a referral to an otolaryngologist for further evaluation for pressure equalization tubes or, if the patient is over 4 years of age adenoidectomy. Other reasons for consultation include any evidence of hearing loss; the presence of any anatomic abnormality, such as a defect of the TM (perforations, cholesteatomas) or intranasal problems (deviated septum, polyp); signs and symptoms of an OM but normal physical examina-tion; and a predisposition to chronic-recurrent OM (e.g., children with a cleft palate or Down syndrome).

PROGNOSIS

Complications associated with OM are much less common with early antibiotic therapy but occasionally occur. They can be divided into two categories: extracranial and intracranial. Extracranial complications include perforation of the TM, conductive and sensorineural hearing loss, cholesteatoma, mastoiditis, facial nerve (cranial nerve VII) paralysis, osteomyelitis of the temporal bone, and Bezold's abscess. Intracranial complications are meningitis, extradural as well as subdural abscesses, lateral venous sinus thrombosis, brain abscess, and hydrocephalus.

Case Resolution

In the case presented at the beginning of the chapter, the child displays the classic signs and symptoms of acute OM: fever, URI, decreased appetite, and an abnormal TM on physical examination. He should be treated for 10–14 days with oral antibiotics and then placed on prophylaxis during the winter and spring months to prevent further infections. The prognosis is good, given his normal speech development.

Selected Readings

Berman, S. Otitis media in children. N. Engl. J. Med. 332:1560–1565, 1995.

Bluestone, C. D., J. S. Stephenson, and L. M. Martin. Ten-year review of otitis media pathogens. Pediatr. Infect. Dis. J. 11:S7–S11, 1992.

Duncan, B., et al. Exclusive breast-feeding for at least four months protects against otitis media. Pediatrics 93:867–872, 1993.

Faden, H., L. Duffy, and M. Boeve. Otitis media: back to basics. Pediatr. Infec. Dis. J. 17:1105–1113, 1998.

Fliss, D. M., A. Leiberman, and R. Dagan. Medical sequelae and complications of acute otitis media. Pediatr. Infec. Dis. J. 13:534–540, 1994.

Giebink, G. S., D. M. Canafax, and J. Kempthorne. Antimicrobial treatment of acute otitis media. J. Pediatr. 119:495–500, 1991.

Klein, J. O. Preventing recurrent otitis: what role for antibiotics? Contemp. Pediatr. 11:44–60, 1994.

Lieberman, J. M. Bacterial resistance in the '90s. Contemp. Pediatr. 11:72–99, 1994.

Maxon, S., and T. Yamauchi. Acute otitis media. Pediatr. Rev. 17:191–196, 1996.

The Otitis Media Guidelines Panel. Managing otitis media with effusion in young children. Pediatrics 94:766–773, 1994.

Paradise, J. L. Managing otitis media: a time for change. Pediatrics 96:712–715, 1995.

Pichichero, M. E., and C. L. Pichichero. Persistent otitis media. I. Causative organisms. Pediatr. Infect. Dis. J. 14:178–183, 1995.

Pichichero, M. E., and C. L. Pichichero. Persistent otitis media. II. Antimicrobial treatment. Pediatr. Infect. Dis. J. 14:183–188, 1995.

Ruuskanen, O., and T. Heikkinen. Otitis media: etiology and diagnosis. Pediatr. Infect. Dis. J. 13:523–526, 1994.

Stool, S., C. Johnson, and A. Stark. Diagnosis and management of otitis media in 1998. Pediatr. Rev. 19CD:1–7, 1998.

Teele, D. W. Strategies to control recurrent acute otitis media in infants and children. Pediatr. Ann. 20:609–616, 1991.

Wright, P. F., J. Thompson, and F.H. Bess. Hearing, speech, and language sequelae of otitis media with effusion. Pediatr. Ann. 20:617–621, 1991.

CHAPTER 53

HEARING IMPAIRMENTS

Monica Sifuentes, M.D.

Hx A 15-month-old girl is brought to the office because the parents are concerned that she has not yet begun to speak. The child was the full-term product of an uncomplicated pregnancy. Her 25-year-old mother, who began to receive regular prenatal care during the second month of gestation, had no documented infections during the pregnancy, took no medications, and has denied using illicit drugs or alcohol. The 27-year-old father is reportedly healthy. There is no family history of deafness, mental retardation, or consanguinity.

The girl, who is otherwise healthy, has never been hospitalized, but she has had three documented ear infections. She rolled over at 4–5 months of age, sat at 7 months, and walked at 13 months. She is able to scribble. The parents report that their daughter smiles appropriately, laughs occasionally, and plays well with other children. As an infant, the girl cooed and babbled, but she now points and grunts to indicate her needs. She does not respond to loud noises by turning her head.

The child's growth parameters, including head circumference, are normal for age. The rest of the physical examination is unremarkable.

Questions

1. When should deafness be suspected in infants or children?
2. What is the relationship between hearing loss and language development?
3. What are the major causes of deafness in children?
4. What neonates are at risk for the development of hearing deficits?
5. What methods are currently available to evaluate hearing in infants and children?
6. What are the important issues to address with families who have infants or children with suspected hearing impairments?

Children may either be born with a hearing deficit or may develop the condition during childhood. A mild hearing deficit occurs with a 26–40 decibel (dB) loss. Severe hearing loss, on the other hand, is defined as 71–90 dB, and profound loss is 90$^+$ dB. The most important period for language and speech development is generally the first 3–4 years of life, and reduced hearing acuity during this time can greatly interfere with this important process. When these crucial years for language and speech development are lost, children's social, emotional, cognitive, and academic development can be affected (see Chapter 15, Language Development). Their potential financial and vocational status may also be influenced. Therefore, primary care physicians must have a clear understanding of when to suspect deafness in infancy and early childhood and must be familiar with its identification and evaluation.

EPIDEMIOLOGY

The prevalence of deafness in children is approximately 0.1% at birth; approximately 1:1000 children is born severely to profoundly deaf. It has been estimated, however, that 3–5:1000 children have mild to moderate hearing loss. The average age at diagnosis of most children who are born deaf is now 2–3 years. Current methods of screening miss approximately 50% of infants who are born with hearing impairments, and lesser degrees of deafness may go undetected for several years. Although early detection and intervention programs are now being implemented in several states, careful assessment of language development is nonetheless essential at each patient encounter.

An estimated 20–30% of children who are hearing impaired developed the condition during childhood. In addition, 70% of children with acquired hearing loss are initially identified by the parents rather than physicians.

Graduates of the neonatal intensive care unit have a significant risk of bilateral sensorineural hearing loss (1–3%); associated factors such as prematurity (birth weight <1500 grams) and neonatal sepsis increase this risk. Other factors associated with deafness in infancy include meningitis, parental consanguinity, craniofacial malformations, congenital viral infections, hyperbilirubinemia, perinatal asphyxia, and a family history of deafness.

CLINICAL PRESENTATION

Children with hearing impairments appear to physicians most commonly with delayed speech. Parents may be concerned that the toddler is indicating his needs by grunting and pointing rather than by using words. Children also may display behavioral problems, such as temper tantrums or aggressive play with other children. In addition, they can present with no intelligible speech (D$_x$ Box).

Hearing impairment is more difficult to recognize in infants less than 6 months of age, since they often have no obvious symptoms of hearing loss. They may startle to moderately loud noises and begin to vocalize just as other infants. With the advent of newborn screening, neonates may present to their health care provider with an abnormal hearing test upon discharge from the hospital (see Newborn Screening).

D$_x$ Hearing Impairment

- Parental concern or suspicion of hearing loss
- Delayed speech and language development
- Associated risk factors including prematurity, exposure to ototoxic drugs, congenital or acquired CNS infections, and cranio-facial abnormalities
- History of behavioral problems and/or poor school performance
- Abnormal hearing test

PATHOPHYSIOLOGY

Mechanism of Hearing

Sounds in the form of pressure waves are carried from the external environment through the external auditory canal to the tympanic membrane (TM). These waves are then converted to mechanical vibrations by the ossicles, and the mechanical vibrations are then transmitted from the TM to the inner ear, where they are transformed to fluid vibrations. Finally, these fluid vibrations are converted into nerve impulses by nerve endings located in the cochlea in the inner ear. These impulses are conducted via the auditory nerve to higher levels (Fig. 53–1).

Hearing impairments can be classified either according to the part of the auditory system affected or as the cause of the hearing loss.

Types of Hearing Loss

The tympanic membrane, the ossicles, or both, are affected in **conductive hearing loss.** Various conditions, infections, or anomalies that affect the middle ear such as otitis media or ossicular discontinuity result in this type of hearing loss. Middle ear effusions rarely cause more than a 20–30 dB loss. The cochlea or inner ear is affected in **sensorineural hearing loss.** Congenital infections, anomalies, and genetic disorders lead to this type of loss. A **mixed disorder** has characteristics of both conductive and sensorineural losses. In a **retrocochlear hearing loss,** the auditory nerve, brain stem, or cortex is affected.

ETIOLOGY OF HEARING IMPAIRMENT (TABLE 53–1)

Severe to profound hearing loss has three main causes: genetic, acquired, and malformative. Genetic causes account for at least 50% of cases; primarily these are isolated, sporadic cases without ready explanation. These genetic mutations may result in different types of deafness with various presentations and outcomes: that is, the hearing loss may be conductive, sensorineural, or mixed, and may be static or progressive with the initial presentation either in infancy or later childhood. Most instances of congenital sensorineural hearing loss are autosomal recessive (75%). The estimated recurrence rate in siblings is 10% if the cause of hearing loss in the initial case is unknown.

Acquired causes include prenatal, perinatal, or postnatal events and exposures such as congenital infections, bacterial meningitis, hyperbilirubinemia, complications of prematurity, and exposure to ototoxic medications. Cytomegalovirus is probably the most frequently unrecognized congenital infection causing deafness; however, toxoplasmosis, rubella, herpes simplex, and syphilis can also be implicated. With bacterial meningitis, where the incidence of hearing loss can be as high as 20%, *Streptococcus pneumoniae* is likely to become the most prevalent cause; the incidence of *Haemophilus influenzae* infection has decreased tremendously in young children with the advent of vaccine administration. The role of steroids in the treatment of

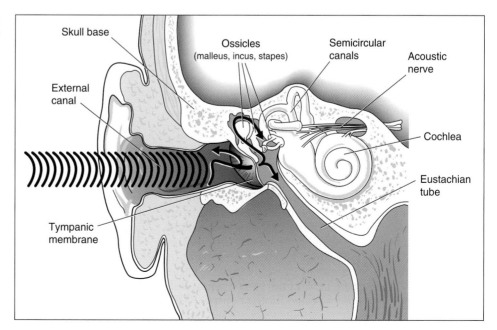

FIGURE 53–1. Sound waves passing through the external ear into the middle ear.

Skull base

Ossicles (malleus, incus, stapes)

Semicircular canals

Acoustic nerve

External canal

Cochlea

Eustachian tube

Tympanic membrane

TABLE 53–1. Major Causes of Childhood Deafness

Genetic (familial or sporadic)
Acquired
  Infections
    Congenital—CMV, rubella, toxoplasmosis, HSV, syphilis
    Acquired—bacterial meningitis, mastoiditis, recurrent and chronic otitis
      media, mumps
  Complications associated with prematurity
  Ototoxic medications and chemicals
  Hyperbilirubinemia
  Head trauma
  Acoustic trauma
Malformations/Syndromes
Unknown

Modified, with permission, from Rapin, I. Hearing disorders. Pediatr. Rev. 14:44, 1993.

bacterial meningitis has also contributed greatly to the decrease in sensorineural hearing loss in survivors. The problem of untreated significant hyperbilirubinemia in term newborns is rare in the United States and other developed countries. Prematurity, however, is not uncommon, but it is still unclear which of the associated complications are responsible for the higher rates of severe hearing loss in this group compared to full term infants. Some antibiotics, such as the aminoglycosides, and other medications like furosemide can be irreversibly ototoxic; other drugs cause only transient effects.

Any head injury causing significant middle ear trauma may also lead to deafness in children. Repeated acoustic trauma such as that associated with continuous or significant exposure to loud noise can also cause irreversible hearing loss.

Malformations are the least common cause for severe to profound hearing loss in infants and children. These include ear malformations in neonates and children with midfacial anomalies, such as a cleft lip or palate. In contrast, profound malformations of the external and middle ears, such as microtia or absence of the external canal and tympanic membrane and fusion of the ossicles, can cause a maximum loss of about 60 dB if the cochlea is normal. Specific syndromes like Down syndrome and Goldenhar's syndrome frequently are associated with hearing impairment. In addition, multiple syndromes with and without anomalies of the head and neck may be associated with hearing impairment, and affected children must be evaluated on an individual basis.

DIFFERENTIAL DIAGNOSIS

In addition to hearing loss, communication disorders should be considered in infants or children with delayed speech and language development. These include problems with speech perception, language comprehension, formulation of language output, and speech production. Unrecognized conditions such as mental retardation can be responsible for some of these disorders. Other etiologies include specific central nervous system deficits as well as impairments of fine motor control of the oropharynx.

EVALUATION

Newborn Screening

In 1994, the Joint Committee on Infant Hearing, composed of representatives from several professional organizations, endorsed universal newborn screening. Their goal was the early identification of hearing loss in infants before 3 months of age, and the implementation of intervention services by 6 months of age. As a result of these recommendations, some states have implemented legislation mandating newborn hearing screening and intervention programs. For those neonates for whom universal screening is not available, the clinician should maintain a high index of suspicion and be familiar with the high-risk factors associated with sensorineural and/or conductive hearing loss.

History

Because the primary symptom of deafness is failure to learn to speak at the appropriate age, the most important aspect of the history in children with possible hearing loss is determining whether speech is developing normally (Fig. 53–2). Even deaf infants may begin cooing and babbling in infancy, and these early attempts at verbalization are not useful milestones for assessment of hearing loss. It helps to ask parents whether they are at all suspicious or concerned about their children's speech or hearing. Guidelines to assess language development are found in Table 53–2. (See Chapter 15, Language Development.) An assessment of risk factors for deafness, such as history of prematurity, hyperbilirubinemia, neonatal sepsis, and asphyxia is also important (Questions Box).

Physical Examination

A complete physical examination should be performed on all children. In particular, any dysmorphic facial features that may suggest the presence of a syndrome with an associated hearing deficit should be noted. Other anomalies of the head and neck should be noted as well. The size and shape of the pinnae and external ear canals should be carefully inspected for abnormalities and patency, respectively. In addition, the tympanic membranes should also be visualized and assessed for the presence of a middle ear effusion that may influence subsequent audiologic tests. The oropharynx should be examined for a cleft palate or a bifid uvular, which may be associated with a submucous cleft. The manner in which children communicate with parents should be noted, if possible.

Laboratory Tests

Although tympanometry is not a hearing test, it can be useful to assess the presence of fluid in the middle ear as well as the mobility of the tympanic membrane. Tympanometry can be particularly helpful with uncooperative, crying children in whom the detection of any

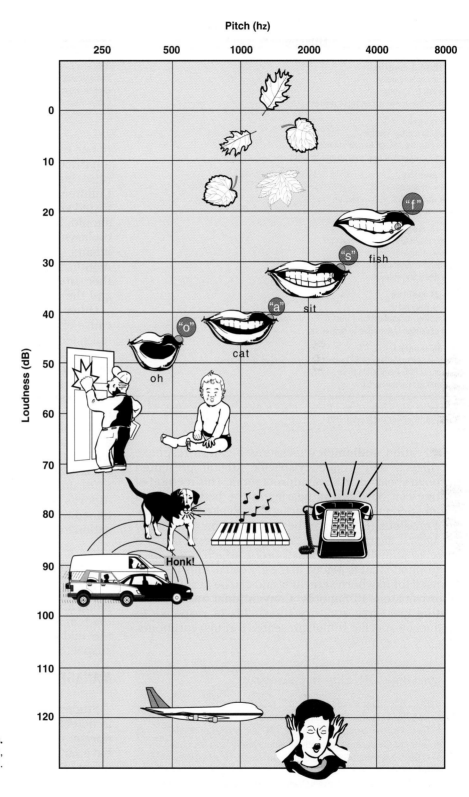

Pitch (hz)

Loudness (dB)

FIGURE 53–2. Loudness of everyday sounds. (Reproduced, with permission, from Northern, J., and M. Downs. Hearing in Children, 4th ed. Baltimore, Williams & Wilkins, 1991.)

problems based solely on the appearance of the TM and insufflation is difficult. Different types of hearing tests for evaluating infants and children for possible hearing deficits are available to general pediatricians (Table 53–3). **Automated Auditory Brainstem Response (ABR)** and **Brainstem Auditory Evoked Response (BAER)** are electrophysiologic measurements of activity in the auditory nerve and brain stem pathways. Electrodes are placed on the infant's head to record brain wave activity while a specific auditory stimulus is presented through earphones to one ear at a time. The ABR is used for newborn screening and only takes approximately 10 minutes, whereas a BAER is much more comprehensive and can take up to 90 minutes to perform. **Behavioral**

TABLE 53–2.   Expected Speech-Language-Auditory Milestones*

Birth to 3 months
Startles to loud noise
Awakens to sounds
Blink reflex or eye widening to noises

3–4 months
Quiets to mother's voice
Stops playing, listens to new sounds
Looks for source of new sounds not in sight

6–9 months
Enjoys musical toys
Coos and gurgles with inflection
Says "mama"

12–15 months
Responds to his/her name and "no"
Follows simple requests
Expressive vocabulary of 3–5 words
Imitates some sounds

18–24 months
Knows body parts
Expressive vocabulary minimum of 20–50 words (uses two-word phrases)
50% of speech intelligible to strangers

By 36 months
Expressive vocabulary of 500 words (uses 4–5 word sentences)
Speech is 80% intelligible to strangers
Understands some verbs

---

*Adapted, with permission, from Northern J., and M. Downs. Hearing in Children. *4th ed.* Baltimore, Wililams and Wilkins, 1991.

observation audiometry measures a child's response to speech and frequency-specific stimuli presented through speakers in a soundproof room. This method of testing can only assess hearing in the better ear and cannot detect unilateral hearing loss. **Evoked Otoacoustic Emissions (EOAE)** can be performed on children of all ages. It measures cochlear function in response to a specific stimulus via a small probe which contains a microphone that is placed in the ear canal. This test can be used for newborn screening and can be performed in approximately 10 minutes. **Conventional audiometric testing** measures auditory thresholds in response to frequency-specific stimuli presented through earphones

---

Questions: Hearing Impairment

- Does the infant seem to respond to sounds?
- Does the infant attempt to repeat sounds?
- How does the young child indicate his/her desires or needs?
- How are the parents currently communicating with the child?
- Is there any evidence of a congenital infection, structural anomaly of the head and neck, or syndrome?
- Is there a history of prematurity or other prenatal or perinatal problem?
- Have there been any serious bacterial infections such as meningitis?
- Has the child had a history of repeated ear infections or exposure to ototoxic drugs?
- Aside from the hearing problem, is the child developmentally normal?
- Is there a family history of deafness, consanguinity, or multiple miscarriages or stillbirths?

TABLE 53–3.   Tests to Evaluate Hearing

Automated auditory brainstem response (ABR): used for newborn screening
Behavioral observation audiometry
Brainstem auditory evoked response (BAER)
Evoked otoacoustic emissions (EOAE): newer type of newborn screening
Conventional audiometric testing

---

to one ear at a time. The patient is instructed to perform a particular task, such as put a block in a container or raise his or her hand, when the stimulus is heard. Children as young as 4 or 5 years of age can usually be tested via conventional audiometric testing. These tests should be used in conjunction with audiologic and otolaryngologic consultations. In the case of high-risk infants, testing should be repeated at least every 6 months until 3 years of age, and at appropriate intervals thereafter depending on the etiology of the hearing loss and the hearing test results.

Other diagnostic tests to consider in infants whose cause of deafness is unknown include titers for congenital infections such as toxoplasmosis and rubella and fluorescent treponemal antibody absorption (FTA-ABS) tests for syphilis. There are a number of genetic syndromes in which hearing impairment is associated with other medical conditions. Thyroid function tests are used to rule out Pendred's syndrome in school-age children with goiters. One-third of affected children have an associated sensorineural hearing defect. Proteinuria and hematuria should also be ruled out by urine dipstick, especially in boys with a positive family history of deafness and renal failure, which is suggestive of Alport's syndrome. An electrocardiogram can be obtained to detect conduction defects such as QT prolongation in Jervell and Lange-Nielsen syndrome.

Imaging Studies

A renal ultrasound should be obtained in infants with pinna abnormalities. Occasionally, a CT or MRI scan of the temporal bone may be used to view the anatomy of the middle and inner ear, particularly in cases of a suspected cochlear/vestibular malformation or fistula.

MANAGEMENT

Studies have shown that the earlier the hearing loss is detected and rehabilitation begun in the otherwise normal infant, the greater the likelihood the child will have language development close to that of a hearing infant. School performance and the development of intelligible speech also have been shown to be better in those identified at a younger age.

Once infants or children are found to have a hearing impairment, careful follow-up is necessary so that no further hearing loss occurs. The role of primary care providers thus becomes even more crucial. Both parents and other family members may initially be devastated by the diagnosis of a hearing impairment, especially if the loss is severe to profound, and they probably will have multiple questions about children's medical prognosis and educational future. The possibility of further speech and language development may also be a foremost concern in their minds. In addition to providing patients with comprehensive care, all of the parents' questions and concerns must be addressed and anticipated.

Future Audiologic Evaluations

In newly diagnosed patients with sensorineural hearing loss, **audiograms** should be repeated every 3 months in the first year and then every 6 months when children are in preschool. The test should be repeated at least annually after children have begun school. Continued monitoring is essential to detect any progression of hearing loss, especially in the less affected ear.

Assistive Devices

Although **hearing aids** do not restore hearing, all children with conductive as well as sensorineural hearing loss benefit from amplification. Several different types of hearing aids are available for children; these devices should be fitted appropriately and adjusted regularly. In addition, it is also recommended that all patients receive bilateral hearing aids to improve auditory localization and training, particularly in the context of different learning situations. In reality, unfortunately, many children do not use bilateral hearing aids, either because their families do not have the necessary financial resources or because one is lost, damaged, or malfunctioning. **Closed-caption television** (signed or subtitled) is another method of auditory training. In addition, **teletype telephone systems** are available for children who can read.

At one time, **cochlear implants** were considered purely experimental and perhaps even dangerous because of a significant risk of permanent damage at implantation. However, they are currently being used in children with profound sensorineural hearing loss, particularly those who have acquired postlingual deafness. A majority of patients with implants show significant improvement in communication skills.

Education and Communication

Much controversy exists regarding the optimal method of communication for deaf children. **Oral communication (lip reading)** and **sign language** each have their advantages as well as disadvantages depending on children's age, the type of deafness, and whether the deficit is congenital or acquired. Whether the children already know a language is also important to consider. The preferred methods seem to vary from region to region; therefore schools, other institutions, and resource groups often use the most popular communication method in a particular area. In general, some authors recommend that children with minimal hearing loss may do better with lip reading than those with greater hearing loss who will most likely benefit more from sign language.

Whether to "mainstream" children with severe hearing loss in a regular classroom with an interpreter or place them in a school for deaf children is another controversial issue. Parents should be encouraged to explore the possibilities of each option and to make a decision based on the individual needs of their children and not current trends. The expertise of an educator who is knowledgeable in this field can also be helpful when making this decision.

Outside Resources and Referrals

Newly diagnosed children should be evaluated by **otolaryngologists** with pediatric experience, **audiologists,** pediatric **ophthalmologists** and medical **geneticists**. Any refractory error should be treated and followed closely, because children with severe hearing difficulties are so dependent on vision. A complete eye examination may also reveal retinal lesions that contribute to diagnosing the etiology of the hearing loss. A genetics evaluation is important for diagnostic reasons as well as for providing families with information and counseling about recurrence.

Support groups and referrals to national organizations for hearing impaired individuals can be valuable resources for parents and families. Resources for financial support should also be explored. Agencies with multidisciplinary teams are particularly important in infants or children with other associated handicaps.

PROGNOSIS

The goal of early recognition and treatment of hearing loss is to minimize the possible long-term sequelae of persistent speech and language problems. An additional goal is to prevent the development of learning disabilities. Most children, however, do well with early recognition and intervention, and learn to communicate using sign language, lip reading, or a combination of both methods.

Case Resolution

In the case presented at the beginning of the chapter, the child clearly has a hearing deficit. She does not turn to loud noises, she has not developed any specific words, and she indicates her needs nonverbally. Although there are no obvious historical risk factors for hearing loss, a behavioral audiogram or BAER should be performed. The physician's suspicion should be discussed with the family, and a follow-up visit should be arranged to review the hearing test results as soon as possible.

Selected Readings

Bachman, K. R., and J. C. Arvedson. Early identification and intervention for children who are hearing impaired. Pediatr. Rev. 19:155–165, 1998.

Brookhouser, P. E. Sensorineural hearing loss in children. Pediatr. Clin. North Am. 43:1195–1216, 1996.

Combs, J. T. Office screening for hearing loss. Contemp. Pediatr. 12:132–142, 1995.

Gerhardt, K. J. Prenatal and perinatal risks of hearing loss. Semin. Perinatol. 14:299–304, 1990.

Joint Committee on infant hearing 1994 position statement. Pediatrics 95:152–156, 1995.

Lotke, M. The sounds of silence. Contemp. Pediatrics 12:104–130, 1995.

Rapin, I. Hearing disorders. Pediatr. Rev. 14:43–49, 1993.

Roizen, N. J., and Diefendorf, A. O. (eds.). Hearing loss in children (entire issue). Ped. Clin. North Am. 46:1–166, 1999.

Schuman, A. J. Universal newborn hearing screening: the time is right. Contemp. Pediatr. 15:49–60, 1998.

U.S. Department of Health and Human Services. Early identification of hearing impairment in infants and young children. NIH Consensus Statement 11:1–20, 1993.

Wright, P. F., J. Thompson, and F. Bess. Hearing, speech, and language sequelae of otitis media with effusion. Pediatr. Ann. 20:617–621, 1991.

CHAPTER 54

SORE THROAT

Stanley H. Inkelis, M.D.

H$_x$
An 8-year-old girl has had a sore throat and fever for 2 days. She also has pain on swallowing, a headache, and a feeling of general malaise but no stridor, drooling, breathing difficulty, or rash. Other than the current illness, the girl is in good health. Although she has had sore throats in the past, she has never had one this severe. One week ago both her mother and father had a sore throat and fever that resolved after 5 days with no medication.

The child has a temperature of 102.2° F (39.0° C). The physical examination is normal except for red tonsils with exudate bilaterally, palatal petechiae, and tender cervical lymphadenopathy.

Questions

1. What are the causes of sore throat in children?
2. What is the appropriate evaluation of children with sore throat? What laboratory tests are necessary?
3. What is the appropriate management for children with sore throat?
4. When should otolaryngologic consultation be obtained?

Sore throat, one of the most common illnesses seen by the primary care physician, is a painful inflammation of the pharynx, tonsils, or surrounding areas. In most cases, children with sore throat have mild symptoms that require little or no treatment. However, sore throat may be the presenting complaint of a severe illness such as epiglottitis or retropharyngeal abscess. Small children are not able to define their complaints very well, which makes a careful history from parents or other care givers and a good physical examination essential for correct diagnosis. Optimal management of sore throat, especially if group A beta-hemolytic streptococcus is suspected, is still very controversial.

EPIDEMIOLOGY

Five percent of all pediatric visits are for pharyngitis. Sore throats are most common in children 5–8 years of age, and they continue to occur during later childhood. They are uncommon in children under 1 year of age. Like other respiratory infections, sore throats occur most often in the late fall and winter months. Approximately 11% of all school-age children receive medical care for pharyngitis. Fifteen to 20% or more of cases of pharyngitis in these children are caused by group A beta-hemolytic streptococcus.

The organisms that cause bacterial and viral pharyngitis, are present in saliva and nasal secretions and are almost always transmitted by close contact. Spread from child to child in school is the common mode of transmission.

CLINICAL PRESENTATION

The clinical presentation of sore throat is variable and often depends on etiology (D$_x$ Box and see Differential

D$_x$ **Sore Throat**

VIRAL
- Pain in throat
- Fever (variable)*
- Rhinorrhea (common)
- Cough (common)
- Erythema of pharynx or tonsils
- Follicular, ulcerative, exudative lesions of pharynx or tonsils*

BACTERIAL
- Pain in throat
- Fever
- Marked erythema of pharynx, tonsils, or uvula
- Tonsillar and posterior pharyngeal wall exudate
- Tender, swollen cervical lymphadenopathy
- Positive rapid antigen test or throat culture

*Dependent on etiology (see Differential Diagnosis).

Diagnosis). Most children with sore throat present with sudden onset of pain and fever. The height of the fever is variable and is typically higher in younger children. In older children, especially if the sore throat is associated with a common cold, fever is minimal or absent. The throat or tonsils are red, and the breath may be malodorous. Headache, nausea, vomiting, and abdominal pain may occur, especially if children are febrile. The appetite may be decreased. Children may be less active than usual.

In children with the common cold, rhinorrhea and postnasal discharge are present. A pharyngeal and tonsillar exudate is not typical. Although the cervical lymph nodes may be enlarged, they are usually not very tender. In contrast, children with streptococcal pharyngitis typically have high fever, pharyngeal and tonsillar exudate, and tender cervical lymph nodes.

PATHOPHYSIOLOGY

Various bacterial and viral organisms lead to sore throat by causing inflammation in the ring of posterior pharyngeal lymphoid tissue that consists of the tonsils, adenoids, and surrounding lymphoid tissue. This ring of tissue, called Waldeyer's ring, drains the oral and pharyngeal cavity and defends against infection of the mouth and throat. Other host defenses that protect against infection include the sneeze, gag and cough reflexes, secretory IgA, and a rich blood supply.

Viral sore throats may be acquired by inhalation or self-inoculation from the nasal mucosa or conjunctiva. The local respiratory epithelium becomes infected with the virus, and inflammation occurs. In some instances, inflammatory mediators may be responsible for the pain of sore throat. Group A streptococcus and other bacterial organisms directly invade the mucous membranes. Enzymes produced by this organism, streptolysin O and hyaluronidase, aid in the spread of infection.

DIFFERENTIAL DIAGNOSIS

Although most children who present with sore throat have common viral or bacterial pharyngitis, other less common disorders such as infectious mononucleosis, epiglottitis, retropharyngeal abscess, or peritonsillar abscess should be considered.

Viral Infection

Viral infection, the most common cause of sore throat in children, is most often associated with a URI caused by a rhinovirus. Cough and rhinorrhea associated with a sore throat suggest this etiology.

Adenovirus often leads to exudative pharyngitis, frequently in children less than 3 years old. Pharyngoconjunctival fever, caused by adenovirus 3, is characterized by a high fever (temperature: >102.2° F [39.0° C]) for several days, conjunctivitis, and exudative tonsillitis.

Coxsackie virus and **echovirus** (enteroviruses) are the usual cause of herpangina. Vesicles and ulcers are generally apparent on the anterior tonsillar pillars and soft palate. They may also be found on the tonsils,

pharynx, or posterior buccal mucosa. Children may have a high fever (temperature: >102.2° F [39.0° C]), irritability, and refuse to eat or drink; dehydration may result. Coxsackie virus A16 causes hand-foot-and-mouth disease, which is characterized by ulcerative oral lesions on the tongue and buccal mucosa and, less frequently, on the palate and anterior tonsillar pillars. Vesicular and papulovesicular lesions are evident on the hands and feet and occasionally on other parts of the body. Enteroviral infections typically occur in the late spring, summer, and early fall.

Herpes simplex virus (HSV) may lead to pharyngotonsillitis but can be distinguished from most of the enteroviral infections because HSV almost always involves the anterior portion of the mouth and lips, and is associated with a gingivitis (herpes gingivostomatitis). The lesions often appear as whitish-yellow plaques with an erythematous base, and are sometimes ulcerative. This illness is characterized by a high fever (temperature: 102.2° F [39.0° C]) for up to 7–10 days and frequent refusal to eat or drink because of the painful lesions. Dehydration may occur.

Epstein-Barr virus (EBV) may cause exudative pharyngotonsillitis either alone or as part of the infectious mononucleosis syndrome that includes fever, malaise, lymphadenopathy, and hepatosplenomegaly.

Bacterial Infection

Group A beta-hemolytic streptococcus is the most common cause of bacterial sore throat in children over 3 years of age. The pharynx is typically very red and sometimes edematous, and the tonsils are red, enlarged, and covered with exudate. Occasionally, the uvula is very inflamed as well. Children may also have dysphagia, fever, vomiting, headache, malaise, and abdominal pain. Swollen anterior cervical lymphadenopathy and petechiae on the soft palate and uvula are usually apparent. In addition, the occurrence of a scarlatiniform rash, "strawberry tongue," and Pastia's lines (petechiae in the flexor skin creases of joints) indicates scarlet fever, which is diagnostic of Group A streptococcal infection (see Chapter 101, Maculopapular Rashes). Sore throat from group A beta-hemolytic streptococcus typically occurs in the winter and spring. Rheumatic fever and glomerulonephritis are nonsuppurative complications of group A streptococcal infection.

Peritonsillar abscess or cellulitis and cervical lymphadenitis are suppurative complications of group A beta-hemolytic streptococcus. Children with peritonsillar abscess often experience trismus and drooling and speak with a "hot potato" voice. The abscess in the affected tonsil causes a bulge in the posterior soft palate and pushes the uvula away from the midline to the unaffected side of the pharynx. On palpation, the abscess may feel fluctuant. Peritonsillar cellulitis typically produces a bulge in the soft palate but does not cause deviation of the uvula.

Group B, C, and G beta-hemolytic streptococci (non-group A beta-hemolytic streptococci) have all been isolated from children with pharyngitis. *Streptococcus pneumoniae* and *Arcanobacterium haemolyticum* infrequently cause pharyngitis in children. The latter organism is associated with a scarlatiniform rash in some patients and is most common in adolescents and young adults. Although *Corynebacterium diphtheriae* (diphtheria) rarely causes sore throat in immunized children, this organism should be considered in nonimmunized children who have exudative pharyngotonsillitis and a grayish pseudomembrane that bleeds when removal is attempted.

Chlamydia trachomatis may lead to pharyngitis and tonsillitis in adolescents and young adults, through sexual transmission. The role of *Chlamydia pneumoniae* as a cause of sore throat in children remains unclear. *Mycoplasma pneumoniae* does not usually produce sore throat in children unless they have lower respiratory tract disease. *Neisseria gonorrhoeae* may lead to sore throat in sexually active adolescents. Its occurrence in prepubertal children is often secondary to sexual abuse. The appearance of the throat is not characteristic, and diagnosis is made by cultures when the degree of suspicion is high. **Tularemia** is a rare cause of exudative pharyngitis in children but should be suspected if contact with wild animals has occurred.

Other Causes

Candida albicans may be responsible for sore throat in infants and in children who are immunocompromised or taking antibiotics. Children with oral candidiasis usually present with whitish plaques on the labial or buccal mucosa that do not wipe off easily. When the pharynx and tonsils are involved, some discomfort or dysphagia, but usually not significant pain, may occur.

Retropharyngeal abscess typically occurs in children less than 4 years of age. Sore throat is associated with this condition, but it is usually more evident when swallowing. Fever, refusal to swallow, drooling, stridor, and meningismus in toxic-appearing children suggest this diagnosis.

Epiglottitis (supraglottitis), may present as sore throat. This condition typically affects children 2–7 years of age who present with signs of toxicity, stridor, difficulty swallowing, and drooling. In relatively well-appearing children with sore throat but no stridor, neither epiglottitis nor retropharyngeal abscess is a likely cause of sore throat. In the past, epiglottis was almost always caused by *Haemophilus influenzae* type b. With the widespread use of the *H influenzae* type b (Hib) conjugate vaccine, this organism is now rarely the etiology. *S pneumoniae*, *Staphylococcus aureus* and group A, B, and C beta-hemolytic streptococci are unusual but reported causative agents of epiglottitis.

Children with croup may have sore throat and stridor, but they do not usually appear toxic and do not have difficulty swallowing. Affected children are usually between 6 months and 3 years of age (see Chapter 38, Stridor and Croup).

Trauma from penetrating objects, burns, or exposure to caustic materials may cause sore throat in children. Household smoking may also lead to pharyngeal irritation. In addition, allergic rhinitis with postnasal drip may result in sore throat. Tumor rarely causes sore throat in children but should be considered if a mass is present or pharyngeal inflammation persists. Persistent sore throat may also be a symptom of Kawasaki disease.

EVALUATION

History

A thorough history often reveals the etiology of the sore throat (Questions Box). Questions regarding duration, fever, headache, vomiting, pain on swallowing, rash, oral lesions, abdominal pain, and history of contact with other family members or classmates with similar symptoms suggest the most common causes of sore throat (infections with viruses and group A beta-hemolytic streptococcus). A history of rapid onset of fever, toxicity, difficulty swallowing, drooling, and respiratory distress suggest epiglottitis and retropharyngeal abscess. Voice changes suggest peritonsillar abscess or tonsillar hypertrophy associated with infectious mononucleosis (EBV). Immunization history or history of immigration from a developing country helps assess the risk of diphtheria. Oral sexual activity suggests the possibility of an STD. A history of allergies, trauma, and environmental smoke may help diagnose other causes of sore throat. Red or pink eye with a rash, persistent fever (>5 days), and sore throat suggest Kawasaki disease.

Physical Examination

A general physical examination should be performed. It is important to note whether children appear toxic. The skin should be examined for a scarlatiniform, sandpaper-like rash, a vesicular rash involving the hands and feet, or a generalized maculopapular rash. The eyes should be evaluated for conjunctivitis and the nose for rhinorrhea (serous or purulent). The mouth, pharynx, and tonsils should be examined for vesicular lesions, ulcers, and gingivitis. The pharynx should be checked for redness, exudate, vesicles, edema, and foreign bodies. The tonsils and uvula should be examined for these same findings as well as asymmetry, and the neck should be checked for nuchal rigidity. The lymph nodes should be evaluated for enlargement

---

Questions: Sore Throat

- How long has the child had a sore throat?
- Does the child have fever, headache, or vomiting?
- How rapid was the onset of fever?
- Does the child have pain on swallowing?
- Are there any voice changes?
- Does the child have a rash or oral lesions?
- Does the child have abdominal pain?
- Does the child have any ill contacts?
- Are the child's immunizations up-to-date?
- Is the child having any difficulty breathing?
- Does the child have a history of allergies?
- Has the child suffered any trauma to the throat or neck?
- Has the child been exposed to environmental smoke?
- (For sexually active adolescents or children with a history of sexual abuse with nonresponding sore throats) Has there been any oral sexual activity?

(adenopathy) and inflammation (adenitis). The abdomen should be examined for hepatosplenomegaly.

Laboratory Tests

Although many signs and symptoms may suggest streptococcal pharyngitis, diagnosis can be confirmed only with laboratory tests. The **throat culture** is the "gold standard" for diagnosis. However, it has a false-negative rate of 10% and a false-positive rate of up to 50%, because streptococcal carriers are not infected with the organism at the time they present with sore throat. Nevertheless, throat culture is the most reliable way to confirm streptococcal infection.

Rapid streptococcal antigen detection tests are available for "on-the-spot" diagnosis. False-positive results are uncommon (specificity: 95% or greater), but false-negative results for the most rapid antigen tests occur commonly (sensitivity: 80–90%). Because a negative test may not exclude a streptococcal infection, it is currently recommended that this result should be confirmed by throat culture. However, newer rapid antigen detection tests using optical immunoassay (OIA) and chemiluminescent DNA may be as sensitive as throat cultures. Recent data suggest that a negative OIA rapid streptococcal antigen detection test may not always need routine confirmation with a throat culture. An antistreptolysin-O titer and an anti-DNAase-B titer may help diagnose a recent streptococcal infection if the throat culture is negative.

Differentiating between viral and bacterial pharyngitis is often difficult, and the rapid streptococcal antigen tests and throat cultures should be reserved for patients who have signs and symptoms common for both illnesses. For example, afebrile children with a sore throat, runny nose, and cough who have slight pharyngeal erythema almost certainly have viral pharyngitis and do not need further workup. On the other hand, children with fever, exudative tonsillitis, red pharynx and tonsils, or exposure to an individual with streptococcal pharyngitis may need further confirmation by rapid streptococcal antigen detection test or throat culture to determine if the pharyngitis is bacterial.

Viral throat cultures and acute and convalescent titers to determine viral pharyngitis are rarely indicated unless systemic infection occurs (e.g., herpes encephalitis). EBV infection can be determined by specific serologic assays, but a heterophil agglutination test is the test of choice for diagnosing infectious mononucleosis. However, it may be negative in children younger than 4 years of age or early in the course of the infection. Only 75% of infected children between 2 and 4 years of age are identified by this test, and less than 30% of children under 2 years of age are identified. The monospot test, a rapid slide test for heterophil antibodies, may remain positive for months after the infection and may suggest the diagnosis of infectious mononucleosis in children who do not have this disorder. A CBC with more than 50–60% lymphocytes or more than 10% atypical lymphocytes is suggestive of mononucleosis.

Culture or fluorescent antibody evaluation of the pseudomembrane may be used to diagnose diphtheria.

Culture or presence of serum agglutinins confirms tularemia. Thayer-Martin culture plates should be used to diagnose suspected gonorrheal sore throat.

Imaging Studies

If epiglottitis or retropharyngeal abscess is suspected but is not clinically apparent, a lateral neck x-ray may be obtained. The x-ray should be performed with a physician in attendance who is capable of performing endotracheal intubation in case the child has respiratory difficulties (see Chapter 38, Stridor and Croup).

MANAGEMENT

The management of children with sore throat is based on the etiology of the condition. The early recognition of potentially serious conditions based on history and physical examination is essential to providing optimal care. **Otolaryngologic consultation** should be obtained in children with peritonsillar abscess, retropharyngeal abscess, epiglottitis, significant pharyngeal trauma, or pharyngeal tumor. Recurrent tonsillitis, especially in children who miss school, may be a reason for referral to an otolaryngologist.

Outpatient Treatment

In most cases of children with sore throat, the physician must differentiate between viral and streptococcal pharyngitis. Viral sore throat can be managed symptomatically. Treatment of pain and discomfort with **analgesics** and maintenance of **hydration** are the mainstays of therapy for young children with viral sore throat. Gargling with warm water and sucking on hard candy may provide additional symptomatic relief for older children.

The pain from lesions of herpes stomatitis sometimes responds to acetaminophen. For those children with persistent pain, acetaminophen with codeine may be helpful. **Anesthetics** such as lidocaine may also decrease the pain. Lidocaine can be placed on a gloved finger and applied directly on the oral lesions of the tongue, labial, and buccal mucosa. It is best used about 30 minutes before feeding or drinking, especially in children who refuse to drink. Lidocaine should be used cautiously because it can suppress the gag reflex. The dose should never exceed 3 mg/kg/dose. Too much lidocaine may result in seizures. Antacids to coat the mucosa or a mixture (1 part each) of lidocaine, diphenhydramine (Benadryl), and kaolin-pectin (Kaopectate), either gargled or applied are alternative analgesics.

In children without clear-cut evidence of streptococcal pharyngitis, a positive rapid streptococcal antigen test helps direct antibiotic treatment. A negative test in the presence of positive symptoms should be accompanied by a throat culture. However, the OIA rapid test may preclude the need for culture confirmation. Patients can await the results of culture before beginning antibiotic therapy. **Antibiotics** are indicated in children without confirmation from rapid streptococcal tests or cultures, who appear toxic, who have scarlet fever or peritonsillar cellulitis/abscess, or who have a past history of rheumatic fever. Most evidence suggests that early treatment results in more rapid clinical improvement, although this is controversial. The experienced physician may treat children with antibiotics on clinical grounds alone. Rheumatic fever can be prevented if treatment is started within 9 days of sore throat symptom development. Glomerulonephritis probably is not affected by antibiotic therapy.

Children with streptococcal pharyngitis should be treated with antibiotics to relieve symptoms; shorten the course of their illness; and prevent disease dissemination, suppurative complications, and rheumatic fever. Penicillin is the antibiotic of choice. It may be administered orally as penicillin V (phenoxymethyl penicillin) in a dose of 250 mg two to three times a day for 10 days for children and 500 mg two to three times a day for adolescents and adults. Most patients will feel better after 2–3 days, but it is important to stress to parents that their children need to complete the full 10-day course. Amoxicillin, which tastes better, is frequently used to treat streptococcal pharyngitis, but offers no bacteriologic advantage over penicillin.

If the risk of noncompliance is high or if the risk of complication is great (e.g., children have a history of rheumatic fever), the penicillin should be administered intramuscularly. Intramuscular penicillin has two disadvantages: (1) pain associated with the injection and (2) increased incidence of a potentially more severe allergic reaction. The dose of benzathine penicillin for children weighing less than 60 lb (27.3 kg) is 600,000 U. The dose for larger children and adults is 1,200,000 U. Bicillin CR, which contains 900,000 U of benzathine penicillin and 300,000 U of procaine penicillin, is the preferable form of delivering penicillin intramuscularly in children because it causes less pain and less severe local reaction. This preparation has not been determined to be effective in heavier patients (adolescents and adults) and therefore the benzathine preparation noted above is recommended. The injection of benzathine penicillin is less painful if it is given after it reaches room temperature. (See Table 54–1 for dosage information). Erythromycin may be substituted in children who are allergic to penicillin. A first-generation oral cephalosporin is also an acceptable alternative. Some of the newer macrolides, clarithromycin and azithromycin, offer the benefit of less gastrointestinal side effects than erythromycin. Azithromycin has the added advantage of once-a-day dosing and a shortened course of therapy of only 5 days. Tetracyclines and sulfonamides are not recommended for the treatment of streptococcal pharyngitis.

Recent studies have shown that a 5-day course of many of the oral cephalosporins, including cefpodoxime proxetil, cefadroxil, and cefuroxime axetil, may be used in place of penicillin with equal efficacy. These agents are more costly, have a broader microbiologic spectrum, and are therefore not recommended as first-line therapy. These antibiotics, however, may be beneficial in children with recurrent streptococcal tonsillopharyngitis, especially those in whom compliance is an issue.

TABLE 54–1. Antibiotics Used in the Management of Sore Throat in Children

Drug (for Streptococcal Pharyngitis)	Dosage
Penicillin V	250 mg x 2–3/d for children and 500 mg x 2–3/d for adolescents PO for 10 days
Benzathine penicillin	600,000 U (<27 kg or 60 lb); 1.2 million U (>27 kg or 60 lb) as single IM injection
Bicillin CR	900,000 U benzathine penicillin and 300,000 U procaine penicillin for children as single IM injection
Erythromycin estolate	20–40 mg/kg/d in 2–4 divided doses PO for 10 days
Erythromycin ethyl succinate	40 mg/kg/d in 2–4 divided doses PO for 10 days
Clarithromycin	15 mg/kg/d in 2 divided doses PO for 10 days
Azithromycin	12 mg/kg/d, once a day PO for 5 days (1 hr before or 2 hrs after a meal)
Cefadroxil*	30 mg/kg/d, in 2 divided doses PO for 5 days
Cefuroxime axetil*	20 mg/kg/d, in 2 divided doses PO for 4–5 days
Cefpodoxime proxetil	10 mg/kg/d, in 2 divided doses PO for 5 days
Rifampin	10 mg/kg/dose PO q12h for 4 days (started with benzathine penicillin or bicillin CR for chronic streptococcal carriers)
Clindamycin	20 mg/kg/d in 3 divided doses (maximum 450 mg/d) PO for 10 days (for chronic streptococcal carriers)
Drug (for Gonococcal Pharyngitis)	**Dosage**
Ceftriaxone	125 mg (45 kg or <100 lb) IM in a single dose
	250 mg (45 kg or ≥100 lb) IM in a single dose
Plus Erythromycin	40 mg/kg/d (maximum 2 g/d) PO q6h for 7 days
or Azithromycin	20 mg/kg (maximum 1 g) PO in a single dose
or (if ≥9 yrs) Doxycycline	100 mg PO 2 times a day for 7 days

*Short course regimen not FDA approved as yet

Many children are asymptomatic carriers of group A streptococci. In general, these children do well, and eradication of the bacteria is not necessary. Cultures after treatment are generally not recommended, except for children with recurring or persistent symptoms or those with a previous history of rheumatic fever. If cultures remain positive, these children may be treated with benzathine penicillin and oral rifampin for 4 days in an attempt to eradicate the organism (see Table 54–1 for dosages). Clindamycin may be more effective in eradication of the organism from symptom-free carriers (see Table 54–1 for dosages).

M. pneumoniae pharyngitis is usually associated with a generalized infection. Because it is often a self-limited illness, it does not require antibiotic therapy unless symptoms persist. Erythromycin (30–50 mg/kg/day) is the drug of choice. Clarithromycin and azithromycin are costlier alternatives which have fewer side effects and are likely to produce better compliance.

Diphtheria is a life-threatening infection that requires prompt diagnosis and treatment. Penicillin G or erythromycin must be given to kill *C. diphtheriae* and, in addition, equine antitoxin must be administered to neutralize the exotoxin. Tularemia is treated with streptomycin or gentamicin.

For gonococcal pharyngitis caused by *N. gonorrhoeae,* intramuscular ceftriaxone is the drug of choice (see Table 54–1 for dosages). Oral doxycycline or azithromycin should also be given to children 9 years of age or older to cover associated *C. trachomatis* infection (see Table 54–1 for dosages). Erythromycin or azithromycin may be used for younger children. Children should be examined and cultured for STDs in other sites and should have a serologic test for syphilis at the first visit and have a repeat test 6–8 weeks later. They should also be evaluated for concurrent hepatitis B and HIV infection. Sexual abuse should be considered in all cases of gonococcal pharyngitis, particularly in prepubertal children. (See Chapter 76, Sexually Transmitted Diseases, and Chapter 105, Child Sexual Abuse.)

Children with croup usually respond to cool mist. Oral nystatin can be used in children with oral candidiasis. Adolescents with uncomplicated peritonsillar abscess may be managed as outpatients in selected cases with needle aspiration and oral antibiotics.

Inpatient Treatment

Children with sore throat should be admitted to the hospital if they have airway obstruction or need intravenous hydration or antibiotics. Children with retropharyngeal abscess and epiglottitis require intravenous antibiotics. Preadolescent children or adolescents with complicated peritonsillar abscess also require intravenous antibiotics. Incision and drainage is indicated if the abscess is fluctuant, the child is toxic, or if there is no resolution within 48 hours. Needle aspiration may be acceptable in selected cases. Intravenous hydration is occasionally needed for patients with severe herpes stomatitis who will not drink because of pain and who become dehydrated.

The role of tonsillectomy in recurrent sore throat is still controversial. Indications are not clearly defined, and in many cases, surgery is not indicated.

Education

Both patients and families should receive general education about sore throats. Medication for pain with drugs such as acetaminophen or ibuprofen is useful, especially if children are having difficulty swallowing. Gargling with warm salt water or sucking on hard candy may soothe the pain of sore throat. Children with bacterial pharyngitis may return to school after 24 hours of antibiotic therapy and the disappearance of fever. The practitioner should recommend that symptomatic family members see a physician. Parents should call or return to the physician if their children have respiratory or swallowing difficulties, drooling, severe pain, or fever (temperature: >101.0° F [38.3° C]) for more than 48 hours after the initiation of appropriate antibiotics.

PROGNOSIS

The prognosis for children with viral sore throat is excellent because of its self-limited nature. The outlook for children with streptococcal sore throat is also excellent. If the infection is not diagnosed and treated appropriately, however, suppurative (e.g., peritonsillar abscess) and nonsuppurative complications (e.g., rheumatic fever, acute glomerulonephritis) may occur. With early diagnosis and prompt treatment, the prognosis for unusual, life-threatening causes of sore throat is also very good.

Case Resolution

In the case presented, the child has palatal petechiae and tonsillar exudate, which are signs and symptoms consistent with streptococcal pharyngitis. A rapid streptococcal antigen detection test or throat culture should be performed, and if positive, the child should be treated accordingly. If the test is negative and the child is ill-appearing, treatment may be started and either continued or stopped, depending on the results of the throat culture. Parents who have sore throat symptoms should be evaluated with a rapid streptococcal detection test or throat culture. If either test is positive, the parent should be treated with antibiotics.

EBV infection can present in a similar manner. If the child continues to be ill after a negative throat culture, workup for EBV should be considered.

Selected Readings

American Academy of Pediatrics. Group A streptococcal infections. *In* Peter, G., ed. 1997 Red Book: Report of the Committee of Infectious Diseases. 24th ed. Elk Grove Village, IL. American Academy of Pediatrics, 1997, pp. 483–494.

Barkin, R. M., and P. Rosen. Pharyngotonsillitis (sore throat). *In* Barkin, R. M., and P. Rosen (eds.). Emergency Pediatrics, 5th ed. St. Louis, Mosby, 1999, pp. 604–608.

Bisno, A. L. Acute pharyngitis: etiology and diagnosis. Pediatrics 97(suppl.):949–954, 1996.

Cherry, J. D. Pharyngitis (pharyngitis, tonsillitis, tonsillopharyngitis, and nasopharyngitis). *In* Feigen, R. D., and J. D. Cherry (eds.). Textbook of Pediatric Infectious Diseases, 4th ed., Philadelphia, W. B. Saunders, 1998, pp. 148–156.

Dajani, A. S. Current therapy of group A streptococcal pharyngitis. Pediatr. Ann. 27:277–280, 1998.

Dajani, A., et al. Treatment of acute streptococcal pharyngitis and prevention of rheumatic fever: a statement for health professionals. Pediatrics 96:758–764, 1995.

Gerber, M. A. Diagnosis of group A streptococcal pharyngitis. Pediatr. Ann. 27:269–273, 1998.

Koomson, B., and D. M. Jaffe. Pharyngeal disease. *In* Reisdorf, E. J., M. R. Roberts, and J. G. Wiegenstein. Pediatric Emergency Medicine, Philadelphia, W. B. Saunders, 1993, pp. 623–628.

Niederman, L. G., and J. F. Marcinak. Sore throat. *In* Dershewitz, R. A. (ed.). Ambulatory Pediatric Care, 3rd ed. Philadelphia, J. B. Lippincott, 1999, pp. 482–485.

Pichichero, M. E. Sore throat after sore throat after sore throat. Are you asking the critical questions? Postgrad. Med. 101:205–225, 1997.

Pichichero, M. E. Group A streptococcal tonsillopharyngitis: Cost effective diagnosis and treatment. Ann. Emerg. Med. 25:390–403, 1995.

Shulman, S. T. Evaluation of penicillins, cephalosporins, and macrolides for therapy of streptococcal pharyngitis. Pediatrics 97(suppl.):955–959, 1996.

Tanz, R. R., and S. T. Shulman. Streptococcal pharyngitis: The carrier state, definition and management. Pediatr. Ann. 27:277–280, 1998.

CHAPTER 55

NOSEBLEEDS

Stanley H. Inkelis, M.D.

H$_x$ A 3-year-old boy is brought to the office one winter day. He has had four nosebleeds in the past week as well as a cold with a runny nose and cough, which began the day before the first nosebleed. The nosebleeds occurred either at night or during sleep and stopped spontaneously or with gentle pressure. Other than the cold and nosebleeds, the boy is in good health. He is active, with bruises over both tibias but none elsewhere. The many cuts and scrapes he has had in the past resulted in minimal bleeding. His family has no history of a bleeding disorder or easy bruisability.

The child's physical examination is entirely normal, except for a small amount of blood in the left anterior naris.

Questions

1. What are the common causes of nosebleeds in children?
2. What systemic diseases are associated with nosebleeds?
3. How should nosebleeds be evaluated in children?
4. How should minor and severe nosebleeds be managed in children?

Nosebleed, or epistaxis, occurs commonly in children, especially in those between the ages of 2 and 10 years. In most cases, nosebleeds are secondary to local trauma and can be cared for by primary care physicians. In rare instances, however, a nosebleed may be difficult to control or may be a manifestation of a serious systemic illness. Referral to an otolaryngologist or a hematologist/oncologist is usually not required except in these situations, and hospitalization is generally unnecessary. Parents and children, who are often frightened by nosebleeds, frequently overestimate the amount of blood lost. Understanding and reassurance are important in allaying anxiety.

EPIDEMIOLOGY

Thirty percent of children have one nosebleed by the time they are 5 years of age. In children between the ages of 6 and 10, the frequency increases to 56%. Nosebleeds are rare in infancy and infrequent after puberty. They occur much more frequently in the late fall and winter months, when URIs are common, environmental humidity is relatively low, and the use of heating systems results in dryness. Nosebleeds are also more common in children who live in dry climates, especially if they have a URI or allergic rhinitis.

CLINICAL PRESENTATION

Most children with nosebleeds have a history of bleeding at home and have minimal or no bleeding at the time of presentation (D$_x$ Box). With anterior nosebleeds, blood exits almost entirely from the anterior portion of the nose. With posterior nosebleeds, most of the bleeding occurs in the nasopharynx and mouth, although some blood exits through the nose as well. Posterior nosebleeds are heavier and more difficult to control, and children may present in a hemodynamically unstable condition.

Children with bleeding disorders may have recurrent nosebleeds and a history of prolonged bleeding, easy bruisability, or multiple bruises in unlikely locations. In unusual situations, children with GI or respiratory tract bleeding may present with blood exiting through the nose. Alternatively, some children who present with hematemesis have vomited swallowed nasal blood.

PATHOPHYSIOLOGY

Nosebleeds may be either anterior or posterior in origin. The large majority of nosebleeds in children (90%) are anterior and are more easily controlled than posterior nosebleeds. The anteroinferior portion of the nasal septum, about 0.5 cm from the tip of the nose, known as Kiesselbach's plexus or Little's area, is the

---

D$_x$ Nosebleeds

- Blood in anterior nares, nasopharynx, or mouth
- History of any of the following:
  - Frequent digital manipulation (nose picking)
  - URI (recent)
  - Allergic rhinitis
  - Dry climate
  - Foreign body in nose
  - Trauma to nose
  - Prolonged or difficult to stop bleeding or easy bruisability
- Physical examination consistent with any of the following:
  - Rhinorrhea
  - Dry, cracked nasal mucosa
  - Foreign body in nose
  - Trauma to nose
  - Multiple bruises

most common part of the nose involved in anterior nosebleeds. This area is supplied by the anterior and posterior ethmoidal arteries, the sphenopalatine artery, and the septal branches of the superior labial artery (Fig. 55–1). The mucosa covering the area is thin and friable, and the small vessels supplying the nasal mucous membrane have little structural support. Congestion of the vessels caused by conditions such as a URI or drying of the mucosa from low environmental humidity makes this area susceptible to bleeding.

Posterior nosebleeds generally arise from the turbinate or nasal wall. Significant bleeding, usually from a branch of the sphenopalatine artery, may occur.

DIFFERENTIAL DIAGNOSIS

Trauma from nose picking and **inflammation** of the nasal mucosa from a URI are by far the most common causes of nosebleeds in children. Repetitive, habitual nose picking results in the formation of friable granulation tissue that bleeds when traumatized (epistaxis digitorum). Mucosal inflammation predisposes children to bleeding because of erosion of congested blood vessels. As the nasal mucosa dries, it may lead to crust formation and cracking. Bleeding may occur spontaneously, but more often it results from forceful nose blowing and sneezing that increases venous pressure in the more vascularized nasal septum.

Viral respiratory infections, such as measles, infectious mononucleosis, and influenza, may also predispose children to nosebleeds because of their local inflammatory effect. Nosebleeds in children with these infections are more common in areas of low environmental humidity. Many children with no URI-like symptoms also suffer from nosebleeds in such environments, usually in winter, when inhaling dry hot air from heating systems causes desiccation of the nasal mucosa (rhinitis sicca). **Allergic rhinitis** with inflammation and subsequent drying may also lead to nosebleeds. Children with allergic rhinitis who take decongestants may be more likely to suffer from nosebleeds.

Foreign bodies may cause direct trauma or pressure necrosis to the vessels of the nasal mucosa. **External trauma** can cause either tears to the nasal mucosa or nasal fractures. If bleeding from mucosal vessels occurs but the mucosa remains intact, a septal hematoma may develop. Abscess formation or septal perforation may occur if the septal hematoma is not drained.

Although nosebleeds are usually benign conditions, they may be the first sign of serious illness. Persistent or recurrent nosebleeds with no obvious cause should raise the suspicion of **bleeding disorders.** Thrombocytopenia is the most common coagulation defect causing nosebleeds. Idiopathic thrombocytopenic purpura is the most frequent thrombocytopenic disorder associated with nosebleeds. Leukemia, aplastic anemia, and

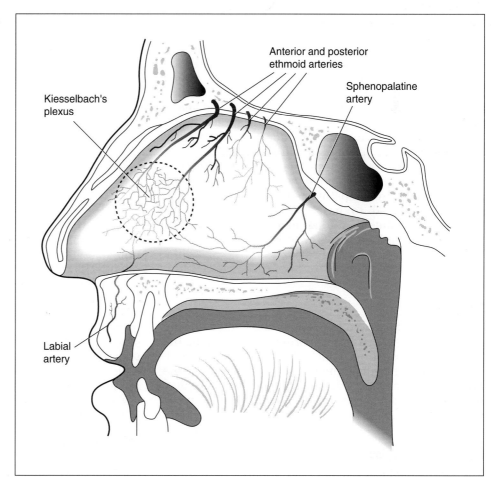

FIGURE 55–1. Vascular supply of nasal septum. Note the confluence of vessels that forms Kiesselbach's plexus.

Anterior and posterior ethmoid arteries

Sphenopalatine artery

Kiesselbach's plexus

Labial artery

HIV infection must be strongly considered and ruled out in children with nosebleeds and thrombocytopenia.

The most commonly inherited bleeding disorder associated with nosebleeds is von Willebrand's disease, an autosomal dominant bleeding disorder characterized by varying degrees of factor VIII deficiency and platelet dysfunction (decreased platelet adhesiveness). Hemophilia (factor VIII, IX, or XI deficiency) and Glanzmann's thrombasthenia are other inherited bleeding disorders that may lead to nosebleeds. Hepatic disease, severe vitamin K deficiency, or malabsorption syndrome is associated with an acquired coagulopathy, which may present with nosebleed.

Nosebleeds may be a manifestation of **blood vessel disorders,** either hereditary or acquired. Osler-Weber-Rendu syndrome (hereditary hemorrhagic telangiectasia) is an inherited autosomal dominant disease with multiple mucosal telangiectasias, especially in the nose. Because telangiectasias are deficient in muscular and connective tissue, these telangiectasias may rupture spontaneously and bleed profusely. An acquired blood vessel disorder, from vitamin C deficiency is a rare cause of nosebleeds.

Neoplasms, particularly malignancies, are uncommon causes of nosebleeds in children. Polyps are usually present in association with cystic fibrosis or allergies. Capillary, cavernous, and mixed hemangiomas may occur in the nose. Juvenile nasopharyngeal angiofibroma occurs almost exclusively in adolescent males, who present with nasal obstruction and bleeding. Rhabdomyosarcomas, lymphomas, and squamous cell carcinomas of the nose, sinuses, or nasopharynx are rare causes of nosebleeds.

Drugs such as aspirin and NSAIDs, which interfere with platelet function, and warfarin and heparin, which inhibit clotting factors, increase the risk of nasal hemorrhage with minor trauma, infection, or inflammation. Accidental ingestion of these medications should be suspected if they are available. Cocaine snorting may cause nasal septal perforation and nosebleeds.

Hypertension is rarely associated with nosebleeds in children. Wegener's granulomatosis and lethal midline granuloma are rare idiopathic inflammatory diseases in children that lead to nasal tissue destruction and bleeding. Nosebleeds during menstruation may be secondary to endometriosis with ectopic endometrial tissue implants in the nasal cavity.

EVALUATION

History

A thorough history often reveals the etiology of the nosebleed (Questions Box). Information concerning the side of the nose from which the bleeding occurred, the amount of bleeding, the measures used to stop the bleeding, and the time required to stop the bleeding may be helpful to quickly assess the severity of the nosebleed.

Physical Examination

A general physical examination should be performed. In children with significant blood loss, particular atten-

---

Questions: Nosebleeds

- Does the child pick his or her nose?
- Has the child suffered any trauma recently?
- Has the child recently had a URI?
- Has the child recently had any systemic viral or bacterial illness?
- Does the child have any allergies?
- Is the child exposed to dry conditions (e.g., dry climate, dry heat, dehumidified air)?
- Has the child put or tried to put foreign objects in his or her nose?
- Is there a history of easy bruisability or prolonged, difficult-to-stop bleeding in the child or family?
- Does the child or anyone in the family use any aspirin, aspirin-containing medications, NSAIDs, or warfarin?
- Which side of the nose was bleeding?
- How extensive was the bleeding?
- Did the child spit out or swallow blood? Was there blood in the mouth?
- What measures were used to stop the bleeding? How long did it take to stop the bleeding?
- Was this the first nosebleed? If the nosebleeds are recurrent, how often do they occur and how long do they last?

---

tion should be directed toward the mental status and vital signs to determine hemodynamic stability. If vital signs are normal, these children should also be evaluated for orthostatic changes. If the blood pressure is elevated, it should be reassessed at a time when the anxiety related to the nosebleed has dissipated.

In addition, the skin and mucous membranes should be checked carefully for petechiae, purpura, and ecchymosis, which are signs of easy bruisability. The abdomen should be examined for hepatosplenomegaly and the child should be evaluated for lymphadenopathy. Telangiectasias in the oropharynx or mucous membranes suggest Osler-Weber-Rendu syndrome. The oropharynx and nasopharynx should be examined for masses and blood dripping downward from a posterior bleed. The nose should then be inspected for the site of bleeding with special attention directed toward Kiesselbach's plexus in the anterior septum.

Diagnostic Studies

Laboratory tests are rarely indicated in most children with nosebleeds. A hematocrit/hemoglobin should be obtained if the nosebleeds are severe or recur frequently. Blood for type and cross-match should be sent in children who have signs or symptoms of hypovolemia (increased pulse; cool, clammy skin; increased capillary refill; decreased blood pressure; etc.) or a marked drop in hematocrit. If the history or physical examination suggests that a coagulopathy may be present, a CBC with platelet count, PT, and PTT should be obtained and a bleeding time considered if the other laboratory tests are negative.

X-rays and other imaging studies are rarely necessary in children with nosebleeds.

MANAGEMENT

Children who present to primary care physicians with a history of a nosebleed or nosebleeds that have resolved spontaneously or with application of pressure to the nose need no further treatment in the office setting, provided that the history and physical examination are consistent with a benign cause of the nosebleed. These children or their parents should be instructed to apply **petroleum jelly** (Vaseline) or an antibiotic ointment inside the septal portion of the involved naris twice a day for 3–5 days with a cotton-tipped swab (Q-tip) or with the little finger. Often the child's little finger is used because it is nonthreatening and it "knows where to go." Further nose picking should be discouraged, and fingernails should be trimmed to minimize trauma. In addition, a bedside **humidifier** helps to moisturize the air, especially in dry climates or during the winter when forced hot air heat is used. Children whose nares moisten from rhinorrhea and then dry and crack also benefit from humidified air. Buffered saline nasal spray may also be helpful in humidifying the nose. Those children who are prone to recurrent nosebleeds in whom serious causes have been ruled out, may benefit from regular use of some of the above measures when they have URIs, allergic manifestations, or are in a dry season or environment. In addition, for those children with allergic rhinitis and recurrent nosebleeds, topical corticosteroid or cromolyn sodium nasal spray may reduce vascular inflammation and decrease the number of recurrences.

Children or parents should be given advice about how to care for nosebleeds at home. These instructions can also be given to parents who seek advice over the telephone about how to stop children's nosebleeds. Practitioners should reassure parents and children that most nosebleeds are easily controlled. Children should sit upright and lean forward slightly while **direct pressure** is applied to the nose. External compression of the nares between two fingers for 5 to 10 minutes should be sufficient. Pressure applied to the anterior and midportion of the nose rather than at the base is more effective in stopping the bleeding because most nosebleeds occur in these parts of the nose.

Children who are actively bleeding through the nose when seen by primary care physicians should be positioned sitting upright and leaning forward slightly, and they should be given a basin and facial tissue. Direct pressure should be applied by a nurse or physician to the anterior and midportion of the nose while following universal precautions. A cotton dental roll may be placed under the upper lip to compress the labial artery in older children in whom concern about displacement and possible aspiration of the cotton is minimal. If the bleeding continues after external compression, children should be instructed to blow their nose to remove as much clot as possible. Fresh blood should be removed with suction. Cotton pledgets moistened with a few drops of a topical **vasoconstrictor,** such as 0.05% oxymetazoline (Afrin), 0.25% phenylephrine (Neo-Synephrine) or epinephrine (1:1000) mixed with lidocaine if local anesthesia is needed, or topical thrombin, should be inserted into the side of the nose involved. Pressure should then be applied for an additional 10 minutes.

If the bleeding persists, **cauterization** of the bleeding site with a silver nitrate stick is indicated. Continued bleeding is slowed by first cauterizing a small ring around the bleeding point to interrupt flow from surrounding vessels and then rolling the tip of the applicator onto the bleeding site. Cauterization is often difficult in children, and consultation with an otolaryngologist is advisable. Cauterization should not be performed in children with a bleeding diathesis.

If the bleeding continues, an absorbable **nasal sponge** made from oxidized cellulose (Oxicel, Surgicel) may be directly applied to the bleeding site to form an artificial clot. Alternatively, a **nasal tampon** (Merocel) made from a dehydrated material that expands when it becomes moist, may be inserted to tamponade the area of bleeding. Applying antibiotic ointment to the tampon allows for easier insertion and removal. Avitene, a microfibrillar collagen material, provides for platelet aggregation and clot formation when applied to the bleeding site. Continued uncontrolled bleeding requires anterior **nasal packing** with antibiotic-impregnated, one-inch petrolatum gauze strips, which should remain in place for approximately 2–3 days. Prophylactic **antibiotics** should be started because sinusitis is a complication of anterior nasal packing.

Posterior nosebleeds, which are more difficult to control, should be suspected if (1) the measures described previously are ineffective, (2) bleeding is vigorous and the cause cannot be identified, or (3) most of the bleeding is into the nasopharynx and mouth. A posterior nasal pack using a Foley catheter or an intranasal balloon is indicated to control posterior nosebleeds. This pack is left in place for 2–5 days, and children should be started on antibiotics to prevent sinusitis.

The need for **otolaryngologic consultation** depends on the experience of the individual physician and the availability of consultation. Prompt consultation, if available, should be obtained for children with severe nosebleeds who need volume replacement, for children with nosebleeds that do not stop or recur after the above measures have been taken, for children who may need anterior or posterior nasal packing, and for children with recurrent, difficult-to-stop nosebleeds. In some cases, obtaining consultation before cauterization with silver nitrate is advisable. Children with septal hematomas, tumors, polyps, and telangiectasias should be referred to an otolaryngologist for further care. Children with a documented or suspected bleeding disorder should be referred to a hematologist.

Children with severe nosebleeds should have an intravenous line started early; blood sent for type and cross-match; and fluids replaced, depending on the amount of blood loss and physical evidence of hypovolemia. In children who are frightened or in whom certain procedures (e.g., cauterization of bleeding site, drainage of septal hematoma) are performed, sedation should be strongly considered. Pain medication should be used in children who need anterior or posterior packing. If procedures that cause undue pain or discomfort are necessary, general anesthesia in an operating room setting may be indicated.

Hospitalization is not often necessary for children with nosebleeds. However, children who are hemodynamically unstable on presentation or who need placement of a posterior nasal pack usually require inpatient treatment. Hospitalization may be necessary for children with difficult-to-stop bleeds who need an anterior nasal pack or who have a bleeding disorder or underlying chronic illness such as leukemia, aplastic anemia, or HIV infection.

PROGNOSIS

The prognosis for nosebleeds in children is excellent. Almost all nosebleeds are easily controlled with a minimal amount of home care or medical management. Surgery is rarely indicated. Complications associated with significant nosebleeds include hypovolemia from blood loss, and sinusitis and toxic shock syndrome from anterior or posterior nasal packs. Even for rare causes of nosebleeds, the prognosis is very good with prompt diagnosis and treatment.

Case Resolution

In the case presented, the boy has experienced several nosebleeds of short duration associated with a URI and winter dryness. His history and physical examination are unremarkable for a bleeding disorder or chronic illness. The small amount of blood in his nose is consistent with an anterior nosebleed originating from Kiesselbach's plexus with inflammation and drying of the nasal mucosa. Laboratory tests are not indicated. The parents should be instructed to apply petroleum jelly to the septal portion of the left side of the child's nose twice a day for 3–5 days and to humidify the child's bedroom. They should also be reassured that their child has a common condition that he will outgrow.

Selected Readings

Friedman, E. M. Epistaxis. *In* Dershowitz, R. A. (ed.). Ambulatory Pediatric Care, 2nd ed. Philadelphia, J. B. Lippincott, 1993, pp. 308–310.

Henretig, F. M. Epistaxis. *In* Fleisher, G. R., and S. Ludwig (eds.). Textbook of Pediatric Emergency Medicine, 3rd ed. Baltimore, Williams & Wilkins, 1993, pp. 175–177.

Josephson, G. D., F. A. Godley, and P. Stierna. Practical management of epistaxis. Med. Clin. North Am. 75:1311–1320, 1991.

Katsanis, E., et al. Prevalence and significance of mild bleeding disorders in children with recurrent epistaxis. J. Pediatr. 113:73–76, 1988.

Kost, S. I., and J. C. Post. Management of epistaxis. *In* Henretig, F. M., and C. King (eds.). Textbook of Pediatric Emergency Procedures. Baltimore, Williams & Wilkins, 1997, pp. 663–673.

Manning, S. C., and M. C. Culbertson Jr. Epistaxis. *In* Bluestone, C. D., S. E. Stool, and M. A. Kenna (eds.). Pediatric Otolaryngology, 3rd ed. Philadelphia, W. B. Saunders, 1996, pp. 781–786.

Mulbury, P. E. Recurrent epistaxis. Pediatr. Rev. 12:213–217, 1991.

Potsic, W. P., and S. D. Handler. Otolaryngology emergencies (epistaxis). *In* Fleisher, G. R., and S. Ludwig (eds.). Textbook of Pediatric Emergency Medicine, 3rd ed. Baltimore, Williams & Wilkins, 1993, pp. 1377–1379.

Roberson, D. W. Epistaxis. *In* Dershowitz, R. A. (ed.). Ambulatory Pediatric Care, 3rd ed. Philadelphia, Lippincott-Raven, 1999, pp. 475–477.

Santamaria, J. P., and T. J. Abrunzo. Ear, nose, and throat (epistaxis). *In* Barkin, R. M. (ed.). Pediatric Emergency Medicine, 2nd ed. St. Louis, C.V. Mosby, 1997, pp. 713–716.

Wallace, L., and M. R. Clark. Epistaxis. *In* Reisdorff, E. J., M. R. Roberts, and J. G. Wiegenstein (eds.). Pediatric Emergency Medicine. Philadelphia, W. B. Saunders, 1993, pp. 629–634.

Walton, S. A., et al. Miscellaneous wounds (epistaxis and septal hematoma). *In* Dieckman, R. A., D. H. Fiser, and S. M. Selbst (eds.). Pediatric Emergency and Critical Care Procedures. St. Louis, Mosby, 1997, pp. 696–699.

Werner, E. J., et al. Prevalence of von Willebrand disease in children: a multiethnic study. J. Pediatr. 123:893–898, 1993.

CHAPTER 56

STRABISMUS

Geeta Grover, M.D.

H_x The mother of an 8-month-old infant complains that every time her son looks to either side his eyes seem "crossed." Otherwise, he is growing and developing normally. A symmetric pupillary light reflex, bilateral red reflex, and normal extraocular eye movements in all directions are noted on physical examination of the eyes.

Questions

1. What is strabismus?
2. What conditions make infants' eyes appear "crossed"? What is the differential diagnosis?
3. What tests are used in the office evaluation of children suspected of having strabismus?
4. Which infants with "crossed" eyes require referral for further evaluation and treatment?

Strabismus refers to any abnormality in ocular alignment. It is one of the most common eye problems observed in infants and children. The pediatrician plays an important role in the early detection and prompt referral of children with suspected ocular alignment abnormalities.

EPIDEMIOLOGY

Strabismus affects approximately 3% of the population, and the condition is seen most commonly in children under 6 years of age. About 50% of all affected children have a positive family history of strabismus, although the exact genetic mode of inheritance is unclear. Up to 75% of normal infants have transient intermittent strabismus during the first 3 months of life.

CLINICAL PRESENTATION

Children with ocular misalignment have an asymmetric corneal light reflex test. Eye movement is noted with cover testing. Children with paralytic strabismus may present with torticollis or head tilting in an effort to avoid diplopia (D_x Box).

PATHOPHYSIOLOGY

Normal binocular vision is the result of the fusion of images from both eyes working synchronously across the visual field. Six extraocular muscles control all eye movements. Orthophoria is proper alignment of the eyes, and strabismus results from an imbalance in muscle movements.

Strabismus

The classification of strabismus is complex. Based on etiology, it may be considered nonparalytic (comitant) or paralytic (noncomitant). Strabismus may also be classified as congenital or acquired, intermittent or constant, alternating or unilateral, and convergent or divergent.

In **nonparalytic strabismus,** the extraocular muscles and the nerves that control them are normal. The degree of deviation is constant or nearly constant in all directions of gaze. Nonparalytic strabismus is the most common type of strabismus seen in children, and congenital or infantile esotropia is usually of this kind. Ocular or visual defects such as cataracts or high refractive errors occasionally cause nonparalytic strabismus.

In **paralytic strabismus,** paralysis or paresis of one or more of the extraocular muscles produces a muscle imbalance. The deviation is asymmetric, and characteristically the degree of deviation is worse when gazing in the direction of the affected muscle.

D_x Strabismus

- Head tilt
- Blurred vision
- Double vision (diplopia)
- Squint
- Asymmetric corneal light reflex
- Eye movement with cover testing

Paralytic strabismus may be congenital or acquired. **Congenital strabismus** may result from birth trauma, muscle anomalies, abnormal development of the cranial nerve nuclei, or congenital infections affecting the eyes. Congenital strabismus may be seen in association with neurodevelopmental disorders such as cerebral palsy. **Acquired strabismus** due to extraocular muscle palsies usually indicates the presence of a serious underlying condition, such as an intracranial tumor, a demyelinating or neurodegenerative disease, myasthenia gravis, a progressive myopathy, or a CNS infection. Children may present with a complaint of double vision or a compensatory torticollis (head tilt) to avoid double vision (diplopia).

Intermittent (latent) misalignment of the eyes is referred to as **heterophoria.** Under normal conditions, the fusional mechanisms of the CNS maintain eye alignment. Eye deviation is appreciated only under certain conditions, such as illness, fatigue, stress, or when fusion is interrupted by occluding one eye (e.g., during cover testing). Some degree of heterophoria may be found in almost all individuals and it is usually asymptomatic. Larger degrees of heterophoria may give rise to troublesome symptoms such as headaches, transient diplopia, or asthenopia (eye strain).

Constant misalignment of the eyes is referred to as **heterotropia.** This condition occurs because normal fusional mechanisms are unable to control eye deviation; children are unable to use both eyes together to fixate on an object. Heterotropias may be alternating and involve either one or both eyes. In alternating tropias, both eyes appear to deviate equally, and vision generally develops normally in each eye because children have no preference for fixation. If strabismus affects one eye, the other eye is always used for fixation, and there is danger of amblyopia or loss of vision in the deviating eye.

Convergent deviation, a "turning in" or "crossing" of the eyes, is called an esodeviation (e.g., esotropia or esophoria). Divergent deviation, a "turning out" of the eyes, is an exodeviation. The prefixes hyper- and hypo- are used for upward and downward vertical deviations, respectively. Esodeviations are the most common type of ocular misalignment, accounting for 50–75% of all cases of strabismus. Vertical deviations represent less than 5% of all cases of strabismus.

Amblyopia

Amblyopia, a potential complication if strabismus is not corrected in a timely manner, refers to poor vision in one eye, or rarely both, despite correction of any refractive errors. If children have no significant refractive error and the visual acuity of one eye is worse than the other, they probably have amblyopia. To be considered amblyopia, visual acuity, as measured by reading an eye chart, should differ by at least two lines (e.g., 20/20 in one eye and 20/40 in the other). It is the leading cause of preventable visual loss in children.

Amblyopia may be classified into three major categories. **Deprivational amblyopia** generally results when a unilateral lesion or developmental defect in one of the structures of the eye or its visual pathways obstructs vision. Causes of deprivational amblyopia include congenital cataract, ptosis, corneal scarring or opacity, orbital tumors, and retinal detachment. These conditions cause a lack of formation of a retinal image or a blurred retinal image, usually in one eye. **Refractive amblyopia** refers to a blurring of the retinal image due to bilateral large or asymmetric refractive errors. In **strabismic amblyopia,** the immature or developing brain suppresses images from the deviating eye to prevent diplopia. Strabismic amblyopia is most commonly associated with strabismus that develops in children who are younger than 4 years of age. If the condition leading to the amblyopia is not corrected while the brain's visual pathways are still malleable (e.g., before approximately 6–7 years of age), children may have some degree of permanent visual loss.

DIFFERENTIAL DIAGNOSIS

The differential diagnosis of strabismus may be divided into three categories: transient neonatal strabismus, congenital or infantile strabismus, and acquired strabismus. True strabismus must be differentiated from the illusion of deviation created by facial asymmetry or anatomic variations.

Transient Neonatal Strabismus

Eye alignment in normal infants during the first 2–3 months of life may vary from normal to intermittent esotropia or exotropia. These deviations are believed to result from CNS immaturity and resolve spontaneously in the vast majority of children by 4 months of age. If such deviations are constant or persist beyond this age, children should be referred to an ophthalmologist for further evaluation.

Congenital or Infantile Strabismus

This type of strabismus is defined as a deviation that occurs during the first 6 months of life. Because the deviation may not always be present at birth, the term "infantile" may be more accurate. The differential diagnosis of infantile strabismus is presented in Table 56–1. **Pseudoesotropia** is an illusion or apparent deviation and not a true deviation. In many infants, the broad, flat nasal bridge and prominent epicanthal folds may obscure a portion of the sclera near the nose and create the appearance of esotropia (Fig. 56–1). This illusion resolves as children mature. Symmetric corneal light reflexes or normal cover tests differentiate pseudoesotropia from true esotropia.

Esotropia is one of the more common types of childhood strabismus. The constant deviation of infantile esotropia is usually readily apparent because of the large angle of deviation. Affected children usually have good bilateral vision because of the alternation of fixation from one eye to the other. Cross-fixation, in which children look to the left with the adducted right eye and to the right with the adducted left eye, may be

TABLE 56–1. Differential Diagnosis of Strabismus

Congenital or Infantile Strabismus
Esodeviations
Infantile esotropia
Pseudoesotropia
Möbius syndrome
Exodeviations
Congenital exotropia
Congenital third nerve paralysis
Abnormalities of the bony orbit (Crouzon's disease)
Both Esodeviations and Exodeviations
Duane's syndrome (esotropia more common than exotropia)

Acquired Strabismus
Esodeviations
Accommodative esotropia
Benign sixth cranial nerve palsy
Exodeviations
Intermittent exotropia
Overcorrection after surgery for esotropia
Both Esodeviations and Exodeviations
Poor vision
Orbital trauma causing entrapment of extraocular muscles
Intracranial tumors or tumors involving the orbit (e.g., retinoblastoma)
Myasthenia gravis
Central nervous system (CNS) infection (e.g., meningitis)
CNS tumor
Orbital cellulitis

evident because of the large angle of deviation. Rarely, esotropia may be due to palsy of the sixth cranial nerve either in isolation (Duane's syndrome) or in association with other cranial nerve palsies (Möbius' syndrome).

Infantile exotropia is less common than esotropia. Like esotropia, exotropia develops within the first 6 months of life and is characterized by a large angle of deviation. Other causes of infantile exotropia include congenital third nerve palsy (paralytic strabismus) and abnormalities of the bones of the orbit (e.g., Crouzon's disease).

Acquired Strabismus

Acquired strabismus may result from a variety of causes (see Table 56–1). Accommodative esotropia and

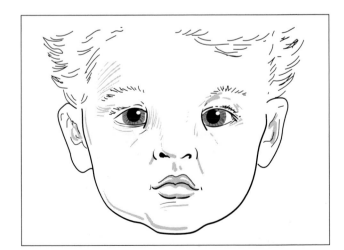

FIGURE 56–1. Child with pseudoesotropia. Note the wide nasal bridge and prominent epicanthal folds.

intermittent exotropia are two common types of acquired strabismus. **Accommodative esotropia** typically develops in children between 2–3 years of age but may appear as early as 6 months or as late as 8 years. Children with hyperopia use accommodation (alteration in the shape of the lens) to see clearly. The accommodative reflex is closely linked to convergence; when accommodation occurs, so does convergence. If children have severe hyperopia (farsightedness), the amount of convergence that occurs with accommodation may be severe and lead to the development of esotropia. Such esotropia is usually intermittent initially and only gradually becomes constant.

Intermittent exotropia, the most common form of exodeviation seen in children, develops between birth and 4 years of age. Although it begins as an intermittent condition in which children's eyes appear to deviate outward, especially when they are tired, ill, or fixating at a distance, the exotropia can become constant with time. Children may also close one eye in bright sunlight, presumably in an effort to prevent diplopia.

EVALUATION

History

The evaluation of infants or children suspected of having strabismus should begin with a thorough family history; strabismus often runs in families (Questions Box). Parental description of the ocular deviation is useful, because misalignments, especially intermittent deviations that may only become manifest when children are tired, may not always be evident during the office visit. A history of head or orbital trauma may help in the evaluation of acquired strabismus.

Physical Examination

On physical examination, the presence of any dysmorphic features and structural abnormalities of the face or neck (e.g., torticollis) should be noted. Children with paralytic strabismus may compensate for their paretic lesion by tilting their head to avoid diplopia.

It is important that visual screening of children begin during the neonatal period. Newborn screening should emphasize the presence of a bilateral red reflex. An abnormal red reflex or a white reflex may indicate the presence of a cataract or retinoblastoma. Evaluation for ocular alignment should begin at the 4-month health maintenance visit. Intermittent misalignment of the eyes is often seen in normal infants who are younger than 4

months of age. However, constant misalignment requires immediate attention at any age.

Vision Testing

Testing visual acuity is essential in the evaluation of children with suspected strabismus. Such testing may be performed as early as 3 years of age, if children are cooperative. Charts with symbols, figures, or letters can be used. The traditional Snellen eye chart with letters can generally be used in children who are 4 years of age. Decreased vision in one eye may be indicative of ocular abnormalities, including ocular deviations.

Tests for Strabismus

The two basic tests for strabismus that can be easily performed in the office are the corneal light reflex test, or Hirschberg test, and the cover tests. The pediatrician should be comfortable performing both tests.

The **corneal light reflex test** is the simplest and quickest test for the evaluation of strabismus. In this test, a penlight is projected simultaneously onto the corneas of both eyes as the child looks straight ahead. The examiner compares the placement of the corneal light reflex in each eye with respect to the center of the pupil. If the eyes are straight, the reflection appears symmetrically in the center of both pupils or on the same point on each cornea. If the light reflex appears off center in one eye as compared to the other, an ocular deviation or tropia is present. Nasal deviation of the light reflex on the cornea indicates exotropia on that side; temporal deviation signifies esotropia; and superior or inferior deviation indicates hypo- and hypertropia, respectively.

Unlike the corneal light reflex test, which may be performed even in uncooperative children, the **cover tests** require children's cooperation and ability to fixate on a specified object. These tests are used to detect heterophorias. Two types of cover tests, alternate-cover and cover-uncover, are used. Only the alternate-cover test detects both heterophorias and heterotropias. This test may be preferred by the primary care physician as a screening tool; the cover-uncover test detects only manifest deviations or heterotropias. In the alternate-cover test, one eye and then the other is covered as the child fixates on an object at a distance. If neither eye moves as the cover is moved rapidly between the eyes, the eyes are in alignment or orthophoric. With heterotropia, the deviating eye moves when the fixating eye is occluded; in heterophoria, the deviating eye moves when it is uncovered (Fig. 56–2).

The alternate-cover test may be illustrated with the following example. A child presents with constant esotropia of the left eye. When the right or fixating eye is occluded, the left eye is forced to fixate so that the child can see, and the left eye moves outward as the right eye is occluded. In the case of a child with an esophoria or latent deviation of the left eye, the eye deviates inward when it is occluded, because it is not being forced to fixate. As the occluder is removed from

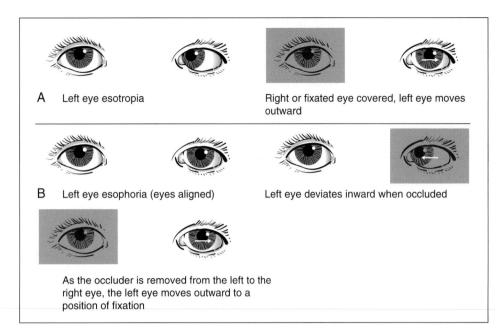

A Left eye esotropia   Right or fixated eye covered, left eye moves outward

B Left eye esophoria (eyes aligned)   Left eye deviates inward when occluded

As the occluder is removed from the left to the right eye, the left eye moves outward to a position of fixation

FIGURE 56–2. Alternate-cover test in the detection of strabismus. Normally, both eyes appear to be aligned and centrally fixed.

A. Detection of esotropia. The right eye is fixating and a left esotropia is present. When the right or fixating eye is covered, the left eye moves outward (away from the nose).

B. Detection of esophoria. The eyes are aligned with a left esophoria. When the left eye is covered, it deviates inward. As the occluder is moved from the left eye to the right eye, the left eye moves outward to a position of fixation.

the left eye to the right, the left eye moves outward and returns to a position of fixation.

The alternate-cover test may be more difficult to interpret in children with bilateral or alternating strabismus who use both eyes in turn for fixation. It is not necessary for the pediatrician to identify exactly what type of strabismus is present; abnormal movement should be noted and children should be referred for further evaluation. An ophthalmologist is able to perform a more detailed examination.

MANAGEMENT

The goal of management is the attainment of the best possible vision in each eye. The sooner deviations are corrected, the better are children's chances for equal bilateral vision. Treatment includes correction of any underlying refractive error with **corrective lenses.** Such lenses, which remedy the refractive error and minimize the need for accommodation, are used to treat accommodative esotropia.

Children who do not see equally well from both eyes may be at risk for amblyopia if they preferentially fixate with only one eye. If detected, amblyopia should be corrected with occlusion therapy of the fixating "good" eye. **Occlusion therapy** forces children to use the amblyopic eye. This treatment is best accomplished by constantly patching the eye with better vision during waking hours. Children require repeat evaluations and close monitoring during this therapy.

If nonsurgical methods fail to align the eyes, surgical correction may be necessary. **Surgery** may be used to achieve the best possible ocular alignment and is usually required for treatment of infantile esotropia. It is generally performed in children between 6 months and 2 years of age, while the visual system is still pliable enough to allow for development of postsurgical binocular vision. Surgery also may be needed in children with intermittent exotropia if the frequency or deviation is increasing.

PROGNOSIS

Certain conditions, such as pseudoesotropia or infrequent intermittent exotropia, may resolve as children mature. Others, such as infantile esotropia, require early detection and treatment to achieve the best binocular vision. Amblyopia and permanent vision loss may result if correction of strabismus is delayed.

Case Resolution

The infant in the case history has pseudoesotropia. Although the boy's eyes appear to deviate, the corneal light reflex and cover tests are normal. Physical examination reveals prominent epicanthal folds and a broad, flat nasal bridge.

Selected Readings

Bacal, D. A. Don't be lazy about looking for amblyopia. Contemp. Pediatr. 15:99–107, 1998.

Catalano, J. D. Strabismus. Pediatr. Ann. 19:289–297, 1990.

Cheng, K. P., A. W. Biglan, and D. A. Hiles. Pediatric ophthalmology. In Zitelli, B. J., and H. W. Davis. Pediatric Physical Diagnosis, 3rd ed. St. Louis, Mosby-Wolfe, 1997, pp. 563–601.

Crouch, E. R., and E. R. Crouch. Pediatric vision screening: why? when? what? how? Contemp. Pediatr. 8:9–30, September 1991. (Special issue.)

Lavrich, J. B., and L. B. Nelson. Diagnosis and treatment of strabismus disorders. Pediatr. Clin. North Am. 40:737–752, 1993.

Spencer, R. F., et al. Botulinum toxin management of childhood intermittent exotropia. Ophthalmology 104:1762–1767, 1997.

CHAPTER 57

INFECTIONS OF THE EYE

Geeta Grover, M.D.

H$_x$ A 10-day-old infant has a 1-day history of red, watery eyes and nonproductive cough with no fever. The girl is breast-fed and continues to eat well. She was the 7 lb, 2 oz (3238 g) product of a term gestation, born via normal spontaneous vaginal delivery without complications to a 26-year-old woman. The pregnancy was also uncomplicated. No one at home is ill.

On examination, the infant is afebrile with normal vital signs. Examination of the eyes reveals bilateral conjunctival injection with only a mild amount of purulent discharge. Bilateral red reflexes are present. The rest of the physical examination is within normal limits.

Questions

1. What is the differential diagnosis of conjunctivitis both during and following the neonatal period?
2. What laboratory tests, if any, should be performed?
3. When is a chest x-ray indicated in the evaluation of neonates with conjunctivitis?
4. What are management strategies for eye infections?

Infections of the eye and surrounding structures are commonly seen by pediatricians. Such infections range in severity from more common problems such as blepharitis and conjunctivitis, which lack serious sequelae, to more severe and less common infections such as periorbital and orbital cellulitis. The presenting complaint in many children with eye infections is a red-appearing eye. Familiarity with the common causes of a red eye makes prompt diagnosis and treatment possible.

EPIDEMIOLOGY

Conjunctivitis, which affects children of all ages, is perhaps the most common eye infection of childhood. The incidence of conjunctivitis in the newborn period is estimated to range from 1.6–12%. The incidence of chlamydial conjunctivitis is about 8:1000 live births. About two thirds of acute childhood conjunctivitis has a bacterial etiology, and one third is viral. *Haemophilus influenzae* and *Streptococcus pneumoniae* are the most common bacterial agents and account for about 40% and 10% of culture-proven cases, respectively. *Staphylococcus aureus* is isolated from the conjunctivae of children with acute conjunctivitis, but it is found with about the same frequency in the eyes of children without conjunctivitis. Adenovirus is the most common viral isolate. Most cases of acute conjunctivitis in young adults have a viral etiology. Serious eye infections such as periorbital and orbital cellulitis occur far less often.

CLINICAL PRESENTATION

Red eyes are a common presenting sign of infections of the eyelids and conjunctivae. Eyelid edema and erythema surrounding the eye characterize periorbital and orbital cellulitis. Proptosis, abnormal extraocular movement, or loss of visual acuity may signal spread of the infection beyond the orbital septum (orbital cellulitis) (D$_x$ Box).

D$_x$ Eye Infections

EYELID INFECTIONS

- Redness
- Itching (blepharitis)
- Burning (blepharitis)
- Scales at the base of the lashes (seborrheic blepharitis)
- Swelling (external hordeolum and chalazion)
- Pain (external hordeolum)

CONJUNCTIVITIS

- Conjunctival injection and edema
- Excessive tearing
- Discharge or crusting
- Itching (allergic conjunctivitis)

UVEITIS

- Conjunctival injection
- Pain
- Blurred vision
- Photophobia
- Headache

PERIORBITAL CELLULITIS

- Unilateral eyelid edema
- Erythema surrounding the eye
- Pain
- Fever

ORBITAL CELLULITIS

- Eyelid edema
- Proptosis
- Decreased extraocular movements
- Loss of visual acuity
- Fever
- Ill appearance
- Associated sinusitis

PATHOPHYSIOLOGY

Eye infections may be divided into two types: those affecting the structures surrounding the orbit and those involving the orbital contents themselves (Fig. 57–1). Although all structures surrounding the eye may potentially become inflamed or infected, the eyelids, nasolacrimal drainage system (dacryocystitis; see Chapter 58, Excessive Tearing), conjunctiva, and cornea are most commonly involved. Orbital cellulitis is defined as an infection of the orbital structures posterior to the orbital septum. The orbital septum, an extension of the periosteum of the bones of the orbit, extends to the margins of both the upper and lower eyelids, and provides an anatomic barrier to the spread of most infectious and inflammatory processes. Preseptal, or periorbital, cellulitis is localized to structures superficial to the orbital septum, whereas septal, or orbital, cellulitis implies that the disease process involves orbital structures extending beyond the septum.

DIFFERENTIAL DIAGNOSIS

Infections of the eye are included in the differential diagnosis of conditions presenting with red eye (Table 57–1). Also included in the differential diagnosis are congenital, inflammatory, traumatic, and systemic processes. Although infection and irritation are by far the most common causes of an acute onset of red eye, other possibilities, especially trauma, glaucoma, or underlying systemic disease, must be considered.

Eyelid Infections

Common conditions affecting the eyelid and its related structures are blepharitis, hordeolum, and chalazion.

Blepharitis is an inflammation of the lid margins.

TABLE 57–1.   Differential Diagnosis of Red Eye

Congenital Anomalies
Nasolacrimal duct obstruction
Congenital glaucoma

Infection
Keratitis
Conjunctivitis
Dacryocystitis
Periorbital and orbital cellulitis

Inflammation
Blepharitis
Hordeolum
Chalazion

Trauma
Corneal abrasion
Foreign body
Blunt trauma: hyphema, perforating injuries
Exposure to chemicals or other noxious substances

Systemic Illnesses
Kawasaki syndrome
Varicella
Measles
Lyme disease
Stevens-Johnson syndrome
Ataxia-telangiectasia
Juvenile rheumatoid arthritis

This condition, which is often bilateral, may be chronic or recurrent. The two most common causes of blepharitis are staphylococcal infection and seborrheic dermatitis. Children with staphylococcal blepharitis often present with scales at the base of the lashes, ulceration of the lid margin, and loss of lashes. The infection may spread to the conjunctiva or cornea, producing conjunctivitis or keratitis. In contrast, seborrheic blepharitis is characterized by greasy, yellow scales attached to the base of the lashes. In addition, associated seborrhea of the scalp or eyebrows may be present. Mixed staphylococcal-seborrheic infections, which oc-

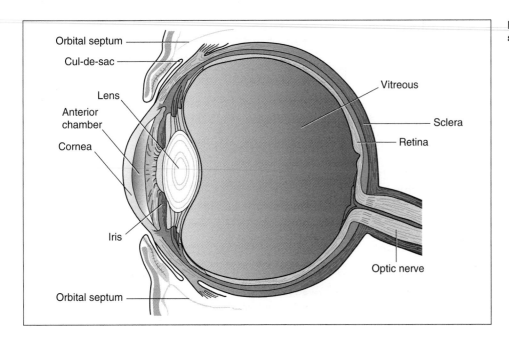

FIGURE 57–1. The eye and surrounding structures.

Orbital septum
Cul-de-sac
Lens
Anterior chamber
Cornea
Iris
Orbital septum
Vitreous
Sclera
Retina
Optic nerve

cur as staphylococcal superinfection, may complicate seborrheic blepharitis. Less commonly seen forms of blepharitis are parasitic blepharitis, which results from infestation of the lids by the head louse, *Pediculus capitis,* or crab louse, *Pediculus pubis,* and primary or recurrent herpes virus type 1 infections that may manifest as clusters of vesicles on the eyelids.

The glands of the eyelid can also be infected. *S. aureus* is the most common organism. An external **hordeolum,** or common stye, results from an infection of the glands of Moll or Zeis located along the lid margins. Affected children present with a well-circumscribed, painful swelling along the lid margin that generally ruptures spontaneously and resolves without complications. An internal hordeolum, on the other hand, is an acute infection of the meibomian glands that tends to be larger and ruptures through either the skin or the conjunctival surface.

A **chalazion** is a chronic granulomatous inflammation of the meibomian glands that is caused by retention of secretions. The resulting firm, nontender, slow-growing mass within the upper or lower eyelid may be painful if secondary infection is present.

Infections of the Conjunctiva

Conjunctivitis refers to any inflammation of the conjunctiva. The condition may be allergic, chemical, viral, or bacterial in etiology. In addition, it may be a sign of systemic disease such as Kawasaki syndrome or Stevens-Johnson syndrome.

Acute conjunctivitis, or pink eye, is common during childhood and can be extremely contagious. The usual signs are conjunctival injection, tearing, discharge, crusting of the lashes, and conjunctival edema (chemosis). Pain and decreased vision are uncommon symptoms and may signal corneal involvement.

In general, it is difficult to distinguish bacterial conjunctivitis from viral conjunctivitis on clinical features alone. Certain clinical characteristics may guide the diagnosis. The average age of children affected with **bacterial conjunctivitis** tends to be younger than for viral conjunctivitis, which is more frequent in adolescents; however, considerable overlap occurs. Children with bacterial conjunctivitis typically present with an acute onset of unilateral or bilateral injection and edema of both the palpebral and bulbar conjunctiva, minimal to copious purulent discharge, and crusting of the eyelashes. Children may have difficulty opening their eyes on awakening in the morning because of the crusting of the exudate. An association between conjunctivitis and concomitant otitis media has been well described. *H. influenzae,* which is often resistant to ampicillin, is the pathogen most commonly isolated from affected children.

The diagnosis of **viral conjunctivitis** is considered if signs of viral URI (e.g., low-grade fever, cough, rhinorrhea) are evident. Viral infection is associated with unilateral rather than bilateral mild conjunctival injection, watery or thin mucoid discharge, and only mild lid edema and erythema. Adenoviral infection is usually bilateral, with significant conjunctival injection and chemosis of the lids, and is often accompanied by a tender preauricular lymph node. Epidemic keratoconjunctivitis is a highly contagious form of adenoviral conjunctivitis. Affected children often complain of foreign body sensation beneath the lids or photophobia due to corneal involvement. Pharyngeal conjunctival fever, another presentation of adenoviral conjunctivitis, usually manifests as conjunctivitis in association with pharyngitis and fever.

Infants who suffer from **chronic or recurrent conjunctivitis** may have an obstruction of the nasolacrimal duct, whereas older children with chronic conjunctivitis may have allergic diseases, recurrent blepharitis, or chlamydial infections. Blepharitis is the most common cause of chronic conjunctivitis in older children. *S. aureus* is frequently implicated in these infections.

Itching, tearing, and conjunctival edema are the hallmarks of **allergic conjunctivitis,** a noninfectious form of conjunctival inflammation often seen in children with other allergic disorders such as asthma or hay fever. Conjunctival injection tends to be mild, bilateral, and seasonal. The etiology is most often a hypersensitivity to pollens, dust, or animal hair. Vernal conjunctivitis is a particularly severe form of allergic conjunctivitis seen primarily during childhood. Usually bilateral, it occurs more frequently in boys. The majority of cases occur during the spring and summer. Severe itching and tearing are the most frequent complaints. The conjunctivae of the upper eyelid may have a cobblestone appearance due to the accumulation of inflammatory cells, or there may be small, elevated lesions of the bulbar conjunctiva at the corneal limbus. The pathogenesis is unclear, but atopy appears to play a role.

Chlamydial conjunctivitis frequently affects both neonates and adolescents. Inclusion conjunctivitis is an acute infection of the eyes caused by sexually transmitted *Chlamydia trachomatis* (usually serotypes D through K). This condition may be seen in neonates or sexually active adolescents. Trachoma, the most common cause of impaired vision and preventable blindness worldwide, is a chronic conjunctivitis usually caused by *C. trachomatis* serotypes A, B, and C. Although this disease is rarely seen in North America, it is endemic among certain populations, especially Native American. Inclusion conjunctivitis and endemic trachoma are both characterized initially by conjunctivitis with small lymphoid follicles in the conjunctiva.

Neonatal conjunctivitis, or ophthalmia neonatorum, occurs during the first month of life. The major causes of neonatal conjunctivitis are chemical, chlamydial, and bacterial (in decreasing order of frequency). Ophthalmia neonatorum may be produced by the same bacteria that cause childhood conjunctivitis but also results from organisms such as *C. trachomatis* or *Neisseria gonorrhoeae.* Newborns may acquire these latter pathogens following premature rupture of membranes or passage through an infected or colonized birth canal. *C. trachomatis* is the organism most commonly identified. It has been isolated from 17–40% of neonates with conjunctivitis. Infants born to mothers with active cervical chlamydial infection have a 20–50% chance of developing chlamydial conjunctivitis. Viruses are uncommon causes of neonatal ocular infections. Herpes simplex virus (HSV) is the primary viral agent involved in neonatal conjunctivitis. The presence of characteristic vesicular skin lesions or corneal dendritic lesions helps in the diagnosis.

The time of onset of symptoms is related to the etiologic agent. Inflammation secondary to the silver nitrate drops instilled at birth to prevent gonococcal infection presents as mild conjunctivitis 12–24 hours after birth in 10–100% of treated newborns. This condition usually resolves spontaneously in 24–48 hours. Conjunctivitis due to *N. gonorrhoeae* appears 2–5 days after birth and is associated with copious purulent discharge. Conjunctivitis due to *C. trachomatis* occurs at 5–14 days, a result of a longer incubation period. The time of onset and the severity of symptoms of these two conditions may overlap, however. The presentation of gonococcal infection may be delayed for 5 days or more because of the partial suppression of the infection by the prophylactic drops instilled at birth. Chlamydial infection can vary in severity from mild erythema of the eyelids to severe inflammation and copious purulent discharge. Chlamydial infection is primarily localized to the palpebral conjunctiva and only rarely affects the cornea. Gonococcal conjunctivitis is considered a medical emergency because the gonococcus can penetrate the cornea, resulting in corneal ulceration and perforation of the globe within 24 hours if untreated.

Concomitant nasopharyngeal chlamydial infection is commonly seen. Spread of the organism from the nasopharynx to the lungs is a sequela of colonization. Ten to 20% of infants with conjunctivitis have chlamydial pneumonia. It may occur either simultaneously with the conjunctivitis or up to 4–6 weeks later. Affected infants are usually afebrile and present with symptoms of increasing tachypnea and cough.

Anterior uveitis may be confused with conjunctivitis. The uvea consists of the iris, the ciliary body, and the choroid. Inflammation of the iris, or ciliary body may produce conjuntival infection which may be associated with decreased visual acuity, pain, headache, and photophobia. Systemic conditions associated with uveitis include Kawasaki syndrome, juvenile rheumatoid arthritis, Lyme disease, tuberculosis, sarcoidosis, toxocara infection, toxoplasmosis, and spondyloarthropathies.

Infections of the Eye and Surrounding Tissues

Preseptal cellulitis and **orbital cellulitis** are two serious infections of the eye and surrounding structures. Although these infections are not as frequent as those that are limited to the eye, they have serious sequelae. The preseptal space is defined by the skin of the eyelid on one side and the orbital septum on the other. Children with preseptal, or periorbital, cellulitis usually present with acute onset, and unilateral upper and lower eyelid edema, erythema, and pain. The condition is often associated with systemic signs and symptoms such as ill appearance, fever, and leukocytosis. The eye itself usually appears normal. Infection may follow hematogenous seeding of the preseptal space, most often with *H. influenzae* type b or *S. pneumoniae*, or traumatic breaks in the skin that usually lead to *S. aureus* infection.

Orbital cellulitis is an infection of the contents of the orbit posterior to the orbital septum. Usually an insidious onset of eyelid edema, proptosis, decreased extraocular movements, and loss of visual acuity occurs. As with periorbital cellulitis, children are often febrile and ill-appearing. Contiguous spread of infection from adjacent sinusitis (most often ethmoid) is the most common cause. The organisms most often involved are the same as those in acute sinusitis (*S. aureus*, *S. pneumoniae*, nontypeable *H. influenzae*, and *Staphylococcus pyogenes*). Untreated, the infection may progress to orbital abscess formation.

Primary herpes simplex infection can affect the skin surrounding the eyes as well as the eye itself. Most such infections are caused by HSV type 1, although type 2 infections may be seen in newborns. Children with **herpetic infections of the eye** usually present with unilateral skin vesicles and a mild conjunctivitis or keratitis. Herpetic keratoconjunctivitis can recur following fever, exposure to sunlight, or mild trauma. The characteristic corneal lesion of herpes keratitis is the dendritic corneal ulcer, which appears as a tree-branch pattern on fluorescein staining of the cornea. Although this lesion may be seen with primary infection, it is more common in recurrent infections. Skin vesicles may not appear with recurrences, which makes it difficult to distinguish herpetic infection from other causes of conjunctivitis. Empiric topical steroid treatment for presumed viral conjunctivitis should be avoided for this reason; steroids may lead to progression of the herpetic infection and permanent corneal scarring.

Neonatal herpetic infections of the eye primarily result from HSV 2. Infections may be isolated to the eye or the eye may be infected secondarily due to CNS or disseminated disease. Proper diagnosis is important, because disseminated herpetic disease has a mortality of about 85%, and CNS disease has a mortality of 50%. Isolated herpetic eye disease is actually quite rare in neonates.

EVALUATION

History

A careful history taken from the parent or primary caregiver as well as the child can guide the diagnosis (Questions Box). It is important to exclude the possibility of ocular trauma or exposure to noxious chemicals when evaluating children with red, irritated eyes.

Physical Examination

A thorough examination of the eyes should be performed. The eyelids, conjunctiva, and cornea should be inspected for evidence of inflammation or foreign bodies. The presence of any discharge or crusting of the eyelids as well as light sensitivity or pain should be noted. Extraocular movements should be checked, and their symmetry should be noted. Visual acuity should be determined, and an ophthalmoscopic examination of the retina should be performed whenever possible. A slit lamp examination of the eye is indicated if uveitis is suspected. In addition, it is important to perform a thorough head and neck examination, noting the presence of associated sinusitis, otitis media, or pharyngitis.

Laboratory Tests

Laboratory assessment is guided by the history and physical examination. Although clinical differentiation between a bacterial and viral etiology is difficult, cultures are usually not required, because acute conjunctivitis in children is a self-limited disease. In neonatal conjunctivitis, however, the time of onset of illness and the clinical findings overlap, and Gram stain and cultures are essential. Gonococcal infection is assessed by both Gram stain and culture. Treatment may be initiated on the basis of Gram stain alone because of the serious potential for corneal involvement and subsequent loss of visual acuity.

If HSV is suspected, viral cultures should be obtained. If chlamydial infection is suspected, a nasopharyngeal culture should be sent in addition to conjunctival scraping. Purulent material may be examined for gonococci, but conjunctival scrapings are required for chlamydia, because chlamydia is an obligate intracellular organism.

Laboratory assessment of periorbital cellulitis includes a CBC, blood culture, and a lumbar puncture in young infants or in children with signs of meningeal irritation. The reported prevalence of meningitis is 1% in children with periorbital cellulitis, and it is 10% in children with bacteremia and periorbital cellulitis. As with periorbital cellulitis, laboratory assessment of orbital cellulitis includes a CBC and blood culture.

Imaging Studies

Imaging studies are required infrequently in the assessment of eye infections. A chest x-ray to detect pneumonia should be taken if infants with neonatal conjunctivitis have respiratory symptoms. Characteristic features on chest x-ray include hyperinflation and diffuse or patchy interstitial infiltrates. In orbital cellulitis, a CT scan of the orbit and sinuses may be useful for assessing the degree of involvement.

MANAGEMENT

The majority of common eye infections either resolve spontaneously or respond readily to **hygiene** and **topical antibiotics.** Treatment of both staphylococcal and seborrheic blepharitis consists of daily lid hygiene (usually at bedtime), including application of a warm compress and removal of the scales and crusts with a moistened, warm washcloth. The eyelashes and lid margins may also be scrubbed with a cotton-tipped applicator soaked in a 50:50 mixture of baby shampoo and water. When staphylococcal blepharitis is present, an ointment containing an antistaphylococcal antibiotic agent such as erythromycin may be applied to the eyelids after cleansing. Treatment of parasitic blepharitis consists of application of petrolatum ophthalmic ointment several times a day for one week, followed by removal of the remaining parasites and their ova with tweezers or forceps.

Treatment for both external and internal hordeolum consists of application of warm compresses several times a day and local application of an antistaphylococcal ointment. Once the infection comes to a head or point, the hair at the center of the external hordeolum can sometimes be removed with tweezers, thereby creating an opening and allowing the infection to drain. Occasionally, surgical excision and drainage may be required if the abscess does not resolve (more common for internal hordeolum than external hordeolum). Unlike the hordeolum, a chalazion generally requires surgical excision, because spontaneous resolution is uncommon.

The vast majority of cases of acute childhood conjunctivitis can be managed successfully by primary care physicians. Acute conjunctivitis in childhood is generally a self-limited disease. However, antibiotic treatment of bacterial conjunctivitis hastens recovery and may help prevent secondary cases by eradicating the bacterial pathogen. It is helpful to determine clinically whether the infection is bacterial and initiate empiric treatment with topical antibiotic preparations. Trimethoprim and polymyxin B sulfate (Polytrim), sodium sulfacetamide (Bleph-10), gentamicin (Garamycin), and tobramycin (TobraDex) are some of the commonly prescribed antibiotics. Avoid neomycin-containing products because sensitivity to neomycin occurs frequently. Antibiotic ointments may be easier to instill in infants and young children. Antibiotic drops should be used in older children during the day because these preparations do not interfere with vision. Ointments may be used at bedtime. Systemic therapy can be considered for concomitant conjunctivitis and otitis media. If symptoms persist for more than 7–10 days or if the diagnosis is in question, appropriate cultures should be taken. Complicated cases such as suspected herpetic or gonococcal infection, foreign bodies that cannot be removed easily, loss of visual acuity, presence of significant pain, those involving children with a history of recent penetrating ocular trauma or surgery, and those involving children who use contact lenses should be referred to an ophthalmologist immediately.

Chronic conjunctivitis can be managed with cool compresses. Topical decongestant drops may provide symptomatic relief if treatment is indicated. Vernal conjunctivitis may be treated with topical cromolyn sodium drops. Corticosteroid therapy may be considered. Caution should be used when prescribing corticosteroid preparations for the eye, however, because they may lead to progression of an undiagnosed herpetic eye infection.

Treatment of neonatal conjunctivitis depends on the diagnosis. If gonococcal infection is suspected and Gram stain is positive for gram-negative diplococci, immediate parenteral therapy with ceftriaxone should be initiated. Chlamydial conjunctivitis should be managed with systemic rather than topical treatment to prevent systemic disease. Oral erythromycin is the drug of choice. Although oral treatment provides adequate local antibiotic levels, topical erythromycin ointment may be used in conjunction with systemic therapy to provide more prompt relief of ophthalmic symptoms.

Empiric parenteral antibiotic therapy (e.g., cefuroxime) should be initiated for periorbital cellulitis. Repeat evaluations for signs of progression should be performed frequently during the initial 24–48 hours. If orbital cellulitis is suspected, an ophthalmologist should be consulted, and hospitalization and systemic antibiotics should be instituted. Surgical drainage of the sinuses or of an orbital abscess is sometimes necessary.

Children with suspected herpetic infection should be referred to an ophthalmologist. Intravenous acyclovir is often recommended for the treatment of isolated herpetic eye infections in neonates.

PROGNOSIS

The majority of common eye infections such as blepharitis, hordeolum, and acute childhood conjunctivitis resolve without sequelae. Recurrence is common for hordeolums, and periorbital cellulitis may be a potential complication in rare or untreated cases. Unlike acute conjunctivitis, chronic conjunctivitis may not be self-limited. Appropriate diagnosis and management are extremely important to prevent serious sequelae in some children. For example, endemic trachoma may progress to produce conjunctival scarring, pannus

formation, and even blindness if not appropriately treated with systemic erythromycin or tetracycline. (In general, systemic tetracycline should not be used in children under age 8 years to avoid discoloration of the teeth.)

Periorbital cellulitis generally resolves without sequelae if treated promptly with systemic antibiotics. Orbital cellulitis should be considered a true ophthalmologic emergency because the potential for complications is high. The optic nerve may become involved, resulting in loss of vision or spread of the infection into the cranial cavity. This spreading may lead to meningitis, cavernous sinus thrombosis, or brain abscess.

Case Resolution

The infant presented in the case history has neonatal conjunctivitis. A Gram stain of the purulent discharge should be examined, and cultures should be taken from the eye and nasopharynx. If the Gram stain is negative for gonococci, empiric treatment may begin with oral erythromycin.

Selected Readings

Gigliotti, F. Acute conjunctivitis. Pediatr. Rev. 16:203–207, 1995.

King, R. A. Common ocular signs and symptoms in childhood. Pediatr. Clin. North Am. 40:753–766, 1993.

O'Hara, M. A. Ophthalmia neonatorum. Pediatr. Clin. North Am. 40:715–725, 1993.

Persaud, D., W. J. Moss, and J. L. Munoz. Serious eye infections in children. Pediatr. Ann. 22:379–383, 1993.

Powell, K. R. Orbital and periorbital cellulitis. Pediatr. Rev. 16:163–167, 1995.

Wagner, R. S. Eye infections and abnormalities: issues for the pediatrician. Contemp. Pediatr. 14:137–153, 1997.

Wagner, R. S. The differential diagnosis of the red eye. Contemp. Pediatr. 8:26–48, 1991.

Weiss, A. H. Chronic conjunctivitis in infants and children. Pediatr. Ann. 22:366–374, 1993.

CHAPTER 58

EXCESSIVE TEARING

Geeta Grover, M.D.

Hx A 4-week-old infant girl has had a persistent watery discharge from the left eye since birth. Her mother has noticed white, crusty material on her daughter's eyelids for the past few days. The infant's birth and medical history are unremarkable. Examination of the eyes, including bilateral red reflexes and symmetric extraocular movements, is normal, except that the left eye appears "wetter" than the right.

Infants or young children with excessive tearing or epiphora in one or both eyes are a common pediatric ophthalmologic concern. The pediatrician must be capable of differentiating benign causes of this common childhood condition from other more serious illnesses, such as glaucoma, that potentially threaten vision.

EPIDEMIOLOGY

Congenital obstruction of the nasolacrimal duct or dacryostenosis, which occurs in 1–6% of newborn infants, is the most common cause of excessive tearing in infancy. Spontaneous resolution of this obstruction before 6 months of age is common.

In contrast, congenital or infantile glaucoma, a serious cause of excessive tearing, is quite rare; the incidence is about 1:10,000 live births. Although glaucoma may be present at birth, onset during the first few weeks to months of life is more common. Approximately 25% of cases are diagnosed at birth and 80% by 1 year of age. The majority of affected infants are male; the male: female ratio in older infants is 2:1. Infantile glaucoma appears to have a multifactorial inheritance pattern, but the majority of cases are sporadic. In families with one affected child or a parental history of infantile glaucoma, the chance of having a child with glaucoma is about 5%. Although glaucoma may be unilateral or bilateral, the vast majority of children (75–90%) who present before 3 months of age have bilateral glaucoma.

CLINICAL PRESENTATION

Infants with dacryostenosis usually present with a history of a mucoid eye discharge and crusting along the eyelid margins. The affected eye appears "wetter" than the normal eye, and a small pool of tears may be noted along the lower eyelid. Infants with glaucoma characteristically present with excessive tearing, rhinorrhea, photophobia, and corneal haziness (D$_x$ Box).

D$_x$ Excessive Tearing

- Conjunctival injection or edema
- Crusting of the eyelids
- Rhinorrhea
- Photophobia
- Corneal haziness
- Reflux of tears with gentle pressure on medial canthus
- Wetness of eye

PATHOPHYSIOLOGY

Tears serve many important functions within the visual system. As well as lubricating the eyes, they provide them with oxygen and antibacterial substances. The tear film is composed of three layers: oily, mucoid, and aqueous. The lacrimal system (Fig. 58–1) produces and drains tears away from the eyes and into the nose. The accessory lacrimal glands of Krause and Wolfring, located behind the upper and lower eyelids in the conjunctival cul-de-sac, are responsible for the basal secretion of tears necessary to keep the eyes moist and lubricated, and the lacrimal gland itself produces reflex tears or tears due to emotions. Reflex tearing is usually present shortly after birth but may be delayed for several weeks to months until the lacrimal gland begins to function. Tears drain away from the eyes through the superior and inferior puncta into the superior and inferior canalicula and finally into the nasolacrimal duct, which drains beneath the inferior turbinate in the nose.

Excessive tearing during infancy may result from either increased production of tears or obstruction of drainage. Outflow obstruction, most often due to obstruction of the nasolacrimal duct or dacryostenosis, is the most common cause of excessive tearing in infancy. The obstruction is usually unilateral and occurs during fetal development. Most commonly, a congenital narrowing of the duct or a persistent, thin membrane obstructs it. The membrane is usually located in the distal or nasal segment of the duct rather than in the proximal portion. The term "dacryocystitis" is used if acute infection or inflammation is associated with the obstruction. If both the canaliculi and the nasolacrimal duct are obstructed, a mucocele over the nasolacrimal sac may be noted at birth. This sac appears as a bluish, firm mass located below the medial canthus. Atresia of

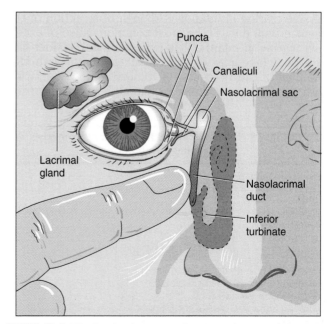

FIGURE 58–1. The lacrimal system, showing massage of the lacrimal sac.

some portion of the drainage system may also occur, but this is extremely rare.

The most common reason for excessive production of tears is **eye irritation** (e.g., due to a foreign body in the eyelid or corneal abrasion). The congenital paradoxical gustolacrimal reflex, or **crocodile tears,** is a rare disorder that may also produce epiphora. In this disorder, an abnormal connection between the salivary and lacrimal glands produces unilateral and sometimes bilateral tearing with salivation. This condition may also be acquired secondary to facial trauma.

Glaucoma is the most serious and potentially sight-threatening etiology for excessive production of tears. Glaucoma refers to an increase in intraocular pressure that is severe enough to damage the eye and alter vision. In infants and children, glaucoma is usually a result of a developmental abnormality of the iridocorneal angle interfering with drainage of aqueous humor from the anterior chamber. Young infants differ from adults in that the globe in infants' eyes is distensible; the increased intraocular pressure not only produces corneal enlargement and edema but also expands the globe itself. Breakdown of the corneal epithelium and resultant irritation of the eyes produce reflex tearing. Untreated glaucoma may lead to optic nerve damage with resultant loss of visual acuity and even blindness.

Glaucoma in children younger than 3 years of age is referred to broadly as infantile glaucoma, and glaucoma that occurs in children between 3 and 20 years of age is called juvenile glaucoma. Infantile glaucoma is further classified as being primary or secondary. Primary glaucoma refers to isolated abnormalities of the iridocorneal angle, whereas secondary glaucoma may be associated with other ocular or systemic diseases. Juvenile glaucoma is a form of open-angle glaucoma.

DIFFERENTIAL DIAGNOSIS

Table 58–1 outlines the differential diagnosis of excessive tearing in infancy. Although obstruction of the nasolacrimal duct is the most common cause of excessive tearing in infants, it is important to consider and rule out glaucoma when evaluating infants with this complaint. The presence of rhinorrhea in association with epiphora distinguishes infantile glaucoma from dacryostenosis. Rhinorrhea is not associated with dacryostenosis because the nasolacrimal duct is obstructed, and no tears drain out of the nose. Unlike dacryostenosis, which is usually unilateral, infantile glaucoma is very commonly bilateral.

Acute onset of excessive tearing in older children is usually due to ocular irritation. Any irritation of the conjunctiva, cornea, or eyelids may produce tearing. Conjunctivitis and corneal abrasion, usually secondary to a retained foreign body or herpes simplex keratoconjunctivitis, are the two most common causes. Eye infections are discussed in Chapter 57.

EVALUATION

History

Evaluation of excessive tearing should begin with a thorough history. The nature of any discharge (e.g., watery, mucoid, or purulent) should be noted. Parents or other care givers should be questioned about the appearance of the child's eyes (Questions Box). The excessive mucoid discharge in the medial canthal region and on the eyelashes is usually more noticeable to the family than the increased tearing. Crusting along the eyelashes caused by drying of the mucoid material is usually noted when children awaken in the morning or after a nap. Mucopurulent discharge may be noted if an associated acute infection is present (dacryocystitis).

Physical Examination

A careful examination of the eyes in infants includes inspection, evaluation of extraocular movements, and funduscopic examination. Funduscopic examination may be difficult in this age group, but bilateral red reflexes should at least be elicited. Signs of **dacryostenosis,** which usually appear days to weeks after birth, include tearing, mucoid discharge, and crusting of the eyelids. Tearing may be as mild as an increased wetness of the affected eye; this is best evaluated prior to disturbing children. Visible overflow of tears from the affected eye is unusual, and is typically seen only when the eye is irritated (e.g., due to cold or wind). If dacryostenosis is present, associated conjunctival injection, erythema, and edema of the eyelids or systemic signs of infection such as fever may be noted. Dacryocystitis may also spread to the surrounding tissues, producing a periorbital cellulitis. Gentle pressure along

---

TABLE 58–1. Differential Diagnosis of Excessive Tearing in Infants

Increased Production
Infantile glaucoma
Irritation
    Conjunctivitis
    Corneal abrasion
    Foreign body under the eyelid
Congenital paradoxical gustolacrimal reflex (crocodile tears)
Outflow Obstruction
Nasolacrimal duct obstruction (dacryostenosis)
Anomalies of the lacrimal drainage system
    Mucocele of the lacrimal sac
    Atresia of the lacrimal punctum or canaliculus
Nasal congestion
Craniofacial anomalies involving the midface

Questions: Excessive Tearing

- How old was the child when the excessive tearing appeared?
- Are one or both eyes affected?
- How does the eye appear? How has its appearance changed?
- Is there a family history of infantile glaucoma?
- Is the child photophobic or light-sensitive (e.g., closes the eyes in bright sunlight)?
- Has the child had any persistent, watery discharge?
- Does the child have difficulty opening the affected eye on awakening in the morning or after a nap?

the medial canthal region over the lacrimal sac may produce a reflux of tears or mucoid discharge onto the surface of the eye, thus confirming the diagnosis of obstruction. If the diagnosis is uncertain, fluorescein dye should be placed in the eye and observed for a few minutes. If an obstruction of the duct is present, the fluorescein will not disappear as expected, and no dye will exit through the nose. The cornea may be examined after instillation of fluorescein dye if an ocular foreign body or corneal abrasion is the suspected cause of the excessive tearing.

In addition to excessive tearing, other clinical signs of infantile glaucoma include blepharospasm (spasmodic winking of the eyelids), photophobia, corneal enlargement and corneal haziness due to corneal edema, progressive enlargement of the eye (buphthalmos), and cupping and atrophy of the optic nerve. A corneal diameter greater than 12 mm in infants is suggestive of infantile glaucoma. Corneal edema is more common in younger infants (<3 months of age) and may cause the red reflex to appear dull in the affected eye. The optic cup may be enlarged. A cup-to-disk ratio greater than 0.3 or an asymmetry of the ratio between the eyes may indicate glaucoma.

As in adults, loss of visual fields occurs in children with glaucoma. Visual fields are difficult to evaluate in young children because of their inability to cooperate with the examination. Suspected cases of glaucoma should be referred to an ophthalmologist for further evaluation, including measurement of intraocular pressure. Pressures greater than 20 mm Hg are suggestive of glaucoma (normal pressures are 10–20 mm Hg in infants and young children as well as in adults).

Laboratory Tests

Routine laboratory assessment is generally not necessary.

MANAGEMENT

Spontaneous resolution of dacryostenosis is common by 6–8 months of age. The primary medical treatment of uncomplicated nasolacrimal duct obstruction consists of **local massage** and **cleansing** beginning when the symptoms are noted. Parents are instructed to massage the nasolacrimal duct several times a day by applying firm, downward pressure over the medial canthal region with their finger and then sliding the finger down towards the mouth (Creiger maneuver) (see Fig. 58–1). This maneuver attempts to move fluid trapped within the nasolacrimal sac down through the duct in an attempt to break the obstruction with hydrostatic pressure. Parents may be asked to cleanse the eyes with warm water before performing this maneuver. Antibiotic ointments and drops should be prescribed only if the discharge is purulent or associated conjunctivitis is evident.

Controversy exists regarding when probing of the nasolacrimal duct should be performed. Many ophthalmologists prefer probing the duct before children are 6 months of age, because prior to this time the procedure may be performed in the office without general anesthesia. Others state that over 90% of obstructions resolve with conservative medical management by 12 months of age and prefer to delay probing until the age of 12–15 months. At this age the procedure needs to be performed under general anesthesia. Deciding when to proceed with the probing depends on the standard of practice within the community, the severity of symptoms, the response to medical management, and the level of parental concern.

Ophthalmologic referral is necessary for affected infants by 6 months of age if the obstruction has not resolved. Referral should be made sooner if symptoms are severe or infections recur. Suspected cases of infantile glaucoma should be immediately referred to an ophthalmologist because if the condition is left untreated, it may progress to blindness. **Surgery** is the primary treatment. The goal is to normalize intraocular pressure and minimize irreversible corneal and optic nerve damage.

PROGNOSIS

The majority of cases of dacryostenosis resolve spontaneously during the first year of life without further sequelae. Infantile glaucoma, if left untreated, may progress to blindness. The visual prognosis depends on several factors, including the age at onset of glaucoma (the earlier the onset, the worse the prognosis) and the degree of myopia caused by the enlargement of the eye. In addition, amblyopia, secondary to either deprivation due to corneal opacities or unequal refractive errors, is often seen (see Chapter 56, Strabismus).

> ### Case Resolution
>
> The infant presented in the case history at the beginning of the chapter has dacryostenosis. She can be managed with medical treatment such as local massage and cleansing at this stage. If her symptoms persist beyond the age of 6 months, consultation with an ophthalmologist is recommended.

Selected Readings

Calhoun, J. H. Disorders of the lacrimal apparatus in infancy and childhood. *In* Nelson, L. B., J. H. Calhoun, and R. D. Harley. Pediatric Ophthalmology, 3rd ed. Philadelphia, W. B. Saunders, 1991.

Howard, C. W. The baby with too many tears: what to do and how to do it. Int. Pediatr. 5:239–242, 1990.

Isenberg, S. J., et al. Development of tearing in preterm and term neonates. Arch. Ophthalmol. 116:773–776, 1998.

Lavrich, J. B., and L. B. Nelson. Disorders of the lacrimal system apparatus. Pediatr. Clin. North Am. 40:767–776, 1993.

Wagner, R. S. Glaucoma in children. Pediatr. Clin. North Am. 40:855–867, 1993.

NECK MASSES

Stanley H. Inkelis, M.D.

Hₓ A 2-year-old boy is brought to the office with a one-day history of an enlarging red, tender "bump" beneath his right mandible. He has a fever of 101.6° F (38.5° C) and sores around his nose, upper lip, and cheek. These sores have been present for 3 days and have not responded to an over-the-counter antibiotic ointment. He had a URI 1 week ago, which has almost entirely resolved. He is otherwise in good health. The family has no history of tuberculosis or recent travel, and the child has not been playing with cats or other animals.

The physical examination is completely normal except for fever, mild rhinorrhea, honey-crusted lesions on the nares and upper lip, and a 4 x 5-cm, right submandibular neck mass that is erythematous, warm, and tender to palpation.

Questions

1. What are the common causes of neck masses in children?
2. What steps are involved in the evaluation of children with neck masses?
3. What clinical findings suggest that neck masses are neoplasms? When should neck masses be biopsied or removed?
4. What is involved in the treatment of the different types of neck masses in children?
5. When should children with neck masses be referred for further consultation?

Neck masses are any swellings or enlargements of the structures in the area between the inferior mandible and the clavicle. Normal variants, such as the angle of the mandible or tip of the mastoid, may occasionally appear as swellings, and parents sometimes confuse these with neck masses. If the swelling is not a normal structure, a well-directed history and physical examination usually determine the etiology.

Lymphadenopathy from viral or bacterial throat infections is the most common cause of neck mass in children. Therefore, neck masses are common because children frequently have sore throats. Most parents know about "swollen lymph glands," and they usually do not seek medical advice unless the glands become very large or do not recede in a few days. Neck masses in children may have many other causes besides lymphadenopathy. Most of these masses may be categorized as inflammatory, neoplastic, traumatic, or congenital in origin.

EPIDEMIOLOGY

Most neck masses are benign. Almost 50% of all 2-year old children have palpable cervical lymph nodes. Although more than 25% of malignant tumors in children are found in the head and neck region (this is the primary site in only 5%), less than 2% of suspicious head and neck masses are malignant.

The epidemiology of neck masses of infectious origin depends on the infectious agent itself, geographic location of the child, and the child's socioeconomic status. Neck masses of viral origin may be related to focal infection of the oropharynx or respiratory tract but are often associated with generalized adenopathy. Neck masses of bacterial origin typically occur from normal bacterial flora of the nose, mouth, pharynx, and skin. These organisms are not usually transmitted from person to person. Pathologic flora such as group A streptococcus and *Mycobacterium tuberculosis* that result in neck masses can spread by human-to-human contact, however.

CLINICAL PRESENTATION

Children with neck masses present in a variety of different ways depending on the etiology of the mass. Typically a swelling or enlargement in the neck, which parents often notice more than children, is evident. Associated signs and symptoms include fever, upper respiratory tract infection, sore throat, ear pain, pain or tenderness over the mass, changes in skin color over the mass, skin lesions of the head or neck, and dental caries or infections (Dₓ Box). Malignant tumors are usually slow-growing, firm, fixed, nontender masses. Congenital neck masses and benign tumors, which have frequently been present since birth or early infancy, are soft, smooth, and cystlike and may be recurrent. Neck masses associated with trauma are often rapidly evolving and may lead to airway obstruction.

PATHOPHYSIOLOGY

The pathophysiology of neck masses in children is dependent on etiology. Most neck masses are related to inflammation or infection of lymph nodes. Enlargement of lymph nodes usually results from proliferation of intrinsic lymphocytes or histiocytes already present in the lymph node (e.g., lymphadenopathy caused by a viral infection) or from infiltration of extrinsic cells (e.g., lymphadenitis, metastatic tumor). Neck masses from trauma occur from leakage of fluid into the neck, and

D_x Neck Masses

INFLAMMATORY/INFECTIOUS

- Swelling or enlargement in the neck
- Fever
- Sore throat, dental infection, skin infection of head or neck
- Pain or tenderness over the mass (usually)

NEOPLASTIC

- Slowly enlarging mass
- Unilateral, discrete
- Firm or rubbery
- Fixed to tissue
- Deep within the fascia
- Nontender (usually)

CONGENITAL

- Enlargement in neck (usually present since birth or soon after)
- Soft, smooth, cyst-like
- Nontender (unless infected)
- Recurrent

adenopathy may be seen in children with systemic illness (e.g., Kawasaki syndrome, sarcoid, HIV). Cat-scratch disease, toxoplasmosis, fungal infection, and mycobacterial and atypical mycobacterial infections may be associated with lympadenopathy that may later progress to lymphadenitis. Viral illnesses, including EBV (mononucleosis), adenovirus, enterovirus, herpes simplex virus, human herpes virus 6 (HHV-6), and CMV, commonly cause lymphadenopathy and lymphadenitis.

Lymphadenitis is infection or inflammation of the lymph node, that occurs when neutrophils infiltrate the node, leading to necrosis and abscess formation. This condition is usually associated with proximal bacterial infection that drains to the affected nodes by connecting afferent lymphatic channels. Lymphadenitis is often a progression of disease, resulting in enlarged nodes that measure 2–6 cm. These nodes, which are typical of bacterial disease, are often termed "hot" nodes, and they are erythematous, warm, tender, and sometimes fluctuant. "Cold" nodes or "cold" lymphadenitis usually represents subacute or chronic inflammation of lymph nodes typical in illnesses such as cat-scratch disease,

congenital anatomic abnormalities become apparent because of fluid collection or infection of the defect. The parotid gland may be enlarged from inflammation (e.g., blocked salivary gland duct), infection (e.g., mumps), or tumor (e.g., pleomorphic adenoma), but the swelling primarily involves the face rather than the neck and obscures the angle of the jaw.

DIFFERENTIAL DIAGNOSIS

Neck masses in children are usually the result of inflammation or infection of lymph nodes, tumors of lymph nodes and other neck structures, trauma, and congenital lesions. The location of the mass is often a clue to its etiology (Fig. 59–1).

Lymphadenopathy/Lymphadenitis

Lymphadenopathy is lymph node enlargement or hyperplasia secondary to localized infection or antigenic stimulation proximal to the involved node or nodes. Because lymphoid tissue steadily increases until puberty, palpable lymph nodes, including those in the cervical area, are a common, normal finding in children. Any lymph node in the neck larger than 10 mm qualifies as cervical lymphadenopathy.

The most common cause of cervical lymphadenopathy is a viral infection of the upper respiratory tract. Lymphadenopathy usually begins and resolves with the acute infection. Occasionally the swelling remains for several days or months, however, and children present because of parental concern. Bacterial pharyngitis, usually from infection with group A beta-hemolytic streptococcus, is often associated with cervical lymphadenopathy. Cervical as well as generalized lymph-

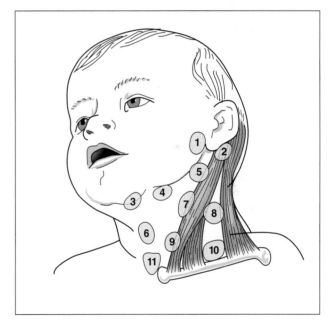

FIGURE 59–1. Differential diagnosis of neck mass by location. 1: Parotid—cystic hygroma, hemangioma, lymphadenitis, parotitis, Sjögren's and Caffey-Silverman syndromes, lymphoma. 2: Postauricular—lymphadenitis, branchial cleft cyst (1st), squamous epithelial cyst. 3: Submental—lymphadenitis, cystic hygroma, thyroglossal duct cyst, dermoid, sialoadenitis. 4: Submandibular—lymphadenitis, cystic hygroma, sialoadenitis, tumor, cystic fibrosis. 5: Jugulodiagastic—lymphadenitis, squamous epithelial cyst, branchial cleft cyst (1st), parotid tumor, normal-transverse process C2, styloid process. 6: Midline neck—lymphadenitis, thyroglossal duct cyst, dermoid, laryngocele, normal-hyoid, thyroid. 7: Sternomastoid (anterior)—lymphadenitis, branchial cleft cyst (2nd, 3rd) pilomatrixoma, rare tumors. 8: Spinal accessory—lymphadenitis, lymphoma, metastasis from nasopharynx. 9: Paratracheal—thyroid, parathyroid, esophageal diverticulum. 10: Supraclavicular—cystic hygroma, lipoma, lymphoma, metastasis, normal-fat pad, pneumatocele of upper lobe. 11: Suprasternal—thyroid, lipoma, dermoid, thymus, mediastinal mass. (Reproduced, with permission, from Fleisher, G. R., and S. Ludwig [eds.]. Textbook of Pediatric Emergency Medicine, 3rd ed. Baltimore, Williams & Wilkins, 1993, p. 321.)

mycobacterial infection, or toxoplasmosis. Unlike hot nodes, cold nodes are not warm to the touch and are usually not as tender. They are usually not suppurative and may be difficult to distinguish from nodes that are simply enlarged (Fig. 59–2).

Staphylococcus aureus and group A streptococcus are responsible for 60–85% of cases of acute unilateral cervical lymphadenitis. These organisms spread from a primary site to the lymph nodes draining those sites. Common primary sites of infection are the throat; teeth and gums; and skin (lesions), particularly on the scalp or ears. Infections at these sites may result from trauma, such as scratches or scabs, or from primary infection, such as impetigo. *S. aureus* or group B streptococcus usually causes cervical lymphadenitis in neonates or very young infants. Such staphylococcal infections, which are often nosocomially spread from contact in the newborn nursery, present as discrete masses. Group B streptococcus causes the "cellulitis-adenitis" syndrome, which presents as cervical adenitis associated with a facial cellulitis. *Pseudomonas aeruginosa* is an unusual cause of cervical adenitis in newborns.

Mycobacterial disease must always be considered in children of all ages who present with cervical adenitis. Nodes are often multiple, sometimes bilateral, usually nontender, and are not erythematous or warm. Atypical mycobacterial infection usually occurs in children between 1 and 5 years of age with unilateral rather than bilateral lymph node enlargement.

Cat-scratch disease should be considered in children who have cats or kittens or who play with them. The infection may result from a cat scratch or from a cat's licking a child's broken skin. If the inoculum is near the head and neck area, cervical adenitis develops. Occasionally, generalized lymphadenopathy is present. An associated papule or papules where the cat scratch or lick occurred may be apparent. *Bartonella henselae* has been identified as the organism causing cat-scratch disease.

Toxoplasmosis may be accompanied by adenitis, usually in the posterior cervical area. Nodes are painless and may fluctuate in size, and children are often asymptomatic. Multiple lymph nodes are involved in about one third to one half of cases.

Less common bacterial, viral, and fungal causes of cervical adenitis are listed in Table 59–1.

Tumors

Compared to other neck masses, **malignant neck tumors** occur rarely; nevertheless, they should be considered in any children with rapidly enlarging or persistent neck masses. Hodgkin's disease and lymphosarcoma account for approximately two thirds of malignant neoplasms of the head and neck in children. Age is an important factor in determining the likelihood of specific tumors. Neuroblastoma, lymphosarcoma, rhabdomyosarcoma, and Hodgkin's disease are the most frequent tumor types in children under the age of 6 years. Hodgkin's disease and lymphosarcoma occur with almost equal frequency in preadolescent children, followed by thyroid malignancies and rhabdomyosarcoma. Hodgkin's disease is the most common malignancy in adolescents.

Benign neck tumors, with the exception of those mentioned later in the discussion of congenital lesions, are uncommon. They include epidermoid inclusion cysts, lipomas, fibromas, neurofibromas, keloids, goiters, and ranulas (intraoral mucocysts).

Trauma

Trauma to the neck may be associated with bleeding and edema. Large hematomas that affect vital structures are potentially life-threatening. Significant trauma and structural injury usually accompany neck hematomas. In children with mild injuries and neck hematomas, bleeding disorders are a possible cause of the

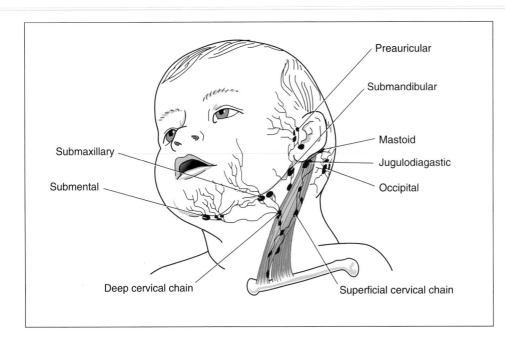

FIGURE 59–2. The lymphatic drainage and lymph nodes involved in infants and children with cervical lymphadenitis. (Reproduced, with permission, from Feigin, R. D., and J. D. Cherry [eds.]. Textbook of Pediatric Infectious Diseases, 4th ed. Philadelphia, W. B. Saunders, 1998, p. 171.)

TABLE 59-1.   Differential Diagnosis of Neck Masses

Cervical Lymphadenopathy/Lymphadenitis
Bacterial origin
  Staphylococcus aureus
  Group A beta-hemolytic streptococcus
  Mycobacterium tuberculosis
  Atypical mycobacteria
  Cat-scratch disease *(Bartonella henselae)*
  Anaerobes
  Gram-negative enteric bacteria
  Haemophilus influenzae
  Plague
  Actinomycosis
  Diphtheria
  Tularemia
  Brucellosis
  Syphilis
  Group B streptococcus (neonates)
Viral origin
  Epstein-Barr virus (infectious mononucleosis)
  Adenovirus
  Cytomegalovirus
  Herpes virus
  Enterovirus
  Human immunodeficiency virus
  Measles
  Rubella
  Human herpes virus
Fungal origin
  Histoplasmosis
  Coccidioidomycosis
  Aspergillosis
  Candidiasis
  Sporotrichosis
  Cryptococcosis
Parasitic origin
  Toxoplasmosis

Tumor
Malignant
  Hodgkin's disease
  Non-Hodgkin's lymphoma
  Lymphosarcoma
  Rhabdomyosarcoma
  Neuroblastoma
  Leukemia
  Histiocytosis X
  Thyroid tumors
  Nasopharyngeal squamous cell carcinoma
  Salivary gland carcinoma
Benign
  Epidermoid cyst
  Lipoma
  Fibroma
  Neurofibroma
  Keloid
  Goiter
  Osteochondroma
  Teratoma (may be malignant)
  Ranula

Congenital Disorders
Hemangioma
Cystic hygroma (lymphangioma)
Branchial cleft cyst
Thyroglossal duct cyst
Laryngocele
Dermoid cyst
Cervical rib
Sternocleidomastoid tumor

TABLE 59-1.   Differential Diagnosis of Neck Masses
Continued

Trauma
Hematoma (acute or organized)
Subcutaneous emphysema
Foreign body
Arteriovenous malformation

Immunologic Disorders
Local hypersensitivity reaction (sting or bite)
Pseudolymphoma (from phenytoin)
Serum sickness
Sarcoidosis
Caffey-Silverman syndrome
Kawasaki syndrome
Systemic lupus erythematosus
Juvenile rheumatoid arthritis
Kikuchi's disease (necrotizing lymphadenitis)

Miscellaneous
Storage disorders
  Niemann-Pick disease
  Gaucher's disease
Obstructive airway disease (asthma, cystic fibrosis)

hematoma. Twisting injuries to the neck may lead to muscle spasm of the sternocleidomastoid muscle (torticollis) and an apparent mass that is the contracted muscle. Child abuse should also be considered in children who have neck injuries that do not agree with their histories.

A foreign body in the neck may present as a mass because of the foreign body itself (e.g., piece of glass or metal, bullet) or surrounding inflammation. A "crepitant" neck mass following trauma to the neck or chest suggests subcutaneous emphysema from tracheal injury or a pneumomediastinum. Crepitant neck masses may also be seen secondary to pneumomediastinum in children with obstructive lung diseases such as asthma or cystic fibrosis.

Congenital Lesions

Children with congenital neck lesions can present with a neck mass in early infancy or later in childhood. Some congenital lesions are not discovered until adulthood. The most common of these benign lesions are thyroglossal duct cysts, branchial cleft cysts, cystic hygromas (lymphangiomas), and hemangiomas (Fig. 59-3).

Thyroglossal duct cysts are almost always midline in the neck and inferior to the hyoid bone. They usually move upward with tongue protrusion or swallowing. Most branchial cleft cysts occur anterior to the middle one third of the sternocleidomastoid muscle. Branchial cleft sinus tracts appear as slit-like openings anterior to the lower third of the sternocleidomastoid muscle and may present as neck masses if they become infected. Thyroglossal duct cysts and branchial cleft cysts may also present for the first time as infected neck masses.

Cystic hygromas are usually large, soft, easily compressible masses found in the posterior triangle behind the sternocleidomastoid muscle in the supraclavicular fossa. They transilluminate well. Two thirds of cystic hygromas are present at birth, and 80–90% are identi-

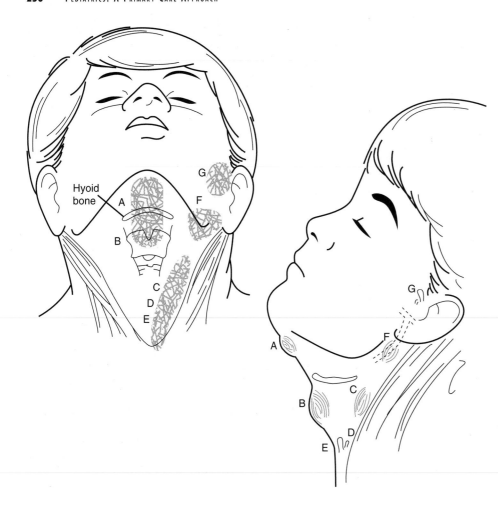

FIGURE 59–3. Head and neck congenital lesions seen in children in frontal and lateral views. The shaded areas denote the distribution in which a given lesion may be found. A, dermoid cyst; B, thyroglossal duct cyst; C, second branchial cleft appendage; D, second branchial cleft sinus; E, second branchial cleft cyst; F, first branchial pouch defect; G, preauricular sinus or appendage. (Reproduced, with permission, from Fleisher, G. R., and S. Ludwig [eds.]. Textbook of Pediatric Emergency Medicine, 3rd ed. Baltimore, Williams & Wilkins, 1993, p. 1301.)

fied before 3 years of age. They are more common on the left side of the neck. Cystic hygromas occasionally become secondarily infected, with findings of erythema, warmth, and tenderness.

Hemangiomas are usually not present at birth but appear in early infancy and may enlarge rapidly. In most cases, they recede spontaneously by 5–6 years of age. They are usually much smaller than cystic hygromas, do not transilluminate, and may be recognized by their reddish color (capillary or strawberry hemangioma) or by a bluish hue of the overlying skin (cavernous hemangioma).

Small infants who present with torticollis should be examined for a sternocleidomastoid mass ("tumor"), which represents fibrosis and contracture of that sternocleidomastoid muscle so that the head tilts toward the affected side. Contusion of the sternocleidomastoid muscle from traumatic extraction of the head during delivery with subsequent hemorrhage and healing has been implicated as the cause of the fibrotic mass. However, it is more likely that this mass occurs prior to birth, since it contains mature fibrous tissue. In addition, the mass may be present following cesarean section and is associated with hip dysplasia and other congenital lesions, suggesting that the condition is related to abnormal positioning *in utero*. Venous occlusion of the sternocleidomastoid muscle either *in utero* or at the time of delivery has also been proposed as a cause.

EVALUATION

History

A thorough history is important in establishing the etiology of the neck mass (Questions Box).

Physical Examination

A general physical examination should be performed. The neck mass should be examined for anatomic location, color, size, shape, consistency, tenderness, fluctuance, and mobility. The mass should also be measured.

Questions: Neck Masses

- How old is the child?
- How long has the neck mass been present?
- What signs and symptoms are associated with the neck mass?
- Has the child been exposed to tuberculosis?
- Has the child ever drunk any unpasteurized cow's milk?
- Has the child been in contact with any cats or kittens?
- Has the child traveled to areas where endemic diseases such as histoplasmosis or coccidioidomycosis are prevalent?
- Has the child suffered any trauma recently?
- Does the child have any allergies?
- Does the child have any risk factors for HIV?

The head, neck, and face should be examined for lesions, most often infections, that drain into neck lymph nodes. Lesions can frequently be found on the scalp, neck, face, ears, mouth, teeth, tongue, gums, and throat. Hair styles such as tight braids can sometimes provide ports of entry for bacteria. Occasionally, sinus tracts or fistulas may be the entry point of infection.

In addition, other lymph node groups should be examined to determine if the lymphadenopathy is local or generalized. Particular attention should be paid to the supraclavicular area, because enlarged supraclavicular nodes are more frequently associated with malignant pathology such as Hodgkin's disease.

The chest should be examined for use of accessory muscles, equality of breath sounds, and wheezing. The abdomen should be examined for hepatosplenomegaly.

Laboratory Tests

Laboratory tests are rarely indicated in children with cervical lymphadenopathy or lymphadenitis of acute onset. Although a rapid streptococcal antigen detection test or throat culture is helpful in children with suspected streptococcal sore throat, it may be unnecessary if antibiotic therapy is empirically prescribed for the lymphadenitis. If the adenitis is fluctuant, aspiration and culture may be helpful in determining the specific bacteriologic diagnosis. A PPD test should be applied to all children who present with lymphadenitis.

If the adenitis does not resolve or improve after two to three days of observation or therapy, laboratory tests directed by the history and physical examination should be considered. A CBC with differential and a monospot or heterophil test may be helpful in the diagnosis of infectious mononucleosis. If the mass in the neck is a hematoma and a bleeding disorder is suspected, a CBC with platelet count, PT, and PTT should be obtained. Possible additional tests include an ESR and, if indicated, serologic tests for toxoplasmosis, EBV, CMV, HHV-6, coccidioidomycosis, histoplasmosis, tularemia, *Bartonella henselae,* and syphilis should be performed. Skin tests for fungi should be considered in those patients coming from endemic areas. These tests should be placed after serologic tests are performed so that false-positive serologic test results are not obtained.

Similar laboratory tests should be considered for children who present for the first time with enlarged or enlarging lymph nodes of long duration or those who do not respond after 2 weeks of antibiotic therapy. The physician may choose to do more of these laboratory tests at the initial evaluation or after a therapeutic trial, as the likelihood of viral lymphadenopathy decreases and the possibility of a more unusual etiology increases. HIV testing should also be considered.

Thyroid function tests and thyroid scans should be considered in children with a thyroid mass or suspected thyroglossal duct cyst.

Unless cat-scratch disease is very likely, immediate lymph node biopsy is indicated for enlarged supraclavicular nodes or lymph nodes in the lower half of the neck, rapidly progressive and enlarging nodes, fixed nodes, nodes deep within the fascia, or firm or hard nodes. Children who have a persistent fever or weight loss despite antibiotic therapy should have a biopsy at 1 week if a diagnosis has not been established. Asymptomatic children without an established diagnosis should have a biopsy at 2 weeks if the node increases in size, at 4–6 weeks if the node is not increased in size but is persistent, and at 8–12 weeks if the node has not regressed to a normal size. In some cases, the initial biopsy is nondiagnostic but on subsequent biopsy a specific diagnosis may be made. Consequently, children with persistent adenopathy should be followed closely and be biopsied again if indicated. Fine needle aspiration biopsy in children is controversial. If malignancy is a consideration, consultation with an oncologist is advisable to determine the biopsy method of choice.

Imaging Studies

A chest x-ray should be obtained in all children with suspected tuberculosis or tumor (e.g., enlarged supraclavicular nodes) as well as in children with crepitant neck masses. If a foreign body in the neck is suspected, both anteroposterior and lateral neck x-rays should be obtained.

Ultrasonography is helpful in differentiating cystic from solid masses. In addition, demonstration of a normal thyroid gland by ultrasound in patients with thyroglossal duct cysts confirms a source of thyroid hormone. Consequently, a thyroid scan is not necessary. MRI may be useful in very select cases where soft tissue detail is necessary for diagnostic purposes.

MANAGEMENT

Neck masses are rarely acutely life-threatening. If neck masses impinge on the airway, children may experience stridor, hoarseness, drooling, increased effort of breathing, unequal breath sounds, or evidence of shock. Resuscitation and stabilization should be initiated immediately. The algorithm in Figure 59–4 outlines the management of cervical lymphadenitis.

Children with lymphadenitis who do not appear toxic and have no evidence of sepsis may be treated empirically with **oral antibiotics** that cover *S. aureus* and group A beta-hemolytic streptococcus. A first-generation cephalosporin such as cephalexin (50 mg/kg/d), dicloxacillin (50 mg/kg/d), or amoxicillin-clavulanic acid (40 mg/kg/d [amoxicillin]), provides satisfactory coverage. Treatment should be continued for a minimum of 10 days but for no less than 5 days after resolution of acute signs and symptoms. Lack of clinical improvement after 36–48 hours suggests that the diagnosis and proposed therapy need to be re-evaluated.

Infants and small children, as well as those older children who do not respond to oral antibiotic therapy, may require admission for **intravenous antibiotics** such as oxacillin or a cephalosporin. Incision and drainage of large, fluctuant nodes that are clearly from bacterial disease should be done, in consultation with an otolar-

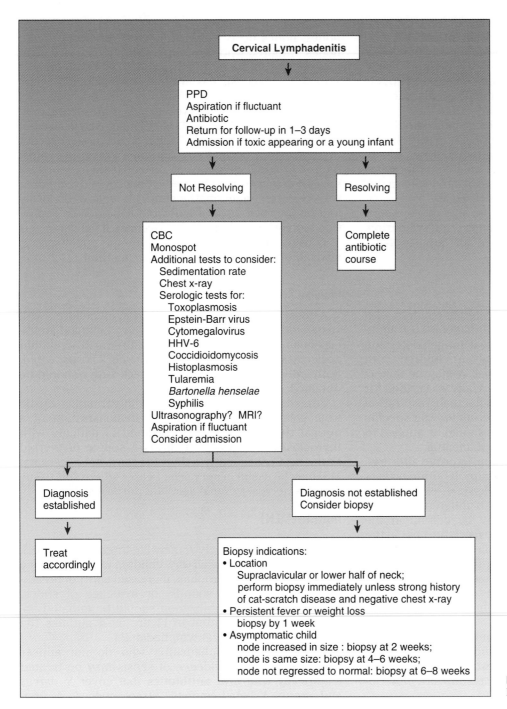

FIGURE 59–4. Management of cervical lymphadenitis.

yngologist or surgeon to promote resolution of the lymphadenitis. Alternatively, treatment by needle aspiration instead of incision and drainage has been advocated by some physicians. If *M. tuberculosis* or atypical mycobacterial infection is suspected, incision and drainage should not be done because persistent sinus tracts may result.

Atypical mycobacterial infection is virtually always unresponsive to treatment with antituberculous medications. **Surgical excision** of all visibly affected nodes, deep as well as superficial, is required. Tuberculous mycobacterial adenitis (scrofula) usually responds to short-course medical therapy. Antituberculous medication for 6–9 months is recommended.

Lymphadenitis from cat-scratch disease usually resolves on its own. Antibiotic therapy is usually not indicated, but if children are toxic-appearing or admitted for a suppurative adenitis, treatment with oral antibiotics such as rifampin or trimethoprim-sulfamethoxazole for young children and ciprofloxacin for adolescents may be beneficial. If there is no improvement, the addition of parenteral gentamicin to the regimen may be considered. If the node is fluctuant, **aspiration** is indicated. Total removal of the node is sometimes necessary to effect a cure.

There is no specific therapy for lymphadenitis caused by *Toxoplasma gondii*. Excision of the affected node may be indicated if the diagnosis is questionable.

If a tumor is suspected, consultation with a pediatric oncologist is recommended. The mass should be biopsied for a definitive diagnosis. If it is malignant, a treatment plan should be generated with the appropriate consultants.

Congenital torticollis from fibrosis of the sternocleidomastoid muscle is best treated with nonoperative intervention. Repetitive passive range-of-motion exercises over several weeks usually result in loosening the tight muscle and increasing the range of motion.

Hemangiomas usually resolve by the time children are 5 years of age, and surgical intervention is rarely indicated. For life-threatening hemangiomas, or those which may cause complications such as vision loss, corticosteroids and interferon alfa-2a are effective medications. Surgical excision is usually indicated for cystic hygromas (lymphangiomas), branchial cleft cysts, and thyroglossal duct cysts. A thyroid ultrasound should be performed before removal of a thyroglossal duct cyst to confirm that other thyroid tissue is present. Endocrinologic consultation is recommended in these cases. Thyroid nodules in children may be cancerous, especially in children who have had irradiation to the head and neck region. Consultation with an endocrinologist and surgeon should be obtained. Goiters in children should be evaluated by an endocrinologist.

PROGNOSIS

The prognosis for children with neck masses is generally excellent but differs depending on the cause. Children with an infectious etiology do very well if diagnosed and treated with appropriate antimicrobials. Mycobacterial lymphadenitis may result in sinus tract formation or disseminated disease. Surgical excision usually cures atypical mycobacterial infection. Cat-scratch disease is usually benign and self-limited. Encephalopathy is a rare complication of this disorder.

The prognosis for benign tumors of the neck is excellent. The outlook for children with malignant neck tumors depends on etiology of the tumor and the spread of the malignancy to other organs. Early diagnosis and treatment are clearly important in improving outcome.

Children with neck masses from trauma usually have had significant injury. The outcome often depends on establishment of an airway, provision of ventilatory support, and management of hemodynamic instability. Availability of surgical support is often essential to a good outcome.

Children with congenital lesions of the neck usually have an excellent prognosis. Some lesions resolve spontaneously, while others require simple surgical excision. Cystic hygromas may require multiple operations for complete removal because of their diffuse nature.

Case Resolution

In the case presented, the boy has signs and symptoms consistent with submandibular bacterial cervical lymphadenitis. The location of the neck mass in relation to the honey-crusted lesions (nonbullous impetigo) implicates spread of bacteria from the primary site of infection to the lymph nodes. Laboratory tests are unnecessary because the child does not appear septic. Culture of the impetigo is of academic interest only because the child will be started empirically on antibiotics directed against *S. aureus* and group A beta-hemolytic streptococcus. If the affected lymph node is fluctuant, aspiration of fluid for culture is indicated, and incision and drainage should be considered. The child should be treated as an outpatient with an oral antibiotic such as cephalexin, amoxicillin-clavulanic acid, or dicloxacillin as well as an analgesic for pain as needed. If the child is toxic-appearing, or if there is marked lymph node enlargement, the child should be admitted for intravenous antibiotics. A PPD skin test should be placed. The child should be followed in 1–3 days for clinical improvement depending on the severity of the infection.

Selected Readings

Benson-Mitchell, R., and G. Buchanan. Cervical lymphadenopathy secondary to atypical mycobacteria in children. J. Laryngol. Otol. 110:48–51, 1995.

Bergman, K. S., and B. H. Harris. Scalp and neck masses. Pediatr. Clin. North Am. 40:1151–1161, 1993.

Brown, R. L., and R. G. Azizkhan. Pediatric head and neck lesions. Pediatr. Clin. North Am. 45:889–905, 1998.

Butler, K. M., and C. J. Baker. Cervical lymphadenitis. *In* Feigin, R. D., and J. D. Cherry (eds.). Textbook of Pediatric Infectious Diseases, 4th ed. Philadelphia, W. B. Saunders, 1998, pp. 170–180.

Clary, R. A., and R. P. Lusk. Neck masses. *In* Bluestone C. D., S. E. Stool, and M. D. Scheetz (eds.). Pediatric Otolaryngology, 3rd ed. Philadelphia, W. B. Saunders, 1996, pp. 1488–1496.

Karmody, C. S. Developmental anomalies of the neck. *In* Bluestone, C. D., S. E. Stool, and M. D. Scheetz (eds.). Pediatric Otolaryngology, 3rd ed. Philadelphia, W. B. Saunders, 1996, pp. 1497–1511.

Kelly, C. S., and R. E. Kelly, Jr. Lymphadenopathy in children. Pediatr. Clin. North Am. 45:875–888, 1998.

Knight, P. J., A. F. Mulne, and L. E. Vassy. When is lymph node biopsy indicated in children with enlarged peripheral nodes. Pediatrics 69:391–396, 1982.

Park Y. W. Evaluation of neck masses in children. Am. Fam. Phys. 51:1904–1912, 1995.

Rosenfeld, R. M. Cervical adenopathy. *In* Bluestone, C. D., S. E. Stool, and M. D. Scheetz (eds.). Pediatric Otolaryngology, 3rd ed. Philadelphia, W. B. Saunders, 1996, pp. 1512–1524.

Ruddy, R. M. Neck mass. *In* Fleisher, G. R., and S. Ludwig (eds.). Textbook of Pediatric Emergency Medicine, 3rd ed. Baltimore, Williams & Wilkins, 1993, pp. 318–322.

Smith, K. M., and B. M. Malone. Neck masses. *In* Reisdorff, E. J., M. R. Roberts, and J. G. Wiegenstein. Pediatric Emergency Medicine. Philadelphia, W. B. Saunders, 1993, pp. 636–639.

Triglia, J. M., et al. First branchial cleft anomalies. Arch. Otolaryngol. Head Neck Surg. 124:291–295, 1998.

Zitelli, B. J. Neck masses. *In* Dershewitz, R. A. (ed.). Ambulatory Pediatric Care, 3rd ed. Philadelphia, J. B. Lippincott, 1999, pp. 497–503.

CHAPTER 60

ALLERGIC DISEASE

Julie E. Noble, M.D.

H$_x$ A 3-year-old girl is rushed to the office by her mother after her daughter develops a pruritic rash, facial swelling, and hoarseness shortly after eating a peanut butter sandwich. Previously she has been well except for recurrent nasal congestion every spring that has responded to antihistamines. She has also had an intermittent skin rash that has been treated with topical steroid creams. She has never had an acute reaction before and has no history of asthma. Her father had asthma as a child, however.

Physical examination reveals a well-developed, 3-year-old girl with marked facial swelling who is in mild respiratory distress. Vital signs, including blood pressure, are normal. Growth parameters are at the 50th percentile. The girl has a diffuse blotchy erythematous rash with central wheals, a hoarse voice, and a mild expiratory wheeze on auscultation of her chest. The remainder of the examination is normal.

Questions

1. What are the various symptoms of allergic disease?
2. What is the appropriate evaluation of children with manifestations of allergic disease?
3. What allergens are common triggers for allergic symptoms?
4. What management is helpful in treatment of children with manifestations of allergic disease?
5. Can allergic disease be prevented?

Allergic disease, which occurs frequently in the general population, is manifested in many ways. Asthma, atopic dermatitis, allergic rhinitis, allergic conjunctivitis, urticaria, angioedema, anaphylaxis, and vomiting and diarrhea (with food allergies) are all types of allergic diseases. These reactions generally result from the production of immunoglobulin E (IgE) on exposure to a foreign antigen. Similar non–IgE-mediated symptoms may occur, but these are not true allergic reactions. The reader should refer to Chapter 61, Wheezing and Asthma, for details concerning asthma, and Chapter 100, Papulosquamous Eruptions, for a review of atopic dermatitis. This chapter focuses on the remaining manifestations of allergies, including food allergies.

EPIDEMIOLOGY

Allergic disease or some form of allergic symptoms is found in 12–20% of the general population. The prevalence of symptoms varies depending on the population being investigated. Factors such as age, genetic background, and place of residence are significant. Allergic

rhinitis occurs in 10% of children, as does asthma. Up to 8% of children under 3 years of age develop food allergies. Urticaria occurs at some time in about 2% of children.

It is generally accepted that if neither parent is atopic (has the allergic tendency to manufacture IgE on antigen exposure), then the chance that children will develop allergic symptoms is less than 1:5. If one parent is atopic, the risk doubles. If both parents are atopic, the chance is greater than three in five.

CLINICAL PRESENTATION

Children with allergic disease frequently present with persistent, clear rhinorrhea, sneezing, postnasal drip, or injected pruritic conjunctiva. Skin manifestations include dry, scaling, erythematous rashes, wheals, or subcutaneous swelling (D$_x$ Box). A recurrent cough or wheezing on chest examination is further evidence of allergic disease.

PATHOPHYSIOLOGY

Allergic rhinitis, like all allergic manifestations, is caused primarily by an antigen-antibody reaction involving IgE. Antigen-specific IgE is produced by the B lymphocytes of allergic patients on exposure to a particular antigen. The IgE attaches to mast cells in the conjunctiva and mucous membranes of the respiratory tract. On reexposure, the antigen reacts with this specific IgE on the mast cells, releasing vasoactive mediators including histamine, leukotrienes, kinins, and prostaglandins. These mediators produce vasodilatation and edema, and they also stimulate neural reflexes

---

D$_x$ Allergic Disease

- Chronic, clear rhinorrhea
- Conjunctival tearing and pruritus
- Skin findings of atopic dermatitis or urticaria
- Seasonal variability
- Occurrence of symptoms after exposure to an antigen
- Family history of allergic disease
- Conjunctival injection
- Wheezing
- Chronic cough
- Postnasal drip
- Repetitive sneezing
- Acute onset of symptoms following exposure to possible allergen

to produce mucous hypersecretion and sneezing. Eosinophils, induced by chemotactic factors, pour into nasal secretions and release proteins that worsen the edema. Other immunologic mechanisms can also be involved.

Urticaria, the clinical rash produced by vasodilatation and edema of the skin, is the allergic condition that occurs when histamine is released from the dermal mast cells. The antigen-specific IgE is located on these mast cells. Otherwise, the pathophysiology is similar to that of allergic rhinitis. Exposure to that antigen causes release of chemical mediators from the mast cells. Other mechanisms, including physical stimuli, can produce nonallergic urticaria.

Angioedema is the extension of the urticarial process deeper into the dermis of the skin, producing circumscribed swelling. The mucous membranes may be affected. The pathophysiology is the same as for urticaria. A hereditary type of angioedema, which is not allergy-related, is caused by the inherited deficiency of C1 esterase inhibitor.

Anaphylaxis is an acute, systemic allergic reaction resulting from antigen-specific IgE on mast cells and basophils. The pathophysiology is similar to allergic rhinitis but it occurs in mast cells in many locations simultaneously, and prior sensitization to an allergen is essential. Anaphylactic reactions may be life-threatening. Vasodilatation may be so severe that decreased venous return can lead to acute myocardial infarctions and arrhythmias. Reactions can occur in seconds or as late as 1 hour after exposure. Common antigens that precipitate anaphylactic reactions include injections of foreign serum, drugs, and venous contrast material, and foods or food additives. The drug most frequently implicated is penicillin. Patients initially experience tightness and intense itching of the skin. Nausea, vomiting, and abdominal pain may ensue. Subsequently, the full spectrum of anaphylaxis appears.

A **food allergy** may produce any of the previously described allergic manifestations, including atopic dermatitis and asthma, as well as vomiting, diarrhea, and FTT. Food intolerance, which has a nonimmunologic pathogenesis, should be differentiated from food allergy, which is an IgE-mediated, allergic reaction. The localization of the IgE-sensitized mast cells to that specific antigen determines the symptoms produced by the allergy. The antigen enters through the GI mucosal barrier. Intact food proteins may enter the circulation, stimulating the production of antigen-specific IgE.

Major food allergens are usually glycoproteins (Table 60–1), but any food can be sensitizing. Sensitized GI

TABLE 60–1. Highly Allergenic Foods

Egg white
Cow's milk
Nuts
Tomatoes
Fruits (citrus)
Fish and shellfish
Wheat
Soy
Corn

---

mast cells release mediators, causing vomiting and diarrhea. As a result of the edema and vasodilation, the mucosa becomes more permeable to enteric antigens, resulting in more hypersensitivity and inflammation.

DIFFERENTIAL DIAGNOSIS

In evaluating children with possible allergic disease, other etiologies for the symptoms should be considered and explored. Allergic rhinitis is most often confused with a URI but may also resemble vasomotor rhinitis, sinusitis, or a nasal foreign body. Unlike allergic rhinitis, infectious etiologies of rhinitis result in inflammatory nasal mucosa and possible fever. Foreign bodies elicit a unilateral, purulent, often foul-smelling discharge. Vasomotor rhinitis is usually transient.

Urticaria can resemble insect bites, erythema multiforme, papular urticaria, mastocytosis, or contact dermatitis. Distinct features of urticaria include pruritus and a transient nature, without any epidermal break. It may result from an allergic reaction or may occur secondary to an infectious etiology. Parasitic, bacterial, fungal, and viral infections can all cause urticaria. Physical stimuli (e.g., sun, cold), exercise, or anxiety can also produce the reaction. In addition, a deficiency in factor H in the complement system may cause a genetic form of urticaria.

Anaphylaxis is usually associated with edema, wheezing, and fever, although it presents like other forms of shock. A history of an acute exposure is more likely to be seen with anaphylaxis.

Food allergies may resemble food intolerances, which are nonallergenic, with regard to clinical presentation. Food intolerances include toxic contamination, metabolic disorders (e.g., lactose intolerance), and reactions to pharmacologic properties of the ingested food. Associated allergic findings (e.g., asthma, atopic dermatitis) may be seen with true allergies. Specific testing of the food, stool, or patient may be necessary to differentiate allergic reactions from food intolerance.

EVALUATION: HISTORY AND PHYSICAL EXAMINATION

Allergic Rhinitis and Conjunctivitis

Practitioners should determine if children with possible allergic rhinitis have a history of symptoms of sneezing, itching, and nasal discharge. The eyes, ears, palate, and throat may itch. Children may also have a history of mouth breathing and snoring at night from nasal obstruction. These symptoms may be seasonal or associated with a specific stimulus. In addition, systemic symptoms of fatigue, headache, anorexia, and irritability may be present.

The history should also include a search for other manifestations of allergies (e.g., wheezing, atopic dermatitis) as well as a family history of atopy. An environmental history of allergen exposure, including pets, is also important to obtain.

The physical examination should be thorough. The skin should be inspected for atopic dermatitis and the lungs for evidence of asthma. The nasal mucosa should be examined with an otoscope. In children with allergic rhinitis, the nasal mucosa is swollen, pale, and sometimes cyanotic with copious clear discharge. Nasal polyps, if present, should be noted. Although polyps are most often present on an allergic basis, they may occur with cystic fibrosis. A transverse crease across the nose ("an allergic salute") can occur from repeated rubbing of the nose. Dark circles under the eyes, termed "allergic shiners," may be present from venous stasis. If affected, the conjunctivae are erythematous with a clear discharge and may have a follicular appearance. The mouth may reveal a high arched palate from chronic mouth breathing, and the pharyngeal follicular lymphoid tissue may be increased (Fig. 60–1).

Complications of chronic allergic rhinitis may be evident on examination. If children have one of these conditions, such as chronic serous otitis, recurrent otitis media, hearing loss secondary to otitis, sinusitis, sleep apnea, or dental malocclusion, the possibility of allergic disease as a cause should be explored.

Urticaria and Angioedema

When children present with an acute rash, questions should include recent exposures, including drugs, dietary changes, new soaps or detergents, and environmental agents. An urticarial rash is acute in onset, extremely pruritic, and typically evanescent. Evidence of infection and a history of chronic disease or any other allergic disease should be explored.

The rash should be evaluated carefully. An urticarial rash appears as erythematous lesions of various sizes with pale, papular centers. Lesions may coalesce, the rash blanches on pressure, and the skin is intact.

The physical examination should also assess whether other contributing problems, such as infection, are present.

Anaphylaxis

An acute exposure to a foreign antigen (e.g., medication, food, venom) should be elicited in the history of any patient who presents with anaphylaxis.

On physical examination, vital signs indicate hypotension and tachycardia. The skin is erythematous with diffuse edema. Airway edema may produce hoarseness with stridor and wheezing noted on auscultation of the chest. Patients may have severe difficulty breathing. Cardiac examination may reveal arrhythmias.

Food Allergies

An accurate diet diary is essential in diagnosing a food allergy. The timing of symptoms associated with a specific food must be obtained. Personal as well as family history of atopy is important. An elimination diet followed by a challenge helps the diagnostic evaluation. The double-blind, placebo-controlled food challenge is the most accurate assessment for diagnosis.

EVALUATION: LABORATORY TESTS

With allergic rhinitis, as with any allergic disease, the diagnosis can usually be made with a thorough history and physical examination. Frequently, therapy can be initiated with no laboratory data.

Screening tests may include a nasal smear for eosinophils. A result of greater than 10% eosinophils is considered confirmatory data for allergic rhinitis. Although serum IgE levels are sometimes performed, they are not sensitive or specific and have limited value. A multiallergen screening test, which gives reliable results when checking for the presence of allergic disease, is currently available.

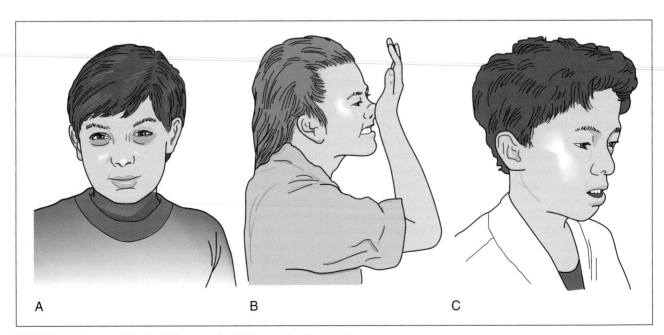

FIGURE 60–1. Characteristic facial features in children with allergic diseases.
A. Allergic shiner.
B. Nasal crease.
C. Open-mouth facies.

Skin testing for specific antigens should be performed if desensitization shots or environmental changes are being considered in the management plan. Skin tests are sensitive and accurate. Positive tests indicate the presence of an antigen-specific IgE. Prick tests are used initially. They may be followed by intradermal tests for allergens that are negative on prick testing. Although skin testing may be less reliable in infants because their skin is less reactive, the tests have been performed in children as young as 4 months of age.

Radioallergosorbent testing (RAST) of sera, which is also available for the laboratory assessment of allergies, provides a semiquantitative measure of the amount of IgE specific for individual allergens. RAST is much more expensive than skin testing and has no advantage unless skin testing cannot be performed.

Objective testing with skin tests by the prick method may be helpful in diagnosing food allergies. Negative tests are accurate for excluding food allergies, but positive tests may occur in patients without symptoms related to a particular food. Intradermal skin tests are not indicated. They do not give additional information, and they increase the risk of a serious reaction. RAST of sera may be used for specific foods.

MANAGEMENT

The first line of therapy for all allergic diseases is **avoidance of any precipitants.** For allergic rhinitis, this begins with environmental control, because the most frequent precipitants are inhalant allergens. Reducing exposure to the dust mite, a common allergen, can help control allergic rhinitis. Environmental humidity, which increases the dust mite population, should be decreased. Specifically, parents should be instructed to remove carpets, drapes, and upholstered furniture, which can harbor dust mites, from the house. They should cover mattresses with plastic covers and remove furry pets. Decreasing humidity also helps reduce mold counts, another important allergen, and air-conditioning units can lower pollen and mold counts. Nonspecific irritants such as smoke should be avoided because they can also precipitate any allergic symptom.

Anaphylaxis is considered a **medical emergency.** The first step in management is to establish an airway. Oxygen therapy should be instituted, and intravenous access established. Epinephrine is the drug of choice because of its potent vasoconstrictive and myocardial stimulating effects. The dose is 0.01 mL/kg of 1:1000 aqueous solution, up to 0.5 mL, given subcutaneously. If the blood pressure is decreased, epinephrine may be given intravenously, with normal saline fluid boluses to expand intravascular volume. Intravenous administration of an antihistamine, such as diphenhydramine, at 5 mg/kg/24 h is used as well as a steroid, such as methylprednisolone, at 2 mg/kg.

The management of urticaria should begin with the **identification of the causal agent** and its elimination. Children who have experienced anaphylaxis should be instructed to avoid future exposure to the precipitating allergen. In addition, they should be instructed to wear a Medic Alert tag that notifies others of the potential for a severe allergic reaction and carry an epinephrine kit for immediate treatment.

A maintenance diet that does not contain the allergen is the basis for management of food allergies. It is essential that the prescribed diet be nutritionally sound. Families should be instructed by a nutritionist and taught to read food labels appropriately to avoid all exposure to the antigen. They should also be advised about what foods children can consume.

Medications should be used in allergic disease when additional management is indicated by persistent symptoms. H_1-receptor antagonists or **antihistamines** are frequently indicated in the treatment of allergic rhinitis. Diphenhydramine, chlorpheniramine, and brompheniramine have all been useful in relieving symptoms but may be very sedating. The newer antagonists, terfenadine, astemizole, and loratadine, do not readily cross the blood-brain barrier and are less sedating. They are approved for use in children over the age of 6 years. Oral decongestants have been effective in decreasing nasal congestion. Pseudoephedrine has been used in children. Topical nasal decongestants, which can cause dependence and rebound swelling, should not be used on a long-term basis.

Antihistamines are also used in the symptomatic treatment of urticaria and angioedema. These agents can relieve the rash as well as the itching of the rash. Diphenhydramine, 5–7 mg/kg/d in four doses, and hydroxyzine, 2–4 mg/kg/d in four doses, are both used. If the urticaria is extensive or severe, epinephrine or Sus-Phrine (epinephrine in oil) may be used subcutaneously. This often provides immediate relief of symptoms and is diagnostic as well as therapeutic.

Cromolyn sodium nasal spray is the next line of treatment for allergic rhinitis in children over the age of 6 years. A very effective mast cell stabilizer, it suppresses mediator release. Cromolyn spray should be used prophylactically on a regular basis two to four times per day, one spray per nostril, to prevent symptoms.

Steroids have an anti-inflammatory effect and work well topically for allergic rhinitis. Beclomethasone, triamcinolone, and flunisolide are available as nasal sprays. None of these agents is recommended in children under the age of 6 years, and all three agents may cause stinging and nasal irritation. Systemic steroids may also be utilized for treatment of urticaria, angioedema, and anaphylaxis.

Immunotherapy should be considered for children with allergic rhinitis when medications are not controlling symptoms or when there is a history of anaphylaxis, depending on the allergen. This treatment has been effective in relieving symptoms due to dust mites, pollens, animal dander, molds, insect stings, and drug reactions. Immunotherapy involves a series of injections with extracts of allergens specific for individual patients, producing tolerance to particular antigens. The results of skin testing dictate which allergens to use. Initially, injections are given weekly. Then they are tapered and given on a maintenance schedule. Although immunotherapy can be performed at any age, the injections are painful and expensive. They necessitate frequent visits. Patients risk an allergic reaction with each injection.

PREVENTION

The cost of medical care, lost school and work days, disability from complications, and actual lives lost from allergic disease takes a great toll on the population. Many investigators have questioned whether the symptoms of allergies can be prevented.

No research indicates that maternal avoidance of allergens during pregnancy has any effect on subsequent development of allergies in children. Evidence currently suggests that sensitization to certain pollens and foods is more likely to occur in the first 6–12 months of life. Avoidance of these allergens at this age may decrease the subsequent development of allergic disease. For children at high risk for the development of allergic disease, which is usually determined by family history, the following steps are recommended:

- Keep the home free of dust.
- Keep pets out of the home.
- Keep humidity below 35% in the home.
- Prevent smoking in the environment.
- Limit infectious exposures.

To reduce the incidence of food allergies, it is recommended that mothers breast-feed infants exclusively for the first 6 months of life. When infants are 6 months old, foods can gradually be introduced. Cow's milk, wheat, corn, and citrus should be avoided until after the age of 1 year. Peanuts, eggs, fish, and shellfish should be delayed until 24 months. Postponing the introduction of food allergens may reduce the rate of sensitization in high-risk infants, but this is a controversial issue. Recent studies demonstrate that such postponement may only delay the sensitization.

PROGNOSIS

The prognosis for children with allergic disease is good when the diagnosis is made correctly. Allergic rhinitis, urticaria, and anaphylactic reactions tend to persist throughout life on exposure to antigens. However, with appropriate management with medication and avoidance of allergens, children with allergic disease can thrive and live a normal life without restrictions on activity. Immunotherapy can be effective in alleviating the allergic response to inhalants in allergic rhinitis and to bee venoms in anaphylaxis. The chance for resolution of food allergies is very good. Many foods that initially elicit an allergenic reaction can be tolerated after the age of 3–4 years, presumably as a result of maturation of the GI mucosa.

Case Resolution

In the case presented at the beginning of the chapter, the girl's symptoms of rash, swelling, and wheezing after exposure to an antigen suggest a systemic allergic reaction of angioedema and asthma. Treatment with epinephrine and antihistamines is clearly indicated. Because of the presence of pulmonary symptoms, admission for observation is warranted. The child and family should be counseled to avoid peanut butter in the future.

Selected Readings

Burks, A. W., and H. Sampson. Food allergies in children. Curr. Probl. Pediatr. 23:230–252, 1993.

Drugs for asthma. Med. Lett. Drugs Ther. 41:5–10, January 15, 1999.

Ferguson, A. Definitions and diagnosis of food intolerance and food allergy: consensus and controversy. J. Pediatr. 121:S1–S11, 1992.

Fireman, P. Diagnosis of allergic disorders. Pediatr. Rev. 16:178–183, 1995.

Murphy, S. J., and H. W. Kelly. Advances in the management of acute asthma in children. Pediatr. Rev. 17:227–234, 1996.

Nash, D. R. Allergic rhinitis. Pediatr. Ann. 27:799–808, 1998.

Rooklin, A. R., and S. M. Gaqchik. Allergic rhinitis—it's that time again. Contemp. Pediatr. 11:19–41, 1994.

Rosen, F. S. Urticaria, angioedema, and anaphylaxis. Pediatr. Rev. 13:387–390, 1992.

Solomon, W. R. Prevention of allergic disorders. Pediatr. Rev. 15:301–309, 1994.

Virant, F. S. Allergic rhinitis. Pediatr. Rev. 13:323–333, 1992.

Weston, W. L., and J. T. Badgett. Urticaria. Pediatr. Rev. 19:240–244, 1988.

Wood, R. A. Diagnosing allergies: when to test, when to refer. Contemp. Pediatr. 11:13–28, 1994.

CHAPTER 61

WHEEZING AND ASTHMA

James S. Seidel, M.D., Ph.D.

Hx A 7-year-old boy is referred to the office after being seen in the emergency department for wheezing. He has been treated in the emergency department for wheezing four times in the past month and was once hospitalized for 3 days. The boy's father and paternal grandmother both have asthma.

The child's physical examination is remarkable for end-expiratory wheezing on forced expiration.

Questions

1. What are the most common causes of wheezing in infants and children?
2. What are the causes of reversible bronchospasm?
3. What is the pathophysiology of reversible bronchospasm?
4. How should children with asthma be managed?

Recurrent wheezing is a frequent symptom of obstructive airway disease in children that may be caused by intrinsic or extrinsic compression of the airway, bronchospasm, inflammation, or defective clearance of secretions. Reactive airway disease (asthma) is the most common cause of wheezing in childhood. This is a chronic illness and requires longitudinal care by a primary care provider to ensure optimal treatment and reduction in costly emergency department visits and hospital admissions.

The site of the airway obstruction may be in the large or small bronchioles, and the audible "musical or squeaking sounds" noted with obstruction are caused by the turbulence of the air as it is forced through a narrowed airway. Infants and young children are more prone to wheezing when they have airway obstruction because air forced through smaller airways is more turbulent than air forced through the larger airways of older children and adults. Wheezing in children under 1 year of age is most commonly due to bronchiolitis, an infectious disease caused by RSV; pneumonia; and asthma. Less common causes include congenital structural anomalies, gastroesophageal reflux and aspiration, cardiac failure, cystic fibrosis, and foreign bodies (Table 61–1).

Infants may present with apnea, inspiratory and expiratory wheezing, fever, and respiratory distress.

TABLE 61–1. Causes of Wheezing

Infection	**Cardiac Disease**
Bronchiolitis	**Defective Secretion Clearance**
Pneumonia	Cystic fibrosis
Toxocariasis	Immotile cilia syndrome
Ascariasis	**Tumor**
Foreign Body	Mediastinal tumors (lymphoma, tera-
Reactive Airway Disease	toma, neuroblastoma, thymoma)
Asthma	**Chronic Aspiration**
Exercise-induced asthma	Gastroesophageal reflux
Anaphylaxis	Bulbar palsy
Nighttime cough asthma	Tracheoesophageal fistula
Toxic exposure (smoke,	**Other Causes**
organophosphate poisoning)	Bronchopulmonary dysplasia
Allergic aspergillosis	α_1-Antitrypsin deficiency
Congenital Structural	Pulmonary hemosiderosis
Anomalies	Sarcoidosis
Vascular rings	
Bronchiectasis	
Lung cysts	
Laryngotracheoesophageal cleft	
Tracheobronchomalacia	

Treatment is symptomatic, including hospitalization for apnea and severe respiratory distress. Infants with "recurrent bronchiolitis" may have reactive airway disease.

In older children, asthma is the most common cause of persistent or recurrent wheezing, although foreign body aspiration should also be considered in children who present with new onset wheezing. Asthma is a lung disease with the following characteristics: (1) increased airway responsiveness to a variety of stimuli, (2) reversible airway obstruction (reversibility may be incomplete in some children), and (3) inflammation of the airways. Less common causes of wheezing include α_1-antitrypsin deficiency, tumors, and pulmonary hemosiderosis. Most children with recurrent reversible bronchospasm have asthma.

EPIDEMIOLOGY

Asthma is the most common chronic childhood illness. The disease affects 5–15% of all children and has increased by 29% in recent years. One third of patients first experience symptoms in the first year of life, and 80% are diagnosed by the time they reach school age. One percent of all outpatient visits (6.5 million visits per year) are for asthma; the condition is the fourth most common reason for visits to emergency departments by children. In the United States, asthma is the most frequent admitting diagnosis to children's hospitals. Hospitalization for children under 15 years of age with asthma has increased by 10% in the last several years. In addition, asthma is a major cause of school absence; 23% of school days missed can be attributed to asthma.

In recent years more serious disease in younger children and adolescents has increased. Inner-city African Americans are most at risk. At present, about 4500 individuals die annually from asthma in the United States, which represents an increase of over 30% from a decade ago.

CLINICAL PRESENTATION

Children with asthma may present with acute symptoms of cough and shortness of breath. Wheezing may be audible and detected by the parent or not appreciated until the child is examined by a physician. There may be no wheezing in children with severe bronchoconstriction, because the flow of air is impeded. Some children have cough, which may be nocturnal or recurrent as a predominant symptom. Some pediatric patients have symptoms such as cough or wheezing that are precipitated or exacerbated by exercise (D_x Box).

PATHOPHYSIOLOGY

Asthma is a chronic inflammatory disorder of the airways. The immunohistopathologic features of asthma include denudation of the airway epithelium, collagen deposition beneath the basement membrane, edema, mast cell activation, and inflammatory cell infiltration. These changes lead to airway hyperresponsiveness,

---

D$_x$ Asthma

- Recurrent wheezing
- Shortness of breath
- Exercise intolerance
- History of allergies
- History of atopic dermatitis
- Nasal polyps
- History of nighttime cough

---

airflow limitation, respiratory symptoms, and disease chronicity. The limitation to the flow of air includes acute bronchoconstriction, airway edema, mucus plug formation, and airway wall remodeling. Atopy, the genetic predisposition to the development of IgE—mediated response to common aeroallergens, is the strongest predisposing factor for developing asthma. Environmental changes such as wind, temperature fluctuations, and increased exposure to allergens or air pollutants such as tobacco smoke may precipitate clinical attacks. Emotional stress may also play a role in the exacerbation of asthma. The changes in the airway are thought to be due to inflammatory changes that are the result of complex interactions between inflammatory cells and mediators and the target cells of the airway. Damage to the epithelial cells varies from mild loss of cilia to total destruction of the bronchioles.

The physiologic changes involved in asthma occur in two phases. An immediate response to the offending agent causes edema and bronchial smooth muscle constriction that lead to narrowing of the airway and plugging with secretions. Air is trapped behind the narrowed airways, resulting in altered gas exchange, increased respiratory rate, decreased tidal volume, and increased work of breathing. The late response, which occurs 4–8 hours after the initial symptoms, primarily involves infiltration of the airways with inflammatory cells. The end pathway in the disease process is obstruction to airflow. The pathophysiology of asthma is reviewed in Figure 61–1.

DIFFERENTIAL DIAGNOSIS

An extensive differential diagnosis is listed in Table 61–1. Most conditions are differentiated from asthma by the presence of associated symptoms or the child's response to bronchodilators.

In 1997, The National Institutes of Health (NIH) published the "Guidelines for the Diagnosis and Management of Asthma." These guidelines, which offer a new classification system for asthma severity, are divided into four steps based upon symptoms before treatment (Table 61–2): step 1: mild intermittent; step 2: mild persistent; step 3: moderate persistent; and step 4: severe persistent. The mildest form of the disease is not associated with school absence, sleep disturbance, or loss of pulmonary function. The moderate and severe cases are associated with daily symptoms, limited physical activity, school absence, and sleep disturbances. Pulmonary function is always affected.

EVALUATION

An acute asthmatic attack is always considered a medical emergency because it has the potential to deteriorate into respiratory failure. Initially only a brief history should be obtained. If children have recurrent asthma, critical interventions should be begun during the evaluation. The initial assessment should include an estimation of the severity of the attack. This can be accomplished by a rapid assessment of the ventilation, oxygenation, and perfusion of the patient (Table 61–3).

Signs of respiratory distress include rapid respiratory rate, decreased breath sounds, shortness of breath, use of accessory muscles of respiration, retractions (intercostal, sternal, and supraclavicular), nasal flaring, altered mental status, increased expiratory-inspiratory ratio, changes in skin color, and oxygen saturation. Pulsus paradoxus, the difference between systolic arterial blood pressure during inspiration and expiration, is normally less than 10 mm Hg. During an acute asthmatic attack this difference may be increased; however, this measurement may be difficult to obtain in young children. Children who are older than 6 years of age and are not in extreme respiratory distress should have their pulmonary function measured; this may include an estimation of peak expiratory flow rate or forced expiratory volume in one second (FEV_1).

If signs of a moderate or severe attack are present, children need to be monitored continuously. A severe attack may be heralded by the signs of respiratory distress listed above. In addition, patients may be unable to speak in sentences or have altered mental status. Therapy includes placing patients in a position of comfort and giving oxygen by mask, nasal prongs, or having oxygen blown in front of the face. Initiation of drug therapy may also be indicated.

History

If children are not in respiratory distress, a history should be taken (Questions Box). Practitioners should also find out how children and their families perceive the illness.

Physical Examination

Vital signs should be obtained and breath sounds, work of breathing, and the inspiratory-expiratory ratio should be carefully assessed. The nose and associated nasal passages should be examined for secretions, edema, pallor, and polyps. The skin should be assessed for eczema and other rashes. The chest should be carefully checked for increased anteroposterior diameter of the chest wall, use of accessory muscles, presence of retractions, decreased quality of breath sounds, and presence of prolonged expiration.

Laboratory Tests

The laboratory assessment of children with recurrent wheezing is still somewhat controversial. In older children air flow should be assessed by some objective

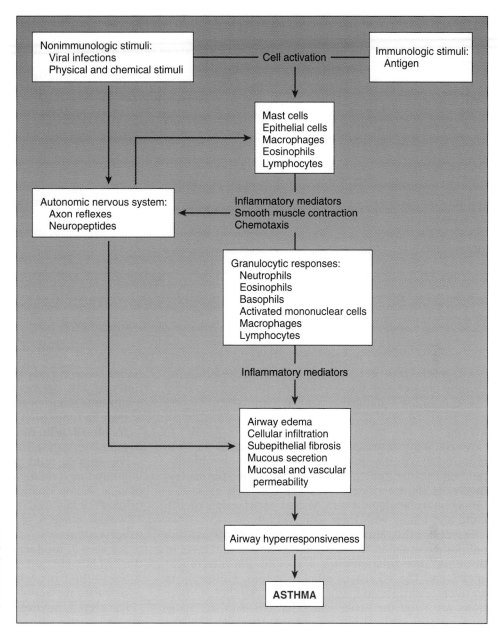

FIGURE 61-1. Proposed pathways in the pathogenesis of bronchial inflammation and airway hyperresponsiveness. (Reproduced from the National Asthma Education Program Expert Panel Report, Guidelines for Diagnosis and Management of Asthma, NIH Publication No. 91-3042, 1991.)

measure such as peak expiratory flow or FEV$_1$. A CBC with a differential count may suggest infection or allergies. Nasal swabs for eosinophils and serum IgE antibodies may identify patients with asthma who may benefit from management of specific allergies. Pulse oximetry assesses the degree of oxygen saturation. Arterial blood gases are indicated for children with acute asthma attacks who are not improving with therapy or who may have possible respiratory failure. Extensive laboratory testing should be reserved for children with severe disease who may benefit from consultation with an allergy specialist.

Imaging Studies

Although some physicians recommend routine chest radiographs in children with asthma, such films are probably not indicated unless there is clinical evidence

of infection or a foreign body or if another cause of wheezing is suspected. Sinus radiographs should be obtained in children with clinical evidence of acute sinusitis.

MANAGEMENT

The goals of asthma therapy are as follows:

- prevent chronic and disabling symptoms (e.g. coughing, sleep disturbances, exercise intolerance, shortness of breath)
- maintain (near) normal pulmonary function
- maintain normal activity levels
- prevent recurrent exacerbations and minimize the need for emergency department visits and admission to the hospital
- provide drug therapy that is effective with minimal side effects

TABLE 61–2. Classification of Asthma Severity

Clinical Features Before Treatment*

	Symptoms†	Nighttime Symptoms	Lung Function
STEP 4 Severe Persistent	Continual symptoms Limited physical activity Frequent exacerbations	Frequent	FEV_1 or PEF <60% predicted PEF variability >30%
STEP 3 Moderate Persistent	Daily symptoms Daily use of inhaled short-acting β_2-agonist Exacerbations affect activity Exacerbations ≥2 times a week; may last days	>1 time a week	FEV_1 or PEF >60%–<80% predicted PEF variability >30%
STEP 2 Mild Persistent	Symptoms >2 times a week but <1 time a day Exacerbations may affect activity	>2 times a month	FEV_1 or PEF ≥80% predicted PEF variability 20–30%
STEP 1 Mild Intermittent	Symptoms ≤2 times a week Asymptomatic and normal PEF between exacerbations Exacerbations brief (from a few hours to a few days); intensity may vary	≤2 times a month	FEV_1 or PEF ≥80% predicted PEF variability <20%

*The presence of one of the features of severity is sufficient to place a patient in that category. An individual should be assigned to the most severe grade in which any feature occurs.
The characteristics noted in this table are general and may overlap because asthma is highly variable. Furthermore, an individual's classification may change over time.
†Patients at any level of severity can have mild, moderate, or severe exacerbations. Some patients with intermittent asthma experience severe and life-threatening exacerbations separated by long periods of normal lung function and no symptoms.
Reproduced from National Institutes of Health, NHLBI. Guidelines for the Diagnosis and Management of Asthma. NIH Publication No. 97-4051, 1997, p. 20.

- meet the expectations of the child and the family for the care of asthma
- encourage self-management of asthma

Assessment measures for asthma should include monitoring of the following: signs and symptoms, pulmonary function through peak flow or spirometry, quality of life/functional status, acute disease exacerbations, pharmacologic therapy, and satisfaction of the child and family with their asthma care.

Selecting the appropriate therapy for an asthma patient depends on the age and developmental level of the child, the tolerance for a specific pharmacologic agent, and the routes of administration. Following is an overview of these medications. Quick-relief medications are used for acute exacerbations and the long-term control medications for chronic therapy. The NIH

panel recommends that patients be started on "step-down or step up therapy" depending on the severity of symptoms. An overview of asthma medications is shown in Table 61–4.

For **step 1, mild intermittent asthma,** use short-acting β_2-agonists as needed to treat symptoms.

For **step 2, mild persistent asthma,** use daily anti-inflammatory medication; either inhaled corticosteroids at a low dose or cromolyn, or nedocromil. Zalfirlukast or zileuton may be considered for children over 12 years of age. Use short-acting β_2-agonists for acute exacerbations.

For **step 3, moderate persistent asthma,** increase the dose of inhaled corticosteroids to a medium range. Add a long-acting bronchodilator or add nedocromil. Use β_2-agonists for acute exacerbations.

For **step 4, severe persistent asthma,** use high-dose inhaled corticosteroids and a long-acting bronchodila-

TABLE 61–3. Parameters Used to Estimate the Severity of Acute Asthma

Sign/Symptom	Classification		
	Mild	Moderate	Severe
Respiratory rate	Normal	Increased	Increased > 2 S.D.
Breath sounds	Normal (some end-expiratory wheezes)	Wheezing in inspiration and expiration	Decreased ± wheezing
Shortness of breath	None (can speak in sentences)	Can speak in phrases	Speaks only single words
Skin color	Normal (pink)	Pale	Pale to cyanotic
Work of breathing	Normal	Moderate retractions; some use of accessory muscles	Severe retractions; nasal flaring; use of accessory muscles
Pulse	Normal	Normal or increased	Increased
Level of consciousness	Normal	Normal	Diminished; may be lethargic or combative
Pulsus paradoxus	< 10 mm Hg	10–20 mm Hg	20–40 mm Hg
Oxygen saturation	> 95%	90–95%	< 92%
Pulmonary function	80% of predicted	50–70% of predicted	< 50% of predicted

Abbreviations: S.D., standard deviation.

Questions: Asthma

- What symptoms (e.g., wheezing, exercise intolerance) does the child experience?
- Does the child experience any nocturnal awakening or cough?
- What time of day and year do the symptoms occur?
- When did the symptoms begin? How old was the child?
- Are the symptoms associated with any particular activity? Does anything seem to trigger the symptoms?
- Are the child's activities limited in any way?
- How often do the asthma attacks occur?
- What is the child's living situation? Are there pets in the home?
- Does anyone smoke in the home?
- Do the asthma attacks cause the child to be absent from school?
- Does the child manage the condition at home with any particular treatments or medications?
- Has the child visited any urgent care and emergency departments for treatment for asthma or related episodes in the past? Has the child had any hospitalizations?
- Does the child have a history of allergies?

tor. Systemic corticosteroids may also be necessary. Use short-acting β_2-agonists for acute exacerbations.

Specific immediate and long-term management of asthma are indicated.

TABLE 61–4.   Pharmacologic Therapy: An Overview of Medications Used to Treat Asthma

Long-Term-Control Medications

Corticosteroids
Most potent and effective anti-inflammatory medication currently available. Inhaled form is used in the long-term control of asthma. Systemic corticosteroids are often used to gain prompt control of the disease when initiating long-term therapy.

Cromolyn Sodium and Nedocromil
Mild-to-moderate anti-inflammatory medication. May be used as initial choice for long-term-control therapy for children. Can also be used as preventive treatment prior to exercise or unavoidable exposure to known allergens.

Long-Acting β_2-Agonists
Long-acting bronchodilator used concomitantly with anti-inflammatory medications for long-term control of symptoms, especially nocturnal symptoms. Also prevents exercise-induced bronchospasm (EIB).

Methylxanthines
Sustained-release theophylline is a mild-to-moderate bronchodilator used principally as adjuvant to inhaled corticosteroids for prevention of nocturnal asthma symptoms. May have mild anti-inflammatory effect.

Leukotriene Modifiers
Zafirlukast, a leukotriene receptor antagonist, or zileuton, a 5-lipoxygenase inhibitor, may be considered an alternative therapy to low doses of inhaled corticosteroids or cromolyn or nedocromil for patients ≥12 years of age with mild persistent asthma, although further clinical experience and study are needed to establish their roles in asthma therapy.

Quick-Relief Medications

Short-Acting β_2-Agonists
Therapy of choice for relief of acute symptoms and prevention of EIB.

Anticholinergics
Ipratropium bromide may provide some additive benefit to inhaled β_2-agonists in severe exacerbations. May be an alternative bronchodilator for patients who do not tolerate inhaled β_2-agonists.

Systemic Corticosteroids
Used for moderate-to-severe exacerbations to speed recovery and prevent recurrence of exacerbations.

Reproduced from National Institutes of Health, NHLBI. Guidelines for the Diagnosis and Management of Asthma. NIH Publication No. 97-4051, 1997, p. 59.

Short-Term Management

Acute attacks can be managed in the office if the staff is prepared to deal with children in respiratory distress. Otherwise children can be referred to the emergency department. Equipment and supplies for resuscitation of infants and children must be available in offices that care for children with asthma.

The goal of therapy is to relieve airflow obstruction and prevent respiratory failure. All children with moderate or severe asthma should be placed in a **position of comfort** and given **oxygen** by nasal prongs or mask as tolerated. Assessment of work of breathing and the use of pulse oximetry help guide oxygen therapy. Nebulized β_2-agonists such as albuterol are used until symptoms subside. Children may require drug therapy every 20–30 minutes. β_2-agonists may also be given as a continuous nebulized treatment for severe acute attacks. Not only are nebulized beta-adrenergic agonists more effective than oral medications, they are associated with fewer side effects. Methylprednisolone, which helps reduce the inflammation associated with clinical attacks, is indicated in most moderate and severe cases. Response to therapy is determined by clinical assessment of work of breathing, respiratory rate, objective changes in pulmonary function, and pulse oximetry. Children with incomplete responses to initial therapy may require several hours of treatment or hospitalization.

Long-Term Management

Asthma is a chronic condition with a varying number of acute exacerbations. The goals of long-term management are shown in Table 61–5.

Continuous and longitudinal primary care of children with asthma can profoundly affect the course of their disease. Primary care practitioners, children, and their families must work together to achieve good control of symptoms. Prevention of exacerbations may be accomplished by **removal of offending allergens,** giving **appropriate medications,** and participation in **home pulmonary function testing.** Periodic assessment ensures appropriate therapy and compliance with treatment. Practitioners should make sure that families can afford the necessary medications. During routine visits, home monitoring and therapy as well as any diaries and records should be reviewed, children's and families' expectations about the course of the disease should be discussed, and all parties should be allowed to express

---

TABLE 61–5.   Therapeutic Goals for Children With Chronic Asthma

To maintain a normal, age-appropriate activity level
To maintain near-normal pulmonary function
To prevent symptoms such as exercise intolerance, chronic cough, and shortness of breath
To prevent acute exacerbations of the disease that require acute therapy
To minimize adverse effects of the drugs used to treat the disease
To promote self-esteem and a sense of well-being

										Peak Flow			
Date	Wheeze	Cough	Activity	Sleep	Quick Relief: β₂–Agonist	Cromolyn/Nedocromil	Inhaled Steroids	Other—Inhaled	Oral Steroids	Theophylline	AM	PM	Other Times	Comments

Patient Self–Assessment: Example of Patient Diary

Wheeze	None = 0		Some = 1	Medium = 2	Severe = 3
Cough	None = 0		Occasional = 1	Frequent = 2	Continuous = 3
Activity	Normal = 0		Can run short distance or climb = 1 3 flights of stairs	Can walk only = 2	Missed school or work or stayed = 3 indoors
Sleep	Fine = 0		Slept well, slight wheeze or cough = 1	Awake 2–3 times, wheeze or cough = 2	Bad night, awake most of the time = 3

FIGURE 61–2. Patient self-assessment. An example of a patient diary. (Modified, with permission, from Plaut, T. F. One Minute Asthma: What You Need to Know. Amherst, MA, Pedipress, 1991, pp. 12–13.)

their concerns regarding the development of a treatment plan.

Home therapy can be directed by assessment of pulmonary function and respiratory status. (See Figure 61–2, an example of a patient self-assessment chart.) Family members and children should be instructed in the use of peak flow meters to indicate when medical treatment is necessary. Some meters have three color zones: a green zone, which indicates good air flow; a yellow zone, which signals the need for treatment; and a red zone, which suggests that a visit to the emergency department may be indicated. The patient should be encouraged to bring the peak flow meter with him/her to each visit as well as all medications, including metered-dose inhalers and spacers. The NIH Guidelines and the step classification of the child's disease should guide the type of drug therapy used.

PROGNOSIS

Asthma can result in significant morbidity and mortality if children are not managed appropriately. Children without longitudinal primary care generally require expensive therapy in emergency departments or inpatient settings. A significant number of individuals with asthma have fatal outcomes because of lack of timely and appropriate care. Practically all of these deaths are preventable.

Case Resolution

The 7-year-old boy in the case history who visits the office for asthma requires not only medication but also education and longitudinal primary care. It is particularly important to assess possible environmental factors (e.g., pets), exposure to smoke, and poor compliance with previous recommendations, which have contributed to his recurrent symptoms.

Selected Readings

American Academy of Pediatrics, Provisional Committee on Quality Improvement. Practice parameters: the office management of acute asthma exacerbations in children. Pediatrics 93:119–127, 1994.

Buist, A. S., and W. M. Vollmer. Preventing deaths from asthma. N. Engl. J. Med. 331:1584–1585, 1994.

Creer, T. L., et al. Living with asthma. 1. Genesis and development of a self-management program for childhood asthma. J. Asthma 25:335–362, 1988.

Donahue, J. G., et al. Inhaled steroids and the risk of hospitalization for asthma. JAMA 227:887–881, 1997.

Hickey, R. W., et al. Albuterol delivered via a metered-dose inhaler with spacer for outpatient treatment of young children with wheezing. Arch. Pediatr. Adol. Med. 148:189–194, 1994.

Kulick, R. M., and R. M. Ruddy. Allergic emergencies. *In* Fleisher, G. R. and S. Ludwig (eds). Textbook of Pediatric Emergency Medicine. Baltimore, Williams & Wilkins, 1993, pp. 858–866.

Letourneau, M. A., S. Schuh, and M. Gausche. Respiratory disorders. *In* Barkin, R. (ed.). Pediatric Emergency Medicine. Concepts and Clinical Practice. St. Louis, Mosby-Year Book, 1992, pp. 969–1037.

National Institutes of Health, NHLBI. Practical guide to the management and diagnosis of asthma. NIH Publication No. 97-4053, 1997.

National Institutes of Health, NHLBI. Guidelines for the Diagnosis and Management of Asthma. NIH Publication No. 97-4051, 1997.

Schuh, S., et al. High- versus low-dose, frequently administered nebulized albuterol in children with severe asthma. Pediatrics 83:513–518, 1989.

Silverstein, M. D., et al. Long-term survival of community residents with asthma. N. Engl. J. Med. 331:1537–1541, 1994.

Stempel, D. A., and S. J. Szelfer (eds.). Asthma. Pediatr. Clin. North Am. 39, 1992.

CHAPTER 62

COUGH

Julie E. Noble, M.D.

H$_x$ A 3-year-old boy presents with a cough that he has had for 4 weeks. In the past he has had coughs with colds, but this cough is persistent and deeper in quality. The cough seemed to develop suddenly when he was playing at a friend's house. It occurs all day and disrupts his sleep at night. The boy has had no nasal congestion, fever, or sore throat. No one at home is coughing, and the boy has not traveled recently. Neither the boy nor his family have a history of allergies or asthma. Over-the-counter cough preparations have not helped relieve his symptoms.

On examination, growth parameters are normal. The child has a persistent cough with no respiratory distress. Chest examination reveals a normal respiratory rate, no retractions, no use of accessory muscles, but diffuse expiratory wheezing is noted in the right lower lobe. The remainder of the examination is normal.

Questions

1. What are common parental concerns regarding cough?
2. What diagnoses in children with persistent cough should be considered?
3. What historical factors and physical findings are important to determine the etiology of cough?
4. What diagnostic workup is appropriate?
5. How should children with chronic cough be managed?

Cough is an essential protective reflex to ensure airway patency. Its persistence can generate much parental anxiety because of concern about its etiology and frequently associated disruption of sleep patterns.

Cough is either acute or chronic. Acute cough, which may persist up to 2 weeks, is often associated with respiratory tract infections in children. It is important to remember that always chronic cough begins acutely. When the duration is prolonged, cough is considered chronic and etiologic possibilities are expanded. Chronic cough is defined as a cough lasting for more than 2–4 weeks. Parental sensitivity as well as accessibility to medical care influence when in the course of disease children present with this problem.

EPIDEMIOLOGY

Cough is a very common complaint initiating pediatric office visits. In the National Ambulatory Medical Care Survey, 6.7% of pediatric office visits involved children who presented with cough. Typically, preschool children have up to eight URIs with associated cough in a winter season. But many serious diseases, including cystic fibrosis, congenital heart disease, asthma, and immunodeficiency disorders, may result in cough.

CLINICAL PRESENTATION

The presentation varies greatly depending on the etiology of the cough. Children may present in severe respiratory distress or have no evidence of respiratory compromise. They may have conditions such as FTT or appear totally healthy (D$_x$ Box).

PATHOPHYSIOLOGY

Coughing is a complicated reflex process initiated through irritation of one of the multiple cough receptors. These receptors are located in the nose, paranasal sinuses, posterior pharynx, larynx, trachea, bronchi, and pleura. They can also be found outside of the respiratory tract in the ear canal, stomach, pericardium, and diaphragm. Stimulation of any of these receptors by an irritant, whether mechanical, chemical, thermal, or inflammatory, can initiate the cough reflex. The lung parenchymal tissue contains no cough receptors, so pneumonia may not produce a cough. The receptors send the cough message along the vagal and laryngeal nerves to the upper brain stem, where the cough center in the medulla receives the message and coordinates the cough mechanism. The cough center can be voluntarily stimulated or suppressed.

The actual cough experienced by patients may be broken down into three phases. First, the glottis opens with an inspiratory gasp. Second, the glottis closes with forceful contraction of the chest wall, diaphragm, and abdominal muscles. Third, the glottis again opens with release of airway pressure in an expiratory phase. This process expels mucus or irritants from the airways, clearing the passages for normal air flow.

DIFFERENTIAL DIAGNOSIS

The list of differential diagnoses of cough is long (Table 62–1). Narrowing the list of causes can be accomplished by paying attention to several factors.

As with any pediatric symptom, the child's **age** influences the diagnostic possibilities and management of the cough. Congenital anomalies, which are most likely to present in the first few months of life, include tracheoesophageal fistula, laryngeal cleft, vocal cord paralysis, and tracheobronchomalacia. Congenital heart disease can produce a cough from heart failure and pulmonary edema. Congenital mediastinal tumors cause infants to cough if the tumor presses on the bronchial tree.

D$_x$ Cough

- Dry, productive, brassy cough
  - Duration: acute, chronic, recurrent
  - Timing: during day, at night, on awakening, with exercise
- Fever or URI associated with infectious origin
- Allergic findings of rhinorrhea, sneezing, wheezing, atopic dermatitis associated with asthma or allergic rhinitis
- FTT (indicates chronic disease)

TABLE 62–1. Causes of Cough

Congenital Anomalies
Tracheoesophageal fistula
Laryngeal cleft
Vocal cord paralysis
Mediastinal masses
Pulmonary malformations
Tracheobronchomalacia
Congenital heart disease
Infections (e.g., upper respiratory infection, sinusitis, pneumonia)
Viral
  Adenovirus
  Influenza
  Parainfluenza
  Respiratory syncytial virus
  Rhinovirus
Bacterial
  Pertussis
  Pneumococcal
  Staphylococcal
  Tuberculosis
Fungal
  Coccidioidomycosis
Other
  Chlamydial
  Mycoplasmosis
Chronic Disease
Cystic fibrosis
Human immunodeficiency virus infection
Immunodeficiency syndrome
Dyskinetic cilia
Allergic Conditions
Allergic rhinitis
Asthma
Serous otitis media
Mediastinal Tumors
Foreign Body Aspiration
Gastroesophageal Reflux
Environmental Irritants
Psychogenic Cough
Drug-Induced Conditions

The **duration of the cough** also determines its possible cause. Most acute coughs are infectious in origin. URIs can initiate an acute cough through stimulation of the cough receptors in the nose and posterior pharynx. If nasal congestion and cough persist, a diagnosis of allergic rhinitis or sinusitis should be considered. Serous otitis media can also cause a persistent cough and may occur in children with chronic congestion. Children with pneumonia may present with either acute or chronic cough.

The presence of a **nighttime cough** can be important. Pathologic coughs, including those caused by sinusitis with postnasal drip, gastroesophageal reflux, and asthma, are more likely to occur at night.

The **character of the cough** is a fourth factor to consider in the differential diagnosis. Some causes produce a very specific type of cough. A barking cough is consistent with laryngeal edema and croup, whereas an inspiratory whoop is characteristic of pertussis or parapertussis. The psychogenic cough is a strange, honking sound.

Pneumococcus is the most probable causal agent in acute cough with pneumonia, but when the cough becomes chronic, other infectious agents are more likely. Adenovirus and RSV, which occur more commonly in infants, and influenza and parainfluenza, which affect children of all ages, are common viral agents that produce chronic cough. *Bordetella pertussis,* mycoplasma, and chlamydia also cause chronic cough. Other infections such as tuberculosis and coccidioidomycosis should also be considered in endemic areas or high-risk populations. Chronic infectious coughs, such as those associated with influenza and pertussis, can last up to 6 months. Host factors that may predispose to chronic cough should also be investigated. Children with cystic fibrosis, BPD, HIV and other immunodeficiency syndromes, and congenital pulmonary malformations may present with chronic, recurrent cough.

The most common cause of chronic cough is reactive airway disease (asthma) (see Chapter 61, Wheezing and Asthma). In fact, cough with no notable wheezing may be the only manifestation of asthma. In infants or neurologically impaired children, chronic cough may indicate gastroesophageal reflux with recurrent aspiration. An unexplained persistent cough, primarily in toddlers, may be the result of foreign body aspiration if the initial aspiration was not observed. The foreign object acts as a chronic airway irritant that stimulates coughing, and it may be the cause of recurrent infections. Other irritants that initiate cough include dust, smoke, and chemicals. A psychogenic cough should also be considered, especially if the cough is absent at night. Such a cough may be a habit or an expression of anxiety. Drugs such as beta-adrenergic receptor antagonists and angiotensin-converting enzyme inhibitors can also induce a chronic cough, probably by increasing the sensitivity of the cough reflex.

EVALUATION

History

A complete history should be obtained when children present with cough (Questions Box). All symptoms should be noted. Vomiting with cough can indicate phlegm production. In fact, some children present with a chief complaint of vomiting when it is actually the cough that precipitates the vomiting.

Physical Examination

A complete physical examination should be performed on all children who present with cough. Growth parameters and vital signs should be assessed. Skin should be examined for evidence of cyanosis or atopy. Facial petechiae or subconjunctival hemorrhage indicates particularly forceful coughing. Extremities should be evaluated for fingernail clubbing, which is a sign of chronic pulmonary disease. The nose should be assessed for evidence of congestion. Allergic disease produces pale, cyanotic mucosa, whereas infection results in more inflammatory mucosa. TMs should be examined and mobility tested.

The effort of respiration, including the use of accessory muscles, should also be noted. Careful attention should be paid to breath sounds; whether abnormal sounds are in the inspiratory or expiratory phase of

Questions: Cough

- How old is the child?
- How long has the child had the cough?
- How frequent is the child's cough?
- Does the cough occur at night?
- Does exercise make the cough worse?
- Do any factors such as environmental irritants seem to precipitate the cough?
- Does the child have any related infectious symptoms, including fever and nasal congestion?
- Does the child have any other symptoms?
- Has the child had any previous episodes of coughing or associated symptoms?
- Has the child lost weight recently?
- What is the child's birth history?
- Has the child had any pulmonary injuries?
- What is the child's immunization status?
- Does the child have a history of recent travel?
- Has a family member had similar symptoms?
- Does the family have a history of pulmonary disease or allergies?
- Has the child been treated with any medications for the cough? Have they helped?
- Is the child taking any other medications?

respiration should be determined. Stridor is classically an inspiratory sound (see Chapter 38, Stridor and Croup), whereas wheezing is usually an expiratory sound. Prolongation of the expiratory phase also indicates wheezing. Abnormal breath sounds should be localized if possible. Because the character of the cough can establish the diagnosis, listening to the cough is probably the most important part of the physical examination. A parental description of the cough may be less diagnostic.

Laboratory Tests

After a thorough history and physical examination, laboratory data may not be necessary. Laboratory tests should be ordered when more information is needed to help make a reasonable diagnosis. The laboratory data should be directed at proving or disproving the most likely diagnosis in a specific patient.

If after the history, physical examination, and chest x-ray, an infectious etiology for cough is suspected, a CBC with differential and a PPD test should be ordered. Appropriate cultures should be obtained, if possible. Most children swallow their phlegm, so sputum cultures may be difficult to obtain. Gastric aspirates can sometimes yield a reasonable sputum specimen for culture. Nasopharyngeal cultures are useful for diagnosing pertussis and viral etiologies.

If a specific diagnosis is suspected, laboratory tests should be directed toward that diagnosis, e.g., sweat chloride to rule out cystic fibrosis or quantitative immunoglobulins to rule out immunodeficiency.

Imaging Studies

The chest x-ray (anteroposterior and lateral), the mainstay of the laboratory evaluation of cough, should be the first test ordered in the evaluation of a chronic cough or if definite findings are evident on physical examination. A lateral decubitus film can provide additional information about pleural fluid or air trapping. Inspiratory and expiratory films can be obtained if a foreign body is suspected. If a nodular pulmonary lesion is found on x-ray, bronchoscopy may be the next step to further define the lesion. If sinusitis is suspected, x-rays or a CT scan of the sinuses can be performed. An upper GI series of x-rays or a pH probe study would help to define gastroesophageal reflux if the cough occurs after recurrent episodes of vomiting or at night.

In children with asthma, the chest x-ray may be totally normal. Further laboratory testing with peak flow measurements in children over the age of 4 can be done to demonstrate restricted expiratory flow. The most helpful test to diagnose asthma may be a trial of a bronchodilator (see Chapter 61, Wheezing and Asthma).

MANAGEMENT

Cough should not be treated until the cause has been identified by a thorough consideration of the differential diagnoses. Therapy should then be directed toward treating that etiology. If the cough is secondary to a URI or allergic rhinitis, an **antihistamine/decongestant** combination or nasal steroid spray may help decrease postnasal drip and relieve the cough. A cough of an infectious etiology should be treated with the appropriate antibiotics. If the cough is keeping children awake at night, a **cough suppressant** may be indicated so that children and their families can rest. Cough syrups containing dextromethorphan are efficacious. Cough syrups with codeine can also be used. Such medications can be very helpful in interrupting the cough cycle generated by constant irritation of the cough receptors.

Expectorants and mucolytic agents in cough syrups have little effect on relieving coughs.

PROGNOSIS

With thoughtful evaluation, it is usually possible to identify the causes of both acute and chronic cough. Most symptoms resolve with appropriate therapy. If the cough persists with treatment, then alternate diagnoses should be considered.

Case Resolution

In the case presented at the beginning of this chapter, the child's cough began acutely and developed into a chronic cough. The boy has no history of allergies or symptoms consistent with an infectious process. Physical examination reveals localized wheezing. A chest x-ray should be ordered to gain more information. His symptoms and presentation are most consistent with foreign body aspiration.

Selected Readings

Guilbert, T. W., and L. M. Taussig. "Doctor, he's been coughing for a month. Is it serious?" Contemp. Pediatr. 15:155–172, 1998.

Hatch, R. T., G. B. Carpenter, and L. J. Smith. Treatment options in the child with a chronic cough. Drugs 45:367–373, 1993.

Kamei, R. K. Chronic cough in children. Pediatr. Clin. North Am. 38:593–605, 1991.

Katcher, M. L. Cold, cough, and allergy medications: Uses and abuses. Pediatr. Rev. 17:12–17, 1996.

Parks, D. P., et al. Chronic cough in childhood: approach to diagnosis and treatment. J. Pediatr. 115:856–862, 1989.

Richards, W. What's causing that child's chronic cough? Compr. Ther. 19:256–260, 1993.

Rojas, A. R., E. J. O'Connell, and M. I. Sachs. Chronic cough in children: what to do, and why. J. Respir. Dis. 12:891–903, 1991.

HEMATOLOGIC DISORDERS

C H A P T E R 6 3

ANEMIA

Pamela S. Cohen, M.D. and Pamelyn Close, M.D., M.P.H.

H$_x$ An 18-month-old girl is brought to the office with a 36-hour history of increasing scleral icterus and pallor, which are accompanied by symptoms of a viral upper respiratory tract infection (e.g., coughing, nasal discharge, low-grade fever). During her first week of life, the girl had hyperbilirubinemia of unknown etiology that required "bililights." Her family history is significant for mild anemia in her father; the cause of his condition is also unknown. A paternal aunt and grandfather had cholecystectomies while in their thirties.

On physical examination, the girl has tachycardia and mild tachypnea (no respiratory distress), in addition to the scleral icterus and pallor. Except for a spleen palpable 3 cm below the midcostal margin, the rest of the examination is normal.

Questions

1. What hemoglobin/hematocrit values are associated with anemia?
2. What is the appropriate initial evaluation of children with anemia?
3. When should children receive transfusions of red blood cells?
4. What emergency situations in children who present with anemia should be recognized by the primary pediatrician?

Anemia, a very common condition encountered by every pediatrician, is characterized by a hemoglobin or hematocrit value that is less than two standard deviations below the mean normal value for age. These values vary widely during the first year of life as newborn infants' hematopoiesis changes from fetal to adult-type (see Table 63–1 for normal age-related values). From the age of about 6 months through 8 years, a value of hemoglobin less than 11 g/dL or a hematocrit below 33% is considered consistent with the diagnosis of anemia. When evaluating children with suspected anemia, it is very important to ascertain whether only anemia is present or whether the WBC count or platelet count is also affected by the underlying disorder. This information greatly helps determine the diagnosis and dictates the treatment plan.

EPIDEMIOLOGY

Iron deficiency anemia is the leading cause of anemia among infants and children in the United States. The overall incidence of anemia has decreased markedly in the past 15 years as a result of iron supplementation of infant formula and food products. The incidence of iron deficiency anemia in particular, and anemia in general, appears to depend on socioeconomic status, and is about 3% in children under 2 years of age seen in a suburban pediatric office, compared to about 8% among inner-city children not taking iron-fortified formula.

Other epidemiologic factors that contribute to anemia are presented in Table 63–2. Anemias that have a genetic etiology, including hemoglobinopathies (i.e., sickle cell disease and thalessemias), enzyme deficiencies (glucose-6-phosphate-dehydrogenase [G6PD] and pyruvate kinase), and red blood cell membrane defects (hereditary spherocytosis) are commonly diagnosed in childhood. Immune hemolytic anemias are often associated with a preceding viral illness. Dietary factors, such as oxidants (e.g., fava beans), can trigger hemolysis in G6PD deficiency or can cause suppression of hematopoiesis as in iron, folate, or vitamin B$_{12}$ deficiency. Ingestion of toxins such as lead can also result in impaired hematopoiesis.

CLINICAL PRESENTATION

Children who have anemia present with pallor, fatigue, and decreased exercise tolerance. Other signs and symptoms that suggest anemia or its underlying causes include scleral icterus, jaundice, hepatosplenomegaly, and in severe cases, shortness of breath due to congestive heart failure (CHF) (D$_x$ Box).

PATHOPHYSIOLOGY

RBCs develop from pluripotent stem cells in the bone marrow that also give rise to myeloid cells and platelets. These stem cells ultimately differentiate into

TABLE 63–1. Values (Mean and Lower Limits of Normal) for Hemoglobin, Hematocrit, and Mean Corpuscular Volume Determinations

Age, yr	Hemoglobin gm/dL		Hematocrit, %		MCV, μ^3	
	Mean	Lower Limit	Mean	Lower Limit	Mean	Lower Limit
0.5–1.9	12.5	11.0	37	33	77	70
2–4	12.5	11.0	38	34	79	73
5–7	13.0	11.5	39	35	81	75
8–11	13.5	12.0	40	36	83	76
12–14						
Female	13.5	12.0	41	36	85	78
Male	14.0	12.5	43	37	84	77
15–17						
Female	14.0	12.0	41	36	87	79
Male	15.0	13.0	46	38	86	78
18–49						
Female	14.0	12.0	42	37	90	80
Male	16.0	14.0	47	40	90	80

MCV, mean corpuscular volume.

Reproduced, with permission, from Oski FA, Brugnara C, and Nathan DG: A diagnostic approach to the anemic patient. *In* Nathan DG and Orkin SH: Nathan and Oski's Hematology of Infancy and Childhood, 5th ed. Philadelphia, WB Saunders, 1998, p. 376.

mature, enucleated RBCs through interaction with various hematopoietic growth factors, including erythropoietin (whose synthesis requires functioning kidneys), interleukin-3, and stem cell factor. RBCs, which are then extruded through the bone marrow into the peripheral circulation, normally have a life span of about 120 days. They become deformed with age and eventually are trapped in the spleen and destroyed. Iron from RBCs is then recycled via binding to transferrin and returned to the marrow for further use.

Anemia can occur as a consequence of perturbation of any of these steps. Pathophysiologically, it can result from conditions leading to **decreased production** or **increased destruction** (i.e., hemolysis) of RBCs or **increased blood loss.** Deficient production may be caused by either marrow infiltration (e.g., leukemia), bone marrow failure (i.e., Blackfan-Diamond syndrome),

or dietary factors (iron deficiency anemia). Increased destruction of red cells (hemolysis) can be either intracorpuscular (RBC cytoskeleton defects, RBC enzyme deficiencies, or hemoglobinopathies) or extracorpuscular (immune or nonimmune etiologies). Anemia results when the rate of red cell loss exceeds the rate of red cell production.

DIFFERENTIAL DIAGNOSIS

The differential diagnosis of anemia can be assessed either by the production/destruction state or size of RBCs. The clinician can determine whether the anemia is associated with decreased or increased production of red cells or increased blood loss. A differential diagnosis of anemia based on this classification is shown in Table 63–3. A reduced reticulocyte count indicates decreased marrow production in children with suspected anemia. In general, an elevated indirect bilirubin along with a high reticulocyte count is highly suggestive of hemolysis. Various tests indicate increased destruction, depending on the extent and the chronicity of the hemolysis. Excessive blood loss can occur at any mucosal site. Blood may be lost into the stool or urine as well as through menorrhagia or nosebleeds.

RBC size, as assessed by mean corpuscular volume (MCV), is useful for determining the cause of anemia. Table 63–4 lists the acute anemias of child-

TABLE 63–2. Epidemiologic Factors Related to Anemia

Genetic
Autosomal dominant: hereditary spherocytosis
Autosomal recessive: most Embden-Meyerhof pathway enzyme deficiencies (e.g., pyruvate kinase deficiency), most hemoglobinopathies (e.g., sickle cell anemia, beta-thalassemia)
X-linked: glucose-6-phosphate dehydrogenase (G6PD) deficiency
Ethnicity
  Northern European Caucasian: hereditary spherocytosis, pyruvate kinase deficiency
  Mediterranean (Italian, Greek, North African): beta-thalassemia
  African: sickle cell anemia, hemoglobin C, D
  Asian: alpha-thalassemia, hemoglobin E
Dietary
Ingestion of oxidants (e.g., fava beans in G6PD deficiency)
Poor dietary intake (e.g., iron, folate, or vitamin B_{12} deficiency)
Poor gastrointestinal absorption (e.g., vitamin B_{12} deficiency)
Toxins (e.g., lead)
Socioeconomic
Living near highways: increased incidence of lead poisoning
Poverty: associated with pica and lead poisoning
Infectious
Malaria (hemoglobin S confers protection)
Parvovirus (risk of aplastic crisis in patients with hemolytic anemias)

D_x Anemia

- Pallor, fatigue
- Scleral icterus
- Hepatosplenomegaly
- Lymphadenopathy
- Weight loss
- Congestive heart failure

TABLE 63–3. Differential Diagnosis of Anemia Based on Pathophysiology

Pathophysiologic Mechanism	General Diagnostic Features	Specific Diagnostic Features
Decreased Production of Red Blood Cells	Evidence of decreased production: ↓ reticulocytes	**Pancytopenia due to bone marrow infiltration with:**
Marrow infiltration		
Secondary to tumor infiltration		Leukemia, neuroblastoma, etc.
Secondary to infiltration with nonmalignant cells		
Lipidoses		Lipid-filled macrophages
X-linked lymphoproliferative disorder		Erythrophagocytosis
		Hepatosplenomegaly
Decreased production of hematopoietic elements (bone marrow failure)		
Decreased RBC production only		
Constitutional: Blackfan-Diamond syndrome		Multiple physical deformities
Acquired		
Acquired pure red cell aplasia		Associated with thymoma
Transient erythrocytopenia of childhood		Associated with parvovirus infection
Decreased RBC and WBC production		
Constitutional		
Fanconi's anemia		Multiple physical deformities
Shwachman's syndrome		Pancreatic insufficiency
Decreased production of RBC, WBC, and platelets		
Constitutional		
Fanconi's anemia		Multiple physical deformities
Shwachman's syndrome		Pancreatic insufficiency
Acquired: aplastic anemia (idiopathic or secondary to toxins, drugs, or infection [e.g., hepatitis B]		History of hepatitis B, toxin exposure
Dietary deficiency		
Iron deficiency		↓ MCV, ↓ MCH, ↑ RDW, ↓ serum iron, ↓ serum ferritin, excessive milk intake
Folic acid deficiency		↑ MCV, ↑ RDW, megaloblastic marrow, low serum and RBC folate
Vitamin B_{12} deficiency		↑ MCV, ↑ RDW, megaloblastic marrow, low serum B_{12} levels, + Schilling test
Vitamin C deficiency		Clinical scurvy
Protein deficiency		Kwashiorkor
Hypothyroidism		Low T_4, elevated TSH
Increased Production (Hemolysis)	Evidence of hemolysis: ↑ Reticulocytes	
Intrinsic RBC defects		
RBC membrane defects (spherocytosis, elliptocytosis)	Hyperbilirubinemia	+ Osmotic fragility, spectrin deficiency (HS)
RBC enzyme defects (G6PD deficiency, pyruvate kinase)	↑ LDH (RBC)	+ enzyme assays
Hemoglobin defects	MCV may be ↑ if reticulocytes high	
1. Qualitative defects (sickle cell anemia, Hb C, Hb E)		Hb electrophoresis
2. Quantitative defects (thalassemia)		↑ Hb A2 (beta-thalassemia), targets cells, basophilic stippling
Extrinsic RBC disorders		
Immune		
Isoimmune hemolytic anemia (e.g., ABO, Rh incompatibility)		+ Coombs' test
Autoimmune hemolytic anemia		
Idiopathic		
Secondary: postviral, autoimmune disorders, Evans' syndrome		+ ANA
Nonimmune (e.g., DIC, HUS)		Concomitant renal disease (HUS)
Blood Loss	Reticulocytes normal (acute loss)	
Overt (e.g. splenic sequestration, gastrointestinal, or nasal bleeding)	↑ Reticulocytes (chronic loss, not iron deficient)	Sickle cell anemia (splenic sequestration)
Occult (e.g. bleeding Meckel's diverticulum, pulmonary hemosiderosis)	↓ Reticulocytes (chronic loss, iron deficient) May have rapidly falling hematocrit	Pulmonary infiltrates + iron deficiency (pulmonary hemosiderosis)

Abbreviations: RBC, red blood cell; WBC, white blood cell; MCV, mean corpuscular volume; MCH, mean corpuscular hemoglobin; RDW, red cell distribution width; TSH, thyroid-stimulating hormone; LDH, lactate dehydrogenase; HS, hereditary spherocytosis; G6PD, glucose-6-phosphate dehydrogenase; DIC, disseminated intravascular coagulation; HUS, hemolytic-uremic syndrome; ANA, antinuclear antibodies.

Adapted from Lanzkowsky, P. Manual of Pediatric Hematology-Oncology. New York, Churchill Livingstone, 1989, pp. 2–3.

hood by cell size with pertinent clinical and laboratory features. Low MCV anemias usually result from iron deficiency or thalassemia trait. High MCV anemias are usually of nutritional origin (vitamin B_{12} or folate deficiency). The many other causes of anemia commonly fall into the normal MCV category.

Etiology and RBC size, the two systems for classification of anemia, are not mutually exclusive and are not

TABLE 63–4.   Differential Diagnosis of Childhood Anemias Based on Red Blood Cell (RBC) Size

Hypochromic, Microcytic Anemia (low MCV)
Iron deficiency anemia
Thalassemia trait (alpha-, beta-)
Lead poisoning
Anemia of chronic disease (juvenile rheumatoid arthritis)
Normochromic, Normocytic Anemia (normal MCV)
Caused by intrinsic RBC defects
  Hemoglobinopathies (e.g., SS)
  Enzymopathies (e.g., G6PD deficiency, PK deficiency)
  RBC membrane abnormalities
    Nonimmune (e.g., HS, HE [not readily apparent])
    Immune (e.g., autoimmune hemolytic anemia)
  Decreased RBC production (e.g., aplastic anemia)
Caused by extrinsic RBC defects
  Microangiopathic hemolytic anemia (e.g., hemolytic-uremic syndrome)
Hyperchromic, Macrocytic Anemia (increased MCV)
Folate deficiency
Vitamin B_{12} deficiency
Preleukemia

Abbreviations: MCV, mean corpuscular volume; G6PD, glucose-6-phosphate dehydrogenase; PK, pyruvate kinase; SS, sickle cell anemia; HS, hereditary spherocytosis; HE, hereditary elliptocytosis.

equally helpful in all situations. Simultaneous application of these two systems enables the physician to make a primary diagnosis of the anemia and determine its probable causes.

EVALUATION

History

It is important to take a good history from patients with anemia to obtain etiologic clues relating to their condition (Questions Box). Anemia based on marrow failure can be congenital or acquired. Historical clues consistent with all marrow failure syndromes include a prolonged (months) history of increased fatigue and pallor, with occasional history of previous transfusions of RBCs prior to diagnosis. In acquired marrow failure states such as aplastic anemia, the history is occasionally consistent with antecedent hepatitis, a viral syndrome, or, rarely, exposure to toxins such as benzene- and toluene-containing compounds, or oral chloramphenicol use (commonly available over-the-counter in Latin America).

A clinical history consistent with anemia secondary to hemolysis includes hyperbilirubinemia with scleral icterus in the newborn period. If hemolysis is acute, red or cola-colored urine due to hemoglobinuria is evident. If the cause is genetic, a positive family history for anemia as well as for cholecystectomy is often elicited.

Questions: Anemia

- Does the child eat meat?
- Does the child drink too much milk (>32 oz/day)?
- Has the child lost a lot of blood recently?
- Have the child's eyes appeared "yellow"?
- Does the child have a family history of anemia, jaundice, or gallstones?
- Did the child need phototherapy at birth for hyperbilirubinemia?

Physical Examination

In addition to historical features, physical findings can often give the clinician strong clues concerning the pathophysiologic process that has caused the anemia. Severe anemia (hemoglobin < 3 g/dL) secondary to chronic causes and moderate anemia (hemoglobin of 3–7 g/dL) in more acute conditions (e.g., blood loss) can cause CHF regardless of etiology owing to insufficient oxygenation of the anemic blood. Aplastic anemia occurs with concomitant neutropenia and thrombocytopenia. Symptoms consistent with concomitant neutropenia (absolute neutrophil count < 1000/mL), including fever or focal infection, especially pneumonia and perirectal abscesses, may be elicited. Symptoms associated with thrombocytopenia include bruises, petechiae, and mucosal bleeding from the mouth, nose, and GI tract. Absent or bifid thumbs are often indicators of both Fanconi's anemia and amegakaryocytic thrombocytopenia. Children with either Fanconi's anemia or Blackfan-Diamond syndrome may exhibit several other physical deformities, including short stature, cardiac anomalies, and mental retardation. Thinning hair that falls out and koilonychia (nail spooning) may result from chronic, severe iron deficiency.

Some physical findings are particular to individual diseases that lead to increased destruction of RBCs. In infants, sickle cell disease may present as hand-foot syndrome, a form of painful crisis that manifests as swelling of one to four digits associated with pain and sometimes fever. Splenomegaly, a feature of sickle cell anemia in younger children prior to autosplenectomy, thalassemia major, and thalassemia intermedia, is also characteristic of RBC membrane disorders, most commonly hereditary spherocytosis. In children with severe chronic hemolysis, regardless of etiology, classic facies (often called "thalassemia facies") can develop, with frontal bossing and flattened nasal bridge, because of the thinning of the facial bones as a result of brisk intramedullary hematopoiesis.

Laboratory Tests

Initial laboratory tests for patients with suspected anemia include hemoglobin, hematocrit, MCV, and blood smear examination. Screening laboratory findings consistent with hemolysis, regardless of etiology, include an elevated reticulocyte count (if secondary to chronic disease), and mildly to moderately elevated indirect and total bilirubin. If the anemia is secondary to immune causes, Coombs' test is positive. All children with anemia secondary to marrow failure have decreased reticulocyte counts in the peripheral blood. Further tests specific for individual hemolytic diseases or particular diseases secondary to marrow failure are summarized in Table 63–3.

Imaging Studies

Few children routinely require imaging studies to determine the cause of their anemia. Hemolysis is reflected on x-ray by the "hair-on-end" appearance of bones. Patients who have anemia associated with lead poisoning may have lead deposition in their long bones.

MANAGEMENT

Two anemia-related conditions constitute emergencies. Prompt recognition of these conditions is vital if proper treatment is to be initiated. **Splenic sequestration** occurs in patients, usually infants, with sickle cell anemia who sequester large volumes of sickling blood within the spleen over a period of hours. This results in rapidly dropping hemoglobin, clinically resembling anemia due to massive blood loss. The blood pooled in the spleen is not available to the circulation, and affected children are subject to fatal splenic rupture. The clinician should suspect this condition in young African-American or Hispanic infants with severe Coombs-negative anemia, rapidly dropping hemoglobin, tachypnea, tachycardia, and an enlarged spleen, even in the absence of a history of sickle cell anemia. Treatment involves transfusion or exchange transfusion.

Severe autoimmune hemolytic anemia is the second anemia-related emergency. Children with this disorder can occasionally present with severe Coombs-positive anemia and clinical evidence of rapid hemolysis; their hemoglobin may fall as much as 1 g/dL/hr. These patients generally require hospitalization, transfusion, and treatment with prednisone, 2 mg/kg/day.

The treatment of anemia varies depending on the etiology. In **iron deficiency anemia,** the single most common cause of anemia in children, administration of **supplemental iron** may be all that is necessary. In physically normal children with a history of poor iron intake, a therapeutic trial of iron, 6 mg/kg/day divided into two doses, is justified before proceeding with further laboratory tests. Normal-appearing children who drink excessive amounts of milk or eat no meat and have a CBC consistent with iron deficiency (i.e., microcytic anemia with a hemoglobin concentration less than the 10th percentile for age with absent reticulocytes) should be treated with iron supplementation. They should demonstrate a brisk reticulocytosis within 7 days of starting iron. An increase of 1.0 g/dL or more in the hemoglobin concentration in 1 month is considered diagnostic of iron deficiency anemia; this justifies the continuation of therapy for an additional 2–3 months. The therapeutic trial should not be continued if the hemoglobin concentration does not increase. Other diagnoses, particularly those related to microcytic anemia, should be entertained and evaluated with appropriate laboratory tests at this point.

The use of **blood transfusions** in patients with anemia is a complex topic that ultimately should be decided after careful consideration by the physician responsible for the patient's care. Because of the risk of acquisition of blood-borne infection, including hepatitis, CMV, and HIV, blood transfusions should never be given to a patient unless it is deemed necessary. "Necessary" reasons for transfusion include (1) patients who are unable to make their own RBCs (e.g., patients with aplastic anemia) and (2) patients whose cardiovascular status is compromised because of the anemia (e.g., patients with orthostatic hypotension or poor tissue perfusion) or who suffer congestive heart failure.

Before children with acute anemia receive transfusions, the clinician must be sure that all blood tests necessary for making the diagnosis have been obtained. This is very important because in several conditions, such as sickle cell anemia, thalassemia, and RBC enzyme disorders such as G6PD and pyruvate kinase deficiency, transfusion obscures the diagnosis until transfused cells have diminished in number. Packed RBCs should be used slowly in conditions in which anemia has occurred slowly to avoid fluid overload. In children with hemoglobin over 7 g/dL, packed RBCs can be given at 10 mL/kg over 3–4 hours; in children with less than 7 g/dL of hemoglobin, 5 mL/kg of packed RBCs can be given over 3–4 hours and then repeated until the desired hemoglobin level is reached. Children with anemia secondary to acute rapid blood loss should be transfused rapidly to keep pace with loss while maintaining intravascular volume and treating the anemia. Packed red cells are the blood product of choice along with normal saline and/or colloid to replace plasma proteins and coagulation factors as necessary.

PROGNOSIS

The prognosis for a child with anemia depends on the underlying cause. Children with some conditions (e.g., thalassemia trait) require no treatment. Early diagnosis and intervention through newborn screening for children with sickle cell anemia has significantly reduced early mortality for this disease. Some children, such as those with thalassemia major, Blackfan-Diamond syndrome, and aplastic anemia, have a lifelong dependency on transfusions that may result in premature death at age 30–40 years from iron overload. Some conditions normalize after splenectomy (e.g., hereditary spherocytosis).

Case Resolution

The girl described in the case history at the beginning of the chapter has hereditary spherocytosis. Her history is highly suggestive of a hereditary hemolytic disorder, and the combination of spherocytes in the peripheral smear, a negative Coombs' test, and a positive, incubated, osmotic fragility test is diagnostic of the condition. At the age of 5 years, she undergoes a splenectomy and has no more hemolytic episodes that require transfusions.

Selected Readings

Charache, S., B. Lubin, and C. D. Reid (eds.). Management and Therapy of Sickle Cell Disease. NIH Publication No. 96–2117, December, 1995.

McKie, V. C. Sickle cell anemia in children: Practical issues for the pediatrician. Pediatr. Ann. 27:521–524, 1998.

Recommendations to prevent and control iron deficiency in the United States. Centers for Disease Control and Prevention. M.M.W.R. 47 (RR-3):1–29, 1998.

Screening for elevated blood lead levels. American Academy of Pediatrics Committee on Environmental Health. Pediatrics 101: 1072–1078, 1998.

CHAPTER 64

BLEEDING DISORDERS

Pamela S. Cohen, M.D. and Pamelyn Close, M.D., M.P.H.

H$_x$ An 8-year-old girl who has been healthy is brought to the office with a two-week history of increased bruises and nosebleeds. On physical examination, hypertension, petechiae, and ecchymosis are evident, but no lymphadenopathy or hepatomegaly is seen. Dried blood is present around the nares. The initial laboratory evaluation includes a CBC, which is normal, except for a platelet count of 7000/mL. The ESR is 105 mm/hr, and a urinalysis is 2+ for protein.

Questions

1. What conditions should be considered when easy bruisability is the chief complaint?
2. What is the appropriate laboratory workup for children with clinical signs of bleeding disorders?
3. What management is appropriate for the most common pediatric bleeding disorders?

Bruises are a common finding in children and usually reflect their activity level. However, bruises as well as mucosal bleeding may be indicative of a clotting disorder. Such disorders most commonly involve disturbances in number or function of platelets or in one or more of the factors essential in the formation of normal clots.

EPIDEMIOLOGY

Classic hemophilia, an x-linked hereditary deficiency of factor VIII, is the most commonly diagnosed coagulation factor deficiency. Factor IX deficiency, or Christmas disease, another sex-linked disease, is second in terms of prevalence. Other factor deficiencies are quite rare.

Genetics control the occurrence of factor deficiencies. Infections, most often viral, can precede the development of acute ITP and aplastic anemia. Viral or bacterial sepsis or trauma can trigger a rapid consumption of clotting factors (disseminated intravascular coagulation [DIC]). Dietary deficiency of vitamin K, caused by intestinal disease or malabsorption, or failure to provide the breast-fed neonate with exogenous vitamin K, can give rise to a bleeding diathesis.

CLINICAL PRESENTATION

Bleeding disorders can manifest themselves in various ways, depending on etiology. Children with deficiencies of clotting factors that cause diseases such as hemophilia often present with ecchymosis (often multiple), bleeding from mucous membranes (e.g., nasal, oral, vaginal), and bleeding into large joints (e.g., elbows, knees, hips). CNS hemorrhage or retroperitoneal bleeding may also occur. Newborn males with hemophilia who undergo circumcision first come to medical attention because of unceasing bleeding after the procedure. Bleeding disorders involving platelet number or function are also characterized by mucous membrane bleeding but usually lead to petechiae rather than large ecchymoses (D$_x$ Box).

PATHOPHYSIOLOGY

Normally, hemostasis occurs following vascular injury. Platelets adhere via von Willebrand's factor to the exposed vascular endothelium and release thromboxane A$_2$, causing local vasoconstriction and further platelet aggregation. The activated platelets then release granules containing adhesive factors (factor V) and serve as a template for the coagulation factor cascade. This ultimately leads to the formation of thrombin and fibrin (Figs. 64–1 and 64–2). This platelet-fibrin collection, called the hemostatic plug, becomes a permanent barrier to further blood loss at the site of vessel injury.

Effective hemostasis depends on blood platelets, plasma proteins with coagulation factors, and components of the vessel wall. Changes in either the number or function of any of these elements can result in hemorrhaging.

DIFFERENTIAL DIAGNOSIS

Disorders involving coagulation factors can be either hereditary or acquired. **Hereditary deficiencies** include the various factor deficiencies such as factor VIII deficiency (hemophilia), factor IX deficiency (Christmas disease), and other rare factor deficiencies, such as defects or dysfunctional production of factors I (fibrinogen), II (prothrombin), V, VII, X, XI, XIII, α_2-antiplasmin, and α_1-antitrypsin.

D$_x$ | **Bleeding Disorders**

- Easy bruising with minimal or no trauma
- Ecchymosis, petechiae
- Mucosal bleeding (e.g., oral, nasal, vaginal, urinary)
- Anemia (if bleeding has been extensive or chronic)

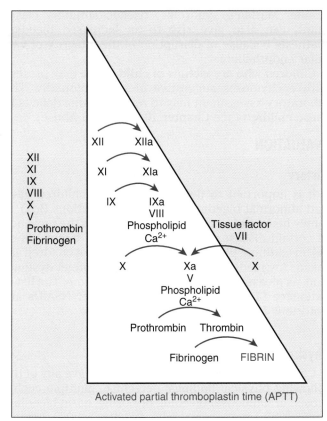

FIGURE 64–1. Activated partial thromboplastin time (APTT). The portion of the coagulation mechanism measured by the APTT is enclosed within the triangle, with the clotting factor to which the APTT is sensitive to the left. (Redrawn, with permission, from Nathan, D. G., and F. A. Oski [eds.]. Hematology of Infancy and Childhood, 4th ed. Philadelphia, W. B. Saunders, 1993, p. 1194.)

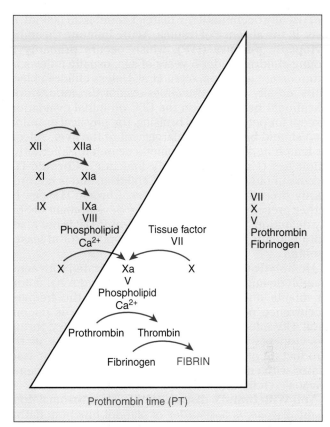

FIGURE 64–2. Prothrombin time (PT). The portion of the coagulation mechanism measured by the PT is enclosed within the triangle, with the clotting factors to which the PT is sensitive listed to the right. (Redrawn, with permission, from Nathan, D. G., and F. A. Oski [eds.]. Hematology of Infancy and Childhood, 4th ed. Philadelphia, W. B. Saunders, 1993, p. 1195.)

Acquired deficiencies may result from vitamin K–dependent conditions, liver disease, blood transfusions, or the presence of certain factor inhibitors. Factors II, VII, IX, and X depend on vitamin K for appropriate synthesis in the liver. Causes of the depletion of vitamin K–dependent factors include antibiotic use (especially for "bowel preps"), obstructive jaundice, malabsorptive states (e.g. cystic fibrosis), parenchymal liver disease, and vitamin K deficiency in the newborn and exclusively breast-fed infant, especially if the mother is a lacto-ovovegetarian. The liver makes the vitamin K–dependent factors II, VII, IX, and X, as well as I and V. In addition, fibrin split products are normally cleared by the liver and therefore may be elevated in parenchymal liver disease, making the coagulation profile difficult to differentiate from DIC. It should be noted that because factor VIII is not made by the liver, normal factor VIII measurement is a way to distinguish liver disease from DIC, in which all factors are consumed.

Massive blood transfusions may also result in wash out of clotting with resultant factor deficiencies. Children who receive large volumes (35 mL/kg) of packed red blood cells may have low levels of platelets and factors V and VIII.

Acquired factor inhibitors are usually only seen in children with hemophilia who receive regular infusions of factor replacement and in children with autoimmune disorders. Autoimmune inhibitors are also seen rarely in children with lymphoma.

Platelet disorders may be classified into two groups: disorders of platelet number (thrombocytopenia) (Table 64–1) and disorders of platelet function (thrombasthenia).

Thrombocytopenia is defined as a platelet count less than 150,000/mL. Spontaneous clinical bleeding does

---

TABLE 64–1. Causes of Most Cases (95%) of Thrombocytopenia in Children

Destructive Thrombocytopenias
Primary platelet consumption syndromes (immunologic)
  Idiopathic thrombocytopenic purpura
  Infection-induced thrombocytopenia
  Autoimmune or lymphoproliferative disorders
  Allergy and anaphylaxis
Impaired or Ineffective Production
Acquired disorders
  Aplastic anemia
  Marrow infiltrative processes
Sequestration
  Hypersplenism

Adapted, with permission, from Nathan, D.G., and F.A. Oski (eds.). Hematology of Infancy and Childhood, 4th ed. Philadelphia, W.B. Saunders, 1993.

not usually occur until the platelet count is 20,000/mL or less, in the absence of trauma. **Acute immune thrombocytopenic purpura (ITP),** which occurs primarily in young children under 5 years of age, usually follows an intercurrent infection, often viral. Unless children bleed substantially, no abnormalities except thrombocytopenia should be evident on the CBC on initial evaluation. Except for petechiae and bruising, the physical examination should be normal. Enlargement of the liver, spleen, or lymph nodes should prompt a search for alternative etiologies (e.g., leukemia, HIV infection). **Chronic ITP** occurs in older, usually female children, and is not ordinarily preceded by a viral illness. Chronic ITP can be either preceded or followed by the development of SLE. By definition, the designation of chronic ITP is not made until patients have had thrombocytopenia for at least 6 months.

Hemolytic-uremic syndrome is associated with acute hemolytic anemia, thrombocytopenia, and renal failure in infants and young children. Despite the frequent occurrence of thrombocytopenia, bleeding is uncommon. HIV infection can often present as isolated thrombocytopenia in children. This occurs because of the production of antiplatelet antibodies and is often associated with concomitant autoimmune hemolytic anemia (Evans' syndrome).

Von Willebrand's disease (vWD), an autosomal dominant disease, is a disorder of platelet function. Pathophysiologically, the plasma von Willebrand's factor (vWF), which is responsible for the adherence of platelets to damaged endothelium, is defective or deficient. In addition, vWF also serves as a carrier protein for factor VIII, so that vWD also results in an effective factor VIII deficiency. Thus in most forms of vWD, the PTT as well as the bleeding time is prolonged. As with factor VIII deficiency, the bleeding diathesis in vWD may be mild, moderate, or severe, depending on the genetic mutation and the extent of deficiency. A large majority of cases of vWD (70–80%) involve a quantitative genetic mutation resulting from a heterozygous deficiency of vWF, resulting in vWF levels between 20 and 40% of normal.

Three other disorders of platelet function are Glanzmann's thrombasthenia, Bernard-Soulier syndrome, and Wiskott-Aldrich syndrome. **Glanzmann's thrombasthenia** results from a defect in Gp IIb/IIIa, the fibrinogen receptor on the surface of platelets that is required for normal platelet aggregation. Patients with this rare disorder can be symptomatic at birth or experience life-threatening bleeding after minor injury. Platelet count is normal in affected individuals, and diagnosis is made by assessment of the platelet Gp IIb/IIIa protein levels.

Bernard-Soulier syndrome results from a defect in platelet glycoprotein Ib, the receptor for vWF, and, like vWD, manifests as a deficiency of platelet aggregation. Platelet counts are slightly lower, but platelet size is somewhat larger than normal.

Patients with **Wiskott-Aldrich syndrome,** which is sex-linked, have severe eczema, a predisposition to opportunistic and pyogenic infections, thrombocytopenia with small platelets, and severe bleeding. The gene affected in this disorder is identified.

Disorders of vascular endothelium, such as diseases of elastic tissue formation (e.g., Ehlers-Danlos syndrome, Marfan's syndrome, pseudoxanthoma elasticum), can also give rise to an increased bleeding diathesis because of disruption of the integrity of vascular endothelium.

Children who are victims of **child abuse** may present with ecchymoses suggestive of a coagulopathy. The laboratory assessment fails to reveal clotting deficits in these children (see Chapter 104, Physical Abuse).

EVALUATION

History

It is important to determine whether children have had abnormal bleeding in the past (Questions Box). A family history of easy bruisability suggests the presence of certain diseases (vWD, deficiencies of factor VIII or IX). In addition, physicians should find out if children are taking any medications that can cause platelet dysfunction, as measured by abnormal bleeding time. The list is extensive (Table 64–2); aspirin and other NSAIDs are notorious for this side effect.

Physical Examination

Children with bleeding disorders may have any of the following physical findings: petechiae, multiple ecchymosis, oral mucosal bleeding or oozing, nasal bleeding, vaginal bleeding, hematuria, swollen joints (hemorrhagic), or limitation of movement in the joints if the condition has been chronic.

Patients with findings related to other organ systems, such as organomegaly, may have a systemic disorder with an associated coagulopathy (e.g., lupus, lymphoma, leukemia). Children with chronic bleeding prior to coming to medical attention may have concomitant iron deficiency anemia from ongoing blood loss. Wiskott-Aldrich syndrome should be considered in male infants with severe eczema and thrombocytopenia. Children with abnormal or absent thumbs may have thrombocytopenia with absent radii (TAR) syndrome or other congenital thrombocytopenic syndromes (amegakaryocytopenic thrombocytopenia, Fanconi's anemia).

Laboratory Tests

Screening tests for children who present with a history of severe bleeding include PT, PTT, fibrinogen, bleeding time, and CBC with platelet count (Tables 64–3 and 64–4). A platelet count of less than 150,000 is abnormal. The bleeding time measures duration of bleeding

---

Questions: Bleeding Disorders

- Has the child ever had any episodes of abnormal bleeding? If so, what sites were involved?
- How long has the child experienced bleeding problems?
- Has the child experienced any recent trauma?
- Has the child had any recent infections?
- Do any other family members have bleeding problems?
- (If appropriate) Is menstrual flow heavy? Is it heavier than usual?
- Is the child taking any drugs that might cause bleeding problems?

TABLE 64–2.   Some Drugs That Inhibit Platelet Function*

Nonsteroidal Anti-inflammatory Drugs
Aspirin†
Beta-Lactam Antibiotics
Penicillins
   Ticarcillin (Ticar, Timentin)
Cephalosporins
   Cefotaxime (Claforan)
Other Drugs
Antibiotics
   Nitrofurantoin (Furadantin, Macrodantin)
Drugs that increase platelet cAMP concentration
   Prostacyclin
Anticoagulants
   Heparin
Cardiovascular drugs
   Propranolol (Inderal)
Psychotropic drugs
   Tricyclic antidepressants
     Imipramine (Tofranil)
   Phenothiazines
     Chlorpromazine (Thorazine)
Anesthetics
   Local
     Dibucaine (Lidocaine)
Narcotics
   Heroin
Oncologic drugs
   Mithramycin
Miscellaneous drugs
   Antihistamines
Foods and Food Additives
Chinese black tree fungus

*This list is by no means exhaustive. Only one drug has been given in each category.
†Used as a therapeutic antithrombotic agent.
Adapted, with permission, from Hoffman, R., et al. Hematology: Basic Principles and Practice. New York, Churchill Livingstone, 1991, p. 1530.

in vivo and assesses platelet function, and vascular endothelial integrity. This may be the only abnormal screening result in children with vWD or bleeding due to uremia.

Mixing studies (i.e., mixing patient plasma 1:1 with normal plasma) are the next step if the PT or PTT is abnormal. If patients have a factor deficiency, the addition of 1:1 of normal plasma to patient plasma corrects a prolonged PT or PTT. If patients have a factor inhibitor, such an addition does not shorten the PT or PTT. Consultation with a pediatric hematologist and the hematology laboratory at this point is necessary to best determine what additional studies are necessary.

TABLE 64–3.   Major Screening Tests in Hemostasis

Test	Hemostatic Functions Measured
Prothrombin time	Extrinsic and common pathways of coagulation: factors I, II, V, VII, X
Partial thromboplastin time	Intrinsic and common pathways of coagulation: factors I, II, V, VIII, IX, XI, XII
Bleeding time	Platelet function and number; vascular endothelial integrity
Platelet count and examination of blood smear	Platelet number and morphology

Reproduced, with permission, from Miller, D.R., and R.L. Baehner. Blood Diseases of Infancy and Childhood, 6th ed. St. Louis, C.V. Mosby, 1990, p. 764.

To avoid treating an unidentified leukemia, a bone marrow aspirate and biopsy is indicated in children with ITP if treatment with intravenous immune globulin (IVIG) has failed and prednisone is being considered. It is also useful in children in whom a marrow failure state (Fanconi's anemia, amegakaryocytic thrombocytopenia) is a possibility.

Imaging Studies

In general, imaging studies are not indicated. Bone films may be taken of the hands and feet in patients with thrombocytopenia to rule out Fanconi's anemia and TAR syndrome.

MANAGEMENT

Management of bleeding disorders in children depends on the diagnosis. In children with classic histories, physical findings, and laboratory features of acute ITP with symptomatic platelet counts less than 20,000/mL, a trial of **IV anti-RhoD** or **IVIG** is warranted and are the treatments of choice where these products are readily available. The speed and ease of administration of anti-RhoD, with a similar efficacy and side effects profile to IVIG, makes this newer product beneficial in the outpatient setting. A short pulse course of prednisone or dexamethasone represents an alternative treatment, especially for patients who do not respond to anti-RhoD or IVIG. This treatment choice should be used only after leukemia is ruled out with a bone marrow examination. The use of **platelet transfusion** is not generally indicated in autoimmune thrombocytopenia (acute and chronic ITP), because the pathophysiology involves the generation of antibodies that recognize all platelets. In children with chronic ITP, **splenectomy** is indicated if severe thrombocytopenia persists, or treatment is prednisone-dependent. Other treatment modalities include **vinblastine.**

In newborn infants with alloimmune thrombocytopenia, washed irradiated maternal platelets can be transfused to correct bleeding.

HIV-associated thrombocytopenia is also immune-mediated and responds well to IVIG at ITP doses. Sometimes monthly IVIG is necessary to control the condition.

Nonimmune thrombocytopenia secondary to either decreased production (e.g., aplastic anemia) or increased destruction (DIC) can be treated with platelet transfusions.

For children with factor deficiencies, treatment requires **factor replacement.** For factor VIII deficient patients there are several highly purified factor replacement products. HIV and other viral infections due to exposure to the blood products of large numbers of donors have effectively been eliminated with new purification procedures. The national standard of care for "PUPS" (previously untreated patients) is to use recombinant factor VIII. Many young children with severe hemophilia currently benefit from three times a week prophylactic treatment programs starting at about 1 year of age and continuing through the elementary school years. These treatment plans are commonly carried out

TABLE 64–4. Screening Test Profiles and Diagnostic Procedures Used in Selected Disorders of Hemostasis

Disorder	Screening Test				Diagnostic Procedures
	PC	BT	PT	PTT	
Vascular Disorders					
Henoch-Schönlein purpura	N	N	N	N	Clinical diagnosis only
Ehlers-Danlos syndrome	N	N*	N	N	Clinical diagnosis only
Platelet Disorders					
Idiopathic thrombocytopenic purpura (ITP)	L	P	N	N	Clinical diagnosis supported by bone marrow examination and, if available, tests for platelet antibodies (positive)
Glanzmann's disease (thrombasthenia)	N	P	N	N	Clot retraction (abnormal) and platelet aggregation studies (defective first-phase aggregation)
Aspirin effect	N	P	N	N	Platelet aggregation studies (defective second-phase aggregation)
Coagulation Disorders					
Classic hemophilia	N	N	N	P	Factor VIII assay (deficient activity)
Christmas disease	N	N	N	P	Factor IX assay (deficient activity)
von Willebrand's disease	N	P	N	P	Assays of factor VIII activity, VIII antigen, and ristocetin cofactor activity (all low in typical cases)
Factor VII deficiency	N	N	P	P	Factor VII assay (deficient activity)
Factor X deficiency	N	N	P	P	Factor X assay (deficient assay)
Vitamin K deficiency	N	N*	P	P	Assay of factors II, VII, IX, X (specific deficiencies with other factors normal)
Disseminated intravascular coagulation	L	P	P	P	Assays of factors I, II, V, and VIII (deficient activities) and FDP titer (increased)

*Bleeding time may be prolonged.
Abbreviations: PC, platelet count; BT, standard bleeding time; PT, prothrombin time; PTT, partial thromboplastin time; N, normal result; L, low; P, prolonged.
Reproduced, with permission, from Miller, D.R., and R.L. Baehner. Blood Diseases of Infancy and Childhood, 6th ed. St. Louis, C.V. Mosby, 1990, p. 771.

using home infusion and central venous catheter techniques. Factor IX replacement is done using similar recombinant, monoclonal and purified-pooled Factor IX concentrates.

Correction of the coagulopathy of vWD depends on the type of vWD (Table 64–5).

In children in whom vitamin K deficiency is strongly suspected as the cause of bleeding, one dose of **vitamin K** should correct the coagulopathy within 12–36 hours.

The coagulopathy of DIC involves both **platelets** and **coagulation factors** as well as factors regulating thrombosis such as **antithrombin II, protein C,** and **protein S.** Children with DIC should be given fresh-frozen plasma, cryoprecipitate (titrate the use of this to the fibrinogen level), and platelets as needed, while the underlying etiology of the DIC (e.g., infection, shock) is treated. In instances where thrombosis also occurs, continuous infusion of heparin may be indicated.

PROGNOSIS

The prognosis of bleeding disorders in children depends on the diagnosis. The most common cause of bleeding, acute ITP, is a time-limited condition that usually resolves uneventfully, although children with platelet counts under 10,000/mL have approximately a 1% chance of life-threatening CNS hemorrhage. Two thirds of patients with chronic ITP go into remission with splenectomy, but one third continue to be at high risk for severe bleeding.

TABLE 64–5. Therapeutic Alternatives in the Treatment of von Willebrand's Disease (vWD)

Type of vWD	DDAVP	vWF or FVIII Concentrate	Platelets
I	Preferred treatment if DDAVP proves effective in therapeutic trial	If DDAVP is not effective or if higher levels are required	Not indicated
IIA	Not usually effective; may cause improvement for 1 or 2 hr	Preferred treatment	Not indicated
IIB	May cause further decrease in platelet count	Preferred treatment	Not usually effective
III (platelet-type vWD)	May cause further decrease in platelet count	May cause further decrease in platelet count	Preferred treatment
Untyped vWD	Use with caution; follow platelet count and vWF levels	Preferred treatment in untyped patient with vWD	Not usually required unless patient has platelet-type vWD

Abbreviations: vWF, von Willebrand's factor; DDAVP, desmopressin.
Reproduced, with permission, from Nathan, D.G., and F.A. Oski (eds.). Hematology of Infancy and Childhood, 4th ed. Philadelphia, W.B. Saunders, 1993.

The prognosis for children with factor deficiencies has markedly improved with viral decontamination technologies and the advent of prophylactic treatment. Many of the quality-of-life issues associated with the pain and incapacitation from chronic, recurrent joint bleeds are being ameliorated through the use of prophylactic treatment programs. Patients with acquired inhibitors after being treated with factor concentrates are now benefiting from new immune-tolerance induction therapies. For those hemophiliacs treated in developing countries or who have had refractory inhibitor problems, chronic arthritis and viral hepatitis remain problems.

Case Resolution

The girl in the case history is found to have SLE with associated ITP. She is started on prednisone after a bone marrow aspirate and biopsy are performed and deemed normal, except for increased megakaryocytes. She ultimately requires a splenectomy before her platelet count rises above 150,000/mL.

Selected Readings

Beardsley, D. B. Platelet abnormalities in infancy and childhood. *In* Nathan, D. G., and F. A. Oski (eds.). Hematology of Infancy and Childhood, 4th ed. Philadelphia, W.B. Saunders, 1993, pp. 1561–1604.

Blanchette, V. S., et al. A prospective, randomized trial of high-dose intravenous immune globulin G therapy, oral prednisone therapy and no therapy in childhood acute immune thrombocytopenic purpura. J. Pediatr. 123:989–995, 1993.

George, J. N., et al. Consensus Panel. Idiopathic thrombocytopenic purpura: a practice guideline developed by explicit methods for the American Society of Hematology. Blood 88:340, 1996.

Hawiger, J., and R. I. Handin. Physiology of hemostasis: cellular aspects. *In* Nathan, D. G., and F. A. Oski (eds.). Hematology of Infancy and Childhood, 4th ed. Philadelphia, W.B. Saunders, 1993, pp. 1494–1533.

Kaspar, C. K. Hereditary plasma clotting factor disorders and their management. Publication of Orthopedic Hospital, Los Angeles, CA, 1996.

Montgomery, R. R., and J. P. Scott. Hemostasis: diseases of the fluid phase. *In* Nathan, D. G., and F. A. Oski (eds.). Hematology of Infancy and Childhood, 4th ed. Philadelphia, W.B. Saunders, 1993, pp. 1561–1604.

Pramanik, A. K. Bleeding disorders in neonates. Pediatr. Rev. 13:163–173, 1992.

Scaradavou, A., et al. Intravenous anti-D treatment of immune thrombocytopenic purpura: experience in 272 patients. Blood 89:2689–2700, 1997.

CHAPTER 65

LYMPHADENOPATHY

Pamela S. Cohen, M.D. and Pamelyn Close, M.D., M.P.H.

H$_x$ An 8-year-old girl is brought to the office with swelling of the anterior cervical nodes, which she has had for 4 weeks. Intermittent fever with temperatures as high as 101° F (38.3° C) and decreased appetite have been associated with the condition. The girl appears pale. On examination, her temperature is 100.4° F (38.0° C), and her other vital signs are normal. Three to four nontender nodes 1–2 cm in diameter are present bilaterally. The remainder of the examination is normal.

Questions

1. When is lymphadenopathy of medical concern?
2. What are the clinical features of childhood diseases that present as cervical lymphadenopathy?
3. What are the diagnostic approaches to the evaluation of children with lymphadenopathy?
4. What is an appropriate therapeutic approach to cervical adenopathy in children?

Lymphadenopathy is a common physical finding in pediatric patients, because lymph node swelling frequently follows the many infections, most often viral, that affect children. Significant lymphadenopathy, which is indicative of a pathologic process requiring diagnosis and intervention, can be defined on the basis of the characteristics of the affected lymph nodes. The nodes must be: (1) greater than 1.0 cm in diameter in children younger than 12 years of age and greater than 0.5 cm in older children; (2) tender, warm, or erythematous; (3) hard, fixed, or matted; and/or (4) located in the supraclavicular area. Lymphadenopathy refers to enlargement of nodes, and adenitis to inflammation. Lymphadenitis is characterized by tenderness, warmth, and erythema.

EPIDEMIOLOGY

Physicians must be able to distinguish significant lymphadenopathy from benign conditions in order to detect underlying causes such as serious bacterial, viral, and protozoal infections; autoimmune disorders; and malignancy. Infections are the most likely cause of tender or unilateral adenopathy. Eighty percent of neck malignancies in children are the result of non-Hodgkin's lymphoma.

CLINICAL PRESENTATION

Cervical lymphadenopathy is the most common type of lymphadenopathy. Most frequently the cause is viral, and the lymphadenopathy is often **bilateral** in the cervical area, or it may be **generalized.** Cervical or generalized adenopathy may be associated with **hepatosplenomegaly** in children with CMV or EBV. Bacterial invasion of lymph nodes produces lymphadenitis, which is often **unilateral.** Bacterial lymphadenopathy may be accompanied by fever, respiratory symptoms, pharyngitis, and skin lesions. Other clues that may suggest bacterial infection include fluctuance, duration greater than 7 days, and dental abnormalities. Lymphadenopathy related to malignancy is often nontender but accompanied by other signs and symptoms such as fever, pallor, and weight loss (D$_x$ Box).

PATHOPHYSIOLOGY

Lymph nodes are the sites at which lymphocytes are exposed to antigens, such as pathogens (e.g., viruses, bacteria, fungi, etc.), which may provoke a cellular or humorally mediated lymphocyte response. Normally, this response involves proliferation of lymphocytes within the nodes; this can result in clinical lymph node enlargement.

Occasionally, lymph nodes themselves become infected, as in tuberculosis (scrofula). Malignancy, most commonly lymphoma and leukemia, can also occur in or invade lymph nodes. This can cause lymph node enlargement and destruction of the normal lymph node architecture, which is a pathognomonic finding in malignant nodal invasion due to lymphoblasts.

DIFFERENTIAL DIAGNOSIS

Cervical lymphadenopathy may be either inflammatory or noninflammatory. Inflammatory lymphadenopathy, which can be infectious, is most commonly either viral or bacterial in etiology. Most cervical adenopathy is viral in etiology, in which case it is often bilateral, or generalized (Table 65–1).

Staphylococcus aureus is the causative agent in 30–40% of cases of bacterial adenitis, followed by group A *Streptococcus pyogenes,* anaerobes, and other species. When the condition appears subacute, cat-scratch disease, tuberculosis, atypical mycobacteria, toxoplasmosis, tularemia, and the more uncommon diseases such as histoplasmosis, brucellosis, and syphilis should be considered.

D$_x$ Lymphadenopathy

- Enlarged lymph nodes
- Fever
- Tenderness or warmth over the lymph nodes (lymphadenitis)
- Antecedent infection (e.g., pharyngitis, URI, otitis media)
- Pallor
- Weight loss
- Bone pain

The cellulitis-adenitis syndrome seen in newborns is consistent with immunodeficiency, especially HIV. HIV, as well as EBV, CMV, and toxoplasmosis, may be associated with diffuse lymphadenopathy.

The noninfectious inflammatory causes of cervical lymphadenopathy include collagen-vascular diseases (e.g., juvenile rheumatoid arthritis, SLE) or other diseases such as chronic granulomatous disease and Kawasaki syndrome. Noninflammatory causes of cervical lymphadenopathy include congenital causes (e.g., thyroglossal duct cyst, branchial cleft cyst, cystic hygroma) and neoplasms. Such neoplasms include Hodgkin's and non-Hodgkin's lymphoma; leukemia and other solid tumors that metastasize to the neck lymph nodes such as neuroblastoma, rhabdomyosarcoma, and fibrosarcoma; and thyroid carcinoma. In both types of lymphomas, nontender, rubbery nodes are usually characteristic. In Hodgkin's disease, the nodes enlarge sequentially, with involvement spreading from one chain to the next, rather than bilaterally. Nodes in Hodgkin's disease are often matted, whereas in non-Hodgkin's disease, the nodes may be large, but they are usually bilateral and not always matted. Supraclavicular adenopathy is particularly worrisome for malignancy.

EVALUATION

History

In patients with lymphadenopathy, physicians should always inquire about the duration of the lymphadenopathy, the rapidity of node enlargement, and the occurrence of associated fever and other constitutional symptoms such as weight loss, itching, or coughing. A history of distant travel; recent immigration from countries with endemic tuberculosis (e.g., Mexico, Central America, Southeast Asia), recent travel to areas with endemic histoplasmosis (southeastern United States) or coccidioidomycosis (San Joaquin Valley, CA); a detailed history of pet contact (cats, which transmit toxoplasmosis and cat-scratch disease); and exposure to ill contacts, particular individuals known to have tuberculosis, are also important (Questions Box).

Physical Examination

The enlarged nodes should be measured and examined at their widest diameter and evaluated for evidence of redness, tenderness, and increased warmth, which are suggestive of infection. The extent of the lymphadenopathy should be assessed, as well as whether there is enlargement of the liver or spleen. Other physical findings depend on the underlying etiology (see Table 65–1).

Laboratory Tests

Laboratory tests used in the evaluation of lymphadenopathy depend on the location and distribution of the adenopathy (unilateral, bilateral, or diffuse). Needle aspirate for a Gram stain and culture is often helpful. CBC, ESR, liver function tests (elevated in EBV and

TABLE 65–1.   Differential Diagnosis of Lymphadenopathy

Diagnostic Category	Clinical Features	Epidemiologic Features	Laboratory Features
Infections			
Viral (EBV, CMV, rubella, HIV)	Usually generalized, not purulent or tender		
Mycobacterial (TB, atypical mycobacteria)	Usually localized; often tender, red, flocculent		
Bacterial (staphylococcal and streptococcal infections, cat-scratch disease, tularemia, plague, diphtheria)	Usually localized; often tender, red, flocculent		
Protozoal (toxoplasmosis)	Generalized		
Spirochete (syphilis)			
Fungal (histoplasmosis, coccidioidomycosis)	May be generalized	Suspicion should be raised based on regional incidence	
Neoplastic Conditions			
Hodgkin's lymphoma	Often associated with "B" symptoms (i.e. fever, weight loss, +/– splenomegaly)	Common among higher socioeconomic groups, only children	↑ ESR (can be >100), ↑ LDH, anergy
Non-Hodgkin's lymphoma	See Hodgkin's lymphoma		
Solid tumors (e.g., rhabdomyosarcoma, neuroblastoma)	Depends on underlying malignancy		
Langerhans cell histiocytosis	Eczema, failure to thrive, bony lesions, diabetes insipidus, proptosis, hepatosplenomegaly all possible		
Sinus histiocytosis with massive lymphadenopathy			
Autoimmune Disorders			
JRA	Generalized lymphadenopathy seen in systemic form (Still's) (i.e., fever, hepatosplenomegaly, evanescent rash, arthritis)	Equal incidence in males and females	↑ ESR, anemia, negative ANA and rheumatoid arthritis in Still's JRA
Lupus	Arthritis, butterfly facial rash, effusions (lung, joint, cardiac), CNS, nephrotic syndrome	Increased incidence in girls, Jewish heritage	↑ ESR, positive ANA, anti-ds DNA, ↓ C3, C4, or CH50, anemia, ↑ platelets, proteinuria
Autoimmune hemolytic anemia	Scleral icterus, splenomegaly +/– hepatomegaly, hemoglobinuria (dark red urine)		Positive Coombs' test, evidence of hemolysis (↑ bilirubin, reticulocytosis)
Granulomatous Disease			
Sarcoidosis	Bilateral hilar lymphadenopathy, noncaseating granulomas (lung, liver)	↑ in those of black and Irish heritage	↑ serum angiotensin-1 converting enzyme (ACE), ↑ serum lysozyme
Chronic granulomatous disease		X-linked	Positive nitroblue tetrazolium test

Abbreviations: ANA, antinuclear antibody; CMV, cytomegalovirus; CNS, central nervous system; EBV, Epstein-Barr virus; ESR, erythrocyte sedimentation rate; JRA, juvenile rheumatoid arthritis; TB, tuberculosis; HIV, human immunodeficiency virus; LDH, lactate dehydrogenase.

CMV), a throat culture, and a PPD are appropriate screening studies. Serum antibody studies (e.g., EBV, CMV, HIV, *Bartonella henselae* for cat-scratch disease) or skin tests for fungal disease may be indicated. In lupus and rheumatoid arthritis, antinuclear antibody (ANA) may be positive and complement levels may be reduced.

Timely lymph node biopsies are needed to diagnose lymphoma. Physicians should consult the pathologist about whether needle or excisional biopsy technique is

preferred for two reasons: (1) in 13–35% of cases in which biopsy is performed, nodes are ultimately malignant; and (2) most pathologists insist on visualizing the entire lymph node to make the diagnosis of lymphoma. In patients with lymphoma, a bone marrow aspirate and biopsy may also be positive.

Imaging Studies

A chest x-ray should be performed in any child with suspected scrofula or malignancy. Other imaging studies are not routinely used, unless the diagnosis of malignant lymphoma is made. In these cases, CT scans of the neck, chest, abdomen, and pelvis, as well as gallium scan, are performed to stage the disease.

MANAGEMENT

Infection is the most common cause of cervical adenopathy. A trial of **antibiotics** with antistaphylococcal coverage is appropriate for tender, unilateral cervical node enlargement. **PPD testing** should also be

---

Questions: Lymphadenopathy

- For how long have the nodes been enlarged?
- Was the child sick before the swelling began?
- Does the child have any symptoms now, such as fever, weight loss, pallor, or anorexia?
- Does the child come in contact with any animals, particularly cats?
- Has the child traveled anywhere?
- Is the child taking any medications?
- Has the child been in contact with anyone who is ill?

carried out. If the adenopathy is unresponsive or progressive and the PPD is negative, a lymph node biopsy should be considered. Other indications for node biopsy include (1) supraclavicular adenopathy of unexplained etiology, (2) fixation of a node to overlying skin, (3) persistent adenopathy with nodes over 3 cm if cat-scratch disease is believed unlikely and cultures and PPD are negative.

Underlying fungal and mycobacterial diseases should be treated with appropriate **antifungal or antibacterial agents,** with the exception of cervical adenopathy due to atypical mycobacteria, which requires **surgical removal.** Malignant disorders such as lymphoma and leukemia require **multimodal therapy** with surgery, chemotherapy, or radiation, depending on the specific disorder and the extent of disease (see Chapter 114, Cancer in Children). Children with HIV are often managed by a multidisciplinary team, with primary care practitioners usually acting as key players in the day-to-day management of these children (see Chapter 115, Pediatric HIV).

PROGNOSIS

The outcome of lymphadenopathy depends entirely on the underlying disorder (see Table 65–1). In the vast majority of cases, the cause is infectious, and the lymphadenopathy resolves completely with the use of appropriate antibiotics.

Case Resolution

In the case history, the bilateral nature of the swelling and the lack of tenderness of the nodes are very worrisome and suggest a noninfectious etiology. The girl had a throat culture, an intermediate PPD, and a chest x-ray, all of which were negative. A CBC reveals leukocytosis with 28,000 WBCs/μL (60% lymphocytes), with a normal hemoglobin and platelet count. A heterophil test for infectious mononucleosis is positive. Bed rest is recommended, and the child makes a complete recovery in 3 weeks.

Selected Readings

Filston, H. C. Common lumps and bumps of the head and neck in infants and children. Pediatr. Ann. 18:180–186, 1989.

Ginsburg, A. M. The tuberculosis epidemic: Scientific challenges and opportunities. Pub. Health Rep. 113(2):128–136, 1998.

Hicks, R. B., and M. E. Melish. Kawasaki syndrome. Pediatr. Clin. North Am. 33:1151–1176, 1986.

Huebner, R. E., et al. Usefulness of skin testing with mycobacterial antigens in children with cervical lymphadenopathy. Pediatr. Infect. Dis. 1:450–456, 1992.

Knight, P. J., A. F. Mulne, and L. E. Vassy. When is lymph node biopsy indicated in children with enlarged peripheral nodes? Pediatrics 69:391–396, 1982.

Knight, P. J., and C. B. Reiner. Superficial lumps in children: what, when and why? Pediatrics 72:147–153, 1983.

Kurtzberg, J., and M. L. Graham. Non-Hodgkin's lymphoma: biologic classification and implications for therapy. Pediatr. Clin. North Am. 38:443–456, 1991.

Leventhal, B. G., and G. J. Kato. Childhood Hodgkin and non-Hodgkin lymphomas. Pediatr. Rev. 12:171–179, 1990.

Marcy, S. M. Infections of lymph nodes of the head and neck. Pediatr. Infect. Dis. 2:397–405, 1983.

Pollock, B. H., J. P. Krischer, and T. J. Vietti. Interval between symptom onset and diagnosis of pediatric solid tumors. J. Pediatr. 119:725–732, 1991.

Zangwill, K. Therapeutic options for cat-scratch disease. Pediatr. Infect. Dis. J. 17(11):1059–1061, 1998.

Zitelli, B. J. Evaluating the child with a neck mass. Contemp. Pediatr. 7:90–112, 1990.

C H A P T E R   6 6

HEART MURMURS

Robin Winkler Doroshow, M.D.

H_x A 6-year-old girl is brought to the office for a physical examination for school. Her past medical history is unremarkable, and her growth and development have been normal. She is asymptomatic. Her physical examination is normal except for a grade II/VI low-pitched vibratory systolic ejection murmur that is loudest at the left lower sternal border, with radiation to the apex and upper sternal border. The murmur increases to III/VI in the supine position.

Questions

1. What is the significance of a heart murmur in asymptomatic children? How reassuring are a negative history and the absence of other physical findings?
2. What workup should be done by primary care physicians?
3. What are the costs of excessive tests and unnecessary consultation? What are the costs of inadequate workup?
4. When should physicians refer children to specialists for consultation?

Asymptomatic children with heart murmurs are commonly encountered by physicians. Murmurs are a finding rather than a medical sign or symptom because they are detected incidentally at an examination conducted for another purpose.

Correct assessment of the significance of a heart murmur is important to ensure appropriate management of children with heart disease. Complications of undiagnosed cardiac disease in children include progressive hemodynamic impairment, endocarditis, and even sudden death.

The misinterpretation of an innocent murmur as organic in nature can also take its toll, primarily on parental anxiety. Unnecessary restriction of activities may result, which can have a negative impact on children's school and social lives as well as self-image. As adults they may be denied health insurance, life insurance, and certain types of employment. In addition, misdiagnosis costs money and utilizes limited re-

sources, with unnecessary tests and doctor visits, as this "non-disease" is evaluated and followed.

EPIDEMIOLOGY

An estimated 50% of healthy children have heart murmurs. The overall incidence of congenital heart disease (CHD), including symptomatic cases, is just under 1%, and some children with CHD have no murmur. Therefore, about 99 out of 100 murmurs noted during childhood are innocent.

CLINICAL PRESENTATION

Heart murmurs are usually detected on routine examination for well child care or on evaluation for an unrelated problem. Innocent murmurs are not associated with signs or symptoms because they are normal findings. The majority of the symptoms sometimes associated with organic murmurs (i.e., murmurs of heart disease) are related to the presence of congestive heart failure (CHF) (see Chapter 68) and usually appear during infancy. Some children with murmurs come to medical attention with complaints of exercise intolerance or chest pain. It is necessary to determine whether these problems are actually referable to the heart.

PATHOPHYSIOLOGY

A murmur is a sustained sound that can be detected with a stethoscope placed on the chest. This sound is produced by turbulence of blood flow in the heart or great vessels. This turbulence may be due to structural abnormalities (e.g., aortic valve stenosis), benign or normal flow patterns (see below), or exaggeration of normal flow patterns (seen in high output states such as fever, exercise, anxiety, or anemia, and sometimes termed "functional").

Not all significant heart disease in children is heralded by a murmur. Structural heart disease may be "silent" and be indicated by other findings. For example, transposition of the great arteries results in cyanosis, anomalous pulmonary venous return in CHF, and hyp-

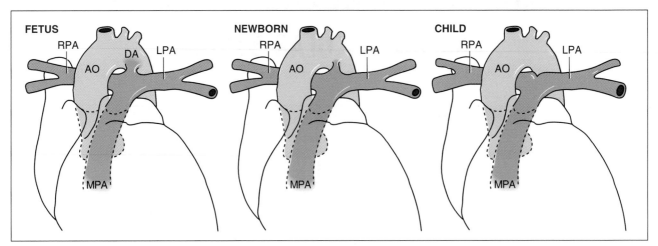

FIGURE 66–1. Configuration of the central pulmonary arteries in the fetus, the newborn, and the child. MPA, main pulmonary artery; RPA, right pulmonary artery; LPA, left pulmonary artery; DA, ductus arteriosus; AO, aorta.

oxia, and anomalous origin of the left coronary artery in CHF. Acquired heart disease such as Kawasaki syndrome, myocarditis, or cardiomyopathy often produces no murmur.

The common innocent murmurs are better recognized than understood. Because they occur in normal, healthy individuals, there are few hemodynamic or anatomic data to correlate with the murmur, and pathophysiology is in some cases conjectural. **Still's murmur,** which was once thought to be due to easily appreciated aortic valve flow, is now believed to result from vibration of normal fibrous bands that cross the left ventricle. This murmur may also be heard in children who have undergone spontaneous closure of a membranous ventricular septal defect, with a small residual aneurysm in the septum. The **pulmonary flow murmur** appears to be caused by normal flow across the pulmonary valve, perhaps made more apparent because of high cardiac output, close proximity to the chest wall, and (in adolescent females) mild anemia. The **venous hum** is attributed to turbulence at the confluence of the innominate veins, which is exacerbated in the upright position by gravity.

The **physiologic peripheral pulmonic stenosis (PPPS) murmur** in newborns is produced by turbulence at the origins of the left and right pulmonary arteries. Because less than 10% of the combined ventricular output of the fetus goes to these branches, they are small and arise at a sharp angle from the main pulmonary artery. When postnatal circulation abruptly requires the entire cardiac output to enter these vessels, a relative stenosis is encountered (Fig. 66–1). This physiologic stenosis resolves gradually with remodeling of the pulmonary artery tree by 2–3 months of age.

DIFFERENTIAL DIAGNOSIS

In healthy children, the differential diagnosis of a heart murmur includes innocent murmurs and murmurs resulting from structural lesions (Table 66–1). The specific features of a particular murmur usually provide the clue to the diagnosis. It is therefore important to develop and maintain auscultatory skills.

Some features may alert examiners to the organic nature of a murmur. Although very loud murmurs (grades IV–VI) are usually not innocent, some innocent murmurs may be as loud as grade III. Diastolic murmurs and continuous murmurs, other than the easily recognizable venous hum, are usually pathologic, as are high-pitched and harsh murmurs, which are better heard with the diaphragm of the stethoscope.

The common innocent murmurs of childhood are recognizable on auscultatory examination. **Still's murmur,** or the **innocent vibratory murmur,** is a low-pitched, vibratory, or musical murmur that sounds like a groan. Because of its low frequency, the murmur is better heard with the bell. It is loudest at the left lower sternal border but is often distributed widely over the precordium. This murmur is often quite loud and is extremely common in school-age children. The characteristics of the murmur are diagnostic, although the absence of other findings is supportive.

The **pulmonary flow murmur,** usually heard in older children, is a short, blowing systolic ejection (i.e., crescendo-decrescendo) murmur localized to the left upper sternal border. It may be louder in the supine position.

The **venous hum** is a soft continuous murmur, similar to the sound heard in a seashell. Because of its constancy, it is often overlooked. This murmur is very

TABLE 66–1. Common Organic Murmurs in Asymptomatic Children

Lesion	Other Clues
Atrial septal defect	Fixed split S_2
Ventricular septal defect (small to moderate)	Loud heart sounds
Patent ductus arteriosus (small to moderate)	Full or bounding pulses
Pulmonic stenosis	Systolic ejection click (SEC)
Aortic stenosis	SEC; suprasternal thrill
Coarctation of the aorta	Weak or absent femoral pulses

commonly heard in preschool and school-age children. Loudest in the right infraclavicular area, it may also be heard on the left. This murmur is highly variable with head and neck position and compression of the neck veins, which may increase or diminish it. It usually disappears in the supine position.

The **PPPS** murmur is an innocent murmur found in newborns. Best heard at the upper sternal border, this blowing systolic ejection murmur radiates strikingly over the lung fields into the back and both axillae.

EVALUATION

History

The history may be helpful in assessment of children with a murmur. If a thorough history shows that children have no symptoms, this suggests the absence of severe heart disease and helps exclude many major or complex defects as well as CHF.

The most common symptom reported by children or parents is easy fatigability (Questions Box). This is difficult to quantitate. Determining exercise intolerance on the basis of history is very subjective; it may be due, of course, to noncardiac causes and may be unrelated to the murmur. Easy fatigability during infancy may be reported as slow or poor feeding. Chest pain, a common symptom in adults with heart disease, is rarely cardiac in origin in children. A history of rapid breathing, excessive sweating, and other complaints referable to CHF suggests organic heart disease. Central cyanosis (i.e., involving the oral mucosa rather than the perioral area or the fingers) may be reported by parents of children with cyanotic CHD but is often not recognized.

Physical Examination

The physical examination often gives strong clues to the cardiac diagnosis beyond the murmur itself. Even in children with known CHD, the nonauscultatory portions of the examination are critical in assessing the cardiac status (i.e., how the patient is tolerating the defect).

Vital signs, preferably obtained with the child at rest or sleeping, yield more information regarding cardiac status than specific diagnosis. Tachypnea and tachycardia are present in CHF. A normal resting respiratory rate (i.e., < 60/minute in infants) argues strongly against CHF. Blood pressure is normal in most

---

Questions: Heart Murmurs

- Is the child easily tired?
  - Does the child keep up with others of his or her age?
  - If the child is having a good time—for example, at a park or a party—how is the child's endurance?
- Does the child have a family history of CHD?
- Was the child exposed antenatally to possible teratogens?
- Does the child ever complain of chest pain? At rest or with activity?
- Does the child ever appear blue?
- Does the child perspire excessively?

---

patients with CHD. It may be useful to measure blood pressure in the legs, especially if coarctation of the aorta is suspected because of diminished pulses in the lower extremities.

The **growth pattern** may reflect the presence of any chronic illness, including hemodynamically significant congenital heart disease. Affected patients, particularly infants and children with large left-to-right shunts (with or without CHF) gain weight poorly. Height and head circumference are usually normal, although in more severe or prolonged situations, height may also be affected.

A complete **cardiac examination** should be performed. Is the chest asymmetric, a sign of long-standing cardiomegaly? Is the precordial impulse hyperdynamic? Are extra sounds (e.g., clicks, rubs, gallops) heard? Is the second sound normal in intensity and in width and motion of splitting (i.e., variation with respiration)?

Additional pertinent findings include lethargy, dysmorphic features suggestive of a genetic syndrome, central cyanosis, and clubbing. Hepatomegaly is found in children with CHF. The peripheral pulses should be normal in volume, neither diminished (e.g., pedal pulses in coarctation) nor bounding (e.g., in patent ductus arteriosus), and equal in all extremities. The temperature and capillary refill of the extremities in children who are not chilled reflect adequacy of the peripheral circulation.

Diagnostic Studies

Routine laboratory studies are not warranted in the evaluation of most murmurs. An **ECG** is indicated when heart disease is known or strongly suspected but a normal ECG may not rule out CHD. In some cases, such as with echocardiography, the manner in which the examination is actually carried out may vary depending on the suspected diagnosis. Such tests are not suitable for screening purposes and should be obtained only after consultation with a pediatric cardiologist.

MANAGEMENT

If a heart murmur is suspected of being organic in origin because of its features or associated findings, referral to a pediatric cardiologist is indicated. In the case of asymptomatic children there is no urgency, but parental and physician anxiety can best be allayed by proceeding to consultation promptly (i.e., within weeks). In some cases, a repeat examination may be useful before deciding whether to consult a specialist, particularly if the murmur is initially heard under nonphysiologic conditions such as fever. Tests are usually best utilized if selected and ordered by specialists. Not all cardiologists perform all tests on all patients.

Management of organic heart disease in infants or children is also best handled by specialists. Treatment may include **medications, interventional catheterization,** or **cardiac surgery.** Communication with pediatricians, however, is essential to delivery of optimal patient care.

If the murmur is innocent, physicians must complete the following steps:

1. Children and their families must be informed about the presence of the murmur. Even if the murmur is benign, children have a right to know that it was heard. In addition, they are likely to be examined by other practitioners who will report it, which may lead to the erroneous suspicion of either a new murmur or negligence on the part of the first examiner.
2. The diagnosis must be clearly explained to parents and children (depending on the age). It is essential that they understand that this is a normal finding rather than a minor abnormality. In some cases, notification of teachers or athletic coaches may be appropriate to prevent misunderstanding. Physicians must stress that no further evaluation is needed and no restrictions are indicated. Printed brochures that explain innocent murmurs are available from organizations such as the American Heart Association.
3. The description of the murmur and the diagnosis itself must be documented in the medical record. A murmur that is clearly and unequivocally innocent, with no evidence of heart disease, should not affect the child's access to insurance, participation in sports, etc. Medical documentation also helps protect patients from unnecessary reevaluations in the future.
4. Physicians should proceed no further. No laboratory studies or consultations need be performed. If the evaluation has been completed by a specialist because of suspicion of CHD by the referring physician, no follow-up with the specialist is indicated. The child is referred back to the primary practitioner.

PROGNOSIS

The prognosis for children with heart murmurs depends on the cause of the murmur. Children with an innocent murmur, who by definition have normal hearts, have a normal prognosis—with one exception. If children or their parents mistakenly believe children to have heart disease, parents may treat the children inappropriately (e.g., unnecessary testing, restriction of activities). As a result, children may develop sedentary habits and inferior self-image.

With appropriate medical attention, the prognosis is normal or near-normal in the majority of cases of CHD. Children with minor defects not requiring intervention (e.g., small ventricular septal defect, mild pulmonic stenosis) need only endocarditis prophylaxis (e.g., for dental procedures) and infrequent cardiology follow-up. With the development of refined cardiac surgery and interventional catheterization, even children with the most complex cardiac anomalies now have a good outlook with respect to both daily living and life expectancy.

Case Resolution

In the case presented, a healthy girl with no history of cardiovascular symptoms has a heart murmur and an otherwise unremarkable physical examination. The murmur is a typical Still's (innocent vibratory) murmur, which is identifiable by its low-pitched, vibratory quality. No further evaluation is necessary. The diagnosis is explained, the girl and her parents are reassured, and the murmur and diagnosis are noted in the medical record.

Selected Readings

Bergman, A. B., and S. J. Stamm. The morbidity of cardiac nondisease in school children. N. Engl. J. Med. 276:1008–1013, 1967.

Danford, D. A., et al. Cost assessment of the evaluation of heart murmurs in children. Pediatrics 91:365–368, 1993.

Helfant, R. H., et al. Role of cardiac testing in an era of proliferating technology and cost containment. J. Am. Coll. Cardiol. 9:1194–1198, 1987.

Hohn, A. R. Congenital heart disease—the first test. West. J. Med. 156:435–436, 1992. (Editorial.)

Liebman, J. Diagnosis and management of heart murmurs in children. Pediatr. Rev. 3:321–329, 1982.

Linde, L. M. Assessing chest pain in children and adolescents. Prim. Cardiol. 19:55–58, 1993.

Mangione, S. and L. Z. Nieman. Cardiac auscultatory skills of internal medicine and family practice trainees. J.A.M.A. 278:717–722, 1997.

Moss, A. J. Clues in diagnosing congenital heart disease. West. J. Med. 156:392–398, 1992.

Newburger, J. W., A. Rosenthal, and R. G. Williams. Noninvasive tests in the initial evaluation of heart murmurs in children. N. Engl. J. Med. 308:61–64, 1983.

Smythe, J. F., et al. Initial evaluation of heart murmurs: are laboratory tests necessary? Pediatrics 86:497–500, 1990.

CHAPTER 67

CYANOSIS IN THE NEWBORN

Robin Winkler Doroshow, M.D.

H$_x$ A 3500-g, term male infant born to a 29-year-old, gravida II para II, healthy mother by spontaneous vaginal delivery is well until 24 hours of age when a nurse notes that he is cyanotic. On examination, he appears blue but in no distress. The vital signs are temperature (axillary), 37° C (98.6° F); pulse, 130; respirations, 40; and blood pressure, 80/60 in the right arm. His general appearance is normal except for the cyanosis. His heart sounds are normal, and no murmur is heard. His liver is not palpable, and the peripheral pulses are normal and equal in all extremities. Capillary refill is normal. Oxygen saturation is 65% by pulse oximetry.

Questions

1. What are the causes of cyanosis in newborns?
2. What is the appropriate evaluation of cyanosis in newborns?
3. How urgent is the assessment? What are the risks and benefits of further evaluation?
4. Which aspects of management should be initiated by a primary physician at a community hospital?
5. Which types of treatment should be undertaken by the consulting pediatric cardiologist at the referral center?

Cyanosis is a bluish appearance of the skin due to the presence of reduced hemoglobin in the tissues. Central cyanosis, which is detected initially in the oral mucosa and nailbeds but is generalized when severe, indicates at least 4–5 grams of reduced hemoglobin per 100 mL blood. Hypoxemia is usually the cause. This condition is frequently present in neonates with pulmonary pathology but is also one of the most common presentations of severe congenital heart disease (CHD).

Because cyanotic CHD in newborns may be life-threatening, it must not go undiagnosed. Most diagnostic studies have minimal risk. Even the risk of cardiac catheterization in this setting is relatively low. Most of the lesions that cause cyanotic CHD can be palliated or corrected, and the prognosis is good.

EPIDEMIOLOGY

Cyanotic CHD occurs in about two to three of every 1000 live born infants. Approximately 80–90% of these cases, usually the most severe ones, are detected in the first 30 days of life. Infants with low pulmonary blood flow or lesions causing poor mixing present most often with obvious cyanosis, although initially they otherwise

---

TABLE 67–1.   Settings With Increased Risk of Congenital Heart Disease

Genetic syndromes (e.g., trisomies, DiGeorge syndrome)
Certain extracardiac anomalies (e.g., omphalocele, forearm anomalies)
Maternal diabetes poorly controlled during first trimester
Exposure to cardiac teratogen (e.g., lithium, isotretinoin)
High incidence of congenital heart disease in family
Fetal or neonatal arrhythmia

---

appear well and comfortable. Those with high pulmonary flow are less blue and often present first with congestive heart failure (CHF) or a murmur.

Most cyanotic CHD is not diagnosed before birth. The antenatal history, gestational age, birth weight, and delivery room examination are unremarkable. CHD is more likely in some situations that can be anticipated prenatally (Table 67–1). In these settings, increased suspicion may lead to antenatal detection using echocardiography.

CLINICAL PRESENTATION

Children with cyanotic CHD often present within the first week of life with blueness of the oral mucosa. In more severe cases, generalized blueness occurs. The abnormal color may be more apparent with effort (e.g., feeding, passing stool) or crying. Respiratory distress, heralded by grunting, nasal flaring, and retractions, is a minor or absent finding in cyanotic CHD. In cases of severe hypoxia, metabolic acidosis leads to poor perfusion and compensatory tachypnea. Additional findings depend on the nature of the causal lesion (D$_x$ Box).

PATHOPHYSIOLOGY

Cardiac cyanosis is due to **right-to-left shunting** so that systemic venous blood bypasses the pulmo-

---

D$_x$ Cyanosis in the Newborn

- Bluish skin
- Heart murmur
- Tachypnea
- Abnormal cardiac silhouette on x-ray
- Abnormal ECG
- Abnormal echocardiogram
- No improvement with oxygen
- Increased perspiration

nary circulation and enters the systemic circulation. Two conditions are necessary to produce this type of shunting: a communication, such as a septal defect, for the blood to shunt across; and some cause, such as pulmonic stenosis, for the blood to be shunted away from the lungs. The most notable exception is simple transposition of the great arteries (TGA), where the fundamental connections are abnormal, and all venous blood is directed to the systemic circulation. Lesions associated with cyanosis may be divided into three groups.

1. The **low pulmonary blood flow (LPBF) group** consists of tetralogy of Fallot, pulmonary atresia with intact ventricular septum, and virtually any combination of defects that includes pulmonary atresia or severe pulmonic stenosis. Pulmonary flow is diminished and may derive entirely from the ductus arteriosus while it remains patent. Aside from obvious cyanosis, infants often appear well.

2. The **high pulmonary blood flow (HPBF) group** includes truncus arteriosus, single ventricle, and combinations of defects that involve mixing of oxygenated and unoxygenated blood and little or no obstruction to pulmonary flow. Although a right-to-left shunt is present, the left-to-right shunt is even greater. Pulmonary venous return is therefore voluminous and contributes disproportionately to systemic output. Cyanosis is less apparent. Pulmonary flow increases over the first days and weeks of life as the pulmonary vascular resistance falls, and CHF develops, as in patients with isolated shunt lesions (e.g., ventricular septal defect). Some children with HPBF lesions also have obstruction to systemic blood flow (e.g., coarctation of the aorta, hypoplastic left heart syndrome) and may depend on the ductus arteriosus to carry some or all of this flow.

3. The **poor mixing group** is limited to TGA and its variants. The right and left circuits are in parallel rather than in series, and survival depends on interchange of oxygenated and unoxygenated blood between them. Most newborns with poor mixing present with marked cyanosis, like patients in the LPBF group.

Severe hypoxemia ($pO_2 < 35$ mm Hg for the average newborn) is not compatible with prolonged survival. Death ensues in a matter of hours. Infants experience tissue hypoxia, anaerobic glycolysis, and metabolic acidosis. Respiratory compensation may occur at first. Even with a normal pH, however, the presence of metabolic acidosis indicates life-threatening hypoxia, necessitating immediate intervention.

DIFFERENTIAL DIAGNOSIS

The major causes of cyanosis are cardiac and respiratory (Table 67–2). Diagnoses in the latter group include problems of the lung, chest, airway, or respiratory drive.

TABLE 67–2. Noncardiac Causes of Neonatal Cyanosis

Pulmonary infection (e.g., group B streptococcal infection)
Aspiration (e.g., meconium aspiration syndrome, tracheoesophageal fistula)
Pulmonary hypoplasia (e.g., Potter's syndrome, diaphragmatic hernia)
Respiratory distress syndrome (e.g., in prematurity)
Thoracic hypoplasia (e.g., thanatophoric dwarfism)
Hypoventilation (e.g., neurologic depression)
Persistent fetal circulation

The syndrome of **persistent fetal circulation** is perhaps most often confused with cyanotic CHD. In this syndrome the heart and great vessels are structurally normal, but high pulmonary resistance, which is often seen in postterm infants with perinatal distress or pulmonary disease, causes blood to shunt away from the lungs at the foramen ovale and ductus arteriosus. Profound cyanosis that is unresponsive to supplemental oxygen may be the only abnormal finding, and echocardiography is required to exclude CHD.

Pulmonary cyanosis may be due to **infection** (e.g., group B streptococcal pneumonia), **aspiration** (e.g., meconium, tracheoesophageal fistula), **pulmonary hypoplasia** (e.g., Potter's syndrome, diaphragmatic hernia), **respiratory distress syndrome** (e.g., prematurity), or a host of other problems of the lung, chest, or airway. Neurologic depression may produce hypoventilation with resultant hypoxia.

EVALUATION

Evaluation of the cyanotic newborn must be expeditious so that management is not delayed. In some cases, therapy may be initiated before the evaluation is complete. All available information, the statistical likelihood of CHD, and the risk-benefit ratio of the treatment must be taken into account.

History

Review of the history may be helpful, particularly in certain situations, such as in children with pulmonary disease (Questions Box). It is important to note that a negative response to any or all of the questions does not make cyanotic CHD unlikely; in fact, negative responses are noted in most cases.

Questions: Cyanosis in the Newborn

- Has the infant been in any distress?
- Has the infant had difficulty feeding?
- Was the infant suspected of having a heart problem prior to birth (e.g., fetal arrhythmia, abnormal heart on ultrasound)?
- Is the mother diabetic?
- Did the mother take any drugs (prescribed or not) during the pregnancy?
- Was the mother ill during the first trimester?
- Is there a positive family history of CHD or other birth defects?
- Did any perinatal problems (e.g., meconium staining) occur?

Physical Examination

Cyanosis may be the only abnormal physical finding in cardiac patients, but a careful, thorough examination often yields information about the underlying cardiac defect and the overall circulatory status.

External anomalies or abnormal phenotypic appearance may indicate a genetic disorder with associated cardiac anomalies. Dyspnea (grunting, nasal flaring, intercostal retractions) is more often seen with lung disease, but tachypnea (rapid respiration) is common with both severe heart disease and pulmonary problems. Tachypnea results either from CHF in HPBF lesions or from metabolic acidosis in severe hypoxia or impaired perfusion. Poor perfusion is also manifested by abnormal color (pallor or a gray or ashen appearance if combined with cyanosis), cool extremities, delayed capillary refill, and generally diminished pulses.

The peripheral pulses are palpated in all extremities. Abnormalities or discrepancies between extremities must be confirmed by measuring blood pressure. Weak pulses may be found in cardiogenic shock, and bounding pulses may be noted with diastolic runoff lesions such as patent ductus arteriosus or aortic insufficiency. Pulse quality and blood pressure may differ in different extremities if an aortic arch abnormality such as coarctation is present. The abdominal examination may reveal hepatomegaly (in CHF) or abnormal situs (as in asplenia syndrome, usually associated with complex cyanotic CHD).

The cardiac examination may disclose a loud murmur if an obstruction such as pulmonary stenosis is present. The physician should note, however, that atresia, being a total obstruction, produces no murmur. Heart sounds may be loud and the precordium hyperdynamic, particularly in children with HPBF. Splitting of the second sound confirms that two patent semilunar valves are present, but this finding is often difficult to appreciate even in normal newborns.

Laboratory Tests

A number of laboratory studies are available (see Chapter 68, Congestive Heart Failure; Table 68–2). As in CHF, it is initially more important to determine whether patients have heart disease than to obtain a precise, complete diagnosis. In cyanotic CHD, sophisticated studies such as echocardiography and catheterization are usually needed to make a detailed diagnosis.

The suspicion of arterial hypoxemia should be confirmed by **pulse oximetry,** an indirect measurement. It is readily available and noninvasive but has shortcomings. Perfusion must be adequate to obtain a reading. Accuracy is diminished at saturations below 75%, although the presence of profound hypoxia can still be confirmed. Cyanotic CHD cannot be ruled out by pulse oximetry, however, because readings of 100% saturation may reflect pO_2 values that range anywhere between 75 and 250 mm Hg (Fig. 67–1). **Arterial blood gases** are more accurate and give important additional information about ventilation and acid-base status. Arterialized capillary gases may suffice if perfusion is adequate.

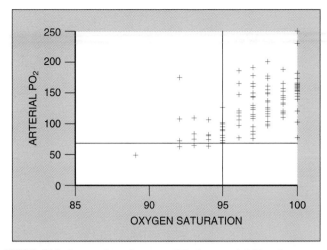

FIGURE 67–1. Comparison between PO_2 by arterial blood gas measurement and oxygen saturation by pulse oximetry. (Reproduced, with permission, from Neihoff, J., et al. Efficacy of pulse oximetry and capnometry in postoperative ventilatory weaning. Crit. Care Med. 16:701, 1988.)

Oxygenation of the extremities may differ in infants with certain lesions (e.g., coarctation). The site of sampling should be noted. If possible, the saturation should be measured at sites both proximal and distal to the ductus arteriosus (i.e., from the right arm and either leg).

A **shunt study,** also known as a hyperoxia challenge, should be performed to determine whether a right-to-left cardiac shunt is present. Pure oxygen (F_IO_2 = 1.00) is given for 5–10 minutes by hood. In patients with LPBF or TGA, increasing the inspired oxygen does not affect the oxygenation of the blood because the blood is unable to enter the lungs; this is a positive result. In patients with pulmonary disease or hypoventilation, oxygenation increases strikingly, often to a pO_2 exceeding 200 mm Hg; this negative result rules out cyanotic CHD.

A "blunted" shunt study, characterized by a rise in pO_2 but rarely to levels above 150 mm Hg, is seen in patients with severe pulmonary disease and in those with HPBF lesions. With such lesions the pulmonary venous blood is high in volume, and the rise in its saturation causes a definite rise in arterial oxygenation. This effect is exaggerated by the further increase in pulmonary flow due to the vasodilating effect of oxygen.

A positive shunt study may be identified with pulse oximetry. It is difficult or impossible, however, to distinguish between a blunted study and a negative one with this tool. The oxyhemoglobin dissociation curve is flattened at the upper end, and the saturation changes very little over a wide range of pO_2 (Fig. 67–2). Capillary gases may be equally inaccurate in this range, but directly measured arterial blood gases are highly reliable. In addition, they may reveal hypercapnia, with or without respiratory acidosis, suggesting a pulmonary cause for the hypoxia.

ECG, a fairly inexpensive test, is readily available and noninvasive. However, it does not often help distinguish

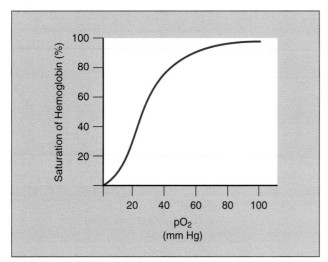

FIGURE 67–2. Oxyhemoglobin dissociation curve. Note that the position of the curve itself may vary with temperature, pH, pCO$_2$, and 2,3-diphosphoglycerate (2,3–DPG).

cyanotic CHD from other causes of cyanosis, particularly for those practitioners who lack experience with neonatal ECGs. The normal range is large in neonates, with much overlap between normal and CHD. Care must also be taken in placing the leads correctly and minimizing artifacts.

Imaging Studies

The **chest x-ray,** a relatively inexpensive and readily available test, is often extremely helpful in differentiating between cardiac and noncardiac disease. Pulmonary disease is often readily apparent on chest x-ray.

The x-ray also helps define the cardiac diagnosis broadly but not precisely. Patients with LPBF lesions have small hearts and diminished pulmonary flow. In contrast, patients with HPBF lesions have large hearts and increased flow, such as is seen in infants with simple left-to-right shunts. With many cyanotic lesions, the cardiac silhouette is abnormal in configuration (e.g., boot-shaped heart in tetralogy of Fallot) or position (e.g., dextrocardia in patients with heterotaxia syndromes). TGA may be more misleading; pulmonary flow may be increased despite the severe cyanosis, and the heart size may be normal. An apparently normal x-ray does not exclude TGA.

Under optimal conditions, **echocardiography** enables the physician not only to recognize CHD but to identify details of anatomy and physiology. Conversely, a properly performed, complete, negative echocardiogram rules out CHD. The performance of a high-quality study requires the appropriate equipment (with high-resolution imaging), an experienced sonographer, and an experienced cardiologist for interpretation. In the absence of these elements, echocardiography may be used cautiously as a screening device as part of the initial assessment to confirm heart disease prior to referral to a specialist. However, referral should not be delayed until echocardiography can be performed.

MANAGEMENT

Initial management prior to cardiac consultation (often with transfer to another institution) includes surveillance, assistance, direct medical management, and supportive care.

Close **surveillance,** including transfer to the highest level of neonatal care available, use of a cardiopulmonary monitor and continuous pulse oximetry, frequent monitoring of vital signs, and repeat physical examinations, is begun as soon as cyanotic CHD is identified. Even if the infant is feeding well, it is best to suspend feedings because of the likelihood of invasive procedures or spontaneous deterioration in the near future. A secure intravenous line should be placed for administration of fluids, glucose, and medications.

While undertaking these measures, the physician should make every effort to seek **assistance** from a pediatric cardiologist. A neonatologist may be consulted if a pediatric cardiologist is not immediately available. Much advice may be obtained over the telephone. In addition, plans for immediate consultation or transfer of patients may be discussed in this way.

The need for **supportive care** depends on the case. In the absence of metabolic acidosis or impaired perfusion, no special care is indicated. In some cases, intravenous fluid boluses, inotropic agents, and other treatments may be needed as part of the early management. Mechanical ventilation should be used in patients with metabolic acidosis, whether compensated or uncompensated, because of the increased oxygen requirement produced by hyperventilation and the tendency for tiring, leading to superimposed respiratory acidosis.

The temptation to give supplemental oxygen for more than the few minutes necessary to perform a shunt study is great but must be resisted. Oxygen is rarely helpful and may be harmful in this setting. In infants with TGA or LPBF lesions, oxygenation is not affected. In infants with HPBF lesions, oxygenation is usually adequate in room air (saturation: > 80%), and an increase in F$_{IO_2}$ may exacerbate the CHF. Oxygen may also constrict the ductus arteriosus on which the patient may depend.

The possibility of ductal dependency should prompt consideration of administering the ductus dilator, **prostaglandin E-1 (PGE-1).** The definitive diagnosis of cyanotic CHD need not be made prior to institution of this lifesaving treatment. In infants who remain adequately oxygenated (no acidosis) and perfused, the drug can be prepared but administration deferred pending consultation. The benefits of giving PGE-1 to severely hypoxic infants or infants with compromised perfusion far outweigh the risks, which include apnea and fever. A dramatic improvement is often seen within seconds to minutes, confirming the diagnosis of a ductal-dependent lesion, and enabling the physician to stabilize the patient until more definitive evaluation and intervention can occur.

PROGNOSIS

If untreated, LPBF lesions and TGA are usually fatal during infancy, most often during the neonatal period, because of severe hypoxia. Untreated HPBF lesions may lead to death in infancy from either CHF or complications such as pneumonia. If the systemic blood flow is ductus-dependent (e.g., interruption of the aortic arch), death occurs shortly after ductal closure, usually during the first week of life.

With prompt recognition and intervention, however, the prognosis for infants with cyanotic CHD is surprisingly good in the absence of a genetic syndrome (e.g., trisomy 18) or a major complicating extracardiac malformation (e.g., neural tube defect). If diagnosed before the onset of severe circulatory compromise, infants can be stabilized and evaluated promptly, and palliative or corrective procedures can be performed. The large majority of such patients can survive for decades with fair-to-good quality of life. Infants with lesions with all four chambers adequate in size (e.g., tetralogy of Fallot) have a better lifetime prognosis than those with a hypoplastic chamber (e.g., tricuspid atresia). Even infants with anatomic abnormalities such as asplenia syndrome or hypoplastic left heart syndrome now have a reasonable outlook with complex reconstructive surgery or heart transplantation.

Case Resolution

In the case presented at the beginning of the chapter, marked hypoxia is present in the absence of other cardiacfindings such as a heart murmur. The oxygen saturation does not rise after the infant breathes 100% oxygen for 10 minutes. The chest x-ray shows a small, boot-shaped heart

and diminished pulmonary blood flow, and the ECG isnormal. Transport is arranged. Because of the marked cyanosis, infusion of PGE-1 is begun, and saturation increases to 80%, with the pO$_2$ rising from 33–48 mm Hg. The infant is transferred to a tertiary care center, where consultation is obtained. An echocardiogram is also performed, which demonstrates tetralogy of Fallot with pulmonary atresia. A Blalock-Taussig shunt is placed in the newborn period, and complete repair using a pulmonary artery homograft is performed at 5 years of age.

Selected Readings

DiMaio, A. M., and J. Singh. The infant with cyanosis in the emergency department. Pediatr. Clin. North Am. 39:987–1006, 1992.

Driscoll, D. J. Evaluation of the cyanotic newborn. Pediatr. Clin. North Am. 37:1–23, 1990.

Freed, M. D., et al. Prostaglandin E-1 in infants with ductus arteriosus dependent congenital heart disease. Circulation 64:899–905, 1981.

Jones, R. W. A., et al. Arterial oxygen tension and response to oxygen breathing in differential diagnosis of congenital heart disease in infancy. Arch. Dis. Child. 51:667–673, 1976.

Lees, M. H., and D. H. King. Cyanosis in the newborn. Pediatr. Rev. 9:36–42, 1987.

Niehoff, J., et al. Efficacy of pulse oximetry and capnometry in postoperative ventilatory weaning. Crit. Care Med. 16:701–705, 1988.

Tateishi, K., and I. Yamanouchi. Noninvasive transcutaneous oxygen pressure diagnosis of reversed ductal shunts in cyanotic heart disease. Pediatrics 66:22–25, 1980.

Victorica, B. E. Cyanotic newborns. In Gessner, I. H., and B. E. Victorica. (eds.). Pediatric Cardiology: A Problem Oriented Approach. Philadelphia, W.B. Saunders, 1993.

C H A P T E R   6 8

CONGESTIVE HEART FAILURE

Robin Winkler Doroshow, M.D.

H$_x$ A 2-month-old infant is brought to the office by his mother, who complains that her son has been eating poorly and breathing oddly for the past few days. The perinatal history is unremarkable. A heart murmur was noted at the 1-month checkup.

The infant is scrawny and irritable. Physical examination shows that the baby's weight, which was at the 50th percentile at birth, is now at the fifth percentile; his height, which was at the 50th percentile, is now at the 25th

percentile. He is afebrile, and his heart rate is 165/min, with respirations 60/min and shallow but without respiratory distress. The skin is pale and diaphoretic, and the mucous membranes are pink. Examination of the head and neck is normal; no jugular distention is present. The lungs are clear. The precordium is hyperdynamic, and the heart sounds are loud; a prominent systolic murmur is audible at the left lower sternal border. The liver edge is palpable 4 cm below the right costal margin in the right midclavicular line, and the spleen is not palpable. The extremities are thin, with normal pulses and no edema. Capillary refill is slightly delayed.

Questions

1. What are acute and chronic signs of cardiac disease in children?
2. What are the signs of congestive heart failure (CHF) in children? How do these signs in children differ from those in adults?
3. What underlying disorders can cause CHF in young infants?
4. What is the appropriate emergent management for infants with CHF? What are the risks of treatment if the diagnosis is incorrect?

Congestive heart failure (CHF) is the most common presentation of serious heart disease in infants. Although this condition also occurs in older children, an estimated 90% of cases of CHF in the pediatric population begin in the first year of life. In children CHF is most often caused by structural congenital heart disease. Compensatory mechanisms are fewer and less successful in small infants. Other causes of CHF are included in Table 68–1.

EPIDEMIOLOGY

The precise incidence of CHF in children is unknown; it is approximately 0.1%. Most cases result from congenital heart disease (CHD), which occurs in 0.8% of live births. The incidence of CHD varies little with geography, ethnic group, or gender. It is far more common in children with recognizable genetic syndromes (e.g., trisomy 21 [Down syndrome], Turner's syndrome).

CLINICAL PRESENTATION

Most commonly, complaints about CHF take the form of queries about an infant's feeding. Comments are

---

TABLE 68–1.   Causes of Congestive Heart Failure in Children

Volume Overload
Left-to-right shunts (e.g., ventricular septal defect)
Bidirectional shunts (e.g., truncus arteriosus)
Valvular insufficiency (e.g., mitral regurgitation)
Extracardiac conditions (e.g., anemia, arteriovenous malformation)
Pressure Overload
Outflow obstruction (e.g., coarctation of the aorta)
Inflow obstruction (e.g., obstructed anomalous pulmonary veins)
Vascular resistance (e.g., hypertension, chronic pulmonary disease)
Myocardial Dysfunction
Intrinsic conditions (e.g., cardiomyopathy, anthracycline toxicity)
Inflammatory conditions (e.g., viral myocarditis, rheumatic fever)
Coronary insufficiency (e.g., anomalous left coronary artery)
Arrhythmias
Tachyarrhythmia (e.g., paroxysmal supraventricular tachycardia)
Bradyarrhythmia (e.g., third-degree atrioventricular block)

Dx   Congestive Heart Failure

- Tachycardia
- Tachypnea
- Hepatomegaly
- Sweating
- Decreased feeding
- Irritability
- Full fontanelle
- Murmur

---

often vague (e.g., "my baby is not a good eater") but may be more precise (e.g., "he is taking less formula with each feeding," "he is taking longer to nurse"). Parents may also describe rapid breathing, excessive sweating, or decreased activity, but usually only on specific questioning.

CHF is also often detected on examination for routine infant checkups or for unrelated complaints. Careful assessment of the physical findings, including vital signs, reveals **tachypnea, tachycardia,** and **hepatomegaly** and frequently signs of underlying structural heart defects, such as a murmur (Dx Box).

PATHOPHYSIOLOGY

High cardiac output may lead to CHF in infants with large left-to-right shunts. Myocardial contractility is relatively normal, and children remain on the "normal" line of the Frank-Starling curve, which relates cardiac output to diastolic volume (also called preload) or pressure (Fig. 68–1). The shunt requires a very large volume of output, primarily to the pulmonary bed. Although the heart may be able to meet this demand, preload is high, leading to "congestive" signs and symptoms (e.g., tachypnea, hepatomegaly). In more severe cases, systemic output may be compromised, resulting in hypotension, renal failure, and metabolic acidosis.

Left-sided failure caused by elevated pulmonary venous pressure produces increased lung water. Initially, this fluid is interstitial, and it does not interfere with gas exchange but does trigger reflex tachypnea. Minute volume is kept normal by decreasing tidal (breath-to-breath) volume, leading to shallow as well as rapid breathing. Only when the ability of the pulmonary lymphatics to drain this fluid is overcome by large volume does fluid accumulate in the alveoli. Rales and respiratory distress, or dyspnea, then result.

Right-sided failure caused by an elevated systemic venous load usually produces more volume than pressure load on this system, possibly as a result of the greater venous compliance in infants as compared with adults. The liver becomes very distended and is easily palpated. As long as the liver can absorb the increased venous volume, the portal pressure does not rise, and splenomegaly does not occur. Because the venous pressure rises very little, jugular distention, which is difficult to detect in young infants in any case, is rarely seen. Edema is also rare.

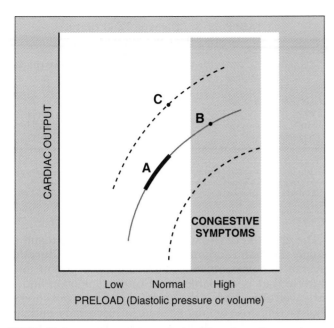

FIGURE 68–1. Graph showing relationship of cardiac output to preload. The solid curve represents normal myocardial contractility, and the dotted curves represent impaired function (shifted downward) and the positive inotropic state (shifted upward). A: Normal range (no heart disease). B: Left-to-right shunt with congestive heart failure (CHF). Note that overall output is high but most of it is shunted. C: Same situation as B but after treatment for CHF. Cardiac output is the same or better, but preload is now out of the range that results in congestive symptoms.

The left and right (systemic and pulmonary) circulations are more interdependent in infants and younger children than they are in older children or adults. As a result, **bilateral heart failure** is much more common than right-sided or left-sided failure alone. Although this means that recognition of bilateral heart failure may be easier, determination of the underlying condition may be more difficult because the clues are less specific. For example, in an adult with left-sided failure, the differential diagnosis includes mitral, but not tricuspid, valve disease.

DIFFERENTIAL DIAGNOSIS

When tachycardia, tachypnea without dyspnea, and hepatomegaly are present, the diagnosis of CHF is straightforward. CHF is most commonly confused with major respiratory infections such as bronchiolitis or pneumonia. Pulmonary infections are frequently associated with dyspnea as well as tachypnea, impaired gas exchange, and other respiratory findings. Rhinorrhea, cough, fever, or wheezing may also be present. Rales may accompany pneumonia but are rare in CHF in infancy or early childhood. Hyperinflation due to lung disease may lead to a false impression of hepatomegaly. In some children, CHD, CHF, and respiratory infections coexist.

Clues to the presence of structural heart disease, such as a murmur or absent femoral pulses, may support the diagnosis of CHF. Severe CHF, with low cardiac output or even shock, has a broader differential diagnosis. In

addition to cardiac causes, sepsis, hypovolemia, and disorders associated with inborn errors of metabolism should be considered.

EVALUATION

History

The history should include specific questions about feeding and growth (Questions Box). Poor feeding, often a nonspecific complaint in chronically or subacutely ill infants, results from tachypnea and fatigability in infants with heart disease. Growth failure may result from poor feeding and increased cardiopulmonary work. The physician should specifically query parents about possible excessive sweating or rapid breathing in infants, because parents may not volunteer this information.

Physical Examination

The diagnosis of CHF is primarily based on clinical findings, and physical examination is essential. The resting respiratory rate must be counted precisely, because infants in CHF most often have tachypnea without dyspnea. The liver edge is palpable more than 1 cm below the right costal margin in the midclavicular line, and the degree of enlargement mirrors the severity of the CHF.

Diagnostic Studies

Many laboratory tests can be performed to assess infants' hearts (Table 68–2), including ECG and echocardiogram. However, some procedures are very costly, and some are invasive and therefore carry risk. The value of most of these tests depends on the expertise of the individuals who perform and interpret them. It is important to remember that although test results and consultation with a pediatric cardiologist may be invaluable in the identification of the underlying lesion, *these procedures are not usually required in the diagnosis of CHF.*

In children with severe CHF, further studies are indicated. **Arterial blood gases** show evidence of metabolic acidosis due to tissue anoxia, with respiratory compensation in early stages and superimposed respiratory acidosis in later stages. A **CBC** shows leukocytosis due to stress. It may not differentiate between heart disease and sepsis.

The most useful supportive study is a **chest x-ray,** preferably in anteroposterior and lateral projections.

Questions: Congestive Heart Failure

- How has the infant been feeding? Does he or she get out of breath or appear exhausted?
- Has the child's growth pattern changed recently?
- Does the child tire easily? With eating? With playing?
- Does the child perspire excessively, especially with efforts such as feeding?
- Does the infant breathe rapidly, even at rest?

TABLE 68–2. Laboratory Tests Used in the Evaluation of Heart Disease in Children

Test	Information
Chest x-ray	Presence and direction of shunt
	Hints concerning specific diagnosis (possible pulmonary disease ruled out)
Electrocardiogram (ECG)	Cardiac rhythm and conduction
	Chamber overload
	Coronary insufficiency
Ambulatory ECG (24-hr ECG)	Subacute rhythm assessment
	Correlation of symptoms with rhythm
Oximetry	Presence and degree of hypoxemia
Arterial blood gases	Hypoxemia
	Acid-base status
Hematocrit	Anemia
	Polycythemia
Exercise test	Quantitation of exercise tolerance
	Provocation of symptoms or arrhythmia
Echocardiogram	Specific structural diagnosis and hemo-dynamics
	Chamber enlargement and function
Cardiac catheterization	Specific structural diagnosis and hemo-dynamics

The chest x-ray may show cardiomegaly, pulmonary venous congestion, and hyperinflation. Cardiomegaly is due not to myocardial dysfunction but to the volume overload from the shunt. In the absence of cardiac enlargement, the diagnosis of CHF must be seriously questioned. (However, CHF may occur in the absence of cardiomegaly in total anomalous pulmonary venous return with obstruction, which usually presents in the first week of life in association with hypoxia.) Pulmonary venous congestion occurs in left heart failure, but increased pulmonary arterial flow from a left-to-right shunt often obscures the congestion. Hyperinflation resulting from peribronchial edema is also a common finding.

MANAGEMENT

Inotropes and **diuretics** are used in the initial management of CHF in children. Inotropic support results in a shift to a higher Frank-Starling curve (see Fig. 68–1), which allows affected patients to maintain the high volume output necessitated by the underlying CHD at lower diastolic pressures, thus alleviating congestive symptoms. **Digoxin,** a form of digitalis, is the drug of choice in such cases, where cardiac output is not severely impaired. This agent is readily available, easily absorbed, safe in the therapeutic range, and easy to administer (elixir for oral administration). If digoxin is initially given at the maintenance dose (10 μg/kg/day), therapeutic levels are not attained for about a week; therefore loading is preferable (Table 68–3). Digoxin is well tolerated and rarely causes side effects. Because of the safety and reliability of absorption, blood levels need not be checked unless overdose is suspected (e.g., history of overadministration, toxic ingestion, unexplained vomiting, or second- or third-degree heart block).

TABLE 68–3. Digoxin: Total Oral Loading Dose in Children*

Age	Dose (μg/kg)
Preterm newborns	20–30
Term newborns and infants	25–35
1–5 yrs	30–40
5–10 yrs†	20–30
10 yrs to adult†	10–15

*IV loading dose = 75–80% of PO dose. Usually given ½, followed 8 hrs later by ¼, followed 8 hrs later by ¼, followed 12 hrs later by initiation of maintenance dose. Assumes normal renal function; dose must be adjusted downward for renal failure.

†In children over 5 yrs of age, loading dose can be calculated by surface area (0.5–1.0 mg/m²).

The elevated diastolic preload of CHF is the result of renally mediated sodium and water retention. **Diuretics** reverse this phenomenon. **Furosemide,** a potent loop diuretic that is available in an oral suspension and is fairly well absorbed, is the most frequent drug of choice. The starting dose is 1 mg/kg once or twice daily. Initially, furosemide may be given intravenously or intramuscularly rather than orally, which reduces the time to onset of action, and is more effective. Such treatment also supports the patient while digoxin loading is in progress.

Fluid and sodium restriction, often used in adults with CHF, is difficult to achieve with infants because their diet is predominantly or exclusively liquid. High-calorie diets using concentrated formulas, complex carbohydrate additives, or medium-chain triglyceride oils may reduce the intake of free water and the effort of feeding without compromising caloric intake.

Breast milk and most proprietary formulas have a low sodium load. In older infants and children with CHF, salt intake is more easily modified and should be minimized.

Children with severe or refractory cases of CHF may require additional medications or interventions. These include **intravenous inotropes** (e.g., dopamine), **vasodilators** for afterload reduction (e.g., angiotensin-converting enzyme inhibitors), **correction of anemia** (e.g., transfusion), **treatment of fever** (e.g., antipyretics), and **reduction of metabolic demands** (e.g., ventilatory support, bed rest, sedation).

Ultimately, the best management for CHF is **treatment of the underlying disorder.** The degree of urgency depends on the nature of the disorder and the severity of the CHF. For example, in neonates with supraventricular tachycardia, conversion to normal sinus rhythm is often the only treatment necessary. CHF caused by severe anemia responds dramatically to correction of hemoglobin levels. When CHF is due to structural CHD (the most common situation), surgery to palliate the problem (e.g., pulmonary artery banding in left-to-right shunts) or correct the defect (e.g., repair of ventricular septal defect [VSD]) usually resolves the CHF. It is rarely necessary to "tolerate" prolonged, uncontrolled CHF in children or to treat the condition aggressively at the expense of a major change in life-style.

Family counseling, which should begin when CHF is identified, is essential. Several important points should be included, in addition to a general description of both the cardiac defect and CHF. The term "heart failure," which is commonly thought to refer to a sudden deterioration of heart function or even cardiac arrest, must be clarified. It is also important to stress that affected infants should be treated as normally as possible, with the exception of administration of medicines and keeping medical appointments. Contrary to popular belief, infants with cardiac conditions are not fragile. Addressing parental concern, assuaging guilt, and normalizing existence are key quality-of-life issues.

PROGNOSIS

In the vast majority of young infants and children with CHF, the prognosis is excellent. CHF responds well to treatment, and the underlying defect can usually be corrected or at least palliated. Without cardiac surgery for CHD, CHF often remits spontaneously over months or years as a result of maturation of compensatory mechanisms, spontaneous improvement in the defect (e.g., decrease in the size of a VSD), or increase in pulmonary vascular resistance because of long-standing high pulmonary artery pressure and flow (Eisenmenger's syndrome). "Catch-up" growth occurs with remission of CHF, and children have the potential to reach their genetically determined height and weight.

Case Resolution

The case presented at the beginning of the chapter is typical of an otherwise normal infant with a large VSD who becomes symptomatic after the development of CHF. The boy's growth failure can be attributed to the chronicity of his illness.

The loud murmur and presentation in infancy strongly suggest the existence of underlying structural CHD as the cause of CHF. The time of onset of CHF also suggests a specific mechanism. When the onset is slightly delayed after birth, a lesion with changing postnatal hemodynamics, such as left-to-right shunt, which has increased as pulmonary resistance has fallen, is suggested. (Note that a ductus-dependent defect would have presented more acutely and severely in the first week of life.)

Selected Readings

Artman, M., and T. P. Graham. Congestive heart failure in infancy: recognition and management. Am. Heart J. 103:1040–1055, 1982.

Friedman, W. F., and B. L. George. Medical progress–treatment of congestive heart failure by altering loading conditions of the heart. J. Pediatr. 106:697–706, 1985.

Kimball, T. R., et al. Effect of digoxin on contractility and symptoms in infants with a large ventricular septal defect. Am. J. Cardiol. 68:1377–1382, 1991.

Soyka, L. F. Pediatric clinical pharmacology of digoxin. Pediatr. Clin. North Am. 28:203–216, 1981.

Talner, N. S. Heart failure. In Emmanouilides, G. C., et al. (eds.). Moss and Adams' Heart Disease in Infants, Children, and Adolescents, 5th ed. Baltimore, Williams & Wilkins, 1995, pp. 890–911.

CHAPTER 69

HYPERTENSION

Sudhir K. Anand, M.D.

Hx A 10-year-old girl is seen in the emergency department with a history of severe headache and generalized seizures lasting 2 minutes. Her past medical history is remarkable for a history of several episodes of unexplained fever as an infant and an episode of urinary tract infection at age 3 years; no radiologic studies were done. She also has a history of headaches for the past 2 years, which have been treated primarily with acetaminophen. There is no known history of drug ingestion or hypertension in the patient or family members.

The physical examination is remarkable for a pulse of 100 and a blood pressure of 210/130 mm Hg in the right arm in supine position. Equal pulses are palpable in all four extremities. Blood pressure is 216/134 mm Hg in the right lower extremity. The funduscopic examination reveals evidence of petechial hemorrhages and mild papilledema. Chest examination finds normal breath sounds and an active precordium with the apical impulse shifted to the left; no murmurs are heard. The liver is palpable one centimeter below the right costal margin. The neurologic examination is remarkable for altered sensorium with lethargy; no focal neurologic deficit is present. A routine urinalysis shows 2+ protein and normal urinary sediment. The hemoglobin is 11.2g/dL and hematocrit is 33%. Sodium is 139 mEq/L, potassium 3.8 mEq/L, chloride 102 mEq/L, and bicarbonate 22 mEq/L. BUN is 35 mg/dL and serum creatinine is 1.8 mg/dL. An electrocardiogram shows left ventricular enlargement. CT scan of the head is normal.

Questions

1. What is the definition of hypertension in children?
2. What are the causes of hypertension in children?
3. What is the appropriate evaluation of hypertension in children?
4. What acute and long-term management is used in hypertensive children?
5. What is the appropriate emergency treatment of symptomatic hypertension?

TABLE 69–1. Definitions of Hypertension

Term	Definition
Normal BP	Systolic and diastolic BPs < 90th percentile for age and sex
High-normal BP*	Average systolic and/or average diastolic BP between 90th and 95th percentiles for age and sex
High BP (hypertension)	Average systolic and/or average diastolic BPs ≥95th percentile for age and sex with measurements obtained on at least three occasions

*If the BP reading is high-normal for age, but can be accounted for by excess height for age or excess lean body mass for age, such children are considered to have normal BP.

Reproduced, with permission, from the Report of the Second Task Force on Blood Pressure Control in Children–1987. Pediatrics 79:1, 1987.

Hypertension is a major public health problem in the adult population. Because of its effects on the heart, central nervous system, kidneys, and eyes, it is one of the leading causes of increased mortality and morbidity. Hypertension is frequently identified in children also. As with adults, the etiology of elevated blood pressure in children may be idiopathic (i.e., essential hypertension); or, more often it may signify the presence of an underlying disorder, especially renal disease.

NORMAL BLOOD PRESSURE

Both systolic and diastolic blood pressures (BP) in children gradually increase, from the newborn period through adolescence; therefore, age-appropriate norms should be used to classify a given BP reading as normal or hypertensive. For example, a BP reading of 132/80 mm Hg would be regarded as normal for a 16-year-old adolescent, but it would signify severe hypertension in a 2-year-old child. BP measurements should be part of routine physical examinations in all children over 3 years of age and in all hospitalized children. Also, an appropriately sized blood-pressure cuff should be used; the cuff width should be approximately 40% of the arm circumference midway between the olecranon and the acromian (D$_x$ Box).

EPIDEMIOLOGY: DEFINITION AND INCIDENCE OF HYPERTENSION

BP values in children are a continuum, with no clear dividing line between normal and high. Despite this limitation, the Report of the Second Task Force on Blood Pressure Control in Children in 1987 defined hypertension to be an average systolic or diastolic BP equal to or greater than the 95th percentile for age and sex, with measurements obtained on at least three occasions (Table 69–1). Readings between the 90th and 95th percentile were regarded as high-normal, and it was suggested that such children should be monitored more closely for future development of hypertension. The Task Force further classified hypertension into two categories: (1) significant hypertension (BP persistently between the 95th and 99th percentiles for age and sex) and (2) severe hypertension (BP persistently at or above the 99th percentile for age and sex). As would be obvious from the above definition of hypertension, 5% of all children (those with BP readings >95th percentile) have hypertension, with 4% having significant hypertension and 1% having severe hypertension. However, most pediatricians and health care workers screening healthy children identify hypertension in only about 1% (or less) of children and not the expected 5%. In 1996, a report from the National High Blood Pressure Education Program updated the 1987 Task Force Report and recommended new blood pressure tables adjusted for height percentiles of children in various age groups (Tables 69–2 and 69–3).

CLINICAL PRESENTATION

Hypertension in most children with mildly elevated BP is usually asymptomatic; the symptoms of headache, dizziness, and nosebleeds occur probably no more frequently in children with hypertension than in those without it. However, children with severe hypertension often complain of headaches, dizziness, and nosebleeds, and these symptoms may be superimposed upon symptoms of primary disorders that led to the hypertension. Children with severe hypertension, especially malignant hypertension, may have signs of heart failure (tachycardia, tachypnea, or enlarged liver), experience seizures, and infrequently suffer seventh nerve paralysis. Also, a fundus examination may show vascular changes, exudates, and papilledema.

D$_x$ Hypertension

- BP elevated > 95th percentile for age on at least 3 consecutive occasions with the child in a quiet, nonapprehensive state and with BP cuff of appropriate size
- BP checked in both upper and at least one lower extremity
- Fundus examination: vascular changes, exudates, and papilledema
- Abnormal urinalysis

TABLE 69–2. Blood Pressure Levels for the 90th and 95th Percentiles of Blood Pressure for Boys Aged 1–17 Years by Percentiles of Height

Age (y)	Blood Pressure Percentile*	Systolic Pressure by Percentile of Height (mm Hg)†							Diastolic Blood Pressure by Percentile of Height (mm Hg)†						
		5%	10%	25%	50%	75%	90%	95%	5%	10%	25%	50%	75%	90%	95%
1	90th	94	95	97	98	100	102	102	50	51	52	53	54	54	55
	95th	98	99	101	102	104	106	106	55	55	56	57	58	59	59
2	90th	98	99	100	102	104	105	106	55	55	56	57	58	59	59
	95th	101	102	104	106	108	109	110	59	59	60	61	62	63	63
3	90th	100	101	103	105	107	108	109	59	59	60	61	62	63	63
	95th	104	105	107	109	111	112	113	63	63	64	65	66	67	67
4	90th	102	103	105	107	109	110	111	62	62	63	64	65	66	66
	95th	106	107	109	111	113	114	115	66	67	67	68	69	70	71
5	90th	104	105	106	108	110	112	112	65	65	66	67	68	69	69
	95th	108	109	110	112	114	115	116	69	70	70	71	72	73	74
6	90th	105	106	108	110	111	113	114	67	68	69	70	70	71	72
	95th	109	110	112	114	115	117	117	72	72	73	74	75	76	76
7	90th	106	107	109	111	113	114	115	69	70	71	72	72	73	74
	95th	110	111	113	115	116	118	119	74	74	75	76	77	78	78
8	90th	107	108	110	112	114	115	116	71	71	72	73	74	75	75
	95th	111	112	114	116	118	119	120	75	76	76	77	78	79	80
9	90th	109	110	112	113	115	117	117	72	73	73	74	75	76	77
	95th	113	114	116	117	119	121	121	76	77	78	79	80	80	81
10	90th	110	112	113	115	117	118	119	73	74	74	75	76	77	78
	95th	114	115	117	119	121	122	123	77	78	79	80	80	81	82
11	90th	112	113	115	117	119	120	121	74	74	75	76	77	78	78
	95th	116	117	119	121	123	124	125	78	79	79	80	81	82	83
12	90th	115	116	117	119	121	123	123	75	75	76	77	78	78	79
	95th	119	120	121	123	125	126	127	79	79	80	81	82	83	83
13	90th	117	118	120	122	124	125	126	75	76	76	77	78	79	80
	95th	121	122	124	126	128	129	130	79	80	81	82	83	83	84
14	90th	120	121	123	125	126	128	128	76	76	77	78	79	80	80
	95th	124	125	127	128	130	132	132	80	81	81	82	83	84	85
15	90th	123	124	125	127	129	131	131	77	77	78	79	80	81	81
	95th	127	128	129	131	133	134	135	81	82	83	83	84	85	86
16	90th	125	126	128	130	132	133	134	79	79	80	81	82	82	83
	95th	129	130	132	134	136	137	138	83	83	84	85	86	87	87
17	90th	128	129	131	133	134	136	136	81	81	82	83	84	85	85
	95th	132	133	135	136	138	140	140	85	85	86	87	88	89	89

*Blood pressure percentile was determined by a single measurement.
†Height percentile was determined by standard growth curves.
Reproduced, with permission, from the Update on the 1987 Task Force Report on High Blood Pressure in Children and Adolescents: A Working Group Report from the National High Blood Pressure Education Program. Pediatrics 98:649–658, 1996.

ETIOLOGY AND PATHOPHYSIOLOGY

An increase in BP results from an increase in peripheral resistance or cardiac output or a mixture of the two. The exact cause of hypertension in 90–95% of adults is still uncertain; hence, the name essential, primary, or idiopathic hypertension. In the past, it was often stated that in more than 80% of children hypertension was secondary to an underlying disorder and that fewer than 20% of cases were idiopathic; however, this is true only in children with severe hypertension. In the majority of children, especially in adolescents, with mild increases in blood pressure (i.e., slightly beyond the 95th percentile), no etiology of hypertension is found, and they are classified as having idiopathic or essential hypertension.

Many factors play a role in the development of essential hypertension; these include **heredity, stress response, salt sensitivity,** and **obesity.** In addition, during investigations of hypertension, alterations to a variable degree have been found in cardiac output, extracellular fluid volume, peripheral resistance, renin-angiotensin system, aldosterone, balance of sodium, potassium, calcium, and chloride ions, catecholamines, sympathetic nervous system, natriuretic hormones, prostaglandins, kinins, antidiuretic hormone, insulin response, endothelins, nitric oxide (endothelium-derived relaxation factors), and others. Whether these abnormalities are primary or secondary and what their exact role is in the pathogenesis of essential hypertension is still uncertain.

The etiology of secondary hypertension varies with the age of the patient and with the nature of the hypertension—i.e., whether the condition is acute or chronic (Tables 69–4 and 69–5). Renal abnormalities account for 70–80% of secondary hypertension in children, the pathogenesis of which may be related to either an increase in extracellular fluid volume (e.g., acute glomerulonephritis or chronic renal failure) or an increase in renin-angiotensin II activity (e.g., renal artery stenosis, renin-producing tumor, or reflux nephropathy) or a combination of both mechanisms (e.g., a patient with chronic renal failure caused by reflux nephropathy).

TABLE 69–3.   Blood Pressure Levels for the 90th and 95th Percentiles of Blood Pressure for Girls Aged 1–17 Years by Percentiles of Height

Age (y)	Blood Pressure Percentile*	Systolic Pressure by Percentile of Height (mm Hg)†							Diastolic Blood Pressure by Percentile of Height (mm Hg)†						
		5%	10%	25%	50%	75%	90%	95%	5%	10%	25%	50%	75%	90%	95%
1	90th	97	98	99	100	102	103	104	53	53	53	54	55	56	56
	95th	101	102	103	104	105	107	107	57	57	57	58	59	60	60
2	90th	99	99	100	102	103	104	105	57	57	58	58	59	60	61
	95th	102	103	104	105	107	108	109	61	61	62	62	63	64	65
3	90th	100	100	102	103	104	105	106	61	61	61	62	63	63	64
	95th	104	104	105	107	108	109	110	65	65	65	66	67	67	68
4	90th	101	102	103	104	106	107	108	63	63	64	65	65	66	67
	95th	105	106	107	108	109	111	111	67	67	68	69	69	70	71
5	90th	103	103	104	106	107	108	109	65	66	66	67	68	68	69
	95th	107	107	108	110	111	112	113	69	70	70	71	72	72	73
6	90th	104	105	106	107	109	110	111	67	67	68	69	69	70	71
	95th	108	109	110	111	112	114	114	71	71	72	73	73	74	75
7	90th	106	107	108	109	110	112	112	69	69	69	70	71	72	72
	95th	110	110	112	113	114	115	116	73	73	73	74	75	76	76
8	90th	108	109	110	111	112	113	114	70	70	71	71	72	73	74
	95th	112	112	113	115	116	117	118	74	74	75	75	76	77	78
9	90th	110	110	112	113	114	115	116	71	72	72	73	74	74	75
	95th	114	114	115	117	118	119	120	75	76	76	77	78	78	79
10	90th	112	112	114	115	116	117	118	73	73	73	74	75	76	76
	95th	116	116	117	119	120	121	122	77	77	77	78	79	80	80
11	90th	114	114	116	117	118	119	120	74	74	75	75	76	77	77
	95th	118	118	119	121	122	123	124	78	78	79	79	80	81	81
12	90th	116	116	118	119	120	121	122	75	75	76	76	77	78	78
	95th	120	120	121	123	124	125	126	79	79	80	80	81	82	82
13	90th	118	118	119	121	122	123	124	76	76	77	78	78	79	80
	95th	121	122	123	125	126	127	128	80	80	81	82	82	83	84
14	90th	119	120	121	122	124	125	126	77	77	78	79	79	80	81
	95th	123	124	125	126	128	129	130	81	81	82	83	83	84	85
15	90th	121	121	122	124	125	126	127	78	78	79	79	80	81	82
	95th	124	125	126	128	129	130	131	82	82	83	83	84	85	86
16	90th	122	122	123	125	126	127	128	79	79	79	80	81	82	82
	95th	125	126	127	128	130	131	132	83	83	83	84	85	86	86
17	90th	122	123	124	125	126	128	128	79	79	79	80	81	82	82
	95th	126	126	127	129	130	131	132	83	83	83	84	85	86	86

*Blood pressure percentile was determined by a single reading.

†Height percentile was determined by standard growth curves.

Reproduced, with permission, from the Update on the 1987 Task Force Report on High Blood Pressure in Children and Adolescents: A Working Group Report from the National High Blood Pressure Education Program. Pediatrics 98:649–658, 1996.

DIFFERENTIAL DIAGNOSIS

In any child in whom hypertension is confirmed, all reasonable effort should be made to identify the cause of hypertension (see Tables 69–4 and 69–5). Even though in children with mild increases in blood pressure, essential hypertension is common, essential hypertension must remain a diagnosis of exclusion. The cause of hypertension is often obvious from a detailed history, complete examination, and simple laboratory tests. However, extensive evaluation is sometimes necessary to determine the etiology of hypertension, especially in cases of renovascular hypertension.

EVALUATION

When a child is identified as having an elevated BP on any occasion, the finding should be verified with at least two additional measurements. The physician should also verify that an appropriately sized cuff is being used

to take the measurements and that efforts have been made to put the child at ease. Many children develop mild increases of BP (which can extend into the hypertensive range) when they visit a doctor's office because of anxiety or apprehension ("white coat hypertension"). Sometimes 24-hour ambulatory BP readings are necessary to confirm whether hypertension is present or not. An isolated finding of a mild increase in BP with normal subsequent readings does not indicate hypertension. Once hypertension is confirmed, a detailed history, complete physical examination, and appropriate laboratory evaluation should be performed.

History

Information should be obtained about the child's symptoms associated with hypertension, such as headaches and visual difficulties (Questions Box). Inquiry should also be made about the child's history of renal disease, especially previous urinary tract infections;

TABLE 69–4.   Causes of Acute or Intermittent Increases in Blood Pressure in Children

Renal Causes
Acute glomerulonephritis
Hemolytic-uremic syndrome
Henoch-Schönlein purpura nephritis
Renal trauma
Renal artery or vein thrombosis
After renal biopsy
Acute obstructive uropathy
Post genitourinary surgery
Blood transfusions in patients with renal failure
After kidney transplant or with transplant rejection
Drug-Induced Causes
Corticosteroids
Amphetamine overdose
Phencyclidine overdose
Cocaine overdose
Anabolic steroids
Oral contraceptives
Excessive erythropoietin use in patients with end-stage renal disease
Cyclosporine A and tacrolimus
Central Nervous System Causes
Increased intracranial pressure (e.g., subdural hematoma, meningitis, tumors)
Encephalitis
Poliomyelitis
Guillain-Barré syndrome
Porphyria
Familial dysautonomia
Miscellaneous Causes
Wrong blood pressure cuff size
Anxiety, apprehension (white coat hypertension)
Pain
Fractures
Orthopedic procedures (especially leg lengthening)
Burns
Leukemia
Stevens-Johnson syndrome
Bacterial endocarditis
Hypernatremia
Hypercalcemia
Heavy metal poisoning

TABLE 69–5.   Causes of Chronic Hypertension in Children

Renal
Scarred kidney: due to pyelonephritis and/or vesicoureteral reflux nephropathy
Chronic glomerulonephritis
Connective tissue disease: systemic lupus erythematosus, HS purpura
Hydronephrosis
Congenital dysplastic kidneys, multicystic kidney
Polycystic kidney disease
Solitary renal cyst
Tumors: Wilms', pericytoma (renin-producing tumor)
Renal Vascular Lesions
Renal artery stenosis (fibromuscular dysplasia)
Renal artery thrombosis (especially in the newborn following umbilical artery catheterization)
Renal vein thrombosis
Renal artery lesions with neurofibromatosis, tuberous sclerosis
Other Vascular Lesions
Coarctation of aorta: thoracic, abdominal
Polyarteritis nodosa and other vasculitides
Endocrine
Corticosteroid treatment
Neuroblastoma or other neural crest tumors
Pheochromocytoma
Congenital adrenal hyperplasia with 11β- or 17α-hydroxylase deficiency
IIβ-hydroxysteroid dehydrogenase deficiency
Liddle's syndrome
Primary hyperaldosteronism
Dexamethasone—suppressible hyperaldosteronism
Hyperthyroidism
Hyperparathyroidism
Cushing's syndrome
Central Nervous System
Intracranial hemorrhage
Intracranial mass
Essential (Primary) Hypertension

unexplained fevers during infancy and early childhood; edema; hematuria; enuresis, or nocturia; and the use of umbilical artery catheterization during the newborn period. Information regarding the child's physical growth; BP recordings during previous physical examinations; eating habits, especially salt intake; use of drugs, especially illicit drugs; and the family's history of hypertension and renal disease should be obtained.

Physical Examination

A thorough examination is essential for determining the etiology of hypertension and the extent of target organ damage caused by hypertension. Poor physical growth or short stature may indicate the presence of some disorder, such as Turner's syndrome or chronic renal disease with or without renal failure; it may also be the consequence of long-standing severe hypertension. Tachycardia may signify heart failure or thyrotoxicosis. The child's pulses should be felt in both the upper and lower extremities, and the BP should be measured in all four extremities to determine whether coarctation of the aorta or other vascular lesions exists. Fundus

examination is essential to determine if hypertension has been severe and chronic leading to arterial changes, exudate, hemorrhages and/or papilledema. Presence of café-au-lait spots or depigmented spots on the skin may signify hypertension secondary to neurofibromatosis or tuberous sclerosis, respectively.

Heart murmur may be present in hypertension due to coarctation of aorta, and heart failure may be present in patients with severe hypertension or in patients with renal disease and fluid retention. The abdomen should be carefully examined for presence of renal or other

---

Questions: Hypertension

- Does the child have any symptoms associated with hypertension, e.g., headache, dizziness, nosebleed, visual difficulty, or shortness of breath?
- Have BP readings been taken during previous routine physical examinations?
- Has the child had any hematuria, generalized swelling of the body (edema), enuresis (nocturia), burning urination, previous urinary tract infection, or other kidney problems?
- How much salt does the child take? Does he or she love to put extra salt on most foods and frequently like to eat salty foods?
- How has the child been growing?
- Is there a history of use of illicit drugs or contraceptives?
- Is there a family history of hypertension or renal disease?

masses caused by, for example, cystic kidneys, Wilms' tumor, or neuroblastoma, and for tenderness especially in the costovertebral angle (CVA). Bruits sometimes may be heard over the CVA in patients with renal artery stenosis.

Laboratory Evaluation

The extent of laboratory evaluation depends upon the clinical findings; the nature of the hypertension (e.g., mild or severe, acute or chronic); and whether an etiology is apparent or obscure. Table 69–6 outlines suggested laboratory workups for a patient with asymptomatic mild hypertension and for a patient with severe hypertension. Presence of hematuria, heavy proteinuria and leukocyturia, and/or elevated BUN or plasma creatinine would clearly signify a renal disorder as the cause of hypertension (unless it is superimposed upon some other disorder) and require appropriate renal evaluation, including renal Doppler ultrasonography, nuclear scans, or renal biopsy to identify scarred kidneys, hydronephrosis, cystic kidneys, renal or other tumors, or glomerulonephritis. The presence of electrolyte abnormalities such as hypokalemia, hypochloremia, or metabolic alkalosis would indicate the presence of an increased mineralocorticoid hormone either on a primary basis (primary hyperaldosteronism, adrenogenital syndrome with 11β- or 17α-hydroxylase deficiency, Liddle's syndrome, 11β-hydroxysteroid deficiency, etc.) or secondary to increased renin activity in renovascular hypertension, renin-producing tumor, or reflux nephropathy; these values would also indicate a need to measure plasma renin activity and urinary or plasma aldosterone levels. Endocrine-based causes of hypertension in children are uncommon, and tests like plasma or urinary catecholamines, plasma cortisol, and T_3 are measured on an individual basis depending on the clinical evaluation of the patient.

Although ECGs and chest x-rays are often requested to evaluate the effects of hypertension on the heart, they reveal normal results until the patient enters the late stages of severe hypertension. Echocardiography showing cardiac hypertrophy is much more sensitive for detecting target organ damage caused by hypertension.

In any child with severe hypertension in whom no etiology is apparent based upon clinical evaluation and the above-mentioned tests, the physician must consider renovascular disease and the necessary tests for it: renal Doppler ultrasonography, captopril-enhanced ^{131}I-MAG-3 renal scan, renal vein renin measurements, and selective renal arteriography (sometimes MRI-angiography may be used as a substitute).

MANAGEMENT

In all children with hypertension, an effort should be made to identify a remediable cause, so that an appropriate medical or surgical treatment can be offered that allows the child to avoid a lifelong regimen of drug treatment.

Patients with mild hypertension should be initially managed with nonpharmacologic measures, including supportive care, reduction in sodium intake to about 80–100 mEq/d, and weight reduction if the child is obese. Some physicians find teaching relaxation and biofeedback techniques helpful in reducing BP. If after a 3–6 month observation period, BP remains persistently elevated or if target organ damage is present, drug treatment should be initiated and a decision should be made whether or not the child needs a more thorough laboratory evaluation. Drug therapy may begin with a beta blocker (e.g., atenolol), an ACE inhibitor (e.g., enalapril) or a diuretic (e.g., hydrochlorothiazide).

Patients with severe hypertension may require combination therapy of the above drugs or additional drugs, such as calcium channel blockers, alpha blockers (e.g., prazocin), combined alpha-beta blockers (e.g., labetalol), peripheral vasodilators (e.g., hydralazine, minoxidil), or centrally acting drugs (e.g., clonidine). The use of one or more of these drugs can control BP in most patients within a satisfactory range and has a limited number of side effects.

Patients with renal artery stenosis can be successfully treated with balloon dilatation of the stenosis. If this procedure is unsuccessful or restenosis occurs, surgical correction of the stenosis is usually successful.

Depending upon their clinical condition, patients with malignant hypertension may be treated initially with oral labetalol or an ACE inhibitor. However, if the condition warrants, they may be started on intravenous labetalol, diazoxide, or sodium nitroprusside. The aim is not to lower BP urgently to a normal range, but to lower BP by about 20–25% of the presenting values. Over the following days to weeks, BP can gradually be controlled to come within normal values for age.

PROGNOSIS

The long-term outcome of hypertension in children depends upon the underlying etiology. In children with severe hypertension, BP control improves growth and overall well-being. The very long-term (30–50 years) prognosis of children with persistent, mild essential hypertension is largely unknown; however, one would anticipate that adequate BP control would prolong life and reduce cardiovascular, central nervous system, renal, and retinal morbidity.

TABLE 69–6. Laboratory Evaluation of Hypertension

A. Mild hypertension
  1. Urinalysis (urine culture if indicated)
  2. CBC, serum electrolytes, BUN, and creatinine
  3. Plasma renin activity along with 24-hour urinary sodium excretion may sometimes be indicated
  4. Sometimes echocardiography, ECG, chest x-ray
B. Severe hypertension (in addition to tests for mild hypertension listed above)
  1. Chem-20 panel
  2. 24-hour urine for creatinine, catecholamines, and aldosterone
  3. Renal Doppler ultrasonography
  4. Captopril-enhanced ^{131}I-MAG-3 renal scan
  5. Renal arteriography (selective if necessary)

Case Resolution

In the case presented above, the child clearly has signs of malignant hypertension. The history of previous urinary tract infection and the laboratory findings of proteinuria and elevated plasma creatinine suggest chronic pyelonephritis or reflux nephropathy with hypertension and chronic renal failure. The elevated creatinine also suggests that both kidneys are affected either by the primary process or as a consequence of severe hypertension. After controlling the initial severe increase in BP, a renal Doppler ultrasound is the appropriate test to determine the kidney size, the extent of kidney damage, and possibly the etiology.

Selected Readings

Adelman, R. D. The hypertensive neonate. Clin. Perinatol. 15:567–584, 1988.

Groshong, T. Hypertensive crisis in children. Pediatr. Ann. 25:368–376, 1996.

Lieberman, E. Hypertension in childhood and adolescence. *In* Kaplan, N. M. (ed.). Clinical Hypertension. 7th ed. Baltimore, Williams & Wilkins Company, 1998, pp. 407–420.

Report of the Second Task Force on Blood Pressure Control in Children—1987. Pediatrics 79:1–25, l987.

Sinaiko, A. R. Hypertension in children. N. Engl. J. Med. 335:1968–1973, 1996.

Update on the 1987 Task Force Report on High Blood Pressure in Children and Adolescents: A Working Group Report from the National High Blood Pressure Education Program. Pediatrics 98:649–658, 1996.

GENITOURINARY DISORDERS

CHAPTER 70

AMBIGUOUS GENITALIA

Monica Sifuentes, M.D.

H$_x$ A term infant is being evaluated in the newborn nursery. The mother received prenatal care from the 8th week of gestation, reportedly had no problems during the pregnancy, and took no medications except prenatal vitamins with iron. She specifically denies taking any progesterone-containing drugs. Her previous pregnancy was uneventful, and her 3-year-old son is healthy.

On physical examination, the infant is active and alert, with normal vital signs. Aside from a minimum amount of breast tissue bilaterally, the physical examination is unremarkable, except for the genitalia. The labia are swollen bilaterally and slightly hyperpigmented with what appear to be rugae. No masses are palpable in the labioscrotal folds. The clitoris is 1 cm in length. The introitus is difficult to visualize, but a vaginal opening and urethra are apparent.

Questions

1. What conditions should be considered in newborns with ambiguous genitalia?
2. What should families of such infants be told regarding the gender of the newborns?
3. What key historical information should be obtained from families of such newborns?
4. What laboratory studies must be obtained to aid in the diagnosis?
5. What psychosocial issues should be addressed with families while infants are in the newborn nursery?

Ambiguous genitalia result from an intersex abnormality in newborns and are classified according to the gonads present. This classification includes: female and male pseudohermaphroditism, true hermaphroditism, and mixed gonadal dysgenesis. Individuals with pure gonadal dysgenesis, another intersex disorder, present with primary amenorrhea during adolescence (see Chapter 77, Menstrual Disorders).

Several health care practitioners are often involved in the care of infants with ambiguous genitalia. In addition to the general pediatrician, nurses, social workers, neonatologists, pediatric endocrinologists, geneticists, and surgeons are all significant members of the health care team. The role of primary care physicians, however, cannot be underestimated since they are always involved in the initial evaluations of the newborns and often have already developed relationships with the families.

EPIDEMIOLOGY

The prevalence of ambiguous genitalia in newborns is approximately 1:3,000–4,000 live births. Female pseudohermaphroditism is characterized by female chromosomes (46,XX), normal ovaries and müllerian structures, and virilized external genitalia. The commonest intersex disorder, female pseudohermaphroditism is most often caused by congenital adrenal hyperplasia (CAH). Neonatal screening studies suggest that the incidence of CAH is 1:5000–1:15,000.

Male pseudohermaphroditism occurs in genetic males (46,XY) who have testes but abnormal masculinization of the external genitalia. This disorder most commonly results from androgen insensitivity.

True hermaphroditism is a rare condition in which both ovarian and testicular tissues are present. Seventy to 80% of affected individuals have the 46,XX karyotype, and the morphology of the external genitalia varies widely.

Mixed gonadal dysgenesis is characterized by one testis and an abnormal streak gonad. Reports indicate that this condition is the second most common form of ambiguous genitalia. Affected newborns often have chromosomal mosaicism (45,X/46,XY).

CLINICAL PRESENTATION

Variability in the phenotypic as well as clinical presentation of these disorders is considerable (D$_x$ Box). The newborn with ambiguous genitalia may have an enlarged phallus and varying degrees of labioscrotal fusion. Signs of virilization in the female infant might include hyperpigmented labia and the presence of labial rugae. Other findings suggestive of an intersex disorder

<table>
<tr><td>

D_x Ambiguous Genitalia

</td></tr>
</table>

D_x Ambiguous Genitalia

- Indeterminate or ambiguous genitalia
- Enlarged phallus
- Hyperpigmented, rugated labia majora that may be fused
- Blind-ending or completely absent vaginal pouch
- Phenotypic male neonate with hypospadias and cryptorchidism
- Phenotypic female neonate with an inguinal hernia or mass

in a female are perineal hypospadias or an inguinal hernia. More dramatic presentations, such as severe dehydration and shock in a neonate, are associated with CAH of the salt-losing form.

PATHOPHYSIOLOGY

In order to appropriately evaluate and interpret laboratory results of neonates with ambiguous genitalia, it is important to understand the physiology of sexual differentiation and how deviations from this process lead to intersex disorders.

Normal Sexual Differentiation

Normally, before embryos are 6 weeks old, undifferentiated bilateral gonads into which germ cells migrate from the yolk sac have developed. Both wolffian and müllerian duct systems are present at this time, making the embryonic gonads of males and females indistinguishable. The tendency of this bipotential fetus, however, is to develop as a female.

If a Y chromosome is present, a testes-determining factor (known as the sex determining region of the Y chromosome) induces differentiation of these gonads into testes, thus blocking female development. This process involves the formation of seminiferous tubules that surround the germ cells. Leydig cells begin to produce testosterone, which in turn acts on the wolffian duct to result in the male internal genitalia: vas deferens, epididymis, and seminal vesicles. Concurrently, regression of the müllerian ducts occurs secondary to testicular production of anti-müllerian hormone (AMH), also called müllerian inhibiting substance (MIS). For normal male external genitalia to form, testosterone must be converted to dihydrotestosterone (DHT) via 5-α-reductase. DHT then combines with a specific androgen receptor, which allows formation of the phallus and scrotum from the previously undifferentiated external genitalia. The process primarily involves growth and fusion. Later in gestation, the testes migrate into the scrotum.

For the undifferentiated gonads to develop into female organs, the Y chromosome must be absent and two intact and normal functioning X chromosomes must be present. Because androgens are not produced and there is no AMH, the wolffian duct degenerates, and the müllerian duct develops into these internal female structures: fallopian tubes, uterus, and upper vagina. Fusion of undifferentiated external genitalia does not occur in the absence of DHT, so folds and swellings become the labia, and the genital tubercle becomes the clitoris.

Development of Ambiguous Genitalia

The adrenogenital syndrome, or CAH, is the most common cause of female pseudohermaphroditism and is a recessively inherited defect. CAH is the result of an enzymatic deficiency in the synthesis of cortisol as well as aldosterone from cholesterol. The most common of these enzymatic defects is 21-hydroxylase deficiency. Other less common defects are 11 α-hydroxylase deficiency and 3 β-hydroxysteroid dehydrogenase deficiency. Prenatally, circulating levels of androgens are abnormally high from the overproduction of intermediate steroids. Hence, the external genitalia of the fetus, which are controlled by androgens, are virilized in the female. Internal female organs, however, are normal, because their development is not influenced by androgens.

The salt-wasting form of 21-hydroxylase deficiency is found in approximately two thirds of patients with classic CAH. As a result of low levels of aldosterone, sodium resorption in the renal tubules is reduced, leading to hyponatremia and hyperkalemia. If this salt-wasting condition goes undiagnosed and untreated, shock and death may result in the first few weeks of life.

Male pseudohermaphroditism is secondary to insufficient testosterone production or insensitivity at the cellular level. Androgen insensitivity, the most common cause of this disorder, is the result of either an abnormality or a reduction in the number of androgen receptors. Not all affected individuals present with ambiguous genitalia at birth because the spectrum of sensitivity is broad. If the androgen receptor is completely nonfunctional or absent, the external genitalia are those of a normal female (complete testicular feminization). This is a recessive condition. In the incomplete forms, which are X-linked recessive, genital ambiguity does occur.

Other causes of male pseudohermaphroditism are (1) inadequate testosterone production secondary to low levels of fetal gonadotropins; (2) defects in testosterone synthesis from enzyme deficiencies; (3) failure to convert testosterone to DHT as a result of 5-α-reductase deficiency; (4) deficient müllerian-duct inhibiting substance, which can be autosomal recessive or X-linked recessive; and (5) intrauterine loss of both testes secondary to torsion or another prenatal event.

Although most causes of ambiguous genitalia are related to chromosomal abnormalities and inherited enzymatic defects, exogenous sources of hormones can affect the differentiation of sexual organs. In most cases, the effect is minimal, and no ambiguity develops. Masculinized female external genitalia can occur, however, depending on the timing and duration of prenatal exposure to androgens or other virilizing drugs. Currently, the most commonly used androgens are probably anabolic steroids. An adrenal tumor or poorly controlled CAH in the mother will also lead to virilization of the female fetus. Birth control pills do not contain sufficient androgens to cause a problem.

DIFFERENTIAL DIAGNOSIS

The differential diagnosis of ambiguous genitalia depends on the classification of the intersex disorder (Table 70–1). Some causes of this condition can be life-threatening and therefore must be recognized immediately (e.g., salt-losing CAH).

EVALUATION

History

The general obstetric history should be reviewed, although it may not be helpful in all cases. Probably the most important source of information on family history can be derived from family pedigrees (Questions Box). Undiagnosed chromosomal disorders, consanguinity, and recurrent medical conditions may be established or inferred from the family background.

Physical Examination

A complete physical examination of newborns must be performed in the nursery, in addition to a detailed assessment of the genitalia. In particular, the presence of dysmorphic features (e.g., microcephaly, low set ears, micrognathia), which suggests the presence of a chromosomal abnormality, should be appreciated. The areola should be examined for any evidence of hyperpigmentation, and the inguinal area should be palpated for any masses or hernias.

A thorough genital examination should then be performed. The appearance and size of the labioscrotal folds should be noted in terms of pigmentation, presence of rugae, and size. Physicians should keep in mind that normal female labia majora may not completely cover the labia minora. Practitioners should determine whether any masses are palpable in what appear to be the labia and whether the testes are palpable in what appears to be the scrotum. The size of the phallus/

Questions: Ambiguous Genitalia

- Did the mother take any medications containing estrogen, progestins, or androgens during the pregnancy? Did she use any other virilizing drugs, such as danazol, during pregnancy?
- Does the mother have poorly controlled CAH or an adrenal tumor?
- What is the mother's prior obstetric history?
- Did she have any problems with any previous pregnancies?
- Is there a history of any unexplained neonatal deaths, particularly in male offspring?
- Are her other children growing and developing normally?
- Is there a family history of ambiguous genitalia, including microphallus, hypospadias, and cryptorchidism?
- Is there a family history of sterility, female hirsutism, or amenorrhea?
- Are the parents or other family members consanguinous?

---

clitoris should be measured; a normal stretched phallus is at least 2.5 cm long, whereas a normal clitoris should not exceed 1 cm in term infants. The labioscrotal folds should then be spread apart to look for a vaginal introitus. The presence of inferior labioscrotal fusion, which may preclude this, confirms the suspicion of indeterminate genitalia. Finally, the location of a urethral meatus should be noted, because if hypospadias and cryptorchidism occur together, the chance of an intersex disorder is approximately 50%. A rectal examination may help detect the presence of a uterus or prostate but may be difficult.

Laboratory Tests

The most important study to obtain is a karyotype, which can be performed in 24–48 hours by many laboratories. Examination of Barr bodies in a buccal smear is not recommended because this test is unreliable. In addition, serum electrolytes should be ordered in the nursery and monitored closely if CAH is suspected.

Certain biochemical studies such as a serum 17-hydroxyprogesterone and a measurement of 17-ketosteroids and pregnanetriol in the urine are mandatory in newborns with ambiguous genitalia, especially in newborns whose gonads are not palpable. If these initial studies are normal, other intermediate metabolites, such as 11-deoxycortisol and dehydroepiandrosterone sulfate (DHEA-S), and sex steroids (e.g., testosterone and dihydrotestosterone) can also be measured at a later date.

A human chorionic gonadotropin stimulation test may be performed when male pseudohermaphroditism is suspected to measure testosterone or if testes are not palpable.

Imaging Studies

Pelvic ultrasonography is effective in determining if müllerian structures are present, but this technique is not as useful for locating the gonads. If the gonads are not palpable, computed tomography or magnetic resonance imaging of the pelvis may be considered. Genitography can aid in visualizing the duct structures under fluoroscopy.

TABLE 70–1. Classification and Causes of Ambiguous Genitalia in the Newborn

Classification of Intersex Disorder	Causes
Female pseudohermaphroditism	Congenital adrenal hyperplasia
	Maternal androgen ingestion
	Maternal virilizing hormones
	Idiopathic, associated with dysmorphic syndromes
Male pseudohermaphroditism	Biochemical defects in testosterone biosynthesis (enzyme deficiencies)
	Androgen insensitivity (receptor defects)
	5α-reductase deficiency
	Persistent müllerian duct syndrome
	Gonadotropic failure
	Dysgenetic testes
	Bilateral vanishing testes syndrome
True hermaphroditism	Chimerism
Mixed gonadal dysgenesis	Chromosomal mosaicism

MANAGEMENT

An interdisciplinary team consisting of a pediatrician, pediatric endocrinologist, medical geneticist, urologist, and psychologist or psychiatrist should be involved in the care of infants with ambiguous genitalia. All aspects of treatment can then be addressed in an efficient and comprehensive manner.

Initial Phase: Delivery Room and Newborn Nursery

If the sex of the newborn is uncertain, it should not be assigned in the delivery room. Parents and nursing staff should be notified immediately of the ambiguity, and a unisex name should be assigned such as "Baby Smith" instead of "Baby Boy Smith" or "Baby Girl Smith." Physicians should then reassure parents that they will soon discuss the issue with them and tell them that until confirmatory tests are done, it is best not to speculate on the sex of the infant.

During the initial hours after birth, parents may have difficulty comprehending the condition. An open line of communication must be maintained with the family, however. Parents should be assured that gender assignment will be made as soon as possible—definitely within 3–5 days. Gender can be assigned even earlier in some institutions because most preliminary laboratory results are reported in 24–48 hours. Necessary radiographic studies should be ordered as soon as possible.

Intermediate Phase: Psychological Issues

Several psychological issues should be addressed at the time of diagnosis. Alleviation of parental anxiety regarding the cause of the condition should be the priority; general questions can also be answered. For example, parents may be unclear about what to tell others about the sex of the infant and find this process very awkward. In addition, parents should be educated about the normal sexual differentiation. Pediatricians must emphasize that during the first 6–8 weeks of gestation, sexual organs are undifferentiated. Ambiguous genitalia should be explained as overdevelopment or underdevelopment rather than as freaky or highly unusual.

Primary care physicians must also assess parents' level of sophistication and their cultural and religious beliefs about gender identity and sexuality. The gender preference for newborn infants should be addressed. Were the parents hoping for a boy or girl? Do they feel strongly about one gender? The medical team can also help families establish a plan for newborns regarding what they want to tell the extended family and in what detail they want to disclose the information. After the initial meeting and while awaiting laboratory data, other questions regarding sexual orientation, puberty, fertility, and self-esteem may arise.

Final Phase: Gender Assignment

After the karyotype is confirmed and the type of intersex disorder has been considered, team members should meet with families to discuss gender assignment before discharge from the hospital. Possible male sex assignment based on factors such as size of the phallus, presence of corporal tissue, and the response to androgen stimulation must be considered. Otherwise, female sex assignment should probably be made regardless of the cause of the intersex disorder. Parents must be involved in this decision and must agree with the final outcome. Some investigators strongly believe that gender reassignment and genital surgery should be discussed with the patient at a later date rather than assigned during the neonatal period. Such an approach involves consistent counseling for the patient, open discussion among the family, and a primary care physician willing to work diligently with both the patient and the family. Support groups should also be offered regardless of the decision regarding sex reassignment.

Detailed information should be given once again regarding the origin of the condition. The timing and nature of any future hormonal treatment and surgical procedures should be addressed as well. Parents should be urged to move beyond the issue of ambiguous genitalia once a decision regarding gender has been made. They must then deal with activities such as birth announcements and inquiries regarding gender from extended family, siblings, and baby-sitters. The entire medical team should offer parents encouragement concerning their parenting ability.

TREATMENT

Hormonal supplementation is indicated for some newborns with ambiguous genitalia. Cortisol replacement is mandatory in infants with CAH at daily physiologic doses of 10–20 mg/m^2/day. In infants with salt-wasting or classic 21-hydroxylase deficiency, mineralocorticoid replacement is indicated. Oral fludrocortisone should be administered at doses that suppress plasma renin activity to normal levels without causing hypertension.

Testosterone or estrogen replacement is needed at puberty in certain intersex disorders. Injections of testosterone cypionate at regular intervals may be used in certain cases to increase the length and width of the phallus. Recombinant human growth hormone replacement may also be considered for short stature in mixed gonadal dysgenesis.

Surgical procedures may be necessary in some cases. Although laparoscopy or laparotomy may be indicated for a gonadal biopsy, this is generally not needed in the neonatal period for gender assignment. A gonadectomy is indicated prophylactically in all phenotypic females with all or part of a Y chromosome because of the potential for malignancy. Clitoral recession, vaginoplasty, and labioscrotal reduction are usually performed if infants are to be raised as females. For children to be raised as males, orchiopexy, hypospadias repair, and chordee release are often indicated, but these surgical procedures may be difficult. In some specific cases, however, surgical procedures should be delayed until response to medical treatment is evaluated. For example, in CAH, clitoral size may decrease with glucocorticoid replacement.

PROGNOSIS

The prognosis for most infants with ambiguous genitalia is excellent. Problems arise with undiagnosed CAH, which may lead to shock and death in the neonatal period if unrecognized and untreated. Otherwise, children should be able to live long healthy lives once their families have come to grips with the diagnosis. Amenorrhea and sterility will need to be addressed with phenotypic females during adolescence, at which time psychological services should be provided.

Case Resolution

In the case described at the beginning of the chapter, the infant has ambiguous genitalia. The parents should be informed immediately of this finding, and all references related to gender should be avoided. A karyotype, in addition to serum electrolyte and 17-OH progesterone analyses, should be performed immediately. The physician should then meet with the family to further discuss intersex disorders and explain the diagnostic workup. General psychological services and information regarding support groups should also be provided.

Selected Readings

Anhalt, H., E. K. Neely, and R. L. Hintz. Ambiguous genitalia. Pediatr. Rev. 17:213–220, 1996.

Diamond, M., and K. Sigmundson. Management of intersexuality. Guidelines for dealing with persons with ambiguous genitalia. Arch. Pediatr. Adolesc. Med. 151:1046–1050, 1997.

Hadjiathanasiou, C. G., et al. True hermaphroditism: genetic variants and clinical management. J. Pediatr. 125:738–744, 1994.

Lee, M. M., et al. Measurements of serum müllerian inhibiting substance in the evaluation of children with nonpalpable gonads. N. Engl. J. Med. 336:1480–1486, 1997.

McCauley, E. Disorders of sexual differentiation and development. Pediatr. Clin. North Am. 37:1405–1420, 1990.

McGillivay, B. C. Genetic aspects of ambiguous genitalia. Pediatr. Clin. North Am. 39:307–317, 1992.

Rubenstein, S. C., and J. Mandell. Ambiguous genitalia in newborns. Contemp. Pediatr. 10:83–94, 1993.

White, P. C., M. I. New, and B. Dupont. Congenital adrenal hyperplasia. N. Engl. J. Med. 316:1519–1524, 1987.

Wright, N. B., et al. Imaging children with ambiguous genitalia and intersex states. Clin. Radiol. 50:823–829, 1995.

CHAPTER 71

INGUINAL LUMPS AND BUMPS

Julie E. Noble, M.D.

H$_x$ A 2-month-old male infant presents to your office for evaluation of a lump in his right groin for a 1-week duration. The lump has been coming and going, and his mother notices that it is larger when he cries. Today, the lump is prominent, and the infant seems fussy. He has been crying more often and vomited once today. His past history is remarkable for having been born at 32 weeks' gestation by spontaneous vaginal delivery. Birth weight was 1500 g, and he did well in the nursery with no respiratory complications. He was sent home at 4 weeks of age and has had no other medical problems. He breast-feeds well and has normal stools.

Physical examination reveals a well-nourished, irritable infant in no acute distress. His vital signs demonstrate mild tachycardia and temperature to 100° F (37.8° C). His abdomen is soft, and the genitourinary examination is significant for a swelling in the right inguinal area that extends into his scrotum. The mass is mildly tender and cannot be reduced. The rest of the examination is normal.

Questions

1. What are the possible causes of inguinal masses?
2. How does age affect the diagnostic possibilities?
3. How do you differentiate between acute and nonacute conditions?
4. What diagnostic modalities can help with the diagnosis?
5. What are the treatment choices for inguinal masses?
6. Are there long-term consequences?

Inguinal masses occur either from disease in normal tissue in the inguinal area or from ectopic tissue, frequently of embryologic origin. A child may present with the chief complaint of an inguinal mass, and the mass may vary in position from anywhere along the inguinal canal to the scrotum or labia (Fig. 71–1). Along the inguinal canal, a mass might be an enlarged lymph node, a

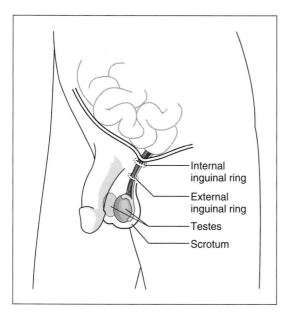

FIGURE 71–1. The inguinal area.

Internal inguinal ring
External inguinal ring
Testes
Scrotum

retractile testis, an ovary, or a synovial cyst. At the inguinal ring, a mass might also be a testis or an ovary, or an inguinal hernia. In the scrotum, swelling could be due to a hernia, hydrocele, varicocele, trauma, or testicular pathology. Labial lesions could be secondary to trauma, an ectopic ovary, mixed gonadal tissue, an actual testis as in testicular feminization, or a Bartholin's gland cyst. The differential diagnosis and the subsequent evaluation will vary not only according to the location of the mass and the patient's age but also with the acuity of presentation of the mass.

EPIDEMIOLOGY

Inguinal masses are a fairly frequent complaint in the office setting. The usual cause is an enlarged lymph node, but hernias and hydroceles are also common. Surgical repair of hernias and hydroceles are the most common surgical procedures performed in children. The incidence of inguinal hernias has been estimated at 10–20 per 1000 live births. Hernias are present on the right side in 60% of cases, on the left in 30%, and are bilateral in 10% of patients. Of affected children, males outnumber females 4:1. Certain conditions are associated with a higher incidence of hernias (Table 71–1). The most significant predisposing factor is prematurity, with

hernias reported in 30% of infants weighing less than 1000 g at birth. Incarcerated hernias are seen in 10–20% of patients presenting for hernia surgery. More than 50% of these incarcerated hernias occur in the first 6 months of life.

The other common acute scrotal lesions—testicular torsion and torsion of the appendix testis—have an incidence of 1:160 males. The peak incidence of testicular torsion occurs in the perinatal period and again at puberty. Torsion of the appendix testis is most likely to occur between ages 7 and 10. Varicoceles occur in pubertal and postpubertal males, with a fairly high incidence of 2–11%. Testicular tumors are rare in childhood. They occur at an incidence of 0.5–2.0 per 100,000 children and account for only 1% of all pediatric solid tumors.

CLINICAL PRESENTATION

The child with an inguinal mass presents either acutely or nonacutely. In the acute presentation, the swelling occurs rapidly and is associated with pain. There may be systemic symptoms of nausea and vomiting. The involved area may be extremely tender. Nonacute masses appear more slowly. Some may be present from birth. They may come and go, especially with crying or straining. Nonacute masses usually are not tender and not associated with systemic symptoms (D_x Box).

PATHOPHYSIOLOGY

Pathophysiologic developmental features of an inguinal mass vary depending on the cause of the mass.

An enlarged lymph node may result from proliferation of intrinsic lymphocytes or inflammatory infiltrate from infection (lymphadenitis). The etiology of lymphadenopathy is extensive (see Chapter 65, Lymphadenopathy). Any of these processes can appear in the inguinal nodes. An enlarged node can also be secondary to metastatic infiltration from another cell line and represent tumor spread.

A hydrocele develops secondary to failure of obliteration of the patent processus vaginalis during embryologic development. During the 27th to 28th weeks of gestation, the testicle, gubernaculum, and processus vaginalis descend from the peritoneum through the inguinal canal into the scrotum. The processus vaginalis begins closing prior to birth and attaches to the testis,

TABLE 71–1.   Conditions Associated with Hernias

Abdominal wall defect
Ascites
Connective tissue disease
Cystic fibrosis
Family history
Low birth weight
Mucopolysaccharidosis
Prematurity
Undescended testis
Urologic malformations

D_x Inguinal Masses	
ACUTE	**NONACUTE**
• Rapid onset	• Slower onset
• Painful	• Not painful
• Tender	• May fluctuate in size
• Nausea and vomiting	• Cremasteric reflex
• Fever	present
• Overlying skin red	
• Cremasteric reflex absent	

forming the tunica vaginalis testis. The closure is complete by 1–2 years of age. Failure of closure results in a hydrocele (a peritoneal connection with fluid) or a hernia, with intra-abdominal contents. Either may bulge into the inguinal canal and scrotum. If the hernia cannot be reduced and abdominal contents are at risk for vascular compromise, the hernia is termed incarcerated. This condition is a surgical emergency.

Sometimes a parent may misinterpret a normal testicle in the process of descent as an abnormal mass. A delay in the normal descent process occurs occasionally, and the testicle may not be in the scrotum at the time of birth. Torsion of the testis after it has reached the scrotum can occur in the newborn if the testis twists upon the spermatic cord. Similarly, the testicle can also twist in the pubertal period upon its own vasculature within the tunica vaginalis. This is frequently secondary to a high attachment of the tunica vaginalis to the spermatic cord, allowing the testis to hang freely, like a "bell clapper." Both types of torsion cause vasculature compromise and an ischemic testis.

Likewise, a vestigial remnant called the appendix testis can twist, resulting in vascular compromise of that localized part of the testis.

Pathologically, a traumatic scrotal mass is usually a hematoma, although testicular rupture may occur if the tunica albuginea is torn as a result of trauma.

Testicular neoplasms in prepubertal children tend to be germ cell tumors. Yolk sac carcinoma, teratomas, and mixed germ cell tumors with infiltration of their respective cell lines are the usual diseases found.

A varicocele, another scrotal mass, is caused by increased pressure within the venous drainage of the testicle with subsequent dilatation of the veins, producing a mass. Because of the anatomy of the veins, 90% of varicoceles occur on the left side. They are a common finding in adolescent males.

Infections of the epididymis or testis can cause an inflammatory infiltrate and swelling. In the female, infection of Bartholin's gland in the labia creates an abscess and leads to an acute, painful mass.

DIFFERENTIAL DIAGNOSIS

Location, acuity, and patient age aid in establishing the differential diagnosis.

Nonacute masses, which have a slow onset and are not painful, include lymphadenopathy, a retractile testis, hydrocele, hernia, varicocele, tumor, and ectopic ovary.

Acute masses that have a sudden onset and are associated with pain include epididymitis, orchitis, testicular torsion, traumatic hematoma, torsion of the appendix testes, lymphadenitis, and incarcerated hernia (Table 71–2).

Skin changes can mimic an acute scrotal mass. Henoch-Schönlein purpura, a vasculitis, can develop in the scrotal area, and idiopathic scrotal edema can also occur acutely.

Testicular torsion occurs most commonly in the newborn period and again at puberty. Incarcerated hernias occur most commonly in the first 6 months of life. Vari-

TABLE 71–2. Differential Diagnosis of Inguinal Masses

Nonacute	Acute
Ectopic ovary	Bartholin's abscess
Hernia	Epididymitis
Hydrocele	Henoch-Schölein purpura
Lymphadenopathy	Idiopathic scrotal swelling
Retractile testis	Incarcerated hernia
Synovial cyst	Lymphadenitis
Testicular tumor	Orchitis
Varicocele	Testicular torsion
Venous aneurysm	Torsion of appendix testis
	Trauma

coceles occur almost always at adolescence and beyond.

The sex of the patient will also influence the differential diagnosis of the lesion as well as the workup.

EVALUATION

History

A thorough, focused history will help narrow down the differential diagnosis (Questions Box). Inquiring about systemic symptoms should always be included and if positive may suggest a more generalized process such as a tumor or systemic infection. Symptoms of dysuria would point to epididymitis or orchitis. A history of trauma or possible sexual abuse should always be sought. Hernias and testicular torsion often have a family history positive for the same condition.

Physical Examination

A complete physical examination should always be performed in assessing any pediatric complaint. With an inguinal mass, a concentrated examination of the inguinal area and lower extremity should be made. If the mass is not apparent on inspection and it comes and goes, ask the parent to point to the location of the mass. Observe the skin for evidence of erythema, swelling, or bruising. Gently palpate the inguinal canal for a mass, then assess the scrotal or labial area. If the mass is acute, observe the scrotum and try to localize the tenderness. An incarcerated hernia, testicular torsion,

---

Questions: Inguinal Masses

- How long has the mass been present?
- Is it painful?
- Does it come and go?
- Was there a history of trauma?
- Does the child have dysuria?
- Is there fever or vomiting?
- Are there any other masses?
- Has the child had any lower extremity infections?
- Is there a history of renal disease?
- Is there a history of preterm delivery?
- Is there a positive family history?

torsion of the appendix testis, epididymitis, and orchitis are extremely tender. If there is torsion of the appendix testis, there may be a classic "blue dot" at the upper pole of the testis. Try to elicit a cremasteric reflex. If present, it virtually eliminates testicular torsion. The pain of epididymitis and orchitis is relieved partially when the testis is elevated (Prehn's sign). Transilluminating the mass may be helpful. A fluid-filled mass such as a hydrocele will definitely transilluminate. Bowel may also transilluminate.

Any mass should be accurately measured. Evaluating the borders of an inguinal mass is important. A hydrocele does not extend into the inguinal canal; therefore, the top border can be felt below the pubis. A hernia will extend into the inguinal canal, so an upper border will not be apparent. Reduction of any hernia with gentle pressure should be attempted. To detect a hernia that is not readily apparent, causing the infant to cry increases intra-abdominal pressure and may demonstrate the hernia. An older child can be asked to stand and cough while the inguinal canal is palpated. A varicocele, which feels like a "bag of worms," is a nontender mass over the spermatic cord and is readily palpated.

Laboratory Tests

The laboratory tests should be directed toward the most likely diagnosis as determined by the history and physical.

If an infection is suspected, a CBC should be obtained. If the infection is thought to be epididymitis or orchitis, a urinalysis and urine culture should also be obtained. If lymphadenopathy is suspected, a CBC, mononucleosis test, cat-scratch disease tests, and possible biopsy may be necessary. If an inguinal mass occurs in a female, chromosomal evaluation is indicated to diagnose testicular feminization syndrome. If a tumor is suspected, the α-fetoprotein (AFP) level, which is elevated in 90% of yolk sac tumors, should be assayed.

Imaging Studies

Ultrasound is the best test to define scrotal contents. It gives accurate information in evaluating tumors. Color Doppler ultrasonography is the test of choice to identify a testicular fracture and also assess blood flow in testicular torsion. If incarceration of a hernia is suspected, a flat plate x-ray of the abdomen is helpful to detect signs of intestinal obstruction.

MANAGEMENT

Many inguinal masses require surgical treatment. The acute scrotum is a surgical emergency. There may not be time to perform diagnostic studies. If there is a high probability of a testicular torsion, the scrotum should be surgically explored immediately. There is only a 6- to 8-hour window of time after presentation to save a viable testis. If the testis is nonviable, it is removed. Torsion of the appendix testis does not need to be explored if the diagnosis is certain.

All hernias require surgical repair at some time. Immediate surgery is indicated for an incarcerated hernia that cannot be reduced. If it is reduced, then elective surgical repair can be scheduled. There is controversy regarding the indications for surgery on the contralateral side. An infant less than 1 year of age has a 20% chance of developing a hernia on the other side, and most surgeons repair both sides at the same time. As a child gets older, the chance is smaller. Currently, some surgeons use laparoscopy at the time of the hernia repair to define a patent processus vaginalis on the opposite side and repair it if patency is found. Hydroceles do not have to be repaired surgically unless they persist beyond 1 year of age. This persistence implies a peritoneal connection and an impending hernia, so repair is indicated. A fracture of the testicle also dictates the need for surgical repair. Varicoceles are removed if the testicle shows growth retardation. All testicular tumors are removed. Additional antitumor therapy is dependent on the stage and cell line of the tumor.

Infectious inguinal masses are treated according to the specific bacteriologic diagnosis.

PROGNOSIS

After surgical treatment, the child generally does well. The most significant long-term complication is subsequent impaired testicular function. Following hernia repair, decreased testicular size is noted in up to 27% of cases. Damage to the vas deferens and testicular vessels may impair spermatogenesis and result in a higher incidence of impaired fertility. Surgery for testicular torsion may also cause infertility, particularly if an affected testis is left in place. Two-thirds of affected testicles demonstrate atrophy.

There may be recurrence of a hernia following repair. A hydrocele may develop following vancocele repair.

Case Resolution

In the case presented at the beginning of the chapter, the infant's history of prematurity associated with a mass that comes and goes most likely indicates a hernia. With the additional symptoms of pain, fever, and vomiting and the findings of an inflamed, nonreducible mass on examination, there is a high likelihood that the hernia is incarcerated. Surgical exploration and repair should be done immediately.

Selected Readings

Cilento, B. G., S. S. Najjar, and A. Atala. Cryptorchidism and testicular torsion, Pediatr. Clin. North Am. 40:1133–1149, 1993.

Ikaguchi, E. F., and T. W. Hensle. The pediatric varicocele. *In* King, L. R. (ed.). Urologic Surgery in Infants and Children. Philadelphia, W. B. Saunders, 1998, pp. 246–253.

Kapur, P., M. G. Caty, and P. L. Glick. Pediatric hernias and hydroceles. Pediatr. Clin. North Am. 45:773–789, 1998.

Kay, R., and J. H. Ross. Testis tumors. *In* King, L. R. (ed.). Urologic Surgery in Infants and Children. Philadelphia, W. B. Saunders, 1998, pp. 255–262.

Nakayama, D. K., and M. I. Rowe. Inguinal hernia and the acute scrotum in infants and children. Pediatr. Rev. 11:87–93, 1989.

Rabinowitz, R., and W. Hulbert. Acute scrotal swelling. Urol. Clin. North Am. 22:101–105, 1995.

Scherer, L. R., and J. L. Grosfeld. Inguinal hernia and umbilical anomalies. Pediatr. Clin. North Am. 40:1121–1131, 1993.

Skoog, S. J., and M. J. Conlin. Pediatric hernias and hydroceles. Urol. Clin. North Am. 22:119–130, 1995.

Yerkes, E. B., and J. W. Brock. Diagnosis and management of testicular torsion. In King, L. R. (ed.). Urologic Surgery in Infants and Children. Philadelphia, W. B. Saunders, 1998, pp. 239–245.

CHAPTER 72

HEMATURIA

Elaine S. Kamil, M.D.

Hx   A 5-year-old boy is brought to the office for a school entry examination. He was the full-term product of an uncomplicated pregnancy, labor, and delivery. Although the boy has had four or five episodes of otitis media, he has generally been in good health. He has never been hospitalized or experienced any significant trauma. He has no known allergies, has been fully immunized, and is developmentally normal.

In addition, the physical examination is completely normal. The boy's height and weight are at the 75th percentile, and his blood pressure is 100/64. Screening tests for hearing and vision are completely normal. The boy's hematocrit is 42. His urinalysis comes back with a specific gravity of 1.025, pH 6, 2+ blood, and trace protein. Microscopic examination shows 18–20 RBCs per high-power field, 0–1 WBC per high-power field, and a rare, fine, granular cast.

Questions

1. What disease entities cause hematuria?
2. How should hematuria be evaluated?
3. How does the approach to hematuria differ in children who complain of "dark" or red urine?
4. What is the appropriate follow-up of children with asymptomatic microscopic hematuria?

Hematuria is a common problem in pediatrics, and primary care physicians should have a clear understanding of its pathophysiology, etiology, evaluation, and therapy. Hematuria can be caused by a serious medical problem, or it may only be an incidental finding with no potential for impairment of patients' health.

In general, hematuria is categorized as either gross or microscopic (microhematuria). The etiology and approach to hematuria vary with its severity. Gross hematuria is defined as red or brown urine caused by the presence of RBCs. Microhematuria is defined as three or more consecutive urine samples with a positive dipstick and six or more RBCs per high-power field in a fresh, spun urine sample.

EPIDEMIOLOGY

The incidence of **gross hematuria** is about 1.3:1000 patient visits (Table 72–1). In about half of these patients, the causes are readily apparent from the intake history or physical examination. The incidence of this type of hematuria may increase in the community as a result of an epidemic of a disease, such as acute glomerulonephritis, that causes hematuria.

Microscopic hematuria is a more common pediatric problem. Prevalence rates for persistent, microscopic hematuria range from 0.5–2.0%, but 4–5% of school-age children have microhematuria on a single voided specimen. The incidence is artificially increased in late

TABLE 72–1. Etiology of Gross Hematuria in an Unselected Pediatric Population

Causes	Percent (%) of Patients
Readily Apparent Causes	
Documented urinary tract infection (UTI)	26
Perineal irritation	11
Meatal stenosis with ulcer	7
Trauma	7
Coagulopathy	3
Stones	2
Total	56
Other Causes	
Suspected UTI	23
Recurrent gross hematuria	5
Acute nephritis	4
Ureteropelvic junction obstruction	1
Cystitis cystica	<1
Epididymitis	<1
Tumor	<1
Unknown	9
Total	44

Modified, with permission, from Ingelfinger, J.R., et al. Frequency and etiology of gross hematuria in a general pediatric setting. Pediatrics 59:557–561, 1977.

summer, because at that time children tend to visit pediatricians for school physicals that typically include a screening urinalysis.

CLINICAL PRESENTATION

Children with gross hematuria present with a sudden appearance of red or brown urine, which may be associated with flank or urethral pain or with a history of trauma.

Children with microscopic hematuria may have urinary complaints (e.g., dysuria). In children who appear well, microhematuria is usually detected on screening dipstick examination.

PATHOPHYSIOLOGY

Gross Hematuria

Gross hematuria occurs because of the presence of large numbers of RBCs in the urine. Blood may enter the urine because of rupture of blood vessels following trauma or inflammation in the glomeruli or interstitial regions of the kidney. It may also occur as a result of severe inflammation of the bladder wall.

Causes of gross hematuria are listed in Table 72–2. The presence of casts in the urine suggests the diagnosis of glomerulonephritis. The most common causes of glomerulonephritis in children include acute poststreptococcal glomerulonephritis, anaphylactoid purpura, IgA nephropathy, membranoproliferative glomerulonephritis (MPGN), and SLE.

Common causes of gross hematuria in the absence of RBC casts include **UTI, renal trauma, bleeding diathesis** (e.g., hemophilia or idiopathic thrombocytopenic purpura), **renal tumors, obstruction of the urinary tract, renal stones**, or perhaps **hemolytic-uremic syndrome (HUS)**. A hemangioma in the urinary tract is an extremely rare cause of gross hematuria.

Microhematuria

Microhematuria occurs when small numbers of RBCs enter the urine via tiny ruptures in the glomerular capillary walls or in the capillaries of the tubular or bladder lining. For purposes of discussion, the following causes of microscopic hematuria are considered: infectious, structural, traumatic, glomerular, and interstitial. Separate consideration of the causes of microscopic and gross hematuria is often helpful, although significant overlap exists.

UTI is one of the most common **infectious causes** of hematuria. Bacterial infections of the bladder or kidney occur much more frequently than viral cystitis. Adenovirus is the most common viral cause of hemorrhagic cystitis and is usually associated with dysuria. Vaginitis in girls and prostatitis in teenage boys may also result in hematuria.

Any type of congenital obstructive uropathy may lead to massive dilatation of the urinary tract, which makes the urinary tract more susceptible to bleeding, even with trivial trauma. **Chronic urinary tract obstruction** in children (e.g., posterior urethral valves or congenital ureteropelvic junction obstruction) is often asymptomatic. In the past, these conditions were typically diagnosed when children presented with UTIs. Now they are commonly diagnosed after a prenatal ultrasound reveals hydronephrosis. Nevertheless, urinary tract obstruction may be detected during an evaluation for asymptomatic microhematuria.

Any **tumor** of the genitourinary tract may be associated with both gross and microscopic hematuria. Pelvic tumors rarely cause urinary obstruction in children, although such tumors frequently cause obstruction in adults. Children with Wilms' tumor, the most common childhood renal tumor, usually present with an abdominal mass, but it may cause hematuria.

Congenital renal malformations are quite common. Any of these may be associated with hematuria and include polycystic kidney disease, renal dysplasia, medullary sponge kidney, and simple cysts. Patients with polycystic kidney disease may even have severe, painful hematuria.

Vascular problems may also lead to hematuria. Hemangiomas of the kidney, bladder, or ureter are very rare. Arteriovenous malformations also occur infrequently. Hematuria may be a sign of a renal artery or vein thrombosis, particularly in sick neonates.

Young children are more susceptible to **renal injury,** which may result in hematuria, than older children or adults because their kidneys are relatively less protected by the rib cage. In addition, children may insert foreign objects into the urethra and bladder that cause pain and hematuria. Microhematuria has also been described after extremely vigorous exercise such as marathon running. Child abuse should be considered if any suspicions are raised on the basis of the history or physical examination.

Hypercalciuria is another cause of microscopic hematuria. Children with hypercalciuria often have a family history of urinary calculi. Calcium oxalate crystals may be present on the microscopic examination of the urine. A urinary calcium-creatinine ratio is best obtained on a first morning, fasting urine sample. Calcium excretion varies with age. Normal values are listed in Table 72–3.

There are two types of hypercalciuria: absorptive and "renal leak." Children with absorptive hypercalciuria overabsorb calcium from the GI tract, probably because

---

TABLE 72–2.   Common Causes of Gross Hematuria in Pediatric Patients

Glomerulonephritis	Structural Causes
IgA nephropathy	Renal trauma
Acute poststreptococcal GN*	Tumor
Lupus nephritis	Obstruction
Membranoproliferative GN*	Renal stones
Anaphylactoid purpura GN*	Vascular abnormality
Hematologic Causes	**Infectious Causes**
Sickle cell disease	Bacterial urinary tract infection
Hemophilia	Viral cystitis
Thrombocytopenia	
Thrombosis (renal arterial or venous)	

*GN, glomerulonephritis.

TABLE 72–3. Normal Values for Urinary Calcium-Creatinine Ratios*

Age	Urine Calcium-Creatinine	24-Hour Urine Calcium
Preterm	≤0.82	≤8.9 mg/kg/d†
< 7 months	≤ 0.86	
7–18 months	≤ 0.60	
19 months–6 years	≤ 0.42	
6 years–adult	≤ 0.22	<4 mg/kg/d

*Samples for calcium-creatinine ratio should be obtained on a fasting, first voided morning specimen. The calcium and creatinine concentrations must be in the same units (e.g., mg/dL) before the ratio is calculated.

†For healthy preterm infants taking no medications. Calcium excretion varies with diet and phosphorus intake, and it is higher if patients are treated with furosemide, xanthines, or glucocorticoids.

of an exquisite sensitivity to vitamin D, and can be treated with a reduced calcium diet. Children with renal leak hypercalciuria have an inherently higher rate of urinary calcium excretion and may require thiazide diuretics to reduce urinary calcium excretion.

Interstitial nephritis, usually from drug exposure, may also cause hematuria. Generally patients with interstitial nephritis may exhibit other signs of tubular disease such as glucosuria or proteinuria.

DIFFERENTIAL DIAGNOSIS

When children complain of gross hematuria or "red" urine, practitioners must first determine if they have hematuria or pigmenturia by using a urine dipstick. If the dipstick is negative for blood, then the dark urine is due to dyes, drugs, or pigments (Table 72–4). If the dipstick is positive for blood, the red color is caused by intact RBCs, hemolyzed RBCs, or myoglobin; the clarification is based on microscopic examination of a fresh, spun urine.

Children whose dipsticks are positive for blood but show no RBCs may have hemoglobinuria or myoglobinuria. Hemoglobinuria may be seen with acute autoimmune hemolytic anemia, drug-induced hemolysis, paroxysmal nocturnal hemoglobinuria, a mismatched blood transfusion, cardiopulmonary bypass, fresh-

TABLE 72–4. Distinguishing Hematuria From Pigmenturia*

	Urine		
Problem	Color	Hemastix	Microscopic Appearance
Hematuria	Red, brown, or red-brown	Positive	Red blood cells
Hemoglobinuria	Red, brown, or red-brown	Positive	Negative
Myoglobinuria	Red, brown, or red-brown	Positive	Negative
Porphyrins	Red	Negative	Negative
Exogenous pigments*	Red or orange	Negative	Negative

*Some common exogenous pigments include phenytoin, beets, rifampin, nitrofurantoin, sulfas, amitriptyline, methyldopa, phenothiazine, and chloroquine.

water drowning, and in some cases, HUS. Myoglobinuria is seen in individuals with rhabdomyolysis. Acute rhabdomyolysis can occur after a crush injury or a very prolonged seizure and in certain susceptible individuals with an inborn error of muscle metabolism. Both free hemoglobin and myoglobin are toxic to the renal epithelial cells, mandating a generous fluid intake and close monitoring.

EVALUATION

Gross Hematuria

History

The history is crucial to an accurate, efficient, and cost-effective evaluation of patients with hematuria (Questions Box). The family should be questioned carefully about trauma (to trunk or perineum), recent skin infection or pharyngitis, dysuria, and abdominal or flank pain. Parents should be asked whether their children appear "puffy." A family history of kidney disease, bleeding diathesis, hemolytic anemia, or inborn error of muscle metabolism may be important.

Physical Examination

A complete physical examination is also essential. Blood pressure should be measured accurately. The skin should be examined thoroughly for rashes or petechiae; the abdomen should be checked carefully for renal masses or tenderness; the genitalia should be examined thoroughly for signs of trauma, masses, or rashes (see Chapter 105, Child Sexual Abuse); and the joints should be checked carefully for signs of arthritis. Fundi should be examined for any hypertensive changes. Children should be assessed for the presence of edema.

A careful cardiac and chest examination is necessary to detect signs of congestive heart failure, a finding sometimes seen in acute glomerulonephritis.

Laboratory Tests

Recent studies have shown that careful microscopic examination of a urine sample can help determine whether bleeding originates from the upper urinary tract or the lower urinary tract. The first morning urine

---

Questions: Hematuria

- Has the child suffered any recent trauma?
- Has the child had fever or dysuria?
- Does the child have any flank or abdominal pain?
- Does the child have any rashes, joint pains, or edema?
- Does the child have a family history of hematuria, kidney disease, kidney stones, or gross hematuria?
- Is there a family history of bleeding disorders or inborn errors of muscle metabolism?

sample is the most reliable but is not appropriate in some settings, such as after an automobile accident. Sometimes the gross hematuria is so substantial that spinning the urine results in a large pellet of debris that is difficult to examine. In such instances, it is prudent to examine an unspun sample. The presence of RBC casts indicates glomerulonephritis, but the absence of such casts does not rule out this condition.

If the urine shows RBC casts, then the evaluation should include an antistreptolysin-O (ASO) titer, antinuclear antibody (ANA), C3, CBC and differential with platelet count, BUN and creatinine, serum albumin, and a random urine for a urinary total protein-creatinine ratio.

If the urine shows only large numbers of RBCs, no RBC casts, and no bacteriuria, a CBC with differential and platelet count, a urine culture, and a PT and PTT should be obtained. A sickle cell test should be considered as well.

Imaging Studies

If the urine has large numbers of RBCs and no bacteriuria, a renal ultrasound should be obtained. With gross hematuria and a history of serious trauma, an abdominal CT scan should be performed. Children with RBC casts should also have a chest x-ray to evaluate for signs of congestive heart failure.

Microhematuria

The evaluation of microscopic hematuria is similar to that of gross hematuria. Figure 72–1 outlines an approach to the evaluation of microscopic hematuria.

History and Physical Examination

Because many conditions may cause either gross or microscopic hematuria, the same historical questions apply to both conditions, and the same careful physical examination is indicated.

Laboratory Tests

Generally, the initial evaluation includes a urine culture and a careful microscopic examination of the urine. If the culture is negative, the hematuria is minimal, and children are otherwise healthy, the urinalysis should be repeated once or twice over the following 2 weeks.

RBC casts always signify a glomerular origin. Casts are best preserved in acidic, concentrated urine. Thus, the first morning urine is the best sample to examine for casts. RBC morphology should be assessed. RBCs originating in the glomerulus are **dysmorphic** and of smaller caliber, whereas those that come from lower downstream appear like normal **biconcave** disks. Although RBC morphology is best appreciated with the use of a polarizing microscope, with experience, dysmorphic RBCs can be recognized using an ordinary microscope. RBCs of glomerular origin have a mean cell volume of 50 μL or less. In contrast, RBCs of nonglomerular origin have a mean cell volume of 80–90 μL. The presence of a newly described, special form of dysmorphic erythrocyte, the G1 cell, is even more specific for glomerular bleeding. These cells are doughnut shaped and contain one or more blebs on their surfaces.

Clotting ability should be determined with a platelet count, PT, and PTT. A sickle cell test should be performed. Renal function should be screened with a BUN and creatinine, and a urine calcium-creatinine ratio

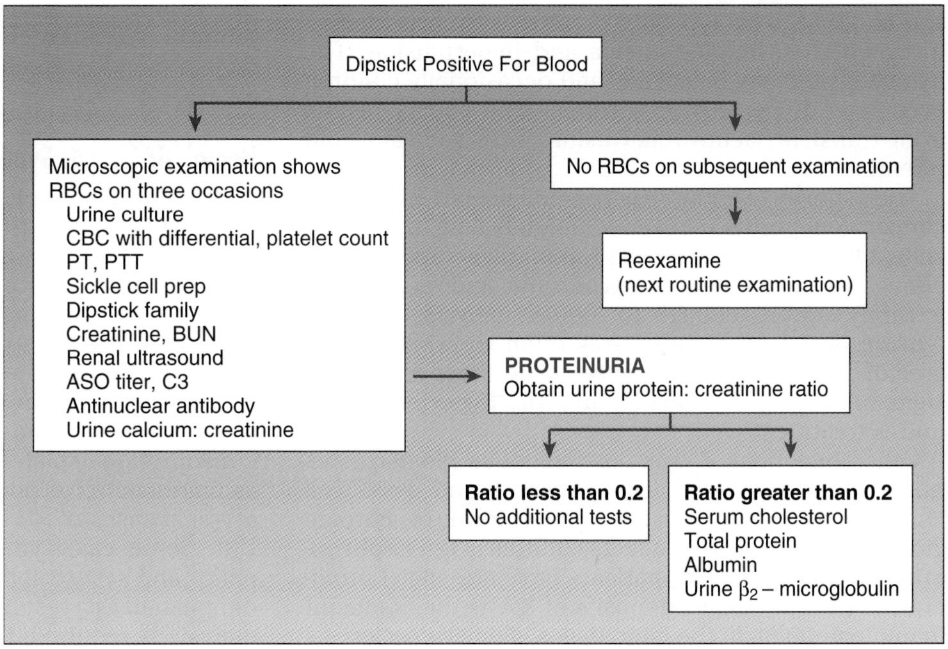

FIGURE 72–1. Evaluation of asymptomatic, microscopic hematuria. ASO, antistreptolysin-O; BUN, blood urea nitrogen; CBC, complete blood count; PT, prothrombin time; PTT, partial thromboplastin time; RBCs, red blood cells.

should be determined. A C3, ANA, and ASO titer should also be checked. If a urine dipstick shows more than a trace of protein, a urinary protein:creatinine ratio should also be determined. If there is a family history of renal disease, a hearing screen should be ordered. All immediate family members should have their urine checked for blood.

If a bloody urine sample is analyzed with a Coulter counter, characteristic distribution curves are seen for glomerular and nonglomerular hematuria. This test is not readily available, however.

Imaging Studies

A renal ultrasound should be performed to rule out structural abnormalities and tumors. Chest x-rays should be obtained if acute glomerulonephritis is suspected.

GLOMERULAR DISEASES ASSOCIATED WITH HEMATURIA

Glomerulonephritis

Both acute and chronic glomerulonephritis are associated with hematuria. The diagnosis of acute poststreptococcal glomerulonephritis requires a "nephritic" urine sediment (RBCs, RBC casts), a low serum complement, and an elevated streptococcal titer (ASO titer, anti-DNAase B, or positive streptozyme). It is important to document that the serum complement returns to normal, because MPGN may present in a similar way. The serum complement is chronically depressed in MPGN.

The most common form of glomerulonephritis in children is **acute poststreptococcal glomerulonephritis.** Many cases are asymptomatic, however, and do not come to the attention of physicians. The resulting hematuria, which may be gross or microscopic, is rarely seen before the age of 2 years. The condition is most commonly diagnosed in preschool-age and school-age children, who typically present with gross hematuria, often with some edema and hypertension. The hypertension may be severe, and occasionally children even have hypertensive seizures. The edema results from transient, acute renal failure with salt and fluid retention.

The majority of children with acute poststreptococcal glomerulonephritis recover completely and have an excellent long-term prognosis. Proteinuria is rarely severe enough to cause nephrotic syndrome, and renal failure is rarely serious enough to require dialysis. If hypertension occurs, the chest x-ray often shows some degree of pulmonary edema, even in the absence of overt signs of congestive heart failure. Any hypertension requires treatment.

Other infections cause postinfectious glomerulonephritis, but they are less common and less well characterized. The most common form of chronic glomerulonephritis that affects children is **IgA nephropathy.** On kidney biopsy, patients have mesangial proliferation with mesangial deposits of IgA as the dominant immunoglobulin. In the later stages, glomerulosclerosis and interstitial fibrosis are apparent. More than one-third of adults with IgA nephropathy develop end-stage renal disease; the percent of children who progress to this point is less well known. Gross hematuria in IgA nephropathy is occasionally so severe that patients may pass clots and have flank pain. The presence of persistent proteinuria is considered a poor prognostic sign.

Other forms of primary chronic glomerulonephritis include **MPGN, mesangial proliferative glomerulonephritis,** and **membranous nephropathy,** which is technically not a form of glomerulonephritis because it usually lacks a significant proliferative component. Children with these diseases present with hematuria, almost always associated with heavy proteinuria.

Secondary forms of glomerulonephritis include the nephritis of SLE, anaphylactoid purpura, and the nephritis associated with various vasculitides such as Wegener's granulomatosis and pauci-immune crescentic glomerulonephritis. Children with lupus tend to present with multisystem disorders but may have only renal manifestations of the disease. ANA is a good screening test for lupus. If ANA is positive, C3, C4, antidouble-stranded DNA, and a Coombs test should be checked.

Anaphylactoid Purpura

This disease is almost always accompanied by the classical cutaneous vasculitis rash, which is prominent over the lower arms and lower extremities. Abdominal pain may be severe, and affected patients are at risk for the development of intussusception. Children with anaphylactoid purpura have microscopic hematuria, which usually clears, but is occasionally associated with heavy proteinuria and nephrotic syndrome. These children are at risk for developing progressive renal disease. All children with anaphylactoid purpura should have their urine monitored for cessation of hematuria or development of proteinuria. Children with heavy proteinuria and suspected anaphylactoid purpura should have a diagnostic renal biopsy.

Hemolytic-Uremic Syndrome

HUS is a disease characterized by microangiopathic hemolytic anemia, thrombocytopenia, and acute renal failure. It typically follows a prodrome of bloody diarrhea from acute colitis caused by a verotoxin-producing strain of *Escherichia coli* (O157/H7). The verotoxin is believed to be toxic to human endothelial cells. The damaged endothelial cells incite the deposition of fibrin within the glomerular capillaries. These fibrin thrombi lead to the shearing of RBCs and consumption of platelets. Several other organisms, such as pneumococcus and *Shigella*, may precipitate HUS. In atypical cases of HUS, the precipitating event may be a URI. Some cases are familial. Children present with pallor and severe abdominal pain. Urine output may be diminished as a result of renal failure, and in many cases dialysis is required. Hypertension may be severe.

Other Glomerular Diseases

Alport's syndrome, thin basement membrane disease (benign familial hematuria), focal segmental glomerulosclerosis (FSGS), minimal change disease (MCD), and nephrosclerosis are also associated with hematuria. **Alport's syndrome** is a disease of the glomerular basement membrane, where thinning and duplication of the basement membrane occur. The renal involvement eventually leads to end-stage renal disease. Patients or their family members often have nerve deafness or keratoconus. The inheritance of Alport's syndrome varies by kindred; it may be either autosomal dominant or sex-linked. Thin basement membrane disease also is characterized by thinning of the glomerular basement membrane, but the glomeruli are otherwise normal, and the clinical course is benign. Patients with MCD and FSGS present with nephrotic syndrome but may also have microscopic hematuria.

MANAGEMENT

Gross Hematuria

The management of gross hematuria depends on the underlying cause. Children with a history of trauma should be placed on bed rest pending surgical consultation (see Chapter 43, Abdominal Trauma). If the evaluation indicates acute glomerulonephritis and if children are not hypertensive, they can be followed carefully as outpatients with monitoring of blood pressure and renal function with consultation with a pediatric nephrologist. Children with coagulopathies require specific treatment of their bleeding disorders (e.g., intravenous gamma globulin for idiopathic thrombocytopenic purpura).

If some degree of renal insufficiency is present, then children should be referred to a pediatric nephrologist to rule out more unusual causes of glomerulonephritis, for consideration of renal biopsy, and for treatment.

Microhematuria

Laboratory tests other than urinalysis may be negative in otherwise healthy children with microscopic hematuria. Some of these children may be recovering from subclinical cases of poststreptococcal glomerulonephritis, which can cause microscopic hematuria for up to 1 year. Others may have early IgA nephropathy and not yet have significant proteinuria, and some may have thin basement membrane disease. As long as children have normal renal function, normal blood pressure, and no significant proteinuria, and all other tests are normal, it is safe to monitor them every 3–6 months until the problem resolves. Healthy children with an otherwise negative workup who show no change in their clinical state for a period of 1 year may subsequently be monitored annually. If hypercalciuria is detected, a low-calcium diet or treatment with thiazide diuretics may be tried.

RENAL BIOPSY

The definitive diagnosis of the etiology of hematuria may require a kidney biopsy. Generally, pediatric nephrologists perform kidney biopsies only in selected instances after ruling out nonglomerular causes for the hematuria. Indications for renal biopsy in a child with hematuria would include an associated abnormal urinary protein excretion, decreased renal function, recurrent macroscopic hematuria, persistently depressed serum complement levels, serological evidence for systemic lupus erythematosus, or a family history of renal insufficiency of unknown etiology.

PROGNOSIS

The prognosis for children with hematuria depends on the underlying cause. Gross hematuria is more often associated with serious renal disease such as acute glomerulonephritis, HUS, or renal trauma. Even so, most children with gross hematuria have a good prognosis, provided the diagnosis is rapidly discovered and appropriate specific therapy is given. Children with persistent microscopic hematuria who have no family history of the condition, have a negative evaluation, and do not develop hypertension or proteinuria have an excellent long-term prognosis.

Case Resolution

The boy in the opening scenario shows no worrisome clinical signs such as hypertension or significant proteinuria. His urine should be rechecked twice more, and if the hematuria persists, his evaluation should follow the algorithm in Figure 72–1.

Selected Readings

Adams, N . D., and J. C. Rowe. Nephrocalcinosis. *In* Bailie, M. D. (ed.). Clinics in Perinatology. Philadelphia, W. B. Saunders, 1992, pp. 179–195.

Feld, L. G., W. R. Waz, L. M. Perez, and D. B. Joseph. Hematuria. An integrated medical and surgical approach. Pediatr. Clin. North Am. 44:1191–1210, 1997.

Ingelfinger, J. R., A. E. Davis, and W. E. Grupe. Frequency and etiology of gross hematuria in a general pediatric setting. Pediatrics 59:557–561, 1977.

Kashtan C. E. Alport syndrome and thin glomerular basement membrane disease. J. Am. Soc. Nephrol. 9:1736–1750, 1998.

Lettgen, B., and A. Wohlmuth. Validity of G1-cells in the differentiation between glomerular and non-glomerular haematuria in children. Pediatr. Nephrol. 9:435–437, 1995.

Lieu, T. A., and H. M. Grasmeder, III. An approach to the evaluation and treatment of microscopic hematuria. Pediatr. Clin. North Am. 38:579–592, 1991.

Piqueras, A. I., R. H. R. White, F. Raafat, N. Moghal, and D. V. Milford. Renal biopsy diagnosis in children presenting with haematuria. Pediatr. Nephrol. 12:386–391, 1998.

Sargent, J. D., et al. Normal values for random urinary calcium to creatinine ratios in infancy. J. Pediatr. 123:393–397, 1993.

Tsukahara, H., et al. Urinary erythrocyte volume analysis: a simple method for localizing the site of hematuria in pediatric patients. J. Pediatr. 115:433–436, 1989.

PROTEINURIA

Elaine S. Kamil, M.D.

H$_x$ A 14-year-old boy is brought to the office for a preparticipation sports physical examination. He has been previously healthy but had one hospital admission at the age of 2 years for treatment of a fractured humerus. He has no acute complaints. The family history is positive for diabetes mellitus in the paternal grandfather and lung cancer in the maternal grandfather. It is negative for renal disease or hypertension. The boy's height and weight are at the 75th percentile for age, and his blood pressure is 110/70.

On physical examination he is a well-developed, well-nourished, athletic teenager. No abnormal findings are present. The CBC reveals a hemoglobin of 14.8 g/dL, a hematocrit of 48.3%, and a WBC of 8400/mm^3 with a normal differential. The urine has a pH of 5, a specific gravity of 1.025, and a 3+ protein on dipstick. The rest of the dipstick is negative. Microscopic examination shows 0–1 WBC per high-power field and 0–2 hyaline casts per low-power field.

Questions

1. What conditions cause proteinuria?
2. When should children with proteinuria undergo further evaluation?
3. What type of evaluation should be carried out to assess proteinuria?
4. When should children with proteinuria be referred to a pediatric nephrologist?

A small amount of protein is normally present in the urine. Protein levels increase somewhat in certain conditions such as vigorous exercise, febrile illnesses, accidental trauma, and congestive heart failure. Most of the protein in the glomerular filtrate is reabsorbed by the tubular cells. Pathologic amounts of protein are present in the urine when the glomerular leak of protein is increased, when the tubules fail to reabsorb the protein filtered by the glomerulus, or if inflammation in the renal interstitium leads to the addition of globulins to the urine.

Urinary protein is initially detected by urine dipstick, but this method is unreliable in alkaline urine. Dipstick protein is also affected by urine concentration. A dipstick for protein of 1+ in a concentrated urine may not correlate with an abnormal 24-hour urinary protein excretion, whereas a dipstick of 1+ in a very dilute urine may be associated with an abnormal 24-hour urinary protein excretion. Proteinuria may be more accurately determined by performing a timed urine collection or a random sample for chemical determination of the total protein concentration divided by the urinary creatinine concentration.

EPIDEMIOLOGY

The prevalence of proteinuria depends on how the condition is defined. In a Texas study, 10 mg/dL of proteinuria was found consistently in the urine of 2–3% of children in three consecutive urine samples. When 50 mg/dL was used as the cutoff for proteinuria, however, only 0.4–0.7% of boys and 0.4–2.5% of girls had proteinuria in two of three consecutive samples. The prevalence of proteinuria increased with age. In Finland, about 11% of school-age children had at least one episode of proteinuria of 25 mg/dL by dipstick when the urine was tested four times. Approximately 2.5% of the children had proteinuria on two of four occasions.

CLINICAL PRESENTATION

Proteinuria is a laboratory finding that may present incidentally on a screening urinalysis or be detected during the evaluation of a complaint, such as edema, that may be caused by renal disease. When proteinuria is detected as an incidental finding in otherwise normal children, the laboratory evaluation of the proteinuria should be delayed until its persistence is confirmed on repeat dipstick (D$_x$ Box). Edematous children with proteinuria certainly have renal lesions. Additional findings on examination could include the presence of hypertension, ascites, pleural effusions, or the rash of SLE or anaphylactoid purpura.

PATHOPHYSIOLOGY

The glomerular capillaries are adapted to permit the filtration of minimal amounts of plasma proteins, particularly those with a small molecular radius. Approximately 320 mg of albumin and 360 mg of lower molecular weight proteins are filtered by the glomerular capillaries each day. Ninety-five percent of this is reabsorbed by the proximal tubular cells. Normally, children may ex-

---

D$_x$ Proteinuria

- Presence of dipstick proteinuria (> 1+ confirmed on three occasions)
- Random urine total protein-creatinine ratio greater than 0.25 *or* 24-hour urine protein greater than 4 mg/m^2/hr
- Orthostatic proteinuria (assessed through separate measurement of afternoon and first-morning urines for total protein-creatinine ratios)

---

crete up to 100 mg/m^2 of protein per day. Urinary protein excretion is increased in newborns to about 240 mg/m^2/day and in adolescents to about 300 mg/day. Adults may normally excrete up to 150 mg of protein per day. Only 10–15% of this is albumin; the rest of the proteins are other plasma proteins and urinary glycoproteins.

When increased proteinuria results from glomerular disease, higher levels of urinary proteins are primarily due to the enhanced filtration of albumin. Protein excretion may be increased transiently by any condition that raises intraglomerular capillary pressure such as congestive heart failure, strenuous exercise, epinephrine use, fever, or surgery.

Orthostatic proteinuria, which affects some children, is a poorly understood, benign condition. Individuals excrete pathologic amounts of protein in their urine while they are upright, but their urinary protein excretion returns to normal when they are recumbent. This condition seems to be more common in athletic individuals. Some investigators believe that orthostatic proteinuria is due to increased pressure in the renal vasculature while patients are upright.

DIFFERENTIAL DIAGNOSIS

The proteinuria may be physiologic (secondary to fever, congestive heart failure), orthostatic, tubular (as seen in allergic interstitial nephritis), or glomerular. Aminoaciduria may occur, as is seen in certain inborn errors of metabolism.

EVALUATION

History

It is important to elicit a complete history (Questions Box) in children with proteinuria. When asking about a history of swelling, the practitioner should note that subtle periorbital edema may be present only in the early morning hours. If the proteinuria is detected at a routine screening examination, the conditions under which the urine was obtained should be determined.

Questions: Proteinuria

- Was the mother's pregnancy remarkable in any way? What was the child's birth like?
- Did the child have any neonatal problems that may indicate possible renal damage?
- Is any swelling apparent in areas such as the ankles, the abdomen, or the periorbital region?
- Has the child had any recent illnesses, particularly pharyngitis or impetigo?
- Does the child have a history of joint pains and skin rashes, especially the adolescent patient who may be at greater risk of having a collagen-vascular disease?
- Has the child had any previous UTIs, urinary abnormalities, or dark urine?
- Does the child have a history of hypertension or weight loss or gain?
- Is there a family history of renal disease?
- Does the child have diabetes mellitus?

Children may have been sick with a high fever or have just participated in an athletic event such as a track meet.

Physical Examination

The physical examination should include a determination of blood pressure and measurement of height and weight. A careful assessment for edema should be made. The skin should be examined for signs of rashes such as Henoch-Schönlein purpura or healing impetigo. The joints should be inspected for any signs of swelling or joint inflammation. The abdominal examination should include a careful search for ascites or organomegaly.

Laboratory Tests

The extent of the laboratory evaluation depends on the child's general health (e.g., is the child ill with another problem?), the amount of proteinuria on dipstick, and whether the child has edema. The suggested evaluation is outlined in Figure 73–1. In nonedematous, otherwise healthy children, it is prudent to examine the urine sediment, and if negative, recheck the dipstick in a few days. If proteinuria of 1+ is consistently present and no hematuria is evident, a first-stage evaluation is indicated. If children are ill with a fever or are hospitalized with a serious illness, it is often appropriate to delay the evaluation of the proteinuria until the acute illness is under control, providing no associated hematuria or azotemia is present.

In healthy ambulatory patients with persistent, isolated, dipstick proteinuria on three occasions, it is important to quantitate the proteinuria (Box 73–1). This may be done simply by ordering a urinary protein-creatinine ratio. If the ratio is abnormal (> 0.25), children need to be evaluated first for orthostatic proteinuria.

Orthostatic proteinuria can be ruled out in several ways. The simplest evaluation involves checking a urine dipstick on a first voided morning sample and again on an afternoon specimen. This procedure should be repeated on 2 different days. It is critical to be sure that children empty their bladders before going to bed, because urine produced when they are nonrecumbent may contain protein and give an inaccurate result. If the dipstick from the morning urine is negative on a concentrated, acid urine, and if the afternoon sample is positive on a concentrated, acid urine, children most likely have orthostatic proteinuria.

A more accurate way of checking for orthostatic proteinuria involves the determination of urine protein: creatinine ratios on the first-morning and afternoon urine samples. A diagnosis of orthostatic proteinuria can be made if the ratio is normal on the "recumbent" sample and elevated on the daytime sample. The most accurate way of diagnosing orthostatic proteinuria entails collecting two timed urine samples, one during the hours that children are up during the day and the other while they are in bed at night. In most instances of orthostatic

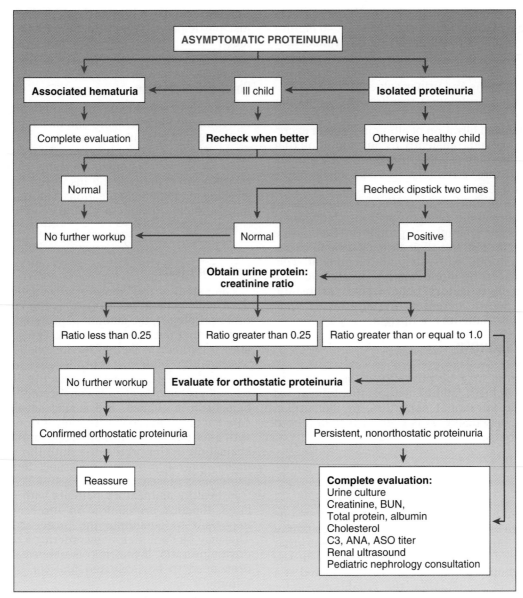

FIGURE 73-1. Suggested evaluation of children with asymptomatic proteinuria.

proteinuria in children, the total urinary protein excretion is less than 1 g. The urine collected in the recumbent period should contain less than 50 mg/m^2 of protein. If these two timed samples meet the criteria for orthostatic proteinuria, they do not need to be repeated. It is important to remember that even in renal disease, proteinuria improves somewhat when patients are recumbent.

If children do not have orthostatic proteinuria, a 24-hour urine protein excretion should be determined. If the collection of a 24-hour urine sample is impractical, the urine protein:creatinine ratio is a reliable alternative. Blood chemistries (e.g., BUN, creatinine) should be obtained to determine renal function. Electrolyte status should be assessed with total carbon dioxide, total protein, albumin, and cholesterol. Serologies should be obtained for antinuclear antibodies, C3, antistreptolysin-O titer, and hepatitis B surface antigen if children come from a population at risk for hepatitis B.

Twenty-four-hour urine protein excretion should be less than 4 mg/m^2/hr. Neonates may excrete as much as 150 mg/m^2/12 hr, however. Table 73–1 gives a summary of normal urinary protein excretion. If children have nephrotic range proteinuria or nephrotic syndrome (heavy proteinuria accompanied by hypoalbuminemia and hypercholesterolemia), they require further evaluation for nephrotic syndrome (see Chapter 112, Nephrotic Syndrome). If they do not have nephrotic range proteinuria, abnormal tubular proteinuria should be ruled out. A normal urinary β$_2$-microglobulin rules out tubular proteinuria.

In general, consultation with a pediatric nephrologist is recommended if children have an abnormal 24-hour urinary protein excretion (see Table 73–1). If the proteinuria exceeds 1 g per day or if any other minor signs of renal dysfunction or hematuria are present, a biopsy is warranted. Often, otherwise healthy children with small amounts of isolated proteinuria of less than 750–1000

BOX 73-1. Methods for Assessment of Urinary Protein

Detection of proteinuria by dipstick is only semiquantitative. This examination is affected by urinary pH and concentration, and therefore more definitive tests are warranted if a patient's urine consistently shows dipstick proteinuria. The sulfasalicylic acid (SSA) turbidity test is also semiquantitative. When SSA is added to an aliquot of urine, it precipitates urinary proteins. The amount of turbidity is graded on a scale of 0 to 4+.

Urinary protein is most accurately quantitated by a chemical determination on a timed urine collection (usually 24 hours). The concentration (measured in mg/dL) is multiplied by the total urine volume to determine the milligrams of protein excreted in 24 hours. Twenty-four-hour urine samples are difficult to collect in young children. However, several studies have shown that a random urine sample for a protein:creatinine ratio correlates well with the 24-hour urinary protein excretion. The ratio is determined by dividing the urine protein concentration (mg/dL) by the urine creatinine concentration (mg/dL). The units must be the same for each component. The urinary protein:creatinine ratio is normally less than 0.25. A ratio of 3.5 or greater in an adult or greater than 1.0 in children indicates nephrotic-range proteinuria.

Occasionally it is important to determine whether proteinuria has a tubular or glomerular basis. In these instances, a urinary β_2-microglobulin is helpful. β_2-microglobulin, a very small protein that is freely filtered at the glomerular level, is nearly completely reabsorbed by the proximal tubules. In instances of tubular injury such as interstitial nephritis, acute tubular necrosis, or nephrotoxic renal injury, urinary β_2-microglobulin is increased. With glomerular proteinuria, urine protein electrophoresis shows a heavy preponderance of albumin.

mg/day are followed by the pediatric nephrologist without a kidney biopsy. However, if this degree of proteinuria persists for 1 year or more, a renal biopsy is warranted.

Imaging Studies

A renal ultrasound should be obtained to rule out any structural abnormalities.

MANAGEMENT

Most children with normal renal function and normal blood pressure whose evaluation reveals physiologic or orthostatic proteinuria should have repeat urinalysis on

an annual basis. If the proteinuria worsens or if hematuria develops, a repeat evaluation of renal function is indicated. Children whose initial evaluation reveals persistent, significant proteinuria require careful follow-up to detect and monitor signs of serious renal disease. This follow-up should include repeat blood pressure measurement and urinalysis every 3 months and repeat chemistries (BUN, creatinine, serum albumin) and urine protein:creatinine ratios every 6 months. These children should be managed in consultation with the pediatric nephrologist, whose experience is helpful in reassessing the need for kidney biopsy.

Children with physiologic or orthostatic proteinuria who have minimal, persistent proteinuria should be able to follow a full school schedule and be allowed to participate in sports, provided there are no other contraindications. The usual immunization schedule should not be interrupted, and children should follow a regular diet. No increase in dietary protein is necessary to compensate for the minimal amounts of protein lost in the urine. Results of recent studies in nephrotic patients have even suggested that a high-protein diet may increase urinary protein losses.

PROGNOSIS

The outlook for children with proteinuria depends entirely on the underlying cause of the proteinuria. Children whose proteinuria is associated with edema or hematuria are more likely to have significant renal disease, such as glomerulonephritis, however, and the prognosis may be less favorable. If the proteinuria is due to a form of chronic glomerulonephritis, children may ultimately develop end-stage renal disease. In individuals with glomerular diseases, persistent proteinuria is a strong risk factor for progressive loss of renal function. If the proteinuria is physiologic or orthostatic, however, the long-term prognosis is excellent. The likelihood that these children will develop renal functional impairment is no greater than for the rest of the general population.

Case Resolution

In the case presented at the beginning of the chapter, odds are that the evaluation of the healthy teenage boy with isolated proteinuria will reveal that he has orthostatic proteinuria, and his long-term prognosis is good.

Selected Readings

Albitol, C., et al. Quantitation of proteinuria with urinary protein/creatinine ratios and random testing with dipsticks in nephrotic children. J. Pediatr. 116:243–247, 1990.

Ginsberg, J. M., et al. Use of single voided urine samples to estimate quantitative proteinuria. N. Engl. J. Med. 309:1543–1546, 1983.

Houser, M. T., M. F. Jahn, and A. Kobayashi. Assessment of urinary protein excretion in the adolescent: effect of body position and exercise. J. Pediatr. 109:556–561, 1986.

Kurtin, P. S. Hematuria and proteinuria. Acute and chronic medical disorders. Adolesc. Med. State Art Rev. 2:649–657, 1991.

Miltenyi, M. Urinary protein excretion in healthy children. Clin. Nephrol. 12:216–221, 1979.

TABLE 73-1. Urinary Protein Excretion by Age

Age	24-hour Urine Protein (mg)	Urine Protein:Creatinine
Premature infant	14–60	—
Full-term infant	15–68	—
2–23 mos	17–85	≤0.50
2–4 yrs	20–121	≤0.25
4–10 yrs	26–194	≤0.25
10–16 yrs	29–238	≤0.25

Reuben, D. B., et al. Transient proteinuria in emergency medical admissions. N. Engl. J. Med. 306:1031–1033, 1982.

Trachtman, H., A. Bergwerk, and B. Gauthier. Isolated proteinuria in children. Natural history and indications for renal biopsy. Clin. Pediatr. 33:468–472, 1994.

Vehaskari, V. M., and J. Rapola. Isolated proteinuria: analysis of a school-age population. J. Pediatr. 101:661–668, 1982.

Vehaskari, V. M. Mechanism of orthostatic proteinuria. Pediatr. Nephrol. 4:328–330, 1990.

Vehaskari, V. M., and A. Robson. Proteinuria. In Edelmann, C. M., et al. (eds.). Pediatric Kidney Disease. Boston, Little, Brown, 1992, pp. 531–551.

Yoshikawa, N., et al. Asymptomatic constant isolated proteinuria in children. J. Pediatr. 119:375–379, 1991.

CHAPTER 74

URINARY TRACT INFECTIONS

Sudhir K. Anand, M.D.

Hₓ A seven-month-old girl is brought to the office with a one-day history of fever (temperature: 103° F [39.4° C]), vomiting, and questionable abdominal pain. The mother has not noticed any change in urination pattern or any unusual urine odor. The child has been somewhat irritable but fully alert.

Physical examination reveals an active infant. The temperature is 102.6° F (39.2° C), the heart rate is 122 beats/min, the respiratory rate is 30 breaths/min, and the blood pressure is 90/60. The neck is supple. The head, eye, ear, nose, throat, chest, heart, abdominal, and genital examination is normal. Urinalysis shows specific gravity 1.025, pH 6.0, leukocyte esterase and nitrite both strongly positive, protein trace, and blood trace; the sediment is 15–20 WBCs per high-power field and 2–4 RBCs per high-power field. Urine is sent for culture.

Questions

1. What are the possible diagnoses of children with positive leukocyte esterase or nitrite on urinalysis?
2. What are the indications for hospital admission of children with UTIs?
3. What antibiotics are used in the treatment of UTIs?
4. What is the appropriate diagnostic workup for children with suspected UTIs? When are renal ultrasound, IVP, 99m-Tc-DMSA renal scan, and voiding cystourethrogram included in the evaluation?
5. If workup reveals vesiculoureteral reflux, how should children be managed over the long term?

Urinary tract infection (UTI) is one of the most common infections that affect infants and children. The disorder may be asymptomatic, associated with urinary symptoms, or occasionally accompanied by sepsis. In most children UTIs resolve completely. In some young children, especially those with vesicoureteral reflux (VUR), obstructive uropathy, or delayed or inadequate antibiotic treatment, however, UTIs may lead to renal scarring and eventual hypertension or end-stage renal failure in later childhood.

UTI is a nonspecific, generic term implying significant bacteriuria, irrespective of the site of bacterial growth in the urinary tract, and includes the heterogeneous group of conditions listed below. In many young children with bacteriuria, clinical findings overlap and precise classification cannot be easily made.

Asymptomatic, covert, and **screening bacteriuria** are synonymous terms usually used when bacteriuria is detected during surveys of healthy children. The term "screening bacteriuria" is preferable because some affected children may have urinary symptoms on close questioning.

Acute pyelonephritis is a symptomatic infection of renal parenchyma characterized by systemic symptoms (e.g., high fever, chills, flank pain, vomiting, and dysuria [burning urination]).

Chronic pyelonephritis is a term that has been used in various ways. Ideally, it should be used in renal biopsy specimens in conjunction with histologic lesions of renal scarring due to infection. Practically, the term often refers to scarred kidneys as demonstrated by radiologic techniques (IVP or nuclear scan) or kidneys with reduced function due to such scarring.

Cystitis implies infection of the bladder. Its major features are voiding symptoms (e.g., dysuria, frequency, urgency, enuresis, and foul-smelling urine). Fever, if present, is usually low-grade.

Recurrent UTI generally refers to reinfection with a new organism (often same species but different strain). This condition is a common problem, especially in the first year after initial infection. Reinfection with the same organism is infrequent and may indicate underlying structural problems of the urinary tract or the presence of stones.

Urethritis implies infection of the urethra, and is usually seen in adolescent children in the context of a venereal infection. The usual symptoms are burning urination and urethral discharge.

EPIDEMIOLOGY

Bacteriuria is detected in approximately 1% of girls and 2% of boys during screening of healthy newborns and young infants. Approximately 1% of girls continue to have screening bacteriuria throughout childhood. In boys over one year of age, however, bacteriuria is uncommon. In most affected infants and children, bacteriuria resolves spontaneously with time, and it does not lead to increased risk of renal damage.

Symptomatic UTI occurs in approximately 0.4–1% of newborns and young infants. In early infancy, UTI is about twice as common in boys than in girls and about 10 times more common in uncircumcised boys than circumcised boys. After the first 6 months of life, the incidence and prevalence of symptomatic UTI become considerably higher in females than males; the difference between circumcised and uncircumcised males disappears. Among febrile infants, UTI is the source of fever in approximately 4–8% of patients, especially in those who do not have an apparent source of infection on physical examination.

CLINICAL PRESENTATION

Symptoms and signs of UTI in newborns and young infants are usually nonspecific and include fever, irritability, poor weight gain (or weight loss), diarrhea, vomiting, and jaundice. Occasionally, severe sepsis with temperature instability, cyanosis, and DIC may occur. Bacteremia may be present in neonates with UTI. In older children, symptoms include fever, abdominal or flank pain, vomiting, dysuria, frequency and urgency of urination, enuresis, foul-smelling or cloudy urine, and occasionally gross hematuria (D_x Box).

PATHOPHYSIOLOGY

The pathogenesis of UTI involves interaction between various bacterial factors and protective host factors.

D_x **Urinary Tract Infection**
• Abdominal pain • Burning urination • Fever • Leukocyturia • Positive urine culture

---

Bacterial Factors

Escherichia coli accounts for 80–90% of first infections. The remainder are caused by other gram-negative enteric bacilli (*Proteus, Klebsiella, Enterobacter*) and gram-positive cocci (enterococci, *Staphylococcus saprophyticus*). Most organisms that cause UTI originate from the fecal flora. *S. saprophyticus* (a coagulase-negative staphylococcus) infections are primarily seen in adolescents with UTI.

Microorganisms that cause UTI usually enter the urinary tract by an ascending route. To initiate colonization and induce UTI, these organisms must first adhere to uroepithelium; otherwise they will be swept away during voiding. Moreover, adherent bacteria come in direct contact with a source of nutrients provided by the host cells. Bacterial adhesion in *E. coli* is mediated by fimbriae, which are fine, hairlike proteins emanating from the bacterial cell wall. One important type of fimbriae, called P-fimbriae, adheres to receptors (Gal-Gal) on uroepithelium. In most young children who have no VUR, acute pyelonephritis is caused by *E. coli* with P-fimbriae. In the majority of patients with VUR and scarred kidneys, however, the infection is caused by *E. coli* which are considered less virulent and lack P-fimbriae. Hence, the role of P-fimbriae in acute pyelonephritis which may lead to renal scarring is uncertain. Other bacterial virulence factors include K and H antigens, colicin, and hemolysin, but their role in the pathogenesis of UTI is not clearly defined.

Host Factors

Host factors that contribute to the pathogenesis of UTI include age, sex, genetic makeup, VUR, abnormal voiding urodynamics leading to incomplete bladder emptying and residual urine, severe constipation, and immune response to infection. The uroepithelium of older girls and adult women who develop recurrent UTI binds *E. coli* more avidly than uroepithelium from nonsusceptible patients, perhaps because of higher density of receptors. In addition, individuals with certain P and Lewis blood groups develop more UTIs than others. Urinary obstruction or other anomalies may contribute to the development of UTIs in about 2% of girls and 5% of boys, especially infants.

VUR signifies retrograde passage of urine from the bladder to the ureter. After passage through the bladder wall, the normal ureter tunnels under the bladder mucosa before it opens into the bladder lumen. Under normal circumstances, when the bladder is filled and during voiding, the submucosal segment is compressed, preventing reflux of urine into the ureter.

Most VURs are primary and caused by a congenital abnormality of the ureterovesical junction, with the ureter having a short submucosal segment and more laterally placed openings. Transient VUR is sometimes believed to follow a UTI, but this finding has not been well substantiated. Reflux may also occur in the presence of normal ureteral anatomy when bladder pressures exceed 40 cm of water, as seen in patients with posterior urethral valves or neurogenic bladders. VUR is

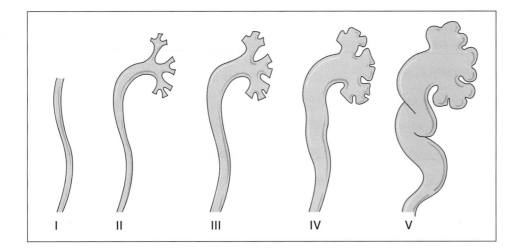

FIGURE 74–1. Grading of vesicoureteral reflux by vesicouretero-gram based on international classification. I, ureter only; II, ureter, pelvis, and calyces, but without dilatation; III, mild or moderate dilatation of ureter and mild or moderate dilatation of renal pelvis, but no or slight blunting of fornices; IV, moderate dilatation or tortuosity of the ureter with moderate dilatation of renal pelvis and calyces and complete obliteration of the sharp angles of fornices, but maintenance of papillary impressions in the majority of calyces; V, gross dilatation and tortuosity of ureters, renal pelvis, and calyces; papillary impressions are no longer visible in the majority of calyces.

graded on a scale of I–V, with stage V being the most severe (Fig. 74–1).

The incidence of VUR in normal infants is less than 2%. In infants with UTI, the incidence of VUR is about 40–50%; in school-age children, about 25–30%; and in adolescents, about 10–15%. These figures suggest that with increasing age and maturation of the bladder wall, VUR spontaneously resolves in the majority of patients. VUR may also be a familial disorder and has been reported in 10–30% of siblings of index cases.

In the presence of VUR, the incidence of UTI is increased, probably because of incomplete emptying of the bladder; the refluxed urine (from the ureters) returns to the bladder at the end of voiding. Furthermore, VUR provides infected urine from the bladder direct access to the ureters and kidneys, leading to pyelonephritis and renal scarring, especially in infants and young children.

The greater the severity of VUR in children with UTI, the greater the likelihood of renal scarring. During the past 8 years, however, it has been clearly recognized that many neonates (especially boys) with antenatal VUR, even in the absence of UTI, have congenital dysplastic renal parenchymal defects which in the past have been misidentified as infective scars. The progression of renal scarring in the latter group, as the infants grow older, may either be the natural history of the congenital defect or result from superimposed UTI.

DIFFERENTIAL DIAGNOSIS

In infants and young children, symptoms of UTI are often nonspecific. Thus a high degree of suspicion for UTI must be maintained. Acute abdomen (e.g., appendicitis, glomerulonephritis, renal stones) may occasionally be confused with UTI. Some children with dysuria may have chemical irritation from exposure to materials such as bubble baths. In these cases, urine culture findings usually help differentiate the disorder.

EVALUATION

In all infants and young children with fever without an apparent source, urinalysis and urine culture must be obtained to verify the presence or absence of UTI.

History

In older children, a history of fever, dysuria, frequency, abdominal pain, and nausea and vomiting is suggestive of UTI (Questions Box). History of previous UTIs, abnormal voiding and constipation should also be sought.

Physical Examination

The abdomen should be examined for masses and tenderness, the genitalia for local lesions, and the lumbosacral area for anomalies such as sinus tracts. Blood pressure should be measured to document the presence of hypertension.

Laboratory Tests

The diagnosis of UTI is established by documenting significant bacteria in a urine specimen sent for culture. In young infants the specimen should always be obtained by bladder puncture or catheterization. Because of the risk of contamination, a "bag urine" sample is reliable only if the urine is sterile. In older children with bladder control, a midstream urine collection is satisfactory. The diagnosis of UTI should never be based on the presence or absence of leukocyturia alone. Although most older children with symptomatic UTI have leukocyturia, many neonates and young infants with UTI (25–50%) may not manifest this finding. Furthermore, leukocyturia may occur in other renal disorders in the absence of UTI. A positive urinary nitrite test is suggestive of UTI, but the false negative rate is nearly 50%.

Questions: Urinary Tract Infection

- Does it hurt when the child urinates? Does the child scream when urinating?
- Does the child void more frequently?
- Does the urine have an unusual odor?
- Has the child had previous urinary infections?
- Does the child have a good urinary stream? Or does the child dribble?

Most patients with UTI (>85%) have urine bacterial counts greater than 100,000/mL on a voided specimen (i.e., significant bacteriuria). Some adult women and teenage girls with symptomatic recurrent UTI have catheterized or "clean catch" urine colony counts less than 1000/mL. In general, this has not been observed in young children. Colony counts between 10,000 and 100,000/mL are generally considered suspect (unlikely to be significant) in clean voided specimens unless children have symptoms of UTI, associated leukocyturia, and cultures that are pure growths of a single organism. Specimens are also considered significant if any growth of organisms is evident in urine samples obtained by suprapubic puncture or if there are more than 10,000 organisms/mL in samples obtained by catheterization. In most children with UTIs, urine collected by either of these techniques grows >50,000 organisms/mL.

C-reactive protein is usually increased in infants and children with high fever and clinical findings suggestive of acute pyelonephritis. Several other laboratory studies, including ESR, urinary lactic acid dehydrogenase isoenzymes, urinary concentrating ability, and antibody-coated bacteria, have been used with varying success to differentiate upper (renal) from lower (bladder) UTI in older children and adults. Overall, the reliability of these studies in pediatric patients, especially infants and young children, is not adequate to recommend their routine use. Furthermore, in young children, both upper and lower tract infections mandate complete evaluation for urinary anomalies and VUR followed by the institution of appropriate treatment.

Imaging Studies

All girls younger than 5 years of age and all boys (irrespective of age) should have renal ultrasonography and voiding cystoureterogram (VCUG) performed following detection of the first UTI. These two studies detect structural renal anomalies and VUR in most patients. In girls, nuclear VCUG instead of contrast VCUG is an acceptable alternative. Renal ultrasound can be performed as soon as feasible after diagnosis. VCUG is generally delayed 4–6 weeks to exclude the possibility of reflux secondary to UTI. This delay, however, entails the administration of antibiotic prophylaxis until completion of the study. An excretory urogram (IVP) is usually not indicated unless a ureteral duplication, a ureterocele, or some other anomaly is suspected.

In recent years, some authorities have recommended a routine 99m-Tc-DMSA renal scan to differentiate upper from lower tract infection. Although the test is positive in 60–90% of children with a clinical diagnosis of actue pyelonephritis, the cost of the nuclear scan, the presence of radiation exposure, and the fact that therapy is usually not altered, preclude the routine use of this study. The scan is most helpful in a child where the diagnosis of acute pyelonephritis is in doubt or when used in follow-up to detect development of renal scars, especially in patients with VUR.

MANAGEMENT

All infants younger than two months of age with UTIs should be treated with parenteral **antibiotics,** starting with ampicillin and gentamicin (or cefotaxime), pending results of sensitivity studies. Children over 2 months of age who are not vomiting and who appear stable and nontoxic may receive oral antibiotics. Most physicians recommend trimethoprim-sulfamethoxazole for the first infection until the results of bacterial sensitivity tests are available. Treatment is continued for 10 days. Children over 2 months of age who have persistent vomiting and appear toxic should be admitted to the hospital and started on parenteral antibiotics until they show clinical improvement. They then can be switched to oral therapy.

In children with VUR, low-dose antibiotics (trimethoprim-sulfamethoxazole) are continued for 1 year following treatment for an acute infection. At the end of this period, a radionuclide VCUG is repeated to determine whether reflux has resolved. Development of new renal scars can be best detected by DMSA scanning.

Surgery is not necessary in most infants with VUR, including many with severe disease (grades IV and V), because most grade I–III and some grade IV–V reflux in infants disappears with increasing age. In older children (>5 years of age) with grade IV or V reflux, the rate of disappearance with medical treatment is much lower (about 20–25%). The results of the International Vesicoureteral Reflux Study Group show no difference in the rate of renal scarring between prophylactic medical treatment and surgery. Surgical reimplantation of the ureter is usually recommended only for those patients who have poor compliance or breakthrough infections, especially if the upper tract is involved. This latter group seems to have benefited the most from surgery. In Europe, endoscopic injection with Teflon has been used with equally good short-term results; the long-term safety of Teflon has not been established, however.

PROGNOSIS

In most children, UTI is a nuisance illness with no or minimal long-term or serious consequences. However, in 25–50% of children, a repeat UTI may occur, especially during the first year following the initial UTI. Repeat urine cultures should be made during follow-up assessments in all children, especially those with VUR, first at 1–2-month intervals and later at 3–4-month intervals for at least 1 year or until disappearance of reflux.

The risk factors for the development of renal scars and eventual hypertension and/or renal failure include: young age, especially less than 1 year, recurrent episodes of acute pyelonephritis, delay in starting effective antibiotic therapy, high grade reflux, and anatomic or neurogenic obstruction. If repeat infection is prevented in these children, however, development of fresh scars is uncommon, and renal function and growth remain normal. As a group, infants and children younger than 3 years of age with UTI and high-grade

VUR are more likely to develop calyceal clubbing and renal scarring, whereas progressive renal scarring as a result of UTI or reflux after age five years is relatively less common.

Case Resolution

In the case history, the young girl is hospitalized because of the vomiting. She is started on intravenous trimethoprim-sulfamethoxazole, and she improves in 48 hours. Renal ultrasound is normal. She is discharged and continued on oral antibiotics, and a radionuclide VCUG is planned in four weeks.

Selected Readings

Belman, A. B. Vesicoureteral reflux. Pediatr. Clin. North Am. 44:1171–1190, 1997.

Crain, E. F., and J. C. Gershal. Urinary tract infections in febrile infants younger than 8 weeks age. Pediatrics 86:363–367, 1990.

Hellerstein, S. Urinary tract infections: Old and new concepts. Pediatr. Clin. North Am. 42:1433–1457, 1995.

Jodal, U., and S. Hansson. Urinary tract infection: clinical. *In* Holliday, M. A., T. M. Barratt, and E. D. Avner (eds.). Pediatric Nephrology, 3rd ed. Baltimore, Williams & Wilkins, 1994, pp. 950–962.

Stark, H. Urinary tract infections in girls: The cost-effectiveness of currently recommended investigative routines. Pediatr. Nephrol. 11:174–177, 1997.

Stokland, E., et al. Renal damage one year after first urinary tract infection: Role of DMSA scintigraphy. J. Pediatr. 129:815–820, 1996.

Weiss, R. A. Update on childhood urinary tract infections and reflux. Semin. Nephrol. 18:264–269, 1998.

CHAPTER 75

VAGINITIS

Monica Sifuentes, M.D.

Hx An 11-year-old girl is brought to your office with vaginal itching that has lasted for 1 week. Her mother has noted a yellow discharge on her panties for the past 4 days. The girl reports no associated abdominal pain, vomiting, or diarrhea. She has no urinary problems and also denies any history of sexual abuse. Although she occasionally bathes with bubble bath, she usually takes showers. Except for the vaginal complaint, she is healthy, and she takes no medications.

The physical examination is remarkable for a soft, nontender abdomen with no organomegaly. Bowel sounds are audible in all quadrants. The girl is at Tanner stage II. The labia majora and minora and the clitoris all appear normal, and the hymen is annular in shape with a smooth rim. A scant amount of yellow discharge, along with minimal perihymenal injection, is noted at the introitus. The anal examination is normal, with an intact anal wink.

Questions

1. What are the most common causes for vaginal discharge in prepubescent and adolescent females? How do they differ?
2. What basic historical information must be obtained from all females whose chief complaint is vaginal discharge?
3. What specific methods are used to perform a gynecologic examination in prepubescent and adolescent females?
4. What is the appropriate laboratory evaluation for prepubescent and adolescent females who complain of vaginal discharge? How does this evaluation differ in adolescent females who are sexually active?
5. What are the various treatment options for females with vaginitis?

A vaginal discharge is not an uncommon occurrence in prepubescent and adolescent females. Practitioners are largely responsible for differentiating between a physiologic discharge, or leukorrhea, and a pathologic discharge, which occurs, for example, with a bacterial or yeast infection. In cases of an abnormal discharge, the possibility of abuse needs to be considered and investigated appropriately (see Chapter 105, Child Sexual Abuse). Therefore, primary care physicians should be familiar with the various causes of vaginal discharge in both prepubescent and adolescent females. In addition, they should be comfortable performing gynecologic examinations in these children. Appropriate treatment can then be initiated.

Vulvovaginitis, which is often used interchangeably with vaginitis or vulvitis, signifies inflammation of the perineal area often accompanied by a vaginal discharge. The discharge may be bloody, malodorous, or purulent, depending on the etiology (Table 75–1).

EPIDEMIOLOGY

Vulvovaginitis is the most common gynecologic complaint in prepubescent girls. Most cases of vulvovaginitis in these girls result from **nonspecific inflammation;** vaginal cultures show normal flora in 33–85% of such cases. The incidence of more specific **bacterial causes,** such as group A beta-hemolytic streptococcus, has been reported in approximately 14% of patients. However, its occurrence appears to be seasonal and diagnosis depends on the use of proper culturing techniques and appropriate media. Other bacterial causes include respiratory pathogens such as *Haemophilus influenzae, Neisseria meningitidis, Streptococcus pneumoniae,* and enteric organisms such as *Shigella.* A positive culture for *Chlamydia trachomatis* or *Neisseria gonorrhoeae* can be found in approximately 5% of children who are evaluated for sexual abuse. Higher figures have been reported from certain centers and when adolescent victims are included. These organisms are not considered part of the normal flora in prepubescent girls. Vaginal and rectal infections with *C. trachomatis* can be acquired perinatally, however.

Parasitic infections may also lead to vaginal symptoms. Twenty percent of females with a rectal infestation of *Enterobius vermicularis,* the organism known as pinworm, have vulvovaginitis. Affected patients often complain of pruritus in addition to the vaginal discharge. **Mycotic infections** with organisms such as *Candida* may also cause symptoms in prepubescent girls, although many of these girls have a previous history of oral antibiotic use.

CLINICAL PRESENTATION

Prepubescent and adolescent females with vulvovaginitis most commonly present with a vaginal discharge, which may be white, purulent (i.e., yellow or green), or serosanguinous. Its consistency can range from smooth and thin to thick and cottage cheeselike. The discharge

TABLE 75–1. Characteristics and Specific Causes of Vaginal Discharge

Color	Consistency	Amount	Cause
Clear/white	Thin	Variable	Physiologic
White	Cottage cheeselike	Moderate	*Candida*
White/yellow	Variable	Variable	Chemical irritation, *Chlamydia*
Yellow/green	Thick	Moderate-profuse	*Neisseria gonorrhoeae,* foreign body, *Trichomonas*
Bloody	Variable	Variable	*Shigella,* group A streptococcus, foreign body

Dx Vaginitis

- Nonphysiologic vaginal discharge
- Perineal erythema
- Pruritus
- Dysuria
- Malodorous vaginal discharge

may also be malodorous. In addition, females may complain of associated pruritus, erythema, urinary problems such as dysuria and increased frequency, and abdominal pain (D$_x$ Box). Sexually active adolescent females with vaginitis from an STD (e.g., gonorrhea) may have a more profuse, purulent discharge.

PATHOPHYSIOLOGY

Prepubescent girls are at risk for developing vulvovaginitis for both anatomic and physiologic reasons. Unlike pubertal adolescents and young women, young girls have no pubic hair and a smaller labial fat pad to protect the introitus. The labia minora are small and tend to open when girls are in a squatting position, thereby exposing the vaginal introitus. The relative proximity of the anus to the vagina in young girls also contributes to vaginal contamination with enteric organisms. More importantly, poor hygienic practices (i.e., wiping back to front after urination or defecation) can further compound the problem.

In addition, the normal physiology of the vaginal epithelium in prepubescent girls predisposes to vaginitis. The unestrogenized vaginal epithelium is relatively thin, immature, and easily traumatized. In addition, the pH of the vagina is neutral to alkaline, as compared to the acidic environment of the vagina in adults. Local antibody production is also believed to be lacking in the vagina of prepubescent girls.

DIFFERENTIAL DIAGNOSIS

A vaginal discharge is normal at two distinct times in prepubescent girls: shortly after birth, secondary to the effects of maternal estrogen, and approximately 6 months to 1 year before the onset of menarche, which occurs, in most girls, after Tanner stage III. The causes of other vaginal discharges in prepubescent and pubescent females are presented in Table 75–2.

EVALUATION

Prepubescent Females

History

A complete history should be obtained in all females with a vaginal discharge (Questions Box). Practitioners should inquire about the appearance of the discharge, its duration, and the relative amount. A profuse, purulent, discharge is probably more consistent with one

TABLE 75–2. Causes of Vaginal Discharge in Prepubescent and Pubescent Females

Prepubescent Females
Estrogen withdrawal (neonates)
Chemical irritation secondary to soaps and detergents
Mechanical irritation from nylon panties or tight-fitting clothes
Foreign body in vagina
Poor hygiene
Pinworms
Yeast infection (e.g., *Candida*)
Bacterial infection (e.g., group A streptococcus, *Shigella*)
Sexually transmitted disease (e.g., gonococcal infection, chlamydial infection, trichomoniasis)
Congenital abnormality (e.g., ectopic ureter [local inflammation])
Acquired abnormality (e.g., labial fusion [pooling of urine in vagina])
Urethral prolapse
Systemic illness (e.g., scarlet fever, Crohn's disease)

Pubescent Females
Physiologic leukorrhea
Foreign body in vagina (e.g., retained tampon)
Yeast infection (e.g., *Candida*)
Bacterial infection (e.g., group A streptococcus, *Staphylococcus aureus*)
Sexually transmitted disease (e.g., gonococcal infection, chlamydial infection, trichomoniasis)
Chemical irritation (e.g., douches, spermicides, latex [condoms])

specific etiology (e.g., *N. gonorrhoeae*) than is a scant, thin discharge that suggests a nonspecific etiology. The existence of urinary problems should also be determined. Pooling of urine in the vagina secondary to labial fusion can lead to vulvovaginitis in addition to a UTI. Changes in bowel or bladder habits and sudden changes in behavior such as nightmares or inappropriate stranger anxiety may also be noted. Such changes in behavior warrant a further inquiry into the possibility of

sexual abuse, regardless of the practitioner's index of suspicion. Depending on the information disclosed, both children and parents should be interviewed independently.

Other points to discuss include the type of detergents or soaps used for laundry as well as for bathing, because these may be irritating. Any recent illnesses should also be documented as a possible source of autoinoculation or, if oral antibiotics were required, as a reason for the alteration of the normal vaginal flora. In addition, patients' hygienic practices should be reviewed.

Adolescent patients should always be interviewed alone (see Chapter 4, Talking to Adolescents). In particular, a reproductive history must be obtained, keeping in mind that puberty and sexual activity both alter vaginal flora.

Physical Examination

Although the genital examination is the priority, a complete physical examination should be performed. This not only allows clinicians to identify other abnormal physical findings, but it also alleviates some of the anxiety often associated with a genital examination. Because most vaginal discharges in prepubescent girls result from nonspecific vulvovaginitis, visualization of the cervix with a speculum is not indicated.

The overall demeanor of young girls at the onset of the genital examination should be noted. Overly compliant, apathetic behavior in children may be a cause for concern regarding abuse, especially in the context of a chronic purulent discharge.

On physical examination, children's Tanner stage or sexual maturity rating must be noted and recorded. In addition, the external genitalia should be examined closely for the presence of any lesions or any evidence of erythema. Chronic changes in labial skin, such as those associated with constant scratching, should also be noted.

Girls should be placed in the modified lithotomy or "frog leg" position, and the labia majora should be gently spread apart to visualize the hymen. The knee-chest position can also be used, depending on the comfort of the practitioner as well as the patient. If the labia cannot be spread apart, the girl may have labial fusion. Perihymenal and periurethral erythema and injection should also be assessed, in addition to any evidence of edema, trauma, or abnormal masses such as urethral prolapse. Hymenal size and appearance should be carefully evaluated for any evidence of abuse (see Chapter 105, Child Sexual Abuse). The appearance, consistency, and amount of the vaginal discharge, including the presence or absence of an odor, should also be noted. These findings may vary depending on the characteristics and cause of the discharge. Finally, the anus should be inspected for tone and any evidence of trauma or abnormal lesions such as venereal warts. An anal wink may normally be elicited. Although not usually indicated, a rectal examination should be performed in an attempt to palpate a foreign body or mass in those patients with a chronic vaginal discharge.

Questions: Vaginitis

Prepubescent Females
- What is the color of the discharge?
- What is the consistency of the discharge?
- How profuse is the discharge?
- Is the discharge malodorous?
- How long has the discharge been apparent?
- How often does the discharge occur (i.e., is it found on the panties daily)?
- Are there any associated problems (e.g., dysuria, abdominal pain)?
- What types of laundry soaps or detergents are used?
- Does the child take bubble baths?
- Has the child had any recent illnesses?
- Does the child clean herself after using the toilet, or does she require help?
- In what direction does she tend to wipe after a bowel movement?

Adolescent Females (all of the above questions plus the following):
- What is the reproductive history (menstrual and sexual)?
- If appropriate, is the adolescent using any form of contraception? When was the last episode of unprotected intercourse?
- If appropriate, how many sexual partners has the patient had?
- Does the patient or partner have any history of a previous STD, including hepatitis B?

Laboratory Tests

Laboratory studies are often unnecessary in prepubescent girls with a nonspecific, nonbloody vaginal discharge, diffuse vulvar erythema, and no suspicion or history of sexual abuse. A vaginal culture for isolation of group A beta-hemolytic streptococcus is indicated in girls with an abrupt onset of a serosanguinous discharge and a history of a systemic illness. The cellophane tape test may be helpful in diagnosing a pinworm infection in girls with associated anal pruritus. A KOH wet mount reveals hyphae if a monilial infection is present.

If the discharge is purulent or malodorous or if abuse is suspected, vaginal cultures should be obtained for gonococcus and chlamydia. A chlamydia culture is preferred because of the risk of a false-positive result with nonculture tests (direct immunofluorescent smears, enzyme immunoassays, ligase chain reaction). With genital and anal specimens, false-positive results can occur because of cross-reaction with fecal flora. In certain cases, a normal saline wet mount to check for mobile trichomonads may be indicated.

Pubescent Females

History

In adolescent or pubescent females with vaginal discharge, physicians should inquire about a history of sexual activity or assault in addition to other information that relates to their condition (Questions Box). Questions concerning the possible acquisition of an STD must also be asked.

Physical Examination

Virginal adolescents with an uncomplicated history should be examined in a similar fashion as the prepubescent female. The external genitalia should be examined to evaluate the Tanner stage of the patient and the presence of any lesions. Perihymenal or periurethral erythema and hymenal size and appearance should also be noted. In the absence of a mucopurulent or bloody discharge, a speculum examination is usually not warranted.

In addition to an overall physical examination, a complete genital examination using a speculum is indicated in the sexually active female. The purpose of the speculum examination is to visualize the cervix, properly obtain cervical specimens, and examine the vagina for lesions (i.e., condylomata acuminata). A bimanual examination must also be performed to check for cervical motion tenderness, which may be associated with pelvic inflammatory disease (PID).

Laboratory Tests

Adolescent females who are not sexually active should have a laboratory evaluation similar to that described for prepubescent girls. The approach to sexually active adolescents, however, warrants modification. A cervical culture for gonorrhea should be obtained in all sexually active adolescents with a vaginal discharge. In addition, a rapid assay for chlamydia should be performed. DNA probes for screening endocervical samples for gonorrhea and chlamydia with a single swab are now available. In addition, ligase chain reaction tests (LCR) have been developed for screening of urine for *N. gonorrhoeae* and *C. trachomatis*. A Pap smear should also be done at this time, not only to screen for cervical dysplasia, but also to detect cellular changes consistent with HPV or trichomoniasis. A culture for herpes simplex is indicated only if the history of exposure is positive and ulcerative or vesicular lesions are present.

A normal saline wet mount should be made, especially if a nonspecific discharge or bacterial vaginosis is a concern. A 10% KOH mount is appropriate in cases of suspected candidiasis. Mixing 10% KOH with the discharge may also produce a "fishy" odor (positive "whiff test"), which is consistent with bacterial vaginosis or trichomoniasis. A Gram stain of any purulent material may lead to an early diagnosis of gonorrhea. Serologies for syphilis should also be obtained in adolescents with suspected or proven STDs. In addition, patients should be offered testing for HIV, with appropriate pretest and posttest counseling.

MANAGEMENT

Management of a **nonspecific vaginal discharge** is aimed at relieving the uncomfortable symptoms associated with this type of inflammation. Prepubescent females should be instructed to **discontinue use of all chemical irritants,** including bubble baths, in the genital area. Warm water **sitz baths** are also recommended twice daily for approximately 1 week or until patients feel better. In addition, females should be instructed in **proper hygiene** (e.g., wiping front to back after a bowel movement). The use of cotton or cotton-crotch panties and loose-fitting skirts or pants should be recommended.

Antifungal medications such as **clotrimazole** (Lotrimin) or **miconazole** (Monistat) cream may be prescribed if a monilial infection is present. Empiric treatment may be warranted in children or adolescents with a previous history of oral antibiotic usage, diabetes mellitus, or other chronic conditions that may alter the normal vaginal flora.

Pinworms are treated with a single oral dose of **mebendazole** (Vermox), 100 mg, or **pyrantel pamoate** (Antiminth), 11 mg/kg/dose (to a maximum of 1 gram). Most authorities recommend repeat treatment after 2 weeks.

If a retained foreign body is suspected in prepubescent girls, then examination under general anesthesia may be necessary. Alternatively, practitioners can attempt vaginal irrigation in cooperative children by placing a small feeding tube at the hymenal opening and injecting warm saline. Toilet paper is

TABLE 75–3. Treatment Recommendations for Adolescents With Infectious Vaginitis

Organism	Treatment*
Neisseria gonorrhoeae	Ceftriaxone, 125 mg IM, once, or Cefixime, 400 mg PO, once, or Ciprofloxin 500 mg PO, once
Chlamydia trachomatis	Azithromycin, 1 g PO, once
Trichomonas	Metronidazole, 2 g PO, once
Bacterial vaginosis	Metronidazole, 500 mg, bid for 7 days or, Clindamycin cream 2%, one applicatorful qhs for 7 days
Candida albicans	1% clotrimazole, cream, one applicatorful vaginally qhs for 7 days; 2% miconazole cream, 1 applicatorful vaginally qhs for 7 days; 0.8% terconazole cream, 1 applicatorful vaginally qhs for 3 days; fluconazole, 150 mg PO once

*For treatment options, refer to Centers for Disease Control and Prevention. 1998 Sexually Transmitted Disease Treatment Guidelines. M.M.W.R. 47:RR–1, 1–118, 1998.

the most commonly retrieved material in prepubescent girls.

Adolescent females who are not sexually active should be treated as outlined above. If the discharge is believed to be physiologic leukorrhea, practitioners should reassure patients and educate them about other issues related to puberty (e.g., menarche, body odor). Sexually active adolescents with positive vaginal cultures or highly suspicious vaginal discharges should receive treatment depending on the causal organism (see Chapter 76, Sexually Transmitted Diseases, for details concerning treatment). Table 75–3 briefly outlines current recommendations.

Any disclosure of molestation by prepubescent or adolescent females must be reported to the appropriate authorities. In addition, abnormal physical findings and positive cultures of STDs in prepubescent females and adolescent females who have never been sexually active must be reported and investigated.

PROGNOSIS

In the majority of prepubescent females, vaginitis resolves spontaneously or after appropriate treatment with no permanent sequelae. In contrast, adolescent females treated for vulvovaginitis or uncomplicated cervicitis from an STD are at some risk for the development of PID, HIV, and pregnancy given their high-risk behavior.

Case Resolution

In the case presented at the beginning of the chapter, the girl and her parents should be assured that the discharge is consistent with a nonspecific process. She should be instructed to take sitz baths for 1 week, discontinue bubble baths and the use of soap in the genital area, and wear loose-fitting clothes with cotton underwear. The girl should be reexamined in 1–2 weeks.

Selected Readings

Altchek, A. Finding the cause of genital bleeding in prepubertal girls. Contemp. Pediatr. 13:80–92, 1996.

Baldwin, D. D., and H. M. Landa. Pediatric gynecology: evaluation and treatment. Contemp. Pediatr. 12:35–60, 1995.

Blake, D. R., et al. Evaluation of vaginal injections in adolescent women: can it be done without a speculum? Pediatrics 102: 939–944, 1998.

Blake, J. Gynecologic examination of the teenager and young child. Obstet. Gynecol. Clin. North Am. 19:27–38, 1992.

Elvik, S. L. Vaginal discharge in the prepubertal girl. J. Pediatr. Health Care 4:181–185, 1990.

Emans, S. J., M. R. Laufer, and D. P. Goldstein (eds.). Vulvovaginal problems in the prepubertal child. *In* Pediatric and Adolescent Gynecology, 4th ed. Philadelphia, Lippincott-Raven, 1998, pp. 75–107.

Pierce, A. M., and C. A. Hart. Vulvovaginitis: causes and management. Arch. Dis. Child 67:509–512, 1992.

Porkorny, S. F. Prepubertal vulvovaginopathies. Obstet. Gynecol. Clin. North Am. 19:39–58, 1992.

Sobel, J. D. Vaginitis. N. Engl. J. Med. 337:1896–1903, 1997.

Vandeven, A. M., and S. J. Emans. Vulvovaginitis in the child and adolescent. Pediatr. Rev. 14:141–147, 1993.

CHAPTER 76

SEXUALLY TRANSMITTED DISEASES

Monica Sifuentes, M.D.

Hₓ A 17-year-old male presents with a small red lesion on the tip of his penis. He noticed an area of erythema a few weeks before, but it resolved spontaneously. He reports no fever, myalgias, headache, dysuria, or urethral discharge. He is sexually active and occasionally uses condoms. He did not use a condom during his last sexual encounter 2 weeks ago, however, because his partner uses oral contraception. The adolescent has never been treated for any sexually transmitted diseases (STDs) and is otherwise healthy.

On examination, he is a Tanner IV circumcised male with a 2- to 3-mm vesicle on the glans penis. Minimal erythema is present at the base of the lesion, and there is no urethral discharge. The testicles are descended bilaterally, and no masses are palpable. Shotty, nontender, inguinal adenopathy is evident.

Questions

1. What conditions are associated with vesicles in the genital area?
2. What risk factors are associated with the acquisition of an STD during adolescence?
3. What screening tests should be performed in patients with suspected STDs?
4. What recommendations regarding partners of patients with STDs should be given?
5. What issues of confidentiality are important to address with adolescents who desire treatment for STDs?

A majority of teenagers in the United States have their first sexual experience before they graduate from high school. In a recent survey conducted by the Centers for Disease Control and Prevention (CDC), nearly half of all students in high school reported having had sexual intercourse during their lifetime. More importantly, nearly 18% of boys and 14% of girls in grades 9 to 12 reported having had four or more sexual partners.

The consequences of such sexual activity in adolescents include increased rates of bacterial and viral STDs, unintended pregnancy, and the emergence of acquired immunodeficiency syndrome (AIDS) as the sixth leading cause of death in the 15- to 24-year age group. Given the dramatic nature of these consequences, the physician must be skilled in obtaining a sexual history in teenage patients and in diagnosing and treating STDs.

Increasing levels of sexual activity directly affect STD trends in adolescents. Other influential factors include multiple (sequential or concurrent) sexual partners; inconsistent use of condoms and other barrier methods; experimentation with drugs, including alcohol, which results in poor judgment concerning sexual activity; poor compliance with antibiotic regimens; and biologic factors, such as an earlier age of menarche and the presence of cervical ectopy in adolescent females. The feeling of invulnerability and the associated risk-taking behavior that occurs during adolescence make sexual activity "spontaneous" rather than premeditated. As a result, preventive measures are hindered, ignored, or simply unheard of, and adolescents deny the consequences of their actions. Other factors influencing STD trends are related to societal norms. Traditionally, educational materials and STD services have not been available to adolescents. In addition, the depiction of casual sexual relationships on television sitcoms, music

videos, and motion pictures may play a major role in glamorizing sex.

EPIDEMIOLOGY

The overall prevalence of STDs in adolescents is difficult to estimate, because not all STDs are reportable, and collected data are often influenced by the particular population studied. It has been estimated, however, that approximately 4% of high school students have had at least one STD. *Chlamydia* remains the most common cause of cervicitis and urethritis in adolescents, with a prevalence rate of 5–40% in females and 8–35% in males. Complications of chlamydial cervicitis occur in 10–30% of cases. Epididymitis, a result of urethral infection, occurs in 1–3% of infected males. It has been estimated that sexually active adolescents are three times more likely to be infected with *Chlamydia* than adults.

Teenagers have the highest incidence of **gonorrhea** of any other population group, although this incidence is decreasing. The highest rates of gonorrhea reportedly occur in adolescent females, young men in their 20s, young adult inner-city minorities, homosexual men, and prostitutes. A large number of sexual partners, intravenous drug use, exposure to prostitutes, and casual sexual contacts also contribute to the risk of infection. In 1996, the CDC reported that the incidence of gonorrhea in the 15- to 19-year age group was 570.8 : 100,000, although in females the incidence was 756.8 : 100,000.

Of the 1 million cases of pelvic inflammatory disease (PID) reported annually in the United States, 20–30% are in sexually active adolescents. The risk of developing PID is increased tenfold in this age group compared with adults for several reasons. Failure to use condoms, new partners within the previous 2–3 months, and a past history of STDs have been cited as risk factors. Complications of PID such as tubo-ovarian abscess formation are also more likely in adolescents as a result of late presentation, delayed diagnosis, and noncompliance with treatment regimens.

CDC data also show that **syphilis** rates have been declining in recent years, a change in direction from the previous ten years. During 1996, the incidence of syphilis in the 15- to 19-year age group was 6.4 : 100,000; 20- to 24-year-olds had the highest rate of primary and secondary syphilis at 10.8 : 100,000. Studies have shown, however, that people with syphilis, as well as other STD-causing genital ulcers, are at increased risk for HIV acquisition.

Human papillomavirus (HPV) may infect 38–46% of adolescent females, a rate reportedly two to three times greater than in older women. The prevalence of HPV in adolescents varies widely for two reasons: (1) infection with HPV is often latent, and (2) HPV is not a reportable condition. Risk factors for HPV infections are similar to those for other STDs: multiple sexual partners, age greater than 25 years, lack of condom use, previous STD infection, pregnancy, sex with an infected partner, and altered immune response.

Infection with **herpes simplex virus type 2 (HSV-2)** is also underestimated. Reportedly, HSV-2 occurs in approximately 4% of whites and 17% of African Americans by the end of their teenage years.

As of June 1998, the number of **AIDS** cases reported in the United States in adolescents aged 13–19 years was 3302; the number of cases in young adults between 20 and 24 years of age was 23,729. Because the incubation period for AIDS is believed to be from 8–10 years for adolescents, estimates of asymptomatic or early HIV infection are often based on reported cases of AIDS in young adults in their 20s. AIDS cases in adolescents occur primarily in males and minorities. Most of these individuals are infected through sexual contact or intravenous drug use.

CLINICAL PRESENTATION

Adolescents with a sexually transmitted disease may go to their physicians with specific complaints related to the genitourinary system, such as painful urination or vaginal discharge. They may also report more generalized complaints, like fever and malaise, especially in cases of primary HSV (D$_x$ Box: STDs). In addition, some teenagers will use a vague complaint to see their primary care practitioner with the hope that the physician asks about sexual activity. It is only then that they will disclose their real concern.

PATHOPHYSIOLOGY

A number of biologic factors contribute to the increased prevalence rates of STDs in adolescents, particularly in females. At the onset of puberty, the columnar epithelial cells in the vagina transform to squamous epithelium while columnar cells at the cervix persist (Fig. 76–1). With increasing age, the squamoco-lumnar junction recedes into the endocervix. In adolescent females, however, this junction, referred to as ectopy, is often located at the ectocervix and is relatively exposed, which places these females at particular risk for gonococcal and chlamydial infections. The infectious organisms preferentially attach to cervical columnar cells and infect them. Of note is that the use of oral contraceptives also prolongs this immature histologic state.

The cytologic changes seen in cervical cells of adolescents with HPV infection are also believed to be age-related. The immature cervical metaplastic or co-lumnar cells appear to be more highly vulnerable to infection and neoplastic changes. In addition, exposure to other cofactors (e.g., tobacco use, multiple episodes of new HPV infections) is likely to promote the development of squamous intraepithelial neoplasia (SIN) and cervical carcinoma. Not all young women exposed to HPV develop lesions or progress to SIN, and most will not remain positive for HPV throughout their lifetime.

The presence of genital ulcers has been shown to facilitate both the transmission and the acquisition of HIV. Such ulcers provide a point of entry past denuded epithelium. In addition, it is hypothesized that many activated lymphocytes and macrophages are located at the base of the ulcer and are therefore "ripe" for infection by HIV.

Pelvic inflammatory disease usually develops from an ascending polymicrobial infection, often an untreated STD of the cervix and vagina, which spreads contiguously upward to the upper genital tract. Inflammation, scarring, and crypt formation in the fallopian tubes result. The most common causal organisms, which account for more than half of the cases of PID in most studies, are *Chlamydia trachomatis* and *Neisseria gonorrhoeae*. Other agents include *Escherichia coli;* other enteric flora; and microbes implicated in bacterial vaginosis, such as *Mycoplasma hominis, Ureaplasma urealyticum, Bacteroides* spp., and anaerobic cocci.

DIFFERENTIAL DIAGNOSIS

Most patients with STDs present with one of five clinical syndromes—urethritis/cervicitis, epididymitis, pelvic inflammatory disease, genital ulcer disease, or genital warts, all of which can be easily diagnosed (Table 76–1). Other conditions that mimic STDs, however, must be considered in certain cases where the adolescent denies sexual activity or where the disorder does not respond to routine treatment. These disorders include **mucocutaneous ulcers** associated with lupus erythematosus and Behçet's disease. Often, systemic disorders such as these can be ruled out historically. **Benign oral lesions** such as aphthous ulcers can also be confused with herpes ulcers. When evaluating an adolescent female with acute lower abdominal pain, surgical conditions such as **appendicitis, ovarian torsion,** and **ectopic pregnancy** must be ruled out. In the sexually active male with testicular pain, **testicular torsion** must be considered before a diagnosis of epididymitis is made.

D$_x$ STDs

MALES

- Dysuria
- Urethral discharge or pain
- Testicular pain
- Presence of any lesions in the genital area such as ulcers, vesicles, or warts
- Sexual partner who has an STD

FEMALES

- Dysuria
- Abnormal vaginal discharge
- Intermenstrual bleeding
- Dysmenorrhea
- Dyspareunia
- Lower abdominal pain
- Systemic symptoms such as fever, nausea, vomiting, malaise
- Presence of any lesions in the genital area such as ulcers, vesicles, or warts
- Sexual partner who has an STD

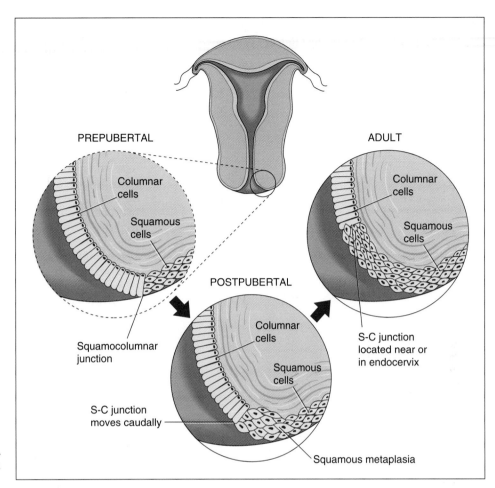

FIGURE 76–1. Development of the cervical squamocolumnar junction, from puberty to adulthood.

EVALUATION

In all sexually active adolescents, a complete history, including a sexual history, should be obtained (Questions Box). A detailed gynecologic history should also be taken in females. The rest of the history should then focus on the particular complaint and any associated symptoms. Sexually active adolescents should have a complete physical examination, including a thorough genital examination. Diagnostic tests should be determined by the adolescent's risk for a specific STD and significant historical and physical findings. One must keep in mind, however, that many patients are asymptomatic and screening for STDs should be based on high-risk behavior.

URETHRITIS AND EPIDIDYMITIS

History

Because urethritis is more common in young men, all sexually active adolescent males should be asked about the presence of dysuria, urethral discharge, and urethral erythema. In females, symptoms such as dysuria may appear more gradually and are reported frequently. Other symptoms like meatal edema, erythema, or urethral discharge are rarely noticed. General urinary symptoms such as acute urinary frequency or urgency are uncommon, especially in males, but all patients should be asked about such symptoms. More often, urethritis is asymptomatic, and the diagnosis is made by routine screening in sexually active adolescents or through known contact with a partner with an STD (e.g., *C. trachomatis* or *T. vaginalis*).

To diagnose epididymitis, sexually active males should be asked about scrotal pain and swelling. Symptoms associated with urethritis may be present or may have preceded the scrotal symptoms.

Physical Examination

In males, the urethra should be the focus of the genital examination. The presence of a urethral discharge and its consistency (i.e., mucoid or purulent) should be noted. Any other urethral or genital lesions should also be assessed. The epididymis, spermatic cord, and testicules should be palpated and may be swollen and tender.

In females, a full pelvic examination should be performed after careful examination of the external genitalia for any ulcerative or wartlike lesions. Urethritis is most often caused by *C. trachomatis,* but HSV and trichomoniasis can be other causes. The urethra should also be inspected for edema, erythema, or any evidence of a discharge. During the speculum examination, the

TABLE 76–1. Differential Diagnosis of Sexually Transmitted Disease by Clinical Syndrome

Urethritis
- *Neisseria gonorrhoeae*
- Nongonococcal disease
  - *Chlamydia trachomatis*
  - *Ureaplasma urealyticum*
  - *Trichomonas vaginalis*
  - Herpes simplex virus
  - Yeasts

Cervicitis
- *C. trachomatis*
- *N. gonorrhoeae*
- Herpes simplex virus

Pelvic Inflammatory Disease
- *N. gonorrhoeae*
- *C. trachomatis*
- Anaerobes
- Gram-negative rods
- Streptococci
- *Mycoplasma hominis*
- *U. urealyticum*

Vaginitis
- *T. vaginalis*
- *Candida albicans* and other fungi
- *Gardnerella vaginalis*

Genital Ulcers
- *Treponema pallidum* (syphilis)
- Herpes simplex virus, types 1 and 2
- *Haemophilus ducreyi* (chancroid)
- *C. trachomatis* (lymphogranuloma venereum)

Genital Warts
- *T. pallidum* (condyloma latum)
- Human papillomavirus (condyloma acuminatum)

Proctitis
- *N. gonorrhoeae*
- *C. trachomatis*
- *T. pallidum*
- Herpes simplex virus
- Particular to homosexual youth (in addition to the above)
  - Hepatitis A and B virus
  - *Shigella* spp.
  - *Campylobacter* spp.
  - *Giardia lamblia*
  - *Entamoeba histolytica*

Pharyngitis
- *N. gonorrhoeae*
- *C. trachomatis*
- Herpes simplex virus, types 1 and 2

presence or absence of a vaginal or cervical discharge should also be noted.

Laboratory Tests

A Gram stain of the urethral discharge may confirm the diagnosis of urethritis in both males and females. The specimen should be obtained using a Dacron or cotton swab because calcium alginate inhibits the growth of *Chlamydia*. The presence of gram-negative, intracellular diplococci with the typical "kidney-bean" morphology is indicative of an infection with *N. gonorrhoeae*. Five or more polymorphonuclear (PMN) leukocytes per high-power field but no organisms indicates the more common type of infection, nongonococcal urethritis, usually found in males. A culture for gonococcus (GC) and *Chlamydia* should still be obtained.

If no PMN leukocytes are seen on Gram stain or if the patient is asymptomatic, assessment for leukocyte esterase with a urine dipstick should be made using the first 10–15 mL of a voided urine specimen. This specimen should also be examined under the microscope for PMNs. A routine urine culture is generally not recommended in males and may be of little help in females.

New screening tests using urine samples are now available for detecting gonorrhea and *Chlamydia*. These nonculture tests rely on amplification of DNA (polymerase chain reaction [PCR] and ligase chain reaction [LCR]) and are highly sensitive and convenient for screening teenagers. A disadvantage is that these tests are costly and may have a greater potential for false-positive results, making a definitive diagnosis questionable. In the adolescent population, however, nonculture screening tests are presumably more acceptable and can be used to initiate treatment for the suspected STD.

A Doppler ultrasound may be necessary to make an accurate diagnosis of epididymitis, especially if there is any question of testicular torsion.

CERVICITIS

History

Cervicitis in females is parallel to urethritis in males. Because cervicitis is a local infection, systemic symptoms may not occur. However, a variety of important historical points and associated complaints should be addressed. Is a vaginal discharge present? If so, does it have an odor? Is the patient experiencing any urinary frequency, urgency, or dysuria? Has she had any nonmenstrual vaginal bleeding, including postcoital bleeding? A known exposure to an STD must also be ascertained. Is the partner symptomatic or currently receiving treatment? Does the patient or her partner have a past history of an STD?

Questions: STDs

Questions to Ask the Patient
- Are you currently sexually active?
- At what age did you begin to have sex?
- Do you have sex with men, women, or both?
- How many partners have you had? When was your last contact?
- Have you even been forced to have sex, or have you ever exchanged sex for food, shelter, money, or drugs?
- Do you or your partner(s) use contraception? What type?
- Do you or your partner(s) use drugs or alcohol?
- Have any of your sexual contacts ever been diagnosed with an STD?
- Do you have abdominal pain, dysuria, increased urinary frequency, or hesitancy?
- Have you noticed any ulcers, blisters, warts, or other bumps in the genital area?
- For females: Do you have a vaginal discharge or itching? Is sex uncomfortable or painful? Do you have bleeding between periods or after intercourse?
- For males: Do you have a discharge from your penis? Any testicular pain? Any associated burning or itching?

More generalized symptoms such as moderate lower abdominal pain (either acute or chronic) and fever may indicate a complication of untreated cervicitis such as PID.

Physical Examination

After completing the full physical examination, the physician should focus on the genitourinary examination. The Tanner stage should first be noted, then the presence of any lesions on the external genitalia or inflammation of the perineum. Any urethral erythema or discharge should also be noted. A vaginal discharge can be assessed more completely when performing the speculum examination, which should be performed in all sexually active adolescent females with vaginal or lower urinary tract complaints.

During the speculum examination, the vaginal mucosa should be inspected and the appearance of the cervical os should be noted. The physician should determine whether a purulent discharge is coming from the os and look for any evidence of cervical friability as opposed to normal adolescent ectopy. A presumptive diagnosis of mucopurulent cervicitis is made when there is a discharge from the cervical os, cervical erosion, or friability. A bimanual examination must also be performed to check for cervical motion tenderness (CMT) and adnexal masses or fullness.

Laboratory Tests

Cultures for GC and *Chlamydia* must be obtained in all sexually active females who, on speculum examination, show symptoms of vaginal discharge or evidence of cervicitis. In addition, a Gram stain of the discharge should be performed to detect the presence of gram-negative diplococci or PMN leukocytes. The presence of ≥ 30 PMNs per oil immersion field is presumptively positive for cervicitis. The culture for gonococcus should be obtained before other cultures because the organisms can be found in the purulent discharge itself. After the cervix is cleaned, the specimen for the chlamydial enzyme immunoassay can be collected. Because *C. trachomatis* is an intracellular organism, the cytobrush should be used to rub the surface of the endocervix, thus enhancing the recovery of organisms. A wet mount to diagnose associated STDs such as trichomoniasis may also be performed, especially if the discharge is foul-smelling or frothy. Although nonculture tests for *Chlamydia* and gonorrhea are available, urine testing is not recommended as the test of choice for symptomatic women but can be used, if available, for screening high-risk inidividuals.

PELVIC INFLAMMATORY DISEASE

History

When considering a diagnosis of PID, the history should include a discussion of known risk factors such as sexual activity, including the number of sexual partners, especially new partners in the previous two months; a previous STD or recent episode of an STD; the type and consistency of contraceptive use; and the timing of the last menstrual cycle, since most women present with PID during the first half of their cycle. The physician should also ask patients about the presence of symptoms associated with PID: the onset, duration, quality, and location of abdominal pain; urinary symptoms that may indicate concomitant urethritis; intermenstrual bleeding; dysmenorrhea or dyspareunia; abnormal vaginal discharge; right upper quadrant pain; and systemic symptoms such as nausea, vomiting, fever, and malaise. The classic symptoms of PID, which include lower abdominal pain, vaginal discharge, fever, and irregular vaginal bleeding, may not be present. More often symptoms are nonspecific, and the practitioner must maintain a high index of suspicion in any sexually active female with abdominal pain.

Physical Examination

Classic signs of acute PID include fever with tenderness of the lower abdomen, cervix, and adnexa. A thorough physical examination should be completed before performing the pelvic examination. Vital signs should be obtained, looking for fever or tachycardia. Blood pressure should also be taken, because hypotension can be seen with a ruptured ectopic pregnancy, which may present with abdominal pain and vaginal bleeding. The abdomen should be assessed for tenderness and guarding. The location of the pain is particularly important, because acute surgical conditions such as appendicitis, ovarian torsion, and ectopic pregnancy are included in the differential diagnosis of PID. In addition, right upper quadrant pain is consistent with perihepatitis, or Fitz-Hugh–Curtis syndrome, which can be seen with a gonorrheal or chlamydial infection.

The speculum examination should then be performed, looking for a purulent discharge or any evidence of cervicitis (cervical friability or erosion). The bimanual examination is the most important part of the physical examination. The cervix should be carefully palpated for any evidence of CMT and the adnexa for tenderness or masses.

Laboratory Tests

A cervical culture for *N. gonorrhoeae,* a cervical specimen for a chlamydial enzyme immunoassay, and a Gram stain of any cervical discharge should be performed. The specimen should be examined microscopically for PMN leukocytes as well as gram-negative, intracellular diplococci. The presence of thirty or more PMNs per oil immersion field is one of the clinical criteria for making a diagnosis of PID. (See D_x Box: Pelvic Inflammatory Disease for additional criteria.) Newer tests using DNA-amplification techniques are now available and can be performed on vaginal, urine, and cervical samples. (See Laboratory Tests section for urethritis and epididymitis.)

Other laboratory studies to be obtained include a complete blood count with differential and a sedimen-

Dx Pelvic Inflammatory Disease

- Lower abdominal pain
- Adnexal tenderness
- Cervical motion tenderness

Additional Findings

- Fever > 38.3° C (101° F)
- Abnormal vaginal or cervical discharge
- Elevated erythrocyte sedimentation rate, or C-reactive protein
- Culture proven infection with *N. gonorrhoeae* or *C. trachomatis*
- Inflammatory mass on palpation, ultrasound,* or laparoscopy*
- Endometritis on biopsy*

---

*CDC definitive criteria for diagnosis

---

tation rate or C-reactive protein. A urine pregnancy test should also be completed to exclude the possibility of a uterine or ectopic pregnancy. Additionally, a urinalysis and urine culture should be obtained, as well as a serologic test for syphilis. HIV testing should also be offered.

Laparoscopy can be performed to make a definitive diagnosis or to obtain diagnostic cultures in cases where the diagnosis is questionable or patients are not responding to standard therapy. A gynecologist should be consulted for these cases.

Imaging Studies

A pelvic ultrasound may help exclude diagnoses such as ectopic pregnancy or ovarian torsion and can also aid in the detection of associated complications of PID such as tubo-ovarian abscess. Fluid in the cul-de-sac may also be seen on ultrasound in these patients.

GENITAL ULCERS

History

Probably the most important information to learn about genital ulcers is whether they are painful. A painless chancre on the penis, around the mouth, in the oropharynx, or on the external genitalia in females is consistent with syphilis. If the lesions are painful or are associated with a grouped vesicular eruption, HSV is the likely cause. The presence of systemic symptoms such as fever, chills, headache, or malaise is also important to determine because these symptoms are seen with a primary infection with either organism. Generalized complaints, however, are associated with secondary syphilis only 50% of the time. A history of adenopathy, either localized or generalized, must also be noted, and dysuria may be present in females with HSV. In addition, a history of a virus-like illness accompanied by a rash should be explored. A diffuse maculopapular rash,

especially on the palms and soles, is a classic sign of secondary syphilis. Known exposure to STDs should also be ascertained.

Physical Examination

All adolescents who present with chancres, or ulcers, should receive a complete physical examination. The skin, including the palms and soles, should be examined closely for any dull red to reddish-brown macular or papular lesions. The orophayrnx should be carefully checked for chancres or blisters. All lymph nodes should be palpated for pain, enlargement, or induration. Suppurative or fluctuant nodes are often associated with chancroid caused by *Haemophilus ducreyi*.

The genital examination should then focus on the appearance of the lesions. The following questions should be asked of the patient: Are the lesions ulcerative, clustered, and painful? (HSV or chancroid.) Are they associated with grouped vesicles on an erythematous base? (HSV.) Is tender inguinal adenopathy present? (HSV or chancroid.) Or is there a single, painless chancre with a clean base and a sharply defined, slightly elevated border? (Syphilis.) The lymph nodes associated with this syphilitic type chancre are often nontender, but enlarged. Other less common STDs produce venereal ulcers that are often painful, deep, and that may be accompanied by some purulence. Adenopathy is also quite impressive with chancroid and lymphogranuloma venereum *(C. trachomatis)*.

Laboratory Tests

The necessary diagnostic tests depend on the patient's clinical picture. However, all adolescents who present with an ulcerative lesion should have darkfield microscopy performed for syphilis. Direct fluorescent antibody testing of the lesions is also available and is very specific. Nontreponemal serologic tests for syphilis, such as the Venereal Disease Research Laboratory (VDRL) or rapid plasma reagin (RPR) tests, should be done if direct examination is not available or the clinical appearance of the ulcer is nonspecific. In cases of early primary syphilis where the VDRL or RPR may not be reactive initially, the test should be repeated in one week. Treponemal tests, such as the fluorescent treponemal antibody absorption test (FTA-ABS), should be used only as confirmatory tests and not for screening purposes.

A viral culture for HSV should also be obtained from the base of an unroofed vesicle. HSV monoclonal antibody can be performed in older lesions that may be culture-negative and can differentiate between types 1 and 2. HSV serology is generally not helpful.

Given the well-described correlation between genital ulcers and HIV, it is recommended that all patients with a diagnosis of syphilis be tested for HIV as well. Conversely, annual syphilis screening is recommended for an adolescent with multiple sexual partners, a history of IV drug use, a history of sex with homosexual or bisexual men, or a diagnosed STD.

GENITAL WARTS

History

Risk factors for HPV infection should be assessed. These include a history of multiple sexual partners; age younger than 25 years; a previous history of an STD; lack of condom use; pregnancy; altered immune response; and tobacco use. Symptoms may include pruritus, pain, or dyspareunia, but often the condition is asymptomatic. Adolescents may inadvertently palpate a papule on the external genitalia and be concerned or may note bleeding from large, traumatized lesions.

Physical Examination

A complete pelvic examination should be performed on all sexually active female adolescents. Before the speculum is inserted, the external genitalia should be carefully inspected for lesions. Genital warts, or condyloma acuminatum, most commonly appear on squamous epithelium as irregular polypoid masses with an irregular, cauliflower-like surface that may coalesce into larger lesions. They are usually located at the posterior introitus, labia minora, and in the vestibule in females, and they may be found on the cervix and vagina as well. In males, warts can be seen more commonly on the penile shaft, glans, or corona. They may also appear as flat, flesh-colored papules on the scrotum and anus. Because this is a common location for lesions, the anus should be inspected carefully in both males and females.

Condylomata planum are subclinical lesions that are not grossly visible but are apparent on colposcopy and histology. Condylomata lata are flat, flesh-colored warts that occur in moist areas (anus, scrotum, vulva) and may be associated with other signs of secondary syphilis.

Laboratory Tests

A Pap smear should be performed on all females with any evidence of condyloma acuminatum. Cytologic findings associated with HPV include atypia, koilocytosis, and dysplasia. When considering referral to a gynecologist, the grade of the lesion should be reviewed. Classification of HPV is often left to the discretion of the specialist, however.

Subclinical HPV infection can be detected using acetic acid, Schiller's iodine, and colposcopy. Suspicious areas of white epithelium or a specific vascular pattern consistent with HPV infection should be biopsied. Females may be referred to a gynecologist for this procedure. Subclinical lesions in males should also be evaluated using 3% acetic acid. Biopsy may be difficult to perform but is indicated if any findings are positive.

A culture for gonorrhea and an enzyme immunoassay for chlamydia should be obtained. A nontreponemal antibody test for syphilis (RPR or VDRL) should also be performed. An HIV antibody test should be offered to all adolescents who are deemed appropriately "at risk" after receiving pretest counseling.

A urinalysis for asymptomatic hematuria is indicated in males with visible condyloma. Its presence would indicate a urethral lesion.

MANAGEMENT

Although many states differ with regard to the details of health care delivery for adolescents, a universal policy allows health care providers to evaluate and treat adolescents for an STD without parental consent. Notification of partners is usually anonymous and carried out by local public health officials. Contacts are informed that a partner has been diagnosed with an STD and are instructed to be evaluated for treatment. The evaluation and treatment of the sexual partners of patients diagnosed with an STD is extremely important to prevent reinfection. Often partners are asymptomatic and would otherwise not seek treatment. The practitioner can also use this opportunity for STD education and prevention. Antibiotic recommendations and dosing schedules are noted in Table 105–5 (Child Sexual Abuse), Table 75–3 (Vaginitis) and Table 76–2. For further details regarding specific conditions and therapies, the reader may consult the selected readings at the end of the chapter.

In addition to antimicrobial therapy, management of an STD should include preventive services. Adolescents with a first-time STD as well as those with recurrent STDs should be educated about disease transmission, consequences of delayed treatment, and methods for prevention. Other associated STDs, such as HIV, should also be addressed. The physician should spend time with adolescents with recurrent STDs and explore the reasons why preventive methods have failed. Several factors are extremely important to consider, including an untreated partner, poor sexual judgment secondary to substance use or abuse, and noncompliance with the treatment regimen, because they are certain to influence current treatment.

PROGNOSIS

If diagnosed and treated in a timely manner, the prognosis for most STDs is good, especially since the advent of single-dose, oral therapies. Sequelae of PID, however, regardless of treatment, include tubo-ovarian abscess and Fitz-Hugh–Curtis syndrome (perihepatitis). Long-term consequences of PID are chronic abdominal

---

TABLE 76–2. Parenteral Regimens for the Treatment of Pelvic Inflammatory Disease

Cefotetan, 2 g IV every 12 h	Clindamycin, 900 mg IV every 8 h
or	*plus*
Cefoxitin, 2 g IV every 6 h	Gentamicin loading dose IV or IM
plus	(2 mg/kg body weight), followed
Doxycycline, 100 mg IV	by a maintenance dose of
or PO every 12 h	1.5 mg/kg every 8 h

The above regimens are continued for at least 48 hours after the patient improves clinically. Upon discharge from the hospital, doxycycline is continued orally for a total of 14 days. Clindamycin, 450 mg PO four times a day, can be used as an alternative to complete 14 days of treatment.

pain, ectopic pregnancy, and infertility. Currently, there is no pharmacologic agent to eradicate HSV or HIV. Although acyclovir is useful in treating the signs of primary herpes and reducing the incidence of recurrences, long-term safety of using acyclovir is unknown. The prognosis for HIV is variable, depending on the individual's progression at the time of diagnosis.

Case Resolution

In the case presented at the beginning of the chapter, a diagnosis of HSV can be made clinically. The adolescent should be counseled with regard to the mode of transmission, the natural history of primary versus recurrent infection, and the role of antiviral agents. A first-void urine sample should be checked for leukocyte esterase or PMNs. An RPR or VDRL test should be performed as well as a thorough assessment for HIV risk. HIV testing should be offered after appropriate pretest counseling has been performed.

Selected Readings

Anderson, M. M., and R. E. Morris. HIV and adolescents. Pediatr. Ann. 22:436–446, 1993.

Centers for Disease Control and Prevention. 1998 Sexually transmitted diseases treatment guidelines. M.M.W.R. 47:RR–1, 1–102, 1998.

Darville, T. Chlamydia. Pediatr. Rev. 19:85–91, 1998.

Ellen, J. M., A. B. Moscicki, and M. B. Shafer. Genital herpes simplex virus and human papillomavirus infection. Adv. Ped. Infect. Dis. 9:97–124, 1994.

Gittes, E. B., and C. E. Irwin. Sexually transmitted diseases in adolescents. Pediatr. Rev. 14:180–189, 1993.

Lappa, S., and A. B. Moscicki. The pediatrician and the sexually active adolescent. A primer for sexually transmitted diseases. Pediatr. Clin. North Am. 44:1405–1445, 1997.

McCabe, E., L. R. Jaffe, and A. Diaz. Human immunodeficiency virus seropositivity in adolescents with syphilis. Pediatrics 92:695–698, 1993.

McCormack, W. M. Pelvic inflammatory disease. N. Engl. J. Med. 330:115–119, 1994.

Oh, M. K., et al. High prevalence of chlamydia trachomatis infections in adolescent females not having pelvic examinations: utility of PCR-based urine screening in urban adolescent clinic setting. J. Adol. Health 21:80–86, 1997.

Pletcher, J. R., and G. B. Slap. Pelvic inflammatory disease. Pediatr. Rev. 19:363–367, 1998.

Scholes, D., et al. Prevention of pelvic inflammatory disease by screening for cervical chlamydial infection. N. Engl. J. Med. 334:1362–1366, 1996.

Shafer, M. B. Sexually transmitted diseases in adolescents: prevention, diagnosis, and treatment in pediatric practice. Adolesc. Health Update 6:1–7. 1994.

CHAPTER 77

MENSTRUAL DISORDERS

Monica Sifuentes, M.D.

H$_x$ A 16-year-old female presents with a 9-day history of vaginal bleeding. She has no history of abdominal pain, nausea, vomiting, fever, dysuria, or anorexia, and she reports no dizziness or syncope. Her menses usually last 4–5 days and occur monthly. Her last menstrual period was 3 weeks ago and was normal in duration and flow. Menarche occurred at 15 years of age. She is sexually active, has had two partners, and reportedly uses condoms. Neither she nor her current partner has ever been diagnosed with or treated for an STD. She has no family history of blood dyscrasias or cancer.

On physical examination, she is an obese adolescent female in no acute distress. Her temperature is 98.4° F (36.9 ° C). Her heart rate is 100 beats/minute, and her blood pressure is 110/60. The physical examination, including a pelvic examination, is unremarkable except for minimal blood noted at the vaginal introitus.

Questions

1. What menstrual disorders commonly affect adolescent females?

2. What factors contribute to the development of menstrual disorders, particularly during adolescence?
3. What relevant history should be obtained in adolescents with menstrual or pelvic complaints?
4. What treatment options are currently available for primary dysmenorrhea?
5. What conditions must be considered in adolescents with abnormal uterine bleeding?
6. How is dysfunctional uterine bleeding managed in adolescent patients?

Gynecologic concerns and complaints are common reasons for visits by adolescent females to their primary care physicians. The challenge for practitioners is to differentiate between an organic etiology, functional condition, and psychogenic complaints. When this cannot be readily done or if the physical examination is equivocal, multiple diagnostic procedures are performed, often with disappointing results. In addition, many pediatricians are uncomfortable dealing with adolescents and performing pelvic examinations, which contributes to this diagnostic dilemma. The purpose of this chapter is to review some of the more common gynecologic conditions affecting the adolescent female and to highlight the significant historical and physical findings associated with each problem. For a discussion of the infectious conditions that cause pelvic pain, the reader is referred to Chapter 76, Sexually Transmitted Diseases.

EPIDEMIOLOGY

The overall prevalence of menstrual disorders during adolescence is estimated to be 50%. The most common gynecologic complaint is dysmenorrhea, or painful menstruation. Dysmenorrhea has been found to be responsible for significantly limiting activity in 10–15% of females. At least 75% of women reportedly have some pain associated with menses regardless of the degree of discomfort. Prevalence estimates regarding premenstrual syndrome (PMS) are difficult to assess because most studies are retrospective and complaints can be exaggerated. Between 30 and 75% of older adolescents reportedly have significant PMS-type complaints. An estimated 20–40% of adult women experience PMS, and 5–10% have debilitating symptoms. Other problems include abnormal uterine bleeding, vaginal discharge, and amenorrhea.

Several factors contribute to the occurrence of gynecologic problems during adolescence. The average age of menarche in the United States is 12.5 years (range: 9–16 years). Bleeding may be irregular or prolonged initially because most early menstrual cycles are anovulatory. Once ovulatory cycles are established, bleeding problems may resolve, but menstrual symptoms such as pain may predominate. Early sexual activity among adolescents and associated STDs may also contribute to the presence of certain gynecologic conditions in this age group, particularly vaginitis and abnormal uterine bleeding.

CLINICAL PRESENTATION

Adolescents with menstrual disorders may present in a variety of ways. They may have specific symptoms, such as heavy bleeding, irregular periods, or painful menses, or more general complaints, such as fatigue, dizziness, and syncope (D_x Box). Adolescents or their parents may have questions or concerns about delayed pubertal development and amenorrhea.

PATHOPHYSIOLOGY

Puberty and the Normal Menstrual Cycle

Figure 77–1 depicts the menstrual cycle, which normally lasts for 21–35 days, with a mean length of approximately 28 days. Normal duration of menses is 4–7 days. Blood loss is usually 30–40 mL per cycle, and most women do not lose more than 60 mL per cycle. Regular ovulatory cycles usually do not occur until 1–2 years after menarche although 10–20% of cycles can remain anovulatory as long as 5 years after menarche.

D_x	**Menstrual Disorders**

PRIMARY DYSMENORRHEA
- Painful menstruation
- Lower abdominal pain associated with menstruation, usually worse on the first few days of bleeding
- Associated back pain
- Pain sometimes accompanied by nausea, vomiting, fatigue, headache, and diarrhea
- Symptoms began 6–12 months after menarche

DYSFUNCTIONAL UTERINE BLEEDING
- Prolonged bleeding (> 8 days) *or*
- Excessive bleeding (> 6 tampons/pads per day) *or*
- Frequent uterine bleeding (≤ 21 days)
- No demonstrable organic etiology
- Normal laboratory studies, except for anemia

PRIMARY AMENORRHEA
- No spontaneous menstruation in a female of reproductive age
- Absence of menarche by age 16 in a female with normal pubertal development *or*
- Absence of menarche by age 14 in a female with no secondary sexual development *or*
- Absence of menarche within 1–2 years of reaching full sexual maturation (Tanner stage V)

One-quarter of females begin menstruating when they reach Tanner stage III of sexual maturation, but approximately two-thirds do not menstruate until they reach Tanner stage IV. It is important to note that several other processes occur before the onset of menstruation. Thelarche, or the beginning of breast development, takes place approximately 2–2½ years before menarche, and growth acceleration usually begins about 1 year before thelarche.

Dysmenorrhea

This condition is often accompanied by other symptoms such as nausea, vomiting, diarrhea, and headaches. It can be classified as either primary or secondary. **Primary dysmenorrhea** occurs in the absence of any pelvic pathology and is most commonly seen in adolescents once ovulatory cycles have developed. **Secondary dysmenorrhea** refers to painful menses associated with some underlying pelvic pathology, such as PID, endometriosis, ovarian cysts or tumors, or cervical stenosis. A complete list of causes of secondary amenorrhea can be found in Table 77–1. In adolescents, endometriosis is the most common cause of secondary dysmenorrhea.

Numerous studies have shown that endometrial prostaglandins play a role in the pathogenesis of primary dysmenorrhea. During menses, prostaglandin $F_{2\alpha}$ ($PGF_{2\alpha}$) is produced locally by the endometrium from arachidonic acid. $PGF_{2\alpha}$ is a potent vasoconstrictor and myometrial stimulant that causes uterine contractions and tissue ischemia. Another prostaglandin, $E_{2\alpha}$, causes hypersensitivity of the pain nerve terminals in the uterine myometrium. The cumulative effect of these

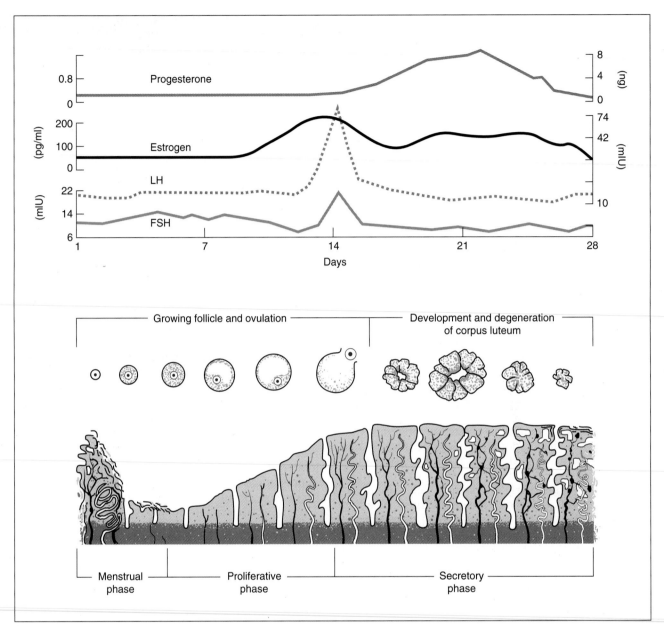

FIGURE 77–1 The normal ovulatory menstrual cycle. FSH, follicle-stimulating hormone; LH, luteinizing hormone.

prostaglandins may cause the pain of primary dysmenorrhea. Hormonal and endocrine factors may also play a role in the etiology of primary dysmenorrhea, because ovulatory cycles with estrogen and progesterone are necessary for development of the condition.

Most cases of primary dysmenorrhea begin 6–12 months after menarche, and symptoms gradually increase until patients reach their mid-20s. Parity and advancing age are associated with a decrease in symptomatology.

Dysfunctional Uterine Bleeding

Dysfunctional uterine bleeding (DUB) is defined as abnormal or excessive endometrial bleeding in the absence of any pelvic pathology. Menstruation is considered excessive if the cycles are short (< 21 days) and

the bleeding is prolonged (8 days or more). Although DUB is relatively common in adolescents, it should be considered a diagnosis of exclusion. Other causes of abnormal bleeding should first be investigated by obtaining a thorough history, performing a complete physical examination and obtaining laboratory studies as indicated.

DUB is usually the result of anovulatory, immature menstrual cycles. In adolescents, 50% of menstrual cycles are anovulatory within the first 2 years of menarche. If menarche occurs later in adolescence (i.e., at Tanner stage V), this period of anovulation reportedly lasts even longer. The majority of cases of DUB in adolescence are thought to result from the delayed maturation of the hypothalamic-pituitary-ovarian axis. Normally, a positive feedback mechanism develops with rising estrogen levels, resulting in a surge in luteinizing

---

TABLE 77–1. Differential Diagnosis of Common Menstrual Disorders

Dysmenorrhea
Primary
Secondary
Endometriosis
Pelvic inflammatory disease
Uterine myomas, polyps, or adhesions
Adenomyosis
Ovarian cysts or tumors
Presence of an intrauterine device
Cervical stenosis or strictures
Congenital malformations (i.e., septate uterus, imperforate hymen)

Abnormal Vaginal Bleeding
Dysfunctional uterine bleeding: anovulation
Complications of pregnancy: threatened/incomplete abortion, ectopic pregnancy, hydatidiform mole
Infections of the lower and upper genital tract: PID, cervicitis/vaginitis
Blood dyscrasias: vWD, ITP, leukemia, platelet defects
Endocrine disorders: hypo- and hyperthyroidism, hyperprolactinemia, late-onset 21-hydroxylase deficiency, Cushing or Addison disease
Vaginal anomalies: adenosis (DES exposure), carcinoma
Cervical/uterine abnormalities: endometriosis, polyps
Ovarian abnormalities: polycystic ovary syndrome, tumors, cysts
Systemic illness: inflammatory bowel disease, malignancy, SLE
Foreign body: condoms, tampons, IUDs
Medications: aspirin, anticoagulants, hormonal contraception
Trauma or sexual assault

Amenorrhea
Pregnancy
Systemic abnormalities: endocrinopathies (hypothyroidism, Cushing syndrome), chronic diseases (IBD, sickle cell disease), poor nutrition (anorexia nervosa), obesity, intense exercise, stress, drugs (opiates, valproate)
Hypothalamic lesions: tumors, infiltrative lesions (TB, CNS leukemia)
Pituitary lesions: prolactinoma, drugs causing elevated prolactins (marijuana, cocaine), cranial irradiation
Ovarian failure: gonadal dysgenesis, autoimmune failure, galactosemia
Congenital abnormalities of the reproductive tract: imperforate hymen, transverse vaginal septum, absence or abnormality of the uterus, complete androgen insensitivity (46, XY-testicular feminization)
Androgen excess: PCOS, benign ovarian androgen excess

Abbreviations: DES, diethylstilbestrol; IUD, intrauterine device; ITP, idiopathic thrombocytopenic purpura; PID, pelvic inflammatory disease; vWD, von Willebrand's disease; SLE, systemic lupus erythematosis; IBD, inflammatory bowel disease; PCOS, polycystic ovarian syndrome.

---

hormone (LH) and follicle-stimulating hormone (FSH), which triggers ovulation. The progesterone-producing corpus luteum then stimulates development of the secretory endometrium, with subsequent shedding after approximately 14 days (menses). With anovulation, there is no progesterone-producing corpus luteum and therefore no development of a secretory endometrium. Thus, estrogen remains unopposed, and proliferative endometrium continues to accumulate. Finally, when the tissue can no longer maintain its integrity, it sloughs. In addition, without progesterone, the normal vasospasm that helps limit endometrial bleeding does not occur. Hence, bleeding is prolonged, frequent, and heavy.

Premenstrual Syndrome

PMS refers to a group of both physical and emotional symptoms that occur prior to menses and resolve following menstruation. A variety of mechanisms have been proposed, including fluctuations in steroid hor-

mones and releasing factors, a deficiency of vitamin B_6, changes in salt and water balance, prostaglandin synthesis, and a release of endorphins and other neurotransmitters. Allergies to environmental agents and foods have also been implicated.

Amenorrhea

Amenorrhea is defined as the lack of spontaneous menstruation in women of reproductive age. Like dysmenorrhea, it can be considered primary or secondary. **Primary amenorrhea** can be further defined by the following criteria: (1) an absence of menarche by age 16 years in females with otherwise normal pubertal development, (2) an absence of menarche by the age of 14 years in females with no secondary sexual development, and (3) an absence of menarche within 1–2 years of reaching Tanner stage V pubic hair. Causes of primary amenorrhea range from congenital anatomic anomalies to genetic and endocrine conditions. A detailed discussion of each of these etiologies is beyond the scope of this chapter (see the references listed at the end of this chapter for more information).

Secondary amenorrhea occurs in females who have already established menstruation but have had no periods for 6 months or the equivalent of three cycles. The most common cause of secondary amenorrhea is pregnancy, which must be ruled out in all adolescents presenting with this complaint, regardless of their acknowledgement of sexual activity. Other causes include infections, systemic illnesses, significant weight loss, stress, exercise, eating disorders (e.g., anorexia nervosa, bulimia nervosa), and certain medications.

Vaginal Discharge

Vaginal discharge can be normal. A thin, white discharge, known as leukorrhea, occurs approximately 1 year prior to the onset of menarche. A purulent, malodorous, or bloody discharge is considered abnormal, however. Etiologies are varied and may be infectious, inflammatory, or traumatic (see Chapter 76, Sexually Transmitted Diseases and Chapter 75, Vaginitis).

DIFFERENTIAL DIAGNOSIS

The differential diagnosis of the disorders described above can be found in Table 77–1. Other etiologies of pelvic pain include midcycle menstrual disorders (e.g., mittelschmerz), UTIs, abdominal conditions such as appendicitis, inflammatory bowel disease, and irritable bowel syndrome. Psychogenic pain should also be considered as a cause of recurrent pelvic pain and may be secondary to depression, anxiety, previous sexual abuse, or another psychological condition.

EVALUATION

History

A thorough history should be obtained in adolescent females with suspected menstrual disorders because many nongynecologic conditions can affect menses. A complete psychosocial assessment should also be performed. The acronym **HEADSSS** (**h**ome environment, **e**mployment and education, **a**ctivities, **d**rugs, **s**exuality/sexual activity, **s**uicide/depression, **s**afety) serves as a useful tool when interviewing adolescents (see Chapter 4, Talking to Adolescents).

The majority of the interview should then focus on the gynecologic history (Table 77–2) and any specific problems (Questions Box). With primary dysmenorrhea, pain that radiates to the anterior thighs or the lower back is not uncommon. The color of the blood may be helpful when assessing abnormal uterine bleeding. Brown or dark blood may be associated with a cervical obstruction or endometriosis, whereas red or pink blood is found with most other conditions. More importantly, the timing of the bleeding is extremely significant. Cyclical bleeding is more consistent with a blood dyscrasia. In contrast, breakthrough bleeding throughout the cycle may indicate an infection, endometriosis, or perhaps a polyp. The passing of blood clots upon rising in the morning is not uncommon secondary to the vaginal pooling of blood while the patient is supine. Clots throughout the day, however, are not normal and require further investigation.

Physical Examination

A complete physical examination, including an evaluation for stigmata of a systemic illness, must be performed in adolescent females with suspected menstrual disorders. Patients' height and weight should be plotted on the growth chart and compared to previous measurements. Depending on the Tanner stage, physicians can then determine if they have experienced their expected growth spurt. Body mass index (BMI = weight, kg/[height, m]^2) should also be calculated and compared to previous values, especially in females with amenorrhea. Vital signs, including orthostatic measurements, are a screen for significant blood loss and are especially important in patients with excessive uterine bleeding. The skin should be inspected for any evidence of androgen excess (e.g., hirsutism, acne), bruis-

Questions: Menstrual Disorders

Dysmenorrhea

- What is the pain like?
- When did the pain first begin?
- How frequently does the pain occur?
- How long does the pain last?
- Are any symptoms associated with the pain (e.g., nausea, vomiting, diarrhea, headache)?
- Does the adolescent miss a lot of school as a result of painful menses?
- Do the painful menses interfere with other activities?
- What does the adolescent do for the pain? Has she tried any medications or home remedies?
- Is there a maternal or sibling history of painful menses?

Abnormal Uterine Bleeding

- Does the adolescent have any symptoms of anemia?
  - Is she fatigued, easily tired, dizzy, or short of breath?
  - Has she experienced any syncopal episodes?
- Does the adolescent have any history of blood loss in the urine or stool?
- Is there any evidence or a family history of a bleeding disorder (e.g., easy bruisability, bleeding from the gums or nares)?
- Does the adolescent have any symptoms of pregnancy (e.g., breast tenderness, nausea, fatigue)?
- Is there any known exposure to STDs?
- Is there a marked change in the adolescent's weight? Has the adolescent been on any diets recently?
- Is the adolescent using any medications such as aspirin, oral contraceptives, or anticoagulants?
- Does the adolescent have a history of trauma?
- Is the bleeding cyclic in nature?
- Is there breakthrough bleeding throughout the cycle?
- Does the adolescent have a family history of bleeding disorders, thyroid disease, or exposure to DES?

Amenorrhea

- Has the adolescent ever had a period?
- Has she noticed any other changes associated with puberty (e.g., breast development, pubic hair)?
- Does she have any other symptoms such as galactorrhea, weight loss, or hirsutism?
- Has the adolescent experienced significant changes in her life (e.g., parental divorce, new school)?
- How often does the adolescent exercise?
- What is the adolescent's diet?

TABLE 77–2.   Gynecologic History

Age at menarche
Last menstrual period
Regularity of menses
Duration of bleeding
Amount of flow (number of pads/tampons used per day and amount of saturation)
Associated symptoms such as bloating, headache, lower abdominal pain and cramping
Sexual activity
    Age at debut
    Number of partners and ages
    Consensual vs. nonconsensual sex
    Date of last encounter
    Protected vs. unprotected sex
    Current method of contraception
Maternal and sibling gynecologic history
    Ages at menarche
    Symptoms with menses
    Treatment of symptoms

---

ing, or petechiae. The thyroid gland should be palpated for masses or any evidence of hypertrophy, and the abdomen and suprapubic area should also be palpated for masses.

In addition, the Tanner stage of the breasts should be noted and compared to the pubic hair development, particularly in adolescents with primary amenorrhea. The presence or absence of galactorrhea should also be noted. The external genitalia should then be carefully inspected for clitoral size and patency of the hymen. A bimanual or rectoabdominal examination should be performed in adolescents who are not sexually active to assure the presence of a normal vagina, uterus, and adnexae. Depending on the findings, a speculum examination is often not necessary. In adolescents who are sexually active or desire contraception, however, complete pelvic and bimanual examinations are indicated.

Laboratory Tests

The performance of laboratory studies depends on the particular menstrual complaint. No laboratory studies are necessary for primary dysmenorrhea because the diagnosis is usually based on history and physical examination. The same is true for PMS. For a discussion of the diagnostic evaluation of amenorrhea, the reader is referred to the article by Neinstein listed in Selected Readings.

In the case of abnormal uterine bleeding, baseline studies mandate a hemoglobin or hematocrit. Initial laboratory studies should also include a CBC to evaluate the red cell indices and platelets, a reticulocyte count, and a pregnancy test. Further studies depend on the severity of the anemia and findings on history and physical examination. These may include coagulation studies (bleeding time, PT/PTT), ESR, and thyroid function tests. If the patient is sexually active, endocervical cultures for *Chlamydia trachomatis* and *Neisseria gonorrhoeae* should also be obtained. Nonculture tests of the urine to screen for gonorrhea and chlamydia are also available (e.g., LCR, PCR), however, a speculum examination is still indicated for abnormal vaginal bleeding. FSH, LH, prolactin, testosterone, and DHEA-S (dehydroepiandrosterone-sulfate) studies should be performed in patients with a history of chronic anovulation or in whom androgen excess is suspected.

Imaging Studies

A pelvic ultrasound or CT scan can be helpful in patients with abnormal uterine bleeding if a mass is suspected or palpated on physical examination.

MANAGEMENT

With each of these adolescent gynecologic conditions, effective treatment is multifaceted and includes patient and parent education, reassurance regarding the ease with which the condition can be treated, and medications. In general, a menstrual calendar or diary can be helpful to gain a more objective idea of the problem and to assess the pattern of the menstrual cycle.

Dysmenorrhea

General measures in the treatment of dysmenorrhea include education about menstruation, proper diet, application of heat, simple exercise, and psychological support.

For mild symptoms of dysmenorrhea, over-the-counter analgesics, such as ibuprofen, aspirin, or acetaminophen, are appropriate. Physicians most often suggest that patients use ibuprofen because it is probably the most efficacious. The dose is 400–600 mg every 4–6 hours. Ibuprofen should be taken at the onset of the menstrual cycle and continued for 24–72 hours.

For moderate to severe dysmenorrhea in patients who are not sexually active and do not desire birth control, a stronger **NSAID,** such as naproxen, is the treatment of choice (Table 77–3). The major mechanism of action of NSAIDs is the inhibition of prostaglandin synthesis. Side effects of these drugs, which most commonly relate to the GI tract, are nausea, vomiting, and dyspepsia. These reactions can be minimized by taking the medication with food or an antacid. Other adverse reactions include renal effects; skin reactions, such as erythema multiforme and urticaria; and CNS effects, including headache and dizziness. Contraindications to NSAID use include peptic ulcer disease, clotting disorders, and renal disease. All NSAIDs should be tried for three to four cycles before their efficacy is judged.

Low-dose combination oral contraceptives are indicated in adolescents with severe dysmenorrhea who are sexually active or in patients whose symptoms are not relieved by NSAIDs alone. Oral contraceptives decrease the production of prostaglandins by inhibiting ovulation as well as endometrial growth. Because the symptoms of dysmenorrhea are prevented only after several cycles, patients should be told not to expect complete resolution of symptoms during the first month of treatment.

Oral contraceptives should be used for a minimum of 3–4 months. If symptoms do not improve, then an NSAID can be added to the treatment regimen. Oral contraceptives are more than 90% effective in cases of severe dysmenorrhea, and physicians should emphasize this benefit to both patients and their parents.

If the patient continues to have dysmenorrhea despite the judious use of NSAIDs and oral contraceptives, a search for other pelvic pathology is warranted.

Dysfunctional Uterine Bleeding (Table 77–4)

The management of DUB depends on the severity of the bleeding. The goal of treatment is threefold: (1) to control the bleeding, (2) to correct the anemia, and (3) to replenish iron stores. Patients with mild or moderate DUB can be treated as outpatients with weekly to monthly follow-up depending on how quickly the bleeding stops. Although **combination oral contraceptives** are appropriate in the treatment of DUB if the condition is moderate or if birth control is desired, **other hormone regimens** such as estrogen (alone) or synthetic progestin (alone) can also be used.

Most adolescent females with severe bleeding and anemia require a more extensive evaluation, and

TABLE 77–3. Nonsteroidal Antiinflammatory Drugs in the Treatment of Primary Dysmenorrhea

Generic Name	Trade Names	Dosage
Ibuprofen	Motrin, Advil	400–600 mg q4–6h for 24–72 h
Naproxen	Aleve, Naprosyn	500 mg at onset, then 250 mg q4–6h
Naproxen sodium	Anaprox	500 mg at onset, then 275 mg q6–8h
Mefenamic acid	Ponstel	500 mg at onset, then 250 mg q6–8h

TABLE 77–4. General Guidelines for the Management of Dysfunctional Uterine Bleeding (DUB) in Adolescents

	Mild DUB	Moderate DUB	Severe DUB
Hemoglobin (g/dL)	> 11	9–11	< 9
Management	Menstrual calendar, oral iron, OBCP (if sexually active)	Initially, 1–4 OBCPs (⅟₃₅) qd to control the bleeding, then cycle with OBCP (⅟₃₅) for minimum of 3 mo; oral iron supplementation	Hospitalization if signs of hypovolemia; consider IV estrogen until bleeding stops; begin 2–4 OBCPs (⅟₅₀) qd and taper over 21 d, then cycle with OBCPs (⅟₃₅) for 3–6 mo; oral iron supplementation
Follow-up	2–3 mo	2–3 wk, then every 2–3 mo	1–2 wk, then every mo

Abbreviations: OBCP, oral birth control pill; (⅟₃₅), monophasic pill with 35 µg ethinyl estradiol; (⅟₅₀), monophasic pill with 50 µg ethinyl estradiol.

such patients usually must be hospitalized for appropriate parenteral therapy. Intravenous conjugated estrogens may be required every 4–6 hours for the first 24 hours to stop the bleeding. This therapy is then followed by a combination oral contraceptive containing 50 µg of estrogen (Ovral); the progesterone component is necessary to stabilize the endometrium. In addition, an antiemetic is often required during the first few days of therapy. Once bleeding is controlled, adolescents can continue Ovral for a total of 21 days and then switch to a low-dose combination oral contraceptive for at least three cycles. Studies have shown that 20–25% of adolescents who require hospitalization for severe anemia within the first year following menarche have an underlying coagulopathy. In cases of DUB where oral contraceptives are used but patients do not desire birth control, oral contraceptives should not be stopped until at least 3 months after the anemia has resolved to ensure restoration of iron stores.

Surgical treatment such as dilatation and curettage is rarely indicated in the adolescent patient and is reserved for patients refractory to medical treatment.

Premenstrual Syndrome

Although various sources have advocated many different treatment regimens for the management of PMS, no single effective treatment has been found. Therapies include diet modification for patients who complain predominantly of bloating, regular exercise, vitamin supplementation with pyridoxine (B₆), and evening primrose oil. Other medications have been used, including the antihypertensive drug clonidine, alprazolam, fluoxetine (Prozac), diuretics such as spironolactone, danazol, and mefenamic acid (Ponstel).

Vaginitis

See Chapter 75, Vaginitis, and Chapter 76, Sexually Transmitted Diseases, for a discussion of the management of vaginal discharge in adolescents.

PROGNOSIS

Most adolescents with common menstrual complaints who receive aggressive, appropriate care are symptom-free after 3–4 months of continuous therapy. Complications associated with oral contraceptive use and NSAIDs are rare in this otherwise healthy population. Symptoms associated with an immature hypothalamic-pituitary-ovarian axis such as anovulatory bleeding and DUB, often resolve spontaneously. The prognosis for adolescents with amenorrhea depends in part on the underlying etiology.

Case Resolution

In the case presented at the beginning of the chapter, more information should be obtained to exclude the numerous other causes of abnormal uterine bleeding in the adolescent before a diagnosis of DUB can be made. Questions about breast tenderness, galactorrhea, weight loss, fatigue, visual changes, prolonged bleeding, and easy bruisability can be particularly important. If the adolescent has no other complaints, a hemoglobin or hematocrit as well as a CBC and a pregnancy test should be performed. Cervical cultures should also be taken to rule out infection. Depending on the degree of anemia and the desire for contraception, the adolescent should then be placed on iron supplementation and hormonal therapy if the bleeding is significant.

Selected Readings

Bayer, S. R., and A. H. DeCherney. Clinical manifestations and treatment of dysfunctional uterine bleeding. J.A.M.A. 269:1823–1828, 1993.

Blythe, M. Common menstrual problems. Part 3, abnormal uterine bleeding. Adolesc. Health Update 4:1–5, 1992.

Braverman, P. K. and S. J. Sondheimer. Menstrual disorders. Pediatr. Rev. 18:17–25, 1997.

Cholst, I. N., and A. T. Carlon. Oral contraceptives and dysmenorrhea. J. Adolesc. Health Care 8:121–128, 1987.

Hertweck, S. P. Dysfunctional uterine bleeding. Obstet. Gynecol. Clin. North Am. 19:129–149, 1992.

Neinstein, L. S. Menstrual problems in adolescents. Med. Clin. North Am. 74:1181–1203, 1990.

O'Connell, B. J. The pediatrician and the sexually active adolescent. Treatment of common menstrual disorders. Pediatr. Clin. North Am. 44:1391–1404, 1997.

Polaneczky, M. M., and G. B. Slap. Dysmenorrhea and dysfunctional uterine bleeding. Pediatr. Rev. 13:83–87, 1992.

Polaneczky, M. M., and G. B. Slap. Menstrual disorders in the adolescent: amenorrhea. Pediatr. Rev. 13:43–48, 1992.

CHAPTER 78

DISORDERS OF THE BREAST

Monica Sifuentes, M. D.

Hx A 2-year-old girl is brought to the office for bilateral breast swelling first noticed 3 weeks ago by her mother. The swelling is nontender and does not appear to be increasing in size. There is no history of galactorrhea. The child is otherwise healthy, takes no medications, and is not using any estrogen-containing creams.

On physical examination, the vital signs are normal, and the child is at the 50th percentile for height and weight. A 1.5-cm firm, nontender mass is palpated below her left nipple. Below the right nipple, a l-cm nontender mass of similar consistency is present. There is no discharge from either nipple and no areolar widening. The abdomen is soft with no masses palpated. The genitalia are those of a normal prepubescent female with no pubic hair.

Questions

1. What is premature thelarche, and how can it be differentiated from true precocious puberty?
2. What are the most common causes of breast hypertrophy in the infant?
3. When does pubertal breast development normally occur in females?
4. What are the most common causes of breast masses in adolescent females, and how should they be managed?
5. How can transient pubertal gynecomastia be differentiated from pathologic causes of gynecomastia in young males?

Breast disorders can occur in all pediatric age groups. The neonate may present to the pediatrician with bilateral breast hypertrophy and galactorrhea or mastitis. A bewildered parent might bring in a young daughter because of early breast development. An anxious adolescent female may notice for the first time that her breasts are asymmetric, or she may feel a lump beneath the skin. An adolescent male can present with unilateral or bilateral gynecomastia that causes him severe psychological distress. Whatever the underlying cause, breast problems can be quite disconcerting at any age. Primary care providers should be equipped to differentiate between normal variants of growth and pathologic conditions in infants, children, and adolescents. Although rare, significant disorders can then be treated appropriately.

EPIDEMIOLOGY

Breast problems range from congenital anomalies and benign disorders related to hormonal stimulation to breast masses and tumors. Serious disorders such as breast cancer are practically unheard of in children and adolescents, although inappropriate breast enlargement or gynecomastia as a sign of another neoplastic process is not uncommon.

Benign breast hypertrophy can occur in 60–90% of neonates and is seen in both male and female term infants. It may occur unilaterally or bilaterally. Occasionally there is a nipple discharge.

Congenital anomalies of the breast include polythelia, athelia, polymastia, and amastia. Breast deformities such as a tuberous breast anomaly also can be thought of as a congenital anomaly, although it is not manifested until puberty when breast growth normally occurs. Polythelia, or extra nipples, can be found anywhere along the embryonic "milk line" from the axilla to the groin and is seen in 2% of the general population (Fig. 78–1). Reportedly, abnormalities of the urologic and cardiovascular systems have been associated with polythelia. Polymastia refers to supernumerary breasts along the "milk line" and is seen less frequently than polythelia (Fig. 78–2). The usual locations for supernumerary breasts are below the breast on the chest or the upper abdomen. Both polythelia and polymastia may be familial and can occur bilaterally as well as unilaterally.

Amastia (absence of a breast) and athelia (absence of a nipple) are rare occurrences, but their presence often is associated with other anomalies of the chest wall such as pectus excavatum. Amastia is also seen in Poland's syndrome (Fig. 78–3), which also includes apla-

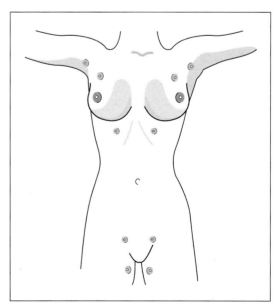

FIGURE 78–1. Polythelia. Supernumerary nipples along the embryonic mammary ridge (milk line).

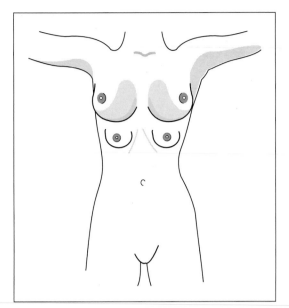

FIGURE 78–2. Polymastia. Supernumerary breasts (accessory breast tissue).

Gynecomastia commonly occurs in males progressing through puberty and is often called transient pubertal gynecomastia (Fig. 78–4). An estimated 70% of adolescent males are said to be affected, with a peak prevalence between ages 12 and 15. This generally corresponds to sexual maturity rating (SMR) (previously termed Tanner stage) 2–3 in the young male. Like breast development in the pubertal female, transient pubertal gynecomastia may be asymmetric, although concurrent or sequential involvement of both breasts can occur.

In the adolescent female, breast masses are not uncommon; however, clinically significant lesions are rare. Breast cancer *per se* has an estimated annual incidence of 0.1 : 100,000 adolescents. In most patient series through age 20, the most common breast tumor is the fibroadenoma, which has been reported in 60–95% of biopsied lesions. Two-thirds of these lesions are located in the lateral quadrants of the breast, with most in the upper outer quadrants. Their peak incidence is in late adolescence (17–21 years of age), and they tend to occur more commonly in African American females. In addition, 25% of cases are multiple fibroadenomas.

Fibrocystic changes are the second most common histologic diagnosis after fibroadenomas. Other breast masses include solitary cysts, abscesses, lipomas, and cystosarcoma phyllodes, a rare, slow-growing, painless breast tumor that is nearly always benign. Malignancy is reported in less than 1% of excised lesions. Rhabdomyosarcoma and lymphoma are among those rarely reported cancers.

NORMAL BREAST DEVELOPMENT

In the female, the first sign of puberty is breast development. This begins with the appearance of a breast bud beneath the areola. Under the influence of estrogen, there is an increase in the adipose tissue along with the beginning of ductal and stromal growth. Progesterone initiates alveolar budding and lobular growth and con-

sia of the ipsilateral pectoral muscles, various rib deformities and upper limb defects such as syndactyly (webbed fingers), and radial nerve aplasia.

Premature thelarche is isolated unilateral or bilateral breast development in girls between 1 and 4 years of age, without other signs of sexual maturation. It has been estimated that 60% of cases occur between 6 months and 2 years of age. In contrast, precocious puberty is the appearance of any sign of secondary sexual maturation before age 8 in girls or age 9 in boys. In young females, this involves both breast and pubic hair development, and in males, pubic hair and genital development.

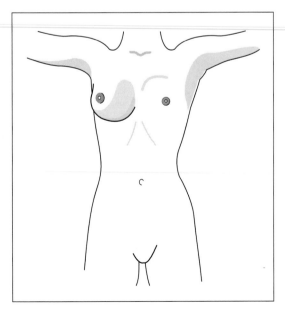

FIGURE 78–3. Amastia. Unilateral (left) complete absence of breast tissue.

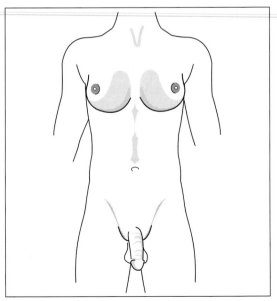

FIGURE 78–4. Gynecomastia. Breast tissue development in a male.

tributes to the development of secretory lobules and alveoli. The alveoli are later lined by milk-secreting cells under the influence of prolactin when full maturation occurs.

The normal progression of breast growth is divided into five stages or SMRs. These descriptions are used to follow normal breast development, which increases in parallel with pubic hair development. It usually takes 2–4 years for the completion of breast development, although as in all aspects of puberty variations do occur. The practitioner should keep in mind that many females will remain in SMR 3 or 4 breast development until pregnancy. Additionally, especially between SMR 2 and 4, significant breast asymmetry can be quite common in the adolescent without indicating a disorder. Once both breasts are fully mature and reach SMR 5, adequate catch-up growth usually has occurred.

CLINICAL PRESENTATION

Infants with breast disorders usually present in the first few weeks of life with bilateral breast enlargement that may be asymmetric (D_x Box). There may be an associated clear or cloudy nipple discharge. If an infection is present, the overlying skin may be warm and erythematous. Fever or other nonspecific symptoms such as poor feeding and irritability also may be present, since mastitis involves the entire breast bud and septicemia can occur.

In prepubertal females, premature thelarche will present as unilateral or bilateral nontender subareolar swelling without other secondary sexual characteristics. Girls with precocious puberty may have axillary hair, nipple and areola enlargement and thinning, and pubic hair in addition to early breast development.

Adolescent females with a breast problem often will complain of a unilateral breast lump noted incidentally by the teenager. It may be tender, fluctuant, firm, rubbery, or nodular. The adolescent may also complain of painful breasts (mastalgia) that can be cyclic in nature. For most breast masses, the overlying skin is normal, but occasionally skin changes occur. An associated nipple discharge may be present.

D_x	**Breast Disorder**

For infants, prepubescent children, and adolescent males:

- Unilateral or bilateral subareolar mass
- Possible associated nipple discharge
- Skin changes such as erythema in infants

For adolescent females:

- Firm, rubbery, freely movable mass
- Possible tenderness
- Breast asymmetry
- Skin changes such as shininess, venous distention, or dimpling (rare)
- Possible associated nipple discharge

Since most breast masses occur in females, gynecomastia is particularly anxiety-provoking in adolescent males. It usually appears as a unilateral or bilateral 2- to 3-cm firm mass beneath the areola, which may or may not be tender. There may be irritation of the skin of the nipple from rubbing against the clothing. Galactorrhea rarely accompanies pubertal gynecomastia and may indicate self-stimulation or illicit drug use, especially marijuana.

PATHOPHYSIOLOGY

Neonatal breast hypertrophy appears to be a response to maternal estrogen exposure *in utero*. Constant stimulation can cause persistent swelling, galactorrhea, and overt infection. In general, preterm infants are less responsive to maternal hormones and therefore have less breast hypertrophy. It also can be delayed for weeks.

True or central precocious puberty is due to early activation of the hypothalamic-pituitary-gonadal axis and the secretion of GnRH-dependent pituitary gonadotropins in a pulsatile pattern. Although a search for an underlying CNS or gonadal abnormality may be undertaken, most cases in females are idiopathic. In contrast, fewer than 10% of males with precocious puberty do not have an identifiable cause. CNS tumors cause precocious puberty by impinging on the neuronal pathways that inhibit the GnRH pulse generator in childhood. Cranial irradiation, received as a part of tumor therapy, also can lead to sexual precocity. Pseudoprecocious puberty is GnRH independent and is caused by the extrapituitary secretion of gonadotropins or the secretion of gonadal steroids independent of pulsatile GnRH stimulation.

Premature thelarche is a variation of normal pubertal development with transient elevations in estrogen levels from either functional ovarian cysts or fluctuations in pituitary gonadotropin secretion. Often the breast enlargement occurs without other estrogen effects such as an increase in uterine size or changes in the appearance of the external genitalia. In addition, no linear growth or bone age advancement is associated with this condition.

The cause of fibroadenomas in adolescent females is postulated to be an abnormal sensitivity to estrogen. Observations supporting this hypothesis include the presence of estrogen receptors in the tumor and an increased incidence of this type of tumor during late adolescence. Thus, prolonged exposure to estrogen may play a role in its development. Enlargement can occur during pregnancy or toward the end of the menstrual cycle.

Transient pubertal galactorrhea is thought to occur from a temporary imbalance of estrogen and androgens. Alterations in the ratio of these hormones leads to an increase in estrogen relative to testosterone. Certain medications can cause elevations in serum prolactin and lead to gynecomastia and/or galactorrhea (Table 78–1). Some drugs, such as marijuana, contain phytoestrogens that can mimic estrogen or stimulate estrogen receptor sites. Others (e.g., spironolactone,

TABLE 78-1. Causes of Galactorrhea*

Mechanical stimulation of the nipple
Drugs
  Estrogenic drugs
    Digitalis
    Marijuana
    Heroin
  Dopamine receptor blockers
    Phenothiazines
    Haloperidol
    Metoclopramide
    Isoniazid
  Dopamine depleters
    Tricyclic antidepressants
    Reserpine
    Methyldopa
    Cimetidine
    Benzodiazepines
Hypothalamic-pituitary disorders

*Reproduced, with permission, from O'Grady, L. F. Nonmalignant breast disease. *In* O'Grady, L. F., et al. (eds.). A Practical Approach to Breast Disease, Boston, MA, Little, Brown and Company, 1995, pp. 9–22.

cimetidine) interfere with androgen receptors or induce inhibition of enzymes needed in steroid synthesis.

DIFFERENTIAL DIAGNOSIS

The differential diagnosis of breast disorders in children and adolescents depends on gender and age at onset. In addition, the presence or absence of other secondary sexual characteristics is helpful to differentiate between a variation of normal pubertal development and a pathologic process.

Infants and Children Under 9 Years of Age

In prepubertal children, the differential diagnosis of isolated early breast development includes exposure to exogenous sources of estrogen such as skin creams, make-up, and medications (oral contraceptives).

For patients with suspected precocious puberty, other etiologies must be considered in addition to exogenous hormones (Table 78–2). Central nervous system tumors, lesions, and insults are among the most common causes. Congenital tumors such as hypothalamic hamartomas are especially important to rule out, since they often present before age 3. Other CNS tumors to consider are neurofibromas, optic gliomas, astrocytomas, and ependymomas. Specific CNS lesions include cysts in the area of the third ventricle and congenital brain defects. Hydrocephalus, postinfectious encephalitis or meningitis, head trauma, and static cerebral encephalopathy also can lead to sexual precocity. Endocrine disorders include hypothyroidism, estrogen-producing tumors of the ovary or adrenal gland, and ovarian cysts.

Adolescents

The differential diagnosis of breast masses in adolescent females is extensive (Table 78–3). Conditions can

TABLE 78-2. Differential Diagnosis of Precocious Puberty*

Central (true)—GnRH-dependent
Idiopathic
  CNS
    Tumor
      Optic and hypothalamic gliomas (often associated with neurofibromatosis), hypothalamic hamartoma, astrocytoma, ependymoma, craniopharyngioma
    Lesion
      Congenital defects, hydrocephalus, cyst in the third ventricle
    Insult
      Postinfectious encephalitis or meningitis, static encephalopathy
    Infection
      Abscess, tuberculous granulomas of the hypothalamus
    Head trauma
    Sequela of cranial radiation
    Sarcoid granuloma
  Endocrine
    Hypothyroidism (mechanism unknown)
  Secondary to GnRH-independent precocious puberty (21-hydroxylase deficiency, McCune-Albright syndrome)
Peripheral (pseudo-)—GnRH-independent
  Adrenal
    Tumor
      21- or 11-Hydroxylase deficiency
  Gonadal
    Tumor
      McCune-Albright syndrome
      Familial testotoxicosis
  Ectopic hCG-secreting tumor
  Exogenous steroids

*Modified and reproduced, with permission, from Kulin, H. E., and J. Muller. The biological aspects of puberty. Pediatr. Rev. 17:84, 1996.

be distinguished from each other based on the location of the lesion; its texture, mobility, and size; and how rapidly it is enlarging.

Gynecomastia is classified as type I or II. Type I is benign adolescent male hypertrophy. The differential diagnosis for type II includes physiologic gynecomastia (no evidence of an underlying disease process), organic disorders, and side effects of medications (Table 78–4). Types I and II also can be differentiated by the size of the breast tissue: enlargement up to 3 cm is type I; enlargement beyond the areolar perimeter is type II.

Persistent galactorrhea can be caused by several conditions in addition to excessive stimulation from sexual activity or jogging without a support bra. Disorders include neurologic, hypothalamic, pituitary, and endocrine causes. Common causes in the adolescent female

TABLE 78-3. Most Common Causes of Breast Masses in the Adolescent Female

Fibroadenoma
Juvenile (giant) fibroadenoma
Cystosarcoma phyllodes
Breast abscess
Breast cyst
Breast carcinoma
Fat necrosis (secondary to trauma)
Lipoma
Hematoma
Papilloma

**TABLE 78–4. Causes of Type II Gynecomastia
in the Adolescent Male***

Idiopathic
Tumors
    Seminomas, Leydig cell tumor, teratoma, feminizing adrenal tumor, hepatoma,
        bronchogenic sarcoma (ectopic HCG production)
Thyroid dysfunction (hyper- and hypothyroidism)
Renal failure and dialysis
Cirrhosis of the liver
Klinefelter's syndrome (XXY)
Testicular feminization syndrome
Drugs
    Marijuana, amphetamines, heroin, methadone
    Anabolic steroids
    Birth control pills
    Cimetidine
    Digitalis
    Spironolactone
    Tricyclic antidepressants
    Isoniazid
    Ketoconazole
Pseudogynecomastia (adipose tissue in obese male)

---

*Modified and reproduced, with permission, from Greydanus, D. E., D. S. Parks, and E. G. Farrell. Breast disorders in children and adolescents. Pediatr. Clin. North Am. 36:634, 1989.

---

are prolactin-secreting tumors and hypothyroidism. Drugs that induce galactorrhea in females are the same ones that cause gynecomastia in males (see Tables 78–1 and 78–4).

EVALUATION

History

In the infant or child, the history should focus on endogenous as well as exogenous sources of estrogen (Questions Box). With teenagers, it is important to rule out drug use and systemic illness. All adolescent patients should be interviewed alone, especially when asked about illicit substance use (see Chapter 108, Substance Abuse). The adolescent male may feel particularly embarrassed given the nature of his visit; thus, the clinician should be especially sympathetic during the interview.

Physical Examination

The physical examination includes an assessment of the patient's growth, especially in cases of suspected precocious puberty. The height and weight should be plotted on the growth curve and compared with previous measurements. Accelerations in height occur in sexual precocity. Excessive weight gain should be noted, since general obesity can stimulate breast enlargement in young females and gynecomastia in males.

The extent of the breast examination depends on the age of the patient. In infants and young children, the breast tissue should be measured and the size recorded so that growth can be monitored over time. Consistency of the tissue and mobility also should be evaluated. Breast growth as a result of neonatal breast hypertrophy and premature thelarche is nontender, firm, and freely mobile. The nipple should be examined for a clear or cloudy discharge by gently compressing each one separately.

In the adolescent female, the breast examination should include visual inspection of the breasts as well as palpation of any lesion and axillary nodes. Ideally this would be performed in the sitting and supine positions as is done in adult women. Most adolescent females, however, would be uncomfortable with so extensive an examination. The physician must take the time to explain the reasons for the examination to help the patient feel less self-conscious.

Visual inspection should assess for SMR, appearance of the skin, breast asymmetry, and evidence of trauma. Shiny skin or superficial venous distention on one breast would indicate the presence of a large mass. A peau d'orange (orange peel) appearance of the skin or erythema and warmth should be noted as a sign of an infiltrative lesion or infection, respectively.

Palpation of the breast mass can be accomplished with the patient in the supine position using one of three methods. Using the second, third, and fourth fingers of one hand, the examiner should gently palpate each breast in a pattern of concentric circles, spokes of a wheel, or vertical and horizontal lines. The location of the mass should be noted; a mass beneath the areola might indicate an intraductal lesion, whereas the upper

---

Questions: Breast Disorder

For prepubertal children:
- How old is the child?
- When was the breast mass first noted?
- Does it seem to be increasing in size?
- Is it tender?
- Is there associated discharge from the nipple?
- Has the child been exposed to any estrogen-containing skin creams or medications?
- In the male patient, is he taking any medications known to cause gynecomastia, such as digoxin?
- Is the child experiencing any neurologic symptoms such a headaches, ataxia, or visual disturbances?
- Is there a past history of head trauma, CNS infection or insult?
- Has the parent noted any other signs of early pubertal development (e.g., pubic hair, acne, sudden inappropriate increase in height)?

For the adolescent:
- When was the breast mass first noticed, and where is it located?
- Does it seem to be increasing in size?
- Is the lesion tender?
- Is there a history of trauma to the breast?
- Is there any discharge from either nipple?
- In the female, when was the last menstrual period?
- Is there a history of headache or visual disturbances?
- Are there any signs or symptoms of systemic illness, such as weight loss?
- Is there a family history of breast cancer in a close relative, particularly the mother?
- In the male, is he taking any medications that can cause gynecomastia, such as cimetidine?
- Is the adolescent male using anabolic steroids?
- Is the adolescent using any other illicit substances such as marijuana or heroin?

outer quadrant is the classic location for a fibroadenoma. The consistency of the lesion is important. Is it firm, rubbery, and fluctuant, or irregular and lumpy? Is it freely movable, or attached to the chest wall? Fibroadenomas tend to be firm, discrete, freely movable, and rubbery. A tender, poorly defined mass is consistent with a contusion; a hematoma is more sharply defined with associated skin ecchymoses. Fat necrosis can develop after trauma and is painless, firm, well circumscribed, and mobile. The size of the mass should be measured and recorded. One must keep in mind that size of tumor does not correlate with malignant potential. Finally, each nipple should be gently squeezed for a discharge. If present, note whether it is clear, milky, or bloody. A serosanguineous or sanguineous discharge would indicate the presence of an intraductal mass. In addition, a retracted nipple indicates involvement of the areolar area.

The examiner should also palpate for axillary lymphadenopathy. Although most clinicians think of its association with breast cancer, it also may be found with infection or necrosis of a benign tumor.

In the adolescent male, in addition to palpation of the breast tissue, it is important to determine the SMR of the genitalia to determine whether it is consistent with pubertal gynecomastia The testicles should be palpated carefully for masses and evidence of atrophy (decrease in testicular size). In addition, findings suggestive of hypo- or hyperthyroidism or liver disease must be noted.

A detailed neurologic examination should be performed, especially in children with sexual precocity.

Laboratory Assessment

The laboratory workup for breast disorders is dictated by the findings on history and physical examination. Isolated neonatal breast hyperplasia and premature thelarche require no laboratory studies. Serum gonadotropin concentrations (LH and FSH) and estradiol level should be obtained in girls with precocious puberty. In addition, a testosterone level should be ordered in boys. Based on these results, further studies may be indicated.

For most breast lesions in adolescent females, no laboratory studies are needed A fine needle aspiration (FNA) of the lesion may be performed for those cases which appear to be cystic or if the diagnosis is uncertain. The aspirated fluid should be sent for cytologic analysis if the mass does not completely disappear with this procedure. Sometimes it is necessary to perform the procedure to relieve patient and parental anxiety. An excisional biopsy of the mass allows for more accurate histologic information but is rarely needed for most lesions.

In the healthy adolescent male with no evidence of systemic illness and no history of drug use, no further laboratory studies are necessary. If pubertal gynecomastia and other systemic illnesses are ruled out, an endocrine workup is appropriate to elucidate the cause of nonpubertal gynecomastia. This should begin with

levels of hCG, LH, and serum testosterone and estradiol. If these laboratory studies are normal, the diagnosis is idiopathic gynecomastia. If they are abnormal, consultation with a pediatric endocrinologist or adolescent medicine specialist should occur.

A pregnancy test and serum prolactin level should be ordered in the adolescent female with galactorrhea, regardless of the menstrual history.

Imaging Studies

Hand and wrist radiographs to determine the child's bone age should be obtained in children with a diagnosis of precocious puberty. In boys with this diagnosis, MRI of the head also should be obtained to evaluate for a CNS lesion. Depending on the history, an MRI may be indicated in some girls. Pelvic ultrasound, although rarely necessary, can be performed to rule out the presence of an ovarian tumor in girls.

Mammograms are not helpful in the pediatric age group, especially in adolescents, and are never indicated in the evaluation of a breast mass. They can be very difficult to interpret because of the dense breast tissue of adolescents. In addition, the risk of breast malignancy is very low. An ultrasound may help distinguish between a cystic lesion and a solid tumor. It can also provide more accurate measurement of the size of the lesion and its location prior to the FNA.

A testicular ultrasound to search for a tumor is indicated in the adolescent male if the level of hCG or estradiol is elevated.

MANAGEMENT

In neonates, mastitis most often is caused by *Staphylococcus aureus* and group B streptococcus. Gram-negative bacilli also have been reported. Parenteral antibiotics should be initiated when the diagnosis is made. Incision and drainage of a breast abscess should only be undertaken by an experienced physician familiar with the anatomy of the breast to minimize the likelihood of injury to the affected breast bud.

Congenital anomalies such as polythelia and polymastia do not require any treatment. If, however, the patient or parent wants the tissue removed for aesthetic or psychological reasons, it is recommended to do so before puberty. Reconstructive surgery for amastia, as in Poland's syndrome, is typically delayed until late adolescence to allow full development of the unaffected breast.

Although no treatment is required for premature thelarche, parents need to be reassured that the condition is self-limited. The patient should be reexamined periodically to check for any further progression of puberty, such as persistent breast growth for the appearance of pubic hair.

The treatment for central precocious puberty is directed at controlling the secondary sexual development with GnRH agonists. When GnRH is administered continuously, gonadotropin secretion decreases. Currently, leuprolide acetate is the only GnRH agonist available for use in the United States. Children should be followed every 1–3 months in conjunction with a pediatric endocrinologist to monitor their progression and response to therapy.

Unless otherwise indicated by the type of tumor, children with a CNS lesion as a cause of precocious puberty usually do not need neurosurgical intervention. Therapy should focus on the degree of growth acceleration and the desire to influence secondary sexual characteristics.

Most breast masses in adolescent females that are small, well-demarcated, firm or rubbery, and nontender benefit from the "wait and watch" approach. The patient can be followed for 2–4 months, preferably allowing a few menstrual cycles to pass. If there is no change in the lesion or just a small increase in its size, no studies or procedures are indicated, since it is most likely a fibroadenoma. As previously noted, a biopsy may be requested to relieve the anxiety that accompanies the presence of a breast lesion. Total excision of the tumor mass and a careful histologic evaluation may be warranted in some cases. Surgical removal of rapidly enlarging tumors such as a giant fibroadenoma is important. When the lesion becomes very large, an acceptable cosmetic result is more difficult. Accordingly, the lesion should be removed shortly after the time of diagnosis rather than "waiting and watching."

The primary treatment for transient pubertal gynecomastia, or type I, is reassurance for the adolescent male and his family that the condition is self-limited and should resolve in 1–2 years. The teenager should be told explicitly that he is not "becoming a girl." In most cases, he should be reexamined periodically until resolution occurs. Type II gynecomastia may need surgical reduction of the mammary gland. Plastic surgery intervention is warranted for cases of persistent breast growth or moderate to severe gynecomastia (SMR 3–4 breasts) with psychological difficulties. Surgical correction involves a combination of liposuction and direct excision of the breast tissue beneath the nipple and areola. The young man may benefit from concurrent psychological counseling as well.

PROGNOSIS

The prognosis of a breast disorder in the child or adolescent depends on the particular lesion. In general, most lesions such as neonatal breast hyperplasia and premature thelarche are self-limited and resolve on their own. Breast development persists for 3–5 years in 50% of cases of premature thelarche, but in one retrospective study, most cases regressed within 6 months to 6 years after the diagnosis. Aside from the short stature that may accompany idiopathic central precocious puberty, these females also tend to have a good prognosis. Fibroadenomas in the adolescent female can recur but typically are benign and have no proven link to the development of breast cancer. Most cases of transient pubertal gynecomastia resolve within 1–2 years.

Case Resolution

The child in the case history has a diagnosis of premature thelarche. She has no known exposure to exogenous sources of estrogen and has isolated breast tissue development with no other signs of pubertal maturation. Her parents should be informed of this diagnosis and reassured that the condition is self-limited and does not indicate that the child is starting puberty. The child should be scheduled for a follow-up visit in 3–4 months to remeasure the breast buds and reexamine the genitalia for the appearance of pubic hair.

Selected Readings

Braunstein, G. D. Gynecomastia. N. Engl. J. Med. 328:490–495, 1993.

Denk, M. J. Topics in plastic surgery. Pediatr. Clin. North Am. 45:1479–1506, 1998.

Hindle, W. H, and E. Y. Pan. Breast disorders in female adolescents. Adolesc. Med. State Art Rev. 5:123–129, 1994.

Greydanus, D. E., D. S. Parks, and E. G. Farrell. Breast disorders in children and adolescents. Pediatr. Clin. North Am. 36:601-638, 1989.

Klein, K. O., et al. Estrogen levels in girls with premature thelarche compared with normal prepubertal girls as determined by an ultrasensitive recombinant cell bioassay. J. Pediatr. 134:190–192, 1999.

Kulin, H. E., and J. Muller. The biological aspects of puberty. Pediatr. Rev. 17:75–86, 1996.

Neinstein, L. S. Breast disorders; Gynecomastia. In Adolescent Health Care: A Practical Guide. Baltimore, MD, Williams & Wilkins, 1996, pp. 840–849; 210–214.

O'Grady, L. F. Nonmalignant breast disease. In O'Grady, L. F., et al. (Eds.). A Practical Approach to Breast Disease. Boston, MA, Little, Brown, 1995, pp. 9–22.

Simmons, P. S. Diagnostic considerations in breast disorders of children and adolescents. Obstet. Gynecol. Clin. North Am. 19:91–102, 1992.

Styne, D. M. New aspects in the diagnosis and treatment of pubertal disorders. Pediatr. Clin. North Am. 44:505–529, 1997.

ORTHOPEDIC DISORDERS

CHAPTER 79

DEVELOPMENTAL HIP DYSPLASIA

Geeta Grover, M.D.

Hx A 4-month-old girl is seen for her routine health maintenance visit. She is doing well and has no complaints. The results of the entire examination are within normal limits except for limited abduction of the left hip, which is approximately 45 degrees, in comparison to that of the right hip, which is almost 90 degrees.

Questions

1. What specific physical maneuvers help in the evaluation of infants with decreased range of motion of the hip?
2. What are the clinical findings of hip dislocation during and after the neonatal period?
3. What are some of the conditions often seen in conjunction with hip dysplasia that may be noted on physical examination?
4. What is the appropriate diagnostic workup of infants with suspected hip dysplasia?

Developmental hip dysplasia (developmental dysplasia of the hip, DDH) defines a range of hip pathology, from frank dislocation to instability. DDH may either exist at birth or develop during infancy. The term DDH has replaced the term congenital hip dysplasia (CHD), because hip dysplasia may not always be apparent or present during the newborn period. DDH is a common pediatric orthopedic concern. When DDH is recognized and treated appropriately, children potentially develop completely normally. If the diagnosis is missed or delayed, however, children may suffer significant morbidity, including severe degenerative hip disease.

EPIDEMIOLOGY

The incidence of neonatal hip instability is estimated to range from 11.5–17:1000 live births. Approximately 50% of these cases resolve by 1 week of age, and 90% resolve by 2 months of age, which gives a true incidence of hip dislocation of 1–1.5:1000 live births. Approximately 60% of affected infants are first-born. Girls are affected six to eight times more frequently than boys.

Incidence is increased among Caucasians (compared to African Americans), with breech presentation (approximately 20% of all dislocations occur in infants born in the breech position), and with a positive family history. The left hip is involved in 60% of children with DDH and the right hip in 20% of cases, and 20% of the time DDH is bilateral. DDH has an increased association with lesions believed to be secondary to mechanical molding such as congenital torticollis (approximately 20% of affected children may have DDH) and metatarsus adductus (approximately 2–10% of these children may have DDH).

CLINICAL PRESENTATION

The clinical presentation and signs of DDH in children vary with age. Diagnosis is made primarily by physical examination (e.g., Ortolani and Barlow maneuvers) during the neonatal period. Asymmetric skin folds, limitation of hip abduction, and a positive Galeazzi's sign are the classic signs of DDH in older infants. Physical signs, which become more obvious once children are walking, include limping and toe-walking (D_x Box).

PATHOPHYSIOLOGY

DDH encompasses a wide variety of conditions ranging from hip instability to dislocation. A dislocated hip is one in which there is complete loss of contact between the femoral head and the acetabulum. The

---

D_x Developmental Hip Dysplasia

- Breech presentation
- Female sex
- Asymmetric skin folds
- Limitation of hip abduction
- Positive Galeazzi's sign
- Limp
- Toe-walking

dislocation may be reducible using the Ortolani test (see below) or nonreducible. Nonreducible dislocations are usually teratologic and associated with other serious malformations such as arthrogryposis or spina bifida. An unstable hip is one in which the femoral head is within the acetabulum but may be dislocated using the Barlow test (see below).

Dysplasia of the acetabulum is also associated with hip instability. The dysplastic acetabular cavity is shallower with a more vertical inclination than normal. An understanding of the pathophysiology that relates primarily to ligamentous laxity and bony abnormalities of the acetabular cavity enables one to see that although most dislocations occur at or near the time of delivery, they can occur later in infancy as well. Late hip dislocations are reported in 3–8% of affected infants.

The etiology of DDH involves mechanical, physiologic, and environmental factors. The primary **mechanical factors** are tight maternal abdominal and uterine musculature, breech presentation (especially frank breech presentation with the knees in extension), and positioning of the fetal hip against the mother's sacrum. *In utero* mechanical factors relate to molding and restriction of fetal movement. It is believed that the tight, unstretched maternal abdomen and uterine musculature of primigravidas may prevent fetal movement, thus predisposing first-born infants to DDH. The increased occurrence of other conditions thought to be secondary to molding (e.g., congenital muscular torticollis) with DDH supports this theory of space restriction. **Physiologic factors** relate to ligamentous laxity. Female infants may be more sensitive to maternal hormones such as estrogen and relaxin, which are present around the time of delivery, resulting in generalized ligamentous laxity, including laxity of the hip capsule. **Environmental factors** that may predispose infants to DDH include swaddling with the legs in extension and adduction, which is still practiced in some societies (e.g., those who use cradleboards, such as Navajos in North America), and muscle contractures secondary to neuromuscular disease such as cerebral palsy.

DIFFERENTIAL DIAGNOSIS

The differential diagnosis of hip dysplasia depends on the age of the child and the presenting complaint. Infants may have a "click" on abduction of the hip that represents the snapping of a ligament rather than the reduction of the dislocated hip into the joint. Infants who have limited abduction may have a neuromuscular disorder such as spastic diplegia. Older children who present with gait disturbances such as limp, waddling gait, or toe-walking may have neuromuscular conditions, fractures, or infection (e.g., osteomyelitis, septic arthritis).

EVALUATION

History

Family history of DDH should be reviewed. A careful neonatal history detailing the type of presentation (e.g.,

---

Questions: Developmental Hip Dysplasia

- Was the infant a breech presentation?
- Does the child have any muscular problems, such as torticollis?
- When did the gait disturbance begin?
- Does anything make the child's gait better or worse?
- Is the child in any pain?
- Did any member of the family have hip dysplasia?

---

breech versus vertex), type of delivery, history of prenatal problems such as oligohydramnios, and presence of congenital torticollis or metatarsus adductus should also be taken (Questions Box).

Physical Examination

It is important to evaluate the hip joint for instability or dislocation throughout the first year of life or until the child begins to walk. The **Ortolani and Barlow maneuvers** may be used in the neonatal period to evaluate for DDH (Fig. 79–1). Both tests are performed with infants in a supine position and the hips and knees flexed to 90 degrees. Infants should be quiet and relaxed. Adequate results are difficult to obtain with crying or fussy infants.

In the Ortolani maneuver, a palpable "thunk" or "clunk" as the examiner relocates a dislocated hip by gentle abduction and lifting of the femoral head anteriorly is a positive result. This "clunk" differs from the audible hip click, which is secondary to nonpathologic processes such as ligamentous snapping. Each leg should be examined separately, not simultaneously. The Barlow maneuver attempts to dislocate the hip by adduction and posterior axial pressure on the thigh. These tests are not useful after approximately 6–8 weeks of age, because the surrounding soft tissues and muscles adapt to the dislocated hip, making it more difficult to reduce.

After the neonatal period, several tests can be used to assess hip stability (Fig. 79–2). Asymmetry of hip abduction is secondary to adductor muscle shortening and contracture on the affected side. This asymmetry is one of the simplest ways to evaluate for hip dislocation. Children under the age of 8 weeks should achieve full abduction (90 degrees) with both knees touching the examination table, often even in the presence of hip dysplasia. After this age, with children supine, hips and knees flexed, and both legs abducted simultaneously, abduction limited to less than 60 degrees or asymmetry between the two sides may indicate dislocation. This test, however, is difficult to interpret with bilateral dislocation because no side is "normal."

As the femoral head dislocates posteriorly, the thigh is shortened on the affected side, producing an asymmetry of skin folds or a discrepancy in knee heights. Asymmetric gluteal folds result from bunching of skin and subcutaneous tissue on the affected side, thus producing extra skin folds. Galeazzi's sign refers to the discrepancy in knee heights noted when infants are supine with the sacrum flat on the examination table and hips and knees bent.

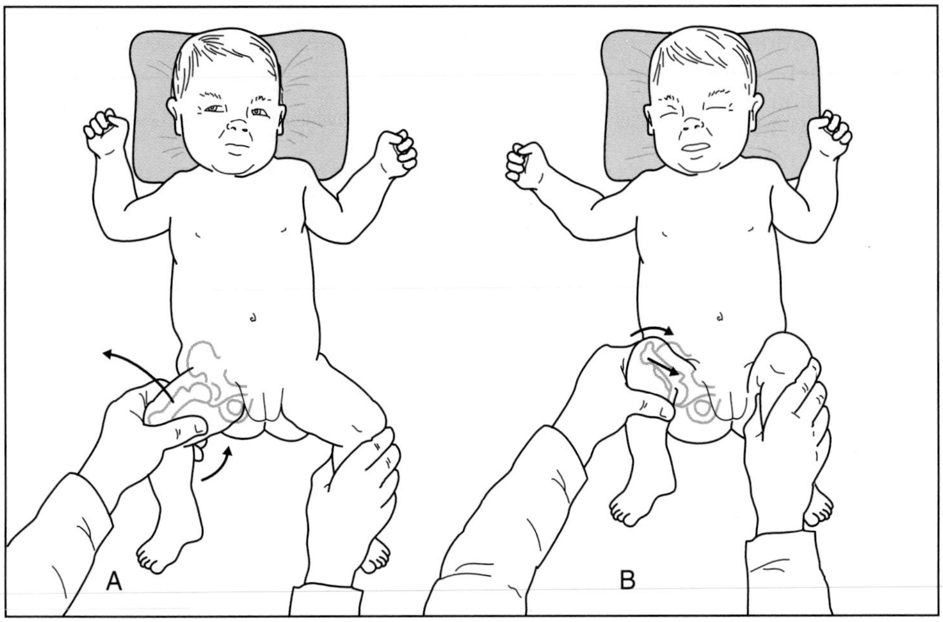

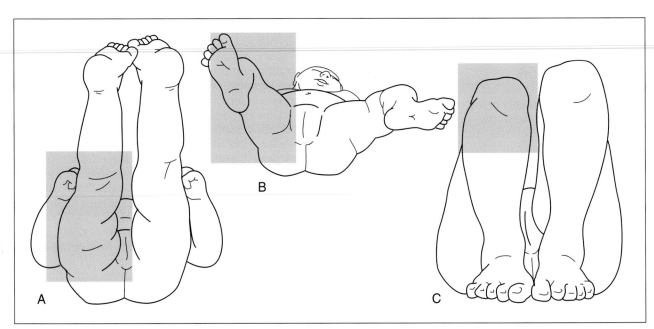

FIGURE 79–1. Ortolani and Barlow tests.
A. Ortolani (reduction) test. **B.** Barlow (dislocation) test.

In children of walking age, the physician may notice a limp secondary to shortening of the leg on the affected side, leading to a leg length discrepancy. (Children may try to disguise the limp by toe-walking.) A Trendelenburg test may be positive. Normally, when a child stands on one leg, the hip abductors straighten the pelvis and keep the center of gravity over the femoral head. If the abductors are weak, the weight shifts to the opposite side, causing it to droop. Children with bilateral dislocations display hyperlordosis of the lumbar spine with a waddling type of gait.

Imaging Studies

Radiologic and ultrasound evaluations may aid in the diagnosis. Ultrasonography can be quite useful in the diagnosis of DDH, especially in the neonatal period when x-ray changes may not be evident because the femoral head is not calcified. Reliable x-ray changes begin to become evident at about 4–6 months of age when the ossific nucleus of the femoral head appears in most infants (Fig. 79–3). A flat, shallow acetabulum and delayed ossification of the femoral head are the simplest, most easily recognized findings.

FIGURE 79–2. Late signs in the diagnosis of developmental dysplasia of the hip. A. Asymmetry of thigh folds. **B.** Asymmetry of hip abduction. **C.** Discrepancy of knee heights.

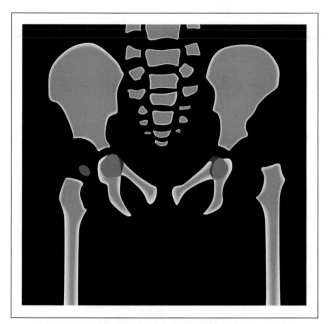

FIGURE 79–3. Radiographic findings associated with developmental dysplasia of the hip. The left hip is dislocated. The femur is lateral and proximal, and the acetabulum is shallow and flat, and there is delayed ossification of the femoral head, as evidenced by the absence of the ossific nucleus on the left.

MANAGEMENT

The need for repeat examinations of the hips during the first year of life cannot be overemphasized. Children suspected of any hip instability or any children with less than 60 degrees of hip abduction should be evaluated with appropriate imaging studies and referred to an orthopedic surgeon for further evaluation and management. An orthopedic surgeon can aid the primary care physician in the management of DDH.

The goal of treatment is to return the femoral head to its normal position within the acetabulum and restore normal hip functioning. The common practice of triple diapering should be discouraged because it is unreliable, often delays definitive therapy, and may produce complications (e.g., avascular necrosis of the femoral head). The **Pavlik harness** is the primary method of treating DDH during infancy. When properly used, the harness holds the hips in a flexed and abducted position while allowing infants to move their legs within safe limits of abduction and adduction until stability is achieved. The harness should be applied and monitored by an orthopedic surgeon, because inappropriate application also may produce adverse outcomes (e.g., avascular necrosis of the femoral head). Treatment should be continued for about 4 weeks in newborns and for a period equal to approximately one to two times the child's age at the time treatment is started in other children.

If this treatment method is ineffective or the diagnosis is not made until after 6 months of age, **traction** followed by either open or closed **reduction and spica cast immobilization** may be used. Good results are more difficult to obtain with increasing age, especially after children are walking. Operative treatment (e.g., open reduction) is usually required in children over the age of 18 months. Additional procedures may be required in older children, especially those over the age of 36 months, including (1) **femoral osteotomy** either to shorten the femur or to correct femoral antetorsion and (2) **pelvic osteotomy** to correct acetabular dysplasia.

PROGNOSIS

The prognosis of DDH depends on age at the time of diagnosis and severity of the deformity. The long-term prognosis for satisfactory hip function is good for children when DDH is recognized early and treated appropriately. Generally, children with DDH that is diagnosed after the first year of life have a poorer prognosis for satisfactory hip function than those with DDH that is diagnosed during infancy. Left untreated, DDH may result in significant disability, ranging from limp to pain and stiffness in the hip.

Case Resolution

The infant presented in the case history has less than 60 degrees of abduction of the left hip, a sign of DDH. An anteroposterior view of the pelvis may be ordered to confirm the diagnosis. Regardless of the radiographic findings, the infant should be referred to an orthopedic surgeon for further evaluation and management. If hip dislocation is confirmed, the initial treatment will probably involve bracing with the Pavlik harness.

Selected Readings

Aronsson, D. D., et al. Developmental dysplasia of the hip. Pediatrics 94:201–208, 1994.

Ballock, R. T., and B. S. Richards. Hip dysplasia: early diagnosis makes a difference. Contemp. Pediatr. 14:108–117, 1997.

Bialik, V., G. M. Bialik, S. Blazer, et al. Developmental dysplasia of the hip: A new approach to incidence. Pediatrics 103:93–99, 1999.

Bond, C. D., W. L. Hennrikus, and E. D. DellaMaggiore. Prospective evaluation of newborn soft-tissue hip "clicks" with ultrasound. J. Pediatr. Orthop. 17:199–201, 1997.

Hensinger, R. N. Congenital dislocation of the hip: treatment in infancy to walking age. Ortho. Clin. North Am. 18:597–615, 1987.

Mooney, J. F., and J. B. Emans. Developmental dislocation of the hip: a clinical overview. Pediatr. Rev. 16:299–303, 1995.

Novacheck, T. F. Developmental dysplasia of the hip. Pediatr. Clin. North Am. 43:829–848, 1996.

Theophilopoulos, E. P., and D. J. Barrett. Get a grip on the pediatric hip. Contemp. Pediatr. 15:43–65, 1998.

ROTATIONAL PROBLEMS OF THE LOWER EXTREMITY: IN-TOEING AND OUT-TOEING

Geeta Grover, M.D.

Hx A 3-year-old girl is brought to the office. Her mother is concerned because beginning a few months ago her daughter's feet appeared to "turn in" when she walked. The girl has never walked like this before, and she has no history of trauma, fever, pain, or swelling in the joints. The physical examination is within normal limits except for the in-toeing gait.

Questions

1. How can observation of children's gaits help determine the etiology of their in-toeing and out-toeing (rotational problems)?
2. What are the common causes of in-toeing and out-toeing?
3. Does evaluation of in-toeing and out-toeing require any laboratory or radiologic studies?
4. What is the natural history of most rotational problems?

Rotational problems of the lower extremities, especially in-toeing, frequently occur during the first several years of life. Although rotational problems that produce in-toeing and out-toeing rarely lead to physical limitations in children, they are a common cause of parental concern during infancy and childhood. The large majority of these problems can be managed adequately by primary care physicians and do not necessitate orthopedic referral. Clubfoot, which is not a rotational deformity but a pathologic one, is included in this discussion because it is often confused with conditions of the feet that produce in-toeing.

EPIDEMIOLOGY

In neonates or young infants, in-toeing is most likely the result of clubfoot (talipes equinovarus), isolated metatarsus adductus, or metatarsus varus. The incidence of clubfoot is 1:1000 live births, with a male-to-female ratio of 2 to 1. The condition is bilateral in approximately 50% of cases. The incidence of metatarsus adductus, a much more common problem, is about 2:1000 live births. It is often bilateral. Medial tibial torsion is the primary cause of in-toeing in the second year of life, and medial femoral torsion (femoral anteversion) accounts for most cases of this condition during early childhood.

Physiologic out-toeing is classically evident in infants who have not yet begun to walk. This condition, which is believed to be secondary to an external rotatory contracture about the hip due to intrauterine positioning, is the most common cause of out-turning in both feet. Lateral tibial torsion may result in out-toeing in older infants and children.

CLINICAL PRESENTATION

Children with congenital clubfoot, metatarsus adductus, and metatarsus varus present with in-toeing during infancy. Congenital clubfoot is usually readily evident at birth. A severe medial, midline, plantar crease is present, and the foot appears C-shaped, with both the heel and forefront turned inward. The affected foot is small, wide, and stiff, and the lower leg appears small due to hypoplasia of the calf muscles. In contrast to clubfoot, only the forefoot turns inward in metatarsus adductus and varus.

Medial tibial torsion is apparent during the second year of life. Children's feet turn inward as they walk, but their knees point straight. Medial femoral torsion is evident at 3–4 years of age. Affected children are usually girls; they can sit in the "W" position with both legs behind them. As children walk, both the knees and the feet appear to turn inward.

Physiologic out-toeing is seen in infancy. Classically, parents note that when they hold their children in a standing position, both feet turn outward. Approximately 5 degrees of out-toeing is normal after age 3. Further degrees of out-toeing may be due to lateral tibial torsion.

PATHOPHYSIOLOGY

Several factors are involved in the etiology of rotational conditions. The majority of these problems are deformations secondary to intrauterine positioning. Metatarsus adductus and medial tibial torsion result from intrauterine positioning, and certain sleeping and sitting positions may perpetuate these problems in infants and children. For example, sleeping in the prone position with the legs internally rotated may lead to continued internal tibial torsion or metatarsus adductus. Heredity is also believed to play a role in the development of rotational problems. Sometimes parents have the same rotational deformity as their children. In addition, **bony and neuromuscular abnormalities** are part of the etiology of clubfoot.

Specific terminology is used to describe the position

of the limb. **Version** is normal variation in limb rotation, whereas **torsion** refers to abnormal conditions (i.e., > 2 standard deviations above or below the mean). **Adduction** is movement toward the midline, in contrast to **abduction,** which is movement away from the midline. **Varus angulation** is deviation toward the midline, whereas **valgus angulation** is deviation away from the midline. An **inverted** foot is one turned toward the midline on its long axis. An **everted** foot is one turned away from the midline on its long axis.

Medial (internal) rotation of the lower extremity brings the big toe to the midline during the early intrauterine period, whereas lateral (external) rotation occurs during the later intrauterine period, infancy, and childhood. Alterations in this normal lateral process caused by either genetic or environmental factors (e.g., intrauterine molding, sleep positions) may lead to rotational problems. Conditions influenced by intrauterine position, such as metatarsus adductus and developmental hip dysplasia, are sometimes found in the same children.

The primary pathology of congenital clubfoot is related to deformity and hypoplasia of the bones of the foot, especially the talus and tarsal bones, and environmental factors such as intrauterine position and molding. In addition, hypoplasia of the calf muscles and thickening of the ligaments contribute to the deformity.

DIFFERENTIAL DIAGNOSIS

In-toeing and out-toeing may be classified according to anatomic level and usual age at presentation (Table 80–1). These conditions may be localized to one of four areas: toe, foot, tibia, and femur. If in-toeing problems are placed in chronological order by age of presentation, the affected area follows a toe-to-femur sequence (see Table 80–1).

IN-TOEING

Searching Toe

Children with a so-called searching toe have a big toe that points medially when they walk. Unlike the other causes of in-toeing, which are structural and present at rest, this condition is a dynamic deformity. Searching toe results from the contraction of the abductors of the

big toe during the stance phase of gait, which pulls the toe toward the midline.

Clubfoot

Congenital **clubfoot,** a pathologic deformity of the foot, may be identified at birth (Fig. 80–1). Clubfoot may be either an isolated deformity or seen in association with other neuromuscular anomalies such as arthrogryposis, myelomeningocele, amniotic band syndrome, cerebral palsy, or poliomyelitis.

The diagnosis of congenital clubfoot is made at birth on the basis of three conditions: forefoot varus, heel varus, and ankle equinus. Clubfoot can range in severity from a rigid deformity, in which the forefoot cannot be brought into a neutral position by passive abduction, to nonrigid deformities, in which the forefoot can be gently brought toward the midline.

Metatarsus Adductus and Metatarsus Varus

These terms, which are often used synonymously to describe an incurving foot, are actually two distinct conditions. **Metatarsus adductus** is a functional deformity in which the forefoot is adducted with respect to the hindfoot. The forefoot can be brought into the neutral position either by stroking the lateral border of the foot or by gently straightening it.

Congenital **metatarsus varus** is a bony abnormality characterized by subluxation of the tarsometatarsal joint with adduction of the metatarsals. The forefoot is inverted and adducted with respect to the hindfoot. Unlike metatarsus adductus, metatarsus varus is a fixed deformity. The foot cannot be bought into the neutral position. The prominence of the base of the fifth metatarsal, the convexity of the lateral border of the foot, and a deep crease along the plantar surface of the tarsometatarsal joints are evident on examination.

TABLE 80–1. Site and Age of Onset of Rotational Problems of the Lower Extremity in Children

Problem	Site of Problem	Age of Onset
In-toeing		
Searching toe	Toe	Infancy
Clubfoot	Foot	Birth
Metatarsus adductus/varus	Foot	Birth/infancy
Medial tibial torsion	Tibia	Toddler stage (12–24 mo)
Medial femoral torsion	Femur	Early childhood (3–5 yr)
Out-toeing		
Physiologic out-toeing	Hips	Infancy
Lateral tibial torsion	Tibia	Childhood

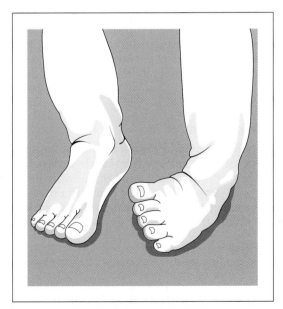

FIGURE 80–1. Congenital clubfoot.

Normal dorsiflexion of the ankle helps distinguish severe forms of metatarsus varus from clubfoot.

Medial Tibial Torsion

This condition is usually first noticed by parents when children begin to walk. Medial tibial torsion is often bilateral; when it is unilateral, it more commonly affects the left leg. Observation of children's gaits reveals that the knees point forward but the feet turn inward. Because the knees are straight, the site of the rotational deformity is below this joint. If the feet are normal and no metatarsus adductus or varus is present, the rotational deformity can be isolated to the lower leg.

Medial Femoral Torsion

This condition can be conceptualized in the following way: When children lie on their backs, the torsion causes the femoral head to protrude instead of lie flat within the acetabulum. The presence of medial femoral torsion causes the entire distal limb to turn inward when the femoral head articulates normally with the acetabulum. The condition is usually bilateral.

Children who are 3–4 years of age present with this classic story: Their parents report that children, who showed no previous in-toeing, have a problem that is becoming severe. Excessive medial femoral torsion, which may have been present at birth, has been masked by the external rotatory forces present during infancy. Thus, the condition is clinically appreciated only as these forces resolve.

OUT-TOEING

Physiologic Out-toeing

Out-toeing of infancy, which is most commonly seen in children who are just learning to walk, is caused by an external rotatory contracture of the soft tissues surrounding the hip seconday to intrauterine position. This condition may be perpetuated in children who sleep in the prone, frog-leg position, which does not allow for stretching of the external rotators of the hips. Although both feet turn outward when infants stand, the lateral rotation of both hips is normal on examination (Fig. 80–2).

Lateral Tibial Torsion

This condition may be suspected in children who are 3–5 years of age and present with out-toeing that worsens with time. Because the tibia normally rotates laterally with development, the condition may become more severe with age. Malalignment between the knee and the direction of gait may produce knee pain.

EVALUATION

History

A family history of any rotational problems should be noted. The age at onset and severity of symptoms in the patient should also be obtained. A thorough develop-

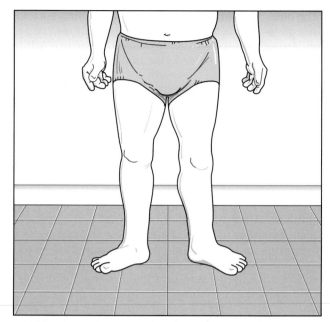

FIGURE 80–2. Physiologic out-toeing of infancy. (Reproduced, with permission, from Staheli, L. T. Torsional deformity. Pediatr. Clin. North Am. 24:799–811, 1977.)

mental history is important, because developmental delays may be a sign of underlying neuromuscular or neurologic disorders (Questions Box).

Physical Examination

A careful, detailed physical examination, including assessment of gait and neurologic and musculoskeletal function, is essential for making the correct diagnosis. This evaluation should include examination of the hips for signs of hip dysplasia, which may be associated with metatarsus adductus (see Chapter 79, Developmental Hip Dysplasia). A rotational profile consisting of four components should be assessed (Fig. 80–3). A negative value indicates in-toeing in these measurements.

The foot progression angle is estimated by watching a child walk (Fig. 80–4). The normal range of the foot progression angle may vary, but more than 5 degrees of in-toeing at any age is considered abnormal. Normal adults walk with their feet externally rotated slightly (approximately 5 degrees). The tibia rotates laterally with growth. In infancy, it is internally rotated and becomes externally rotated at about age 3–5 years. The

---

Questions: In-toeing and Out-toeing

- Is there any family history of in-toeing or out-toeing?
- What is the birth history? Was the child a breech presentation?
- At what age did the child begin walking?
- When did the rotational deformity appear? Is it getting better or worse?
- Does the rotational problem produce any disability (e.g., tripping or falling a great deal when walking or running)?
- Has any previous treatment been tried?
- In what position does the child sleep? In what position does the child sit?

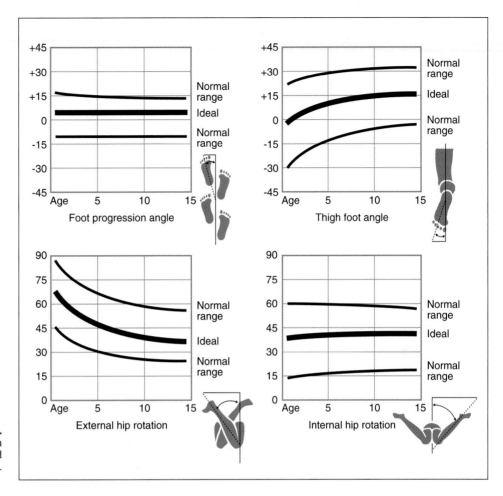

FIGURE 80–3. Rotational profile. (Reproduced, with permission, from Wenger, D. R., and M. Rang. The Art and Practice of Children's Orthopedics. New York, Raven Press, 1993.)

thigh-foot angle can range between –30 and 30 degrees during infancy and 0–30 degrees (average is 10 degrees) during most of childhood. Internal rotation of the hip is normally less than 60–70 degrees. It is greatest during early childhood and gradually declines after this time.

The examination of infants with clubfoot should include a careful examination of the back for signs of possible spinal dysraphism (e.g., skin dimples and hairy patches) and a thorough neurologic examination.

Medial tibial torsion may be diagnosed by having

FIGURE 80–4. Evaluation of foot progression angle. (Reproduced, with permission, from Staheli, L. T. Fundamentals of Pediatric Orthopedics. New York, Raven Press, 1992.)

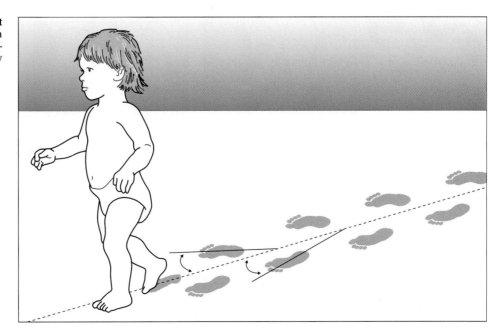

children sit at the end of the examination table with both knees flexed to 90 degrees and palpating the medial and lateral malleoli with the thumb and index finger. Normally, the medial malleolus lies anterior to the lateral malleolus (approximately one fingerbreadth). If the lateral malleolus is on the same plane or anterior to the medial malleolus, internal tibial torsion is indicated.

The diagnosis of tibial torsion can also be made by measuring the thigh-foot angle (Fig. 80–5). Measurement of the thigh-foot angle involves having children lie prone on the examination table and observing the relationship of the long axis of the foot compared to the axis of the thigh as viewed from above. The shape of the foot itself can also be assessed with children in this position. Slight internal rotation is normal as children first learn to walk.

Diagnosis of medial femoral torsion can be made by observing children's gaits and measuring hip rotation. The knees and the feet appear to turn inward when children with medial femoral torsion walk. Internal and external hip rotation are evaluated with the children in a prone position, the pelvis flat, and the knees flexed 90 degrees (Fig. 80–6). The degrees of normal rotation vary with age (see Fig. 80–3). During childhood, internal hip rotation greater than 70 degrees implies medial femoral torsion.

Laboratory Tests

Laboratory tests are generally not required in the assessment of rotational problems.

Imaging Studies

Routine imaging studies are not necessary for rotational deformities. Imaging studies may be considered by the orthopedic surgeon in severe deformities if operative correction is being considered. X-rays are used in clubfoot to assess the relationship and development of the bones of the foot and for monitoring cast correction.

MANAGEMENT

IN-TOEING

Metatarsus adductus generally resolves spontaneously, but stretching exercises for the foot can be advised, particularly if parents are anxious to "do something." Parents are instructed to manipulate the foot with each diaper change. Referral to an orthopedic surgeon for evaluation should be made if the deformity is still present at 3–4 months of age (the majority of cases resolve within the first 3 months of life). Cast correction may be required for rigid deformities or those that persist beyond 3–4 months. Shoe modifications (e.g., putting shoes on the wrong foot) should be avoided because they have not been shown to have any long-term benefits.

Because metatarsus varus may progress when children begin walking, referral to an orthopedic surgeon should be made as soon as the condition is detected. Serial casting followed by corrective shoes or inserts is the first line of treatment. Surgery is only rarely required.

Treatment for medial tibial torsion is rarely required, because this problem generally corrects with time when children learn to walk. Night splinting, although still occasionally instituted, has not been shown to affect the natural history of this condition. If the deformity is severe or persists without improvement beyond the age of 18 months or after children have been walking for 1 year, referral to an orthopedic surgeon for evaluation should be made. Surgical correction (e.g., tibial rota-

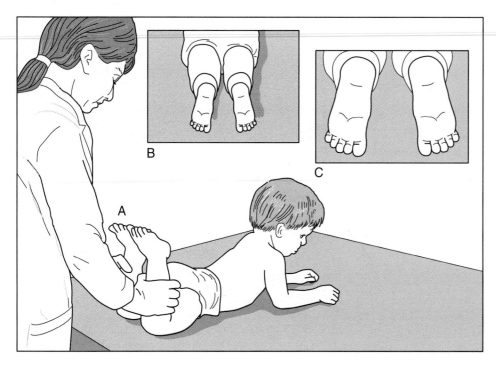

FIGURE 80–5. Evaluation of the thigh-foot axis. A. Observation with the child in the prone position is best. **B.** Determination of the thigh foot axis. **C.** Assessment of the shape of the foot. (Reproduced, with permission, from Staheli, L. T. Fundamentals of Pediatric Orthopedics. New York, Raven Press, 1992.)

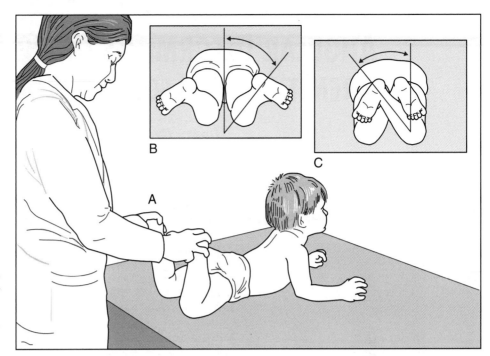

FIGURE 80–6. Evaluation of hip rotation.
A. The child is prone and knees are flexed to 90°. **B.** Medial rotation is measured. **C.** Lateral rotation is measured. (Reproduced, with permission, from Staheli, L. T. Fundamentals of Pediatric Orthopedics. New York, Raven Press, 1992.)

tional osteotomy) may be required if the deformity is severe or persists beyond 8–10 years of age.

Like the other conditions that produce in-toeing, medial femoral torsion generally does not require treatment. Even if it persists into adulthood, it usually produces no disability nor does it increase the risk for degenerative arthritis in the involved joint. Nonoperative treatment is ineffective. Surgical correction may be required if there is a history of repeated falls or severe gait problems. A derotational femoral osteotomy is the only effective method of treatment. It should not be performed until children are at least 8–10 years of age.

Clubfoot, unlike other problems, is a pathologic lesion that requires treatment. Treatment, which should begin during the first week of life, consists of serial manipulations of the foot and casting. Several months of casting may be required to attain full correction. Surgery is often required for resistant or recurrent cases. As many as 50–75% of patients with clubfoot may eventually require surgery. Surgery is usually delayed until infants are 6–12 months of age.

OUT-TOEING

Physiologic out-toeing of infancy is a rotational problem that spontaneously resolves when children learn to walk. Most cases resolve by about 18 months of age. Severe lateral tibial torsion may require surgical correction with a tibial rotational osteotomy.

PROGNOSIS

Because the lower extremity rotates laterally with growth, the natural history of internal rotational problems, such as internal tibial torsion and medial femoral torsion, is resolution over time. In contrast, lateral tibial torsion may become worse with time.

The prognosis for the vast majority of rotational problems is excellent. Parental reassurance and education regarding the natural history of these deformities may decrease anxiety and prevent needless visits to specialists in search of treatments that may not be necessary. Functional disability or degenerative arthritis is not associated with these conditions.

Left untreated, clubfoot often leads to considerable pain and disability. The affected foot can be difficult to fit with shoes. And finally, clubfoot can be unsightly and cause children significant emotional distress.

Case Resolution

The girl described in the case history appears to have medial femoral torsion, because she has no history of rotational problems. Her entire leg turns in when she walks. Internal hip rotation greater than 70 degrees confirms the diagnosis. The mother can be reassured that this is a normal, age-related phenomenon that will most likely resolve over time. The child can be reevaluated in 4–6 months. Orthopedic referral is not required at this time.

Selected Readings

Craig, C. L., and M. J. Goldberg. Foot and leg problems. Pediatr. Rev. 14:395–400, 1993.

Fuchs, R., and L. T. Staheli. Splinting and intoeing. J. Pediatr. Orthop. 16:489–491, 1996.

Hoekelman, R. A. Foot and leg problems. *In* Hoekelman, R. A. (ed.). Primary Pediatric Care, 3rd ed. St. Louis, Mosby-Year Book, 1997, pp. 971–979.

Hoffinger, S. A. Evaluation and management of pediatric foot deformities. Pediatr. Clin. North Am. 43:1091–1111, 1996.

Staheli, L. T. Lower positional deformity in infants and children: a review. J. Pediatr. Orthop. 10:559–563, 1990.

Wenger, D. R., and M. Rang. The Art and Practice of Children's Orthopedics. New York, Raven Press, 1993.

ANGULAR DEFORMITIES OF THE LOWER EXTREMITY: BOW LEGS AND KNOCK KNEES

Geeta Grover, M.D.

Hx During the routine health maintenance examination of a 2-year-old child, you observe moderate to severe bilateral bowing of both legs. The child's mother reports that her son began walking at 10 months. She has noticed no problems with his gait and says he does not trip or fall excessively. On examination, the boy's weight is greater than the 95th percentile for age, but otherwise he appears to be a healthy African American child.

Questions

1. What types of angular deformities affect children's lower extremities?
2. How does children's age help determine whether they have physiologic or pathologic angular deformities?
3. What clinical measurements can help distinguish physiologic from pathologic angular deformities?
4. To what extent are x-rays used in the routine assessment of angular deformities?

With normal growth and development, the angular alignment of children's legs progresses through a series of developmental stages—from relative bow legs to knock knees and eventually straight legs. Rotational problems such as in-toeing and out-toeing are deformities in the transverse plane that occur when a bone rotates either internally or externally along its long axis (Fig. 81–1). Angular deformities such as bow legs and knock knees are deformities in the frontal plane. The legs distal to the knees are angled or tilted toward the midline in bow-leg deformity, whereas they are tilted away from the midline of the body in knock-knee deformity (Fig. 81–2). Variations in the knee angle that fall outside the normal range (e.g., more than plus-or-minus two standard deviations of the mean) are referred to as genu varum for bow legs and genu valgum for knock knees (Dx Box). Appreciation of the normal developmental sequence in conjunction with a careful history and physical examination can help pediatricians identify pathologic cases of bow legs and knock knees and initiate prompt treatment.

EPIDEMIOLOGY

Bow legs and knock knees are common in infants and children. Knock knees occur less frequently than bow legs. Knock knees are seen more often in females and are commonly associated with generalized ligamentous laxity. Pathologic cases of bow legs and knock knees are uncommon.

CLINICAL PRESENTATION

Children with **bow legs** have a characteristic wide-based stance with increased distance between the knees. They may walk with a waddling gait. In-toeing may be noted as a result of associated internal tibial torsion. When the distance between the knees (intercondylar distance) is more than 10 cm when children are laying supine with their hips and knees in extension and their medial malleoli just touching, they require evaluation for pathologic bow legs.

Severe **knock knees** may produce an awkward gait with the knees rubbing. Children may walk with both feet apart in an effort to avoid knee-to-knee contact. They may need to place one knee behind the other to stand with both feet together. When the distance between the ankles (intermalleolar distance) is more than 10 cm when children are laying supine with their hips and knees in extension and their knees just touching, they warrant evaluation for pathologic knock knees.

PATHOPHYSIOLOGY

The normal variation in the angular alignment of the lower extremities changes with age. During the first 2 years of life, relative bowing of the legs is common. Although physiologic bowing of the lower leg may be appreciated at birth, it is most prominent during the second year of life when it most commonly involves both the tibia and the femur. When associated with internal tibial torsion, the deformity may appear more striking. Physiologic knock knees develop between 3 and 4 years of age. The knock-knee stage resolves somewhere between 5 and 7 years of age, when normal adult alignment develops. A slight knock-knee appearance remains in normal adults. Bow legs or knock knees that develop ouside of this sequence require further evaluation for pathologic causes.

The **tibiofemoral angle,** the angle between the long axis of the femur and the long axis of the tibia, is used to assess the angular alignment of the leg. At birth the tibiofemoral angle is approximately 15 degrees varus, and it decreases to 0 between the ages of 18 and 24 months. By 3–4 years, the angle peaks at about 10

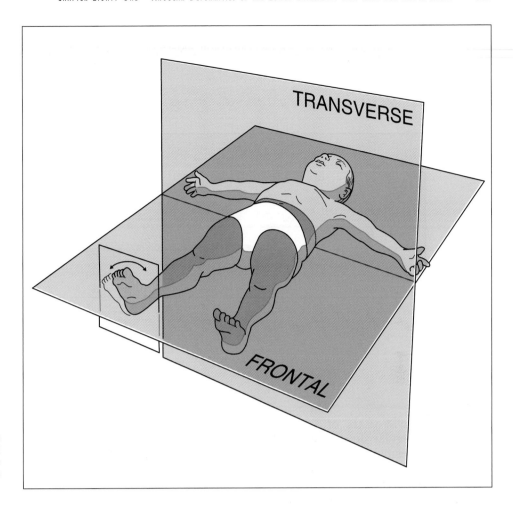

FIGURE 81–1. Select body reference and rotational planes. Rotational problems are deformities in the transverse plane. Angular deformities are in the frontal plane.

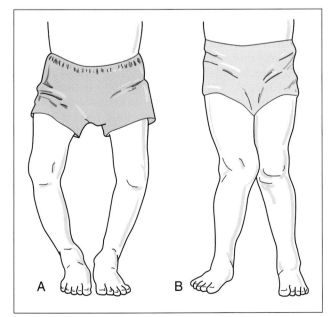

FIGURE 81–2. Varus and valgus deformities of the lower extremities.
A. Bow-leg deformity.
B. Knock-knee deformity.

degrees of valgus angulation. Then between 5 and 7 years it decreases to the normal range of about 7–9 degrees in girls and 4–6 degrees in boys (Fig. 81–3).

DIFFERENTIAL DIAGNOSIS

The most common causes of genu varum and genu valgum are presented in Table 81–1. Physiologic bow legs and knock knees are usually bilateral, and they occur in a sequence that follows the normal developmental pattern. Lateral bowing of the tibia is commonly noted during the first year of life. Bow legs (involving both the femur and the tibia) are pronounced during the second year, and knock knees become prominent

D_x	**Pathologic Bow Legs and Knock Knees**

- Asymmetric deformity
- Inconsistency with the normal sequence of angular development
- Stature less than the fifth percentile for age
- Severe deformity (>10 cm intermalleolar or intercondylar distance)
- History of rapid progression
- Presence of other musculoskeletal abnormalities

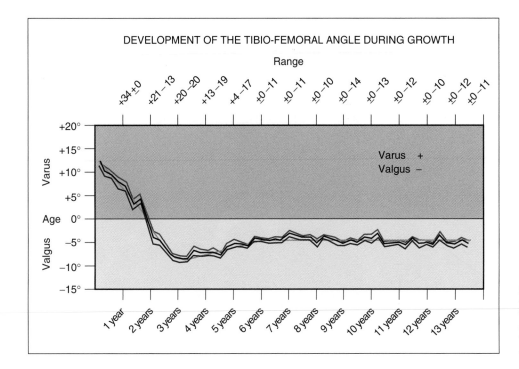

FIGURE 81-3. Development of the tibiofemoral angle. (Reproduced, with permission, from Salenious, P., and E. Vankka. The development of the tibiofemoral angle in children. J. Bone Joint Surg. 57A:259–261, 1975.)

between 3 and 4 years of age. This is the normal sequence of angular development. Most cases of bow legs are the result of normal physiologic processes, Blount's disease (tibia vara), and rickets. Common causes of pathologic knock knees are severe renal rickets and "old" fractures of the proximal tibia.

Blount's disease, a growth disturbance involving the posterior-medial aspect of the proximal tibia (physis, epiphysis, and metaphysis), is the most frequent cause of pathologic bow legs. Both infantile and juvenile forms of the disease are more common in African Americans. The infantile form affects children 1–3 years of age. Usually bilateral, it is associated with internal tibial torsion. The etiology is believed to involve mechanical stress on the growth plate, thus converting physiologic

---

TABLE 81-1. Common Causes of Genu Varum and Genu Valgum

Genu Varum

Physiologic bow legs
Rickets (vitamin D deficiency [nutritional] or vitamin D resistance [hereditary])
Blount's disease (tibia vara)
Achondroplasia
Metaphyseal dysplasia
Trauma, infection, or tumor of the proximal tibia (resulting in malunion or partial physeal arrest)
Excessive prenatal fluoride ingestion

Genu Valgum

Physiologic knock knees
Rickets (renal osteodystrophy)
Trauma, infection, or tumor of the distal femur or proximal tibia (resulting in malunion or partial physeal arrest)
Paralytic conditions (e.g., myelodysplasia, polio, cerebral palsy) leading to contracture of the iliotibial band
Osteogenesis imperfecta
Rheumatoid arthritis of the knee

---

bow legs to pathologic varus. Affected children are often obese and early walkers, which puts early stress on the growth plate. Blount's disease produces a sharp angulation at the proximal tibia, whereas physiologic bow legs lead to a gradual curvature of the legs involving both the femur and the tibia. Six stages of x-ray progression based on the degree of epiphyseal depression and metaphyseal fragmentation at the proximal tibia have been identified (Langenskiöld staging). It may be difficult to distinguish between early stages of Blount's disease and physiologic bow legs.

The less common, juvenile form of Blount's disease occurs in older children and adolescents. Knee pain, rather than deformity, is the most common presenting sign. Usually unilateral, it is more common in males than females. Affected children are generally obese and have a normal height. Although the etiology is unclear, it is believed that in predisposed obese adolescents, the decreased growth of the medial tibial physis is due to the repetitive trauma of excessive weight bearing.

Rickets, a disease of the growing skeleton, produces inadequate mineralization of the bone. The disorder is due to a disturbance in calcium and phosphorus metabolism. Rickets takes several forms, including vitamin D–deficient, or nutritional, rickets; vitamin D–resistant, or hereditary, rickets (the most common form); and severe renal osteodystrophy. Signs of rickets include short stature, poor muscle tone, joint pain, and angular deformities of the lower extremities. The alignment at the time of onset of disease determines the direction of angulation. For example, vitamin D–deficient or vitamin D–resistant rickets generally has an early onset and is more often associated with bow legs. Renal osteodystrophy, which usually has a later onset, results in a valgus deformity.

Pathologic processes, including trauma (fractures), infections, and tumors, involving the proximal tibia are additional potential causes of both bow legs and knock knees. Overgrowth or malunion following fractures of the proximal tibial metaphysis most commonly results in genu valgum rather than genu varum.

EVALUATION

History

A family history, a description of the deformity, its progression, impact, and prior treatment, and an assessment of the child's growth and nutritional history (Questions Box) should be obtained from the parents or caregivers.

Physical Examination

Physical examination begins with a general screening of children's nutritional growth and developmental status. Children's growth parameters (height, weight, head circumference) should be measured and plotted on standard growth curves. The rotational status of the lower limb should be assessed, because internal tibial torsion is often associated with bow leg deformity (see Chapter 80, Rotational Problems of the Lower Extremity). Children should be observed both standing and ambulating to determine the alignment of the legs. The intercondylar and intermalleolar distances can be measured with the child supine to determine the presence of excessive bow legs or knock knees (see Clinical Presentation).

Laboratory Tests

Most children with physiologic angulation do not require any laboratory studies. A general metabolic screening, including hemoglobin, calcium, phosphorus, creatinine, and alkaline phosphatase, may be ordered if a systemic or metabolic abnormality is suspected.

Imaging Studies

X-rays are usually performed in the evaluation of bow legs or knock knees if pathology is suspected. If obtained, x-rays should include the entire leg so that the alignment of the femur and tibia may be assessed. Children should be standing, and a single radiograph of both legs should be taken, if possible. Pathologic conditions such as rickets (osteoporosis, metaphyseal fraying, cortical thinning, widening of the growth plates), Blount's disease (beaking of the medial metaphysis of the femur and tibia), various bone dysplasias, and forms of dwarfism can usually be ruled out by x-rays. An increased uptake of the proximal medial aspect of the tibia on bone scan may help differentiate early infantile Blount's disease from extreme physiologic bow legs.

MANAGEMENT

Angular deformities within normal developmental limits should be managed with continual observation and reassessment. The severity of the deformity should be documented, and children should be followed at three- to six-month intervals until the condition resolves. Physicians should **reassure parents** that bow legs and knock knees are normal developmental variations that will correct spontaneously with time. Special diets, braces or shoe wedges, arch supports, and bars are generally best avoided; they have not been shown to affect the normal developmental sequence.

Children with physiologic varus may be followed clinically until 18 months to 2 years of age. Pathology should be suspected if correction has not begun by this time or if the lesion is progressive. Children with more than 10 degrees of valgus (or an intermalleolar distance >10 cm) after 8–9 years of age may require further evaluation. Children with suspected cases of pathologic bow legs and knock knees require **referral to an orthopedist** for evaluation.

Treatment for children with Blount's disease may consist of **bracing** if the deformity is mild and identified early. **Surgery** may be necessary if the deformity is severe. Medical management, such as administration of vitamin D for nutritional rickets, is of primary importance in the treatment of the various forms of rickets. Surgical correction, such as osteotomies to correct varus or valgus deformities, should be reserved until medical management has been maximized, because even severe deformities may resolve with conservative management.

PROGNOSIS

Physiologic bow legs and knock knees spontaneously resolve without further sequelae. Although knock knees are primarily a cosmetic problem, degenerative arthritis may rarely be a late complication. Surgical correction may be required for adolescents with severe deformity to prevent such late complications.

Questions: Pathologic Bow Legs and Knock Knees

- When was the deformity first noticed?
- Has it changed? If so, how fast?
- Has the problem been treated in any way?
- Does the problem seem to affect how the child walks?
- Has the child had any recent illness or trauma in the affected leg?
- Does anyone else in the family have a similar problem?
- Aside from this condition, is the child growing and developing normally?
- Does the child eat a well-balanced diet?
- Does the child have any chronic medical problems such as kidney disease?

Case Resolution

The boy described in the case history should be evaluated for pathologic causes of genu varum, especially

Blount's disease, for the following reasons: (1) his age is at the upper limit of normal for bow legs and his deformity is severe, (2) he is African American, (3) he has a history of early walking, and (4) he is obese. A standing x-ray of the lower extremities should be obtained, and the boy should be referred to an orthopedist for further evaluation and management.

Selected Readings

Bruce, R. W. Torsional and angular deformities. Pediatr. Clin. North Am. 43:867–881, 1996.

Eggert, P., and M. Viemann, Physiologic bowlegs or infantile Blount's disease. Some new aspects on an old problem. Pediatr. Radiol. 26:349–352, 1996.

Henderson, R. C. Tibia vara: a complication of adolescent obesity. J. Pediatr. 121:482–486, 1992.

Kling, T. F. Angular deformities of the lower limbs in children. Orthop. Clin. North Am. 18:513–527, 1987.

Mankin, K. P., and S. Zimbler. Gait and leg alignment: What's normal and what's not. Contemp. Pediatr. 14:41–70, 1997.

Scoles, P. V. Lower extremity development. *In* Pediatric Orthopedics in Clinical Practice, 2nd ed. Chicago, Year Book Medical Publishers, 1988, pp. 82–121.

Wilkins, K. E. Bowlegs. Pediatr. Clin. North Am. 33:1429–1438, 1986.

CHAPTER 82

ORTHOPEDIC INJURIES AND GROWING PAINS

Geeta Grover, M.D.

H$_x$ A 6-year-old boy has a 1-week history of leg pains. He wakes up at night and cries because his legs hurt, yet during the day he is fine, with no pain or movement limitations. He has no history of trauma, fever, or joint swelling. The family history is negative for rheumatic or collagen-vascular disease. The boy's height and weight are at the 50th percentile for age, he is afebrile, and the physical examination is unremarkable.

Questions

1. What is the differential diagnosis of leg pains in school-age children?
2. What laboratory or radiographic studies are appropriate for children with leg pains?
3. How do musculoskeletal injuries in children differ from those in adults (e.g., the type of injury sustained, the location of the injury, the effect of age on injury, etc.)?

Children by nature are active and explorative. They experience cuts, scrapes, minor injuries, and pain routinely. Because primary care physicians are often the first to examine children with injuries, they play an important role in making the preliminary diagnosis and assessment regarding the need for further evaluation and treatment. The more common complaints and injuries seen in the pediatrician's office are discussed in this chapter: growing pains; nursemaid's elbow; and fractures, including growth plate injuries. The evaluation of children with limp is discussed in Chapter 84.

EPIDEMIOLOGY

The term **"growing pains"** is somewhat misleading, because there is no evidence that these pains are associated with growth. The period of middle childhood, when growing pains are diagnosed, is not the period of most rapid growth in the child. "Leg aches" or "idiopathic leg pain" may be better terms, but "growing pains" is the most widely used term.

Growing pains occur in 15–30% of all children. They are seen most commonly in children between the ages of 3 and 12 years; the reported age range is infancy to 19 years. Girls are affected more frequently than boys.

Nursemaid's elbow or pulled elbow (subluxation of the radial head) is one of the most common ligamentous injuries seen in children. This condition occurs most often in children 1–4 years of age, with a peak incidence between the ages of 2 and 3 years.

Other ligament and tendon injuries are relatively uncommon in children due to the relative strength of these structures as compared to the growth plate of the developing bone. Type I fractures of the growth plate (discussed below) occur before ligamentous injury. When joint dislocations and ligamentous injury occur in children, they are usually secondary to significant trauma.

Trauma and injury, including child abuse or inflicted injury, are significant causes of morbidity and mortality in children. Injuries account for approximately 10–15% of all hospitalizations in children between 1 and 14 years of age and are the leading cause of death in children and adolescents beyond the first year of life. **Fractures,** which account for about 15% of all pediatric injuries, are perhaps the most common significant form of musculoskeletal injury in children who present to physicians for evaluation and treatment.

CLINICAL PRESENTATION (D$_X$ BOX)

Children with **growing pains** present with a history of intermittent night pain in the legs that awakens them from sleep. A feeling of restlessness is sometimes associated with the pain, which most commonly involves the front of the thighs, the calves, and the area behind the knees—never the joints. The pain is usually of short duration and typically bilateral, and it usually resolves after several minutes, with children going back to sleep. Pain may often occur at other sites, such as the abdomen and head. Pain is gone by morning, and children have normal activity during the day.

Nursemaid's elbow is characterized by a sudden onset of elbow pain and a reluctance to use the arm. Children usually cry briefly initially and then are fine except for inability to use the affected arm. Typically, children hold the injured arm close to the body in a position of flexion and pronation.

An underlying **fracture** is strongly indicated by obvious deformity or lack of spontaneous movement in the extremity in question. Localized swelling, tenderness, and limited range of movement may all be signs of a fracture.

PATHOPHYSIOLOGY

Growing pains are recurrent aches or pains localized to the muscles of the legs. The pain is located deep within the extremity and not in the joints. The etiology is unclear. Rapid growth, emotional and psychological stress, and myalgias secondary to exercise or physical activity have been implicated.

Nursemaid's elbow is a subluxation of the radial head caused by rapid extension and pronation of the arm. Typically, the injury occurs when parents suddenly pull children toward themselves, and children resist and want to go in the other direction (Fig. 82–1).

Because of anatomic and physiologic differences (e.g., presence of cartilaginous growth plate as well as thicker periosteum and greater plasticity of the skeleton), **fracture** patterns seen in children often differ from those in adults. Fractures may be more difficult to detect in children and may influence long-term growth and development of affected limbs.

Fractures are classified based on anatomic location, type of fracture, and degree of angulation or displacement. Fracture location may be described as diaphyseal, metaphyseal, or epiphyseal/growth plate depending on the portion of the bone involved (Figs. 82–2 and 82–3). Fractures may be either open or closed. In closed fractures, the skin over the fracture site is intact, whereas in open fractures, the skin is broken. Fractures in which the two bone fragments are displaced relative to each other are described as angulated or displaced; the direction and degree of displacement are based on the distal fragment.

The Salter-Harris classification is used most commonly to classify growth plate injury (Table 82–1, Fig. 82–4). Approximately 15% of all fractures in children involve the growth plate. Type I and type II are the most common fractures involving the growth plate. Type III and IV fractures are intra-articular. Type V fractures are uncommon and are due to a crush injury to the growth plate. Initial x-rays in type I and type V fractures may appear normal, because bone fragments are not displaced. The likelihood of growth arrest associated with type V fractures is high.

DIFFERENTIAL DIAGNOSIS

The diagnosis of **growing pains** is one of exclusion. Leg pain in children has many causes (Table 82–2). If they are limited to vague pains in the legs at night with no associated limp or signs of inflammation, the differential diagnosis may be limited to growing pains, general systemic diseases such as leukemia, benign bone tumors such as osteoid osteoma, and perhaps fibromyalgia. Leukemic infiltration of the bones may cause leg pain before systemic signs such as fever, weight loss, and adenopathy are present. Osteoid osteoma, a benign bone tumor that most commonly occurs in adolescent boys, characteristically causes pain that is worse at night and is usually relieved by anti-inflammatory medications. The pain may be localized in one place, however, unlike with growing pains. Fibromyalgia, which is probably underdiagnosed in the pediatric population, is a well-recognized cause in adults of chronic, generalized limb pain without a clear, organic source. It is seen more commonly in adolescents than in younger children. This benign, intermittent musculoskeletal pain syndrome is

---

D$_x$ Orthopedic Injuries and Growing Pains

GROWING PAINS

- Age between 3 and 12 years
- Normal growth and development
- Intermittent pain or aches in the legs
- Occurrence of symptoms at night
- Pain poorly localized to the anterior thighs, calves, and behind the knees; absence of joint involvement
- Absence of limp, disability, or inflammation
- Response to supportive measures such as heat and massage

NURSEMAID'S ELBOW

- Age between 1 and 4 years
- Elbow pain of acute onset
- History of sudden longitudinal traction on an extended and pronated arm
- Forearm held in a position of flexion and pronation
- Lack of spontaneous movement of the elbow

FRACTURES

- Obvious deformity
- Swelling or tenderness over the fracture site
- Limited range of movement or absence of movement of the affected extremity

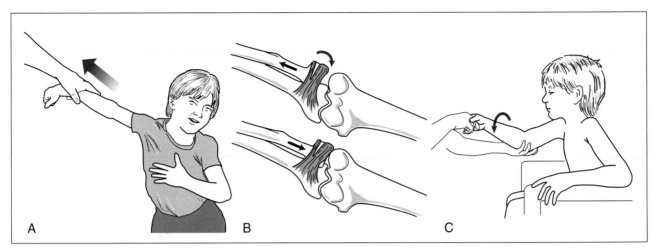

FIGURE 82-1. Nursemaid's elbow. The sudden traction on the outstretched arm pulls the radius distally, causing a tear in the annular ligament at its attachment to the radius. A portion of the ligament becomes trapped within the joint as the traction is released and the arm recoils. A. Mechanism of injury. B. Pathology. C. Method of reduction (hyperpronation).

associated with multiple tender "trigger points," stiffness, fatigue, and a nonrestorative sleep pattern.

When evaluating for **nursemaid's elbow,** an elbow fracture should be ruled out.

Certain **fractures** and specific features of fractures deserve mention (see Fig. 82–3). Fractures that often occur during childhood include clavicular fractures (the most common childhood fracture and the most commonly fractured bone in newborns) and spiral fractures of the distal tibia, or the toddler's fracture. This occurs because of rotational injury to the lower leg and is seen most commonly in early walking children with unsteady gaits. Elbow fractures require careful attention to neurovascular status because of the risk of associated injury to the median or radial nerve, or brachial artery, leading to Volkmann's ischemic contracture. A Monteg-

gia fracture is a dislocation of the radial head in association with an ulnar shaft fracture. Spiral fractures of long bones, especially the femur, multiple rib fractures, and multiple fractures in various stages of healing are highly suggestive of child abuse (see Chapter 104, Physical Abuse).

Because of the relative weakness of the physis compared to the surrounding ligaments, trauma sustained near joints may be more likely to cause a type I Salter-Harris growth plate fracture rather than ligamentous injury (e.g., sprain or strain). Therefore, it is important to include this type of fracture in the differential diagnosis of children with point tenderness near the end of a long bone, because this injury does require cast immobilization.

EVALUATION

Accurate diagnosis of pediatric orthopedic injuries is often challenging, because children may be not only poor "historians" but also uncooperative with examinations, especially if they are experiencing pain.

History

A thorough history is essential for the accurate diagnosis of growing pains and orthopedic injuries (Questions Box: Growing Pains; and Questions Box: Orthopedic Injuries). A complete history of the events related to the injury, including what happened after the injury was sustained, should be obtained.

Physical Examination

The physical examination of children with suspected **growing pains** should include evaluation for signs of systemic disease such as fever, abnormal growth, and generalized weakness or fatigue. Leg length and circumference should be measured. The legs should be palpated and joint range of motion assessed.

FIGURE 82-2. Anatomy of a long bone.

Joint space

Epiphysis

Growth plate (physis)

Metaphysis

Diaphysis

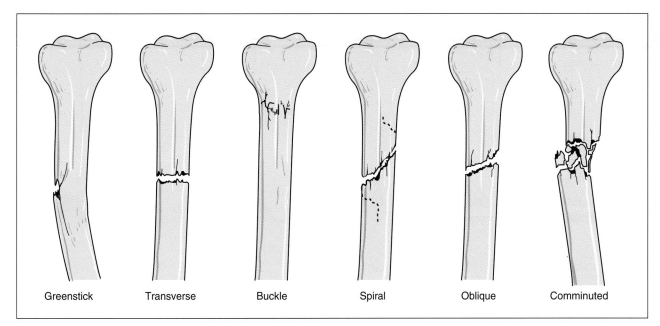

| Greenstick | Transverse | Buckle | Spiral | Oblique | Comminuted |

FIGURE 82–3. Nonepiphyseal plate fractures.

Children with suspected **nursemaid's elbow** should be observed for how they hold the affected arm compared to the unaffected arm. They should be evaluated for limited active motion at the elbow and resistance to attempts at passive movement, especially supination. No swelling or tenderness to palpation should be present.

It is important to undress children with suspected **fractures** and perform a complete physical examination. Simply examining the involved extremity is insufficient. The presence of a deformity, point tenderness, or limitation of motion supports the diagnosis of a fracture. All long bones should be palpated, and the presence of bruises and scars should be noted, because these may indicate child abuse. The examination of the involved extremity includes inspection of the overlying skin for swelling, lacerations, or punctures. The degree of active and passive motion and strength compared to the uninvolved side should be noted. In cases of suspected leg injuries, the child's gait should be observed, if possible. Assessment of neurovascular function distal to the injury includes evaluation of capillary refill, peripheral pulses, and motor and sensory function.

Laboratory Tests

A CBC and ESR may be considered for children with leg pains that do not resolve. Rheumatologic screening tests can be ordered based on abnormalities in these tests (e.g., elevated ESR or WBC count). Routine laboratory studies are not necessary in the evaluation of nursemaid's elbow or fractures. However, because fractures of the femur are often associated with significant blood loss, it is important to monitor the hematocrit in these patients.

Imaging Studies

If leg pains persist and interfere with routine activity, x-rays or bone scans of the legs may be considered. Radiographic evaluation is not required for children with nursemaid's elbow if presentation is typical and reduction is successful. X-rays, if taken in such children, are usually completely negative because the dislocation is often corrected during positioning for x-rays. However, x-rays should be obtained in children with suspected fractures. Fractures involving the growth plate, especially type I and V Salter-Harris fractures, may be

---

TABLE 82–1.   Fracture Patterns Seen in Children

Nonepiphyseal Plate Fractures

Type	Description
Complete	Both sides of the bone fractured; type depends on direction of fracture line
Transverse	Perpendicular to long axis of the bone
Oblique	At an angle to long axis of the bone
Spiral	Zig-zag course around the bone
Comminuted	Fractures with three or more fragments (rare in children)
Buckle or torus	Bone compression causes it to bend or buckle rather than breaking; occurs at junction of metaphysis and diaphysis
Greenstick	Cortex broken on tension side but intact on compression side
Bowing	Deformation of bone due to bending without fracturing

Epiphyseal Plate Fractures (Salter-Harris Classification)

Type	Description
Type I	Horizontal fracture through the physis
Type II	Fracture through the physis, extending into the metaphysis
Type III	Fracture through the epiphysis, extending into the physis
Type IV	Fracture through the epiphysis, physis, and metaphysis
Type V	Crush injury of the physis

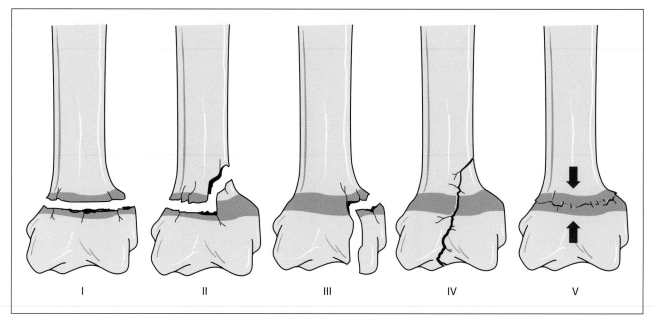

FIGURE 82–4. Salter-Harris classification of epiphyseal plate fractures.

TABLE 82–2. Common Causes of Leg Pain in Children

Growing Pains (leg aches, idiopathic leg pains)

Trauma
Fracture
Compartment syndromes
Soft tissue injury
Muscle strain/sprain

Infection
Cellulitis
Soft tissue abscess
Myositis
Osteomyelitis
Septic arthritis

Neoplasia
Malignant bone tumors (e.g., osteogenic sarcoma, Ewing's sarcoma)
Leukemia
Metastatic disease (e.g., lymphoma, neuroblastoma)

Benign Bone Lesions
Osteoid osteoma
Bone cysts
Histiocytosis X

Collagen-Vascular Disease
Juvenile rheumatoid arthritis
Dermatomyositis
Fibromyalgia
Rheumatic fever

Other Musculoskeletal Causes
Legg-Calvé-Perthes disease
Slipped capital femoral epiphysis
Osgood-Schlatter disease
Transient synovitis of the hip
Osteochondritis dissecans
Patellofemoral stress/chondromalacia patellae
Generalized ligamentous laxity and joint hypermobility

Miscellaneous Causes
Sickle-cell disease pain crisis
Psychosomatic conditions

---

particularly difficult to diagnose radiographically because the growth plate is primarily cartilaginous and hence radiolucent. A bone scan or follow-up x-ray, may be used to diagnose suspected fractures when initial x-rays are negative.

MANAGEMENT

Parental education and reassurance regarding the benign nature of **growing pains** are important. The pains themselves usually respond to **supportive measures** such as heat, massage, and analgesia. Stretching exercises for the legs have also been recommended. Referral to an orthopedist should be considered if the pain is severe and persistent and physical examination and laboratory workup fail to reveal a specific diagnosis.

Nursemaid's elbow is one of the few medical conditions that has a dramatic, immediate cure. Rapid, firm **hyperpronation** of the arm with application of pressure over the radial head usually releases the trapped tissues from the joint and allows for **reduction** of the radial head. A click may be heard or felt as the radial head is reduced. Relief of pain is usually immediate for children treated shortly after injury; return of function may require 15–30 minutes, however. If treatment is delayed,

---

Questions: Growing Pains

- When (i.e., what time of day?) does the pain typically occur?
- Does the pain resolve and then recur in any predictable manner?
- Where is the pain? Does it change location?
- Does anything make the pain better or worse?
- Is the child sick in any other way?
- Does the pain interfere with the child's activities?
- Does the parent notice any changes such as swelling or redness in the child's legs?

such rapid relief of pain and return of mobility may not be seen. Following reduction, **immobilization of the arm** in a sling or splint permits healing of the soft tissues.

Most **fractures** should be referred to an orthopedic surgeon for evaluation and treatment unless the primary care physician is experienced in reducing and casting fractures. Several techniques are used in fracture management. **Closed reduction** is the nonoperative reduction or realignment of fracture fragments. Surgical reduction involves **open reduction** and **internal fixation** with pins to maintain reduction and provide stability. Indications for open reduction include failure of closed reduction; requirement for precise anatomic reduction; intra-articular fractures; Salter-Harris Type III or IV growth plate fractures; and complex, multisystem trauma or multiple fractures.

Certain fractures are common in pediatrics. Most clavicular fractures do not require reduction and can be treated with immobilization in a sling for 4–8 weeks. Elbow fractures (e.g., lateral condyle and supracondylar humeral fractures) are serious and often necessitate open reduction to achieve anatomic reduction. Distal forearm fractures are usually managed with closed reduction and casting. Midforearm fractures may require open reduction, especially in adolescents. Stable metacarpal and phalangeal fractures can be either splinted in an aluminum splint or be taped to an adjacent finger ("buddy taping"). The metacarpophalangeal joints should be maintained in 50–90 degrees of flexion, and the interphalangeal joints should be in about 20 degrees of flexion to minimize stiffness. Unstable finger fractures may require open reduction and pin fixation.

Femoral shaft fractures in infants and children can be managed with either traction and spica cast immobilization or cast immobilization alone. Open reduction and intramedullary rod fixation can be used in adolescents. Closed reduction and cast immobilization are usually used in the management of tibial shaft fractures. Short-cast immobilization may be required for metatarsal fractures, and "buddy taping" is used for stable toe fractures.

Because of the potential for infection, open fractures are orthopedic emergencies that require immediate attention. Careful debridement of the wound is required. External pin fixation may be used to stabilize the fracture because the wound is usually left open. Antibiotics should be administered, and tetanus immunization may be given based on a review of the immunization history.

PROGNOSIS

Growing pains resolve over time without sequelae. Recurrence of nursemaid's elbow is common. Therefore, parents should be cautioned regarding pulling children's arms or lifting them by one hand.

Fractures in children generally heal and remodel (the spontaneous correction of deformity) better and faster than equivalent fractures in adults. Vascular and nerve injuries and growth disturbances are potential complications of fractures and their management. Compartment syndrome, a potentially serious vascular injury, may develop.

Growth plate injuries require special attention because of the potential for growth abnormalities. Prognosis of growth plate fractures depends on the type of injury sustained. Salter-Harris type I and II fractures generally have a good prognosis for long-term healing and growth. The severity of the injury and the accuracy of reduction determine the prognosis of type III and IV fractures; there is also a risk of future degenerative arthritis or growth disturbance. Growth arrest is common following type V fractures because the physis itself is injured.

Case Resolution

The child presented in the opening scenario has the benign condition commonly referred to as growing pains. Management involves parental education and reassurance. Local heat, massage and analgesia (using ibuprofen) may be recommended.

Selected Readings

Davids, J. R. Pediatric knee: clinical assessment and common disorders. Pediatr. Clin. North Am. 43:1067–1090, 1996.

England, S. P., and S. Sundberg. Management of common pediatric fractures. Pediatr. Clin. North Am. 43:991–1012, 1996.

Grogan, D. P., and J. A. Ogden. Knee and ankle injuries in children. Pediatr. Rev. 13:429–434, 1992.

Jackman, K. V. Acute pediatric orthopedic conditions. Pediatr. Ann. 23:240–249, 1994.

Peterson, H. Growing pains. Pediatr. Clin. North Am. 33:1365–1371, 1986.

Teach, S. J., and S. A. Schutzman. Prospective study of recurrent radial head subluxation. Arch. Pediatr. Adolesc. Med. 150:164–166, 1996.

Ward, W. T., et al. Orthopedics. In Zitelli, B. J., and H. W. Davis (ed.). Atlas of Pediatric Physical Diagnosis, 3rd ed. St. Louis, Mosby-Wolfe, 1997.

CHAPTER 83

SPORTS-RELATED INJURIES

Monica Sifuentes, M.D.

H$_x$ A 15-year-old male basketball player complains of 6 months of intermittent pain in his left knee. Occasionally the knee gives out while he is playing ball. The boy denies any associated swelling or erythema over the joint. He is able to walk with no problem and reports no history of direct trauma to the area. He is otherwise healthy.

Upon physical examination, he is a well-developed, well-nourished teenage male in no acute distress. The examination is normal except for mild pain to direct palpation of the left patella. No swelling or erythema of the joint is evident, and the left hip, knee, and ankle have full range of motion. The back is straight.

Questions

1. What are some of the most common orthopedic complaints in adolescent patients, and why do they occur in adolescents?
2. What is the pathophysiology of overuse syndromes?
3. What is the purpose of the preparticipation sports physical examination?
4. What conditions disqualify adolescents from participation in competitive sports?
5. What are the current recommendations for the treatment and rehabilitation of acute soft tissue injuries?

Many adolescents with varying degrees of athletic ability participate in sports during their junior high and high school years. Some choose to continue this participation on the college level. Regardless of the ultimate goal, team sports are an important means by which children and adolescents can experience both winning and losing. Individuals learn the importance of group participation and develop interactive skills with other team members. They are exposed to the concept of physical fitness, which can improve body image as well as self-esteem.

Participation in athletics carries significant risks, however. Accidental injuries, inappropriate coaching, and aggressive training sessions are not uncommon occurrences that have long-term sequelae for young athletes. Primary care practitioners are responsible not only for the evaluation of children prior to their participation in sports but also for the diagnosis, treatment, and prevention of injuries.

EPIDEMIOLOGY

Estimates indicate that as many as 7 million adolescents per year participate in organized sports activities in the United States. Several studies have attempted to quantify the overall injury rate associated with athletic participation. In general, the rate of injury for 13- to 19-year-olds is 7–11%. Approximately 20% of those injured sustain a significant injury. The sport with the highest injury rate in all age groups for boys is football, followed by basketball and soccer. Gymnastics leads to the most injuries in girls. Gender differences between boys and girls have been found in some studies depending on the sport. Overall, boys tend to have more shoulder-related injuries, whereas girls tend to have more knee and ankle injuries and more problems with overuse syndromes. Reports also indicate that girls tend to have more injuries requiring surgical correction.

PREPARTICIPATION SPORTS PHYSICAL EXAMINATION

The goal of the preparticipation physical examination (PPE) is the identification of any physical conditions or abnormalities that may predispose young athletes to injury. Examples include a history of concussion with head trauma or an incompletely healed sprain.

The PPE consists of two parts: (1) a review of the patient's current health, past medical history, including sports injuries, and pertinent family history pertaining to participation in strenuous activities; and (2) a complete physical examination with a focus on the musculoskeletal system. Known as a "two-minute orthopedic examination," the musculoskeletal examination is a detailed assessment of all muscle groups, assessing their strength, tone, and function. Congenital or acquired deformities are also noted. The AAP has developed a form specifically for the PPE visit (see Chapter 18, Health Maintenance in Older Children and Adolescents).

Disqualification from participation in specific sports is appropriate in certain situations. Competitive sports are classified according to their degree of contact or impact and how strenuous they are. Recommendations differ depending on the adolescent's medical condition and the type of sport the athlete desires to play. For details of these recommendations, the reader is referred to the AAP manual *Sports Medicine: Health Care for Young Athletes* and *Sports and the Adolescent,* edited by P. G. Dyment. Fortunately, many young athletes are healthy and rarely need to be restricted from participation.

CLINICAL PRESENTATION

Older children and adolescents with sports-related injuries usually present to the practitioner with specific complaints of pain or swelling in a particular joint

| Dx | **Orthopedic Injury** |

- Joint pain or swelling
- Tenderness to palpation of the affected joint
- Decreased range of motion of the affected joint or extremity
- May or may not have associated bruising of the skin overlying the injury

(D$_x$ Box). In addition, they may complain of nonspecific musculoskeletal pain occurring in certain areas such as the lower back or shoulder. Other complaints may include a limp, decreased range of motion of an extremity, or an inability to participate in a desired activity without pain.

PATHOPHYSIOLOGY

Adolescents, unlike adults, are particularly susceptible to injury because their bones and joints are developing. Most injuries during adolescence involve the epiphysis, which is the weakest point of the musculoskeletal system. In addition, the presence of congenital anomalies such as leg length discrepancies or hip rotation abnormalities puts the young athlete at further risk for injury.

Most orthopedic injuries are the result of either macrotrauma or microtrauma. Sprains are an example of macrotrauma, whereas overuse syndromes can be considered microtrauma. **Macrotrauma** occurs from complete or partial tearing of muscle, ligaments, or tendons, and is often associated with acute injuries. In contrast, **microtrauma** is usually produced by chronic repetitive trauma to a particular area, leading to inflammation and ultimately to pain. This most commonly occurs in soft tissues such as the muscle and tendon but can occur in the bone as well.

Definitions

A **sprain** is a stretching injury of a ligament or the connective tissue that attaches bone to bone. A **strain** is a stretching injury of a muscle or its tendon, which is the connective tissue that attaches muscle to bone. **Tendinitis** is an inflammation of the tendon. **Apophysitis** is an inflammation of the apophysis, which is the site of ligament or tendon attachment to growth cartilage (e.g., Osgood-Schlatter disease [apophysitis of the tibial tubercle], Sever's disease [calcaneal apophysitis]). A **stress fracture** is an incomplete fracture often occurring in the bones of the legs and feet from repetitive trauma to the area. It is believed that the pain associated with shin splints may be due in part to atypical stress fractures of the distal tibia. **Overuse syndromes** occur from repetitive microtrauma to the musculoskeletal system secondary to excessive or biomechanically incorrect activity. They are usually the result of training errors in which athletes are "trying to do too much too fast." Common syn-

dromes in adolescents include Osgood-Schlatter disease, shin splints, and patellofemoral syndrome (chondromalacia patellae).

Grading of Sports Injuries

Sprains can be classified according to the degree of injury and most commonly occur in the knee or ankle. Assigning a grade that describes the injury is useful when considering the prognosis of a particular injury. Consultants also find these grades helpful. Grade I through III is the usual classification used for sprains. Stability of the joint, range of motion, and degree of pain and swelling determine the grade of the sprain. The grading system for strains, on the other hand, is based on an assessment of strength. Because strains do not usually cause joint instability, criteria for grading strains are different than for sprains and may be more subjective. A general description of these two grading systems appears in Table 83–1.

DIFFERENTIAL DIAGNOSIS

The differential diagnosis of orthopedic conditions depends on the anatomic site of the injury or complaint and the mechanism of injury. Table 83–2 lists some of the more common orthopedic conditions by location. Anomalies of skeletal development such as congenital angular deformities of long bones and soft tissue abnormalities like Ehlers-Danlos syndrome should also be considered as possible etiologies for overuse syndromes. Other nonorthopedic conditions such as collagen-vascular diseases, infections and tumors may also present with joint or bone symptomatology.

EVALUATION

History

The history should focus on the musculoskeletal system and how the injury occurred (Questions Box).

TABLE 83–1.   General Classification of Sprains and Strains

	Joint	Range of Motion	Weight Bearing	Pain	Swelling
Sprains					
Grade I	Stable	Normal	Normal	+	+
Grade II	± Stable	↓	↓	++	++
Grade III	Unstable	↓↓	↓↓	+++	+++

	Strength	Palpable Defect	Pain
Strains			
Grade I	$>\frac{4}{5}$	−	+
Grade II	$\frac{3}{5}-\frac{4}{5}$	+/−	++
Grade III	$<\frac{3}{5}$	+/−	+++

TABLE 83–2.   Differential Diagnosis Based
on the Site of Injury

Back Injuries	Injuries to the Lower Extremity
Muscle strain	Iliac crest contusion
Spondylolysis	Iliac apophysitis
Epiphyseal injury	Quadriceps contusion
Herniated disks	Femoral stress fracture
	Medial lateral ligament sprains
Injuries to the Upper Extremity	Anterior cruciate ligament sprain
Acromioclavicular sprains	Posterior cruciate ligament sprain
Sternoclavicular sprains	Patellar dislocation/subluxation
Glenohumeral dislocation	Prepatellar bursitis
Glenohumeral subluxation	Patellofemoral stress syndrome
Impingement syndrome	Patellar tendinitis
Acute elbow injuries	Osgood-Schlatter disease
Olecranon bursitis	Shin splint syndrome
Lateral epicondylitis	Ankle sprains
Flexor-pronator tendinitis	Achilles tendinitis
Wrist sprains	Calcaneal apophysitis
Navicular fractures	Plantar fasciitis
Hamate fractures	
Finger injuries	

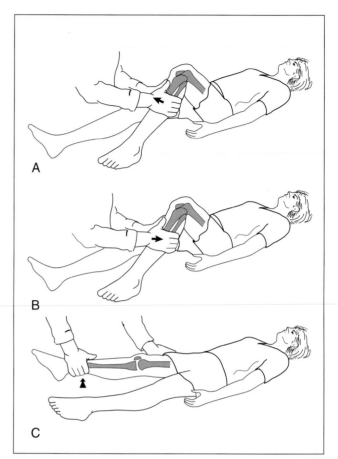

FIGURE 83-1. Maneuvers used to determine stability of the knee joint. A. Anterior drawer test: Anterior force is applied. B. Posterior drawer test: Posterior force is applied. C. Medial ligament stability: Lateral force is applied.

Physical Examination

The physical examination should focus on the musculoskeletal system. If, however, teenagers have not had a physical examination within the past year, a complete physical examination should first be performed to exclude any systemic condition that might manifest itself initially as bone or joint pain. This is especially important in adolescents with chronic complaints.

In general, any pain or swelling of the affected joint or muscle should be noted. If adolescents have a history of acute trauma, an area of ecchymosis may be seen. The affected joint should be tested for range of motion and joint laxity that would differentiate a grade I from a grade II or III sprain. Various maneuvers for testing ligamentous laxity at each joint can be used (Figure 83–1). The most common method is the "drawer test" for anterior and posterior movement of the knee joint. Muscle spasms and diminished range of motion in an adjacent joint should also be noted, because this may indicate a strain injury. Strength of the "strained" muscle(s) and any pain on palpation or contraction of the muscle(s) should be assessed. A palpable defect of the muscle suggests complete rupture of the muscle, whereas muscular contusions are associated with localized pain or hematoma. Pinpoint tenderness over a particular bone may indicate a fracture or, if at the site of a tendon insertion, inflammation. Reviewing the mechanism of injury is often helpful in differentiating between a fracture and tendinitis.

Laboratory Tests

A CBC and ESR may be helpful in adolescents with a history of chronic joint pain or swelling. If the results are abnormal, they suggest a collagen-vascular disease such as lupus, an infection such as osteomyelitis, or rarely, an arthritic disorder such as juvenile rheumatoid arthritis.

Imaging Studies

A radiograph of the involved joint or bone is often the only necessary diagnostic procedure. Other radiographs of joints above and below the symptomatic area are sometimes useful. See Chapter 84, Evaluation of Limp, for a discussion of imaging studies, to help in the diagnosis when limp is the presenting complaint.

Questions: Sports-Related Injuries

- What activity or sport was the patient engaged in at the time of the injury?
- How often has the patient engaged in this sport or particular activity in the past?
- Were there any new additions to the routine this time?
- Did the pain begin after a single injury or after repetitive activity?
  - If the injury is related to a repetitive activity, does the pain occur at a specific time during this activity?
  - Is the pain incapacitating?
  - Has a similar injury ever occurred in the past?
  - How was the injury treated?
    - Was there any pain following the previous injury?
    - Does the patient feel as if he or she has completely recovered?
  - How was this current injury managed acutely?
  - Has the patient altered daily activity in any way to compensate for this problem?

MANAGEMENT

With soft tissue injuries, the aim of acute management is to limit the extent of bleeding and inflammation that occur in the first 48–72 hours following the injury. The mnemonic **RICE** (**r**est, **i**ce, **c**ompression, **e**levation) is helpful. Rest should be explained as "relative rest," since the athletes should be allowed to do whatever they want as long as they are pain free during or within 24 hours of the activity. Ice should be placed in a plastic bag and applied directly to the skin for a continuous 20 minutes. Longer periods of icing are discouraged, since this can result in a peripheral nerve palsy from cryoinjury. Patients should ice the injury three to four times a day for the first 48 hours, and then at least once daily until the swelling or pain is gone. Compression is especially important and should be started as quickly as possible distal and proximal to the injured area. Elevation of the injured extremity should occur as often as possible. The use of this plan for soft tissue injuries facilitates early healing and allows rehabilitation to proceed quickly.

Anti-inflammatory or analgesic medications such as ibuprofen, aspirin, and naproxen are useful in controlling the symptoms of pain and swelling. For adolescent patients, dosages are similar to those used in adults: aspirin, 650–1000 mg every 6 hours; ibuprofen, 400–800 mg every 6–8 hours; naproxen, 500 mg twice daily. To minimize GI side effects, the medication should be administered with a snack or milk. Ideally, these drugs should be used for 7–10 days. Corticosteroids, either oral or parenteral, are not indicated in the management of overuse injuries.

After this acute phase, therapy is aimed at resolution of any edema and hematoma and at rehabilitation (Table 83–3). Athletes should slowly begin range-of-motion exercises as tolerated. Full tissue healing may take 6–8 weeks, but most young athletes do not have to wait that long to return to athletic activity.

Modified activity, depending on the degree of tissue damage, should initially be recommended in athletes who have suffered from overuse syndromes. Complete rest is rarely indicated. Participation in another sport such as swimming or cycling is often preferable to complete immobilization. In addition to the use of anti-inflammatory agents, physical therapy is another important therapeutic modality. Cryotherapy, whirlpool, or alternating heat and ice treatments can be helpful. Reconditioning should be continued after 3–12 weeks of modified activity, depending on the degree of recovery. This entails gradual strengthening and flexibility training as well as a reevaluation of previous modes of training to minimize the risk of reinjury (see Table 83–4).

TABLE 83–3.   Principles of Rehabilitation

Resolution of hematoma
Resolution of edema
Regain full range of motion or flexibility
Regain full muscle strength and endurance
Regain agility and coordination
Regain cardiovascular endurance

TABLE 83–4.   Rehabilitation of Musculoskeletal Injuries

Four Phases of Rehabilitation

1. Limit additional injury, and control pain and swelling (RICE mnemonic)
2. Improve strength and flexibility (range of motion) of the injured structures
3. Progressively improve strength, flexibility, proprioception, and endurance training until near-normal function is attained
4. Return to exercise and sports symptom-free

Modified and reproduced, with permission, from Hergenroeder, A. C. Prevention of sports injuries. Pediatrics 101:1060–1061, 1998.

PREVENTION

Injury prevention is an important aspect of sports medicine with which the primary practitioner should be familiar. Since most injuries are the result of "trying to do too much too soon," proper physical **training and conditioning** is essential, no matter how fit the athlete appears. Stretching, warm-up and cool-down exercises, and the type of equipment used for the sport should be reviewed with the athlete during the sports physical visit. The type of sport to be played should also be reviewed and, if participating in a contact sport, the adolescent should be **matched with other athletes** based on weight and pubertal development rather than age. Some studies suggest that such matching will greatly reduce the risk of injury to the smaller, less mature athlete. Since an old or incompletely healed injury is a significant risk factor for reinjury, all **previous injuries should receive proper treatment and rehabilitation** before the athlete returns to play. **Protective equipment,** especially for collision and contact sports, as well as for those involving a ball or racquet, also should be emphasized to athletes and their parents. In addition, the AAP recommendation of **avoiding strength and weight training** until the athlete reaches SMR (Tanner) stage 5 of pubertal development, to prevent the risk of serious injury, should be endorsed. **Education regarding the hazards of anabolic steroid use** also may be indicated.

PROGNOSIS

Orthopedic injuries in young athletes and active adolescents have a great capacity for healing if given the opportunity. Early medical intervention to prevent irreversible tissue damage assures complete recovery in most cases. Long-term sequelae are associated with repeated trauma, incompletely treated cases, and chronic inflammatory changes. Some conditions, however, such as Osgood-Schlatter disease, will resolve even without treatment and do not lead to any permanent damage to the joint.

Case Resolution

In the case presented at the beginning of the chapter, the teenager has symptoms and physical findings consistent with patellofemoral pain syndrome (traditionally referred to as chondromalacia of the patella). Since radiographs are usually not helpful in confirming the diagnosis, none are necessary at this time. Management should include strength training for the quadriceps muscles, activity modification, nonsteroidal anti-inflammatory medication, and ice compresses after activity. Orthotics such as an elastic cartilage brace may also be considered.

Selected Readings

American Academy of Pediatrics. Sports Medicine: Health Care for Young Athletes, 2nd ed. Elk Grove Village, IL, American Academy of Pediatrics, 1991.

Dyment, P. G., (ed.). Sports medicine. Pediatr. Ann. 26:13–64, 1997.

Dyment, P. G., (ed.). Sports and the adolescent. Adol. Med. State of the Art Rev. 2:1–250, 1991.

Group on Science and Technology, American Medical Association. Athletic preparticipation examination for adolescents: Report of the Board of Trustees. Arch. Pediatr. Adolesc. Med. 148:93–98, 1994.

Hergenroeder, A. C. Acute shoulder, knee, and ankle injuries, II. Rehabil. Adolesc. Health Update 8:1–8, 1996.

Hergenroeder, A. C. Prevention of sports injuries. Pediatrics 101:1057–1063, 1998.

Mankin, K. P., and S. Zimbler. Foot and ankle injuries: solving the diagnostic dilemmas. Contemp. Pediatr. 13:25–45, 1996.

Risser, W. L. Sports medicine. Pediatr. Rev. 14:424–431, 1993.

Rome, E. S. Sports-related injuries among adolescents: when do they occur, and how can we prevent them? Pediatr. Rev. 16: 184–187, 1995.

Ryu, R. K. N., and R. S. Fan. Adolescent and pediatric sport injuries. Pediatr. Clin. North Am. 45:1601–1635, 1998.

CHAPTER 84

EVALUATION OF LIMP

Geeta Grover, M.D.

H$_x$ A 6-year-old boy who has a 2-day history of right knee pain and limp is brought to the office. No history of knee trauma, swelling, redness, or associated fever is present. The past medical history is unremarkable. The boy is afebrile, and his height and weight are at the 10th percentile for age. Examination of the right leg reveals decreased abduction and internal rotation of the hip; the knee is normal. The boy limps when he walks and favors his right leg.

Questions

1. What is the differential diagnosis of painful and painless limps in children?
2. What is the differential diagnosis of knee pain in children?
3. What laboratory and radiographic tests are indicated in the evaluation of children with limp?
4. What is the appropriate management of children with suspected infectious causes of limp?

A limp is an abnormal gait that minimizes weight bearing on the affected leg to reduce pain and instability. Limp may be secondary to muscle weakness, deformity, or pain. Muscle weakness may be due to primary muscle disease, neurologic conditions, or disuse atrophy. Structural causes of limp include leg length discrepancy and joint stiffness, while painful causes of limp include synovitis, trauma, neoplasia, or infection (e.g., bone, joint, or soft-tissue). Because limp can be a sign of significant underlying disease, accurate diagnosis and appropriate management are essential to prevent potentially serious morbidity, including long-term disability.

EPIDEMIOLOGY

Limp, which is not uncommonly seen in children, may be due to pain originating in the leg or referred pain from the abdomen or spine. Age influences the list of diagnostic possibilities, because certain disorders are seen more frequently in one age group than another. Although septic arthritis occurs in children of all ages, it is seen most often in children under 3 years of age and in sexually active adolescents. Transient synovitis, the most common cause of hip pain in young children, is seen mostly in children 3–6 years of age.

Noninfectious causes of limp are more common in school-age children and adolescents than in younger children. Legg-Calvé-Perthes disease (LCPD idiopathic juvenile avascular necrosis of the femoral head) is seen primarily in children 4–8 years of age with a male-to-female ratio of 4–5:1. LCPD has been associated with a history of low birth weight, delayed bone age, and short stature. Bilateral involvement is seen in about 10% of cases. Slipped capital femoral epiphysis (SCFE), the most common hip disorder in adolescents, is seen most often in the 11- to 15-year age group, with a male-to-female ratio of about 2:1. It is bilateral about 20–25% of the time, but many bilateral slips occur sequentially rather than concurrently. SCFE has been associated with obesity and tall stature. Osgood-Schlatter disease is seen most commonly in physically active males between the ages of 10 and 15 years.

- Decreased range of motion of involved extremity
- Knee pain or hip pain
- Abnormal gait (e.g., antalgic, Trendelenburg, toe-to-heel)
- Systemic signs (e.g., fever, irritability)
- Abnormal laboratory results (e.g., leukocytosis, elevated ESR)

CLINICAL PRESENTATION (D_X BOX)

Painful limp usually has an acute onset. It may be associated with systemic signs such as fever or irritability, especially when the etiology is infectious. Toddlers may simply refuse to walk or walk with a slow cautious gait (e.g., characteristic of diskitis) when they are in pain rather than limp. Nonpainful limp often has an insidious onset and is commonly due to weakness (e.g., muscular dystrophy) or deformity (e.g., leg length discrepancy).

PATHOPHYSIOLOGY

An understanding of normal gait and its development is essential to the evaluation of limp. Normal gait has two phases: stance and swing. During the stance phase, either one or both feet are on the ground, whereas during the swing phase, one foot is not touching the ground as the limb is moved forward. Stance phase is shortened in limp to decrease the amount of time spent in weight bearing on the affected side or to minimize instability.

Normal adult gait is smooth and efficient, requiring the coordinated actions of the muscles of the legs and pelvis. Normal gait in children varies according to age and developmental maturity. Toddlers typically walk with a broad-based, tiptoe, "bouncing" gait with arms abducted for balance; they may initiate the stance phase with either toe or heel strike. By 2 years of age, children should initiate the stance phase consistently with heel strike. Children who are 3–4 years of age should exhibit normal adult gait with reciprocating arm swing the majority of the time (Fig. 84–1).

Several types of abnormal gaits are recognized. A shortened stance phase due to pain is characteristic of an **antalgic gait.** Weakness of the hip abductors (gluteus medius) leads to a **Trendelenburg gait,** where the pelvis dips down during stance phase, producing a swaying type of gait. A tiptoe or **toe-to-heel gait** is normal in children for several months after they learn to walk. Persistence of such a gait beyond 2 years of age is abnormal and may result from either idiopathic heelcord contracture or contracture secondary to cerebral palsy.

DIFFERENTIAL DIAGNOSIS

The differential diagnosis of limp may be classified by age group and the presence of associated pain (Table 84–1).

Children Aged 1–3 Years

Infection is the most common cause of painful limp in toddlers. **Septic arthritis** is a significant cause. *Staphylococcus aureus* is the most common etiologic organism in septic arthritis in all age groups. Before the use of *Haemophilus influenzae* type b (Hib) vaccine became widespread, Hib was the most frequently occurring pathogen in children younger than 2 years of age. The hip is involved, most commonly, followed by the knee. Acute onset of pain in the involved joint, fever, limited range of motion of the joint, and an antalgic gait or posturing are common. Often, children appear fine as

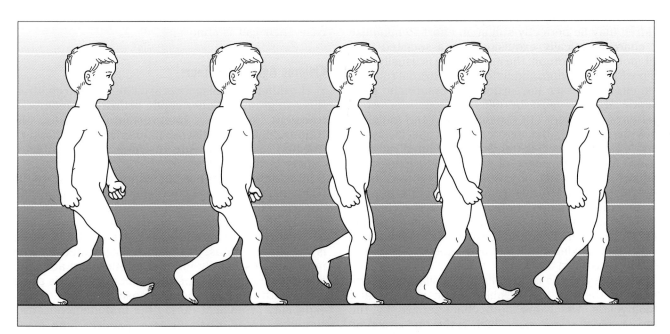

FIGURE 84–1. Phases of gait in a 4-year-old child.

TABLE 84–1. Differential Diagnosis of Limp in Children

Children Ages 1–3 Years
Painful Limp
Septic arthritis/osteomyelitis
Transient synovitis
Intervertebral diskitis
Juvenile rheumatoid arthritis (JRA)
Neoplasia (leukemia, metastatic disease)
Trauma (toddler's fractures)
Child abuse
Painless Limp
Developmental hip dysplasia
Neuromuscular disease (cerebral palsy)
Leg length discrepancy
Children Ages 4–10 Years
Painful Limp
Septic arthritis/osteomyelitis
Transient synovitis
Trauma
Legg-Calvé-Perthes disease (LCPD) (acute phase)
Intervertebral diskitis
JRA
Sickle-cell pain crisis
Neoplasia (leukemia, primary bone tumor, metastatic disease)
Painless Limp
LCPD (chronic phase)
Developmental hip dysplasia
Neuromuscular disease (cerebral palsy, muscular dystrophy)
Leg length discrepancy
Children and Adolescents Ages 11 Years and Older
Painful Limp
Trauma
Septic arthritis/osteomyelitis
Slipped capital femoral epiphysis (SCFE)
Osgood-Schlatter disease
JRA
Sickle cell pain crisis
Neoplasia (leukemia, primary bone tumor, metastatic disease)
Painless Limp
SCFE
Leg length discrepancy
Neuromuscular disease (cerebral palsy, muscular dystrophy)
Scoliosis

---

long as the affected joint is not moved or touched. Children may lie perfectly still in an effort to minimize the characteristically exquisite pain associated with joint motion. In addition, the infected hip is usually kept in a position of flexion, abduction, and external rotation in an effort to lessen intraarticular pressure and pain.

Septic arthritis must be differentiated from **osteomyelitis** (see Chapter 119, Osteomyelitis) and **transient synovitis.** In theory, the absence of joint-specific symptoms (e.g., joint swelling, tenderness, limited range of motion) and the presence of swelling and tenderness localized to the metaphysis of the involved bone distinguish septic arthritis from osteomyelitis. In practice, this differentiation is often difficult. The clinician must maintain a high index of suspicion of simultaneous occurrence of both conditions, especially in joints such as the hip, ankle, shoulder, and elbow, where the metaphysis is intra-articular.

Transient synovitis is a self-limited, unilateral inflammation of the hip joint. Unlike septic arthritis and osteomyelitis, which are both characterized by the acute onset of severe pain, high fever, and systemic signs, transient synovitis is usually associated with a history of low-grade fever, insidious onset of pain, and

antalgic limp or refusal to walk. As in septic arthritis, the hip is maintained in a position of flexion, abduction, and external rotation to minimize pain.

Other significant causes of limp in young children are **intervertebral diskitis, juvenile rheumatoid arthritis (JRA)** (see Chapter 120), and **toddler's fracture.** Diskitis is a benign, self-limited inflammation of the disk, often resulting from infection with *S. aureus*. Low-grade fever, back pain, irritability, and refusal to sit, stand, or walk are often present, depending on age. Although JRA may affect any synovial joint, it commonly begins in the large joints, especially the knee. The occurrence of morning stiffness that gradually resolves as the day progresses, which is characteristic of JRA, may help differentiate it from the other causes of antalgic limp. Occult fractures, especially the toddler's fracture or fracture secondary to child abuse (see Chapter 104), should also be entertained in the differential diagnosis. Toddler's fracture is an oblique or spiral fracture of the mid or distal tibia, which usually develops after a fall or jump with a twist. Toddlers are prone to such injuries because of their unsteady gait. A high index of suspicion is necessary to make this diagnosis because although there is localized tenderness over the tibia, initial x-rays are often negative. Follow-up x-rays or a bone scan will reveal the fracture.

Painless limp in toddlers may be due to **developmental hip dysplasia** (see Chapter 79), **cerebral palsy** (see Chapter 21, Needs of Children With Physical and Sensory Disabilities), or **leg length discrepancy** (anisomelia). As a result of developmental hip dysplasia, children may have a Trendelenburg gait secondary to leg length discrepancy or to weakness of the hip abductors. Children with spastic cerebral palsy often walk on their toes because of increased tone or heelcord contractures. Functional or apparent leg length discrepancies may result from pelvic obliquity or spinal deformity. Children with true leg length inequality compensate by either walking on tiptoe on the shorter side or bending the knee on the longer side; in either case, their gait is abnormal.

Children Aged 4–10 Years

The differential diagnosis of painful limp in children in this age group includes **septic arthritis, osteomyelitis, transient synovitis, intervertebral diskitis, JRA, trauma, sickle cell disease pain crisis** (see Chapter 63, Anemia), and **neoplastic diseases** (see Chapter 114, Cancer in Children).

In addition, **LCPD** is an important cause of limp (both painful and painless). The etiology of LCPD is unclear, but it may result from disruption in blood supply to the femoral head, leading to avascular necrosis. Pain localized to the hip, inner thigh, or knee is usually insidious. The pain is aggravated by movement (e.g., especially internal rotation and abduction) and relieved by rest. Not uncommonly, LCPD is present for months before the diagnosis is made. Pain is especially prominent during the first stage because of synovitis. Later in the disease, painless limp may be more common. In LCPD the hip is kept in a position of flexion and slight external rotation.

Children and Adolescents Aged 11 Years and Older

The differential diagnosis of painful limp in older children and adolescents includes **trauma, septic arthritis, osteomyelitis, JRA, sickle-cell disease pain crisis,** and **neoplastic disease.** In addition to *S. aureus, Neisseria gonorrhoeae* is a common pathogen in sexually active adolescents with septic arthritis. Transient synovitis may develop a few weeks after rubella vaccination, especially in adolescent females. The small joints of the hands are involved more often than larger joints such as the ankles and knees. Other significant causes of painful limp in children aged 11 years and older are **SCFE** and **Osgood-Schlatter disease.**

SCFE is a displacement or slipping of the femoral head from the neck of the femur through the open growth plate. Affected children usually present with a history of dull, aching pain in the hip or knee that increases with activity. The onset of pain is insidious more often than it is acute and children may at times be free of pain. Children with SCFE walk with a Trendelenburg gait. The hip is held in extension and external rotation, and internal rotation is decreased.

Osgood-Schlatter disease, or traction apophysitis of the tibial tubercle, is an overuse syndrome in which repetitive microtrauma causes partial avulsion of the patellar tendon at its insertion on the tibia. Children with this condition present with localized prominence, swelling, and tenderness over the tibial tubercle at the insertion of the patellar tendon.

EVALUATION

History

The history should focus on the time of onset of the limp, its chronicity, and the degree of disability it produces (Questions Box). Delayed motor development may be a sign of neuromuscular disease such as cerebral palsy, whereas a history of loss of motor milestones may indicate muscular dystrophy or spinal cord tumor. It is important to remember that pelvic pain may be referred to the hip, and hip pain is often referred to the knee.

Physical Examination

Physical examination begins with observation for any overt deformities (e.g., leg length discrepancy, fracture, joint swelling). All joints should be palpated, and the presence of swelling, tenderness, erythema, or warmth

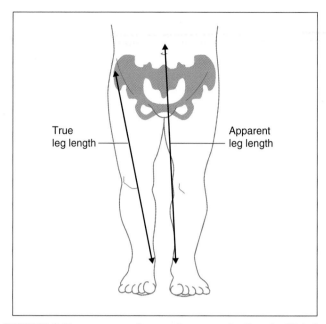

FIGURE 84–2. Measurement of true and apparent leg lengths. With the patient in a supine position, apparent measurement is made from the umbilicus to the medial malleolus (affected by pelvic obliquity and hip position) and true measurement is made from anterosuperior iliac spine to the medial malleolus.

should be noted. A thorough evaluation of the hips is essential in children with knee pain. The type of gait (e.g., antalgic, Trendelenburg) may be determined by observing children walk or run (if possible) up and down corridors.

Children should also be examined both standing and supine, if possible. Standing children can be assessed for pelvic obliquity and spinal deformities. Range of motion of the hips, knees, ankles, and feet can be checked in supine children; one side can be compared to the other. Deep tendon reflexes and muscle strength should be assessed, and leg length measurements should also be made (Fig. 84–2). Children should be supine for a true measurement of leg length from the anterosuperior iliac spine to the medial malleolus. A discrepancy of more than 2 cm is considered significant in adults. The significance of discrepancies can be confirmed by imaging studies.

Laboratory Tests

Laboratory procedures are usually necessary in children with acute onset of limp and may be helpful. CBC, C-reactive protein (CRP), and ESR are useful markers of systemic disease or significant inflammation. A normal CBC, CRP, and ESR may help distinguish transient synovitis from septic arthritis. Blood and local cultures (e.g., joint or bone fluid) may be useful in the evaluation of suspected septic arthritis or osteomyelitis.

Imaging Studies

X-rays are the most commonly required imaging study. If LCPD or SCFE is suspected, x-rays of the hips should include both anteroposterior and frog-leg views.

Questions: Evaluation of Limp

- How old was the child when the limp developed?
- Was the onset acute or chronic?
- Is the limp constant or intermittent (i.e., is it worse in the morning or at the end of the day)?
- Does the limp affect the child's regular activities in any way? How?
- Is the limp painful? Where does it hurt? Is the pain in one place?
- Does the child exhibit any other symptoms associated with the limp?
- Has the child lost any developmental milestones?
- Is there any history of trauma?

Early in the course of LCPD, x-rays may either be negative, or show widening of the joint space. In later stages, radiographic findings include an increased density and decreased size of the femoral head (necrosis), patchy areas of radiolucency near the epiphysis (fragmentation), and flattening of the femoral head (reconstitution). In SCFE, x-rays show the epiphysis slipping posteriorly and inferiorly with respect to the neck of the femur (e.g., like ice cream falling off a cone). In Osgood-Schlatter disease, knee x-rays may show soft tissue swelling over the tibial tubercle and a thickening of the patellar tendon. In children with knee pain, hip x-rays should be taken in addition to knee x-rays. X-rays are usually normal in transient synovitis.

In addition, bone scans may be useful in the early stages of certain diseases (e.g., osteomyelitis or toddler's fracture), when x-rays are typically normal.

MANAGEMENT

Management depends on the specific clinical diagnosis. **Immobilization** and **supportive care** are the backbone of treatment in transient synovitis, diskitis, LCPD, and Osgood-Schlatter disease. Symptoms of transient synovitis usually resolve within 7–10 days with no further intervention. Diskitis is generally a self-limited disease. Symptoms usually resolve within 4–6 weeks with immobilization and supportive care. Antistaphylococcal **antibiotics** may be used if *S. aureus* is suspected. The goals of treatment in LCPD are to maintain full joint mobility and prevent deformity of the femoral head. Bed rest and immobilization decrease the pain associated with synovitis and help restore range of motion. **Traction** and **abduction casts** are used to contain the femoral head within the acetabulum in an effort to maintain its spherical shape. Osgood-Schlatter disease, a self-limited condition, usually resolves when the proximal tibial epiphysis fuses. Symptoms generally resolve over a period of months. Supportive treatment consists of restriction of activity, use of analgesia, and stretching of the quadriceps and hamstring muscles. A knee immobilizer splint may be used.

Surgical treatment is required for SCFE and may be necessary in the management of septic arthritis and osteomyelitis. SCFE requires immediate operative fixation to prevent further slipping of the epiphysis. In septic arthritis, incision and drainage of the affected joint relieve the intraarticular pressure. A culture of the aspirate may allow identification of the organism. Empiric treatment with an antistaphylococcal penicillin (e.g., oxacillin, nafcillin) should be initiated until Gram stain or culture results are available. Typically, 14–21 days of antibiotic treatment is required. Like septic arthritis, osteomyelitis may also necessitate surgical decompression, followed by appropriate intravenous antibiotics (see Chapter 119, Osteomyelitis). Four to six weeks of treatment is usually required.

Management of leg length discrepancy depends on the predicted discrepancy at final adult height. Predicted differences less than 2 cm do not require treatment. Larger discrepancies may be managed either nonsurgically (e.g., heel lifts), especially when the predicted difference is less than 5 cm, or surgically. Surgical treatment may include leg lengthening procedures (e.g., Ilizarov method) of the shorter leg or shortening procedures (e.g., epiphysiodesis to produce growth arrest or osteotomy) of the longer leg.

If history, physical examination, laboratory tests, and imaging studies fail to reveal an abnormality, children should be reassessed weekly until a diagnosis is made or the limp resolves. If any uncertainty remains, **orthopedic consultation** should be promptly obtained, because missed or delayed diagnoses may result in long-term disability.

PROGNOSIS

Prognosis of LCPD is related to the degree of femoral head involvement and age at onset of the disease. Children less than 6 years of age have the best prognosis. The risk of development of degenerative arthritis in adulthood increases in children whose disease is more extensive and whose condition is diagnosed later (i.e., after 8 years of age).

If patients with SCFE are untreated, the potential for further slipping of the femoral head remains until the growth plate closes. Potential treatment-related complications of SCFE include chondrolysis of the femoral head and acetabulum, avascular necrosis, and fracture at the site of pin placement.

In about 5–10% of cases, Osgood-Schlatter disease may become chronic, with persistent swelling and tenderness. In such cases an x-ray may show the formation of an ossicle over the tibial tubercle; this ossicle may require surgical resection.

The prognosis is good in the majority of cases of septic arthritis and osteomyelitis if the infection is diagnosed early and treated appropriately.

Case Resolution

In the case described at the beginning of the chapter, the child's history and physical examination appear to be consistent with LCPD. The child's knee pain is actually secondary to hip pathology. The diagnosis may have been missed if the physician had not examined the hips and noted the abnormality in range of motion. Both anteroposterior and frog-leg x-rays of the hips were taken, which showed widening of the joint space. Orthopedic consultation was obtained, and hospitalization for bed rest and ensured immobilization was recommended.

Selected Readings

Dahl, M. T. Limb length discrepancy. Pediatr. Clin. North Am. 43:849–865, 1996.

Henrickson, M., and M. H. Passo. Recognizing patterns in chronic limb pain. Contemp. Pediatr. 11:33–62, 1994.

Hurley, J. M., et al. Slipped capital femoral epiphysis: the prevalence of late contralateral slip. J. Bone Joint Surg. 78A:226–230, 1996.

Koop, S., and D. Quanbeck. Three common causes of childhood hip pain. Pediatr. Clin. North Am. 43:1053–1066, 1996.

MacEwen, G. D., and R. Dehne. The limping child. Pediatr. Rev. 12:268–274, 1991.

Renshaw, T. S. The child who has a limp. Pediatr. Rev. 16:458–465, 1995.

MUSCULOSKELETAL DISORDERS OF THE NECK AND BACK

Geeta Grover, M. D.

H$_x$ A 4-week-old male infant is brought to the office by his mother, who complains that her son always holds his head tilted to the right. She reports that he has held it in this position for about 1 week and prefers to look mainly to the left. The infant is the 8 lb, 8 oz product of a term gestation born via forceps extraction, and he had no complications in the neonatal period. He is feeding well on breast milk and has no history of fever, upper respiratory symptoms, or vomiting and diarrhea.

On examination, the head is tilted toward the right side with limited lateral rotation to the right and decreased lateral side bending to the left. Except for the presence of a small mass palpable on the right side of the neck, the examination is within normal limits.

Questions

1. What laboratory or radiologic studies are indicated in infants with torticollis?
2. What is the differential diagnosis of torticollis in infants?
3. What are some of the common musculoskeletal abnormalities that may be seen in association with torticollis?
4. What are other common musculoskeletal problems in children and adolescents?

Children with disorders of the spine can present with deformity, back pain, or occasionally both. Nontraumatic congenital and developmental deformities of the spine are frequently encountered in pediatric practice. Torticollis and scoliosis are two of the most common disorders in children that present as spinal deformity. **Torticollis,** or "wry neck," is a positional abnormality of the neck resulting in abnormal tilting and rotation of the head. **Scoliosis** refers to any lateral curvature of the spine. **Back pain** is a far less common complaint in children than in adults. When such pain occurs in children, it usually signals the presence of organic disease. In adolescents, musculoskeletal strain is a common etiology.

EPIDEMIOLOGY

Some degree of spinal asymmetry is seen in about 2–5% of the population.

The most common type of **torticollis** seen in children is congenital muscular torticollis. The incidence of this common neonatal orthopedic complaint is increased in breech presentations and difficult deliveries. It is asso-

ciated with developmental dysplasia of the hip (DDH) in as many as 10–20% of affected infants. Family history may be positive in up to 10% of cases.

Acquired torticollis, usually secondary to infectious or traumatic causes, is much more common in older children. Episodes of benign paroxysmal torticollis, which often begin in the first year of life and generally resolve by 5 years of age, may have a familial basis. An association with benign paroxysmal vertigo and migraines has been noted.

The prevalence of **scoliosis** among school-age children is 3–5%. A right thoracic single curve is the most common curve seen by physicians. Seventy-five to 80% of cases of structural scoliosis are idiopathic, 10% are due to neuromuscular causes, 5% are congenital, and the remaining 5–10% are due to trauma or miscellaneous causes. Scoliosis that begins in childhood affects boys and girls equally, and affected boys actually outnumber girls during the first three years of life. Idiopathic scoliosis that develops after the age of 10 years is seen more frequently in girls than in boys, however. The ratio is approximately 5–7 : 1. In children with cerebral palsy, the incidence of scoliosis is increased and it is found in about 20% of all cases.

Back pain is quite uncommon in preadolescent children. In the majority of cases of back pain in children, it is possible to determine the etiology, unlike in adults, where it is often difficult to identify the cause.

CLINICAL PRESENTATION

Although **torticollis** may be noted at birth, it usually manifests at 2–4 weeks of age. Infants with congenital muscular torticollis present with a characteristic head tilt toward the affected side and the chin pointing toward the opposite side secondary to unilateral fibrosis and contracture of the sternocleidomastoid muscle (Fig. 85–1). Unrecognized or untreated cases of torticollis may present as plagiocephaly (See Chapter 50, Craniofacial Anomalies) or facial asymmetry during infancy. Benign paroxysmal torticollis of infancy may present as recurrent episodes of head tilt that may be associated with vomiting, ataxia, agitation, or malaise (D$_x$ Box).

No obvious deformity may be noted in mild **scoliosis.** Asymmetry of shoulder heights, scapular prominence or position, and waistline or pelvic levelness may all be signs of scoliosis (see D$_x$ Box) (Fig 85–2A). Back pain is uncommon in adolescents with idiopathic scoliosis.

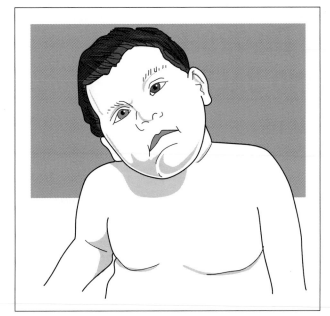

FIGURE 85–1. Torticollis. Infant with congenital muscular torticollis showing head tilt.

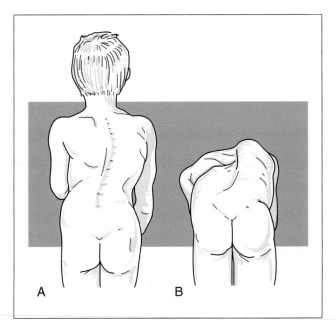

FIGURE 85–2. Scoliosis. A. Child with scoliosis (rear view). B. Child with scoliosis performing bend test.

When pain is present, further examination for some other cause (e.g., bone tumors, spondylolysis, spondylolisthesis) is warranted.

Preverbal children with **back pain** may present with limp or refusal to bear weight or walk.

PATHOPHYSIOLOGY

Torticollis may be either congenital or acquired. The etiology of congenital muscular torticollis is unknown. It is believed to be due to intrauterine positioning or trauma to the soft tissues of the neck during delivery, with resulting ischemia of the sternocleidomastoid muscle secondary to venous occlusion. This leads to edema and degeneration of the muscle fibers with eventual fibrosis of the muscle body. Deformities of the face and skull may result if the condition is left untreated. Plagiocephaly (cranial asymmetry), with flattening of the face on the affected side and flattening of the occiput on the contralateral side, is seen most commonly.

Scoliosis is a lateral curvature of the spine, unlike kyphosis and lordosis, which are curves in the antero-posterior plane. Scoliosis can be either functional (nonstructural) or structural. Because no fixed deformity of the spine is associated with functional scoliosis, the apparent curvature disappears on lying down or forward flexion. Structural scoliosis may be idiopathic or caused by various underlying disorders. In structural scoliosis, as the spine curves laterally, it forces the vertebrae to rotate, resulting in deformity of attached structures. For example, a "rib hump" may be produced due to scoliosis in the thoracic spine (see Fig. 85–2B). Pelvic obliquity or flank prominence may be produced when the curvature is in the lumbar spine.

DIFFERENTIAL DIAGNOSIS

The differential diagnosis of congenital and acquired **torticollis** is presented in Table 85–1. Congenital muscular torticollis is the most common cause of congenital torticollis. Torticollis may appear in association with nystagmus and head nodding, a condition referred to as spasmus nutans. Acquired torticollis is seen primarily in older infants and children. Cervical lymphadenitis is a common cause in children 1–5 years of age, whereas trauma to the soft tissues or muscles of the neck is seen more frequently in school-age children. Acute episodes (e.g., benign paroxysmal torticollis of infancy) must be differentiated from chronic conditions (e.g., Sandifer's syndrome, rheumatoid arthritis).

Functional or nonstructural **scoliosis** may be secondary to poor posture, leg length discrepancies, or muscle spasm. Structural scoliosis can be classified into idiopathic, congenital, neuromuscular, and miscellaneous forms (Table 85–2). Idiopathic scoliosis, which is by far the most common type of structural scoliosis, may be divided into three categories based on age: infantile (0–3 years), juvenile (3–10 years), and adolescent (>10 years). The adolescent form occurs most frequently.

Congenital scoliosis results from anomalies of the spine such as hemivertebrae or failure of vertebral

---

Dx — Torticollis and Scoliosis

TORTICOLLIS
- Head tilt
- Limited range of motion of the neck
- Contracture of the sternocleidomastoid muscle
- Plagiocephaly (congenital torticollis)
- Firm, nontender, mobile mass within the body of the sternocleidomastoid muscle (congenital torticollis)

SCOLIOSIS
- Lateral curvature of the spine
- No pain
- Back or truncal asymmetry

TABLE 85–1.   Common Causes of Torticollis

Congenital
Congenital muscular torticollis
Pterygium coli (skin web)
Occipitocervical spine anomalies (e.g., Klippel-Feil syndrome)

Acquired
Infectious
   Cervical lymphadenitis
   Retropharyngeal abscess
   Osteomyelitis of cervical vertebrae
Traumatic
   Atlanto-occipital, atlas-axis (C1-C2), or C2-C3 subluxation
   Cervical musculature injury (spastic torticollis)
   Cervical spine fractures
Neurologic
   Tumors (posterior fossa or cervical cord)
   Dystonic drug reactions
   Syringomyelia
   Ocular disturbances (strabismus, nystagmus)
Other
   Spasmus nutans
   Sandifer's syndrome (hiatal hernia with gastroesophageal reflux)
   Benign paroxysmal torticollis of infancy
   Rheumatoid arthritis
   Hysteria
   Soft tissue tumors of the neck

TABLE 85–3.   Common Causes of Back Pain in Children

Infectious
Myalgias (e.g., influenza)
Diskitis (more common in children < 5 years of age)
Vertebral osteomyelitis (pyogenic, tuberculosis [Potts disease])
Referred pain (pyelonephritis, pneumonia)
Inflammatory
Rheumatologic diseases (juvenile rheumatoid arthritis, ankylosing spondylitis)
Crohn's disease/ulcerative colitis/psoriatic arthritis
Disk space calcification
Neoplastic
Primary vertebral and spinal tumors (e.g., Ewing's sarcoma, osteosarcoma, neuroblastoma)
Metastatic disease (e.g., neuroblastoma)
Benign tumors (e.g., eosinophilic granuloma, osteoid osteoma)
Developmental
Spondylolysis, spondylolisthesis (adolescents)
Scheuermann's syndrome (adolescents)
Traumatic
Herniated nucleus pulposus (disk herniation)
Ligamentous or muscle strain (e.g., overuse syndromes)
Compression fracture of vertebrae
Other
Sickle cell crisis
Osteoporosis (e.g., rickets, osteogenesis imperfecta)
Child abuse
Psychogenic

segmentation. The incidence of cardiac and renal anomalies is increased. Although neuromuscular scoliosis is most often seen in children with spastic cerebral palsy, it may also be apparent in other conditions such as poliomyelitis, meningomyelocele, muscular dystrophy, Friedreich's ataxia, and spinal muscular atrophy.

The miscellaneous causes of scoliosis are uncommon and include trauma, metabolic disorders, and neurocutaneous diseases.

The most common causes of **back pain** in children may be classified into five categories (Table 85–3). Because the spine of children is smaller and has greater flexibility and ligamentous strength, children have a higher tolerance to trauma and a lower risk of injury than adults do. Infection (e.g., diskitis) and neoplasia are perhaps more common in children. Common causes of back pain in adults, such as herniated disks or musculoskeletal low back pain (usually secondary to muscle strain), are uncommon in children. Only about 2% of all herniated disks occur in children. Predisposed individuals often experience their first episode of musculoskeletal low back pain during adolescence or young adulthood.

EVALUATION

History

A careful history may provide clues to diagnosis and etiology (Questions: Torticollis; Questions: Scoliosis; and Questions: Back Pain).

Physical Examination

In children with suspected **torticollis,** a thorough examination with specific attention to the head and neck region should be performed. Limited head rotation toward the affected side with decreased lateral side bending to the opposite side may occur. During the first 4–6 weeks of life a firm, nontender

TABLE 85–2.   Common Causes of Scoliosis

Functional Scoliosis
Poor posture
Leg length discrepancies
Muscle spasm
   Herniated disk
   Back injury
Structural Scoliosis
Idiopathic
Congenital
Neuromuscular
Miscellaneous
   Trauma (e.g., fractures or dislocations of the vertebrae)
   Intraspinal tumors
   Metabolic disorders (e.g., juvenile osteoporosis, osteogenesis imperfecta, mucopolysaccharidosis)
   Neurocutaneous syndromes (e.g., neurofibromatosis)
   Marfan's syndrome

Questions: Torticollis

- Is there any family history of torticollis?
- What type of delivery did the mother have (e.g., cesarean or vaginal)? Were forceps required?
- When was the head tilt first noticed?
- Does the infant move his or her neck in all directions, or does he or she always prefer to look in one direction?
- Does the infant have any recent history of trauma to the head or neck area?
- Is the head tilt persistent or does it come and go?
- Has the infant been sick or febrile?
- Does the child have nystagmus or head bobbing?

mobile mass, which gradually regresses by 6 months of age, may be palpated within the body of the sternocleidomastoid muscle. The hips should be examined for stability because of the association of torticollis with DDH.

In addition, a neurologic examination should also be performed to look for any neurologic deficits that may be signs of an underlying tumor. Fever or signs of inflammation point to infectious causes. Because torticollis may be secondary to visual disturbances such as strabismus, a careful eye examination is warranted. The presence of nystagmus or head nodding suggests spasmus nutans.

Screening for **scoliosis** should be part of the routine health maintenance examination of school-age children and adolescents. Children should be examined with the back fully exposed. The posture should be observed. The presence of any skin lesions such as café-au-lait spots should be noted. Any midline skin defects such as dimples or hair patches should also be noted, because they are often associated with underlying spinal lesions. The spine should be palpated for any signs of tenderness, and a complete neurologic examination should be performed.

The back should be observed for asymmetry of the shoulders, scapulae, or pelvis. Physicians should have children bend forward at the waist to an angle of 90 degrees. This maneuver accentuates the curvature of structural scoliosis and emphasizes the rotational deformity of the spine. For example, in thoracic scoliosis, a characteristic rib hump is apparent on the convex side of the curve.

Scoliosis is described in terms of the primary or major curve, which is predominantly thoracic. The major curve may be single or compensated by a secondary or minor curve, which is predominantly lumbar. The location is defined by the apical vertebra (e.g., T2–T11 = thoracic, T12–L1 = thoracolumbar), the direction of the curvature by the side of convexity, and the severity indicated by the degree of curvature as measured on the spinal radiograph. Curves greater than 15 degrees are abnormal. Mild scoliosis is defined as curvature of less than 20 degrees, moderate as 20–40 degrees, and severe as greater than 40–45 degrees.

The evaluation of **back pain** begins with observation of children's posture and gait. Any midline skin lesions should be noted. A thorough general physical examination is important because referred pain (e.g., pyelonephritis, nephrolithiasis) may be causing the symptoms in the back. The spine should be palpated for any signs of tenderness. A complete neurologic examination should be performed, and any motor or sensory deficits should be noted. The motor examination should emphasize evaluation of the hips and the lower extremities, including range of motion and strength.

Laboratory Tests

In cases of **congenital torticollis,** laboratory studies are rarely necessary. In acquired torticollis, if any infection is suspected, a CBC and blood and local cultures may aid in the diagnosis.

No specific laboratory tests are required in the evaluation of idiopathic **scoliosis.** Specific laboratory studies may be performed in the evaluation of other forms of scoliosis as indicated by the history and physical examination (e.g., a urine metabolic screen for suspected metabolic disturbances).

Laboratory assessment for **back pain** depends on the history and physical examination. A CBC, blood culture, and ESR may be useful in the evaluation of suspected infectious etiologies. Rheumatologic studies such as a rheumatoid factor or human leukocyte antigen typing may help in the diagnosis of inflammatory conditions. If the back pain is of an acute onset, studies such as a urinalysis or serum amylase would help establish that the pain is referred.

Imaging Studies

X-rays are generally not useful in children with suspected **torticollis** unless bony anomalies are suspected. MRI of the sternocleidomastoid muscle mass may be considered if an underlying condition (e.g., a branchial cleft cyst) is suspected. CT scan or MRI of the head or cervical spinal cord would be indicated if a neurologic tumor is suspected.

Routine x-rays are not required in the evaluation of all children with mild scoliosis (i.e., minor degrees of curvature noted on physical examination). It may be best to obtain x-rays after orthopedic evaluation is complete. A standing anteroposterior spine x-ray is used to determine the location and direction of the curvature, measure the degree of asymmetry (Cobb's angle), and evaluate the vertebrae. Repeat x-rays of the spine are used to follow the progression of the curvature over time. Because the risk of curve progression before skeletal maturity is a primary concern, hand and wrist x-rays should be taken to assess bone age in prepubertal children with scoliosis.

As with scoliosis, routine x-rays are not indicated in all cases of **back pain.** Various radiologic studies may be ordered depending on the suspected diagnosis. X-rays may be useful in the evaluation of suspected vertebral abnormalities such as spondylolysis and spondylolisthesis. However, these conditions may represent incidental findings and not be the source of the back pain. If diskitis is suspected, a bone scan may be more appropriate than x-rays. Similarly, a bone scan or MRI is useful in the evaluation of suspected vertebral tumors.

MANAGEMENT

Treatment of congenital muscular **torticollis** consists of **passive stretching exercises** of the neck. With the neck in a neutral position (i.e., not hyperextended), the head is bent to one side so that the ear on the side opposite to the contracted muscle is brought to the shoulder, or the chin is lowered to touch the shoulder on the affected side. In addition, **changing the placement of the crib** in relation to the nursery door and **repositioning toys and mobiles** in the crib stimulate children to look toward the side opposite the preferred gaze. Torticollis resolves spontaneously in most infants. When the deformity persists beyond the age of one to two years, **surgical release** of the contracted muscle may be indicated.

Management of acquired torticollis depends on etiology. The evaluation and treatment of many of these conditions can be complex and often require consultation with specialists in head and neck surgery, neurology, and orthopedic surgery.

Management of **scoliosis** involves **close follow-up** with careful repeat examinations and radiographic studies. An initial consultation with an orthopedic surgeon is generally advisable, even in minor degrees of curvature. The goal of follow-up is early detection of curvature with implementation of treatment to prevent or reduce curve progression. Children with curves less than 20–25 degrees should be monitored for progression. Curves between 25–45 degrees do not require bracing in skeletally mature individuals but should be braced (e.g., with Milwaukee brace) in growing children. The goal of **bracing** is not to correct any existing curvature but to prevent further curve progression. **Surgery** (e.g., the Harrington rod or posterior spinal fusion) may be indicated for children with curves greater than 45 degrees. These curves have a high likelihood of progression regardless of the patient's age and skeletal maturity.

Although the management of **back pain** is diagnosis-dependent, **rest** and **immobilization** are principles of treatment that apply in many instances. In the management of diskitis, antistaphylococcal antibiotics may be necessary in addition to immobilization. If spondylolisthesis and spondylolysis do not respond to rest and immobilization, operative stabilization may be required. In adolescents with low back pain related to muscular injury, conservative treatment including bed rest, heat, and anti-inflammatory medications may be tried for 1–2 weeks followed by a gradual return to normal activity. It is not advisable to institute such treatment in younger children without pursuing a more extensive evaluation or consultation with an orthopedic surgeon, because the risk of serious disease is significant in this age group.

PROGNOSIS

Congenital muscular **torticollis** responds to conservative management in about 90% of infants. The asymmetry of the face and skull also corrects over time once the contracture of the sternocleidomastoid resolves. Spasmus nutans, a condition which appears between 4 and 12 months, resolves spontaneously by 3 years of age.

The direction and location of the curvature in **scoliosis** do not change with age, but the degree of curvature may remain stable or progress. Factors associated with a high risk of curve progression include female sex, positive family history for scoliosis, younger age at diagnosis (especially before the adolescent growth spurt), and a larger curve at the time of diagnosis. In addition, a double curve is more likely to progress than a single curve, and a thoracic curve is more likely to progress than a lumbar curve. Left untreated, severe scoliosis can produce cardiopulmonary impairment or cosmetic deformity, which may lead to low self-esteem and poor body image.

The vast majority of cases (80–90%) of low **back pain** in adolescents and young adults resolve spontaneously in 2–8 weeks. It is important for patients to learn how to prevent recurrence by improving posture, learning how to lift heavy objects appropriately, and instituting a program of exercises to help strengthen the abdominal and back muscles.

Case Resolution

The history of the infant presented in the opening case scenario is consistent with congenital muscular torticollis. Physical examination helps confirm the diagnosis. The hips should be evaluated thoroughly because of the association of congenital muscular torticollis with congenital hip dysplasia. A program consisting of neck stretching exercises and repositioning of interesting toys and objects in the infant's crib to the side opposite the preferred gaze should be instituted. The infant can be reevaluated in 2–3 weeks to monitor progress.

Selected Readings

Ballock, R. T., and K. M. Song. The prevalence of nonmuscular causes of torticollis in children. J. Pediatr. Orthop. 16:500–504, 1996.

Boachie-Adjei, O., and B. Lonner. Spinal deformity. Pediatr. Clin. North Am. 43:883–897, 1996.

Cheng, J. C. Y., and A. W. Y. Au. Infantile torticollis: a review of 624 cases. J. Pediatr. Orthop. 14:802–808, 1994.

Epps, H. R., and R. B. Salter. Orthopedic conditions of the cervical spine and shoulder. Pediatr. Clin. North Am. 43:919–931, 1996.

Kautz, S. M., and D. L. Skaggs. Getting an angle on spinal deformities. Contemp. Pediatr. 15:111–128, 1998.

Payne, W. K., and J. W. Ogilvie. Back pain in children and adolescents. Pediatr. Clin. North Am. 43:899–917, 1996.

Ramirez, N., C. E. Johnston, and R. H. Browne. The prevalence of back pain in children who have idiopathic scoliosis. J. Bone Joint Surg. 79A:364–368, 1997.

GASTROINTESTINAL DISORDERS

C H A P T E R   8 6

VOMITING

Carol D. Berkowitz, M.D.

H_x A 6-week-old male infant who has been vomiting after each meal for 3 days is brought to the office. He is breast-fed, afebrile, and otherwise well. The history of the pregnancy and birth are normal. His birth weight was 3500 grams, and his current weight is 4500 grams.

The physical examination is unremarkable. The mother nurses the infant in the office. Although he feeds hungrily and well, he vomits about 5 minutes after the feeding. The vomiting is projectile, and the vomitus shoots across the room. The vomitus contains curdled milk. On reexamination of the abdomen, a small mass is felt in the right upper quadrant.

Questions

1. What is the mechanism of vomiting, and how is it different from regurgitation and rumination?
2. What are the common causes of vomiting in infants?
3. What are the common causes of vomiting in older children?
4. What is the significance of bilious vomiting?
5. What are the unique features of vomiting related to increased ICP?
6. What are some strategies for the management of vomiting in older children?

Vomiting is a common complaint of infants and children, and led Thomas Phaire to write "Many times the stomake of ye child is so feble that it cannot retayne eyther meate or drynke" (The Boke of Chyldren, 1553). **Vomiting** is defined as the forceful ejection of the stomach contents through the mouth. The mechanism involves a series of complex, neurologically coordinated events under the control of the CNS. Projectile vomiting is a distinct condition in which central control does not play a role. Instead, an obstruction blocks the egress of food from the stomach. As a result of this blockage (most commonly seen with pyloric stenosis), reverse peristalsis and ejection of food occur.

In contrast, **regurgitation** is the effortless bringing up of one or two mouthfuls of food without distress or discomfort. This is a frequent symptom of gastroesoph-

ageal reflux (GER) (see Chapter 87). **Rumination,** a form of autostimulation, is the voluntary induction of regurgitation. It is most often noted in infants between the ages of 3 and 6 months of age. Rumination occurs in infants with developmental retardation or with a disturbed mother-infant relationship. It is said that affected infants always smell like vomitus, which is on the clothing, but that the vomiting is rarely seen because the presence of another person provides distraction.

Rumination should be considered in infants from deprived environments (e.g., neglectful homes). Cases of rumination have been described in premature infants who were maintained in a neonatal intensive care unit after they no longer needed vigilant care from the nursing staff. Incubators, which were cut off from the outside environment, contributed to the rumination. The condition resolved once the infants were held and nurtured.

EPIDEMIOLOGY

Fifty percent of infants have spitting up or vomiting as an isolated complaint, and fewer than 5% of these infants have significant underlying disease. Vomiting occurs less frequently in older children, who often experience acute, self-limited illnesses such as gastroenteritis.

CLINICAL PRESENTATION

Infants and children may present with vomiting as an isolated complaint or in association with other symptoms, including fever, anorexia, abdominal pain, or diarrhea (D_x Box). When vomiting has persisted over a period of time, weight loss or FTT may occur. Neurologic symptoms, including headache and gait disturbances, may be noted in children with CNS problems. Other neurologic symptoms of altered muscle tone, lethargy, seizures or coma in young infants suggest inborn errors of metabolism.

PATHOPHYSIOLOGY

Vomiting is a reflex reaction that occurs in response to numerous stimuli. The final common pathway involves

D_x Vomiting

- Vomiting
- Nausea
- Abdominal pain
- Anorexia
- Diarrhea
- Headache
- Fever
- Lethargy

stasis of food in the stomach, which is related to the rate of gastric emptying. Anything that delays gastric emptying may be associated with vomiting. Gastric emptying may be retarded by the presence of fat (e.g., a high-fat meal), swallowed mucus (e.g., maternal mucus after birth, nasal mucus with a URI), lax muscle tone, fever, infection, and malnutrition. Delayed gastric emptying may develop with long-standing diabetes mellitus. Vomiting can be divided into three phases: nausea, retching, and emesis.

Nausea, the sensation of the need to vomit, is initiated by afferent fibers in the duodenum that detect stasis in the stomach. Nausea may also be triggered by vestibular or emotional stimuli. Associated autonomic symptoms include faintness, diaphoresis, sweating, pallor, and tachycardia. Anorexia is a key accompanying complaint. The afferent fibers relay the message to the brain to what has classically been referred to as the vomiting center, located in the medulla near the respiratory center. Chemical factors in the cerebrospinal fluid or in the blood stream induce vomiting through their effect on a separate site called the chemoreceptor trigger zone (CTZ) located on the floor of the fourth ventricle in the area postrema. Whether these anatomic sites are specific and localized or the efferent nuclei are scattered is unclear.

In either case, the response to the stimulus is the discharge of efferent fibers that results in **retching,** the second phase of vomiting. Retching involves the contraction of abdominal muscles in conjunction with a patterned series of actions of respiratory muscles, including closure of the glottis and depression of the diaphragm. Duodenal contents move from the small intestine into the stomach through both non-peristaltic and peristaltic contraction. Within the stomach, the fundus remains flaccid, but the antrum and pylorus contract. Relaxation of the lower esophageal sphincter also occurs. The culmination of these reflexes is **emesis** of the gastric contents.

Vomiting related to obstruction does not follow this pattern. With pyloric stenosis, repeated, deep peristaltic waves reverse direction, leading to projectile vomiting. No nausea is associated with the vomiting of pyloric stenosis, and affected infants are frequently eager to eat immediately after vomiting. Vomiting related to elevated ICP is also not associated with nausea. In addition, such vomiting, which frequently occurs first thing in the morning on awakening, is unrelated to meals.

Regurgitation, which may be misdiagnosed as vomiting, is often related to GER (see Chapter 87 for a more detailed discussion).

DIFFERENTIAL DIAGNOSIS

Vomiting may be related to various different GI or extraintestinal (parenteral) conditions. Some conditions respond to medical management, and others mandate surgical intervention (Table 86–1). The presence of bile in the vomitus, referred to as **bilious vomiting,** is a serious sign, usually indicative of intestinal obstruction distal to the ligament of Treitz and of the need for surgical intervention. The presence of blood in the vomitus is another ominous sign and is discussed in Chapter 88, Gastrointestinal Bleeding. In acute gastroenteritis, the most common cause of vomiting, the infectious agent may be a virus, such as enterovirus or rotavirus, or a bacterium, such as *Shigella*. Acute gastroenteritis is discussed in greater detail in Chapter 89, Diarrhea. In cases that are not due to gastroenteritis, the differential diagnosis of vomiting is best approached by considering the age of the patient.

Infants

Vomiting in neonates may be associated with the ingestion of irritants such as maternal **blood** or **mucus**. Either of these substances delays gastric emptying.

Structural anomalies of the GI tract may also cause vomiting in neonates. The higher the structural obstruction, the earlier the onset of symptoms. Lesions of the esophagus, such as esophageal atresia, may be evident in the delivery room, with an unsuccessful attempt to pass a nasogastric tube. Lower GI lesions, such as ileal atresia, may not present for several days. These lesions usually require surgical intervention. Infants with atretic lesions may also have a history of polyhydramnios or a single umbilical artery.

Overfeeding is the most common reason for spitting up in young infants. Frequently, infants who present with vomiting are actually experiencing spitting up or regurgitation. Overfeeding is less likely to occur in breast-fed infants, because they have better control of their

---

**TABLE 86–1. Differential Diagnosis
of Vomiting in Infancy**

Medical Conditions
Gastroenteritis
Ingestion of maternal blood or mucus
Overfeeding
Food allergies
Inborn errors of metabolism
Congenital adrenal hyperplasia
Parenteral infections (e.g., otitis media, urinary tract infection)

Surgical Conditions
Atresia/stenosis of gastrointestinal tract
Pyloric stenosis
Ulcers
Intussusception
Volvulus
Appendicitis

satiation. Mothers of bottle-fed infants may feel that the volume of formula consumed by their infants is insufficient. Nursing mothers, on the other hand, cannot "unscrew" their breasts from their bodies to determine how much milk their infants have consumed. Some nonnursing mothers feel the need to reinsert a nipple in the infant's mouth, and infants who are still interested in sucking (nonnutritive sucking) continue to feed, often exceeding the capacity of the stomach. Vomiting then results. The physician should approach breast-fed infants who are vomiting with care and concern.

Food allergies are another eating-related problem. Infants with cow milk formula intolerance may experience vomiting. Approximately 20% of these infants are also allergic to soy protein. Associated symptoms such as diarrhea, rhinorrhea, eczema, and growth failure frequently occur.

GER is a common cause of regurgitation. Regurgitation may occur with a condition called chalasia, a term that means relaxation. The opposite of this is achalasia, or absence of relaxation. This latter disorder appears to be related to disintegration of the myenteric ganglion. Swallowing may be difficult because of esophageal spasm, and food that is unable to pass into the stomach may be regurgitated. Children with achalasia usually do not present until later in childhood, although they may have a prenatal history of polyhydramnios, a sign suggesting an abnormal swallowing pattern, even in utero.

Metabolic disorders, including inborn errors of metabolism and endocrine problems, may also result with vomiting. For example, children with galactosemia may present with vomiting as well as with jaundice, dehydration, cataracts, and hepatomegaly. Other inborn errors of metabolism include methylmalonic acidemia, disorders of the urea cycle, phenylketonuria, maple syrup urine disease, renal tubular acidosis, hypercalcemia, and diabetes insipidus. Some of these disorders induce symptoms suggestive of sepsis, such as lethargy and seizures.

Male infants with **congenital adrenal hyperplasia (CAH)** may present with vomiting and electrolyte disturbance, symptoms indicative of adrenal insufficiency. Affected male infants usually present at about 10–14 days of age with vomiting and hyperkalemia (which should not be attributed to hemolysis of the specimen); hyponatremia develops later. In females, CAH is usually detected in the newborn nursery because of ambiguous genitalia. Diagnosis of this potentially lethal condition is critical to ensure the institution of replacement therapy and survival of affected infants.

Vomiting may be symptomatic of **infection** in parts of the body other than the GI tract. Most notably, UTIs of young male infants may cause projectile vomiting, a symptom highly suggestive of pyloric stenosis. These infants are usually febrile, and may be jaundiced and the diagnosis is considered when the urinalysis or culture is positive. Otitis media may also be associated with vomiting.

Vomiting, especially if unrelated to meals, may occur with **increased ICP.** In young infants, this suggests the possibility of an intracranial hemorrhage as occurs with inflicted, nonaccidental trauma.

Pyloric stenosis, a condition caused by hypertrophy of the muscle surrounding the pyloric channel, is the most common surgical condition associated with vomiting in infancy. The condition affects males much more frequently than females and usually appears in infants between the ages of 2 weeks and 2 months. The vomitus is projectile, nonbilious, and frequently contains curdled milk, which reflects delayed gastric emptying, a problem caused by failure of the hypertrophied pylorus to relax.

Affected infants have an intact appetite and are eager to eat. In some infants, starvation leads to few bowel movements and constipation; in others there may be small, frequent, mucus-laden stools (starvation diarrhea) that represent succus entericus. If pyloric stenosis is not diagnosed promptly, infants may fail to gain weight or may exhibit FTT. Symptoms suggestive of pyloric stenosis may result from ulcers in the antrum or the pyloric channel.

Children

Vomiting in children is frequently associated with **gastroenteritis.** Infections elsewhere in the body, particularly UTIs, streptococcal pharyngitis, and otitis media, are also associated with vomiting. Labyrinthitis presents with vomiting associated with dizziness.

Diabetes mellitus may result in vomiting in older children. Vomiting may also appear in children who are already known to be diabetic. This is particularly true when ketosis is present. Slow gastric emptying (gastroparesis) is a complication of long-standing diabetes mellitus. Vomiting is also a component of peptic ulcer disease, which is described in more detail in Chapter 91, Abdominal Pain.

Vomiting may be a major symptom of **CNS-related problems,** such as tumors, infections, hydrocephalus, malformations, and other causes of increased intracranial pressure. As previously noted, vomiting in CNS-related conditions is often unrelated to meals and may not be associated with nausea. Autonomic epilepsy and migraine headaches are also associated with vomiting. **Cyclic vomiting** is an unusual condition characterized by recurrent episodes of vomiting with intervals of complete wellness between attacks. Emotional upset can precipitate events, and there may be a history of migraine headaches, seizures, or irritable bowel syndrome.

Vomiting is one of the hallmarks of **Reye syndrome,** a disorder that involves an encephalopathy in association with fatty infiltration of the liver. The etiology of the condition is unclear, but the root of the disorder appears to be related to mitochondrial dysfunction. Affected children usually have a history of an antecedent viral illness, most commonly influenza B or chickenpox. Following a period of recovery, they experience altered consciousness with vomiting. Hepatic enzymes and serum ammonia are elevated. Aspirin, which uncouples oxidative phosphorylation, is apparently linked to Reye syndrome, both epidemiologically as well as theoretically.

Certain **medications,** including theophylline, erythromycin, and digitalis, may also be associated with vomiting. Some of these medications cause transient relaxation of the lower esophageal sphincter and others affect the CTZ.

Familial **dysautonomia,** Riley-Day syndrome, a rare condition that affects Jewish individuals, results in vomiting. The disorder is inherited in an autosomal recessive manner and consists of an imbalance in the autonomic nervous system. Children experience intractable vomiting in addition to excess perspiration, inability to produce tears, difficulty swallowing and chewing, and cold hands and feet. They also have hyperpyrexia and hypertension. These children require fluid replacement and management with antiemetics.

Surgical conditions such as appendicitis, gall bladder disease, and twisted ovarian cysts are discussed in Chapter 91, Abdominal Pain.

Adolescents

Vomiting during the adolescent years may be caused by any of the previously mentioned conditions. In addition, adolescents may develop vomiting in association with intentional **ingestion of illicit drugs or alcohol.** Many adolescents have incorrect notions of the sexual activity needed to initiate pregnancy. Teenage girls who have been vomiting, especially for a period of time, should be evaluated for **pregnancy,** regardless of their disclosed sexual activity status.

Adolescents with **eating disorders,** particularly bulimia, vomit but may not disclose their vomiting. They may ingest emetics, such as ipecac, to help control their weight (see Chapter 109, Eating Disorders).

EVALUATION

History

A complete history is essential for correct diagnosis (Questions Box). A positive family history of vomiting may suggest a diagnosis of migraine, peptic ulcer disease, or familial dysautonomia.

Physical Examination

The examination shows the impact of vomiting on children's growth. The weight may provide evidence of the chronicity of the process; weight loss suggests a protracted course. Evidence of other infections, such

---

Questions: Vomiting

- What is the nature of the vomiting (projectile, bilious, nonbilious, regurgitated)?
- How long has the child been vomiting?
- Are any symptoms such as fever, diarrhea, dizziness, or lethargy associated with the vomiting?
- What is the relationship of the vomiting to meals?
- Does the vomiting occur at night, indicating possible hiatal hernia and gastroesophageal reflux?
- Is there a family history of vomiting?
- Is the child taking any medications?
- Have any measures been taken to relieve the vomiting?

---

as otitis media or pneumonia, may also be apparent. An abnormal neurologic examination would suggest a central nervous system process or an inborn error of metabolism. The fundi of the eyes should be assessed for the presence of papilledema, or retinal hemorrhages. Nystagmus may be noted in children with labyrinthitis or CNS disturbances. The examination of the abdomen may show masses or signs of obstruction and a surgical condition. Distention of the abdomen may be present with an obstruction. Peristaltic waves are an abnormal finding characteristic of pyloric stenosis.

Laboratory Tests

The laboratory assessment is determined by the differential diagnosis. If gastroenteritis is suspected, an examination of the stools for leukocytes and occult blood is appropriate. Specimens for bacterial or viral cultures or viral antigen detection can be submitted. A CBC may support the diagnosis of infection or reveal signs of anemia. In neonates, vomited blood should be evaluated using the Apt test to determine whether it came from the mother or infant.

Electrolytes should be obtained in infants or children with a history of significant vomiting, and may confirm dehydration, acid-base imbalance, or electrolyte disturbance. Infants with pyloric stenosis who vomit stomach contents develop a hypochloremic, hypokalemic alkalosis. A urinalysis also may show evidence of dehydration as well as signs of a UTI. Tests for inborn errors of metabolism, such as urine for amino acid analysis, are appropriate if this is suspected.

Imaging Studies

Radiographic procedures, such as x-rays, ultrasound, and contrast studies, are useful to define obstructive lesions such as pyloric stenosis. A flat plate of the abdomen may show stomach distention, a "double bubble" (air in the stomach and duodenum) or a paucity of intestinal air in cases of high level obstruction. Consultation with a pediatric gastroenterologist may lead to additional diagnostic tests, such as endoscopic evaluation.

MANAGEMENT

The initial step in the management of vomiting infants or children is to ensure adequate hydration and integrity of the cardiovascular bed. This may require the administration of intravenous fluids. **Oral rehydration** is the mainstay of therapy in infants and children whose vomiting is related to gastroenteritis. Small, frequent feedings with clear fluids are better tolerated than large, infrequent feedings, although the latter may be necessary in infants with diarrhea because each feeding may result in a bowel movement. Antiemetics such as phenothiazines are discouraged in children because of the high incidence of side effects, including dystonic posturing. Other emetics, specifically Emetrol, is an over-the-counter medication given to reduce nausea. It is a phosphorated carbohydrate solution that is given to children as 1–2 teaspoons every 15 minutes for up to 1 hour.

Ginger, a perennial plant with thick underground stems, is also used to prevent and treat nausea. Ginger is often given as the beverage ginger ale to soothe an upset stomach.

Further management depends on the diagnosis. Infections should be treated with the appropriate antibiotics. Operative conditions, such as pyloric stenosis or intussusception, should be managed surgically. Inborn errors of metabolism require consultation with a geneticist and dietary manipulation. Congenital adrenal hyperplasia should be managed in consultation with an endocrinologist. This condition necessitates replacement hormonal therapy.

PROGNOSIS

Most cases of acute vomiting resolve spontaneously or are readily managed once the underlying condition is diagnosed. The overall prognosis is therefore quite good.

Protracted vomiting may result in starvation and FTT, however. Severe vomiting may cause tears in the esophagus and lead to hematemesis. Obstructive causes of vomiting in infants respond to surgical intervention. The prognosis for children with Reye syndrome depends on the severity of the disturbance, with the possibility of death in very sick children.

Case Resolution

The infant in the case history exhibits the signs and symptoms consistent with pyloric stenosis. The boy is a healthy, vigorous breast-fed infant, and his weight gain of 1000 grams in 6 weeks (average: 25 g/day) is normal. The vomitus is curdled indicating that it has been in the stomach for over 3 hours. Gastric emptying is delayed. The presence of a mass in the right upper quadrant is also consistent with the diagnosis. An ultrasound would confirm the finding. It would be equally appropriate to keep the infant NPO (nothing by mouth), start intravenous fluids, and obtain surgical consultation.

Selected Readings

Caty, M. G. and R. G. Azizkhan. Acute surgical conditions of the abdomen. Pediatr. Ann. 4:192–201, 1994.

Fleisher, D. R. Functional vomiting disorders in infancy: innocent vomiting, nervous vomiting, and infant rumination syndrome. J. Pediatr. 125(suppl):S84–S94, 1994.

Foley, L. C., et al. Evaluation of the vomiting infant. Am. J. Dis. Child. 143:660–661, 1989.

Gordon, N. Recurrent vomiting in childhood, especially of neurologic origin. Dev. Med. Child. Neurol. 36:463–470, 1994.

Hebra, A., and M. A. Hoffman. Gastroesophageal reflex in children. Pediatr. Clin. North Am. 40:1233–1251, 1993.

Judd, R. H. *Helicobacter pylori.* Gastritis and ulcers in pediatrics. Adv. Pediatr. 39:283–306, 1992.

Murray, K. F. and D. L. Christie. Vomiting. Pediatr. Rev. 19:337–341, 1998.

Sondheimer, J. M. Vomiting. *In* Walker, W. A. et al (eds). Pediatric Gastrointestinal Disease, Pathophysiology, Diagnosis, Management. Vol. 1. St. Louis, MO: Mosby, 1996, pp. 195–203.

CHAPTER 87

GASTROESOPHAGEAL REFLUX

Carlo Di Lorenzo, M.D.

H$_x$ A two-month-old girl has a history of spitting up and vomiting immediately after every meal. Her parents are very anxious and frustrated. The girl's vomiting seems effortless, and the parents have difficulty quantifying the amount of formula that is regurgitated. The child, who has always been in good general health, was the product of a normal pregnancy and delivery and had an uneventful neonatal course. She seems happy, with no apparent abdominal pain, dysphagia, odynophagia, hematemesis, FTT, pneumonia, wheezing, or apnea. The stool is heme-negative, the hematocrit is 40%, and the urinalysis is normal. The physical examination is normal.

Gastroesophageal reflux (GER) is the retrograde movement of gastric contents from the stomach to the esophagus. Such episodes frequently occur physiologically, and the events are brief, asymptomatic, and self-limited. Occasionally, either the overall frequency of reflux or the marked duration of a single episode may cause disease. This is characteristic of pathologic GER. Clinically, pediatric GER takes two forms: infantile and adult. Infantile GER is present during the first months of life and resolves clinically by 18 months of age in at least 80% of affected infants. In contrast, adult GER often manifests initially in children beyond infancy and tends to persist and requires chronic or intermittent therapy.

Understanding of GER in children has been confused by the misuse of terms such as regurgitation, vomiting, and rumination. **Regurgitation** is defined as effortless return of gastric contents to the mouth. **Vomiting** refers to the forceful expulsion of the same material. **Rumination** involves some voluntary effort and contraction of the abdominal muscles, but it is not accompanied by the retching and the retrograde duodenogastric contractions that characterize vomiting.

EPIDEMIOLOGY

The incidence of infantile GER is reported to be 20%, and nearly one-third of affected infants come to medical attention; 80% of these infants (5.4% of all infants) require no workup and only minimal therapy. Of the remaining children who are evaluated, most are successfully treated medically. However, a minority of infants require antireflux surgery. Boys are somewhat more likely than girls to have pathologic GER in infancy and childhood (ratio: 1.27:1). The cause of this male preponderance is unknown. Some children with particular conditions have a higher risk for developing GER disease.

Neurologic Disease

The incidence of pathologic GER in children with severe neurologic disease is 20 to 70%. Reportedly, the incidence of reflux is inversely proportional to mental age. Neurologic disease associated with hypertonia and spasticity may increase the frequency and duration of reflux episodes by raising intra-abdominal pressure. In addition, children with spasticity have a higher incidence of sliding hiatal hernia, a predisposing factor for reflux. Hypotonia, supine position, or abnormal postures facilitate GER episodes. Chronic lying in a horizontal position delays the esophageal clearance of refluxate and increases the risk of esophagitis. Children with neurologic diseases often have a decreased gag reflex, which may lead to life-threatening episodes of aspiration of refluxed material.

In particular, children with Down syndrome are at risk for pathologic GER because they are often hypotonic and have an increased frequency of abnormal esophageal peristalsis. Children with myopathy or systemic sclerosis may also be predisposed to development of esophagitis, because their reflux episodes are poorly cleared by the esophageal peristalsis.

Chronic Respiratory Disease

In children, bronchopulmonary dysplasia (BPD), cystic fibrosis, and asthma are associated with a high prevalence of GER. As many as 20% of premature infants with BPD have pathologic GER, compared with 1 to 2% of preterm infants without BPD. Children with cystic fibrosis have a high incidence of regurgitation, heartburn, and severe esophagitis. The risks for esophagitis are higher in children with severe respiratory disease as compared to those with mild disease. More than 50% of children and adults with asthma have abnormal GER.

Congenital Esophageal Anomalies

Children who have a surgically repaired esophageal atresia have a high incidence of GER disease, which seems to result from an intrinsic abnormality in the esophageal innervation coordinating the esophageal peristalsis. Absence of the intraabdominal segment of the esophagus and damage to the vagus incurred during the surgical repair of the atresia are also believed to contribute to abnormal reflux.

Increased Abdominal Pressure

Increases in intra-abdominal pressure produce higher intragastric pressures that can overcome the opposing pressure of the lower esophageal sphincter (LES). Children who suffer from frequent coughing attacks or are constipated and spend a great amount of time contracting their abdominal muscles in defecatory efforts are at risk for developing GER disease. The chronically increased abdominal pressure in obesity explains the reported 73% prevalence of heartburn in obese adults. The effect of the chronic increase in abdominal pressure during pregnancy is compounded by the effects of progesterone, thus decreasing the LES pressure. Peritoneal dialysis has been shown to increase abdominal pressure and delay gastric emptying, which triggers GER. Placement of a gastrostomy induces abnormal GER by decreasing the LES pressure and length and modifying the gastroesophageal angle. Children with a gastrostomy are also often given rapid bolus feedings that cause a sudden increase in intra-abdominal pressure and induce relaxation of the LES.

D_x Gastroesophageal Reflux

- Regurgitation
- Weight loss or FTT
- Rumination
- Chest pain or heartburn
- Irritability
- Abdominal pain
- Odynophagia
- Dysphagia
- Hematemesis
- Anemia
- Pulmonary failure (aspiration pneumonia, recurrent or chronic pulmonary failure)
- Recurrent apnea or bradycardia

CLINICAL PRESENTATION

In infancy, the most common initial symptom is effortless postprandial regurgitation often accompanied by chronic irritability. The loss of regurgitated calories may lead to weight loss or FTT. GI bleeding and pulmonary disorders, including aspiration pneumonia, asthma, and recurrent apnea, are less common. In addition, children with GER may present with signs and symptoms of neurologic disease. Apparent seizures characterized by apnea and stiffening of the body and abnormal posturing of the head and neck have been associated with GER. The main symptoms of GER in older children are heartburn, chest pain, and eructation (belching) (D_x Box). Odynophagia (painful swallowing), dysphagia (difficulty swallowing) secondary to a stricture, and bleeding are less frequent.

PATHOPHYSIOLOGY

GER disease is a multifactorial process in which different abnormalities may predominate in a single patient. The interaction among the multiple factors that results in GER disease is summarized in Figure 87–1. They include competence of antireflux mechanisms, efficiency of esophageal clearance, volume of gastric contents, aggressiveness of refluxed material, and mucosal resistance to injury.

Reflux may occur by one of three general mechanisms: transient LES relaxation, hypotonic LES, or increases in intra-abdominal pressure. For many years, low LES pressure was believed to be the main cause of reflux. It is now evident that most reflux episodes are due to sudden LES relaxations not associated with swallowing. During these episodes, the LES opens completely for 5 to 35 seconds. The main **antireflux mechanism** disappears, and gastric contents move freely from an area with higher resting pressure (stomach) to one with lower resting pressure (esophagus). The transient LES relaxation explains why more than half of the children with GER disease have a normal LES pressure. Spontaneous reflux without LES relaxation occurs only when the basal LES pressure is extremely low (< 5 mm Hg). Most children with very low LES pressure have severe neurodevelopmental delays.

Esophageal clearance determines the duration of esophageal exposure to the injurious effect of refluxate. Esophageal peristaltic contractions rapidly clear fluid volume from the esophagus, and swallowed saliva neutralizes any small amount of residual acid. In the event that peristalsis is abnormal, gravity promotes esophageal clearance when children are upright but not when they are supine. Children who lie supine most of the time or who reflux during sleep have longer esophageal exposure to acid compared to those who are ambulatory or awake. In some children with reflux esophagitis, abnormal esophageal clearance occurs. Esophagitis can cause either abnormal esophageal peristalsis or esophageal stricture. With abnormal peristalsis, swallowing of both liquids and solids is affected; with a stricture, primarily swallowing of solids is altered. The esophageal inflammation may cause further worsening of the peristalsis, triggering a vicious cycle.

Increased **gastric fluid volume** not only makes more volume available for reflux but also increases the frequency of transient LES relaxations. Some children with reflux disease exhibit delayed gastric emptying, which contributes to the development of reflux disease.

The **aggressiveness of the refluxed material** is also important. The degree of esophagitis correlates with the time of hydrochloric acid exposure. Suppression of acid

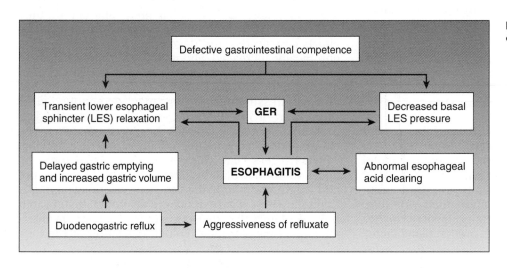

FIGURE 87–1. Pathogenesis of gastroesophageal reflux (GER) disease.

secretion is associated with healing of esophagitis, even when reflux persists. Although acid alone may cause esophageal injury by protein denaturation, pepsin, which becomes an active proteolytic enzyme at pH less than 3.0, contributes substantially to the development of esophagitis. Bile acids and pancreatic enzymes, which may be present in the stomach in patients with duodenogastric reflux, are particularly harmful for the esophageal mucosa.

The mucosal layer, the unstirred water layer, surface bicarbonate, and various aspects of the stratified squamous epithelium affect the **mucosal resistance** to the refluxate. The capacity of the esophageal mucosa to withstand injury and to repair injury appears to be influenced by such factors as age and nutrition.

Children with **hiatal hernias** may exhibit GER. These children lack the intra-abdominal portion of the esophagus, one of the protective mechanisms against reflux. Large, sliding, hiatal hernias may act as fluid traps and promote reflux when the LES opens on swallowing. Although children with large hernias often have severe esophagitis that does not respond to medical treatment, the majority of individuals with hiatal hernias do not have GER. The physician should not equate the presence of a sliding hiatal hernia with the presence of GER disease.

DIFFERENTIAL DIAGNOSIS

The differential diagnosis of reflux symptoms is presented in Table 87–1. **Regurgitation** is a far more frequent symptom in infants than in older children. It is quite easy to diagnose GER as the cause of this symptom. The challenge lies in avoiding inappropriate investigations in children whose only problem is the messiness of regurgitated food. Other causes of vomiting should not be overlooked. Excessive regurgitation causes weight loss, which requires aggressive diagnostic and therapeutic intervention. Poor intake may also contribute to FTT because discomfort due to esophagitis is associated with ingestion of food. In addition, parents may be hesitant to feed infants whose response to eating is regurgitation and irritability. Infantile rumination, which involves regurgitation of previously swallowed food and rechewing and reswallowing of the food, is a particularly ominous presentation of GER disease.

Absence of regurgitation does not rule out GER disease. Esophagitis due to nonregurgitant reflux can present with chest pain or heartburn, abdominal pain, irritability, refusal to feed, dysphagia, hematemesis, and anemia. **Chest pain or heartburn** in response to the acid bathing of the inflamed esophageal mucosa is a common complaint of verbal children. Under the same conditions, infants and younger children are more likely to show irritability or complain of abdominal pain. **Dysphagia** may be a manifestation of esophagitis. **Hematemesis** and **anemia** are a consequence of bleeding due to esophagitis.

Some older children with GER disease may develop **Sandifer's syndrome.** They hold their neck in a twisted position, often without realizing they are doing so. This position disappears when reflux is successfully treated

TABLE 87–1. Differential Diagnosis of Reflux Symptoms

Regurgitation, Vomiting
Stimulation of central vomiting center
Drugs, toxins
Metabolic conditions: diabetic ketoacidosis; diabetes insipidus; lactic acidosis; phenylketonuria; maple syrup urine; methylmalonic acidemia; hereditary fructose intolerance; galactosemia; tyrosinemia; hyperammonemia; fatty-acid oxidation disorders (e.g., medium-chain acyl CoA dehydrogenase deficiency); uremia; renal tubular acidosis

Stimulation of supramedullary receptors
Psychogenic vomiting
Vestibular disease; "motion sickness"
Increased intracerebral pressure: subdural effusion or hematoma; hydrocephalus; cerebral edema or tumor; meningoencephalitis; Reye's syndrome

Stimulation of peripheral receptors
Pharyngeal: gag reflex
Gastric conditions: peptic ulcer disease; dysmotility; obstruction (e.g., bezoar; pyloric stenosis; web)
Intestinal conditions
  Infection; enterotoxin; appendicitis
  Nutrient intolerance (e.g., cow's milk, soy, eosinophilic gastroenteropathy)
  Obstruction (e.g., web; superior mesentric artery syndrome; volvulus; meconium ileus; intussusception; adhesions; meconium plug; Hirschsprung's disease)
Hepatobiliary conditions: hepatitis; cholecystitis
Pancreatic conditions: pancreatitis
Miscellaneous conditions: peritonitis; pyelonephritis; sepsis

Other esophageal diseases
Structural: stricture; ring; etc.
Functional: esophageal body dysmotility, achalasia

Pain, Esophagitis Symptoms
Cardiac pain
Pulmonary or mediastinal pain; chest wall pain (e.g., costrochondritis)
Nonesophagitis upper gastrointestinal inflammation (e.g., peptic ulcer disease)
  Nonesophagitis dysphagia
  Many possible causes of nonspecific irritability in infants (e.g., milk allergy, infantile colic)
  Functional; malingering

Respiratory Symptoms (e.g., Wheeze, Stridor, Cough)
Extrinsic compression (e.g., vascular ring)
Intrinsic obstruction (e.g., malformation, foreign body, cyst, tumor)
Airways reactive to other stimuli (e.g., allergens, infection)
Infection; inflammation; cystic fibrosis; pertussis; asthma
"Central" events (e.g., central apnea)

Neurobehavioral Symptoms (Sandifer's Syndrome, Seizurelike Spells)
Seizures
Dystonic reaction to drugs
Vestibular disorders
Early pertussis

Adapted, with permission, from Orenstein, S.R. Gastroesophageal reflux. *In* Stockman, J.A., III, and R.J. Winter (eds.). Current Problems in Pediatrics 21:223, 1991.

and appears to be the children's way of reducing the discomfort associated with reflux.

Certain **respiratory symptoms** in children may actually result from GER disease. Two mechanisms have been suggested to explain respiratory complications of GER disease: (1) pulmonary aspiration of regurgitated gastric contents and (2) bronchoconstriction triggered by refluxate stimulation of an inflamed esophageal mucosa. Pulmonary aspiration of refluxate causes pneumonia, particularly in neurologically abnormal children, whose airway protective mechanisms can be defective. It may be difficult to distinguish aspiration during reflux from aspiration during swallowing in these children.

Apnea or bradycardia may occur in neurologically immature infants as a response to various stimuli. Reflux may be an important cause of intrinsic asthma. Children with nocturnal asthma symptoms, including cough, are especially likely to have GER disease. Several studies have shown an improvement in bronchospastic symptoms following medical or surgical treatment of reflux. Stridor, croup, hoarseness, otitis, and sinusitis are other respiratory conditions that have been linked to pathologic GER.

EVALUATION

Diagnostic evaluation of reflux should be undertaken only in children suspected of suffering pathologic effects from reflux. Thus infants with regurgitation but no other sequelae are simply managed with conservative antireflux measures.

History

The diagnostic evaluation begins with a complete history (Questions Box). It is important to inquire about the reflux-associated symptoms even if they are not part of the presenting complaint.

Physical Examination

In most children with GER disease the physical examination is normal. Nevertheless, a complete physical examination should be performed to eliminate conditions discussed in the differential diagnosis (see Table 87–1).

Laboratory Studies

Several diagnostic techniques are available to diagnose different aspects of GER disease (Table 87–2). **Monitoring of intraesophageal pH** for 24 hours is considered the gold standard for diagnosing GER. It allows the physician to correlate symptoms with changes in intraesophageal pH. Although the pH probe can quantify frequency and duration of reflux, it cannot detect reflux for at least one hour following feeding with an infant formula because of the buffering effect of the formula on the intragastric pH. A diagnosis of esophagitis can be obtained either through visualization and biopsy of the

esophagus by esophagoscopy or through a blind peroral suction biopsy of the distal esophagus, which provides larger bioptic specimens. Because of the necessarily brief chronology of reflux in infants, children may not have yet developed the pathologic changes diagnostic of esophagitis. Esophageal manometry and intraesophageal acid perfusion have a very limited role in the diagnostic workup of children with GER disease.

All children who present with anemia should undergo hemoccult test of the stools. A hemoccult-positive stool is an important clue that indicates that esophagitis may be causing the anemia.

Imaging Studies

Barium contrast studies of the pharynx, esophagus, and upper GI tract should be performed to rule out anatomic abnormalities such as malrotations, webs, stenoses, and hiatal hernia. The sensitivity of barium fluoroscopy in detecting GER may be poor, and it has a very low specificity; many infants with no clinically significant GER reflux some barium into the esophagus. Scintigraphy measures gastric emptying and diagnoses pulmonary aspiration of gastric contents. This technique involves offering formula containing small amounts of radioactive technetium to children.

MANAGEMENT

A stepwise approach to the treatment of GER disease is summarized in Table 87–3. Most infants with pathologic GER are free of disease within one to two years because of the combined effect of the maturation of the LES function, the introduction of more solid feedings, and the increasing amount of time spent in the upright position.

Optimal positioning for infants with GER disease is prone, with the head of the bed elevated 30 degrees. Although the AAP recommends placing infants in the supine position to decrease the risk of SIDS, this does not apply to infants with GER disease. **Thickening infant formula** with rice cereal decreases the amount of regurgitation, diminishes crying, and increases the caloric density of the formula. When a thickened formula is used, the nipple should be enlarged to allow adequate flow. Second hand cigarette smoke exposure seems to exacerbate GER in infants, by reducing LES pressure, delaying gastric emptying, and favoring development of esophagitis. Thus, strict avoidance of cigarette exposure is strongly recommended.

Medications are usually added to the regimen when pathologic GER has been demonstrated. **Cisapride,** which has recently been approved for use in GER, is the first-line drug for children with pathologic reflux. Cisapride increases LES pressure, improves esophageal peristalsis, and accelerates gastric emptying. Care should be taken to avoid concurrent administration of cisapride with agents which inhibit the hepatic cytochrome P450 3A4, the isoenzyme responsible for the metabolism of cisapride. This can result in an increase in cisapride plasma levels and prolongation of the QT interval, possibly leading to fatal arrhythmias. This list

---

Questions: Gastroesophageal Reflux

- Is the emesis effortless, forceful, or projectile?
- When does the infant regurgitate (i.e., how long after a meal; lying supine or prone; during crying, coughing, or diaper change)?
- Has the child ever vomited blood?
- Is the child losing weight or not gaining weight satisfactorily?
- Does the child cry a lot and refuse to eat?
- Does the child have a chronic cough or asthma that is not responsive to conventional therapy?
- Does the child have heartburn exacerbated by citrus juices and relieved by liquid antacids?

TABLE 87–2.   Diagnostic Techniques in the Evaluation of Gastroesophageal Reflux

Investigation	Sensitivity	Specificity	Advantages	Disadvantages
Radiology	++	+	Availability; illustrates anatomy	Not physiologic; short duration
Intraesophageal pH monitoring	+++	+++	Accurate; correlates with symptoms	Duration 24 hours; misses postprandial reflux
Endoscopy	++	+++	Detects esophagitis; allows biopsy	Invasive; may be normal when biopsy is abnormal
Scintigraphy	+	++	Noninvasive, physiologic; detects aspiration; measures gastric emptying	Does not detect esophagitis; needs patient cooperation
Esophageal suction biopsy	++	+++	Minimally invasive; detects esophagitis	May be normal in early stages of GER disease
Manometry	+	+	Measures peristalsis and LES pressure	Does not detect esophagitis; may be normal in presence of severe GER disease
Acid perfusion	±	++	Available; easy to perform	Needs patient cooperation; does not detect esophagitis

of drugs includes erythromycin, clarithromycin, azythromycin, fluconazole, itraconazole, miconazole, troleandomycin, nefazodone, ritonavir, indinavir and any other medication known to increase the QT interval. Alternative prokinetics are metoclopramide, bethanechol, and domperidone (not available yet in the United States). **Acid-reducing agents** (e.g., H_2-receptor antagonists such as cimetidine, ranitidine, and famotidine; proton pump inhibitors such as omeprazole) should be used when esophagitis is evident.

Infants with rumination may benefit from pharmacologic therapy of GER in combination with any modification of their psychosocial situation, because a problematic parent-infant relationship may play a role in the etiology of infantile rumination.

Surgical therapy is reserved for children who fail to respond to medical treatment or have GER-related, life-threatening events, such as recurrent episodes of apnea or pneumonia. The majority of children who undergo antireflux surgery are neurologically impaired, and 2 to 10% of these infants have Down syndrome. Nissen fundoplication is the most popular and reliable surgical procedure for treatment of reflux. Success rates of 80 to 90% are reported. Both short- and long-term complications are frequent, however, especially in children with neurologic deficits. These complications include gas bloat, inability to burp and vomit, dysphagia, dumping syndrome (overly rapid gastric emptying), small bowel obstruction due to adhesions, and herniation of the wrap through the hiatus.

PROGNOSIS

The prognosis of infantile reflux is excellent. Most cases resolve in the first year of life. GER that occurs beyond infancy has a less benign course and often requires chronic treatment.

TABLE 87–3.   Therapy for Gastroesophageal Reflux*

Conservative
Put in prone or completely upright position
Thicken infant feedings (1 Tbsp. rice cereal/oz)
Fast before bed
Avoid large meals, obesity, tight clothing
Avoid provocative foods and medications
 Fatty foods, citrus, tomato, carbonation, coffee, alcohol
 Smoke exposure
 Anticholinergics, adrenergics, xanthines (theophylline, caffeine), calcium channel blockers, prostaglandins

Pharmacologic (Usual Course, 8–12 Weeks)
Prokinetic
 Metoclopramide (0.1 mg/kg/dose qid)
 Bethanechol (0.1–0.3 mg/kg/dose tid or qid)
 Cisapride (0.2 mg/kg/dose tid)
 Domperidone (not available in the United States)
Antacid
 Cimetidine (5–10 mg/kg/dose qid)
 Ranitidine (2–4 mg/kg/dose tid)
 Famotidine, Nizatidine (adult, 40 mg HS; 300 mg HS)
 Omeprazole (1–3 mg/kg hs, adult, 20 mg HS)
 Antacids (0.5–1 mL/kg/dose, 3–8 times/day: 1–2 hr [PC, HS])
Barrier or miscellaneous mechanism
 Sucralfate slurry (1 g in 5–15 mL solution qid [PC, HS])
 Alginic acid-antacid (2 g 3–8 times/day [PC])

Surgical
Fundoplication
Angelchik prosthesis

*Dosages for children unless otherwise specified.
Adapted, with permission, from Orenstein, S.R. Gastroesophageal reflux. *In* Stockman, J.A., III, and R.J. Winter, (eds). Curr. Probl. Pediatr. 21:224, 1991.

Case Resolution

The girl in the case history has physiologic GER. She requires no diagnostic tests and can be sent home without any pharmacologic intervention. The parents should receive reassurance that the condition is harmless and self-limited. The spitting up will slowly resolve, and the girl should do well.

Selected Readings

Del Rosario J. F., S. R. Orenstein. Common pediatric esophageal disorders. The Gastroenterologist 6:104–121, 1998.

Faubion W. A., N. N. Zein. Gastroesophageal reflux in infants and children. Mayo. Clin. Proc. 73:166–173, 1998.

Herbst, J. J., S. D. Minton, and L. S. Book. Gastroesophageal reflux causing distress and apnea in newborn infants. J. Pediatr. 95:763–768, 1979.

Orenstein, S. R. Prone positioning in infant gastroesophageal reflux: is elevation of the head worth the trouble? J. Pediatr. 117:184–187, 1990.

Orenstein, S. R., P. F. Whitington, and D. M. Orenstein. The infant seat as treatment for gastroesophageal reflux. N. Engl. J. Med. 116:540–543, 1983.

Sondheimer, J. M., and B. A. Morris. Gastroesophageal reflux among severely retarded children. J. Pediatr. 94:710–714, 1979.

Treem, W., P. Davis, and J. Hyams. Gastroesophageal reflux in the older child: presentation, response to treatment and long-term follow-up. Clin. Pediatr. 30:435–440, 1991.

Willinger, M., H. J. Hoffman, and R. B. Hartford. Infant sleep position and risk of sudden infant death syndrome. Report of meeting held January 13 and 14, 1994, National Institutes of Health, Bethesda, MD. Pediatrics 93:814–820, 1994.

CHAPTER 88

GASTROINTESTINAL BLEEDING

Carlo Di Lorenzo, M.D. and Eric A. Vasiliauskas, M.D.

H$_x$ A 4-year-old boy is evaluated for intermittent passing of bright red blood from the rectum for 2 weeks. Blood either coats the stool or appears as a spot after a bowel movement. The mother reports no vomiting, diarrhea, loss of appetite, weight loss, fever, or abdominal pain. The boy has no history of constipation, straining, or pain with defecation and is taking no medications. The family has no pets and has not traveled recently.

On physical examination, the boy is a well-appearing, energetic, interactive youngster. Weight and height are at the 75th percentile for age. The abdomen is soft, flat, and nontender, and bowel sounds are normally active. No organomegaly or masses are evident. No rashes, bruising, or hemangiomas are present. No tags, fissures, or fistulas are seen on close visual inspection of the perianal area. Digital rectal examination reveals normal sphincter tone, and a small, mobile, pealike mass is palpable in the rectal vault. A film of bright red blood is present on the glove after the examination. A CBC with platelet count and a PT/PTT determination yield normal results.

Questions

1. What is involved in the assessment of children with GI bleeding?
2. How are upper and lower GI tract bleeding differentiated?
3. What conditions usually account for upper and lower GI tract bleeding?
4. What management options are available for GI bleeding?
5. How does the physician decide what type of management is appropriate for each individual patient?

Gastrointestinal (GI) bleeding, which is commonly encountered in pediatric practice, is a source of great anxiety for patients and families. GI bleeding ranges in severity, and clinically asymptomatic children with iron deficiency anemia as well as children with acute life-threatening shock from massive hemorrhage may have GI bleeding. Prompt assessment, diagnosis, and treatment are essential. An age-specific differential diagnosis, detailed history, and physical examination indicate the etiology in most patients.

EPIDEMIOLOGY

There are multiple conditions associated with GI bleeding. Studies have evaluated the frequency of conditions in various ages by location of the bleeding (upper versus lower GI bleeding), and hospitalized versus ambulatory patients. In addition, disease frequency varies between developed and developing countries. For instance, peptic ulcer disease is a common cause of upper GI bleeding in Western countries, whereas esophageal varices are the most common cause in India (reported in 95% of cases).

In newborns, maternal blood swallowed at the time of delivery or ingested from the bleeding nipples of nursing mothers accounts for approximately 30% of blood found in their GI tracts. Necrotizing enterocolitis has been reported in 44% of hospitalized neonates with GI bleeding. Newborns also commonly develop gastritis or stress ulcers related to perinatal hypoxia, sepsis, or CNS lesions. Sepsis, vitamin K deficiency, or maternal drugs that crossed the placenta or were passed via the breast milk may result in coagulopathy. Older infants with protein intolerances to cow's milk and soy products may present with hematemesis or rectal bleeding (gross or occult).

Anal fissures are one of the most common causes of lower GI bleeding in ambulatory children, and accounted for GI bleeding in 23% of patients in one study. Juvenile polyps are another common cause.

Hospitalized children suffering from the stress of major trauma, burns, shock, or sepsis commonly develop multiple superficial erosions of the gastric mucosa. The anticipatory use of H₂-blockers and antacids has reduced the incidence of hemorrhage in this group. Current studies report an incidence of upper GI bleeding in the pediatric intensive care unit of only 6–7%. Higher incidence of hemorrhage (20%) is reported in children who have undergone cardiovascular surgery.

Portal hypertension produces esophageal and gastric varices, which may intermittently bleed briskly, resulting in hematemesis or melena. Patients with coagulopathies from infection, hemophilia, idiopathic thrombocytopenic purpura, poor hepatic synthetic function, vitamin K malabsorption, hypersplenism, giant hemangiomas, platelet dysfunction, platelet inhibitors (aspirin), anticoagulants (Coumadin), or iron intoxication are at high risk as well (see Chapter 64, Bleeding Disorders). Patients with hemophila A or B have an incidence of GI bleeding from 10–25%. GI bleeding may also occur in children with chronic renal failure. Patients taking NSAIDs or corticosteroids and those receiving radiation or chemotherapeutic agents such as Cytoxan, methotrexate, and Adriamycin, which can induce mucositis or neutropenic colitis, may also experience GI bleeding. Opportunistic infections with herpes simplex, CMV, or *Candida* should be considered in immunocompromised children. Vascular anomalies are an uncommon cause of GI bleeding in children.

DEFINITIONS (D_X BOX)

- **Hematemesis** is the vomiting of blood. Fresh blood is bright red. Once blood is denatured by gastric acid, it assumes a "coffee-ground" appearance. Hematemesis suggests that the source of bleeding lies proximal to the ligament of Treitz.
- **Hematochezia** is the term used for blood passed out of the rectum. The discharge may be in the form of pure blood, bloody diarrhea, or blood mixed with stool. Bright red blood almost always originates in the left colon, most commonly in the anorectal region.
- **Melena** refers to black, tarry stools, which usually originate in the upper GI tract and rarely the right colon. The color depends on the volume of blood lost and the transit time; the slower the transit, the darker the color of the stool. Melena results from bacterial degradation of hemoglobin.
- **Occult bleeding** refers to the presence of blood in amounts small enough not to be appreciated visually.
- **Hemodynamic changes** are caused by blood loss.

D_x Gastrointestinal Bleeding

- Hematemesis
- Hematochezia
- Melena
- Anemia
- Signs of portal hypertension (splenomegaly, caput medusae, jaundice)
- Rash, purpura, hemangioma
- Abdominal mass or distention

Symptoms include dizziness, dyspnea, tachycardia, and shock. They are the only symptoms that the child with GI bleeding may have on initial presentation.

PATHOPHYSIOLOGY

The body compensates for GI bleeding in a variety of ways depending on the amount of blood lost. When less than 15% of the circulating blood volume is lost, the venous system contracts and extravascular fluid is shifted into the vascular space, thus maintaining both intravascular volume and cardiac output. Very rapid loss of as little as 10% of the blood volume, however, may overwhelm these compensatory mechanisms and lead to shock (See Chapter 41, Shock).

When blood loss exceeds 15%, these homeostatic mechanisms are inadequate. Increased sympathetic output raises the heart rate and force of contraction in an effort to maintain cardiac output. The blood volume is maintained through peripheral vasoconstriction. Oxygen consumption increases. Hyperventilation may result in initial respiratory alkalosis, followed by metabolic acidosis, as blood lactate levels increase secondary to tissue hypoxia.

Blood loss in excess of 30% is associated with hypotension. Decreased cardiac output leads to tissue damage. The resulting metabolic acidosis contributes to the severity of the symptoms. Patients are at risk for acute renal failure, hepatic hypoperfusion, myocardial infarction, and bowel ischemia.

DIFFERENTIAL DIAGNOSIS

Astute clinicians can minimize anxiety and inappropriate diagnostic evaluation by identifying substances that commonly mimic GI blood. Products that are mistaken for hematemesis include cherry or strawberry candy, red licorice, juice pops, Jello, Kool-Aid, tomatoes, cranberries, beets, antibiotics (ampicillin, amoxicillin), and other medications (Tylenol). Urinary sources of blood or redness in the diaper include hematuria, rifampin, beets, and dyes. *Serratia marcescens* may cause a pink discoloration in the diaper. The parent may misinterpret a urinary source as having originated in the GI tract. Chocolate, blueberries, spinach, iron products, and bismuth preparations (Pepto-Bismol) may be mistaken for melena. Menarche should be considered in pubertal females.

Blood may be detected in the stool or emesis, but not originate in the GI tract. Swallowed blood may come from nongastrointestinal sources such as epistaxis or oropharyngeal lesions.

The causes of upper and lower GI tract bleeding vary depending on age (Tables 88–1, 88–2, and 88–3).

EVALUATION

To help guide the workup in children with presumed GI hemorrhage, it is important to look for clues in the history and physical examination that quantify the amount and rapidity of the blood loss and help localize the site of bleeding.

TABLE 88–1. Differential Diagnosis of Upper Gastrointestinal Bleeding

Age Group	Common Causes	Less Common Causes
Neonates (0–30 d)	Swallowed maternal blood	Coagulopathy
	Gastritis	Vascular malformations
	Duodenitis	Gastric/esophageal duplication
		Leiomyoma
Infants (30 d–1 yr)	Gastritis and gastric ulcer	Esophageal varices
	Esophagitis	Foreign body
	Duodenitis	Aortoesophageal fistula
Children (1–12 yr)	Esophagitis	Salicylates
	Esophageal varices	Henoch-Schönlein purpura (HSP)
	Gastritis and gastric ulcer	Vascular malformation
	Duodenal ulcer	Hematobilia
	Mallory-Weiss tear	Caustic ingestion
	Nasopharyngeal bleeding	Foreign body
		Leiomyoma
Adolescents (> 12 yr)	Duodenal ulcer	HSP
	Esophagitis	Thrombocytopenia
	Esophageal varices	Dieulafoy's ulcer
	Gastritis	Hematobilia
	Mallory-Weiss tear	

Adapted, with permission, from Olson, A.D., and A.C. Hillemeier. Gastrointestinal hemorrhage. *In* Wyllie R., and J.S. Hyams (eds.). Pediatric Gastrointestinal Disease. Philadelphia, W.B. Saunders, 1993, p. 259.

TABLE 88–2. Differential Diagnosis of Lower Gastrointestinal Bleeding

Age Group	Common Causes	Less Common Causes
Neonates (0–30 d)	Anorectal lesions	Hirschsprung's enterocolitis
	Swallowed maternal blood	Infectious diarrhea*
	Milk allergy	Coagulopathy
	Necrotizing enterocolitis	Vascular malformations
	Midgut volvulus	Intestinal duplication
Infants (30 d–1 yr)	Anorectal lesions	Vascular malformations
	Midgut volvulus	Intestinal duplication
	Intussusception	Acquired thrombocytopenia
	Meckel's diverticulum	
	Infectious diarrhea*	
	Milk allergy	
Children (1–12 yr)	Juvenile polyps	Henoch-Schönlein purpura (HSP)
	Meckel's diverticulum	Hemolytic-uremic syndrome
	Intussusception	
	Infectious diarrhea*	Vasculitis (systemic lupus erythematosus)
	Anal fissure	
	Nodular lymphoid hyperplasia	Inflammatory bowel disease
Adolescents (> 12 yr)	Inflammatory bowel disease	Arteriovascular malformation
	Polyps	Adenocarcinomas
	Hemorrhoids	HSP
	Anal fissure	Pseudomembranous colitis
	Infectious diarrhea*	

*Infectious etiologies for lower GI bleeding include *Salmonella, Shigella, Campylobacter jejuni, Yersinia enterocolitica,* enteroinvasive *Escherichia coli,* enterohemorrhagic *E. coli, Clostridium difficile, Entamoeba histolytica,* and *Aeromonas hydrophilia.*

Adapted, with permission, from Olson, A.D., and A.C. Hillemeier. Gastrointestinal hemorrhage. *In* Wyllie R., and J.S. Hyams (eds.). Pediatric Gastrointestinal Disease. Philadelphia, W.B. Saunders, 1993, p. 259.

TABLE 88–3. Causes of Occult Gastrointestinal Bleeding

Inflammatory	**Tumors and Neoplastic**
Peptic esophagitis	Polyps
Crohn's disease	Lymphoma
Ulcerative colitis	Leiomyoma
Mild enterocolitis	Lipoma
Celiac disease	Carcinoma
Eosinophilic gastroenteritis	
Meckel's diverticulum	**Drugs**
Solitary colon ulcer	Salicylates
	Other nonsteroidal anti-inflammatory drugs
Infectious	
Helicobacter pylori	**Extragastrointestinal**
Hookworm	Hemoptysis
Strongyloidiasis	Epistaxis
Ascariasis	Oropharyngeal bleeding
Tuberculous enterocolitis	
Amebiasis	**Artifactual**
	Hematuria
Vascular	Menstrual bleeding
Angiodysplasia and vascular ectasias	Nonspecific Hemoccult test positivity
Gastroesophageal varices	**Miscellaneous**
Congestive gastropathy	Long-distance running
Hemangiomas	Coagulopathies
	Irritation from nasogastric or gastrostomy tubes
	Factitial

Adapted, with permission, from Olson, A.D., and A.C. Hillemeier. Gastrointestinal hemorrhage. *In* Wyllie R., and J.S. Hyams (eds.). Pediatric Gastrointestinal Disease. Philadelphia, W.B. Saunders, 1993, p. 262.

History

The physician should first determine whether the blood is actually blood. This can be accomplished using diagnostic tests described below. A thorough history should then be obtained (Questions Box).

Physical Examination

A meticulous examination is important, because the initial signs and symptoms of blood loss such as weakness, dizziness, fatigue, and pain may be nonspecific. Most importantly, the physician should determine

---

Questions: Gastrointestinal Bleeding

- Is the blood loss acute or chronic?
- What is the color and quantity of the blood in the stool or emesis?
- What symptoms preceded the episode of GI bleeding?
- Does the child have a history of vomiting, diarrhea, fever, ill contacts, or travel that may suggest an infectious etiology?
- Has the child experienced any abdominal pain?
- Has the child suffered any trauma recently?
- Has the child ingested any substances that might irritate the GI tract such as NSAIDs, steroids, tetracycline, caustic materials, or foreign bodies?
- Does the child have a history of straining with stooling?
- Has there been recurrent retching or forceful emesis, which could cause a Mallory-Weiss tear?
- Does the child have a history of increased stool frequency, weight loss, poor weight gain, or arthritis?
- Do any family members have a history of inflammatory bowel disease?
- Does the child have risk factors for portal hypertension such as a history of umbilical venous catheterization or liver disease?

whether patients are stable or show any signs of shock or impending shock such as delayed capillary refill, tachycardia, pallor, weak pulse, or dyspnea. Vital signs should be measured to help assess volume loss. A decrease of 10 mm Hg during orthostatic blood pressure measurements represents a 10–20% intravascular volume loss, and syncope or fainting implies either a larger deficit or a rapid 10% loss. Resting tachycardia and hypotension occur with losses in excess of 30%. A very narrow pulse pressure is an ominous sign, suggesting that the body's compensatory mechanisms are overwhelmed and warning of impending vascular collapse.

The physician should carefully examine the anterior nares and oropharynx. Blood draining into the esophagus and stomach from these areas is the most common nongastrointestinal source of blood in the GI tract. Marked tenderness with or without a palpable mass on abdominal examination raises the possibility of ischemia or intussusception. Bowel sounds may be normal, as expected with a lower GI bleed, or hyperactive, the result of rapid transit of blood through the bowel from the upper GI tract. Signs of obstruction should be noted. Jaundice, hepatomegaly, splenomegaly, ascites, or caput medusae suggests possible hepatic disease and portal hypertension. The practitioner should also inspect the perirectal area, looking for fissures, fistulas, tags, skin breakdown, or evidence of trauma. A digital rectal examination should be performed, and the following questions should be asked: Is a large, hard mass of stool or a polyp palpable? What does the stool look like? Is the blood fresh or denatured? The physician should also check for any evidence of child abuse.

In addition, patients should be examined for any rashes, petechiae, purpura, buccal mucosal discolorations, hemangiomas, telangiectasias, or other vascular lesions that suggest inflammatory bowel disease, Henoch-Schönlein purpura, Peutz-Jeghers polyposis syndrome, or coagulopathy. The presence of scars, which suggest prior surgery, should also be determined.

Laboratory Tests

Depending on the clinical scenario, a type and cross-match, CBC, platelet count, reticulocyte count, Coombs' test, PT, PTT, aspartate aminotransferase, alanine aminotransferase, BUN, and creatinine should be obtained. Gastric contents and stool should be checked for occult blood using the appropriate diagnostic test. Stool may be sent for culture and microscopic examination for leukocytes, ova, and parasites.

Hemoccult and **Hematest** are both used to detect blood in stool. A thin smear of stool is applied to the test pad, and a few drops of developing solution are then added. Hemoglobin and its derivatives (oxyhemoglobin, methemoglobin, reduced hemoglobin, carboxyhemoglobin), when exposed to the hydrogen peroxide developer, catalytically oxidize the guaiac or orthotolidine substrates that are impregnated in pads, producing a color change in the substrate, a positive reaction. **Gastroccult** is based on the same principles and uses guaiac as the substrate, but is more reliable at the low pHs encountered in the stomach. It is used to detect blood in emesis or gastric aspirate.

Blood from the GI tract of newborns should be checked using the **Apt-Downey test,** which detects blood of maternal origin. When 1% sodium hydroxide is added to blood, adult hemoglobin is reduced to a rusty, brownish-yellow color, signifying the presence of maternal blood. Fetal hemoglobin, being much more resistant to denaturization, does not undergo any color change and remains pink or bright red. The substance tested must be grossly bloody (red) and not denatured (e.g., coffee-ground emesis or tarry stools, in which the oxyhemoglobin has already been converted to hematin).

Ingested substances that may produce false-positive results include rare, red meat and peroxidase-containing fruits and vegetables such as broccoli, radishes, cauliflower, cantaloupe, and turnips. Ascorbic acid (vitamin C) and hemoglobin that has been changed to porphyrin by intestinal bacteria may give false-negative results.

Diagnostic Studies

If the source of bleeding remains unclear after a complete history and thorough physical examination, a nasogastric (NG) tube should be inserted and the gastric contents aspirated. NG tubes are generally better tolerated than orogastric tubes. The appropriate tube size depends on the size of the child. The largest bore tube that can be tolerated should be used, and the physician should be careful not to induce trauma. Small-bore tubes may suffice for diagnosis, but they obstruct easily and are not useful in removing larger clots. The presence of esophageal varices is not a contraindication to passing an NG tube. Gastric contents are aspirated with a large syringe.

Gastric lavage not only helps localize the site of hemorrhage but also aids in clearing the stomach of blood and clots prior to endoscopic evaluation. In patients with liver disease, it may prevent encephalopathy by avoiding hyperammonemia. Water is as effective as saline for lavage and should be used at room temperature. Cold or iced solutions offer no advantage and may induce hypothermia; large amounts of lavage fluid pass into the intestine and may lower the core temperature. In addition, cooling appears to adversely alter the clotting mechanism, prolonging bleeding time and prothrombin time, and shifting the hemoglobin-oxygen dissociation curve to the left, thereby reducing tissue oxygenation. Antacids are not used for lavage, because they interfere with endoscopic evaluation and do not stop bleeding.

If the aspirate does not show blood, the NG tube can be removed. If the aspirate contains bright red blood or coffee-ground material, however, the NG tube may be left in place to monitor ongoing bleeding. Tests of the NG aspirate for the presence of occult blood are rarely useful, because vomiting alone or trauma induced during passage of the NG tube can produce a positive test in the absence of true hemorrhage.

An aspirate showing blood is highly specific for upper tract bleeding. **Esophagogastroduodenoscopy** using flexible endoscopes, if performed within the first 24 hours, identifies the source of bleeding in approximately 90% of cases. Radiologic studies are not sufficiently sensitive for detection of superficial lesions such as esophagitis, gastritis, and Mallory-Weiss tears. When these studies fail to define the site of hemorrhage and the bleeding is massive (> 0.5 mL/min), **arteriography** or an **erythrocyte-labeled technetium 99m (Tc 99m) pertechnetate scan** (tagged RBC scan) should be performed to detect lesions located distal to the ligament of Treitz. These lesions may include hepatic artery aneurysms, hematobilia occurring after trauma, duplication cysts, arteriovenous malformations, and hemangiomas.

A negative aspirate suggests lower GI tract bleeding but does not rule out an upper tract source that is no longer bleeding or a duodenal lesion in which the blood has not refluxed back through the pylorus. **Careful visual inspection** of the anus, **digital examination,** and **proctosigmoidoscopy** reveal the site of lower tract bleeding about 80% of the time.

In the remainder of cases, the diagnosis is made on the basis of **colonoscopy, barium enema,** or **Meckel's scan.** When bright red blood covers the outside of the stool, the source is usually anorectal, such as a fissure, a distal polyp, or proctitis. The cathartic effect of blood on the GI tract can cause rapid transit in children, however, resulting in bright red blood from an upper GI bleed. Darker blood or blood mixed with the stool suggests a more proximal origin. Melena implies a bleeding site proximal to the ligament of Treitz. Anal fissures, juvenile polyps, and nodular lymphoid hyperplasia are usually associated with minimal bleeding, whereas significant blood loss may be seen with Meckel's diverticulum, a duplication cyst, or an autoamputated polyp. **Plain films** are used to rule out bowel obstruction and perforation. A **barium enema** may be both diagnostic and therapeutic if intussusception is suspected. It can also identify malrotations with secondary intestinal volvulus. In **Meckel's scan,** intravenously injected Tc 99m pertechnetate loosely binds to plasma proteins and accumulates in functional gastric mucosa, including the ectopic mucosa, which is present in the majority of children with bleeding from Meckel's diverticula. A false positive or a false negative scan occurs in 20%. If the diagnosis remains unclear, arteriography or laparotomy may be indicated.

MANAGEMENT

Attention must be focused on stabilizing children prior to initiation of an extensive diagnostic workup. Vigorous cardiovascular resuscitation is essential for orthostatic hypotension, which indicates massive blood loss. Good intravenous access should be established immediately with at least two large-bore lines. Placement of a central venous catheter should be considered. Intravascular volume expansion can be achieved using normal saline, lactated Ringer's solution, whole blood, or a combination of packed red blood cells and fresh-frozen plasma (10–20 mL/kg for 10–20 minutes). In life-threatening circumstances, unmatched blood products are given in an effort to keep patients alive long enough to stop the bleeding.

Once the bleeding has stopped, **packed cells** may be given alone to return oxygen-carrying capacity to normal. Heart rate, blood pressure, and central venous pressure should be carefully monitored to avoid fluid overload. Patients who are at risk for further bleeding should be in a setting where vital signs can be monitored continuously. Coagulopathy should be corrected with **fresh-frozen plasma, platelets,** or **vitamin K** (about 1 mg/yr of age, to a maximum of 10 mg). Hypoxia exacerbates the systemic effects of poor perfusion and resultant metabolic acidosis. All patients suspected of having a massive bleed should receive **supplemental oxygen.** Intubation and ventilator support should be considered. After an acute hemorrhage, equilibration of the hematocrit may take 24–72 hours or more, and initial values may not be an accurate reflection of blood volume.

Consultation with the pediatric surgeon and the pediatric gastroenterologist should be sought from the early moments of the evaluation. Although only few conditions require surgery (e.g., Hirschsprung's disease, Meckel's diverticulum), operative procedures should be considered for children who are bleeding severely or for those with undiagnosed, persistent bleeding. The gastroenterologist may assist in diagnosing the condition causing the bleeding by performing endoscopic studies of the upper and lower GI tract. Methods such as injection of sclerosant solutions or use of thermal, laser, or electrical coagulation allow the gastroenterologist to stop the bleeding from esophageal varices or peptic ulcers. Infusion of vasoactive agents such as vasopressin and somatostatin has successfully controlled upper GI hemorrhage in some patients.

PROGNOSIS

Prognosis for infants and children with GI bleeding depends on the condition causing the bleeding. Early, aggressive treatment of the consequences of blood loss is essential to decreasing morbidity and mortality. Generally, the prognosis is good, and overall mortality is only about 5%.

Case Resolution

The young child in the case history with episodic, painless rectal bleeding has a juvenile polyp. No associated nausea or vomiting is present. The polyp is palpable on digital rectal examination. Full colonoscopy and therapeutic polypectomy are performed. In addition, the polyp is evaluated for dysplasia, although the majority of polyps found in children are benign. He is referred to a pediatric gastroenterologist.

Selected Readings

Ament, M. E. Diagnosis and management of upper gastrointestinal tract bleeding in the pediatric patient. Pediatr. Rev. 12:107–116, 1990.

Gonzalez-Peralta, R. P., and J. M. Andres. Polyps and polyposis syndromes. *In* Wyllie, R., and J. S. Hyams (eds.). Pediatric Gastrointestinal Disease. Philadelphia, W. B. Saunders, 1993.

Olson, A. D., and A. C. Hillemeier. Gastrointestinal hemorrhage. *In* Wyllie, R. and J. S. Hyams (eds.). Pediatric Gastrointestinal Disease. Philadelphia, W. B. Saunders, 1993.

Perrault, J. F., and R. Berry. Gastrointestinal bleeding. *In* Walker, W. A. et al, (eds.). Pediatric Gastrointestinal Disease: Pathophysiology-Diagnosis-Management. 2nd ed. St. Louis, MO, Mosby-Yearbook, 1996, pp. 323–342.

Silber, G. Lower gastrointestinal bleeding. Pediatr. Rev. 12:89–93, 1990.

Squires, R. H., Jr. Gastrointestinal bleeding. Pediatr. Rev. 20:95–101, 1999.

Thompson, E. C., et al. Causes of gastrointestinal hemorrhage in neonates and children. South. Med. J. 89:370–374, 1996.

Yachha, S. K., A. Khanduri, B. C. Sharma, and M. Kumar. Gastrointestinal bleeding in children. J. Gastroenterol. Hepatol. 11:903–907, 1996.

CHAPTER 89

DIARRHEA

Carol D. Berkowitz, M.D.

H$_x$ An 8-month-old male infant is evaluated for a 2-day history of fever and blood-streaked, mucus-laden stools. His appetite is reduced, and he is only taking sips of diluted apple juice. He has had a single episode of vomiting. There are no ill contacts. On examination, the patient is irritable with a temperature of 102.2° F (39.0° C), a pulse of 180, a respiratory rate of 58, and a blood pressure of 90/65. The mucous membranes are dry, the fontanelle is depressed, and the skin turgor is reduced. The abdomen is somewhat scaphoid, and bowel sounds are active.

Questions

1. What are the four major categories of diarrhea?
2. What are the common infectious agents that cause diarrhea in infants and children?
3. What are the characteristics of diarrheal stools caused by different etiologies?
4. What conditions lead to prolonged diarrhea in infants and children?
5. How is diarrhea managed in infants and children?

The word "diarrhea" is derived from Greek and means "to flow through." The disorder is characterized by a greater volume of stool, which is associated with a looser consistency and an increased frequency of stooling. The frequency and consistency of stooling vary from individual to individual. Under normal conditions, stooling frequency is related to genetic factors of muscle function and GI motility. Wide variations in stooling frequency may be seen under certain conditions such as breast-feeding. Some breast-fed infants have a bowel movement every one to two weeks, whereas others may pass stool 12 to 15 times a day.

Diarrhea has several causes, which include infection, inflammation, and exposure to foods, drugs and hormones that affect the absorption of water from the small and large intestines.

EPIDEMIOLOGY

Diarrheal illnesses are very common both throughout the world and in the United States, where diarrhea resulting from acute gastroenteritis is second in frequency only to URIs. An estimated five million children in Latin America, Asia, and Africa die annually from dehydration secondary to diarrhea. In contrast, approximately 500 children die from this condition in the United States each year. These children often come from lower socioeconomic classes.

In the United States, each child experiences an average of 0.9 episodes of diarrhea per year unless enrolled in a daycare facility. In that case, the number increases to up to 4.5 episodes per year, a figure similar to that of children in developing nations. The leading cause of diarrhea in children in developing nations is infection with viruses, bacteria, or parasites. The severity of the infection is influenced by the underlying state of nutrition. An episode of acute gastroenteritis can precipitate severe malnutrition in marginally intact children.

The major route of spread of diarrheal infections is fecal-oral. In developing nations, poor sanitation and contaminated drinking water perpetuate the problem. In the United States, contaminated food supply such as the contamination of eggs and poultry with *Salmonella* is associated with the spread of bacterial gastroenteritis. Puppies have been found to be a reservoir of *Campylobacter* spp.

CLINICAL PRESENTATION

Children with diarrhea present with complaints of frequent, watery stools, which may contain blood or mucus. Affected children may have associated symptoms, including fever, vomiting, bloating, and abdominal pain. Signs and symptoms of dehydration such as decreased skin turgor, dry mucous membranes, depressed fontanelle, diminished tearing, and tachycardia may be pre-

D_x Diarrhea

- Liquid stools
- Frequent stools
- Blood in stool
- Mucus in stool
- Fever
- Poor weight gain or weight loss
- Dehydration
- Vomiting
- Abdominal pain

sent. Persistent diarrhea may be associated with weight loss and failure to gain weight at an appropriate rate (D_x Box).

PATHOPHYSIOLOGY

The consistency of stool depends on the stool's water content. The movement of water into the lumen of the gut is always related to the movement of electrolytes, because no active transport of water occurs. The absorption of water is associated with the active transport of sodium, and the secretion of water is associated with the active transport of potassium. Four different systems influence these processes: (1) the enteric nervous system; (2) the endocrine system; (3) the immune system; and (4) extrinsic factors such as bacterial enterotoxins, drugs, and chemicals. These four systems work by changing the cellular concentration of one or more messengers: cyclic AMP, cyclic GMP, or ionized divalent calcium ion. Medications to counteract diarrhea usually inhibit one of these messengers.

In all cases, diarrhea results when the absorptive capacity of the colon is exceeded. Normal infants excrete 5 to 10 g/kg of stool per day, of which 60 to 95% is water. Adults pass a total of 100 to 200 g of stool per day. Therefore, the infant colon is already functioning near its absorptive capacity. Stool volumes of over 10 g/kg/d in infants and over 200 g/d in older children and adults constitutes diarrhea. In cases of certain infections such as rotavirus or enterotoxic *Escherichia coli,* fluid secretion into the lumen of the gut may increase 20-fold.

Diarrhea can be divided into four major categories: osmotic (malabsorptive), secretory, motility, and inflammatory. **Osmotic diarrhea** may be characterized as general or specific. In general osmotic diarrhea, many components of the diet are not absorbed, whereas in specific osmotic diarrhea, certain substances such as lactose are not absorbed. These failures may be related to reduced absorptive surface or absorptive capacity. Infection with certain agents, such as rotaviruses, or bacteria (*Shigella, Salmonella,* or *Campylobacter*) may damage the villous structure of the small intestine and lead to osmotic diarrhea. Simply speaking, stooling stops with the cessation of eating in cases of osmotic diarrhea.

Secretory diarrhea occurs when the bowel continues to secrete water and electrolytes. This type of diarrhea is believed to be related to the presence of intraluminal substances, which are referred to as secretagogues. The best known of these secretagogues are bacterial toxins such as those associated with infection with *E. coli,* one cause of traveler's diarrhea, and *Vibrio comma,* the cause of cholera. In addition, some chemicals, including certain laxatives, dihydroxy bile salts, and long-chain fatty acids, produce secretory diarrhea. Secretory diarrhea is also seen with certain tumors, such as ganglioneuroblastoma, and congenital disorders of fluid and electrolyte metabolism such as congenital chloridorrhea. Classically, the stooling of secretory diarrhea continues even with cessation of eating.

In reality, both secretory and osmotic components are present in many cases of diarrhea. If the malabsorption of osmotic diarrhea is present, and bile salts or fatty acids remain in the lumen of the gut, their presence may lead to secretory diarrhea. Secretory diarrhea is particularly common in the developing nations of the world, where it is related to infection with organisms such as enterotoxin *E. coli* and *Vibrio comma.* In the United States, vasoactive intestinal peptide-secreting tumors such as ganglioneuroma and neuroblastoma must be considered in the diagnosis.

Motility disorders are the cause of irritable colon syndrome or chronic nonspecific diarrhea. Diarrhea without malabsorption is noted. **Inflammatory diarrhea** occurs acutely with certain infections or chronically with Crohn's disease and ulcerative colitis. **Steatorrhea** refers to the presence of fat in the stools. Approximately 95% of the fat content of food should be absorbed. In infants under the age of 12 months, 10 to 15% of ingested fat may appear in the stool. Fat malabsorption occurs with problems of the small intestine, including giardiasis; liver; and pancreas. Steatorrhea is not related to colonic problems. It may occur in cases of acute gastroenteritis, where the brush border of the small intestine is affected. Fat in the stool is associated with both osmotic diarrhea and secretory diarrhea because the presence of long-chain fatty acids promotes the secretion of chloride and accompanying water.

DIFFERENTIAL DIAGNOSIS

Acute Diarrhea

The major cause of diarrhea in children and infants is related to **acute gastroenteritis,** most commonly with a **viral infection.** The most common virus is rotavirus, which usually occurs during the winter months. This has been referred to as "winter vomiting syndrome." Infants present with an antecedent history of mild upper respiratory symptoms, followed by fever and vomiting. Watery diarrhea, which is usually free of blood or mucus, then occurs. About 10% of infected infants have signs of otitis media. Dehydration may also occur with rotavirus infection. It is typically mildly hypernatremic, with serum sodium values about 150 mEq/L. Enteric adenovirus is the second most common viral pathogen causing diarrhea. In the summer months, enteroviral infections may produce similar pathology.

The most common **bacterial agents** associated with gastroenteritis in the United States are *Shigella, Salmonella,* and *Campylobacter.* Aeromonas, a common pathogen in developing countries, is recovered in <1% of cases of diarrhea in the United States. Both *Shigella* and

Campylobacter produce signs of colitis, with blood and mucus in the stools. Patients are usually febrile. As a rule, children infected with *Shigella* are sicker, with higher levels of fever and more marked leukocytosis. In addition, they are particularly prone to seizures. Infection with *Salmonella* may also be associated with high fever. Stools may be mucus-laden, and inflammation of the small intestine may be evident. Parasitic infections particularly with *Giardia lamblia, Entamoeba histolytica,* and *Cryptosporidium parvum* may be associated with diarrhea and may follow a more protracted course. Infestation with these organisms does not usually result in fever.

Infectious conditions that do not affect the GI tract may also be associated with diarrhea. **Parenteral or secondary gastroenteritis** occurs with infections of the middle ear and urine. Likewise, infectious hepatitis may be associated with diarrhea and right upper quadrant tenderness.

Other conditions may also result in diarrhea. In newborns, infection with *E. coli* may produce epidemic outbreaks of large, explosive watery, green stools without blood. These outbreaks may result in closure of newborn nurseries. Watery stools may herald the onset of **necrotizing enterocolitis** (NEC); blood is usually present, however. NEC most often affects preterm infants with respiratory distress syndrome. The mechanism of disease production appears to be related to hypoxia of the intestinal mucosa. Enterocolitis may also occur in infants with Hirschsprung's disease. Bloody stools and air in the bowel wall, or pneumatosis intestinales, are the hallmarks of the disorder. Adrenal insufficiency, as well as certain inborn errors of metabolism such as galactosemia may lead to diarrhea. In general, other symptoms such as vomiting occur. Infants may present in shock because of hypovolemia related to dehydration.

Food intolerance may result in diarrhea in infants as well as in older children. Overfeeding or the ingestion of large quantities of fruit juices, dried fruits, or sorbitol-containing products can produce an osmotic diarrhea. Food allergies may also be associated with malabsorption.

In infants, cow protein intolerance can produce diarrhea, steatorrhea, growth retardation, anemia, hypoproteinemia, edema, respiratory symptoms, eczema, eosinophilia, and elevated levels of immunoglobulin E (IgE). Because 25–50% of cow protein-allergic children are also soy protein-allergic, symptoms of diarrhea may not abate when soy formula is offered. However, soy formula does help infants with certain disaccharidase deficiencies, such as lactase deficiency. Although lactose intolerance rarely occurs as a congenital deficiency, it is reported more frequently as a transitory condition following a bout of acute gastroenteritis, when the brush border of the small intestine has been disrupted. Acquired lactase deficiency is fairly common, especially in certain racial groups; it is reported in 10% of Caucasians, 70 to 80% of African Americans, and 90% of Asians. The disorder is associated with diarrhea, cramping, bloating, and abdominal pain after consumption of lactose. The stool has an acid pH, floats because it contains air, and is positive for reducing substances.

Chronic Diarrhea

Chronic diarrhea occurs when symptoms last longer than two weeks. Most cases of acute gastroenteritis resolve within two to five days. Four major conditions are associated with chronic diarrhea without evidence of malabsorption.

Infants and children may have a protracted course of loose stools **following** an episode of **acute gastroenteritis.** In most cases, no cause for the diarrhea can be detected, but infestation with *Cryptosporidium* or *E. coli* may be the source of the problem. The possibility of infection with HIV should be considered in infants and children with protracted diarrhea, especially in geographic areas where disease prevalence is high (see Chapter 115, Pediatric HIV). Certain children with acute diarrhea have such a modified diet (e.g., clear fluids) that they develop starvation stools. These slimy, dark green or golden stools represent succus entericus, the secretion of the small intestine. Starvation stools do not have a fecal odor. Insufficient fat in the diet may contribute to starvation diarrhea.

Inflammatory bowel disease, which occurs more commonly in older children and adolescents, is associated with chronic diarrhea. Ulcerative colitis involves inflammation of the mucosa and submucosa with the formation of abscesses. Fever, weight loss, and anorexia are often present. Diarrhea is the hallmark of the disease, and patients experience tenesmus as well as mucus-laden and bloody stools. Evidence of the disease is present on sigmoidoscopy in 95% of affected patients.

Crohn's disease, or regional enteritis, may also lead to chronic diarrhea, although lower abdominal pain relieved by defecation may be a more prominent part of the medical history. Affected individuals frequently experience extraintestinal manifestations of the disease, such as fever, anorexia, weight loss or growth retardation, recurrent stomatitis, uveitis, arthralgia and arthritis, and clubbing. Perianal disease, such as fistulas, may be noted in 70% of patients.

Irritable colon syndrome, which occurs in infants and children between the ages of six months and three years, also results in chronic diarrhea. No stooling during the night, at least a partially formed first stool in the morning, and increased stooling frequency during the day is the classic history. Stooling tends to occur after each meal, suggesting a prominent gastrocolic reflex. Children may have 3 to 10 stools per day, which may be mucus-laden and contain undigested vegetable fiber. Alternating periods of constipation may occur. Affected children appear well throughout this illness, and no evidence of weight loss, growth impairment, fever, leukocytosis, steatorrhea, or protein malabsorption is evident. Their appetite remains good. Treatment of this type of chronic diarrhea involves the use of a high-residue diet to add bulk to the stool and thereby prevent small, frequent stools. The addition of fat to the diet, by the inclusion of foods such as butter, gravy, and whole milk, slow gastric emptying, increase the transit time in the small intestine, and thereby reduce the diarrhea.

Other conditions that lead to chronic diarrhea include intestinal polyposis and the use of certain medications, such as antibiotics, and heavy metals, such as iron. Intestinal polyposis is associated with a history of cramping, and other family members may be affected.

Chronic diarrhea may also be associated with **malabsorption.** The two most common conditions of malabsorptive chronic diarrhea are cystic fibrosis and celiac disease or gluten enteropathy.

Newborns with **cystic fibrosis** may present with meconium ileus or rarely with acute appendicitis. Children with this disease tend to have voracious appetites because the pylorus fails to contract and food rapidly passes from the stomach into the duodenum. Contraction of the pylorus occurs secondary to the release of enterogastrone, whose secretion depends on the presence of free fatty acids. Children with cystic fibrosis have pancreatic insufficiency and do not produce lipase. Hence, they do not experience a surge in free fatty acids in the serum. Malabsorption occurs because the body fails to digest food effectively. Weight gain is therefore poor. Stools are large, bulky, and foul-smelling secondary to the bacterial overgrowth related to fat and protein malabsorption. Isolated GI complaints are reported in 10 to 15% of patients with cystic fibrosis, but most affected children are also prone to pulmonary infections. Rectal prolapse is another complication (see Chapter 118, Chronic Lung Disease).

Celiac disease is related to an allergy to the gliadin portion of the wheat protein, gluten. This protein is also found in barley, rye, and oat. Characteristically, villous flattening is apparent on small intestinal biopsy. This flattening restricts the absorptive capacity of the intestine and leads to malabsorption. Children with celiac disease have protuberant abdomens, appear bloated, and are frequently irritable because of GI discomfort. Their rate of growth is retarded. Symptoms usually appear when grains are introduced into the diet, usually between the ages of 6 and 12 months. Stools are mushy, bulky, and foul-smelling. Fat content in the stool may be two to three times the normal level.

EVALUATION

History

A careful history should be obtained (Questions Box).

Physical Examination

Children should be assessed for the presence of dehydration as evidenced by altered vital signs, delayed capillary refill, decreased skin turgor, a sunken fontanelle, dry mucous membranes, and reduced tearing. Skin changes in the perianal area or diaper dermatitis would indicate the irritative nature of the stools. Perianal fissures may be present in Crohn's disease, along with extraintestinal findings such as clubbing and uveitis. Evidence of growth retardation should be determined by assessing the growth parameters, particularly weight. Failure to gain weight over a period of months signifies a chronic diarrheal condition with malabsorption.

Questions: Diarrhea

- How long has the diarrhea been present?
- How frequent is the stooling?
- What is the consistency of the stools?
- Is stooling related to eating, which is a sign of osmotic diarrhea, or does it occur even if the child does not eat, which is a sign of secretory diarrhea?
- Do the stools contain any blood or mucus, which suggests a bacterial or parasitic infection?
- Is the child febrile?
- Does the child have any symptoms associated with the stooling problems?
- Does the child have a recent history of travel or exposure to animals?
- Is anyone at home ill?
- Has the child experienced any change in the frequency of urination, which is an important measure of the state of hydration?
- What is the child's diet now? What has it been?

Laboratory Tests

Stool assessment, a major component of the evaluation, involves four steps. First, the stool is evaluated for its quantity as well as its gross appearance. Undigested pieces of fruits and vegetables in the stool of toddlers are often a sign of poor chewing. Small, threadlike bodies that resemble worms are concretions of bile and are common in the stool of infants. The change in stool volume with fasting can also be checked. Reduced volume in the face of fasting is consistent with osmotic diarrhea.

Second, the stool is subjected to chemical and microscopic analyses to detect the presence of unabsorbed nutrients such as carbohydrates and fats. The presence of carbohydrates may be detected using a small amount of stool liquefied in about one milliliter of water. A Clinitest tablet is added to the sample, and a change in color from blue to green or orange is indicative of the presence of undigested carbohydrate. If the main source of dietary sugar is sucrose, as determined by the history, the specimen must be hydrolyzed by heating with hydrochloric acid. If the specimen sits around for too long a time, the presence of bacteria in the stool may break down the carbohydrate and lead to a false-negative result. The presence of fat can be determined both qualitatively and quantitatively. The stool may be examined under a microscope with just water or using a Sudan or Carmine red stain. If there are 10 or more globules of fat per high-power field, a quantitative fat analysis over a three-day period should be undertaken. Ten percent of children with an abnormal stool fat on microscopic assessment have a normal three-day quantitative stool fat value.

Third, the stool is examined for the presence of blood and leukocytes. Blood may be present in the stool but originates from excoriations in the diaper area rather than from the GI tract. To assess for leukocytes in the stool, the mucous component of the stool should be smeared on a glass slide and stained with methylene blue. More than two to four leukocytes per high-power field is abnormal and suggests a bacterial infection. The sensitivity of the fecal leukocyte test is 85% but the specifity is only 50–60%. If there are neither fecal leukocytes nor blood, the likelihood of an invasive bacterial pathogen is very low (predictive value of a negative test, 95%). A stool specimen should be submitted for culture and may be evaluated for ova and parasites. Stool analysis using Rotazyme will detect rotavirus.

Fourth, the stool is assessed for levels of sodium and potassium and for stool osmolality. These values may be helpful in distinguishing between osmotic and secretory diarrhea.

Additional studies, especially in the face of dehydration or fever, include serum electrolytes, CBC, urinalysis, and urine culture. Sigmoidoscopy or barium enema should be considered after consultation with a gastroenterologist if inflammatory bowel disease or familial polyposis is suspected.

MANAGEMENT

Initial management of children with gastroenteritis involves **adequate hydration and replacement of any fluid or electrolyte deficits** (see Chapter 46, Fluid and Electrolyte Disturbances). Bolus therapy may be necessary in children with significant dehydration. Children with significant dehydration may require admission to the hospital and the administration of intravenous fluids. Less severely affected children may be managed as outpatients using oral rehydrating solutions such as Pedialyte or Infalyte. Alternatively, parents can be advised to make oral rehydrating solutions by using water (1 liter), sugar (4–8 teaspoons), and salt (½ teaspoon).

Dietary manipulation in the treatment of diarrhea is somewhat controversial. Traditionally, affected children have been placed on clear fluids for one or two days, with a gradual return to a more regular diet with time. A **BRAT diet** (**b**ananas, **r**ice or rice cereal, **a**pplesauce, **t**ea or toast) was often recommended because of the intrinsic binding properties of the particular food. Recent studies recommend a full resumption of a normal diet, including dairy products, as the way to ensure adequate nutrition during the acute illness. A high-fat, low-carbohydrate diet accelerates improvement.

Antimicrobial therapy is indicated for infection with certain pathogens such as *Campylobacter*, *E. histolytica*, *G. lamblia*, and *Shigella*. Antimicrobial agents are used to treat *Salmonella* infection in certain populations such as neonates, immunodeficient children, and children with sickle cell anemia. **Antidiarrheal agents** are not usually recommended for the management of diarrhea in children. Diarrhea is believed to be the body's way of eliminating a toxic substance that has been ingested. In addition, the diarrhea often progresses in spite of the medication, which has its most binding effect after the illness has subsided, leading to constipation.

Children with chronic diarrhea secondary to a specific condition should be managed as dictated by the particular disorder.

PROGNOSIS

Most cases of diarrhea in infants and children in the United States are self-limited and resolve without problems. More chronic cases may lead to malnutrition. Enteral feedings or hyperalimentation may be used to ensure a good outcome. Some children require consultation with a pediatric gastroenterologist.

Case Resolution

In the case history, the presence of blood and mucus in the stools suggests a bacterial etiology. The stool should be examined microscopically for the presence of leukocytes using methylene blue. Their presence supports a bacterial etiology. A stool specimen as well as a blood specimen should be sent for culture. Because the infant appears dehydrated (i.e., sunken fontanelle, poor skin turgor, tachycardia), admission to the hospital should be considered to allow for rehydration and the administration of parenteral antibiotics.

Selected Readings

Cohen, M. B. Etiology and mechanisms of acute infectious diarrhea in infants in the United States. J. Pediatr. 118:534–539, 1991.

Gastanaduy, A. S. and R. E. Begue. Acute gastroenteritis. Clin. Peditr. 38:1–12, 1999.

Huicho, L., and D. Sanchez. Occult blood and fecal leukocytes as screening tests in childhood infectious diarrhea. An old problem revisited. Pediatr. Infect. Dis. J. 12:474–477, 1993.

Judd, R. H. Chronic nonspecific diarrhea. Pediatr. Rev. 17:379–386, 1996.

O'Gorman, M., and A. M. Lake. Chronic inflammatory bowel disease in childhood. Pediatr. Rev. 14:475–480, 1993.

Rhodes, J. M., and D. W. Powell. Diarrhea. *In* Walker, W. A., et al (eds.). Pediatric Gastrointestinal Disease. Philadelphia, B. C. Decker, 1991, pp. 62–76.

Richards, L., M. Claeson, and N. E. Pierce. Management of acute diarrhea in children: lessons learned. Pediatr. Infect. Dis. J. 12:5–9, 1993.

Sondheimer, J. M. Office stool examination: a practical guide. Contemp. Pediatr. (Supplement to Residents):5–14, 1994.

Talusan-Soriano, K. and A. M. Lake. Malabsorption in childhood Pediatr. Rev. 17:135–142, 1996.

Vanderhoof, J. A. Chronic diarrhea. Pediatr. Rev. 19:418–422, 1998.

CONSTIPATION

Carol D. Berkowitz, M.D.

H$_x$ A 5-month-old infant is brought to the office for a routine examination by his mother, who complains that her son is constipated. He grunts with each bowel movement, and his face turns bright red. He has soft bowel movements every 5 days. The infant is breast-feeding and has not yet started other foods. The mother reports that she and her husband are regular and have bowel movements every day.

On examination, the infant's vital signs are normal, and the infant is at the 75th percentile in height and weight. The remainder of the physical examination, including a visual inspection of the anal area, is normal.

Questions

1. What is the definition of constipation?
2. How is the stooling pattern of infants related to their diet?
3. What diseases and medical conditions may be associated with constipation in infants and children?
4. What familial factors relate to constipation?
5. How is routine functional constipation managed?

Constipation refers to the ease of passage of stool. In individuals with constipation, stools are dry, hard, and difficult to pass. Reduced frequency of stooling is sometimes characteristic of constipation, but infrequent passage of soft stool is not considered constipation.

Many factors influence the frequency of stooling in normal children, including familial patterns of intestinal motility and sensitivity, diet, medication, degree of hydration, and disease. In addition, children's reaction to the passage of stool may be misinterpreted as a sign of constipation when in fact it simply represents their physiologic effort to facilitate the passage of stool. Parent-child interactions around the time of toilet training may be associated with resistance on the part of children, resulting in withholding of stool and functional constipation. Assessment of the etiology of constipation requires a careful medical history to determine the age of onset of the symptoms and the presence of contributing factors.

EPIDEMIOLOGY

Complaints related to constipation or fecal soiling account for 3% of all outpatient visits and 10–25% of visits to gastroenterologists. Young boys are more frequently constipated than young girls, but women are more likely to be constipated than men. The normal frequency of stooling ranges widely. Many people do not have a bowel movement on a daily basis and are not constipated. Ninety-five percent of preschool children have bowel movements every other day, every day, or two or three times a day. The average amount of the stool is 5–10 g/kg/day, with most adults excreting about 200 g of stool per day. The average number of daily bowel movements decreases from 4 each day during the first week of life, to 1–7 times a day by age 2 years. Transit time increases with age, which means that the frequency of stooling decreases as one gets older (Table 90–1). Longer transit times are associated with harder, drier stools that may lead to bleeding and subsequent withholding of stool.

CLINICAL PRESENTATION

Many infants and children who are constipated present with complaints of infrequent stooling (D$_x$ Box). Some parents are concerned that facial grimacing and grunting during defecation are indicative of constipation in infants. Infants with "Grunting Baby Syndrome" are usually 1- to 10-weeks-old and may cry for 5–10 minutes as a means of increasing abdominal pressure to initiate defecation. Fecal soiling, which represents overflow incontinence, may also occur in some constipated children. About 60% of constipated children experience recurrent abdominal pain. Poor appetite and poor growth may also be noted secondary to maintenance of a sense of fullness from the feces-filled colon. Some children maintain a withholding posture, where they keep their legs clamped together and contract their gluteal muscles in an effort to suppress the urge to defecate (Fig. 90–1).

PATHOPHYSIOLOGY

To understand the pathophysiology of constipation, the mechanics of the normal passage of stool must be understood (Fig. 90–2). The rectum is the sensing organ that initiates the process of defecation. As stool moves from the sigmoid colon into the rectum, pressure is

TABLE 90–1. Intestinal Transit Time
in Infants and Children

Age	Transit Time
1–3 mo	8.5 hr
4–24 mo	16 hr
3–13 yr	26 hr
>13 yr	30–48 hr

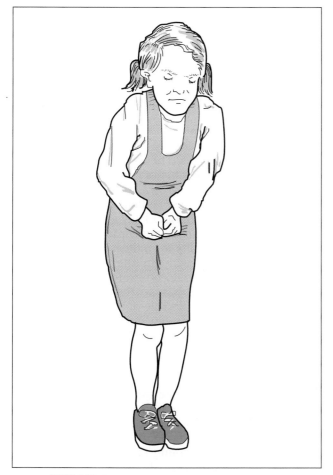

D$_x$ **Constipation**

- Hard, dry stools
- Infrequent stooling
- Abdominal pain
- Hematochezia (bleeding with stooling)
- Painful defecation
- Anorexia
- Fecal soiling

exerted on both the walls of the rectum and the rectal valves. This pressure initiates a nervous impulse that triggers relaxation of the internal anal sphincter, which is sensed as urgency and the need to defecate. If it is convenient, defecation occurs. If it is not convenient, the urge to defecate is consciously repressed by voluntary contraction of the external anal sphincter. Subconscious reflex inhibition as well as repression by the contraction of the puborectalis muscle may be involved. Colonic peristalsis may move stool into the anal canal. Voluntary contraction of the somatic abdominal musculature increases intra-abdominal pressure and facilitates expulsion of stool.

FIGURE 90–1. Child exhibiting retentive posture.

If the urge to defecate has been suppressed, defecation is sometimes difficult. The urge to defecate may be suppressed if stooling has been painful, a condition referred to as dyschesia and noted in infants and toddlers who change from breast milk to formula or cow's milk. Suppression of defecation is also an important factor in the pathogenesis of constipation in some school-age children who have an urge to defecate during the school day. These children choose not to go to the restroom for several reasons related to school bathrooms.

A similar phenomenon occurs during toilet training and may lead to chronic functional constipation. In an attempt to maintain independence and a sense of control, children withhold stool. The stool then becomes harder and drier, and attempts to defecate at a later time are associated with pain. This leads to further withholding, and a vicious cycle develops. To accommodate retained stool, the rectum enlarges and loses its propulsive ability. A decrease in sensory sensitivity and subsequent stool retention result.

Other factors may lead to transitory constipation. These include dietary changes; rectal fissures; medications such as aspirin and codeine; intercurrent illness, especially those associated with dehydration such as pharyngitis and URIs; and environmental changes such as vacation travel, a new home or school, birth of a sibling, and family stress. Changes in routine may also contribute to changes in stooling patterns.

Some families are predisposed to constipation. Concordance for constipation is four times more common in monozygotic twins than in dizygotic twins. Physiologic factors are believed to be related to stooling difficulties. Absorption of water may be increased, leading to drier, harder stools. In other cases, the bowel is unusually long or poorly motile. In some families, sensitivity to critical rectal volumes appears to be decreased, or particularly large rectal volumes are necessary for initiation of the process of defecation.

Constipation may be related to disorders of innervation of the intestine, thereby not allowing for the normal peristaltic wave. Hirschsprung's disease, a condition reported in 1:5000 individuals, involves absence of ganglion cells from the distal rectum and other areas of the more proximal large intestine. It accounts for fewer than 1% of children presenting with constipation for the first time.

DIFFERENTIAL DIAGNOSIS

The differential diagnosis of constipation is age-related and depends on assessment of the factors that have led to the conclusion that constipation is occurring. For example, infrequent though soft stools are common and normal in breast-fed infants who may have initially experienced frequent, watery stools. This change in stooling may be misinterpreted as constipation. Similarly, older children may defecate every 3–4 days and pass soft-formed stools. This is not constipation.

Four conditions should be considered in the differential diagnosis of constipation in infants under the age of 6 months.

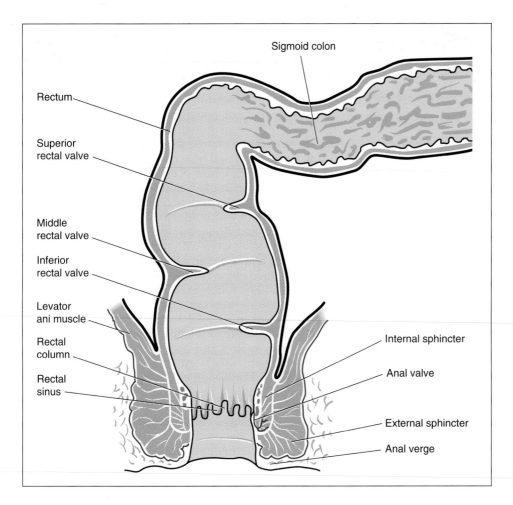

Sigmoid colon

Rectum

Superior
rectal valve

Middle
rectal valve

Inferior
rectal valve

Levator
ani muscle

Rectal
column

Rectal
sinus

Internal sphincter

Anal valve

External sphincter

Anal verge

FIGURE 90–2. Diagram of anus, rectum, and sigmoid colon.

1. **Hirschsprung's disease** may be suspected in young infants in whom the initial passage of meconium has been delayed over 24 hours. Forty percent of affected infants have not passed their first stool by 48 hours. Early recognition of this condition may prevent the development of enterocolitis and toxic megacolon, two conditions with high morbidity and mortality. Hirschsprung's disease may not be diagnosed until children are older (age 5–6 years), however. Hirschsprung's disease may be seen in conjunction with other syndromes including Trisomy 21, Smith-Lemli-Opitz, and Waardenburg's.

2. **Hypothyroidism** is also associated with constipation. Infants with hypothyroidism secondary to hypopituitarism are not diagnosed through the newborn screening process because of normal levels of thyroid-stimulating hormone. These children may either appear clinically normal or display some of the features of hypothyroidism (e.g., large anterior and posterior fontanelles; umbilical hernia; coarse facies; large, protruding tongue).

3. **Imperforate anus** can also lead to constipation. Some infants with imperforate anus with perineal fistula may not be recognized immediately in the newborn period because of the subtlety of the condition. These infants may have an anteriorly displaced anus, which does not allow for the easy egress of stool. Anorectal malformations occur in 1:7000 births.

4. **Infantile botulism** may result in constipation in infants who are usually between the ages of 6 weeks and 6 months. These infants are most often breast-fed or have a history of exposure to honey, corn syrup, or home-grown herbal teas. In addition to constipation, these infants are often febrile, hypotonic, and lethargic. They may be admitted to rule out sepsis. Clinical appearance, with flattened facies and an inability to smile or to gaze away from a light shined directly in the eye, is a clue to diagnosis. Care should be exercised when managing these infants because the administration of gentamicin as part of a rule-out sepsis regimen may potentiate the neuromuscular blockade of the botulinum toxin and precipitate respiratory arrest.

Constipation that begins prior to toilet training indicates possible organic etiology such as **Hirschsprung's disease** or **pseudo-obstruction.** Pseudo-obstruction may also present in older children, who may have a history of abdominal distention, pain, and intestinal paresis. The onset of constipation around the time of toilet training, when stooling has been normal in the past, suggests functional constipation.

Constipation may develop in some children in association with the use of **medications** such as aspirin and codeine, **chemotherapeutic agents** (e.g., vincristine), **heavy metals** (e.g., iron, bismuth [Pepto-Bismol]), and **agents with anticholinergic properties** (e.g., imipramine). A medication history should be obtained in all children with constipation of recent onset. Likewise, **intercurrent illnesses,** particularly those in which children's hydration has been poor (e.g., sore throat, URI), may also be associated with constipation. A diet low in bulk and fiber may be the reason for hard, infrequent stools in some children.

Children with **neurologic disorders** are frequently constipated. This may be secondary to spinal cord dysfunction, as in meningomyelocele, and to the inactivity and low-fiber diet of these children.

EVALUATION

History

The evaluation involves a careful history (Questions Box).

Physical Examination

A complete physical examination should be performed. Although the physical examination is frequently normal, palpation of the abdomen may indicate the presence of stool-filled intestines. Inspection of the anal area may reveal fecal soiling, dermatitis secondary to fecal soiling, an anteriorly placed anus or rectoperineal fistula, abnormal anal tone, or skin changes over the lower spine suggestive of spina bifida occulta. A rectal examination should be performed to assess the location and tone of the anus. In the face of a spinal cord problem, the tone may be decreased. A short anal canal and a dilated rectal segment may be revealed by rectal examination. In other conditions (e.g., Hirschsprung's disease), a tight sphincter or a tight rectal segment may be found. The passage of a large liquid stool after a digital examination is also suggestive of Hirschsprung's disease.

Laboratory Tests

If the history and physical examination suggest hypothyroidism or infantile botulism, appropriate studies should be ordered (e.g., thyroid function studies, stool tests for botulinum toxin). Anorectal manometry may also be carried out by a gastroenterologist to diagnose Hirschsprung's disease. Rectal biopsy may be performed to determine whether ganglion cells are present and whether acetylcholinesterase is increased. Similar studies that monitor the peristaltic wave can be conducted to diagnose pseudo-obstruction.

Imaging Studies

GI assessment may include the use of radiographic studies, including flat plates of the abdomen. Diagnostic radiographs using contrast material such as barium enemas help establish the diagnosis of imperforate anus and Hirschsprung's disease. It is suggested that the barium enema be attempted without prior cleanout to better document the presence of a dilated, stool-filled rectum. Radiopaque markers may be swallowed and their rate of passage determined by x-rays. This allows for the calculation of transit time, or the detection of areas of outlet obstruction or delay.

MANAGEMENT

Most cases of constipation can be evaluated and managed by primary care physicians. The precise management depends on the etiology, with conditions such as Hirschsprung's disease requiring surgical intervention. Children with pseudo-obstruction may show some improvement with cisapride. Parents of normal infants who grunt and grimace during defecation should be reassured that these symptoms resolve over time. In cases of familial or functional constipation, the mainstay of management involves **dietary manipulation** and use of **medications** to soften and increase the bulk of the stool. Parental reassurance and dispelling fears about the dangers of fecal retention (e.g., fevers, toxins entering the blood stream, bad breath) should also be addressed.

Many physicians alter the formula of young infants if the formula contains iron. Controlled trials with infant formula have not shown a relationship between iron in the formula and constipation, however. Management of infants with constipation may involve increasing the fluid in their diet or adding fruits or fruit juices, including prune juice or pear nectar. Raw fruits and vegetables provide soluble fiber, whereas bran provides insoluble fiber that increases water retention in the intestine. Changing from rice cereal to barley cereal may improve constipation. The nonabsorbable carbohydrate Maltsupex may also be effective. The initial dose of one teaspoon per bottle three times a day can be increased to obtain the desired results. Corn syrup should not be given to infants under 1 year of age because of the risk of infantile botulism.

Management of functional constipation in older children frequently involves dietary manipulation. **Bulk** should be added to the diet. Certain fruits, including

---

Questions: Constipation

- What is the child's stooling pattern? How often does the child have a bowel movement? What is the appearance and consistency of the stool?
- What was the child's age when the problem began?
- What makes up the child's diet?
- Does the child take any medications?
- Does the child have any symptoms associated with constipation, such as recurrent abdominal pain? If so, how long have these been occurring?
- Has the child been sick recently with any illnesses that might cause constipation?
- Has the child recently experienced any changes in routine that could cause constipation?
- Is there a family history of constipation?
- How old was the child when he or she was toilet-trained?
- Is there any bleeding with stooling?
- Is there pain with stooling?
- Have any remedies such as laxatives, enemas, or suppositories been used to relieve the symptoms?

papaya and cantaloupe, are very high in fiber. Popcorn is a readily acceptable and effective stool stimulant in children over 5 years of age. It can be offered as an after-school snack. Neurologically disabled children who are on nutritional supplements may respond to products such as Pediasure with fiber. Some children may need to take **mineral oil.** The dose should be adjusted to produce soft stools without leakage of excess mineral oil from the rectum. There is no evidence that daily use of mineral oil for up to 6 months interferes with absorption of lipid soluble vitamins such as vitamins A and E. Colace adds bulk to the stool. **Laxatives** such as milk of magnesia, which is available over-the-counter, and lactulose (Cephulac), which can be obtained by prescription only, can also be used. Laxatives should not be used on a regular basis, however. They are more appropriate in the management of acute constipation, or briefly, with chronic constipation.

In cases of chronic constipation, management may involve aggressive cleanout, especially if the colon is dilated. **Cleanout** involves the use of **enemas.** The need for enemas is reported in only 2% of children during the initial cleanout. Fleet enemas, which are small in volume, may not be as successful as soapsuds enemas, which cause irritation with subsequent peristalsis. Softening the stool using mineral oil enemas is useful. Retraining of the chronically dilated rectum may be accomplished by employing the strategies used in the treatment of encopresis (see Chapter 34, Encopresis). These modalities include the use of stool softeners and laxatives coupled with sitting on the toilet for 15 minutes after meals and assisting with the egress of stool using enemas or suppositories. Cisapride, in a dose of 0.2 mg/kg per dose TID to a maximum of 10 mg per dose has been used successfully in some children with intractable constipation. Behavior modification sometimes is effective. Success is rewarded with positive reinforcement as with the use of star charts or other reward systems. Biofeedback is particularly useful in children with paradoxical contraction of their external anal sphincter, and in some children with central nervous system disorders.

The symptoms of children with predisposing conditions are more refractory to routine treatment, and they should be managed in consultation with specialists such as pediatric gastroenterologists and child psychiatrists.

PROGNOSIS

The prognosis varies with the etiology. Functional constipation is usually amenable to routine management although treatment failures are reported in 20% of children with functional fecal retention. Long duration of symptoms, poor self-esteem and prior sexual abuse are associated with a poorer prognosis. Even in these cases, functional retention is uncommon after the age of 12 years. With appropriate surgical treatment, the prognosis for children with Hirschsprung's disease and imperforate anus is excellent.

Case Resolution

The infant in the case scenario has a normal stooling pattern for a breast-fed infant. Stooling frequency is decreased, but the consistency of stools is normal. No diagnostic interventions are warranted at this time.

Selected Readings

Abi-Hanna, A. and A. M. Lake. Constipation and encopresis in children. Pediatr. Rev. 19:23–31, 1998.

Di Lorenzo, C. Constipation. In Hyman, P. E. (ed.). Pediatric Gastrointestinal Motility Disorders. New York, Academy Professional Information Services, Inc., 1994, pp. 129–143.

Di Lorenzo, C., and A. F. Flores. Use of colonic manometry to differentiate causes of intractable constipation in children. J. Pediatr. 120:690–695, 1992.

Green, M. Constipation and encopresis. In Green, M., and R. J. Haggerty (eds.). Ambulatory Pediatrics IV. Philadelphia, W. B. Saunders, 1990, pp. 417–419.

Johanson, J. F. Geographic distribution of constipation in the United States. Am. J. Gastroenterol. 93:188–191, 1998.

Murphy, M. S. Constipation. In Walker, W. A., et al (eds.). Pediatric Gastrointestinal Disease. Philadelphia, B. C. Decker, 1991, pp. 90–110.

Potts, M. J., and J. Sesney. Infant constipation: maternal knowledge and beliefs. Clin. Pediatr. 31:143–148, 1992.

Rosenberg, A. J. Constipation and encopresis. In Wyllie, R., and J. S. Hyams (eds.). Pediatric Gastrointestinal Disease. Philadelphia, W. B. Saunders, 1993, pp. 198–208.

Rudolph, C., and L. Benaroch. Hirschsprung disease. Pediatr. Rev. 16:5–11, 1995.

Wald, A. Evaluation and management of constipation. Clin. Perspect. Gastroenterol. 1:106–115, 1998.

ABDOMINAL PAIN

Carol D. Berkowitz, M.D.

H$_x$ An 8-year-old girl has a 3-month history of intermittent abdominal pain. The pain is present prior to eating and is intensified by food. Vomiting often follows and relieves the pain. The pain also occurs at night. As a result of her symptoms, the child has missed 1–2 days of school each week. The family moved to the area 6 months ago, and initially the child seemed to be adjusting to her new school and environment. In addition, the girl has a history of a 5 lb weight loss. She has a positive family history of abdominal pain; her father has been diagnosed with a peptic ulcer.

On physical examination, the vital signs are normal. The weight is at the fifth percentile and the height is at the 25th percentile. There are no abnormal physical findings, and the patient is quiet and cooperative. The rectal examination is normal, and the stool is negative for occult blood.

Questions

1. What are the different types of abdominal pain?
2. What characteristics distinguish functional from organic abdominal pain?
3. What are the common organic causes of recurrent abdominal pain in children?
4. What are two etiologies for functional pain?

Abdominal pain is a common pediatric complaint. Pain may be acute or occur on a recurrent basis. Acute abdominal pain in association with vomiting or diarrhea in febrile children is frequently secondary to acute gastroenteritis, whether viral or bacterial. Recurrent or chronic abdominal pain is defined as pain that has occurred on three or more occasions in a 3-month period and interferes with the patient's activities.

An organic etiology is found in less than 10% of school-age children with recurrent abdominal pain (RAP). The three leading organic causes of RAP are genitourinary problems such as UTIs and hydronephrosis, peptic ulcer disease, and inflammatory bowel disease. In other cases, constipation is believed to contribute to the symptomatology. When no organic etiology can be established, the term functional abdominal pain is used. This term should not suggest that affected children are malingerers or are confabulating their symptoms. Rather GI function may be disturbed or children may have increased sensitivity to the normal degree of gastric discomfort and distention that all individuals experience.

EPIDEMIOLOGY

Abdominal pain, one of the most common symptoms of childhood, is often fleeting and therefore not brought to medical attention. Acute pain may be related to multiple etiologies, which occur with variable frequency in different age groups. RAP, also a common problem, is reported in 10–25% of school-age children. Primary peptic ulcers, which affect 4–8 million adults, are uncommon in children. Even large pediatric centers see only five cases per year.

CLINICAL PRESENTATION

Children who experience abdominal pain may present with pain that may be characterized as persistent or intermittent, waxing and waning or steady and unrelenting, sharp or dull, and worsened or unaffected by movement. They may have associated complaints, including vomiting, diarrhea, constipation, fever, weight loss, headache, and anorexia (D$_x$ Box).

PATHOPHYSIOLOGY

Abdominal pain has two major causes: **inflammation** and **smooth muscle distention.** Pain from inflammation results from inflammation of the mucosa, serosa, and peritoneal lining. Guarding and rigidity are distinguishing features. Inflammatory pain is characteristically well-localized and constant. Motion makes the pain worse. The pain of acute appendicitis, which is localized to McBurney's point and intensified by movement (e.g., hopping on one foot), is classic inflammatory pain.

Inflammation of the peritoneal lining may result in two different types of pain. Pain from inflammation of the parietal peritoneum travels along the somatic sensory pathway and is referred to the dermatome with the same innervation, because the parietal peritoneum has the same innervation as the abdominal musculature. Inflammation of the visceral peritoneum (i.e., that surrounding the viscera) is innervated by the autonomic nervous system. Pain that results from inflammation of the visceral peritoneum produces symptoms similar to

D$_x$ Abdominal Pain

- Abdominal pain
- Abdominal wall rigidity
- Abdominal tenderness
- Vomiting
- Alterations in bowel sounds
- Diarrhea or constipation
- Anorexia
- Fever

those of distention of the viscera. The pain is vague and poorly localized, waxes and wanes, and is usually felt in the midepigastrium.

Pain from distention of smooth muscle also waxes and wanes, is poorly localized, and is unaffected by motion. Distention of any hollow viscus, including the stomach, intestines, biliary tree, fallopian tubes, or ureters, can result in such symptomatology. A classic example of such pain is renal colic, where the patient is writhing because of the discomfort.

DIFFERENTIAL DIAGNOSIS

In assessing the possible disease entities that may account for abdominal pain, patient age and duration of symptoms are the key differential components. As previously mentioned, acute gastroenteritis is a major diagnostic category when children have abdominal pain and fever, particularly if vomiting or diarrhea is associated with the pain.

The location of the pain may provide a clue to the etiology. Disease affecting the stomach is usually appreciated in the epigastrium. Duodenal problems are noted between the xiphoid and the umbilicus, small intestinal pathology is appreciated in the periumbilical area, and cecal inflammation may be felt from the epigastrium to McBurney's point. Disease in the colon is less specifically noted but is usually felt in the hypogastrium. Bladder and colon problems may be suprapubic or sacral. Pain may also be referred to the back. Classically, biliary colic is noted in the high midback, and pancreatic inflammation noted in the lower midback. Renal colic is also noted in the back, but more in a lateral or costovertebral angle (CVA tenderness) site.

Acute and Recurrent Abdominal Pain

Young Infants: Medical Conditions

A unique disorder of infants, **colic** has been referred to as paroxysmal fussiness of infancy (see Chapter 27, Crying and Colic). The onset of symptoms is usually between 2 and 4 weeks of age, with resolution by 3–4 months. Although recurrent abdominal pain appears to be present, abdominal pain has never been established as the cause of colic. Colic is characterized by fussiness and crying. Symptoms usually appear after feeding, particularly late in the day around dinner time. Infants cry, clench their fists, and flex their legs. A gas-cry–air swallowing cycle seems to occur. The symptoms may respond to a number of measures, including rhythmic motion and antigas medications. Infants with colic usually appear well otherwise and often have accelerated weight gain secondary to repeated feeding made in efforts to quiet them.

Abdominal pain may also occur with **food allergy,** particularly cow's milk protein allergy. Generally, symptoms such as vomiting, diarrhea, Hemoccult-positive stools, FTT, rhinitis, eczema, pallor, irritability, and a positive family history of allergies are associated with food allergies. Congenital disaccharidase deficiency may result in abdominal pain, but diarrhea is also usually present.

Young Infants: Surgical Conditions

Intussusception occurs in infants between the ages of 6 and 24 months. Children may have been previously well or have experienced a recent bout of diarrhea. Vomiting is reported in about 50% of patients, and pallor is frequently present. An etiology is noted in less than 2.5% of affected infants, although a lead point (lymphoma or Meckel's diverticulum) may be found in 5–10% of older children. The intussusception most often involves the area around the ileocecal valve. Compression of the vessels within the bowel wall may lead to necrosis and gangrene. The presence of blood and mucus in the stools gives a "currant jelly" appearance, although the initial stool is often normal, having been the stool that was present in the rectum prior to the intussusception.

The abdominal examination of affected children may be benign except for pain over the area of the intussusception or may reveal the presence of a mass. Bowel sounds may be increased secondary to the obstruction. The rectal examination may reveal blood and the presence of a mass. Fever and leukocytosis may also be noted. A flat plate of the abdomen may show an obstructive pattern, with distended loops of bowel and air fluid levels. Intussusception is both diagnosed and managed by a barium enema, which reduces the intussusception using hydrostatic pressure. In some countries, such as China and Canada, air rather than barium may be used to reduce the risk of barium peritonitis should gangrene of the bowel be present.

School-Age Children: Medical Conditions

Peptic ulcers may develop in children in three situations. One, acute infantile ulcers may occur in newborns secondary to stress and hypoxia. Two, stress ulcers may occur in children who are the victims of trauma, including burns and hypoxia (e.g., after submersion). The routine use of H_2 receptor antagonists has reduced the incidence of ulcers in hospitalized critically ill children. Third, adult or chronic primary ulcers may develop in children with no apparent precipitating factors. A positive family history of peptic ulcer disease is reported in 25–50% of children. Unlike the classic ulcer symptoms of adults, in which pain occurs on an empty stomach and is relieved by eating, younger children may find that ulcer-related pain is exacerbated by eating and relieved by vomiting. Hematemesis and Hemoccult-positive stools are clues to the diagnosis. There is clear evidence linking ulcer disease and infection with *Helicobacter pylori* in adults. The relationship between *H. pylori* and peptic ulcer disease in children is not so strong, though one-third of pediatric patients with endoscopic evidence of peptic ulcer disease have infection with *H. pylori*. Ulcers may also develop in children taking both NSAIDs and corticosteroids.

Primary peritonitis is secondary to infection with *Streptococcus pneumoniae* and is seen in children with nephrotic syndrome, cirrhosis, sickle cell disease, and in young girls with fever, abdominal pain, and vaginal discharge.

Mesenteric adenitis may produce symptoms indistinguishable from appendicitis (see below), although children may not be so ill-appearing. Nausea and vomiting and a history of an antecedent URI are often present.

Parenteral infections such as tonsillitis or pneumonia may present with fever and abdominal pain. In addition, hepatitis may result in pain and tenderness localized to the right upper quadrant in association with anorexia. Hepatitis in children is usually due to hepatitis A, and many infected children are anicteric (see Chapter 93, Hepatitis).

Pancreatitis produces abdominal pain that is often referred to the back. In the past, mumps was the most common cause of pancreatitis. At present, certain medications (e.g., steroids, chemotherapeutic agents) induce pancreatitis as a side effect. Familial and recurrent forms of pancreatitis are also reported. Trauma, particularly from injuries sustained as a result of impact against handle bars of bicycles, is a common cause. In children with pancreatitis and no apparent etiology, trauma related to child abuse should be considered.

Parasitic infestations, particularly with *Giardia lamblia,* may produce abdominal pain, often with bloating and diarrhea.

Genitourinary problems may result in abdominal pain. An abnormal urinalysis provides clues to the etiology. Renal stones occur infrequently in children, and boys are more often affected than girls. In two-thirds of affected children, stones are detected incidentally or in association with a urinary tract infection. Stones may be composed of calcium phosphate or oxalate, magnesium, uric acid, cystine, or xanthine. In addition to flank or abdominal pain, patients may also experience hematuria, fever, recurrent UTI, and persistent pyuria.

Hematologic and vascular disorders such as sickle-cell disease, rheumatic fever, and Henoch-Schönlein purpura (HSP) may also present with abdominal pain. Sickle cell anemia should be considered in African-American children with abdominal pain. Pain may be related to vaso-occlusive events including bowel ischemia and splenic infarction or cholecystitis. HSP, which is also referred to as anaphylactoid purpura, is characterized by a hemorrhagic skin rash, joint pain, and renal abnormalities in addition to abdominal pain. This pain may result from a number of processes, including vasculitis and ischemia of the bowel wall, edema of the bowel wall, and intussusception of the small intestine. The intussusception which occurs in 10% of affected children, may be difficult to diagnose because the colon is unaffected and a barium enema is normal.

Diabetes mellitus may lead to abdominal pain secondary to cramping of accessory muscles of respiration during a bout of ketoacidosis.

Acute intermittent porphyria is an uncommon cause of abdominal pain in children. The pain is often colicky and may be associated with constipation, nausea, and vomiting. Neurologic symptoms such as pain or paresthesia in the extremities may be present. Often symptoms are precipitated by the ingestion of medications (e.g., barbiturates, sulfa drugs). Some antispasmodic medications such as Donnatal elixir contain phenobarbital and can precipitate an attack. The diagnosis is made by evaluating the urine for the presence of protoporphyrins.

School-Age Children: Surgical Conditions

Appendicitis is the most common surgical condition that produces abdominal pain in school-age children. Appendicitis may even occur in newborns, where it is seen in association with conditions such as cystic fibrosis and Hirschsprung's disease that lead to diminished passage of stool. The condition is frequently difficult to diagnose in children under the age of 3 or 4 years for two reasons: (1) examination of such young children for pain is difficult and (2) symptoms are similar to those of acute gastroenteritis (i.e., fever, abdominal pain, anorexia). Classically, patients complain of periumbilical pain that localizes to the right lower quadrant in 1–5 hours. They often have a low-grade fever, with a temperature of 100.4° F (38° C). Vomiting and increased urinary frequency may occur. Stooling is variable.

The physical examination may reveal guarding and localized pain as well as rebound tenderness. A positive psoas or obturator sign may be present, indicating inflammation of these muscles. Tenderness may also be noted on rectal examination. Leukocytosis over $10,000/\mu L$ is also noted. An x-ray of the abdomen may reveal one of four signs: a fecalith in the appendix (appendicolith), air in the cecum (sentinel loop), blurring of the shadow of the psoas muscle, or edema of the abdominal wall on the right side. A chest x-ray is also useful to rule out the presence of pneumonia, which may produce symptoms that mimic appendicitis.

Meckel's diverticulum may be responsible for abdominal pain in a number of ways. It may serve as the lead point for an intussusception, may cause symptoms of ulcer disease (pain or hemorrhage) secondary to the presence of ectopic gastric mucosa, or may become acutely inflamed as in appendicitis. Meckel's diverticulum follows the rule of twos: it affects 2% of the population, is 2 feet from the ileocecal valve, is 2 inches in length, and is two times more common in males than in females.

Adolescents

In female adolescents, **gynecologic problems** such as torsion of the ovary, mittelschmerz, dysmenorrhea, and pelvic inflammatory disease must be considered as causes of abdominal pain (see Chapter 77, Menstrual Disorders). In addition, pain may result from gall bladder disease secondary to cholelithiasis or cholecystitis. Cholelithiasis is also a consideration in previously pregnant adolescent patients with abdominal pain and fatty food intolerance.

Recurrent Abdominal Pain

As noted previously, most children with RAP do not have a diagnosable condition that accounts for their pain. Much has been written about the family dynamics of these children and the reactions of families to children's pain. Pain in these children is functional rather than structural. Motility disturbances or visceral hypersensitivity may account for symptomatology. Although many children seem to outgrow the pain, some investigators believe that a percentage of these children experience irritable bowel syndrome as adults. Other children with abdominal pain may have nonulcer dyspepsia. The association of nonulcer dyspepsia with infection with *H. pylori* is speculative. Lactose intolerance may account for abdominal pain in another subset of children.

EVALUATION

History

A thorough history should be obtained (Questions Box). Pain made worse by eating is characteristic of both peptic ulcer disease in children and cholecystitis. Pain relieved by defecation is suggestive of inflammatory bowel disease. An organic etiology is suggested by pain that awakens children at night and is lateral rather than periumbilical. Associated symptoms such as fever, weight loss, anorexia, vomiting, diarrhea, leukocytosis, and an elevated sedimentation rate also suggest an organic etiology.

Physical Examination

The physical examination should include an assessment of the severity of the pain. Children should be observed when they do not suspect that they are being watched. For example, a child who stands up and hops around when the physician leaves the room may have pain with a psychosomatic basis. Detection of abdominal tenderness may be ascertained during auscultation of the abdomen by pressing down with the stethoscope. In young children suspected of having an acute abdomen, sedation with a non–pain killer may be necessary to assess the presence of tenderness. Sedated children with an acute abdomen awaken with palpation of the abdomen.

A rectal examination is also an integral part of the evaluation. In prepubescent girls with genitourinary symptoms or adolescent females, a genital assessment should be included.

Growth parameters should be evaluated for evidence of impairments, especially in children with RAP. Abnormal findings such as abdominal masses or perianal skin tags are clues to an organic etiology. Children who appear vigilant and keep their eyes open during the examination often have organic problems.

Laboratory Tests

The laboratory assessment is determined by the differential diagnosis. In general, laboratory tests include a CBC, a urinalysis, and an ESR (in recurrent cases). In children with suspected lactose intolerance, a hydrogen breath test is recommended by some physicians, although a trial of dietary manipulation or use of exogenous lactase (e.g., Lactaid) may be more cost-effective. Other laboratory tests, such as serum amylase or liver function studies, are appropriate if pancreatitis or hepatitis is suspected. Serologic studies may support the diagnosis of *H. pylori*. Stool evaluation for occult blood and parasites is also helpful. Consultation with a gastroenterologist should be considered in patients suspected of having ulcer disease or inflammatory bowel disease. Specialists may order diagnostic procedures such as endoscopy to arrive at the diagnosis.

Imaging Studies

In general, a flat plate of the abdomen should be obtained, especially if an acute surgical condition is suspected. A chest x-ray may also be ordered in children with acute symptoms consistent with appendicitis. Barium enema is indicated to diagnose intussusception. Technetium scans help detect Meckel's diverticulum if ectopic gastric mucosa is present. Ultrasonography is useful in suspected cases of cholelithiasis and cholecystitis. It may also detect pancreatic edema or pseudocyst, hydronephrosis, or abdominal masses.

MANAGEMENT

Management depends on the suspected cause of the abdominal pain. Medical conditions warrant treatment with **pharmacologic agents.** Peptic ulcer disease requires H_2-blockers such as cimetidine, proton pump inhibitors such as omeprazole, or cytoprotective agents like sucralfate. Infection with *H. pylori* is managed with amoxicillin and Pepto-Bismol. Urinary tract infections should be treated with antibiotics. Conditions such as appendicitis mandate **surgical intervention.**

The management of children with RAP is challenging. A three-tiered empiric trial has been suggested for children in whom no distinct cause is identified. First, a high-fiber diet should be implemented. This helps alleviate the abdominal pain symptoms of children with irritable bowel syndrome. Second, antacids or H_2-blockers are used empirically to see if symptoms respond to decreased acid levels. The use of H_2-blockers is currently very popular for the treatment of adults with abdominal pain. Third, a trial of Lactaid or a lactose-free period may also be implemented. Psychological referral has been suggested, but it is more appropriate for the primary care physician to explore and address some of the psychosocial concerns that may be contributing to children's symptoms.

Questions: Abdominal Pain

- What is the nature of the pain? Is it sharp or dull, well or poorly localized, intermittent or relentless, worsened or unaffected by movement?
- How often does the pain occur?
- How long has the pain been present?
- Do any maneuvers, such as eating or lying down, reduce the symptomatology?
- Is the pain related to meals in any way? Is it worse after eating?
- Are any symptoms such as fever, weight loss, anorexia, vomiting, diarrhea, constipation, dysuria, or headache associated with the pain?
- Does any one else in the family have similar symptoms?
- Does the pain occur at night and on weekends?
- Is there a history of travel?

PROGNOSIS

In general, the prognosis for children with acute abdominal pain is good, although it varies depending on the condition. In 30–50% of children with RAP, the symptoms resolve within 2–6 weeks of diagnosis. Thirty to 50% of affected children experience abdominal pain as adults, however, although the pain does not limit their activities. As adults, these individuals may experience irritable bowel syndrome or other chronic nonspecific complaints, such as headache, backache, and chronic pelvic pain.

Case Resolution

In the case history, the girl has the classic symptoms of peptic ulcer disease. Her symptoms are exacerbated by eating and relieved by vomiting. In addition, the family history is positive. Further evaluation may include a serologic test for *H. pylori*, an upper GI series, or consultation with a gastroenterologist. Management involves the institution of H_2-blockers.

Selected Readings

Boyle, J. T. Recurrent abdominal pain: An update. Pediatr. Rev. 18: 310–320.

Boyle, J. T. Abdominal pain. *In* Walker, W. A., et al (eds.). Pediatric Gastrointestinal Disease: Pathophysiology—Diagnosis—Management. 2nd ed. St. Louis, Mosby-Yearbook, 1996, pp. 205–227.

Gartner, J. C. Recurrent abdominal pain: who needs a workup? Contemp. Pediatr. (Supplement to Residents) 11:28–34, June 1994.

Hamilton, A. B., and L. K. Zeltzer. Visceral pain in infants. J. Pediatr. 125:S95–S102, 1994.

Hirsch, B. Z. Recurrent abdominal pain. *In* Snyder, J. D., and W. A. Walker (eds.). Common Problems in Pediatric Gastroenterology and Nutrition. Chicago, Year Book Medical Publishers, 1989.

Hyams, J. S., and P. E. Hyman. Recurrent abdominal pain and the biopsychosocial model of medical practice. J. Pediatr. 133:473–478, 1998.

Mezoff, A. G., and W. F. Balisteri. Peptic ulcer disease in children. Pediatr. Rev. 16:257–265, 1995.

Oberlander, T. F., and L. A. Rappaport. Recurrent abdominal pain during childhood. Pediatr. Rev. 14:313–319, 1993.

Silverberg, M. Chronic abdominal pain in adolescents. Pediatr. Ann. 20:179–185, 1991.

Stevenson, R. J., and M. M. Ziegler. Abdominal pain unrelated to trauma. Pediatr. Rev. 14:302–311, 1993.

Walker, L. S., et al. Recurrent abdominal pain: A potential precursor of irritable bowel syndrome in adolescents and young adults. J. Pediatr. 132:1010–1015, 1998.

CHAPTER 92

JAUNDICE

Carol D. Berkowitz, M.D.

H$_x$ A 2-month-old male infant is brought to the office for a routine well child checkup. He was the product of a full-term, normal, spontaneous, vaginal delivery, with a birth weight of 3600 g. He has been feeding well, exclusively at the breast. Loose stools follow each nursing.

On physical examination, the infant weighs 4900 g. The examination is normal except that the boy appears jaundiced. On further questioning, the mother states that her son has been jaundiced since shortly after birth, and she feels that his appearance has not changed. The color of the stool is yellow.

Questions

1. What are the common causes of unconjugated hyperbilirubinemia in young infants?
2. What are the common causes of conjugated hyperbilirubinemia in young infants?
3. What are the usual causes of jaundice in older children and adolescents?
4. What is the appropriate management of hyperbilirubinemia in breast-fed infants?

Jaundice is a condition that occurs when bilirubin reaches a level in the blood that makes it visibly apparent. In newborn infants, this level is 5 mg/dL. In older children and adolescents, jaundice becomes apparent at serum bilirubin levels of 2 mg/dL. The term **physiologic jaundice** is used to denote the jaundice that normally occurs following birth. In full-term infants, bilirubin reaches its peak of about 6 mg/dL between the second and fourth days of life. Levels above 10 mg/dL are probably not physiologic. Bilirubin generally returns to a normal level (<1 mg/dL) by 12 days of age. Premature infants experience their peak level of bilirubin, which may be up to 10–12 mg/dL, between the fifth and seventh days of life. Levels over 14 mg/dL are probably not physiologic. Levels may be elevated in premature infants for up to 2 months.

Although physiologic jaundice, a benign finding, affects all infants, other more serious disorders may present with similar symptomatology. The physician must be able to differentiate between these conditions to ensure appropriate intervention and management. New-onset jaundice in older children and adolescents is caused by other disorders.

EPIDEMIOLOGY

Jaundice is nearly universal in neonates because of the rapid turnover of red blood cells and the relative immaturity of the liver. Breast milk jaundice affects about 1% of breast-fed infants. Various illnesses, particularly bacterial infections, also may precipitate jaundice in newborns. Neonatal cholestasis (conjugated hyperbilirubinemia), which is seen in a small number of cases of neonatal jaundice, is due to neonatal hepatitis or extrahepatic biliary atresia 70–80% of the time. Jaundice occurs much less frequently in the postneonatal period and is most often secondary to viral hepatitis (see Chapter 93, Hepatitis).

CLINICAL PRESENTATION

Children with jaundice have yellow skin, conjunctiva, and mucous membranes. In newborns, the coloration may not be appreciated by parents because of its gradual onset and the parents' inexperience. The finding may be apparent in otherwise asymptomatic infants during routine health maintenance visits.

In addition to the yellow color, children with jaundice may also present with symptoms related to the cause of the jaundice, including vomiting, anorexia, FTT, acholic (white) stools, dark urine, fatigue, and abdominal pain or fullness (D_x Box).

PATHOPHYSIOLOGY

Bilirubin, a yellow pigment found primarily in bile, forms from the breakdown of heme-containing compounds, mainly hemoglobin, but also muscle myoglobin, cytochromes, catalases, and tryptophan pyrrolase. Blockage along any point in the physiologic or anatomic pathway may result in increased levels of bilirubin and the appearance of jaundice (Fig. 92–1). After the breakdown of hemoglobin, unconjugated bilirubin is taken up by the hepatocyte plasma membrane carrier, bilitranslocase. Once within the hepatocyte, bilirubin is bound to intracellular proteins (Y proteins or ligandin). Uptake depends on hepatic blood flow and the presence of the necessary binding proteins. Once in the liver, unconjugated bilirubin is conjugated by the enzyme glucuronyl transferase. Conjugated bilirubin, which is water-soluble, can be eliminated through the kidneys. Following conjugation, bilirubin passes into the bile through the bile canaliculi. It then moves to the GI tract, where

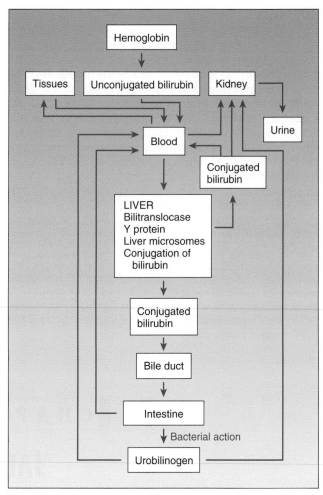

FIGURE 92–1. The bilirubin pathway.

some of it may be reabsorbed (enterohepatic circulation), or be acted on by bacteria to form urobilinogen, which may appear in the urine or stool.

In neonates, a number of factors contribute to physiologic jaundice. Increased destruction of red blood cells occurs, because the red blood cell survival in infants is only 70–90 days, as opposed to 120 days in older children. Hepatic uptake is lower, perhaps as a result of decreased levels of hepatic proteins as well as decreased hepatic blood flow. Levels of glucuronyl transferase do not reach adult values until the second week of life. These decreased levels of glucuronyl transferase mean that conjugation of bilirubin occurs at a slower rate. In some infants, glucuronyl transferase levels remain low; these individuals remain prone to jaundice at times of illness, stress, and starvation (Gilbert's syndrome). Some breast-fed infants also experience prolonged jaundice. Jaundice in breast-fed infants may be related to poor caloric or fluid intake, weight loss, slow passage of meconium, or the type or number of bacteria in the intestine. It is believed that some unknown substance in the mother's milk, perhaps pregnanetriol, blocks glucuronyl transferase. Reabsorption of bilirubin is increased through the enterohepatic circulation because of the diminished number of bacteria in the GI tract in young infants.

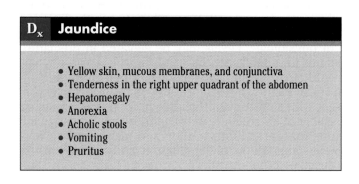

D_x **Jaundice**

- Yellow skin, mucous membranes, and conjunctiva
- Tenderness in the right upper quadrant of the abdomen
- Hepatomegaly
- Anorexia
- Acholic stools
- Vomiting
- Pruritus

In older children, similar mechanisms may act to cause an increase in the bilirubin level. Hemolytic anemias (e.g., glucose-6-phosphatase or pyruvate kinase deficiencies) may lead to increased red blood cell destruction. Inflammatory or infectious processes involving the liver, such as hepatitis, may impair the ability of the liver to excrete bilirubin. Pharmaceutical and toxicologic agents may also interfere with the ability of the liver to metabolize bilirubin.

DIFFERENTIAL DIAGNOSIS

The differential diagnosis of jaundice in children involves three criteria: (1) age, (2) the type of hyperbilirubinemia (conjugated or unconjugated), and (3) if the hyperbilirubinemia is conjugated, the nature of the obstruction (intrahepatic or extrahepatic). The latter two factors are particularly important in determining the etiology of jaundice in young infants. A diagrammatic representation of the differential diagnosis of jaundice in children is shown in Figures 92–2, 92–3, and 92–4.

Infants Under Eight Weeks of Age
Unconjugated Hyperbilirubinemia

Jaundice occurs universally in all newborns, but marked elevation of bilirubin levels or persistence of jaundice beyond 2 weeks of age warrants assessment. When less than 15% of the total bilirubin is direct, unconjugated hyperbilirubinemia is present. This is best determined by measuring the levels of total and direct bilirubin in the blood. **Physiologic jaundice** is associated with unconjugated hyperbilirubinemia. The hematologic workup of affected infants is normal. Jaundice related to breast-feeding is called breast-feeding jaundice, which may resemble physiologic jaundice and occurs during the first week of life, or breast-milk jaundice, where bilirubin levels rise during the second week of life when physiologic jaundice is improving. In breast-fed infants, levels may reach as high as 25–30 mg/dL. Breast milk jaundice usually peaks by the age of 4 weeks and decreases by 10 weeks.

Conditions associated with slow intestinal transit

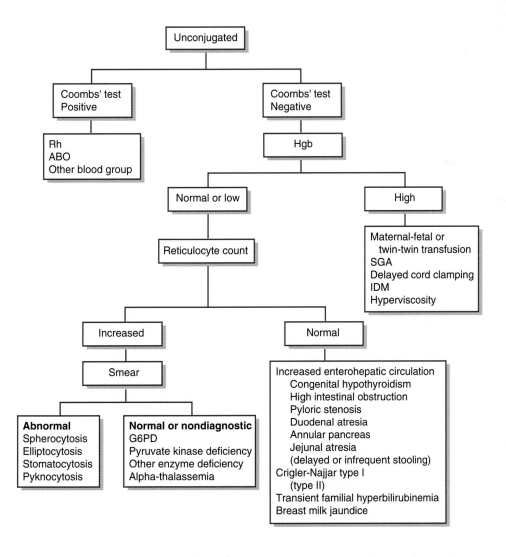

FIGURE 92–2. Differential diagnosis of jaundice in neonates (during the first 8 weeks of life). Unconjugated hyperbilirubinemia.

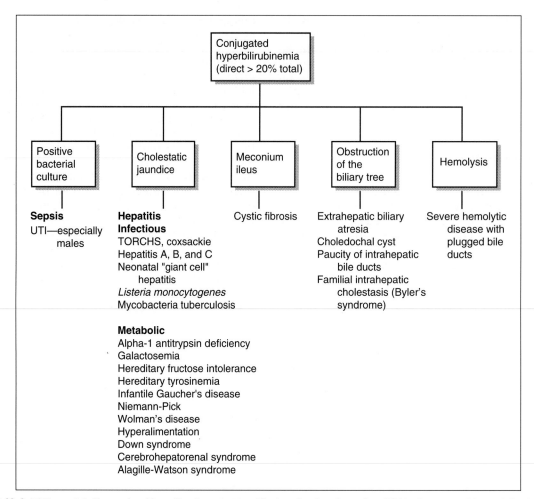

FIGURE 92–3. Differential diagnosis of jaundice in neonates (during the first 8 weeks of life). Conjugated hyperbilirubinemia.

time and increased enterohepatic circulation, such as hypothyroidism, also may result in jaundice. As with physiologic and breast milk jaundice, the hematologic workup is normal. High intestinal obstructions, such as pyloric stenosis, duodenal atresia, annular pancreas, and jejunal atresia may lead to jaundice, perhaps because of starvation and decreased levels of glucuronyl transferase.

Crigler-Najjar syndrome type I, which involves a deficiency in glucuronyl transferase, is associated with neonatal jaundice. Because of very high bilirubin levels, type I disease may lead to kernicterus unless managed with exchange transfusion. Phototherapy, cholestyramine, and eventual liver transplantation are additional therapies. The disorder is inherited in an autosomal recessive manner.

Hematologic problems may also produce jaundice in the neonatal period. Such problems are most often associated with blood group (usually Rh or ABO) incompatibility between mothers and infants, but some minor blood group determinants can precipitate similar problems. Jaundice occurs in affected infants because of the rapid destruction of red blood cells. Other infants may have a hemolytic anemia such as spherocytosis.

Jaundice may also occur if excess blood is present in the infant's system. Situations in which elevated hemo-globin is associated with jaundice include maternal-infant or twin-twin transfusions, infants who are small for gestational age, delayed clamping of the umbilical cord, infants of diabetic mothers, and infants with hyperviscosity syndrome.

Conjugated Hyperbilirubinemia

When over 15% of the total bilirubin is direct, the jaundice is categorized as conjugated hyperbilirubinemia. Conjugated hyperbilirubinemia is always pathological. Total parenteral nutrition is the most common cause of conjugated hyperbilirubinemia in the neonatal intensive care unit but does not usually present a diagnostic dilemma. The institution of oral feedings helps reverse the process. In other cases, determination of whether the problem is intrahepatic or extrahepatic is the major consideration. Some conditions of intrahepatic involvement represent a spectrum involving progression from inflammation of bile canaliculi (hepatitis) to their destruction (biliary atresia).

Inflammation of the hepatocytes is hepatitis. This disease may be caused by an infection in the liver or elsewhere in the body (e.g., sepsis and UTIs in young infants). UTIs are usually caused by *Escherichia coli.* Three mechanisms of action for jaundice in bacterial infections have been postulated: (1) increased hemolysis, with an increased reticulocyte count; (2) toxic hepatitis, with inflammation and lymphocytic infiltration in the liver; and (3) poor nutrition secondary to fever and illness. The common pathway seems to be some degree of hepatocellular necrosis, with pericholangitis, bile duct proliferation, and mild amounts of portal fibrosis. The hepatic involvement resolves with appropriate antibiotic therapy of the primary infection.

Primary liver infection may be due to hepatitis A, B, or C, or other so-called **TORCHS** agents (**t**oxoplasma, **r**ubella, **c**ytomegalovirus, **h**erpesvirus, **s**yphilis). Infants infected prenatally often have low birth weights, hepatosplenomegaly, petechial rashes, and ocular findings such as cataracts and chorioretinitis. **Other infectious causes** include coxsackie B virus, echovirus II, adenovirus 2, *Listeria monocytogenes,* and tuberculosis.

Differentiating among these conditions is usually done on the basis of culture or serology. Certain physical and epidemiologic findings may help to distinguish these entities, however. Syphilis is more common in the developing nations of the world. Jaundice may appear within the first 24 hours of life or be of later onset. Infection with *L. monocytogenes* infection may be associated with the presence of focal granulomas on the posterior pharynx. Similar granulomas in the liver are evident.

Metabolic diseases and **inborn errors of metabolism** may also lead to hepatitis. Most of these conditions are inherited in an autosomal recessive manner. In addition to jaundice, infants may present with vomiting, irritability, lethargy, anorexia, hepatomegaly, hypoglycemia, FTT, bleeding, or cataracts. Galactosemia may be detected through neonatal screening. Infants with hereditary fructose intolerance present after exposure to fructose, sucrose, or sorbitol. Alpha-1 antitrypsin deficiency may account for 20–30% of cases of idiopathic neonatal liver disease.

Other metabolic conditions that lead to jaundice in newborns include hereditary tyrosinemia, infantile Gaucher's disease, Niemann-Pick disease, and Wolman's disease. Cystic fibrosis may also cause cholestatic jaundice because of the presence of inspissated bile in the bile canaliculi. Fifty percent of these infants have meconium ileus, meconium peritonitis, or intestinal atresia. "Plugged" bile ducts may be seen with severe hemolytic anemia where bilirubin production is markedly elevated. Drugs may also induce intrahepatic cholestasis.

A number of syndromes are associated with persistent intrahepatic cholestasis. Alagille syndrome (arteriohepatic dysplasia) is characterized by unusual facies, skeletal and cardiovascular anomalies, and a paucity of intralobular bile ducts. The incidence is 1:100,000 live births.

Extrahepatic biliary atresia accounts for about 30% of cases of cholestasis in newborns. Obliteration of the biliary tree is apparent. Infants are often well until 3–6 weeks of age, when they develop conjugated hyperbilirubinemia. The incidence is 1:14,000 live births. Choledochal cysts appear as dilatations of the biliary tree and obstruct the passage of bile.

FIGURE 92–4. Differential diagnosis of jaundice in older infants, children, and adolescents.

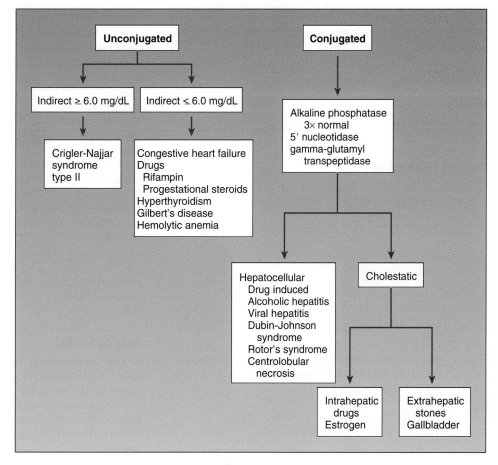

Older Infants, Children, and Adolescents

The approach to the differential diagnosis of jaundice in older infants and children is similar to the process in young infants. In cases of unconjugated hyperbilirubinemia, the level of indirect bilirubin helps clarify the differential diagnosis. Patients whose indirect bilirubin is greater than 6 mg/dL may have **Crigler-Najjar syndrome type II** and respond favorably to phenobarbital. Patients with levels under 6 mg/dL may have hemolytic anemia. **Congestive heart failure** and **hyperthyroidism** may also produce unconjugated hyperbilirubinemia. **Gilbert's disease,** a benign condition in which the bilirubin rises in response to stress and starvation, may result in jaundice. The prevalence of Gilbert's syndrome is 6%. **Drugs,** including rifampin and birth control pills, may also be associated with unconjugated hyperbilirubinemia.

Conjugated hyperbilirubinemia may result from two different processes: (1) cholestasis and (2) hepatocellular inflammation or injury. Signs of cholestasis are high levels of alkaline phosphatase (three times normal), increased 5′ nucleotidase, and increased gamma glutamyl transpeptidase. Cholestatic jaundice, related to drugs (estrogens) and alcohol, may occur on an intrahepatic basis. **Byler's syndrome** is a familial disorder characterized by intrahepatic cholestasis. Extrahepatic cholestasis is seen with cholelithiasis or other obstructions of the biliary tree. Cholelithiasis may occur in individuals with hemolytic anemia and in female adolescents who have been pregnant. Hepatocellular injury most often results from hepatitis (discussed in Chapter 93, Hepatitis), including infectious, alcoholic, and drug-induced hepatitis. Rarer disorders include Dubin-Johnson syndrome and Rotor's syndrome.

EVALUATION

History

A careful history must be obtained (Questions Box).

Physical Examination

Patients should be evaluated for evidence of organomegaly, ocular anomalies, rashes, hearing deficits, and unusual facial features. The unique facial features are pathognomic for certain genetic disorders such as Byler's or Alagille syndromes. Rashes and lymphadenopathy are associated with certain infectious conditions, including congenital infections (TORCHS) in newborns and infectious mononucleosis in adolescents. Patients should also be checked for the presence of any cardiac anomaly, which may suggest a genetic syndrome or congestive heart failure.

Laboratory Tests

In the newborn nursery, noninvasive methods are used to measure the level of jaundice. The "jaundice meter" uses reflectance spectrophotometry to determine the skin color and correlates highly with serum bilirubin levels. An icterometer is another noninvasive method, which uses an acrylic plastic color chart that is placed against an infant's nose.

The aim of the laboratory assessment is to discover where the bilirubin metabolism is abnormal. The total bilirubin as well as the fractionated bilirubin levels should be determined. The presence of elevated levels of direct-reacting bilirubin represents conjugated hyperbilirubinemia. The demonstration of a yellow color to the foam of a shaken specimen of urine is a rapid test for conjugated hyperbilirubinemia. Urine test strips also readily detect conjugated bilirubin in the urine.

In children with unconjugated hyperbilirubinemia, a CBC with reticulocyte count and evaluation of the peripheral smear confirm hemolytic anemia. Serum haptoglobulin levels are diminished in hemolytic disorders. In neonates, the Coombs test should be performed, and infant and maternal blood types should be determined. The hemoglobin should also be obtained. A normal or low hemoglobin may be seen in the face of hemolytic anemia. An elevated reticulocyte count or an abnormal peripheral blood smear indicates hemolysis. Hemolytic anemias with abnormal peripheral smears include spherocytosis, elliptocytosis, stomatocytosis, and pyknocytosis.

In children with conjugated hyperbilirubinemia, tests should be performed to determine if infections such as bacteremia, UTI, congenital infection, or hepatitis are present. Evaluation for metabolic diseases should also be obtained by assessing the urine for the presence of reducing substances (e.g., Clinitest tablet) or amino acids. The status of liver function can be determined by evaluating aspartate aminotransferase, gamma-glutamyl transpeptidase, alkaline phosphatase, or 5′ nucleotidase.

Imaging Studies

The anatomy of the biliary tree can be evaluated using ultrasound. Choledochal cysts may be visualized using this modality. Other imaging tests, including excretion studies (radioisotope scans), can be used to help differentiate hepatitis from biliary atresia. Consultation with a pediatric gastroenterologist may be appropriate.

Questions: Jaundice

- What associated symptoms are present?
- How long have the symptoms been present?
- Does the child have a fever, which may suggest the presence of an infection?
- What is the color of the stools (acholic stools suggest obstruction)?
- Does the child have a family history of jaundice or consanguinity?
- What makes up the child's diet? If the child is an infant, is he or she breast-fed or bottle-fed?
- When did the parents first notice the jaundice?
- Has the child been jaundiced previously?
- Has the child been vaccinated against hepatitis B?
- Is there a history of foreign travel or shellfish ingestion?

MANAGEMENT

The management of jaundice depends on the cause of the condition. Physiologic jaundice and jaundice secondary to breast-feeding frequently require no intervention. Interrupting breast-feeding for 24–48 hours will successfully lower bilirubin levels, but support and counselling are mandatory to ensure that breast-feeding resumes. Studies suggest that the use of a casein-hydrolysate formula such as Nutramigen may lead to a greater degree of reduction in the level of bilirubin than the use of a whey-predominant formula such as Enfamil. Some practitioners use **bilirubin-reducing lights,** but other clinicians believe that breast-fed infants can tolerate bilirubin levels as high as 25–30 mg/dL without danger of kernicterus. Newer phototherapy techniques involve the use of woven fiberoptic pads that can be used in the home. Increasing the exposure of the infant to phototherapy by using standard phototherapy above and a fiberoptic pad below is more effective than either modality alone. Recent studies have demonstrated the efficacy of a single intramuscular dose of Sn-mesoporphyrin in treating neonatal hyperbilirubinemia. Sn-mesoporphyrin, a **metalloporphyrin,** blocks heme oxygenase, the first step in the production of bilirubin. Infants who are preterm, ill, or have jaundice as a result of hemolysis may be at a greater risk from elevated bilirubin levels. **Exchange transfusion** may be indicated in addition to placement under bilirubin-reducing lights. A rule of thumb: Preterm infants should receive exchange transfusions when the bilirubin reaches the infant's weight (e.g., 11 mg/dL in an 1100-g infant).

Medications play a limited role in the management of jaundice. **Phenobarbital** may speed up the liver's excretion of bilirubin, even in cases of hemolytic anemia. This drug is also useful in the management of jaundice due to certain genetic conditions such as Crigler-Najjar syndrome type II. The appropriate **antibiotics** should be used to combat infections associated with jaundice.

Infants with biliary atresia may require **surgery.** Surgery links the surface of the liver to the intestinal tract, allowing for passage of bilirubin directly into the lumen of the small intestine. Adolescents with gallbladder disease may also require surgical intervention (i.e., a cholecystectomy).

PROGNOSIS

The majority of infants with elevated bilirubin levels have physiologic jaundice or jaundice related to breast milk. The prognosis is excellent in these children. In recent years, concern has arisen about a recrudescence of kernicterus, including cases in breast-fed, healthy term infants. Early discharge from the nursery may have contributed to this debilitating complication. Physicians should pursue an appropriate assessment of hyperbilirubinemia in jaundiced infants and not ascribe the symptoms to breast-feeding. Conditions other than physiologic jaundice or breast milk jaundice may be less amenable to therapy and may require ongoing medical or surgical intervention. Children with metabolic abnormalities usually require lifelong nutritional intervention, those with hepatic disease may succumb to their hepatic dysfunction, and those treated with surgical correction of biliary atresia may have recurrent episodes of cholangitis leading to cirrhosis and the eventual need for liver transplantation.

In contrast, older infants, children, and adolescents with jaundice often have self-limited conditions that spontaneously resolve.

Case Resolution

In the case history, the infant is breast-fed, which raises the possibility of breast milk jaundice. Bilirubin and hemoglobin determination are appropriate to assess the bilirubin level and confirm the absence of hemolysis. One approach to the diagnosis of breast-feeding as the etiology of the jaundice is to stop breast-feeding for a day or two to see if the bilirubin level decreases. (Sometimes an infant may not resume breast-feeding.) Biliary atresia or metabolic or infectious hepatitis should be also be considered because of the infant's age.

The presence of normal-colored stools is reassuring, however, and excludes biliary atresia. The urine should be checked for the presence of reducing substances, which is a noninvasive way of evaluating the infant for galactosemia. The birth record should be obtained. Knowledge of the maternal and infant blood types would allow evaluation for mother-infant blood group incompatibility.

Selected Readings

Gartner, L. M. Neonatal jaundice. Pediatr. Rev. 15:422–432, 1994.

Gourley, G. R. Bilirubin metabolism and kernicterus. Adv. Pediatr. 44:173–229, 1997.

Heubi, J. E., and C. C. Daugherty. Neonatal cholestasis: an approach for the practicing pediatrician. Curr. Probl. Pediatr. 20:239–295, 1990.

Martinez, J. C., et al. Control of severe hyperbilirubinemia in full-term newborns with the inhibitor of bilirubin production Sn-mesoporphyrin. Pediatrics 103:1–5, 1999,

Mews, C., and F. R. Sinatra. Cholestasis in infancy. Pediatr. Rev. 15:233–240, 1994.

Mowat, A. P. Liver Disorders in Children, 3rd ed. London, Butterworth, 1994.

Newman, T. B., and M. J. Maisels. Evaluation and treatment of jaundice in a term newborn: a kinder, gentler approach. Pediatrics 89:809–818, 1992.

Suchy, F. J. Liver Disease in Children. St. Louis, Mosby, 1994.

CHAPTER 93

HEPATITIS

Monica Sifuentes, M.D.

Hx A 7-year-old boy is brought to the office with a 1-week history of intermittent fever, vomiting, diarrhea, and diffuse abdominal pain. His mother reports the appearance of "yellow eyes and skin" on the day before the visit. Her son was previously in good health. He is taking no medications and has no ill contacts. The boy came to the United States 5 years ago. The pregnancy and delivery in El Salvador were normal. He has no history of recent travel outside the United States.

The physical examination is significant for a temperature of 100.4° F (38.0° C), pulse of 100, and blood pressure of 110/63. The child is a well-developed, well-nourished male with yellow skin and sclera. The abdomen is soft, with minimal diffuse tenderness and normal bowel sounds. The liver edge is palpated 5 cm below the right costal margin, and no splenomegaly is present. The rectal examination is normal, with guaiac-negative stool.

Questions

1. What conditions could account for symptoms of jaundice and GI upset?
2. What is the appropriate evaluation for children with suspected hepatitis?
3. What are the most common causes of hepatitis in children?
4. What complications are associated with viral hepatitis?
5. What treatments are currently available for viral hepatitis, and how does treatment differ depending on the specific etiology?

Hepatitis is an inflammation of the liver that can occur as the result of an exposure to a toxin, such as a chemical or drug, or an infectious agent. Viruses are the most common cause in children, and a majority of cases are the result of hepatitis A or B infection. Other common viruses that can cause hepatitis in children are EBV, varicella-zoster virus, and herpes simplex virus. However, their contribution to the overall morbidity and mortality associated with infectious hepatitis is minimal. Recent public health efforts have been aimed at immunizing infants, adolescents, and other high-risk individuals against hepatitis B, thus reducing the incidence of this illness as well as its long-term consequences.

EPIDEMIOLOGY

Approximately 60,000 cases of viral hepatitis are reported each year in the United States, the majority of which are hepatitis A and hepatitis B. Other etiologies include hepatitis C (formerly called non-A, non-B hepatitis) and unidentified causes. The total number of hepatitis cases is probably underestimated as a result of underreporting.

Certain situations are associated with increased risk for infection with hepatitis A. These include crowded living conditions, chronic care facilities, military institutions, prisons, day care centers, and homosexuality. Poor personal hygiene and sanitation are also risk factors. In approximately 50% of cases, however, the source of infection is unknown. Hepatitis A is found worldwide, but specific locations are associated with an increased incidence of the disease: Central and South America, Africa, the Mediterranean region, and Asia. Children less than 15 years of age have the highest incidence of the disease, and both sexes are equally affected.

Groups at high risk for hepatitis B include illicit parenteral drug users, homosexuals, heterosexuals with multiple sexual partners, health care workers, recipients of hemodialysis, household contacts of carriers of hepatitis B virus (HBV), and immigrants from HBV-endemic areas. Individuals who live in crowded environments with poor hygienic standards, such as institutions for the developmentally disabled or correctional facilities, are at risk for hepatitis B. No risk factors are identified in 40% of cases. Areas with the highest incidence of hepatitis B include Southeast Asia, most of Africa, the Pacific Islands, China, and parts of the Middle East.

Approximately 10–15% of primary infections with HBV result in a chronic carrier state. The younger children are when they are infected with HBV, the more likely they are to become chronic carriers. Between 70 and 90% of infants born to infected mothers become carriers, and at least 50% of children infected before the age of 5 years become carriers. Boys have a greater risk of becoming carriers than girls.

Hepatitis C accounts for 20–40% of all viral hepatitis. High-risk individuals are recipients of transfusions of blood or blood products, recipients of organ or tissue transplants, intravenous drug users, health care workers with blood exposure, hemodialysis patients and, infrequently, sexual or household contacts of infected persons. No identifiable source can be found in at least 35% of cases. In the pediatric population, recipients of blood and blood products before 1992, clotting factor concentrates before 1987 (e.g., hemophiliacs), dialysis patients, institutionalized children, and "high-risk" infants (e.g., maternal history of intravenous drug abuse, STDs, HIV coinfection) are most likely to be at risk for hepatitis C.

Because hepatitis D only occurs as a coinfection with hepatitis B, high-risk groups are the same, with the exclusion of health care workers and homosexual males.

High prevalence rates occur in eastern Europe, Central Africa, southern Italy, and the Middle East.

No cases of hepatitis E acquired in the United States have been reported, although the disease is endemic in developing countries such as Mexico, Central and Southeast Asia, North Africa, China, and India. In these regions, hepatitis E is the most common cause of symptomatic hepatitis in children. Young and middle-aged adults are most commonly affected.

CLINICAL PRESENTATION

Children with hepatitis have diffuse abdominal pain, decreased appetite, nausea, and vomiting. Additional symptoms may include fever and malaise. Unlike adults in whom jaundice is a common finding, pediatric patients, particularly infants and young children, are frequently anicteric. Hepatomegaly is not universally found on physical examination, along with varying degrees of right upper quadrant discomfort (D_x Box). A nonspecific macular rash and arthralgias can also occur early in the course of hepatitis B.

PATHOPHYSIOLOGY

Hepatitis A

Hepatitis A, formerly called infectious hepatitis, is caused by a picornavirus composed of single-stranded RNA with only one serotype. The most common modes of transmission are through close personal contact and contaminated food and water. This generally occurs by fecal contamination and oral ingestion. Shellfish, such as raw oysters, clams and mussels, are a frequent source of infection. Infected food handlers may also transmit the disease.

The average incubation period for hepatitis A is 28–30 days (range: 15–50 days). Peak viral secretion occurs before the onset of jaundice. The virus is shed in the stool 2–3 weeks before the onset of jaundice and up to 1 week after its appearance. Most young children, however, are anicteric, and so infections often go unnoticed during this highly contagious period (Fig. 93–1). The duration of illness is usually 2–4 weeks. A prolonged course or relapse occurs in 10–20% of adult cases.

A chronic carrier state for hepatitis A does not exist, although fulminant infections can occur. Lifelong immunity is conferred after a single infection. Mortality is rare, especially in children.

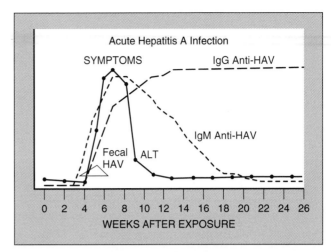

FIGURE 93–1. Course of acute hepatitis A infection. (Reproduced, with permission, from Tabor, E. Etiology, diagnosis and treatment of viral hepatitis in children. In Aronoff, S.C., et al. [eds.]. Advances in Pediatric Infectious Diseases. Chicago, Year Book Medical Publishers, 1988.)

Hepatitis B

Hepatitis B, formerly called serum hepatitis, is caused by a double-stranded DNA virus. The disease is usually spread by contact with infected blood or blood products, but it can also occur through close interpersonal contact. Although hepatitis B surface antigen (HBsAg) is found in numerous body secretions such as blood and blood products, feces, urine, tears, saliva, semen, breast milk, vaginal secretions, cerebrospinal and synovial fluid, only serum, semen, vaginal secretions, and saliva are contagious. No fecal-oral transmission occurs. Transmission is facilitated through percutaneous inoculation (e.g., tattooing, intravenous drug use) and exposure of cuts in the skin and mucous membranes to contaminated fluids on objects such as razors and utensils. Sexual transmission occurs via semen, vaginal secretions, and saliva. Perinatal vertical transmission occurs in mothers who are acutely infected or chronic carriers. Although the exact mode of transmission is unclear for household contacts, postnatal infection from household exposure is reported.

The average incubation period for hepatitis B is 3–4 months (range: 1–6 months). Figure 93–2 depicts the typical course of acute hepatitis B, along with the course of the chronic carrier state.

Hepatitis C

Hepatitis C results from infection with a single-stranded RNA virus that is able to rapidly mutate and thus escape detection by the host's immune system. Like HBV, the hepatitis C virus (HCV) can be spread through contact with contaminated blood and blood products. Conditions associated with hepatitis C infection in children include hemoglobinopathies such as thalessemia and sickle-cell disease, hemophilia, a history of malignancy, administration of hemodialysis or solid organ transplantation, and intravenous drug use. Contaminated immune globulin administered between

---

D_x	**Hepatitis**

- Diffuse abdominal pain
- Nonspecific symptoms (fever, malaise, anorexia, nausea, and vomiting)
- Jaundice (not necessarily in all cases)
- Dark urine and light-colored stool
- Pain or tenderness over the liver area
- Hepatomegaly

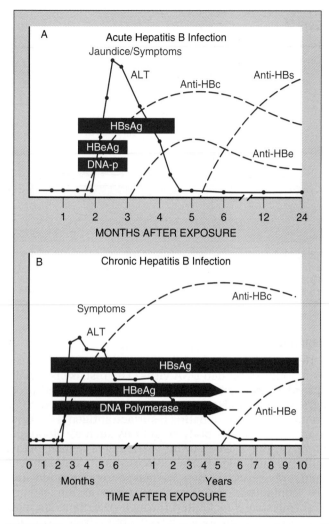

FIGURE 93–2. Course of hepatitis B infection. A. Acute hepatitis B infection. B. Chronic hepatitis B infection. (Reproduced, with permission, from Tabor, E. Etiology, diagnosis and treatment of viral hepatitis in children. In Aronoff, S.C., et al. [eds.]. Advances in Pediatric Infectious Diseases. Chicago, Year Book Medical Publishers, 1988.)

enclosed in an envelope of HBsAg. Transmission is similar to hepatitis B, but vertical transmission is uncommon.

Hepatitis D occurs either as a coinfection with HBV or a superinfection in a chronic carrier of HBV. Acute disease is usually more severe and carries a higher risk of fulminant hepatitis than hepatitis B infection alone.

Hepatitis E

Hepatitis E is caused by an enterically transmitted RNA virus. Transmission is primarily through contaminated drinking water and fecal-oral spread, especially during rainy or monsoon seasons.

The incubation period ranges from 2–9 weeks, with most cases of acute infection being self-limited. Mortality is low in endemic populations, except in pregnant women.

DIFFERENTIAL DIAGNOSIS

The differential diagnosis of hepatitis depends on patient age. Possible causes in neonates include congenital infections such as toxoplasmosis, CMV, and syphilis, in addition to hepatitis B. Anatomical abnormalities causing biliary obstruction (e.g., biliary atresia) should also be considered (see Chapter 92, Jaundice).

In infants and children, viral etiologies include EBV, CMV, herpes simplex, varicella-zoster, rubella, rubeola, coxsackie B, adenovirus, and HIV. Acute or chronic anemias such as sickle cell disease can also cause hepatomegaly and jaundice. Other rarer conditions to consider include cystic fibrosis, α_1-antitrypsin deficiency, drug-induced hepatitis (e.g., treatment with isoniazid, phenytoin), and congenital disorders such as Caroli's disease (intrahepatic dilation of the bile ducts).

In adolescents, specific drugs that cause liver toxicity include oral contraceptives, alcohol, acetaminophen, and tetracycline. Viral etiologies to consider in this age group are the same as those listed for children.

EVALUATION

History

A comprehensive history should be obtained in children of all ages (Questions Box). A dietary and travel history may also be helpful when considering hepatitis A.

A complete maternal and obstetrical history, which includes the following questions, should be taken. Does the mother have any history of intravenous drug use? Does the mother come from an area where hepatitis is highly endemic, such as Southeast Asia? Did the mother receive prenatal care? Was hepatitis B screening performed prenatally or at delivery? Did the mother have any known sexual contacts with hepatitis B, or did she have multiple sexual partners?

The physician should ask adolescents about sexual activity, STDs, and the number of sexual partners. In addition, it is important to inquire about parenteral drug use and tattoos.

April 1, 1993, and February 23, 1994, also has been implicated as a source of hepatitis C. Studies indicate that perinatal transmission does occur and may be related to the maternal titer of HCV RNA. Transmission of infection via household and sexual contact has been demonstrated as well.

The incubation period is variable, ranging from 2 weeks to 6 months, and can average 6–7 weeks. Most affected children are anicteric as well as asymptomatic. If symptomatic infection is present, it is usually mild, insidious, and indistinguishable from hepatitis A or B. Jaundice occurs in only 25% of patients. Fulminant hepatitis is extremely uncommon.

Hepatitis D

Acute delta hepatitis, or hepatitis D, is caused by a distinct single-stranded RNA virus that requires HBsAg for replication. Both the virus and a delta antigen are

Physical Examination

Because most children with viral hepatitis are asymptomatic, and all forms of the disease are clinically indistinguishable, a complete physical examination should be performed to rule out other etiologies. Growth parameters, particularly weight, should be obtained and compared to previous measurements. The temperature should be recorded, especially if children have a recent history of fever. In children who are vomiting, signs of dehydration (e.g., tachycardia, evidence of orthostatic hypotension, dry mucous membranes, tenting of the skin, sunken eyes, lethargy) should be noted.

In addition, the skin should be examined for jaundice, evidence of pruritus (e.g., excoriations), or a nonspecific rash. Icterus of the sclera, tympanic membranes, and palate should also be noted. The abdomen should be palpated for tenderness and organomegaly, particularly hepatomegaly. The liver span should also be measured because it will help monitor the patient's progress. Splenomegaly, which is not typically found in hepatitis, indicates a different diagnosis, such as leukemia, or another infectious cause, such as CMV. A rectal examination should also be performed to look for masses or blood in the stool, which may indicate a neoplastic etiology.

A neurologic examination is important to document any signs of encephalopathy from hyperammonemia, which occurs more commonly in chronic liver disease or fulminant hepatic failure.

Laboratory Tests

A limited number of laboratory studies are initially needed. These include liver function tests (LFTs) (alanine aminotransferase [ALT], aspartate aminotransferase [AST], gammaglutamyl transferase [GGT], and total bilirubin) and coagulation studies (PT/PTT).

A PT is particularly useful because of its rapid turn-around time and predictive utility; if the value is greater than 3 seconds above the upper limit of normal (INR >1.5), the prognosis is poor. A urinalysis for bilirubin should be done. Serologies for hepatitis A (HAV-IgM and HAV-IgG) and hepatitis B (HBsAg, anti-HBs, HBeAg, anti-HBe, and anti-HBc) should also be performed.

In patients at high risk for hepatitis C, serum antibody to HCV (anti-HCV) should be sent. A confirmatory test such as a recombinant immunoblot assay, which measures antibody to various regions of the HCV genome, is always run after a screening enzyme immunoassay is performed. Both assays detect IgG anti-HCV antibody; IgM tests are not available. Polymerase chain reaction (PCR) can also be considered; however, its cost and limited availability preclude its use outside of the research setting. Serologic markers for hepatitis D (IgM and IgG anti-HDV) can be sent when concurrent HBV infection is evident. Isolation of the hepatitis D antigen (HDAg) in the liver, however, is the "gold standard" test for diagnosis of hepatitis D.

MANAGEMENT

For most cases of acute hepatitis A, B, C, and D, therapy consists of general **supportive care.** No specific therapy is available, and the illness is usually self-limited. Adequate nutrition and hydration are of primary importance. Therefore, the **intake of sufficient food and fluids** should be ensured. A low-protein diet during the acute phase of the illness may be considered as well. The use of **antipyretics** such as acetaminophen or ibuprofen for fever usually does not pose a problem in patients with acutely elevated LFTs and mild disease. Physical activity should be limited until patients feel better and LFTs return to normal. Children and adolescents can return to school when they are no longer jaundiced; they can resume a normal diet at that time.

In children with more severe symptoms, intravenous hydration and an antiemetic, such as promethazine (e.g., Phenergan), are indicated. Hospitalization is required for children who are moderately to severely dehydrated, are unable to keep fluids down, or have evidence of fulminant liver failure. Treatment is aimed at correcting any metabolic abnormalities or electrolyte disturbances, including hypoglycemia. Coagulopathies should be corrected with vitamin K, fresh-frozen plasma, and cryoprecipitate. Total parenteral nutrition may be required to maintain caloric needs. Consultation with a pediatric gastroenterologist is important for children with acute fulminant liver failure or chronic, active hepatitis.

Treatment of chronic, active hepatitis B and C with recombinant interferon (IFN) alfa-2b has been effective in adults. Approximately 40–50% of patients have responded with normalization of LFTs, particularly ALT, and histologic improvement. Only 10–15% of patients, however, have a sustained response. Currently, no approved treatments exist for children. Although limited numbers of clinical trials of IFN in children show response rates similar to those in adults, interferon is not approved by the U. S. Food and Drug Administration for use in individuals <18 years of age. Fortunately, most pediatric patients with chronic HCV infection are asymptomatic.

Patients with hepatitis C should be counseled to avoid hepatotoxic medications and alcohol. Their parents should be informed of the possibility of transmission to others, and patients should refrain from donating blood, organs, tissue, or semen. Specifically, sexually active adolescents should be informed of the possible risk to sexual partners. Toothbrushes and razors should not be shared among household contacts. Children with HCV should not be excluded from child care centers because of their infection.

All children should receive the hepatitis B vaccine, and those with chronic HCV infection should also receive hepatitis A vaccine to prevent the risk of additional liver damage. Since children with chronic HCV infection are at risk for the development of serious liver disease, they should be followed regularly by their physician in conjunction with a pediatric gastroenterologist experienced in caring for children with HCV.

PREVENTION

Hepatitis A

Handwashing by food handlers, medical personnel, and day care workers is a primary method for prevention of the spread of hepatitis A. **Enteric precautions** should be used for infected patients. **Immune globulin** (IG) is recommended as postexposure prophylaxis for all people who have had intimate exposure to infected individuals. It is indicated for all household and day care contacts but not for contacts at school or work. The dose is 0.02 mL/kg within 48 hours of exposure, given no later than 2 weeks after exposure. IG is 80–90% effective in prevention of clinical HAV disease. Preexposure prophylaxis is recommended for travelers to endemic areas. If the stay is less than 3 months, the dose is the same as for postexposure prophylaxis, and for longer stays, the dose is 0.06 mL/kg every 5 months. Two inactivated hepatitis A vaccines have been licensed for use in the United States. Both have been approved for children 2–18 years of age and for adults. Factors to consider for immunization include the interval before departure if traveling, cost of vaccine versus that of immune globulin, duration of stay, and likelihood of reexposure.

Specific groups for whom hepatits A vaccine is recommended include children 2 years and older living in communities with high endemic rates or periodic outbreaks of HAV infection; patients with chronic liver disease; homosexual and bisexual men; users of injection and illicit drugs; and those at occupational risk of exposure. Other potential recipients include child care center staff and attendees, hospital personnel, food handlers, and patients with hemophilia. The vaccine dose is 360 EL.U. IM for children aged 2–18 years. Two initial injections should be given 1 month apart, followed by a booster 6–12 months after the first injection. Side effects include soreness at the site of injection and headache.

Hepatitis B

Preventive strategies for hepatitis B include preexposure and postexposure prophylaxis and universal immunization of all infants beginning shortly after birth. In addition, the vaccination of all adolescents, especially those at high risk, and other selected individuals is recommended.

Hepatitis B immune globulin (passive immunization) is recommended for infants born to known HBsAg-positive mothers or mothers considered at risk for the disease (history of intravenous drug use, STDs, or multiple sexual partners). Passive immunization is also recommended for susceptible individuals who are sexual partners of persons with acute hepatitis B infections, household contacts (especially children less than 1 year of age) of persons with acute infection, and those who experience mucosal or percutaneous exposure to HBsAg-positive blood. Simultaneous active immunization with the hepatitis B vaccine is recommended in these cases.

Immunization with the hepatitis B vaccine (active immunization) is currently recommended for all infants, adolescents not previously immunized, intravenous drug users, homosexual males, children receiving blood or blood products regularly (e.g., hemophiliacs), children in chronic care facilities, household contacts of chronic carriers, and health care professionals. The schedule consists of three doses. Infants should receive the first dose before discharge from the nursery or shortly thereafter, the second dose 1–2 months later, and the third dose at 6–18 months of age. Intervals for other individuals should be similar.

Perinatal vertical transmission of hepatitis B can be prevented by giving newborns hepatitis B immune globulin (0.5 mL intramuscularly) within 12 hours after birth and hepatitis B vaccine concurrently (at a different site) prior to discharge. This practice prevents approximately 90% of chronic infections in infants born to mothers with HBsAg and hepatitis Be antigen (HBeAG). Postimmunization serologic screening is recommended, however, for these infants at 1 year of age, since approximately 5% become carriers despite appropriate preventive vaccination.

Hepatitis C

No vaccine exists for the prevention of hepatitis C infection. Since immune globulin is manufactured from plasma that is anti-HCV-negative, it is not recommended for prophylaxis.

Current recommendations include screening individuals with risk factors for HCV infection (see pathophysiology section); infants born to HCV-infected women; recipients of IG between April 1993 and February 1994; and children with clinical hepatitis found not to be hepatitis A or B.

Hepatitis D

Prevention of HBV infection through universal vaccination is the most important means of controlling HDV infection.

PROGNOSIS

The prognosis for children with viral hepatitis depends on etiology as well as age. For hepatitis A, the outcome is generally good, with an uneventful recovery. Infants and children infected with hepatitis B, on the other hand, are at high risk of becoming chronic carriers especially if infected at a young age. Approximately 25% of carriers develop chronic, active hepatitis, which often progresses to cirrhosis. In addition, the risk of developing hepatocellular carcinoma is 12–300 times higher in these patients compared to the rest of the population.

Chronic hepatitis also occurs with hepatitis C, although it is unknown whether chronic infection and subsequent complications are higher for neonates. Autoimmune complications such as arthritis, serum sickness, and erythema multiforme are common, however, with chronic disease. Approximately 70% of patients with acute disease later develop chronic hepatitis, and 10–20% progress to cirrhosis and hepatic failure. Hepatocellular carcinoma has also been described in a small proportion of patients.

Likewise, complications of hepatitis D, such as cirrhosis and portal hypertension, are not uncommon. They occur more frequently than with hepatitis B, however, and progress more rapidly. Infection with hepatitis E does not result in a chronic condition.

Fatal hepatitis A is a rare occurrence. The overall mortality associated with hepatitis B, C, and E is also low (approximately 1–2%). For hepatitis D, however, it is more variable, ranging from 2% to 20%. Figures increase to 30% for hepatitis B with coinfection with hepatitis D. In addition, hepatitis E can be fatal in 20% of infected pregnant women.

Case Resolution

In the case history, the boy has a classic presentation of viral hepatitis despite no history of travel to an endemic area. Because he does not appear to be dehydrated or seriously ill, he can be managed as an outpatient. Statistics point to probable infection with hepatitis A. Serologies for both hepatitis A and B should be performed, however, in addition to LFTs and coagulation studies. The parents should be informed of the probable diagnosis and receive prophylaxis with immune globulin. They should also be educated regarding the infectivity of the disease and counseled about supportive therapy. The boy should be scheduled for a follow-up visit in a few days for repeat LFTs and coagulation tests. The prognosis is good.

Selected Readings

American Academy of Pediatrics, Committee on Infectious Diseases. Hepatitis C virus infection. Pediatrics 101:481–485, 1998.

American Academy of Pediatrics, Committee on Infectious Diseases. Prevention of hepatitis A infections: guidelines for use of hepatitis A vaccine and immune globulin. Pediatrics 98:1207–1215, 1996.

American Academy of Pediatrics, Committee on School Health. Prevention of hepatitis B virus infection in school settings. Pediatrics 91:848–850, 1993.

American Medical Association. Prevention, Diagnosis, and Management of Viral Hepatitis. Chicago, American Medical Association, 1995.

A-Kader, H. H., and W. F. Balistreri. Hepatitis C virus: implications to pediatric practice. Pediatr. Infect. Dis. J. 12:853–866, 1993.

Centers for Disease Control and Prevention. Recommendations for prevention and control of hepatitis C virus (HCV) infection and HCV-related chronic disease. M.M.W.R. 47(RR-19), 1998.

Fishman, L. N., et al. Update on viral hepatitis in children. Pediatr. Clin. North Am. 43:57–74, 1996.

Frymoyer, C. L. Preventing the spread of viral hepatitis. Am. Fam. Physician 48:1479–1486, 1993.

Krugman, S. Viral hepatitis: A, B, C, D, and E—infection. Pediatr. Rev. 13:203–212, 1992.

Krugman, S. Viral hepatitis: A, B, C, D, and E—prevention. Pediatr. Rev. 13:245–247, 1992.

Lee, M. A., and H. C. Meissner. Hepatitis in adolescents. Adolesc. Med. State Art Rev. 2:499–507, 1991.

Nowicki, M. J., and W. F. Balistreri. The Cs, Ds, and Es of viral hepatitis. Contemp. Pediatr. 9:23–42, 1992.

Shapiro, C. N. Epidemiology of hepatitis B. Pediatr. Infect. Dis. J. 12:433–437, 1993.

Shapiro, C. N., and S. C. Hadler. Hepatitis A and hepatitis B virus infection in day-care settings. Pediatr. Ann. 20:435–441, 1991.

Stevens, C. E., et al. Prospects for control of hepatitis B virus infection: implications of childhood vaccination and long-term protection. Pediatrics 90:170–173, 1992.

CHAPTER 94

HYPOTONIA

Kenneth R. Huff, M.D.

H$_x$
A 6-month-old girl is brought to the office because she does not reach for her toys anymore. The pregnancy was full term, but the mother remembers that the fetal kicking was less than with an older brother. Delivery was uncomplicated, and the infant fed well. The girl began to show visual attention at 2–3 weeks, smiled socially at 1 month, and pushed up while prone at 2 months. Although she turned over at 4 months, she has not done this in the last month. She no longer reaches up to the mobile over her crib.

On examination, the girl lies quietly on the table and watches the examiner intently. Her growth parameters, including head circumference, are normal. After she has been undressed, it is apparent that she "see-saw" breathes (i.e., abdomen rises with inspiration) and has a "frog leg" posture. Her cranial nerve examination is normal except for head-turning strength. When she is pulled to a sitting position, her head lags far behind and her arms are straight at the elbows. She cannot raise her arms off the table. When a rattle is placed in her hands, she manipulates the toy, which she regards from the corner of her eye. Her deep tendon reflexes are absent, but her pain sensation is intact.

Questions

1. How is the level of nervous system involvement determined in infants with hypotonia? What levels of the nervous system are usually involved in the infant with hypotonia?
2. What is the significance of the loss of developmental milestones or abilities?
3. How are clinical management issues related to prognosis?
4. When is genetic counseling appropriate for children with hypotonia?

Infants with decreased tone are referred to as hypotonic, or "floppy." Hypotonia is most simply defined as lower than normal resistance to passive motion across a joint. Although this resistance has other components, muscle strength is a key component. Tone can be used effectively as a measure of strength in infants who cannot cooperate with testing. Identification of the level of the nervous system affected (e.g., upper motor neurons, spinal cord, anterior horn cell, peripheral nerve components, myoneural junction, or muscle fibers) is most important in determining the etiology of hypotonia in infants and children.

EPIDEMIOLOGY

Hypotonia is not unusual in neonates, and nonneuromuscular causes of hypotonia are more common than neuromuscular conditions. Nonneuromuscular causes include hypoxic ischemic encephalopathy and brain lesions related to premature birth, such as intraventricular hemorrhage and periventricular leukomalacia. Spinal muscular atrophy is a common genetic condition with an incidence similar to cystic fibrosis, about 1:5000. Duchenne's muscular dystrophy is the most common neuromuscular condition in childhood, with an incidence of 1:1700–3500 male births. The Duchenne's gene has been found to spontaneously mutate in approximately 50% of the cases. Among nongenetic disorders, the incidence of acute postinfectious polyneuritis or Landry-Guillain-Barré syndrome is 2–8 per 100,000.

CLINICAL PRESENTATION

Hypotonic infants have delayed motor milestones, decreased movements, and poor head and trunk control (Fig. 94–1). Older children may have decreased ability to resist with strength testing of individual muscle groups as well as impaired functional strength in sitting, standing, walking, climbing, or running (D$_x$ Box).

PATHOPHYSIOLOGY

Tone is a product of connective tissue structural elements, including ligaments, tendons, and joint capsules; muscle fiber number and integrity; and nerve fiber input to muscle. Nerve input to the muscle includes the number and myelination of axon fibers, trophic factors from the nerve, and the frequency of action potentials depolarizing the muscle membrane. The control of tone through the anterior horn cell is complex and involves

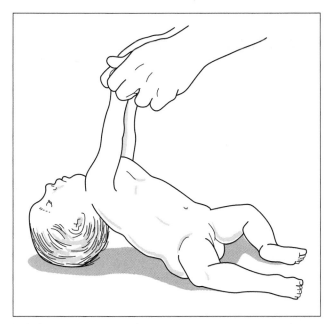

FIGURE 94–1. Hypotonic infant being pulled into sitting position. Arms are completely extended, head control is poor, and legs are abducted at the hip.

TABLE 94–1.   Differential Diagnosis of Infantile Hypotonia

Level	Specific Lesion
Cerebral hemisphere	Static encephalopathy related to perinatal or prenatal insults
	Dysgenesis (e.g., Down syndrome)
	Degenerative conditions (e.g., storage disease)
Spinal cord	Traumatic transection
	Dysraphism or other malformation
Anterior horn cell	Spinal muscular atrophy
	Poliomyelitis
Peripheral nerve	Leukodystrophy
	Type III hereditary sensory-motor neuropathy
	Acute polyneuritis (rarely occurs in infancy)
Myoneural junction	Myasthenia gravis
	Toxin (botulism or "mycin" antibiotic)
Muscle	Congenital structural myopathy
	Congenital myotonic dystrophy
	Congenital muscular dystrophy
	Mitochondrial myopathy
Systemic	Amino and organic acidopathies, hypercalcemia, renal acidosis, rickets, scurvy, celiac disease, hypothyroidism, collagen disease, congenital heart disease

more than just corticospinal tract influences. Lesions of the neuromuscular apparatus, which includes muscle, nerve, nerve sheaths, and anterior horn cell, can most directly decrease tone, but lesions of any of the other structures at many levels of the nervous system can affect tone.

The nature of the lesion is quite variable. Ultrastructural abnormalities occur in congenital myopathies including those related to respiratory chain defects. Anterior horn cell apoptosis occurs in spinal muscular atrophy and may also occur with ischemic insults. Stripping of myelin by macrophages occurs with acute postinfectious polyneuritis.

DIFFERENTIAL DIAGNOSIS

It is useful when assessing the hypotonic child to separate upper motor neuron or brain causes from neuromuscular causes (Table 94–1). The former include perinatal hypoxia-ischemia, intracranial hemorrhage, and cerebral dysgenesis. These problems may present with hypotonia in infancy but later present as a static encephalopathy. A child with a central cause may have a below normal level or range of attention and may lack age-appropriate social skills. Fine motor coordination, quality and repertoire of movements, and language may

Dx | **Hypotonia**

- Decreased resistance to passive movement of a joint
- Muscular weakness in older children
- Etiologic diagnosis related to the nervous system level of the lesion

be affected in an older child. The deep tendon reflexes may be brisk or easily elicited. On the other hand, neuromuscular causes include congenital myopathy, spinal muscular atrophy, muscular dystrophy, and acute postinfectious polyneuritis. A child with a neuromuscular cause for the hypotonia may have an interested and visually attentive facial appearance in the presence of severe weakness that allows only sparse or nearly absent limb movements. Deep tendon reflexes may be difficult to elicit or absent in many neuromuscular lesions.

Older children may display a pattern of weakness that gives a clue to the level of involvement. If the weakness is preferentially in upper extremity extensor and lower extremity knee flexor, ankle dorsiflexor, and ankle everter muscle groups, the lesion may involve the upper motor neuron. This differential weakness from CNS causes may be present and contribute to hypotonia for a long period before spasticity intervenes and affects tone. If the weakness involves limb agonist and antagonist muscles equally, however, it may represent a neuromuscular process.

EVALUATION

A methodical assessment using clinical and laboratory features in children to localize the lesion to a level of the nervous systems can help narrow a wide differential diagnosis (Table 94–2).

History

Particular areas of the history are especially important (Questions Box). Level of fetal movements relative to other pregnancies and possibilities of toxic or infectious fetal exposures should be obtained. Relatively decreased fetal movements may signify an early degenerative condition. Birth events should be investi-

TABLE 94–2. Approach to the Diagnosis of Hypotonia

Clinical Feature	Cerebrum	Spinal Cord	Anterior Horn Cell	Neuromuscular Junction	Muscle
Alertness	Decreased	Normal	Normal	Normal	Normal
Cry	Decreased	Normal	Normal/weak	Weak	Normal/weak
Eye movements	Sometimes abnormal	Normal	Normal	Abnormal	Normal
Tongue fasciculations	Absent	Absent	Present	Absent	Absent
Muscle bulk	Normal	Normal	Decreased	Normal	Decreased
Deep tendon reflexes	Normal/increased	Decreased/increased	Absent	Normal	Normal/decreased

gated for sources of possible trauma to the neonatal nervous system, such as prematurity or birth asphyxia. The physician should determine whether any developmental skills have been lost. Any associated loss of tone or strength could signify a progressive condition rather than a static problem as would occur with a birth injury. The acuity of the developing weakness is an important clue in the differential diagnosis also.

In addition, the family history should be determined. The presence of weakness or hypotonia in other family members, or the presence of early unexplained neonatal deaths in the family, may indicate a genetic or maternal basis for the patient's hypotonia.

Physical Examination

Dysmorphic features should be noted in developmentally delayed children because they may suggest cerebral dysgenesis in some instances, or neuromuscular conditions in other instances (e.g., hypoplastic mandible, high arched palate, thin ribs with deformed rib cage). Age-appropriate cognitive abilities should be assessed as a measure of cerebral function. This assessment may range from primarily observation of visual attention in very young infants to evaluation of language and academic skills in older children. Cranial nerve examination with regard to eye movements, facial strength, and presence of tongue fasciculations is important, especially in the differential diagnosis of many neuromuscular conditions (e.g., spinal muscular atrophy, congenital myopathies).

Tone and strength should be examined carefully in both trunk and limbs. Individual joint movements should be observed and agonist-antagonist strengths should be tested bilaterally looking for asymmetries and focal discrepancies. The presence of deep tendon reflexes should also be carefully noted. Sensory testing is important in suspected neuropathies, radiculopathies, and myelopathies. In the case of the hypotonic neonate, the mother may also need to be examined for the presence of signs of myotonic dystrophy or myasthenia gravis.

Observation rather than formal neuromuscular testing is often easier and more revealing, particularly in infants and pre–school-age children. Useful activities to observe include walking, running, climbing stairs or stepping onto a stool, lying on the floor and coming to a standing position unassisted, smiling, closing the eyes tightly, and speaking.

Laboratory Assessment

One purpose of laboratory tests in children with neuromuscular conditions is to confirm the level of the nervous system involved (Table 94–3). Serum **creatine phosphokinase (CPK),** a screen for muscle fiber necrosis, should be requested when the history suggests a degenerative condition or the examination indicates the cause of the hypotonia is in the neuromuscular unit. CPK is one to two orders of magnitude higher than normal in children with muscular dystrophy, and it may also be mildly elevated in female carriers of the mutant dystrophin gene early in life. The serum CPK level may be less markedly elevated in children with inflammatory myopathies such as dermatomyositis and polymyositis and to some extent following muscle trauma.

Useful information about the presence of neuropathic, myopathic, and neuromuscular junction disorders can be obtained from the **nerve conduction velocity (NCV)** and **electromyography (EMG).** Demyelinating neuropathies slow nerve conduction or produce signs of a segmental conduction block. If the problem is a motor neuropathy, an axonal neuropathy may have depressed amplitude of the nerve action potential or fibrillation potentials on EMG. In some myopathies, bizarre or small amplitude potentials and myotonia may be seen on EMG. Decremental response to stimulation and other abnormalities are evident with myasthenia gravis and neuromuscular junction blockade caused by the botulinum toxin. An intravenous edrophonium (Tensilon) test can confirm the diagnosis of myasthenia gravis in children with easy fatigability on history or by examination.

Questions: Hypotonia

- Were the fetal movements of the child abnormal or less than those of previous pregnancies?
- Was the pregnancy full term? Was the delivery complicated?
- Do the mother, any siblings, or other family members suffer from a similar weakness?
- Has the child lost any developmental skills? Is the problem getting worse?
- If the weakness is worsening, how rapidly is it progressing?

TABLE 94–3   Laboratory Tests Useful in the Diagnosis of Hypotonia Caused by Neuromuscular Lesions

Test	Anatomic Site		
	Anterior Horn Cell	Neuromuscular Junction	Muscle
Muscle enzymes	Normal	Normal	Normal/increased
Tensilon test	Normal	Abnormal	Normal
Electromyography (EMG)	Neuropathic	Decremental	Myopathic
Muscle biopsy	Group atrophy	Normal	Myopathic

When properly handled, the **muscle biopsy** gives useful diagnostic information about neuromuscular disorders that may cause hypotonia. A large portion of the tissue should be frozen for histochemical studies. Histochemistry can differentiate neuropathic changes from myopathic changes related to fiber type specificities as well as disclose structural abnormalities pointing to dystrophy or congenital myopathy. Histochemical stains can also give information about metabolic myopathic disorders. Another portion of the muscle should be fixed in glutaraldehyde for electron microscopy to determine if ultrastructural abnormalities such as those seen in specific congenital or mitochondrial myopathies are present.

Metabolic and molecular genetic studies can sometimes be done on blood samples, but if a genetic disorder is preferentially expressed in muscle tissue and direct gene analysis is not feasible, a muscle biopsy specimen must be analyzed. Tissue can be subjected to specific analyses such as dystrophin protein levels, glycolytic enzyme activity, respiratory chain enzyme complex assays, carnitine levels, or fatty acid transport assays to confirm the diagnosis. Tissue or blood sample molecular techniques, including use of specific nucleic acid probes, restriction fragment length polymorphism analysis, and linkage analysis can sometimes be used to help make specific diagnoses for genetic disorders (e.g., Duchenne's or other X-linked muscular dystrophies, myotonic dystrophies, mitochondrial cytopathies, and spinal muscular atrophy). Cytogenetic analysis may be useful when Down or Prader-Willi syndrome is suspected as a cause of nonparalytic hypotonia.

Imaging Studies

An MRI scan is helpful in three situations: (1) when deficits in mental status, cognitive function, or attention are apparent in children with hypotonia; (2) when the neurologic examination suggests an upper motor neuron component to the weakness or hypotonia such as active deep tendon reflexes or persistent ankle clonus; and (3) when children have hypotonia as part of a multiorgan system dysgenesis such as with a chromosomal aberration, because of the relatively higher likelihood of a CNS component to the dysgenesis. A CT scan is also sometimes helpful in evaluating the presence of calcification in brain structures as might occur in metabolic abnormalities and necrotizing brain insults if these are part of the clinical differential.

MANAGEMENT

Specific management depends on diagnosis but ranges from supportive respiratory measures to anti-inflammatory therapies to physical and orthopedic therapy and devices to improve function practically. The potential for recovery is an important factor sometimes in determining the management of children with neuromuscular conditions. An infant with a congenital myopathy may gradually increase in strength and should therefore receive intensive supportive care including long-term ventilatory support and gastrostomy feeding. On the other hand, the family of an infant with a degenerative terminal condition such as the severe infantile type of Werdnig-Hoffmann anterior horn cell disease may elect not to undertake respiratory support after they understand the course of the disease and lack of curative therapy. Such families benefit from the information provided by the physician and the support of paramedical personnel and lay groups. Affected children can benefit from palliative therapies and hospice care.

Children with profound weakness easily succumb to respiratory infections and have difficulty with recovery from anesthesia; therefore, they require vigilance and early intervention and intense **respiratory support.** Children with long-term neuromuscular weakness can sometimes benefit from **orthopedic** procedures to improve limb function by joint stabilization or equalizing of muscle strengths across joints. **Physical and occupational therapy** can accelerate recovery and maximize function.

Children with acquired acute hypotonic weakness (Table 94–4) may require therapies more directed at the underlying pathophysiologic process. Acute postinfectious polyneuritis requires careful frequent monitoring of respiratory status and artificial ventilation when

TABLE 94–4.   Specific Etiologies of Hypotonia Caused by Acute Generalized Weaknesses

Acute postinfectious polyradiculoneuritis (Landry-Guillain-Barré syndrome)
Postinfectious myositis
Enteroviral poliomyelitis
Acute myasthenia gravis
Infantile botulism
Tick paralysis
Periodic paralysis (hyperkalemic, hypokalemic, and normokalemic)
Metabolic myopathy

significant loss of vital capacity has occurred. In addition, children should be considered for **plasmapheresis** when their condition rapidly worsens early in the course of the disorder. **Intravenous immunoglobulin** is an alternative therapy that may be particularly useful in a child too small for the venous access required for pheresis. Specific antisera are used for botulinum toxin. Dysimmune myasthenia can be treated with anticholinesterase medication, intravenous immunoglobulin, or thymectomy when it is resistant or only partly responsive to medication. In addition to the more acute disorders, chronic relapsing polyneuritis and myositis can be treated effectively with anti-inflammatory agents such as prednisone and immunoglobulin during periods of exacerbation.

Treatment and care of children with muscular dystrophy is presently directed individually toward maintaining mobility and preventing contractures through physical therapy, bivalved casts, braces, and surgical repair. Inactivity increases disability. Adjunctive corticosteroid therapy is useful in children with Duchenne's dystrophy, but beneficial effects are temporary and must be weighed against steroid toxicity. Many new hardware technologies (e.g., long leg braces, electric wheelchairs, battery operated ventilators, and noninvasive positive pressure ventilation for some circumstances of respiratory insufficiency) have allowed affected children to overcome previously insurmountable disabilities.

PROGNOSIS

The course of many genetic conditions can be quite variable, and is related to different alleles at the disease gene locus or other loci that may have a modifying effect on either disease gene expression or the pathophysiology of the disease. For example, both the spinal muscular atrophy and dystrophin genes have multiple alleles with different prognostic implications for rapidity of progression. Type I SMA, over a couple of years, and Duchenne's muscular dystrophy, over 15–20 years, generally progress to death, however. The weakness of congenital myopathies sometimes improves slowly. Toxin-mediated infant botulism and immune-mediated disorders, particularly Guillain-Barré, generally have a good outcome.

Case Resolution

The 6-month-old girl in the case history is judged to have hypotonia caused by a neuromuscular condition, in part because of her alert appearance and absent deep tendon reflexes. Neuropathic abnormalities on EMG and muscle biopsy were also present. A blood test for the survival motor neuron gene did not detect normal exons, confirming the diagnosis of spinal muscular atrophy. The family received genetic counseling, became involved in a support group, and eventually reached a decision to forego intubation with eventual respiratory failure for their daughter. The physician coordinates hospice services for the family.

Selected Readings

Brooke, M. H. A Clinician's View of Neuromuscular Diseases, 2nd ed. Baltimore, Williams & Wilkins, 1986.

Buist, N. R. M., and B. R. Powell. Approaches to the evaluation of muscle diseases. Int. Pediatr. 7:320–326, 1992.

Dubowitz, V. Muscle Disorders in Childhood, 2nd ed. (1995) Philadelphia, W. B. Saunders, 1995.

Fenichel, G. M. Clinical Pediatric Neurology, 2nd ed. Philadelphia, W. B. Saunders, 1993, pp. 169–195.

Goebel, H. Pediatric neuromuscular disorders. Semin. Pediatr. Neuromus. Dis. 3:51–161, 1996.

Iannaccone, S. Rehabilitation for pediatric neuromuscular patients. Semin. Pediatr. Neurol. 5:77–131, 1998.

Shapira, Y. Clinical aspects of mitochondrial encephalomyopathies. Int. Pediatr. 8:225–232, 1993.

CHAPTER 95

HEADACHES

Kenneth R. Huff, M.D.

H$_x$ A 12-year-old girl is brought in with a history of headaches. Although she has been sent home from school twice in the last 6 weeks, she has experienced headaches for at least a year. The last episode, 1 week ago, was typical. The headache began as a dull feeling over both eyes, radiated up to the top of her head, and eventually became pounding. She had no preliminary visual symptoms or other warning signs prior to the head pain. The episode began during an afternoon class after she had been outside on a hot, sunny day for physical education. The headache worsened after she walked home from school. Once she got home, she went to her room, drew the curtains, and lay down on her bed. She experienced some nausea and loss of appetite but no vomiting. She did not get up for dinner. She denied diplopia, vertigo, ataxia, or limb weakness, and her speech was observed to be articulate and coherent. She took two 80-mg children's acetaminophen tablets without significant relief but eventually fell asleep. The following morning she felt fine.

Between headaches, her behavior has not changed, and she has continued to make above average grades. She has not experienced any major changes in her home environment. When initially questioned, her mother denied having "migraines," but she admits to needing to lie down because of headaches about once a month. A detailed neurologic examination of the girl is completely normal.

Questions

1. What are the major types of headache?
2. How do the symptoms help differentiate the types?
3. How does family history influence the etiology of headache?
4. What is the appropriate treatment for the problem headache?

Headaches, which are very common in adolescents and older children, frequently prompt parents to bring their children to the physician's attention. The physician must differentiate headaches that are symptomatic of a progressive intracranial process from those which may possibly be intermittently disabling but do not necessitate surgery. The cornerstone of this determination is obtaining key historical information and noting abnormalities on examination of the nervous system. Decisions about management strategies are most influenced by etiology and the impact the headaches are having on the child's life.

EPIDEMIOLOGY

Chronic recurrent headaches in children that are not related to a self-limited condition are frequently lumped together as "migraine," which includes classic and common migraine. The prevalence of "migraine" that comes to a physician's attention is about 3% for all children, but as many as 30% of children by age 15 admit to having experienced a headache in the last year. The initial symptoms begin most often between ages 6 and 12 years, but many adolescents come to medical attention for the first time, especially girls whose headache prevalence is double that of boys in that age range. Headaches are also commonly associated with trauma, acute intercurrent infection, or systemic illness. The contribution of symptomatic headaches (those related to tumors, vascular abnormalities, or meningitis) to the overall prevalence of headache is relatively small, however.

A multigenerational family history of "sick headaches" is a frequent finding in the child with migraine. This history must be specifically elicited by the physician, however, because its significance is often discounted by the parents.

CLINICAL PRESENTATION

Younger children may complain of head pain or present with nausea or vomiting. Adolescents may report persistent, dull, aching or pounding head pain. The

Dx Headaches

- Head pain, often pounding in character, over the eyes, at the vertex, or in the occipital region
- Pain frequently accompanied by nausea and anorexia
- Pain sometimes preceded by visual symptoms such as scotomata
- Presence of "trigger" factors, including bright light, intercurrent illness, or stress
- Family history of headaches (often)

pain may be episodic, stable in frequency, and similar to that experienced by other family members to some degree (Dx Box). Alternatively, it may be increasing in intensity or frequency and be associated with neurologic signs, suggesting an intracranial mass lesion. Classic migraine, which is relatively unusual in children, is distinguished from common migraine by the presence of an aura and sensory symptoms that precede the headache. Both types of headache may be associated with lethargy, slowness of movement and response, intolerance of intense sound or light, and loss of appetite.

PATHOPHYSIOLOGY

Pain fibers are carried in the trigeminal nerves from the scalp, skull, meninges, and vessel walls within the brain. Traction on these fibers or inflammation at the endings produces the pain that is associated with mass lesions or meningeal inflammation. The usual distinction between migraine and tension headache pathophysiology is more difficult to make in the younger child and may involve the types of "trigger factors" (Table 95–1) that occur at different ages. Several different mechanisms that involve one or many environmental factors may "trigger" headache in genetically predisposed individuals. The pathogenic neurotransmitter at the nerve endings may be serotoninergic (perhaps emanating from platelet stores), but release may be precipitated by a cascade of local cytokines in and around vessel walls owing to these triggers. The role of genetic susceptibility and environmental agents is under investigation.

DIFFERENTIAL DIAGNOSIS

Acute Headaches

Emergent causes should be considered if headaches have an abrupt onset, develop rapidly, or are especially

TABLE 95–1. Triggers of Migraine

Glare, dazzle, bright sunlight, or fluorescent lighting
Physical exertion, fatigue, lack of sleep, hunger
Change in ambient temperature or humidity
Allergic reactions, pungent odors
Certain foods, alcoholic beverages, and cold foods or beverages
Anxiety, stress, and worry
Head trauma
Menstruation and oral contraceptives
Refractive errors (rare)

severe or if children describe them as "the worst of my life." **Intracranial hemorrhage** from a ruptured aneurysm, an arteriovenous malformation, or rarely as a secondary effect of hypertension is foremost on the list of such causes. If children have a condition that may potentially lead to stroke, such as coagulopathy, hemoglobinopathy, or heart disease, the stroke may become hemorrhagic and produce acute, severe headache.

Nonhemorrhagic meningeal irritation, such as the inflammation produced by bacterial or viral meningitis, may also cause acute headaches. These conditions may render patients confused and lethargic while still conscious and are often associated with fever. Both types of meningitis produce signs of meningeal irritation: nuchal rigidity (stiff neck) and Kernig's and Brudzinski's signs.

Chronic Progressive Headaches

Children with brain tumors frequently have a "crescendo" history of increasing severity or frequency of headaches. Many children with brain tumors do not complain of a localized headache and may present with vomiting without headache as a prominent symptom. The headache may awaken the patient from sleep, presumably related to relative shift in intracranial traction forces due to gravity and the horizontal position.

Chronic Recurrent Headaches

Sinus infection may be a cause of either chronically recurring headaches or acute headaches, especially if children relate that the pain is more facial than cranial. Symptoms of chronic nasal congestion, allergies, and postnasal drip may be associated with **sinus headaches.**

Other types of headaches may recur. **Tension headaches** in the adolescent may produce the feeling of a tightening band around the head, occur late in the day, and be associated with a stressful environment. **Posttraumatic headaches** may recur with decreasing severity up to several months following head trauma. **Cluster headaches** that occur infrequently are associated with lancinating pain, unilateral tearing, and nasal stuffiness. The pain of **migraine headaches** is dull in character, and if headaches are severe, patients shun other intense sensory stimuli.

EVALUATION

History

Information should be obtained from patients, parents, and other caregivers concerning the quality, intensity, and location of the headache as well as associated symptoms before and during the headache (Questions Box). The duration, clinical course, and conditions that evoke, intensify, or alleviate the pain are also important. It is useful to have children describe a typical episode (perhaps the most recent), including the circumstances of when and where the headache began and how it affected activities at the time. The degree to

---

Questions: Headaches

- Where is the child, what time of day is it, and what is the child doing when a typical headache begins?
- Where is the pain located? How severe is the pain? How long does the pain last?
- Is nausea, vomiting, or photophobia associated with the headache?
- What does the child do after getting the headache? Does the episode require cessation of activities?
- Does the child take any medication for the pain? Does this or anything else make the child feel better?
- How long ago did the first headache occur? Are the headaches becoming more frequent or severe?
- Have headaches ever awakened the child at night?
- Have there been any changes in speech, vision, gait, or personality, or any loss of skills or abilities between headaches?
- Does the child have any warning symptoms before the pain? Does unilateral visual loss, weakness or numbness, diplopia, confusion, or loss of consciousness occur with the headache?
- How often does the child miss school because of a headache?
- Do other members of the family have headaches? Do they ever need to lie down with these headaches?

---

which the headache problem affects the child's life-style influences the management plan.

Physical Examination

A thorough examination is needed to determine if neurologic findings suggest an emergent problem such as meningitis or potential neurosurgical condition such as intracranial hemorrhage, or brain tumor. The examination should assess for the presence of sinus tenderness by palpation, nuchal rigidity, funduscopic abnormalities and any focal neurologic signs. A brain tumor or other space-occupying lesion may present with ataxia and cranial nerve signs for a posterior fossa lesion, loss of visual fields or hypothalamic dysfunction (endocrine abnormalities) for a suprasellar lesion, and hemiparesis, hemisensory deficit, or language dysfunction for a cerebral hemispheric lesion. Increased intracranial pressure (ICP) may lead to papilledema, general hypertonicity, positive Babinski sign, spastic gait, loss of continence, or confusion or stupor owing to blockage of CSF by the tumor.

Rarely, children in the midst of a migraine headache may display confusion, aphasia, unilateral numbness, or, less commonly, weakness, hemianopsia, or ophthalmoplegia. In these circumstances, the diagnosis of migraine is reached only after other diagnostic tests have eliminated more emergent conditions.

Laboratory Tests

If stiff neck is present and focal or lateralized neurologic signs are absent, an immediate CSF examination is indicated to diagnose the cause of meningeal inflammation. When hemorrhagic fluid is encountered, it is often useful to centrifuge a specimen to check for xanthochromia and to count cells in a subsequent sample to differentiate a traumatic spinal tap from subarachnoid hemorrhage.

Imaging Studies

If signs or symptoms of increased ICP are apparent, a CT or MRI scan must be obtained to diagnose the etiology of the headaches. Focal neurologic signs also suggest the need for a CT or MRI scan. Radiologic studies, including CT or plain films, are helpful with the diagnosis of chronic or recurrent sinus headaches. Cerebral angiography may be necessary to locate a focal source of subarachnoid hemorrhage.

MANAGEMENT

After a careful assessment has revealed no acute or progressive conditions, the appropriate management is often just **reassurance.** Frequently, concern about a potential surgical lesion or worsening neurologic state far outweighs the morbidity produced by the headache symptom itself. Sometimes pointing out the familial component of the child's headache problem (and similarities to the parent's own headaches) will help put the minor headache condition in a more benign context and even sometimes lead parents to nonpharmalogic strategies to help alleviate their child's discomfort.

However, it may be apparent that the headaches have produced significant pain and suffering for the child. The duration, severity, and frequency of the headache may have adversely affected the child's lifestyle. In such cases, symptomatic or prophylactic treatment, or a combination, is warranted (Table 95–2). **Symptomatic treatment** often begins with a trial of an adequate dose of **acetaminophen.** If this is not effective, **NSAIDs** may be beneficial. If severe headaches resolve with sleep, then a short-acting **barbiturate** such as butalbital may be effective. Headaches in adolescents are often helped by **isometheptene mucate.** For severe, recurrent headaches, serotonin receptor agonists are useful. **Sumatriptan** has proved beneficial and has relatively mild side effects. Refractory headaches may require intravenous **dihydroergotamine** or **dexamethasone.** A newer preparation of dihydroergotamine given intranasally shows promise.

The decision to begin a **prophylactic medication** should be based on a combination of frequency and severity of the headaches. The virtues of potentially controlling headache-related symptoms must be weighed against the risk of side effects. In younger children, anticonvulsants such as **diphenylhydantoin** have been found to be successful antimigraine agents. **Valproic acid** is useful for more chronic headaches in older children. The beta-blockers including **propranolol,** have demonstrated efficacy as prophylactic agents. The antihistamine **cyproheptadine** has also been successful in many patients. **Amitriptyline** is an effective preventive treatment in older children and adolescents; a single bedtime dose should be used at first. A 1- to 2-week trial is necessary before concluding the initial treatment has been ineffective. Amitriptyline can be combined with propranolol if necessary. Calcium channel blockers, such as **verapamil,** and serotonin reuptake inhibitors, such as **fluoxetine,** are also useful in older children and adolescents.

TABLE 95–2. Drugs Useful in Childhood Headaches

Abortive (Symptomatic)	
Acetaminophen, PO	325–975 mg q4h (15 mg/kg/dose) (max. 5 doses/24 h)
Ibuprofen, PO	200–800 mg q6h (10 mg/kg/dose) (max. 40 mg/kg/24 h)
Naproxen, PO	5–7 mg/kg/dose q8–12 h (max. 15 mg/kg/24 h [age > 2 yr])
Butalbital (Fioricet), PO	50 mg q6h (1.5 mg/kg/dose) (max. 9 mg/kg/24 h)
Ergotamine, PR	¼ rectal suppository (2 mg), repeat ¼ suppository q30min prn (max. 4 mg/d [older children and adolescents])
Sumatriptan, SC or IN	6 mg SC or 20 mg intranasal (may repeat after 1 h) (max. 2 doses/24 h [older children and adolescents])
Isometheptene mucate with dichloralphenazone and acetaminophen, PO	1–2 caps at onset (may repeat q1h to 3–5 caps/d [adolescents])
Dihydroergotamine, IN or IV	4 mg intranasal (1 spray each nostril, repeat once after 15 min) or 0.25–1 mg at onset and 1 mg/h × 2 (max. 6 mg/wk [older children and adolescents])
Dexamethasone, IV	4–16 mg single dose (0.25 mg/kg) or rapidly tapering q6h
Prophylactic	
Diphenylhydantoin	2–4 mg/kg/dose bid (max. 5 mg/kg [follow serum level])
Propranolol	10–40 mg bid to qid (max. 40–80 mg/24 h if ≤ 35 kg; 120–160 mg/24 h if > 35 kg; no more than 320 mg/24 h)
Cyproheptadine	1–4 mg bid to qid (0.25–0.5 mg/kg/24 h) (max. 16 mg/24 h)
Amitriptyline	10–75 mg qhs (max. 150 mg/24 h [older children and adolescents])
Verapamil	40 mg q8h (age 1–5 yr); 40–80 mg q8h (age > 5 yr) (max. 240 mg/24 h)
Valproic acid	10–15 mg/kg/d initial, 30–60 mg/kg/d maintenance, divided bid (max. 60 mg/kg/d [follow clinical signs of toxicity and serum level])
Fluoxetine	10 mg qAM initial (max. 40 mg/d [adolescents])

PROGNOSIS

Many children with headaches have a good prognosis and do not require ongoing intervention after families are reassured of the benign nature of the problem. For the remainder of children, symptomatic medications are frequently effective. Prophylactic medication is necessary in a few cases. For patients receiving prophylactic therapy, periodic withdrawal of the medication should be attempted to establish its continued necessity. Pediatric patients frequently experience remission of their headaches by late adolescence, and by adulthood, the incidence of headaches is decreased, particularly for males.

Case Resolution

In the case history, the child's symptoms and the circumstances of the headache suggest a diagnosis of migraine. No laboratory tests or imaging studies are necessary. The girl is begun on amitriptyline and instructed to keep a calendar of headache occurrences. She has two headaches in the first 2 weeks, which are aborted effectively with ibuprofen. Following these episodes, she has no further recurrences, and the amitriptyline is withdrawn successfully after 3 months.

Selected Readings

Diamond, S. Diagnosing and Managing Headaches, 2nd ed. Caddo, OK, Professional Communications, Inc., 1998.

Forsyth, R., and K. Farrell. Headache in childhood. Pediatr. Rev. 20:39–45, 1999.

Jensen, V. K., and A. D. Rothner. Chronic nonprogressive headaches in children and adolescents. *In* Headaches in Children and Adolescents, Semin. Pediatr. Neurol. 2:151–158, 1995.

Moskowitz, M. A. Neurogenic versus vascular mechanisms of sumitriptan and ergot alkaloids in migraine. Trends Pharmacol. Sci. 13:307–311, 1992.

Raskin, N. H. Headache. West. J. Med. 161(special issue):299–302, 1994.

Rothner, A. D. The evaluation of headaches in children and adolescents. *In* Headaches in Children and Adolescents. Semin. Pediatr. Neurol. 2:109–118, 1995.

Solomon, G. D. The pharmacology of medications used in treating headache. *In* Headaches in children and adolescents. Semin. Pediatr. Neurol. 2:165–177, 1995.

CHAPTER 96

TICS

Kenneth R. Huff, M.D.

H$_x$ An 8-year-old boy has unusual recurring behaviors that began 2–3 months ago. He stretches his neck or raises his eyebrows several times a day. Sometimes he is able to suppress these actions. The boy's parents report that in the last 2 years he has displayed repetitive behaviors, including blinking, grimacing, rubbing his chin on his left shoulder, making a "gulping" sound, and sniffing. Originally they thought the sniffing was related to hay fever, but the boy has no other allergic symptoms. He does not use profane words. In conversations, he sometimes repeats the last phrase of a sentence that was just used whether by himself or someone else. In addition, he must touch each light switch in the hallway every time he leaves his room, and he must retie his shoelaces several times until they are exactly the same length. Although his schoolwork has not deteriorated, he has always had trouble completing tasks and finishing homework. Both his teacher and his best friend have asked about his strange behavior. His mother has a "psychological" problem with her son's gulping sounds (i.e., they recur in her own mind), and she recalls that her father had a habit of frequently looking over one shoulder for no apparent reason.

Although during examination the boy does not exhibit any unusual behaviors, he raises his eyebrows twice and places his hand over his crotch several times while his parents are interviewed. Except for mild fine motor dyscoordination, the neurologic examination is normal.

Questions

1. What are the characteristics of tics?
2. What are the social implications of tics?
3. Should pharmacologic treatments be part of the management of tic disorders?
4. What other problems are associated with the tic disorder that also should receive intervention?

Tics are brief, abrupt, nonpurposeful movements or utterances. They occur in a background of normal activity and are repetitive and involuntary but can be suppressed. Movements usually involve the face, neck, or shoulders and sometimes muscles in the limbs or other parts of the body. Tics may either mimic normal, sometimes complex movements or involve a series of orchestrated simple movements. In contrast, habits are complex, voluntary, purposeful, repetitive behaviors that involve several movements and suggest more directed actions.

Tourette's syndrome is a common etiology of tics in children. It is defined by multiple types of tics displayed over time. These include both motor tics and vocal tics produced by some sudden movement of air or saliva within the larynx, nasopharynx, or oropharynx, causing a perceptible sound.

EPIDEMIOLOGY

Tics are relatively common in children but often go unrecognized as movement disorders. The onset of tics associated with Tourette's syndrome is generally between 6 and 12 years of age but can be as late as 21. The prevalence of tics is higher in males than in females. By one estimate, Tourette's syndrome occurs in 1:2000 males and 1:10,000 females. Many cases of Tourette's syndrome are familial, although other family members may have symptoms so mild that they never seek medical attention. The only manifestation in some family members may be obsessive-compulsive symptoms.

CLINICAL PRESENTATION

Children with tics display sudden repetitive movements of the face, neck, shoulders, or hands in the

D$_x$ Tics
• Sudden, brief uncontrolled movements • Repetitive sounds from the vocal apparatus • Behaviors occurring in the context of or mimicking normal behaviors but having no purpose

---

TABLE 96–2. Misconceptions in Diagnosing Gilles de la Tourette's Syndrome

Attributing the unusual tic symptom to attention-getting or emotionally based behavior

Diagnosing the episodic behavior as a seizure on the basis of inadequate historical information

Attributing a vocal tic to an upper airway, sinus, or allergic condition

Attributing an ocular tic to an ophthalmologic problem

Requiring tics to be observed in the office before making the diagnosis

Waiting for coprolalia to be present before making the diagnosis

Assuming severe tics are necessary for the diagnosis, or assuming tics are a normal developmental phase

---

context of normal behaviors. Although generally uncontrolled, sometimes these actions can be suppressed for periods of time. Some examples are blinking, eye rolling, grimacing, neck stretching, head turning or shaking, shoulder shrugging, and wrist flicking. Tics may either mimic normal, sometimes complex, movements or involve a series of orchestrated simple movements such as sequential finger flexing, wrist bending, and arm stretching.

Tics associated with Tourette's syndrome will vary in their manifestations over periods of weeks to months and will include sudden repetitive sounds from the vocal apparatus (D$_x$ Box). The sounds may include throat clearing, sniffing, sucking, or blowing. In addition, children with Tourette's syndrome may also have socially inappropriate words or gestures or repeat what they have just said or heard. Tourette's syndrome also includes comorbid conditions of attention deficit disorder and obsessive compulsive disorder. Children may have learning problems of distractibility and inability to finish school work or may have intrusive repetitive thoughts or ritualistic actions that may involve touching, cleanliness, counting, symmetry, or checking.

Different types of tics have been described as part of Tourette's syndrome (Table 96–1). Many affected children describe a "sensory tic," which is an indescribable, uncomfortable feeling that is relieved by a motor tic. In addition to tics, patients may rarely have other unusual behaviors including echopraxia (repetitive gestures), copropraxia (obscene gestures), and coprographia (obscene writing). Unusual speech patterns include irrelevant or nonsense words, pallilalia (repeating one's own words), echolalia (repeating another's words), and coprolalia (obscene speech). Diagnosis is often delayed because of misunderstandings about the common and uncommon manifestations of Tourette's syndrome (Table 96–2).

PATHOPHYSIOLOGY

Tics are thought to be generated from a functional abnormality in deep brain nuclei that might include the striate nuclei, the globus pallidus, the subthalamic nuclei, and the substantia nigra. The frontal cortex and limbic systems may also be involved.

Dopaminergic systems are likely to be involved because of the profile of types of drugs effective as treatments. In patients with Tourette's syndrome, the cerebrospinal fluid contains low levels of homovanillic acid, a dopamine metabolite. In addition, amphetamines and methylphenidate increase dopamine release, and in some instances, these agents precipitate tic symptoms. Haloperidol blocks the dopamine receptor and therefore may block some of the negative feedback from a potentially hypersensitive receptor for dopamine. This then allows for more dopamine release and subsequently higher levels of homovanillic acid. The observations of clinical response and side effects with low amounts of haloperidol and the finding of homovanillic acid levels remaining high long after disappearance of the neuroleptic drug both support this hypothesis.

DIFFERENTIAL DIAGNOSIS

The duration, frequency, and appearance of the movement, and circumstances of occurrence of tics help distinguish them from several other episodic movement disorders. Myoclonus is a lightninglike, nonsuppressible jerk of a small group of muscles, and chorea involves nearly constant, small amplitude movements of the fingers, hands, and feet that are often accompanied by grimacing movements of the face. Tremor is an oscillatory movement of an extremity or the head. Hemiballismus is an uncontrollable episodic throwing movement of an extremity. Hyperexplexia is a hyperactive startle response provoked by touch or sudden noise. Torticollis, or neck writhing, may be paroxysmal but is part of either a benign transient disorder or a chronic degenerative disorder, such as dystonia musculorum deformans. Paroxysmal kinesiogenic choreoathetosis, an unusual episodic condition precipitated by a sudden movement, is characterized by a twisted trunk and limb posture lasting a few seconds

---

TABLE 96–1. Types of Tics Seen in Children With Gilles de la Tourette's Syndrome

Simple Tics
Clonic
Dystonic
Complex Tics
Series of different or similar simple tics
More complicated coordinated movement
Copropraxia and coprographia
Vocal Tics
Oropharyngeal, nasopharyngeal, or laryngeal sounds
Consonants or syllables
Meaningful or nonsense words or phrases
Coprolalia
Pallilalia and echolalia
Sensory Tics

TABLE 96–3. Conditions Necessary for Diagnosis of Gilles de la Tourette's Syndrome

---

Multiple motor and vocal tics variably manifested over time
Tics present for at least 1 year
Onset of tics before 21 years of age
Tics not due to another known condition or substance

---

and not accompanied by loss of consciousness. Hypnogogic jerks and bruxism are persistent normal variant behaviors that occur in sleep.

Tic disorders are sometimes divided into three groups: (1) **simple transient tics,** which are monomorphic (always the same appearance over a period of months), last less than 12 months, and may be caused by particular environmental situations or psychological states; (2) **chronic tics,** which last longer than 12 months but are a single type; and (3) the **tics of Tourette's syndrome** (Table 96–3). However, all three types of tic disorders are sometimes found in the same family.

EVALUATION

History

A thorough history should be taken when evaluating children with potential tic disorders. The physician should find out as much as possible about the duration, circumstances of occurrence, and frequency of the movements (Questions Box). Parents may imitate the behavior or, if possible, bring in a videotape of the child's behavior. This may give the physician more telling information than verbal descriptions.

Physical Examination

Frequently tics are not seen by the physician when confronting the child directly, but the physician may still be able to see the child's tics. The physician might be able to observe the child unobtrusively while the child and family are still in the waiting room, and the child should be observed for tics "out of the corner of one's eye" during the course of the parent interview and physical examination. A screen of cognitive abilities and fine motor coordination should be included in the examination.

Questions: Tics

- How long and how often has the child been displaying the unusual behaviors?
- In what circumstances do the unusual behaviors occur? For example, do the behaviors occur when the child is eating or sleeping, engrossed in an activity, or excited? Or do they occur when attention is on the child or after a startle or other triggering behavior?
- Can the parents or other caregivers imitate the child's unusual behavior?
- Is the child having difficulty at school (cognitively or socially)?

Laboratory Tests

Children with suspected movement disorders should be screened for potential metabolic abnormalities. The evaluation should include routine determinations of calcium, magnesium, glucose, liver function enzymes, and ceruloplasmin levels. Thyroid function tests should also be requested. Treatable endocrine hormone problems can produce tic-like movements and may produce low calcium, magnesium, or glucose as well as abnormal thyroid functions. Wilson's disease affects liver enzymes and ceruloplasmin levels and is associated with many movement problems, including tics.

Imaging Studies

MRI of the brain may be helpful in the consideration of metabolic abnormalities that might produce a characteristic image or the rare circumstance of a structural lesion in the basal ganglia producing a tic-inducing movement disorder.

MANAGEMENT

Goals of management should include (1) reduction in the frequency of tics during critical circumstances with a minimum of medication side effects and (2) attention to the other coexisting learning or behavioral disabilities. Before physicians prescribe drug treatment, they must consider the severity of the tic disorder and the potential for possible psychosocial effects. Some children do not need medication for the movement disorder, and they and their families can be reassured by an understanding of the problem. Other patients may experience remission for weeks or months, during which they can reduce or discontinue their medications.

Several classes of drugs are useful in the treatment of tic disorders. A first-line medication is the **Catapres** transdermal skin patch containing clonidine, an α-adrenergic agonist. Dosage is titrated using the minimally effective size and strength of the patch. Another useful medication is the neuroleptic **Pimozide** (Orap). An ECG is recommended before beginning this medication because it has been associated with electrocardiographic abnormalities. **Haloperidol** has been useful in divided doses starting as low as 0.5 mg/d up to 2–6 mg/d. Children should begin with a low dose that is then titrated up to maximum efficacy or development of intolerable side effects. The primary disadvantage of haloperidol is cognitive sedation and the possibility of tardive dyskinesia. Other medications that may be beneficial include the α₂-adrenergic agonist **guanfacine,** the neuroleptic **fluphenazine,** and the atypical neuroleptic **risperidone.**

Treatment for children with Tourette's syndrome should be multimodal and address all problematic aspects of the syndrome (Table 96–4). Children with Tourette's syndrome should be assessed for learning disabilities including ADHD. Interventions may include **individualized instruction** and also **pharmacologic therapy** with a stimulant such as methylphenidate, the Catapres patch, or a tricyclic antidepressant. Methyl-

TABLE 96–4. Therapies Useful in Gilles de la Tourette's Syndrome

Tics
Clonidine (Catapres transdermal patch): α-adrenergic agonist
Haloperidol (low dose): dopamine receptor blocker
Pimozide (Orap): dopamine receptor blocker
Fluphenazine: dopamine receptor blocker
Guanfacine (Tenex): α-adrenergic agonist
Attention Deficit/Hyperactivity Disorder and Learning Disability
Clonidine (Catapres transdermal patch): α-adrenergic agonist
Methylphenidate: if tics are not worsened
Desipramine: tricyclic antidepressant
Education interventions: individualized or small-group instruction
Obsessive-Compulsive Disorder
Fluoxetine (Prozac): Serotonin uptake inhibitor (nontricyclic)
Clomipramine (Anafranil): tricyclic antidepressant
Depression and Adjustment Problems
Psychotherapy (individual and family)
Imipramine: tricyclic antidepressant
Support group

phenidate is not necessarily contraindicated in children with Tourette's syndrome; the drug does not worsen tics in all patients. Children with Tourette's syndrome are also susceptible to obsessive-compulsive symptoms. **Fluoxetine** and **clomipramine** are most useful for this comorbid problem.

Children with Tourette's syndrome and their families also frequently benefit from **lay educational materials** about the disorder. **Support groups** composed of other families having children with the syndrome and local chapters of the Tourette's Syndrome Association may help. Referral for psychologic or psychiatric counseling for patients and their families may be necessary because in its severe form, Tourette's syndrome may be socially devastating and may provoke secondary emotional problems as well as primary handicapping psychobehavioral aberrations.

PROGNOSIS

The prognosis in the majority of children with tics is good, and these children can have a productive educational experience and appropriate peer relationships. The physician must often individualize and optimize the management strategy to realize this prognosis in more difficult cases, however. Because the movements may remit for long periods of time, the psychologic adjustments allowed by appropriate therapy become very important in the long-term prognosis.

Case Resolution

The boy in the case history is diagnosed as having Tourette's syndrome. After a discussion with his family about the disorder, he is treated with Catapres patches. A questionnaire is sent to his teacher concerning attention deficit symptoms at school. At a 6-week follow-up visit, he has fewer tics and is doing better in school (classroom situation of 15 students for most of the day).

Selected Readings

Calderon-Gonzalez, R., and R. F. Calderon-Sepulveda. Tourette syndrome: Current concepts. Int. Pediatrics 8:176–188, 1993.

Chappell, P., J. Leckman, and M. Riddle. The pharmacologic treatment of tic disorders. Child Adolesc. Psychiatr. Clin. North Am. 4:197–216, 1995.

Comings, D. E., and B. G. Comings. A controlled family history study of Tourette syndrome. I. Attention deficit hyperactivity disorder, learning disorders and dyslexia. J. Clin. Psychiatry 51:275–280, 1990.

Pranzatelli, M. Antidyskinetic drug therapy for pediatric movement disorders. J. Child Neurol. 11:355–369, 1996.

Schuerholz, L., H. Singer, and M. Denckla. Gender study of neuropsychological and neuromotor function in children with Tourette syndrome with and without attention-deficit hyperactivity disorder. J. Child Neurol. 13:277–282, 1998.

Shapiro A., E. Shapiro, J. G. Young, et al. Gilles de la Tourette Syndrome, 2nd ed. New York, Raven Press, 1998.

Singer, H. S. Neurobiologic issues in Tourette's syndrome. Brain Dev. 16:353–364, 1994.

The Tourette Syndrome Classification Group: Definition and classification of tic disorders. Arch. Neurol. 50:1013–1016, 1993.

DERMATOLOGIC DISORDERS

CHAPTER 97

ACNE

Monica Sifuentes, M.D.

H$_x$ A 15-year-old adolescent male seeks a preparticipation sports physical. He is healthy, and he has no questions, complaints, or concerns.

The adolescent is well developed and well nourished, with normal vital signs, including blood pressure. The physical examination is entirely normal except for the skin. Erythematous papules and pustules are present across the hairline, and over both cheeks. Scattered blackheads are located over the nose and cheeks as well. The chest and back are clear, with no lesions.

Questions

1. What is the pathogenesis of acne vulgaris?
2. What are some contributing factors in the development of acne?
3. What are the different types of acne lesions?
4. What management options are available for the treatment of mild, moderate, and severe acne in adolescents?
5. What are the indications for the use of isotretinoin (Accutane)?
6. What is the prognosis for adolescent patients with acne?

Acne vulgaris is a common condition that most frequently occurs in adolescents. The spectrum of disease varies from individual to individual and may be caused by a variety of factors. Regardless of the etiology and extent of acne, the disease can be devastating to adolescents both physically and psychologically. Primary care physicians should therefore acknowledge acne as a medical problem even when patients do not mention it and should treat the condition accordingly.

EPIDEMIOLOGY

Most cases of acne that require treatment occur in individuals 9–19 years of age, although the condition can also affect young infants and young adult women. Boys and girls are equally affected, but the condition is usually more severe in boys. Certain individuals may be genetically susceptible to acne. No ethnic groups are predisposed to acne, but certain cultural practices, such as the use of oily grooming agents by some African Americans, can lead to a specific pattern of lesions. Estimates indicate that more than 85% of adolescents in the United States are affected with acne and that more than $124 million dollars is spent annually on acne treatments.

Several factors contribute to the development of acnelike eruptions. Internal agents include endogenous hormones (e.g., androgens, progesterone) and specific drugs (e.g., oral contraceptives, isoniazid, phenytoin, corticosteroids, lithium-containing compounds). External agents include skin bacteria, especially *Propionibacterium acnes;* industrial chemicals (e.g., petroleum, animal and vegetable oils); oil- or wax-containing cosmetics; greasy sunscreen or suntan preparations; and local pressure from objects such as headbands, shoulder pads, or helmets. Excessive perspiration and emotional stress can also aggravate acne. Specific foods such as chocolate, soda, and french fries have not been shown to cause or worsen acne.

CLINICAL PRESENTATION

The lesions of acne vulgaris primarily affect the face, especially the cheeks, forehead, and chin; the chest; back; and shoulders; and can be noninflamed or inflamed (D$_x$ Box). Noninflamed lesions, or comedones, can be opened or closed to the environment. Closed

D$_x$ Acne

- Occurrence predominantly during puberty
- Lesions more severe in males
- Location on face, chest, back, and shoulders
- Noninflamed open comedones ("blackheads") or closed comedones ("whiteheads")
- Inflamed papules or pustules
- Nodules or cysts may be present
- Possible exacerbation around menses

comedones ("whiteheads") are small, flesh-colored bumps, and open comedones ("blackheads") contain central, dark material. Inflamed lesions are typically erythematous papules or pustules and may be more cystic in appearance.

PATHOPHYSIOLOGY

Although the exact etiology of acne remains unclear, the pathogenesis of acne involves certain processes.

1. **Abnormal follicular keratinization.** The earliest change in the formation of acne occurs in the horny cells that line the sebaceous follicle. A disturbance in the differentiation of these cells leads to excessive shedding of the cells into the lumen. Impaction of the follicle occurs as these horny cells stick together.

2. **Overproduction of sebum.** The sebaceous gland is highly responsive to hormonal stimulation, namely androgens. With the rise in androgens during puberty, hypertrophy of the sebaceous gland occurs, and the production of sebum is increased. The flow of sebum is obstructed by the above follicular hyperkeratosis, resulting in retention of all material.

3. **Proliferation of *P. acnes.*** The overproduction of sebum in acne provides a ripe environment for the proliferation of *P. acnes,* an anaerobic diphtheroid that, along with *Staphylococcus epidermidis* and *Pityrosporum ovale,* is part of the microflora of the sebaceous follicle. In addition, *P. acnes* possesses a lipase that hydrolyzes sebum triglycerides into free fatty acids. These acids irritate the follicular wall and cause inflammation.

4. **Inflammation.** The expulsion of sebum into the dermal layer of the skin occurs as a result of the rupture of the pilosebaceous follicle. This initiates an inflammatory process and the formation of inflammatory lesions such as pustules and cysts. In addition, *P. acnes* produces biologically active extracellular materials, which increase the permeability of the follicular epithelium. The bacterium also produces chemotactic factors that are responsible for the migration of inflammatory cells to the area.

5. **Comedones.** The above processes can lead to a number of noninflammatory and inflammatory lesions (Table 97–1). Comedones are early noninflammatory lesions made up of sebum, horny cells, and bacteria. They can be closed or open. A **closed comedo,** or "whitehead," is a dilated plugged sebaceous follicle that is closed to the surface of the skin. An **open comedo,** or "blackhead," occurs as a result of dilatation of the follicular orifice at the surface of the skin and open communication with the outside environment. The dark color at the surface of the skin is believed to result from melanin in the horny cells, not dirt.

6. **Pustules** and **papules** are inflammatory lesions. Pustules lie in the superficial epidermal layer of the skin, and papules occur in the lower dermal layer. Because of their deeper location, they are often accompanied by a more severe inflammatory reaction, and scarring may result. **Nodules** or **cysts** are suppurative inflammatory lesions located deep within the dermis. Associated with the most severe form of acne, nodules are the result of deep pustules that rupture and then become lined with epithelium. When nodules are present, significant scarring is a major problem.

EVALUATION

History

The primary historical issues to explore in patients with acne vulgaris are both medical and psychological (Questions Box). From a medical standpoint, practitioners should determine how long the acne has been present and if the condition has ever been treated. Psychological aspects should include questions to assess the patient's overall self-esteem. Expectations regarding treatment and recovery should also be assessed at the initial visit before therapy is begun.

Physical Examination

The physical examination should focus on the primary sites of acne: face, chest, back, and shoulders. The entire skin should be inspected closely at the first visit, however. Individual lesions should be checked for signs of inflammation and infection at each follow-up visit.

Questions: Acne

Medical Aspects
- How long has the adolescent had acne?
- Has the adolescent ever received treatment for acne?
  - How long did treatment continue?
  - What treatment methods were used?
  - For what reasons was the therapy discontinued?
- Is the adolescent currently using any treatment products?
  - Do the lesions seem to be getting better or worse?
- If the acne has never been treated, is treatment desired?
- Do any activities, medications, or environmental agents seem to exacerbate the lesions?
- Does the adolescent have a family history of acne?
- Is the adolescent taking any oral medications?

Psychological Aspects
- Is the adolescent bothered by the lesions?
- Is the adolescent embarrassed about his or her appearance? If so, does this embarrassment prevent the adolescent from participating in certain activities?
- Is the adolescent ever ridiculed by his or her peers because of the acne?

TABLE 97–1.   Classification of Acne

Grade I	Noninflammatory acne → open and closed comedones
	Closed comedones then lead to any of the next three levels of inflammatory acne
Grade II	Early inflammatory acne → presence of comedones and papules (obstructed follicles)
Grade III	Moderate, localized inflammatory acne → pustules or larger, more inflamed papules
Grade IV	Severe, more generalized inflammatory acne → cystic, nodular lesions

Their distribution should also be recorded along with their response to treatment. The presence or absence of scarring should also be assessed as a measure of the severity of acne and a predictor of outcome.

Young women with very irregular menses should be examined for hirsutism, which might indicate excessive adrenal or ovarian androgen production as a cause of acne.

Laboratory Tests

No laboratory studies are needed either at the time of the initial evaluation or during the treatment of mild to moderate acne. In the case of severe acne, however, when isotretinoin is indicated, several pretreatment studies are necessary. A CBC, liver function tests, and a fasting lipid profile are recommended. In addition, a pregnancy test must be performed within 2 weeks of starting isotretinoin in sexually active female adolescents. These studies should be obtained in consultation with a dermatologist, who is generally responsible for prescribing isotretinoin.

MANAGEMENT

The general management of acne should include patient education regarding the pathophysiology of the condition to dispel any myths regarding its etiology and treatment. In addition, the patient's motivation should be assessed to better individualize therapy. Parental involvement is optimal in cases of severe acne.

All adolescents with acne should follow these general recommendations:

1. Wash skin with mild soap and water once or twice daily.
2. Use cosmetics sparingly or switch to oil-free products.
3. Avoid picking and excessive scrubbing.
4. Note that dietary modifications are not indicated.
5. Follow the prescribed regimen carefully (Table 97–2).

The specific therapies prescribed depend on the severity and duration of the acne, the type of lesions, and patients' ability to comply with the proposed treatment. The most effective regimens include topical products such as benzoyl peroxide, retinoic acid, and antibiotics; systemic antimicrobials; hormonal agents; and isotretinoin. Most often, however, combination therapy is used and later modified according to patients' responses. Physicians should remember that the acne often looks worse before it gets better. Noticeable improvement usually takes at least 4–6 weeks.

Topical Therapy

Several topical products are available for the treatment of acne. **Benzoyl peroxide** is bactericidal for *P. acnes* and acts as a comedolytic agent as well. Although over-the-counter lotions are available, the more effective gel preparations are preferable. The lowest concentration possible should be used initially. Higher concentrations should be used in cases in which the trunk or back are involved.

Therapy should be initiated gradually, especially if used in combination with retinoic acid, because benzoyl peroxide is inherently irritating and drying. Initially, a thin application should be made once a day every other day, and the frequency should be increased as tolerated. Allergic contact dermatitis rarely develops, but if it does, treatment must be discontinued.

Tretinoin or retinoic acid (Retin-A) is the mainstay of therapy for noninflammatory acne. This vitamin A derivative reduces microcomedo formation by normalizing follicular keratinization and decreasing the adhesiveness of horny cells shed into the follicular lumen. It is available by prescription as a gel, cream, or liquid in several different concentrations.

Like benzoyl peroxide, retinoic acid can be very irritating and may cause some peeling. Therefore therapy should be initiated cautiously with a cream or gel, which is less potent and drying than the liquid preparation. To further reduce irritation, patients should be instructed to wash with a mild soap no more than two times a day and to wait at least 20–30 minutes for the skin to dry completely before applying the product. Physicians often recommend that patients apply retinoic acid before bedtime rather than in the mornings, which tend to be more hectic. A small, pea-sized dot of tretinoin should be used each time and divided into three smaller dots on the skin before rubbing it gently into the area. Patients should also be cautioned against excessive sun exposure while using retinoic acid, because this agent lowers the sunburn threshold. Alternate daily treatment with benzoyl peroxide is warranted in cases of inflammatory acne.

Azelaic acid, a naturally occurring derivative from wheat, has both antibacterial and antikeratinizing activity. It inhibits the growth of *P. acnes* and has an antiproliferative effect on keratinocytes. Although less potent than tretinoin, azelaic acid may be useful in patients with mild to moderate acne who cannot tolerate topical tretinoin or benzoyl peroxide, since it appears to be less irritating. Pruritus, burning, stinging, tingling, and erythema have been reported, however. It is available by prescription as a 20% cream and should be applied twice daily.

TABLE 97–2.   Treatment of Acne

Classification	Recommended Treatment Regimen
Grade I	Benzoyl peroxide 2.5–5% every other day or at bedtime May increase to twice a day, if tolerated or retinoic acid at bedtime
Grade II	Benzoyl peroxide or retinoic acid as above *plus* topical antibiotics once or twice a day if inflammation present
Grade III	Benzoyl peroxide in the morning and retinoic acid at bedtime *plus* oral antibiotics
Grade IV	Above treatment for grade III acne, *plus* referral to a dermatologist for possible treatment with isotretinoin

Modified with permission, from Strasburger, V. C. Acne: what every pediatrician should know about treatment. Pediatr. Clin. North Am. 44:1514, 1997.

Antibiotic Therapy

Both topical as well as systemic antibiotics can be used in the treatment of inflammatory acne. The choice of which to use usually depends on the extent of skin involvement and severity of inflammation. **Topical antibiotics** are often useful in patients with inflammatory lesions that are unresponsive to benzoyl peroxide or retinoic acid alone. Such antibiotics act by inhibiting the growth of *P. acnes* and reducing the number of comedones, papules, and pustules. Erythromycin, tetracycline, clindamycin, and meclocycline are available as topical preparations. The **erythromycin gel** is most popular; the recommended dosage is twice daily. Allergic reactions from topical formulations rarely occur. Compared to systemic antibiotics, topical preparations have fewer systemic side effects because of decreased absorption. A combination benzoyl peroxide and erythromycin gel is now available and is effective against *P. acnes.*

Systemic antibiotics are the mainstay of therapy in patients with nodular or cystic inflammatory acne and in patients who have not responded to topical antibiotics. However, systemic agents have not been shown to be effective with comedonal acne. The success of oral antimicrobial therapy relates to the suppression of *P. acnes* and the inhibition of bacterial lipases. As a result free fatty acids and other byproducts are reduced, thereby decreasing inflammation.

Tetracycline and **erythromycin** are probably the most frequently prescribed oral antibiotics. Other systemic antibiotics that can be used to control inflammatory acne include clindamycin, doxycycline, and minocycline. These agents are particularly beneficial when lesions fail to respond to tetracycline. Tetracycline and doxycycline are not recommended in children less than eight years of age or in pregnant females. The most common side effects include candidal vaginitis, especially in females who also take oral contraceptives, and GI disturbances. The ultimate goal of oral antibiotic therapy is use of the minimum dose to control lesions and minimize side effects. Most patients require prolonged or frequent intermittent courses of antibiotics however before remission occurs. In general, the dose of the antibiotic should not be reduced before 2–4 months, at which time topical antibiotic treatment may also be given.

Hormonal Therapy

Hormonal therapy is indicated in females over 16 years of age who are unresponsive to other forms of treatment and who are not candidates for isotretinoin. **High-dose estrogen** (>50 mcg of ethinyl estradiol or equivalent doses of other estrogens) suppresses sebum production. It cannot be used in males because of its feminizing effects. Estrogen is usually prescribed in the form of oral contraceptives and administered for 21 days. It must be given for 2–4 months before any improvement is seen, with relapses occurring if treatment is discontinued. Ortho-Tri-Cyclen has been approved by the FDA specifically for its antiandrogen effects.

Low-dose glucocorticoids (dexamethasone) are indicated in females with acne accompanied by virilization or any other evidence of excessive androgens. These agents work by decreasing adrenal androgen production. Low-dose glucocorticoids in combination with oral contraceptives can also be extremely effective.

Systemic Therapy

Since sebaceous glands are androgen-dependent, antiandrogens such as spironolactone can reduce sebum production, and therefore improve acne. Doses range from 100–200 mg per day, however, lower doses may also be effective. Several months of spironolactone therapy are needed for maximum benefit, with prolonged therapy often required. Gynecomastia occurs not infrequently. Agranulocytosis is a rare complication.

Isotretinoin Therapy

Isotretinoin (Accutane), a systemic oral analog of vitamin A, is currently the most effective treatment available for severe pustulocystic acne that is resistant to conventional therapy. This agent is also useful in patients with a propensity for scarring. It influences all aspects of acne formation: sebum secretion, skin microflora, and inflammatory responses.

Because isotretinoin has numerous potentially serious side effects, referral to a dermatologist is recommended for patients who require isotretinoin therapy. The most significant of these side effects is teratogenicity. Therefore, isotretinoin should be used cautiously in women of childbearing age, and the drug should not be prescribed in pregnant or nursing women. Compliance with effective contraception must be established before the initiation of treatment. Isotretinoin can also elevate triglyceride levels, particularly in patients with diabetes mellitus, obesity, alcohol abuse, and familial hyperlipidemia. To ensure informed consent as well as avoid potential complications, patients must receive careful instructions prior to the initiation of therapy and must be followed closely during the course of their treatment.

PROGNOSIS

Fortunately, the large majority of uncomplicated cases of acne (approximately 90%) resolve in the third decade of life. For those individuals with pustulocystic lesions, however, acne and significant scarring can continue to be a problem. Therefore, aggressive treatment is imperative.

> ### Case Resolution
>
> In the case history, the adolescent should be offered treatment for his acne. This may include benzoyl peroxide, retinoic acid (Retin-A), and oral antibiotics. The common side effects of the medications (e.g., dry skin, peeling) should be reviewed. A follow-up appointment should be arranged after 3–4 weeks to assess compliance with and tolerance of the treatment regimen.

Selected Readings

Hurwitz, S. Acne treatment for the 90's. Contemp. Pediatr. 12:19–32, 1995.

Hurwitz, S. Acne vulgaris: pathogenesis and management. Pediatr. Rev. 15:47–52, 1994.

Hurwitz, S. Clinical Pediatric Dermatology: A Textbook of Skin Disorders of Childhood and Adolescence, 2nd ed. Philadelphia, W. B. Saunders, 1993.

Leyden, J. J. Therapy for acne vulgaris. N. Engl. J. Med. 336:1156–1162, 1997.

Medical Letter: Azelaic acid—a new topical drug for acne. Med. Lett. Drugs Ther. 38:52–53, 1996.

Strasburger, V. C. Acne: what every pediatrician should know about treatment. Pediatr. Clin. North Am. 44:1505–1523, 1997.

CHAPTER 98

DISORDERS OF THE HAIR AND SCALP

Geeta Grover, M.D.

H$_x$ A 6-year-old child presents with a 1-week history of a swelling on the right side of her scalp that is associated with hair loss. She has previously been in good health, and she has no history of fever. On examination, she is afebrile, has normal vital signs, and appears well. An area of non-tender, boggy swelling 2 × 2 cm with associated alopecia is apparent over the scalp in the right temporal area. Small pustular lesions are scattered over the involved area. Generalized scaling of the scalp and occipital adenopathy are evident.

Questions

1. What are the common causes of circumscribed hair loss in children?
2. What are the common causes of diffuse hair loss in children?
3. What features distinguish tinea capitis from alopecia areata?
4. What is the treatment for tinea capitis? Is there a role for topical antifungal agents?

Disorders of the scalp may be either congenital or acquired during childhood or adolescence. Conditions may be further classified according to the presence or absence of hair loss (alopecia) and whether the hair loss is diffuse or circumscribed.

EPIDEMIOLOGY

Acquired circumscribed hair loss is more commonly seen than diffuse hair loss. The vast majority of cases of acquired circumscribed hair loss result from tinea capitis, alopecia areata, or trauma.

Tinea capitis is a fungal infection of the scalp most often caused by the dermatophytes *Microsporum canis* or *Trichophyton tonsurans*. *T. tonsurans* accounts for about 90–95% of all cases. Tinea capitis, which is rare in infants and postpubertal adolescents, is seen primarily in prepubertal children between the ages of 2 and 10 years. Boys are affected more often than girls.

Human-to-human transmission is rare with *M. canis* but does occur with *T. tonsurans*. Children who handle dogs or cats, which harbor *M. canis*, are susceptible to infection. While random culture studies of asymptomatic school children report a 4% carriage rate for *T. tonsurans*, about 30–50% of adults living with infested children are silent carriers as well.

Alopecia areata is an idiopathic disorder with an incidence of about 17/100,000 population. The cause is unknown, but an autoimmune mechanism has been suggested. Family history is positive in 10–20% of affected patients. Although alopecia areata may develop at any age, it generally begins before the age of 25.

Trichotillomania may be seen in association with other compulsive disorders such as thumb sucking and nail biting (see Chapter 32, Thumb Sucking and Other Habits). Usually the scalp hair is involved, but eyebrows or eyelash hair may also be affected. Although trichotillomania may be seen at any age, it primarily occurs in adolescents and children who are 4–10 years of age.

CLINICAL PRESENTATION

Children may present with specific complaints, including localized baldness, pruritus, scaling, or inflammation (D$_x$ Box). Occasionally, lymphadenopathy, particularly in the occipital area, is the major presenting symptom.

PATHOPHYSIOLOGY

An understanding of the physiology of the normal hair growth cycle helps in the evaluation of hair and scalp disorders. The scalp of an average human being con-

| Dx | Disorders of the Hair and Scalp |

- Circumscribed or generalized hair loss (alopecia)
- Scaling
- Pruritus
- Erythema of the scalp
- Localized or generalized swelling of the scalp

tains about 100,000 hairs. Average healthy terminal hair grows at about 2.5 mm per week or approximately 1 cm per month.

The hair follicle is responsible for the majority of disturbances of hair growth because the hair shaft itself is a nonliving structure. Normal hair growth is a cyclical process composed of three stages. The anagen phase, the period of active hair growth, lasts for an average of 3 years (range: 2–6 years). Normally, about 85–90% of scalp hair is in this phase at any one time. The catagen phase, the transition period, lasts for about 10–14 days. The telogen phase, the final resting phase, lasts for about 3–4 months. The average individual loses about 50–100 telogen hairs per day.

Infection begins when the dermatophytes *M. canis* and *T. tonsurans* invade the hair follicle. The initial stage of infection with either organism is noninflammatory and may last 2–8 weeks. *M. canis* spores remain on the hair surface (ectothrix). In contrast, *T. tonsurans* spores are located inside the hair shaft (endothrix) and may cause the involved hairs to break easily. In some children, the noninflammatory stage may be followed by the inflammatory stage, or kerion, which represents a delayed hypersensitivity reaction to the organism. Histologically, the kerion consists of a mononuclear cell infiltrate.

In alopecia areata, histologic examination of a scalp biopsy reveals a dense, lymphocytic infiltrate around the hair follicle in areas of alopecia. The hairs at the margins of alopecia are easily plucked. They have clubbed or attenuated ends when examined under a low-power microscope. This appearance is pathognomonic, and these hairs are often referred to as "exclamation mark" hairs.

DIFFERENTIAL DIAGNOSIS

Scalp Disorders Without Associated Hair Loss

These conditions are divided into those disorders seen most often in neonates and young infants and those seen more frequently in children and adolescents (Table 98–1). **Caput succedaneum,** a generalized edema involving the soft tissues of the scalp, and **cephalhematoma,** a subperiosteal hematoma, are two of the most common lesions of the scalp that occur during the neonatal period. A cephalhematoma does not extend beyond the suture lines of the affected bone, which distinguishes it from caput succedaneum. Both conditions result from birth trauma and generally resolve spontaneously within a few weeks to months without further complications.

Other common neonatal scalp conditions include infections such as **scalp abscess** and **herpes simplex infection.** When fetal scalp electrode monitors are used, a scalp abscess at the site of the monitor is seen in about 1 : 200 births. The most commonly implicated pathogens are staphylococci, gram-negative enteric bacteria, and gonococci. Management depends on the severity of the infection (e.g., associated cellulitis or signs of systemic involvement). Herpes simplex infections of the scalp are not uncommon in neonates, because the scalp usually has the longest contact with the cervix, the site of infection transmission. Herpes lesions are typically vesicular, but petechial, purpuric, or bullous lesions may also be apparent. Although skin lesions may be present at birth, they typically develop between 5 and 10 days of life.

Seborrheic dermatitis is an erythematous, greasy, scaly eruption that occurs mainly on the scalp, face, and postauricular and intertriginous areas (see Chapter 100, Papulosquamous Eruptions). This condition is seen primarily in infants under the age of 6 months and in adolescents. Seborrheic dermatitis that involves the scalp of neonates is known as cradle cap. This noninflammatory, diffuse, greasy scaling of the scalp usually develops during the first several months of life.

Unlike atopic dermatitis, seborrheic dermatitis is generally nonpruritic. Occasionally the inflammatory process is severe enough to result in diffuse hair loss. Psoriatic lesions of the scalp can mimic seborrhea, and skin biopsy may be required for definitive diagnosis.

Head lice (pediculosis capitis) are an extremely common childhood infestation that affects girls more often than boys. Lice are spread by direct contact with infected individuals or infested clothing, combs, or brushes. Pruritus is the primary symptom. The ova or nits may be visible as small, oval, whitish specks found most commonly in the hair above the ears and the occipital region. They are difficult to remove. Unlike nonspecific scales, nits fluoresce under Wood's light examination.

Scalp Disorders Associated With Hair Loss

Table 98–2 lists the common scalp disorders associated with hair loss. When evaluating hair loss in children, it is important to determine whether the loss is diffuse or circumscribed.

TABLE 98–1. Common Disorders of the Scalp Without Associated Hair Loss

Neonatal Period and Early Infancy
Birth trauma to the scalp (e.g., caput succedaneum, cephalhematoma)
Scalp abscess (at fetal scalp electrode site)
Herpes simplex infection
Cradle cap/seborrheic dermatitis

Childhood and Adolescence
Seborrheic dermatitis*
Head lice (pediculosis capitis)
Psoriasis*

*May occur with or without associated hair loss.

**TABLE 98–2.   Common Disorders of the Scalp
With Associated Hair Loss**

Circumscribed Hair Loss
Congenital
    Aplasia cutis congenita
    Nevus sebaceus
    Epidermal nevus
Acquired
    Tinea capitis
    Alopecia areata
    Traction alopecia
    Trichotillomania
    Discoid lupus erythematosus
    Secondary syphilis

Diffuse Alopecia
Congenital
    Congenital hypothyroidism
    Hair shaft defects (e.g., Menkes' kinky-hair syndrome)
    Ectodermal dysplasias
Acquired
    Seborrheic dermatitis
    Psoriasis
    Telogen effluvium
    Anagen effluvium (secondary to toxins or chemicals)
    Endocrine
        Hypothyroidism-hypoparathyroidism-hypopituitarism
        Diabetes mellitus
        Androgenic alopecia (e.g., male pattern baldness)
    Other
        Nutritional (e.g., acrodermatitis enteropathica)
        Systemic lupus erythematosus

Nevus sebaceus is a common cause of congenital circumscribed hair loss. Lesions are solitary, well-circumscribed plaques on the scalp that may be yellow or tan and round or oval. They can sometimes occur on the face as well. Nevus sebaceus should be differentiated from epidermal nevi. Epidermal nevi tend to occur more on the extremities but may develop anywhere on the body, including the scalp. They range in appearance from oval, hyperpigmented wartlike lesions to linear lesions that consist of a series of confluent papules.

Aplasia cutis congenita is a congenital skin defect with localized areas of epidermal, dermal, and subcutaneous tissue loss. Lesions can occur anywhere on the body, but the majority are found along the midline of the scalp. At birth, the lesions usually appear as small, depressed, hairless areas with associated ulceration or erosion of the skin. Etiology is unknown, and other developmental defects such as cleft lip or palate and syndactyly may be seen. Small defects generally heal well, whereas larger defects may require surgical excision and eventual skin grafting.

Tinea capitis, a fungal infection of the scalp, is one of the most common causes of acquired hair loss in children. This condition is characterized by patchy alopecia with broken-off hairs and scaling of the scalp. *T. tonsurans* infection sometimes appears as a series of black dots within the affected area due to the presence of fragmented hairs. The diagnosis can be difficult in children who present with either diffuse scalp scaling or a diffuse pustular eruption without significant alopecia. Occasionally, an intense hypersensitivity response may result in a boggy swelling of the scalp known as a **kerion.**

The surface of the kerion may be smooth or covered with small pustules, mimicking a bacterial infection. Uncomplicated tinea capitis leaves no scars, but kerions may result in permanent hair loss.

Alopecia areata, which frequently leads to hair loss, is characterized by well-defined areas of complete hair loss without associated scaling, irritation, or inflammation of the scalp. Hairs at the periphery of bald patches can usually be easily plucked. Associated nail defects, including nail pitting and ridging, may be seen in about 20% of affected individuals. Occasionally, alopecia totalis (loss of all scalp hair) or alopecia universalis (loss of all body and scalp hair) may result. Onset at younger age and more extensive involvement are poor prognostic signs.

Common traumatic causes of alopecia are traction alopecia and trichotillomania. **Traction alopecia** often occurs along the margins of the hairline secondary to having the hair pulled back in tight ponytails or braids. **Trichotillomania** is a self-induced form of traction alopecia in which children twist or pull out their hair either consciously or subconsciously (see Chapter 32, Thumb Sucking and Other Habits). The frontal and temporoparietal areas, which are most accessible to children's hands, are most commonly involved. Trichotillomania may mimic other types of alopecia, but the diagnosis can usually be made on the basis of the bizarre patterns of hair loss with hairs broken at differing lengths. Children occasionally eat the hairs as they are pulled out, resulting in the formation of a **trichobezoar** (hair ball) in the stomach.

Discoid lupus erythematosus and **secondary syphilis** are uncommon causes of localized hair loss from the scalp in children. The patches of alopecia in discoid lupus erythematosus often appear hypopigmented with surrounding erythema, whereas those of secondary syphilis are numerous and small in size, with distinct margins.

A variety of structural defects, endocrine and metabolic disorders, and toxins may be associated with diffuse loss of scalp hair (see Table 98–2). **Intrinsic structural defects of the hair** may cause hairs to break, thus resulting in failure of hair growth. In some forms of **ectodermal dysplasia,** the number of hair follicles is reduced or they are altogether absent, giving the appearance of sparse or thinning hair.

Telogen effluvium is a common cause of diffuse hair loss that may occur 2–4 months after a variety of events, including pregnancy, discontinuation of oral contraceptives, severe febrile illness, or severe emotional stress. Hair loss results from the abrupt conversion of numerous scalp hairs from the anagen (growth) phase to the telogen (resting) phase. Loss of more than 100 hairs per day is considered abnormal. Patients may complain of losing several hundred hairs a day, but the occurrence of clinically significant baldness is rare. Estimates indicate that individuals must lose about 25% of their hair before thinning becomes clinically apparent. The hair loss may continue for several weeks, but complete regrowth usually occurs within 6–12 months.

Anagen effluvium results in the loss of growing hairs due to a sudden cessation of the growing phase. It occurs most commonly after systemic chemotherapy.

EVALUATION

History

The age of the child guides the differential diagnosis, because some lesions are more common at one age than another (Questions Box).

Physical Examination

The scalp should be examined to see if the hair loss is diffuse or circumscribed and whether scalp hairs can be plucked easily. Signs of irritation, inflammation, or scaling of the scalp should also be noted, as well as the presence of adenopathy, nail changes, or hair loss elsewhere on the body.

Wood's light examination of the scalp for fungus is helpful if positive. A negative examination does not rule out the possibility of fungal infection, however, because *T. tonsurans,* the most common cause of tinea capitis, does not fluoresce. *M. canis,* which causes about 5–10% of cases, fluoresces yellow-green under the Wood's light.

Laboratory Tests

Laboratory assessment is useful in some cases. If fungal infection is suspected, a KOH examination should be performed by the primary care physician. Scales and broken hairs can be obtained from involved areas by brushing, scraping (e.g., with a No. 15 scalpel blade), plucking, or by rubbing a moistened 4×4 gauze over affected areas and then removing broken hairs and scale from the gauze with forceps. The scrapings should be placed on a glass slide, dissolved in KOH solution, and examined under the microscope. Hyphae and spores within the hair shaft (e.g., *T. tonsurans* infection) or surrounding the hair shaft (e.g., *M. canis* infection) should be noted.

In addition to microscopic examination, many dermatologists recommend routine fungal cultures in all cases of suspected tinea capitis. Hair or scalp scrapings are inoculated onto Sabouraud's agar or dermatophyte test medium (DTM). Within 5–14 days, a distinctive growth seen on the Sabouraud's agar or a color change from yellow to red in the DTM confirms the diagnosis. A

negative KOH examination in addition to a lack of inflammation and scaling may be required for differentiating trichotillomania or alopecia areata from tinea capitis.

The diagnosis of telogen effluvium is usually suggested by the history and counting the number of hairs lost each day. If the diagnosis is in question, the patient may be referred to a dermatologist for examination of the involved hair roots and determination of the anagen-telogen ratio, which is usually about 85:15. A telogen count of more than 25% is considered to be diagnostic of telogen effluvium. The ratio of anagen to telogen hairs is normal in trichotillomania.

A more extensive laboratory workup may be required if the hair loss is persistent or the history or physical examination are suggestive of systemic disease (see Table 98–2). Studies that may be considered include liver function tests, thyroid function studies, a serum Venereal Disease Research Laboratory (VDRL) test or antinuclear antibodies (ANA), and serum electrolytes.

MANAGEMENT

Management depends on the diagnosis. Herpetic infection in a newborn requires immediate attention and systemic antiviral therapy, because the risk of systemic infection is significant.

Children suspected of nevus sebaceus should be referred to a dermatologist. Early identification and excision are important, because 10–15% of lesions undergo secondary neoplastic changes during puberty or adulthood.

Infantile **seborrheic dermatitis** usually resolves spontaneously by the age of 6–8 months. **Mineral oil** can be massaged into the scalp to soften the scale in children with thick scaling of the scalp due to seborrheic dermatitis or cradle cap. A soft brush may be used to loosen the scale before shampooing. An **antiseborrheic shampoo** or a **topical corticosteroid solution** may be required for more severe cases. In adolescents, seborrhea of the scalp may be treated with **shampoos containing zinc or selenium** such as Head & Shoulders or Selsun, respectively. **Tar shampoos** or topical corticosteroid solutions can be used if pruritus is significant.

Head lice may be treated with **pyrethrin products** such as permethrin 1% cream rinse (Nix). A fine-toothed comb or tweezers may be required after rinsing to remove the ova or nits of head lice. An application of vinegar after shampooing may also facilitate removal of nits. Heat, such as that associated with blow-drying the hair, also kills the lice.

Oral griseofulvin administered for at least 6–8 weeks is given for **tinea capitis.** Although griseofulvin can have many side effects, including GI disturbances, hepatotoxicity, and leukopenia, it is generally well tolerated by children. Hematologic, renal, and liver function studies can be monitored in children on high doses or prolonged treatment. Topical antifungal agents are not effective on the scalp. Twice a week shampooing with the sporicide selenium sulfide 2.5% shampoo has been shown to reduce infectivity. A course of oral **prednisone** may be required in conjunction with the griseofulvin if a kerion is present. Children with kerions are often

---

Questions: Disorders of the Hair and Scalp

- Is the child losing any hair?
  - If so, is the child losing hair from all over the scalp or only from localized areas on the scalp?
  - Has the child lost any body hair (e.g., eyebrows, eyelashes) in addition to the scalp hair?
  - How long has the child been losing hair?
- Is the scalp pruritic or scaling?
- Have the parents noticed the child twisting or pulling the hair?
- Is the child's hair often in ponytails or braids?
- Has there recently been any significant stress in the child's life?
- Do any pets live in the home?
- Is the child taking any medications?
- Is anyone else in the home or anyone in close contact with the child having similar symptoms?

misdiagnosed as having a bacterial infection of the scalp and treated with oral antibiotics. However, the pustules in kerions are generally sterile, and even when secondary bacterial infection is present (e.g., about 30–50% of patients), antibiotics do not alter the course of the condition.

Children believed to have alopecia areata should be referred to a dermatologist immediately. Therapy for **alopecia areata** consists of **both topical and intralesional corticosteroids.** Many psychosocial factors should be considered when treating children with this condition. Children with severe forms of the disease may benefit psychologically from wearing a wig. The National Alopecia Areata Foundation is available as a support group for affected children and their families.

PROGNOSIS

Common disorders of the scalp such as seborrheic dermatitis, head lice, and tinea capitis generally respond well to treatment and result in no long-term sequelae. The course and prognosis of alopecia areata is quite variable and may be difficult to predict. Generally, the prognosis for regrowth is good if hair loss has occurred in only a few patches. The prognosis for complete regrowth of hair is usually poorer with younger age at onset and more widespread involvement.

Case Resolution

The child presented in the case scenario exhibits physical findings of a kerion. Diagnosis can be made clinically on the basis of the appearance of the lesion. The diagnosis is established by microscopic evidence of hyphae and culture confirmation. Treatment with griseofulvin should be initiated. The child should be examined in two weeks to ascertain the response to therapy and check for any adverse reactions.

Selected Readings

Atton, A. V., and W. W. Tunnessen. Alopecia in children: the most common causes. Pediatr. Rev. 12:25–30, 1990.

Goldgeier, M. H. Fungal infections of the skin, hair and nails. Pediatr. Ann. 22:253–259, 1993.

Honig, P. J. Treatment of kerions. Pediatr. Dermatol. 11:69–71, 1994.

Hurwitz, S. Disorders of hair and nails. *In* Hurwitz, S. Clinical Pediatric Dermatology, 2nd ed. Philadelphia, W. B. Saunders, 1993. pp. 481–514.

Levy, M. L. Disorders of the hair and scalp in children. Pediatr. Clin. North Am. 38:905–919, 1991.

Rasmussen, J. E. Cutaneous fungus infections in children. Pediatr. Rev. 13:152–156, 1992.

Smith, M. L. Tinea capitis. Pediatr. Ann. 25:101–105, 1996.

Vasiloudes, P., J. G. Morelli, and W. L. Weston. Bald spots: remember the "big three." Contemp. Pediatr. 14:76–91, 1997.

CHAPTER 99

DIAPER DERMATITIS

Geeta Grover, M.D.

H$_x$ A 6-month-old infant has a 3-day history of a rash in the diaper area. The mother has been applying cornstarch, but the rash has gotten worse and has spread to the inner thighs and the abdomen. The infant has no history of fever, upper respiratory tract symptoms, vomiting, or diarrhea. He was seen in the emergency department 1 week ago for acute gastroenteritis, which has since resolved.

On examination, a poorly demarcated, shiny, erythematous rash is noted over the convex surface of the buttocks, lower abdomen, and genitalia, with relative sparing of the intertriginous creases. The rest of the physical examination is within normal limits.

Questions

1. What are the common causes of rashes in the diaper area (diaper dermatitis)?

2. What are the features that distinguish one type of diaper dermatitis from another?

3. What systemic diseases may present with diaper dermatitis?

4. What are some common treatments for diaper dermatitis?

Diaper dermatitis is used to describe a wide variety of skin disorders that present with a rash in the area covered by the diaper. The most familiar form of diaper rash, irritant contact diaper dermatitis, is one of the most common skin disorders of infants and young children. Successful management requires making the correct diagnosis and identifying the etiology and associated factors.

EPIDEMIOLOGY

Diaper dermatitis occurs in infants and young children between birth and 2 years of age, with a peak incidence at 7–9 months. Its estimated prevalence is approximately 10% in children under 2 years of age.

CLINICAL PRESENTATION

The lesions of diaper dermatitis primarily affect the skin of the buttocks, lower abdomen, perineal area, and proximal thighs. Irritant contact dermatitis, the most common type of diaper dermatitis, presents as a poorly demarcated, glistening erythema over the convex surfaces, with relative sparing of the intertriginous folds (Fig. 99–1A). Candidal infection is characterized by a beefy red, sharply demarcated eruption with small, satellite papules and pustules along the margins. The eruption is primarily concentrated within the skin folds (D_x Box) (Fig. 99–1B).

PATHOPHYSIOLOGY

Many factors are involved in the pathophysiology of diaper dermatitis. Prolonged contact with urine, feces,

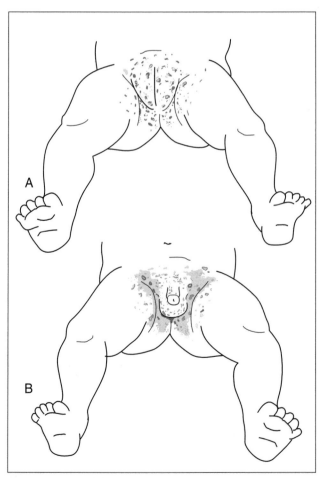

FIGURE 99–1. Diaper dermatitis. A. Diaper dermatitis secondary to contact. Convex surface areas are affected. B. Diaper dermatitis secondary to *Candida*. Intertriginous areas are affected, and satellite lesions are present.

D_x	Diaper Dermatitis

- Age less than 2 years
- Erythematous rash over anogenital region
- Associated gastroenteritis, antibiotic therapy, or oral thrush

---

or irritating chemicals plays an important role in the initiation of these disorders. Friction generated as the infant tries to move around may further aggravate the condition and lead to maceration of the skin. Secondary infection, most often with *Candida albicans,* may be seen in many cases.

For many years it was believed that ammonia produced by bacterial breakdown of urea was the causative factor in the majority of cases of diaper dermatitis. Recent studies have refuted this finding. Currently it is thought that wetness increases the skin's permeability to irritants such as fecal proteases and lipases, which are the major irritants responsible for diaper dermatitis. Although ammonia in the urine is not enough to initiate the dermatitis, it may aggravate existing inflammation.

Whether diaper type (e.g., cloth or disposable) plays any role is controversial. Experts agree that leaving wet diapers on infants for prolonged periods may increase skin damage.

DIFFERENTIAL DIAGNOSIS

Technically, any rash that occurs in the area covered by the diaper can be called diaper dermatitis, but certain rashes occur primarily in this area in infants and young children. The differential diagnosis of diaper dermatitis is presented in Table 99–1.

Irritant contact dermatitis, the most common cause of diaper dermatitis, is most prominent on the skin of the buttocks, perineal area, lower abdomen, and inner thighs. The skin of the creases is relatively unaffected. Exposure to proteolytic enzymes and irritant chemicals in the face of excessive heat or moisture is believed to lead to this condition. Friction with the diaper at sites of contact may aggravate it. Such a rash is poorly demarcated and gives the skin a glistening, red appearance.

Candidal diaper dermatitis, due to infection with *C. albicans,* typically begins in the creases (intertriginous areas) and then spreads to other surfaces. Some-

---

TABLE 99–1. Differential Diagnosis of Diaper Dermatitis

Most Common Causes
Irritant contact dermatitis
Candidiasis
Seborrheic dermatitis
Less Common Causes
Allergic dermatitis
Impetigo
Perianal streptococcal disease
Atopic dermatitis
Psoriasis
Acrodermatitis enteropathica
Histiocytosis X

times associated with oral thrush, it is also a common sequelae to systemic antibiotic therapy. The rash appears bright, beefy red with sharp, raised borders and small satellite papules, vesicles, and pustules along its margins. Scales may also be noted along the edge. *C. albicans* can be a cause of secondary infection of already inflamed skin as well as a primary causative factor in some cases of diaper dermatitis.

Seborrheic diaper dermatitis, like candidal diaper dermatitis, also primarily affects the intertriginous areas of the groin. The lack of pruritus distinguishes it from atopic dermatitis. The rash has a characteristic salmon-colored, greasy appearance with a yellowish scale. Satellite lesions are not evident. Seborrheic dermatitis of the face, scalp, neck, and postauricular areas are usually seen in association with the seborrheic dermatitis of the diaper area.

Less common causes of diaper dermatitis are **allergic dermatitis, impetigo,** and **perianal streptococcal disease.** True **allergic contact dermatitis** in the diaper area is rare in the first two years of life, but irritation caused by harsh soaps or cleansing agents may be commonly seen.

Impetigo, especially bullous impetigo, is a not uncommon eruption in the diaper area. Bullous impetigo is usually caused by *Staphylococcus aureus.* The rash presents as bullae 1–2 cm in diameter within the diaper area. Characteristically, the bullae rupture, leaving superficial erosions with thick, honey-colored crusts. The lesions may spread outside the diaper area, and fever and regional lymphadenopathy may be noted later in the course of the disease.

Perianal streptococcal disease due to group A beta-hemolytic streptococcus manifests as a well-demarcated, erythematous, pruritic, and usually tender perianal rash. Rectal bleeding and painful defecation may also be noted.

Systemic diseases that may present as rashes in the diaper area include psoriasis, atopic dermatitis, acrodermatitis enteropathica, and histiocytosis X. **Psoriasis** may occur anywhere on the body, but lesions typically occur on the scalp, face, elbows, and knees. In infants psoriasis may involve the diaper area. Unlike lesions elsewhere on the body, which are typically well-circumscribed, erythematous plaques with a thick, silvery scale, psoriatic lesions in the diaper area may be difficult to differentiate from seborrheic dermatitis or candidal infection. Psoriasis should be considered in the differential diagnosis of a diaper rash that persists despite seemingly adequate therapy. Skin biopsy, family history of psoriasis, or nail involvement may help confirm the diagnosis.

Atopic dermatitis is rare in the diaper area, even in infants who have lesions elsewhere on the body. The relative sparing of the diaper area is perhaps a result of the increased moisture of the skin in this area (see Chapter 100, Papulosquamous Eruptions, for a discussion of atopic dermatitis).

Acrodermatitis enteropathica is a rare, inherited disorder of zinc metabolism that presents in early infancy with diarrhea, failure to thrive, and skin lesions involving the distal extremities, perioral, and perineal

areas. Erythematous, moist, vesicular, pustular, and eczematoid skin lesions may be apparent. Lesions in the diaper area are often mistaken for candidiasis. The etiology appears to be impaired gastrointestinal zinc absorption. Treatment consists of oral zinc supplementation.

Histiocytosis X, another rare cause of diaper dermatitis, refers to a group of disorders characterized by proliferation of histiocytes within the bone, liver, spleen, lungs, lymph nodes, and skin. Skin lesions may involve the diaper area but more commonly affect the scalp and neck. The lesions appear as small, reddish-brown, scaling papules and pustules; ulceration may be apparent in the inguinal and perineal areas. Diagnosis can be confirmed by skin biopsy.

EVALUATION

History

A thorough history should be obtained (Questions Box). Candidal diaper dermatitis should be suspected if oral antibiotic therapy has recently been used.

Physical Examination

On physical examination, the presence of skin lesions elsewhere on the body should be noted. This is particularly important in the case of a persistent, resistant, or recurrent diaper rash, where systemic diseases such as psoriasis must be considered. The distribution of the rash within the diaper area itself may provide clues to the diagnosis. Candidal dermatitis occurs primarily in the creases, whereas irritant contact dermatitis usually affects the convex areas of the skin with relative sparing of the intertriginous areas. Streptococcal disease manifests primarily as marked perianal erythema.

Laboratory Tests

Although the diagnosis of candidal diaper dermatitis is usually evident clinically, microscopic examination of skin scrapings with KOH may be performed to establish the diagnosis. Typically, budding yeast with hyphae and pseudohyphae is seen. The diagnosis of perianal streptococcal disease or bullous impetigo may be confirmed by bacterial cultures from the perianal area or bullous lesions, respectively.

Questions: Diaper Dermatitis

- When did the rash begin?
- Does the rash resolve and then recur?
- Is the rash pruritic?
- Have any home remedies or previous treatments been used? Which ones?
- Does the child have a family history of atopic dermatitis or psoriasis?
- Is the child taking antibiotics now or been using them recently?
- What type of diapers are used?
- How frequently are the diapers changed?

MANAGEMENT

The mainstay of therapy and the key to prevention is **good hygiene**, which involves keeping the diaper area clean and dry. Gentle but thorough cleansing of the diaper area with water alone or water and a mild soap is usually sufficient. The area should then be patted dry and allowed to air dry completely if possible. Too frequent cleansing with harsh soaps or scrubbing too vigorously can actually aggravate skin that is already damaged and inflamed.

In addition, the diaper should be **changed frequently.** The diaper area should be exposed to as much air as possible (e.g., by allowing the infant to sleep without a diaper). In the absence of any inflammation, **dusting powders,** such as cornstarch powder, may be used to minimize friction and moisture. **Moisture-resistant barrier ointments or creams** such as zinc oxide or petrolatum are usually not needed if the above hygiene measures are carried out routinely. The role of hygiene in all forms of diaper dermatitis cannot be overemphasized. Topical application of medicated creams and ointments is not effective in the presence of poor hygiene.

Irritant contact dermatitis usually responds to hygienic measures and the application of barrier ointments and low-potency **topical corticosteroids** such as 0.5% or 1% hydrocortisone cream. Seborrheic dermatitis usually resolves spontaneously but can also be treated with low-potency topical corticosteroids. Candidal diaper dermatitis responds to **topical antifungal creams** such as nystatin, miconazole, or clotrimazole. In addition, a low-potency corticosteroid may be required if inflammation is severe. Oral penicillin usually clears perianal streptococcal disease, but the relapse rate is high. The topical antibiotic mupirocin may be used to treat bullous impetigo only if the lesions are few and isolated. Oral antibiotics (e.g., erythromycin, cephalexin) may be required for more extensive disease. Combination creams containing both a corticosteroid and an antifungal should not be recommended routinely because they usually contain high-potency corticosteroids.

PROGNOSIS

Although recurrence of diaper dermatitis is common, the usual varieties respond well to measures aimed at keeping the diaper area clean and dry and to medicated creams.

Case Resolution

The infant presented in the case scenario has irritant contact dermatitis. He has a recent history of gastroenteritis, and stool is known to be particularly irritating to the skin. Treatment includes keeping the diaper area clean and dry and topical application of a low-potency corticosteroid cream.

Selected Readings

Arnsmeier, S. L., and A. S. Paller. Getting to the bottom of diaper dermatitis. Contemp. Pediatr. 14:115–129, 1997.

Hurwitz, S. Skin lesions in the first year of life. Contemp. Pediatr. 10:110–128, 1993.

Liptak, G. S. Diaper Rash. *In* Hoekelman, R. A. (ed.). Primary Pediatric Care, 3rd ed. St. Louis, Mosby-Year Book, Inc., 1997, pp. 1277–1280.

Pride, H. B. Pediatric dermatoses commonly seen, uncommonly recognized. Pediatr. Ann. 27:129–135, 1998.

Schuman, A J. Disposable diapers? Definitely! Contemp. Pediatr. 14:131–139, 1997.

CHAPTER 100

PAPULOSQUAMOUS ERUPTIONS

Carol D. Berkowitz, M.D.

H$_x$ A 6-month-old female infant presents with an erythematous, confluent, and scaly rash on the cheeks. The extremities are also covered with a fine papular rash. The infant has had some scaling behind the ears and on the scalp since birth, but the symptoms have recently increased. The mother has been applying baby oil to the scalp to relieve the scaliness. Except for some intermittent rhinorrhea, the infant has otherwise been well. Immunizations are deficient; she received only the first set when she was 2 months old. The family history is positive for bronchitis. The infant's weight is at the 75th percentile, and the height is at the 50th percentile. Vital signs are normal. The physical examination is normal except for the presence of the rash.

Questions

1. What are the characteristics of papulosquamous eruptions?
2. What are the common conditions associated with papulosquamous eruptions in children?
3. What are the appropriate treatments for the common papulosquamous eruptions?

Rashes, a common problem in children, can be classified in ways that help to establish a diagnostic approach. First, rashes are assessed in terms of appearance, whether macular (flat), papular (raised), squamous (scaly), vesicular (fluid-filled), or bullous (large, fluid-filled). Next, the extent of the rash is determined. Rashes may be described as generalized or localized. Location is also important. The site of a localized rash may be consistent with certain diagnoses, for instance, diaper dermatitis.

Alternatively, rashes that are associated with fever can be differentiated from those that are not. Rashes seen in febrile children are called exanthems. Exanthems may be associated with enanthems, or lesions in the oral cavity (see Chapter 101, Maculopapular Rashes).

Papulosquamous eruptions, the subject of this chapter, are raised, scaly lesions. They are often localized to certain parts of the body, but the site may vary according to the age of the child. The rashes are frequently pruritic, but children are usually afebrile. The presence of a secondary infection may lead to fever, however.

EPIDEMIOLOGY

Although a large number of conditions may cause papulosquamous eruptions in children, a select number of diagnoses account for the majority of problems. Two of the most common causes of papulosquamous eruptions in children are atopic dermatitis and scabies. Atopic dermatitis affects about 3–5% of children under age 5 years and accounts for about 4% of pediatric emergency department visits. The world-wide prevalence of the condition varies from 4% to 20%. Males and females are affected with equal frequency. The itching associated with atopic dermatitis and other pruritic rashes is worse at night, which is one reason for the frequent visits. Symptoms are also worse during winter months.

Scabies is believed to affect 300 million persons worldwide, making it a frequent complaint of children seen in general pediatric practices. Although the existence of epidemics and pandemics of scabies has been suggested, the disorder does not appear to occur in regular cycles. Reports of infestations rise when populations are forced into close proximity (e.g., during wars). Increased reporting of scabies is related to increased physician recognition of the disorder. When one family member is affected, scabies is noted in another family member in about two-thirds of cases. When the infection is absent in household contacts, physicians should not be dissuaded from diagnosing scabies, however.

CLINICAL PRESENTATION

Papulosquamous eruptions consist of erythematous raised, scaly lesions that may involve the face, trunk, or extremities. The lesions are often highly pruritic, and scratching may lead to excoriation or secondary infection. Sometimes multiple family members are affected (D_x Box). Chronicity may lead to thickening or lichenification of involved skin.

PATHOPHYSIOLOGY

The pathophysiology of atopic dermatitis has not been definitively established. The disorder, which is attributed to immune dysfunction, is characterized by IgE overproduction and diminished cell-mediated immunity. Elevated IgE is reported in 43–82% of patients with atopic dermatitis. Non-IgE immune factors, particularly T helper cells and the cytokines IL-4 and IL-5, also play a role. Disturbances in fatty acid metabolism, particularly deficiencies in omega-6 fatty acid are noted in some affected infants. Inflammatory hyperactivity of the skin and other sites, including the lungs and nasal tissues, results.

The inflammatory response in scabies is triggered by an infestation with a mite, *Sarcoptes scabiei*. The adult female burrows under the skin and lays her eggs. After 2 weeks, the eggs become adults. Affected individuals may be asymptomatic on first exposure. With time, usually 10–30 days after infestation, signs and symptoms including pruritus and rash become apparent. This reaction relates to the development of cellular or humoral immunity to the mite, feces, or eggs. In infants, rashes may develop in areas away from the site of infestation as a sign of an allergic reaction to foreign material.

DIFFERENTIAL DIAGNOSIS

The major conditions that are associated with papulosquamous eruptions in children are atopic dermatitis, seborrheic dermatitis, allergic contact dermatitis, scabies, xerosis, lichen planus, psoriasis, papular urticaria, flea bites, fungal infections of the skin, and infantile acropustulosis dermatosis.

Eczema is a general term that is used to denote a papulosquamous eruption. The two most common eczematous conditions seen in children are atopic eczema or dermatitis and seborrheic dermatitis. **Atopic dermatitis** is a disorder of infancy and childhood. Sixty percent of affected individuals become symptomatic with a pruritic rash during the first year of life, and 85%

D_x Papulosquamous Eruptions

- Raised, scaly papules
- Pruritus
- Afebrile, unless secondary infection is present
- Allergic personal or family history
- Intertriginous rash

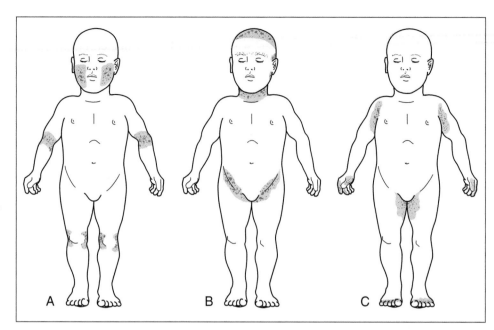

FIGURE 100–1. Typical distribution of papulosquamous eruptions in children. A. Atopic dermatitis: usually located on cheeks, creases of elbows, and knees. B. Seborrheic dermatitis: usually located on scalp, behind ears, thigh creases, and eyebrows. C. Scabies: usually located on axillae, webs of fingers and toes, and intragluteal area.

develop symptoms during the first 5 years. The area of involvement changes with age. In infancy and childhood, the face and extensor surfaces are involved, and the diaper area is often spared (Fig. 100–1A). By adolescence, the flexor surfaces show the characteristic changes of chronic inflammation with lichenification and accentuation of the flexure folds. Clinically, erythema and a pruritic papular eruption are apparent. Scratching and rubbing leads to excoriation, weeping, and eventually lichenification. Changes in coloring, including hypo- and hyperpigmentation, may also occur. Hypopigmented areas that are usually noted on the face are called pityriasis alba. Xeroderma, or dry skin, is a frequent coexisting condition. Lesions around mucosa (Dennie-Morgan infraorbital fold under the eye and cheilitis around the mouth) may also be seen. Symptoms of other allergic conditions, such as rhinorrhea, wheezing, or food-related allergies, may occur. A positive family history is usually elicited. Forty percent of affected children have at least one first-degree relative with atopic dermatitis.

Seborrheic dermatitis, which develops during the first 3 months of life, is characterized by scaliness, particularly of the scalp. Scalp eruptions are referred to as cradle cap. In addition, seborrheic dermatitis has a predilection for intertriginous areas, including the folds in the diaper region and the area behind the ears (Fig. 100–1B). A scaly eruption involving the eyebrows and around the nose may also be apparent. The reddish or pinkish rash may have a greasy quality. Use of baby oil often exacerbates the condition, and secondary infections may occur either with *Candida,* particularly in the intertriginous areas, or with *Pityrosporum,* in the scalp. Seborrheic dermatitis is less pruritic than atopic dermatitis, and this feature can be used to distinguish between the two conditions. The intertriginous involvement and the onset shortly after birth also differentiate these two types of dermatitis.

Contact dermatitis occurs when individuals come into physical contact with an irritant or a specific allergen. Diaper dermatitis and Rhus dermatitis (poison ivy/oak) are two common types of contact dermatitis. The disorder is more commonly observed in individuals with atopic dermatitis, and one study noted that 77% of sensitized patients were atopic. Hands and exposed areas are frequently affected. Although the rash is papulosquamous, it is often also oozing and subsequently lichenified.

Scabies may resemble atopic or seborrheic dermatitis in infants and young children. The lesions may be papules, pustules, or vesicles. The characteristic burrow, which is only about 1 cm long, is often difficult to appreciate unless certain diagnostic maneuvers are undertaken. The lesions are most often noted on the skin of the hands and feet, including the palms and soles in infants and young children. Intertriginous areas such as the intragluteal region, groin, and fingerwebs are commonly infected (Fig. 100–1C). In infants, the face and head may be involved. Scratching and secondary infection may alter the appearance of the rash. Reddish-brown nodules may be characteristic of chronic infection. These nodules are believed to be an immune reaction to the dead mite. In institutionalized or immunosuppressed individuals, the rash may become covered with thick crusts, a condition referred to as "Norwegian scabies."

Xerosis, or xeroderma, refers to dry skin. This condition is frequently noted in patients prone to atopic dermatitis, but it may be seen in other individuals under drying conditions, such as low humidity and frequent bathing with drying soaps. The skin may be scaly and pruritic, and scratching may result in excoriations. A papular eruption is usually absent.

Lichen planus is an uncommon papulosquamous eruption. The polygonal, brownish-pink, scaly lesions are located on flexor surfaces.

Psoriasis, although a papulosquamous eruption, is more plaquelike. In older children the face and scalp are affected, but in infants the eruption is frequently noted in the diaper area, where it is very erythematous. The white, silvery scale, usually noted when the eruption affects the extensor surfaces, is milder because of the hydrating effect of occlusive diapers. Like seborrheic dermatitis, psoriasis may become secondarily infected by *Candida*. In general, psoriasis is only mildly itchy.

Papular urticaria is noted in children between the ages of 3 and 10 years. The eruption may be triggered by the presence of insect bites, particularly **flea bites.** The papular, extremely pruritic lesions are usually confined to the extremities.

Fungal infections (tinea corporis and tinea pedis) may also appear as papulosquamous eruptions. Sometimes the lesions assume a characteristic distribution, with the papules grouped in a circle, and central clearing of the scaliness.

Infantile acropustulosis consists of very pruritic papules and vesicles on the sides of the hands and the feet. Lesions become scaly and hyperpigmented and often show evidence of secondary infection. The lesions may be mistaken for scabies. African-American and Native American children under the age of 3 years have a predilection for this condition.

EVALUATION

History

A thorough history should be obtained (Questions Box). The presence of a rash in other family members suggests a contagious condition such as scabies or a familial disorder such as atopic dermatitis or psoriasis. An onset in the first few weeks of life is consistent with seborrheic dermatitis. It is important to determine if any medications have been used, because these may modify the appearance of the rash.

PHYSICAL EXAMINATION

The physical examination helps define the exact nature of the eruption and its distribution, which is often the clue to its etiology. The entire body should be examined, and particular attention should be paid to the intragluteal region and web spaces between fingers and toes. Certain rashes have characteristic appearances. For example, a circular cluster of scaly papules with central clearing signifies tinea corporis, and the presence of burrows characterizes scabies. Burrows appear

---

as a small, thin, serpiginous line with a black dot at the end. The dot represents the female mite. Vesiculopustules and nodules may also be present. White dermatographism is noted in atopic dermatitis. Scratching the skin results in an erythematous line which quickly becomes white.

Laboratory Tests

Certain diagnostic tests may help clarify the etiology. Skin or radioallergosorbent (RAST) testing is recommended by some to identify offending food allergies (see Chapter 60, Allergic Diseases). The burrow of the mite that causes scabies may not be readily apparent, but a number of studies make it more easily detectable. The ink test helps visualize the burrow. A washable felt tip marker is rubbed across the web spaces, and excess ink is removed with water or alcohol. The ink penetrates through the stratum corneum, thus outlining the burrow. Scrapings should also be taken to identify the mite, eggs, or feces. The yield is reported to be as high as 90–95% if proper technique is followed. Alternatively, mineral oil may be placed on the web space or on a No. 15 scalpel blade. Multiple burrows or web spaces are scraped. The material is then spread on a glass slide and viewed under low power.

Scrapings of skin also assist in diagnosing candidal or tinea infections. These scrapings should be mixed with KOH, which facilitates the dissolution of epithelial debris, and allows for identification of the yeast or fungus.

If a secondary bacterial infection is suspected, cultures of the skin are indicated. No other specific diagnostic tests, short of a skin biopsy, assist in the diagnosis.

MANAGEMENT

The management is determined by the diagnosis. **Topical steroids** are used to treat various papulosquamous eruptions. These drugs are the mainstay of therapy designed to minimize inflammation. The agents usually prescribed in cases of atopic as well as seborrheic dermatitis are triamcinolone 0.1% and hydrocortisone 1% (cream or ointment). Sometimes brief courses of systemic steroids (4–5 days of prednisone) may be needed during more severe exacerbations. Psoriasis does not usually respond to hydrocortisone 1% alone and may require a combination tar-hydrocortisone preparation.

Management of atopic dermatitis involves the **reduction of dryness and irritation.** Children may bathe, but they should avoid using drying soaps. Within 3 minutes of leaving the bath tub they should apply moisturizers to ensure that the skin is hydrated. Seborrheic dermatitis may respond to topical steroids, but additional scalp treatment may be necessary. Baby oil may be applied to help loosen the scales. Parents should be told to massage the child's scalp gently. The scalp should then be washed using either a mild baby shampoo or an over-the-counter antiseborrheic shampoo (usually containing sulfur and sialic acid). The scalp may be brushed

---

> **Questions: Papulosquamous Eruptions**
>
> - How long has the child had the rash?
> - What did the rash look like when it first appeared?
> - Are other family members affected?
> - Have any medications been used to treat the rash?
> - Is pruritus present?
> - Does the child have any other symptoms such as wheezing or rhinorrhea?
> - Does the child have a history of any contact between the affected skin and any irritating substance?
> - Has the child been febrile?

with a soft-bristle tooth brush to loosen scales further while the shampoo is on the scalp.

If specific **allergens** have been identified, these should be eliminated from the child's diet. Human milk, or hydrolyzed casein protein formula help reduce the incidence of atopic dermatitis in young infants.

Antibiotics are indicated if secondary infection is present. The most common pathogen involved is *Staphylococcus aureus.* Staphylococcal antigens also exacerbate the inflammation of atopic dermatitis. A 5-day course of erythromycin may be adequate to treat the infection. Some children are colonized with erythromycin-resistant organisms, however, and they should therefore be treated with a cephalosporin, dicloxacillin, or amoxicillin-clavulanate. Topical antibiotics such as mupirocin, bacitracin, or 3% iodochlorhydroxyquin in 1% hydrocortisone may be used in localized secondary infections.

If children with atopic dermatitis develop infection with **herpes simplex** (eczema herpeticum), they should be treated with **acyclovir.** Atopic children are also prone to infection with warts and molluscum contagiosa. These conditions should be appropriately managed. Other measures in the management of atopic dermatitis include the use of tars and sunlight.

Coinfection with *Candida,* which occurs with seborrheic dermatitis and psoriasis, requires the use of **topical medications** such as nystatin, clotrimazole, or miconazole. Antifungal shampoos may also help in reducing the scaling due to fungal agents such as *Pityrosporum. Tinea corporis* also responds to topical antifungal agents.

Three major medications are used to treat scabies. They all work by killing the mites causing the infestation. **Lindane (Kwell),** which has been used for over 50 years, is a 1% cream. It is generally applied from the neck down and left in place for 8–12 hours. At the end of this time it should be removed by bathing. Because of concern about the absorption of lindane and its potential neurotoxicity, the drug should not be used in young infants or patients with a seizure disorder. Aplastic anemia, urticaria, and muscle spasm have also been reported with lindane. It is recommended that a repeat application of the drug be administered in 7 days in all symptomatic patients. A mild topical steroid, such as hydrocortisone 1% cream, may be used in between applications to decrease the inflammatory response to the mites.

Crotamiton 10%, an antiscabies medication, lacks the neurotoxic effects of lindane. However, the efficacy of crotamiton is low—reportedly only 40–50% after 2 daily applications. Five days of daily applications are therefore recommended, which is both less convenient and more costly for patients. **Permethrin** (Elimite), a newer product, requires only a single application and is safe for individuals of all ages, even those as young as 2 months. An over-the-counter treatment for lice, permethrin is currently the drug of choice for the treatment of scabies. The lotion is applied for 8–12 hours and then removed. The overall cure rate with a single application is 89–92%, though some physicians recommend a reapplication after 1 week.

The effective elimination of scabies necessitates that all affected household members be treated simultaneously and that bed linens and clothing be washed in hot water.

Antihistamines may play a role in reducing the pruritus, especially during the night. Hydroxyzine seems to have the best effect in part because it allows patients to sleep comfortably. If drowsiness is to be avoided, cetirizine or loratadine are non-sedating antipruritics. Clipping fingernails decreases the risk of excoriation from scratching.

Children with recalcitant atopic dermatitis may benefit from referral to an allergist or dermatologist. A trial course of newer immunomodulatory medications may be warranted. Dermatologists also use ultraviolet light as an adjunct to therapy.

PROGNOSIS

In general, the prognosis for children with papulosquamous eruptions is excellent with appropriate management, which is contingent on accurate diagnosis. Both atopic dermatitis and seborrheic dermatitis tend to improve as children get older although 20–40% of atopic children remain atopic as adults. Children with atopic dermatitis frequently face remissions and exacerbations, particularly associated with seasonal changes. Scabies also improves with appropriate management. Psoriasis may have a more prolonged course, and children with this condition often require medical intervention into adulthood.

Case Resolution

The infant's presentation in the case history is characteristic of seborrheic dermatitis. The infant experienced the onset of symptoms shortly after birth, and the involvement of the scalp with scaling and crusting supports the diagnosis of seborrheic dermatitis. The mother should be advised that although she may use the baby oil to loosen the scale on the scalp, she should shampoo immediately afterwards using an antiseborrheic or antifungal shampoo. A mild topical steroid, such as hydrocortisone 1%, may also be recommended. If skin scrapings reveal secondary infection with *Candida,* an antifungal cream should be added to the regimen.

Selected Readings

Birmhall, C. L., and N. B. Esterly. Summertime, and the critters are biting. Contemp. Pediatr. 11:62–77, 1994.

Eichenfield, L. F., and S. F. Friedlander. Coping with chronic dermatitis. Contemp. Pediatr. 15:53–66, 1998.

Friedlander, S. F. Contact dermatitis. Pediatr. Rev. 19:166–172, 1998.

Halbert, A. R. The practical management of atopic dermatitis in children. Pediatr. Ann. 25:72–78, 1996.

Hogan, D. J., L. Schachner, and C. Tanglertsampan. Diagnosis and treatment of childhood scabies and pediculosis. Pediatr. Clin. North Am. 38:941–957, 1991.

Hurwitz, S. Skin lesions in the first year of life. Contemp. Pediatr. 10:110–128, 1993.

Johr, R. H., and L. A. Schachner. Neonatal dermatologic challenges. Pediatr. Rev. 18:86–94, 1997.

Knoell, K. A., and K. E. Greer. Atopic dermatitis. Pediatr. Rev. 20:46–51, 1999.

Mallory, S. B. Neonatal skin disorders. Pediatr. Clin. North Am. 38:745–761, 1991.

Nigro, J. F., and N. B. Esterly. Psoriasis—chronic but controllable. Contemp. Pediatr. 10:114–130, 1993.

Peterson, C. M. and L. F. Eichenfield. Scabies. Pediatr. Ann. 25:97–100, 1996.

Rabinowitz, L. G., and N. B. Esterly. Atopic dermatitis and ichthyosis vulgaris. Pediatr. Rev. 15:220–226, 1994.

Rasmussen, J. E. Scabies. Pediatr. Rev. 15:110–114, 1994.

Stein, D. H. Tineas—Superficial dermatophyte infections. Pediatr. Rev. 19:368–372, 1998.

Woodmansee, D., and S. Christiansen. Atopic dermatitis. Pediatr. Ann. 27:710–716, 1998.

CHAPTER 101

MACULOPAPULAR RASHES

Carol D. Berkowitz, M.D.

H$_x$ A 10-month-old infant girl is brought to the office with a history of rhinorrhea, cough, and fever for 3 days prior to the onset of a confluent, erythematous rash. The rash started on her face. She has been irritable, and her eyes are red and teary. Her immunizations include three sets of diphtheria-pertussis-tetanus (DaPT), oral polio, *Haemophilus influenzae* type B and hepatitis B vaccines. No one at home is ill. The girl was seen in the emergency department 2 weeks before because she caught her finger in a car door.

On physical examination, the girl's temperature is 102° F (39° C). A confluent maculopapular rash is evident on the face, trunk, and extremities, with prominent bilateral posterior cervical nodes. Rhinorrhea and conjunctivitis are also present.

Questions

1. What are the common causes of febrile maculopapular rashes in children?
2. What features distinguish one disease from another?
3. What are the public health considerations concerning viral exanthems in children?

More than 50 different viruses in addition to bacteria and rickettsia cause childhood exanthems. These exanthems may be macular, papular, or vesicular. In most cases, these rashes are seen in conjunction with fever, and sometimes other symptoms, including rhinorrhea, conjunctivitis, and lymphadenopathy. Although many of the common childhood illnesses of the past are now prevented by immunizations, not all segments of the population are adequately immunized. In addition, some children are not eligible for immunization because of their young age. Allergic reactions to medications, particularly antibiotics, may also result in eruptions, although these often have no associated symptoms. Differentiating viral exanthems from allergic reactions may be difficult in febrile children who have empirically been started on antimicrobial agents.

EPIDEMIOLOGY

In most children, the viruses that cause maculopapular exanthems produce mild disease without significant morbidity or long-term sequelae. Of greater concern is that some diseases are a public health risk because of potential spread through the population. Maculopapular eruptions are a common presenting complaint, particularly in certain age groups and at certain times of the year.

Measles, a viral disease, had been virtually eliminated in the United States. Periodic resurgences have occurred, particularly among unimmunized preschoolers and 15- to 19-year-old adolescents. In addition, young infants are also at risk because of decreased levels of passively transferred maternal immunity related to lack of maternal natural infection or immunization. Vaccine-related immunity apparently wanes more rapidly in mothers than does naturally acquired immunity. In a recent outbreak of measles in the Los Angeles area, Hispanic children of poorer immigrant parents were 12.6 times more likely to develop measles than nonimmigrant children. WHO has targeted the year 2010 for the global eradication of measles. The incubation period of measles is about 1 week. Individuals are infectious during the second half of this week, before the rash erupts, and then for several days following its appearance.

Rubella now rarely occurs, but sporadic outbreaks are reported, particularly during the springtime. Adolescents and young adults are at greatest risk for the disease. Congenital rubella syndrome may develop in the offspring of pregnant women who have rubella. The incubation period is 15–21 days.

Erythema infectiosum, also called fifth disease, is most commonly seen in children aged 5–15 years during the spring. The disease is caused by parvovirus B19 and spread through respiratory secretions. The incubation period is generally 4–14 days but may be up to 20 days.

Roseola may affect children from 6 months to 3 years

of age, although the majority are under the age of 1 year. The illness is due to infection with human herpesvirus (HHV) 6 or 7, and the virus is shed in the saliva, even among healthy, previously infected infants. Nearly 100% of toddlers 2–3 years of age have antibodies to HHV-6. The incubation period is 5–15 days.

Enteroviruses are the most common cause of exanthems during August, September, and October and account for two thirds of all exanthems that occur during the summer. Sixty-eight different types of enteroviruses are recognized. Previously these viruses were categorized as coxsackievirus, echovirus, or poliovirus, but now newly identified strains are grouped under picornavirus. Infection is spread through the fecal-oral route. Exanthems are more common in young children, and infection of the central nervous system is more common in older children. Echoviruses are responsible for these two syndromes. The incubation period is 3–7 days, with an absent or brief prodrome.

Kawasaki syndrome is of uncertain etiology, although a bacterial toxin with superantigen properties may be involved. Data do not support toxic shock syndrome toxin-1(TSST-1)–producing staphylococci as the offending organisms. Most patients are under the age of 2 years, and 80% are below the age of 5 years. Males outnumber females by a ratio of 1.5 to 1. The incidence of the disorder among Asians is higher than in other populations. Caucasians and African Americans in the United States are also affected. The incubation period is unknown.

Scarlet fever is a bacterially transmitted illness that can produce a maculopapular eruption. The rash and illness are due to an exotoxin produced by group A beta-hemolytic streptococcus. A resurgence of disease related to exotoxin A, which causes more severe cases, has occurred. These cases may be associated with a toxic shock–like picture, with the classic rash of scarlet fever. Scarlet fever is usually seen in young children with pharyngitis. The incubation period is 2–5 days.

CLINICAL PRESENTATION

Maculopapular eruptions may involve the face, trunk, or extremities. The rash is usually erythematous, and the lesions are flat or slightly raised. Occasionally, lesions within the mouth, referred to as enanthems, are evident. Most children are febrile (D_x Box).

PATHOPHYSIOLOGY

The mechanism for development of a rash is variable. In some cases, the rash is the reaction of the body to

D_x **Maculopapular Rashes**
• Macular, papular, or maculopapular rash • Fever • Enanthems (lesions in the mouth) • Lymphadenopathy • Respiratory symptoms

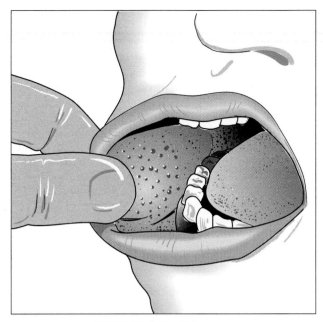

FIGURE 101–1. Koplik's spots.

infection or to the presence of a toxin. In general, the sequence involves exposure to an infectious agent and then acquisition of the agent either through droplet infection or fecal-oral contamination. The agent, usually a virus, then replicates, perhaps in the reticuloendothelial system. Lymph nodes enlarge, reflecting the involvement of the reticuloendothelial system. Associated viremia may be present.

In Kawasaki syndrome, vasculitis affects multiple organ symptoms. Various cytokines and autoantibodies play a role in the inflammatory response.

In a toxin-mediated rash (e.g., scarlet fever), previous exposure to the toxin is believed to sensitize the individual. An antibiotic-related rash may represent an allergy to the antibiotic itself, or not infrequently, a reaction to one of the ingredients in the antibiotic preparation. Reactions to ampicillin and amoxicillin are especially common in patients infected with EBV.

DIFFERENTIAL DIAGNOSIS

Maculopapular rashes are associated with several diseases, such as measles, rubella, erythema infectiosum, roseola, enterovirus-caused diseases, Kawasaki syndrome, and scarlet fever.

The rash associated with **measles** is preceded by rhinorrhea, conjunctivitis, cough, and fever (temperature: 103° F [39.4° C]) , which last for several days before the eruption of the exanthem. Lesions within the oral cavity, called Koplik's spots, are well-circumscribed white lesions (Fig. 101–1) that usually resolve after 2–3 days, with the appearance of the rash. Other oral lesions, referred to as Forschheimer spots, are pinpoint, rose-colored, petechial spots on the soft palate. The conjunctivitis associated with measles is purulent, which distinguishes it from Kawasaki syndrome.

The measles rash itself usually begins on the head, particularly behind the ears and around the margin of the scalp and then spreads over the rest of the body. Initially the lesions are discrete papules that coalesce and become pruritic. As the rash resolves the lesions become brawny, and desquamation occurs.

As with other viral exanthems, the measles rash is associated with lymphadenopathy, particularly in the posterior cervical region. The major complications of measles in children in developed nations are pneumonia, encephalitis, and secondary bacterial infections. In developing nations, children with marginal nutritional status are at high risk of dying from measles or its complications. Arthritis has been reported as a complication in adults. In individuals who were initially immunized with killed measles vaccine (1963–1967), acquisition of measles results in atypical measles, which is characterized by a papular or vesicular eruption that may be hemorrhagic. Pneumonia is always present, and associated findings include hepatosplenomegaly and weakness.

Rubella produces a relatively minor illness in children, although adults, particularly women, may experience a painful arthritis. The rash consists of fine macules and papules, starting on the face and progressing caudally. Lymphadenopathy, particularly of the postauricular nodes, is characteristic of the disease.

Erythema infectiosum is characterized by a sudden onset of the rash. Prodromal symptoms are mild, and may include low-grade fever, headache, and malaise. The rash is variable, and the classic pattern of the markedly erythematous "slapped cheek" appearance is present in only 50% of cases. If involved, the extremities may initially have a discrete maculopapular eruption, which then assumes a fine, lacy quality. The rash on the extremities usually appears 1–4 days after the malar eruption but may last for weeks, waxing and waning. Physical factors such as activity, sun light, and hot baths exacerbate the intensity of the rash. Most children are only mildly ill, but children with underlying hematologic disorders may experience aplastic crises because of the affinity of parvovirus B19 for developing red blood cells. Adults with parvovirus infection frequently develop arthritis though only 10% of children experience this symptom. Neurologic disturbances including encephalitis and neuropathies may follow parvovirus infection.

Roseola is another viral exanthem that usually causes a mild illness in children. Defervescence usually accompanies the rash, which consists of fine pink macules or papules on the neck and trunk. On average, the rash lasts about 4 days, although it may be very evanescent, lasting from a few hours to 1–2 days. Infants may appear sickest during the prodromal phase, when the fever is high (temperature: often 102.2° F [39° C] or above) and infants are irritable. Workups to rule out sepsis are often warranted. During the prodromal phase, as well as following the eruption of the rash, lymphadenopathy is seen in the occipital, cervical, and postauricular nodes.

The rashes associated with **enterovirus infections** are highly variable. They may resemble measles or rubella or may be distinct and characteristic, such as hand-foot-and-mouth disease, usually seen with coxsackievirus A16. The rash of hand-foot-and-mouth disease may be vesicular or maculopapular. Lesions may be anywhere in the mouth and progress from vesicles to sharply demarcated ulcers. Often low-grade fever, anorexia, sore throat, and malaise are present. Other enteroviral infections may have similar systemic symptoms, and some may cause gastroenteritis or aseptic meningitis.

The rash of **Kawasaki syndrome** is also highly variable; it may be morbilliform, urticarial, scarlatiniform, or resemble erythema multiforme. The rash is often pruritic and intensified in the perineal area, where it peels, like the rash of scarlet fever. Other signs and symptoms in addition to the rash characterize Kawasaki syndrome. Temperature over 103° F (39.4° C) occurs for at least 5 days. A nonpurulent conjunctivitis is present, and erythema of the mucous membranes of the mouth, fissuring of the lips, and hypertrophy of the papillae of the tongue are also evident. Cervical lymphadenopathy, which is often unilateral, is present. The distal extremities are also involved; erythema or edema of the palms and soles and desquamation of the tips of the fingers or toes, often around the nails, is apparent. The presence of this symptom complex should suggest the diagnosis. The major complication of Kawasaki syndrome is coronary artery aneurysms, which are reported in 15–20% of affected children. This problem can be averted with appropriate management, but the diagnosis must be considered before the necessary therapy is instituted.

Scarlet fever is the most common bacterially caused exanthem. Symptoms of fever (temperature: 103° F [39.4° C]), headache, vomiting, malaise, and sore throat appear suddenly. The tonsils are covered with a white exudate, and palatal petechiae are seen. The tongue initially has a white coating. Edema of the papillae make them appear prominent, and the finding is referred to as strawberry tongue (Fig. 101–2). The face is flushed, except around the mouth (circumoral pallor), but a discrete facial rash is absent. The fine rash is concentrated on the trunk and it is intensified in flexor folds.

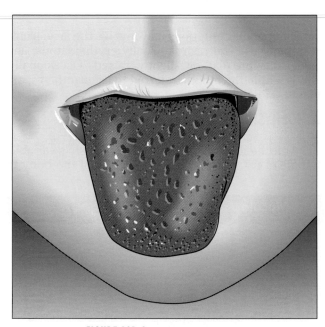

FIGURE 101–2. Strawberry tongue.

The bright red lines noted in the antecubital fossa are called Pastia's lines. As the scarlet fever rash resolves, desquamation begins in 4–5 days.

Adenoviruses account for 2–4% of rashes and occur more commonly in winter and spring. This usually mild rash has nonspecific characteristics. Conjunctivitis, rhinitis, pharyngitis, lymphadenopathy and, occasionally, pneumonia accompany the rash.

Infection with EBV is associated with rash in young children and in adolescents on antibiotics. The eruption is morbilliform, and the lesions may be erythematous or copper-colored. Fever, upper respiratory symptoms, lymphadenopathy, hepatosplenomegaly, and facial and peripheral edema, including unilateral periorbital edema may be noted.

EVALUATION

History

A thorough history should be obtained (Questions Box).

Physical Examination

The focus of the physical examination is to help define the characteristics of the eruption such as location, extent, and degree of coalescence. The presence of any associated physical findings such as fever, lymphadenopathy, enanthem, desquamation, rhinorrhea, conjunctivitis, organomegaly, or CNS symptomatology should be determined.

Laboratory Tests

Laboratory assessment may be helpful in certain conditions. Serologic testing is most valuable for defining a community outbreak of a specific disease such as measles. In most viral exanthems, the results of serologic studies are not available until the condition has resolved and the patient has recovered. Tests may include acute and convalescent titers for specific viruses. Alternatively, IgM levels of antibodies against certain infections may be used to document that the infection was recent. Newer modalities such as PCR may expedite the identification of enterovirus. Viral cultures are costly and are not usually obtained unless aseptic meningitis is diagnosed. Because neutropenia and lymphocytosis characterize many viral illnesses, such findings are not helpful in differentiating specific causal agents. Lymphocytosis, with characteristically atypical lymphocytes, distinguishes EBV infection. Although a mononucleosis spot test is usually positive in older children and adolescents, it may be nonreactive in young children, where infection is documented by specific EBV serology.

Scarlet fever is characterized by leukocytosis. In addition, a throat culture or antigen assay reveals the presence of group A beta-hemolytic streptococci. If the pharyngitis has resolved, serologic studies such as antistreptolysin O or anti-DNAase provide evidence of the recent infection.

Kawasaki syndrome is associated with specific laboratory abnormalities, including an elevated platelet count, erythrocyte sedimentation rate (ESR), C-reactive protein, α-antitrypsin, and IgE. Hypoalbuminemia is associated with prolonged fever. Pyuria is noted in 60% of the cases. A slit lamp examination of the eye may show uveitis.

Imaging Studies

Ultrasound, if performed in children with suspected Kawasaki syndrome, may reveal hydrops of the gallbladder. An echocardiogram to check for evidence of coronary artery aneurysm is a mandated part of the evaluation in this disorder. Electrocardiograms should be obtained to detect cardiac arrhythmias.

MANAGEMENT

The management of most viral exanthems is supportive and symptomatic. In cases where complications such as encephalitis or pneumonia develop, hospitalization is indicated. Spread of infection such as measles to susceptible contacts can be reduced through the use of vaccine within 72 hours of exposure, or immune globulin (IG) within 6 days. IG is given in a dose of 0.25 mL/kg IM (0.5 mL/kg in immunocompromised children). Measles vaccine should be administered 5 months after the IG in children who have received the lower dose and after 6 months in children receiving the higher dose. In developing nations, administration of vitamin A is recommended to all children with measles if vitamin A deficiency is present in the community and mortality from measles is ≥1%. Antibiotic therapy should be initiated if bacterial coinfection is suspected. Antibiotics in the form of penicillin should be given when patients have scarlet fever.

The management of Kawasaki syndrome includes the administration of intravenous immune globulin (IVIG), which should be started within 10 days of onset. The current recommendation is to administer a single dose at 2 g/kg given as an infusion over 1- to 12-hours. IVIG may work by binding to the toxin that is suspected of precipitating the illness. Aspirin is initially administered at 100 mg/kg until several days after defervescence to prevent coronary thrombosis. Dosage is reduced to 3–10 mg/kg until the ESR and platelet count normalize, which usually takes 3 months.

PROGNOSIS

The prognosis for most maculopapular rashes of childhood is excellent, with full resolution of symptoms

---

Questions: Maculopapular Rashes

- What does the rash look like?
- What symptoms, if any, are associated with the rash?
- How long has the child had these symptoms?
- Is the child taking any antibiotics?
- Does the child have any ill contacts?
- What is the child's immunization status?

unless children are very young or have some underlying condition. In some young infants, viruses that cause exanthems may produce severe complications such as pneumonia and encephalitis.

The prognosis for Kawasaki syndrome is excellent with appropriate management. Otherwise, 20% of all children not treated with IVIG develop coronary artery aneurysm. Even with IVIG, infants <1 year may exhibit such coronary artery abnormalities.

Case Resolution

The infant in the case scenario has the classic symptoms of measles. Normally such a young infant would not yet have received immunization against measles. She should be evaluated for evidence of complications, including pneumonia. Unimmunized household contacts should receive IG to reduce the severity of their disease.

Selected Readings

Atkinson, W., L. Furphy, J. Gantt, M. Mayfield, and G. Rhyne (eds.). Epidemiology and Prevention of Vaccine-Preventable Diseases. Department of Health and Human Services, 1996.

Beutner, K. R. Cutaneous viral infections. Pediatr. Ann. 22:247–252, 1993.

Committee on Infectious Disease, American Academy of Pediatrics. 1997 Redbook: Report of the Committee on Infectious Disease. Elk Grove Village, IL, American Academy of Pediatrics, 1997.

Farrar, W. E., et al. Infectious Disease. Text and Color Atlas. London, Gower Medical Publishing, 1992.

Frieden, I. J., and S. D. Resnick. Childhood exanthems, old and new. Pediatr. Clin. North Am. 38:859–885, 1991.

Gold, E. Almost extinct diseases: Measles, mumps, rubella, and pertussis. Pediatr. Rev. 17:120–127, 1996.

Makhene, M. K., and P. S. Diaz. Clinical presentations and complications of suspected measles in hospitalized children. Pediatr. Infect. Dis. J. 12:836–840, 1993.

Mancini, . J. Exanthems in childhood: An update. Pediatr. Ann. 27:163–170, 1998.

Melish, M. E. Kawasaki syndrome. Pediatr. Rev. 17:153–162, 1996.

Zaoutis, T., and J. D. Klein. Enterovirus infections. Pediatr. Rev. 19:183–191, 1998.

CHAPTER 102

VESICULAR EXANTHEMS

Monica Sifuentes, M.D.

H$_x$ A 2-year-old toddler is evaluated for a 2-day history of fever (temperature: 103° F [39.5° C]), runny nose, decreased appetite, and a rash over the abdomen. The boy has had no previous known exposures to chickenpox (varicella) and no history of varicella vaccination. He attends day care daily. No one at home is ill. The boy is currently taking no medications except for acetaminophen for fever, and he has no past history of dermatologic problems.

On physical examination, the heart rate is 120 beats/min, the respiratory rate is 20 breaths/min, and the temperature is 100° F (38.0° C). The toddler's overall appearance is nontoxic. The skin examination is significant for a few scattered erythematous vesicular lesions over the abdomen and one papule on the back. The rest of the examination is normal.

Questions

1. What are the most likely causes of vesicular exanthems in febrile children?
2. How can types of vesicular rashes be differentiated on the basis of patient history?
3. What are the key historical questions to ask?
4. What is the natural course of varicella?

5. What treatment options are available for children with varicella? What options are available for other vesicular exanthems?

Exanthems are generalized, erythematous rashes that often accompany viral or bacterial illnesses. These eruptions have different physical appearances and can be macular, papular, vesicular, or petechial. Vesicles are elevated, fluid-filled lesions that measure 0.5 cm or less in diameter. Bullae are quite similar but are more than 0.5 cm in diameter. Vesicles may be grouped, generalized, or linear depending on their etiology, and their specific distribution is often helpful in formulating a differential diagnosis. This chapter will focus on common vesicular exanthems in children.

EPIDEMIOLOGY

Epidemiologic factors help differentiate infectious from noninfectious etiologies. Patient age, season of the year, presence or absence of similar cases in the community, regular attendance at day care or school, and lower socioeconomic class, which may contribute to exposure, should all be considered. Gender and ethnicity, on the other hand, are not usually helpful from an epidemiologic standpoint.

Varicella, or chickenpox, is by far the most common vesicular exanthem seen in childhood. Approximately 3.9 million cases occur annually in the United States, with most infections occurring in late winter and early spring. Males and females are equally affected. Most reported cases are in children less than 10 years of age, although infections in adolescents and young adults may now become more common with the routine administration of the varicella vaccine at one year of age.

CLINICAL PRESENTATION

Vesicular exanthems are distinctive lesions that are raised and fluid-filled (D_x Box). They may be located anywhere on the child's body and, depending upon the etiology, may or may not be pruritic. Other symptoms that may accompany such rashes include fever, upper respiratory symptoms, and decreased appetite.

PATHOPHYSIOLOGY

Vesicles and bullae arise from a cleavage at various levels of the skin either within the epidermis (intraepidermal) or at the epidermal-dermal junction (subepidermal). Sometimes the two types of lesions can be differentiated based on the amount of pressure required to collapse the lesion, especially if the lesion is a large bulla. In addition, the thickness of the wall of a bulla can be estimated by its translucency or flaccidity. A biopsy of the lesion, however, is the only way to reliably differentiate between the two areas of separation.

Specific changes occur in the epidermis depending on the etiology of the vesicular exanthem. For example, with certain viral infections such as varicella, herpes simplex, and herpes zoster, a "ballooning degeneration" of epidermal cells occurs. In dyshidrotic eczema, vesicles result from intracellular edema, also termed spongiosis. Intradermal vesication also is seen in delayed hypersensitivity reactions of the epidermis (e.g., contact and *Rhus* [plant] dermatitis).

DIFFERENTIAL DIAGNOSIS

Numerous infectious conditions cause vesicular eruptions (Table 102–1). Parasites such as the tiny mite,

D_x	**Vesicular Exanthems**

- Raised, fluid-filled vesicles on the skin
- Lesions may be pruritic
- Possible associated fever, URI symptoms, myalgias
- History of affected contacts
- Lesions on mucous membranes

TABLE 102–1. Common Causes of Acute Vesicular Exanthems

Infectious
Viral
Varicella-zoster virus
Herpes simplex virus
Enterovirus: coxsackievirus A16

Bacterial
Staphylococcus aureus

Parasitic
Sarcoptes scabiei

Fungal
Trichophyton rubrum
T. mentagrophytes

Noninfectious
Contact dermatitis
Rhus (plant) dermatitis
Dyshidrotic eczema

Sarcoptes scabiei, can cause an intensely pruritic vesicular eruption in combination with papules and linear burrows (see Chapter 100, Papulosquamous Eruptions). Fungal pathogens that cause vesiculopustular lesions that appear on the feet and toes include *Trichophyton rubrum, T. mentagrophytes,* and less commonly, *Epidermophyton floccosum.* A delayed hypersensitivity reaction secondary to contact with an oleoresin of the poison ivy or poison oak plant causes the classic linear vesicular lesions of *Rhus* dermatitis. Contact with other allergenic substances may also produce a vesicular rash. The etiology of dyshidrotic eczema, a vesicular eruption involving mainly the hands and feet, is unknown.

The differential diagnosis of acute vesicular exanthems also can be organized according to the distribution of the lesions. Distinctive locations as well as specific patterns are important to consider in each individual case. The presence or absence of fever (a temperature ≥ 101° F [38.3° C]) can also be key to developing the appropriate differential (Figure 102–1). Epidemiologic, as well as historic, information may suggest the diagnosis. For example, known exposure to varicella (chickenpox) 10–21 days prior to a vesicular eruption facilitates diagnosis of this disease. A history of hiking or camping suggests possible contact with poison ivy or poison oak. In addition, the presence of a specific prodrome can often be elicited with primary or recurrent herpes simplex. Pain on swallowing often occurs with coxsackie virus infection. A past history of similar lesions lessens the likelihood of acute primary infection and suggests a chronic condition such as the recurrent disorder pompholyx (dyshidrotic eczema).

EVALUATION

History

A thorough history should be obtained (Questions Box). Practitioners must inquire about the current state of general health, as well as the specific details about the eruption.

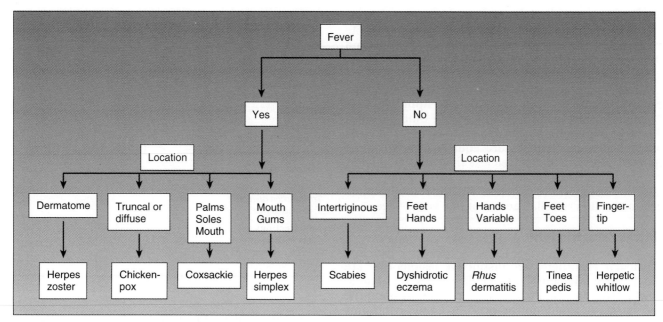

FIGURE 102–1. Approach to the evaluation of vesicular eruptions.

Physical Examination

Although the physical examination focuses on the skin, other aspects of the examination are helpful diagnostically. Vital signs should be taken to verify the presence or absence of fever. The oropharynx should be examined closely for vesicular or ulcerative lesions on the tongue, gingiva, buccal mucosa, anterior tonsillar pillars, and posterior pharynx. The lips should also be examined for any evidence of vesicular lesions that may occur with a primary or recurrent herpes simplex infection.

Patients should be completely unclothed to permit a thorough examination of the skin. The distribution of the lesions should be noted. Physicians should determine whether the vesicles are grouped in a particular dermatomal distribution, as with zoster (shingles), or more generally distributed and in various stages of development, as with varicella. A linear distribution may suggest contact with poison ivy or poison oak. Physicians should also ask the following questions: Do the lesions include or exclude the palms and soles? Are the buttocks involved? Are the lesions concentrated on one specific part of the body, such as the feet and toes or the hands? Are the sizes of the lesions uniform? If not, are other larger bullous-like lesions present in addition to vesicles?

It is also helpful, if at all possible, to examine the skin of family members for similar lesions.

Laboratory Tests

Few, if any, laboratory studies are usually needed in healthy children with vesicular eruptions because the diagnosis is often made clinically. Serologies are indicated in immunocompromised patients with an unknown history of varicella and a definite exposure to the virus. This information may be helpful when considering prophylaxis with varicella-zoster immune globulin (see Chapter 17, Immunizations).

Definitive confirmation of scabies can be made by microscopic examination of skin scrapings from suspicious lesions. The presence of the adult mite or ova, larva, or feces is diagnostic. For children with suspected tinea pedis, a skin scraping mixed with potassium hydroxide can be performed and examined under the microscope. Fungal cultures can also be taken. A Tzanck smear showing multinucleated giant cells that contain intranuclear viral inclusions may be useful in making a preliminary diagnosis of a herpesvirus, but commercially available monoclonal antibody tests are more accurate. A culture for herpes simplex can also be done in specific cases that pose diagnostic dilemmas.

MANAGEMENT

The mainstay of treatment for most vesicular eruptions is parent and child education as well as reassur-

---

Questions: Vesicular Exanthems

- How long has the child had the rash? Where is it located?
- Does the child have associated symptoms such as fever, runny nose, cough, or sore throat?
- Does the child have nonspecific symptoms such as decreased appetite?
- If the child has any symptoms accompanying the rash, did these develop at the same time as the rash?
- Is there any reason to suspect that the patient is relatively immunocompromised from chronic steroid use, chemotherapy, or an acquired immunodeficiency?
- Does the child have a history of similar lesions?
- Does anyone else in the family have a similar rash?
- Has the child been camping or hiking in the woods?

ance. Conditions are usually self-limited and require only **supportive therapy.** For example, hand-foot-and-mouth disease is self-limited and no treatment except parental reassurance and education regarding adequate hydration is necessary. Depending on the etiology of the vesicular rash, immunocompromised children such as those with HIV or AIDS and patients who are receiving chemotherapeutic agents or systemic corticosteroids may require specific intervention.

Topical agents such as calamine lotion, oatmeal soaks, or Aveeno baths should be used in children with intense pruritus or multiple lesions. Topical products, which are potentially sensitizing (e.g., diphenhydra-mine-containing agents) should not be used. Cool wet compresses with plain water or Burow's solution can be quite soothing in cases of *Rhus* dermatitis. Wet compresses may also be helpful with open, macerated lesions of dyshidrotic eczema.

Antipyretics (acetaminophen, ibuprofen) may be used to treat otherwise healthy children with varicella. Aspirin-containing medications should be avoided in children with varicella because of the association with Reye syndrome. Antipyretic therapy may also be indicated for symptomatic relief of pain associated with herpetic gingivostomatitis or coxsackie virus mouth lesions.

Oral antihistamines (diphenhydramine or hydroxy-zine) may be used in children with varicella or scabies for treatment of pruritus. These drugs are also helpful in *Rhus* dermatitis.

Steroids may be effective in the control of some vesicular rashes however, the practitioner must first be certain the lesions are not secondary to varicella or herpes simplex. Topical steroids can be used for outbreaks of vesicles of dyshidrotic eczema on the palms, soles, and lateral aspects of the hands. Although these agents are used by many practitioners to treat *Rhus* dermatitis, their role is minimal. In severe cases of *Rhus* dermatitis, a course of systemic steroids, such as prednisone, 1–2 mg/kg/day, may be warranted.

Oral acyclovir is not recommended routinely for the treatment of uncomplicated varicella in otherwise healthy children, but should be considered when the risk of developing moderate to severe disease is increased. According to the Committee on Infectious Diseases of the American Academy of Pediatrics (AAP), acyclovir is indicated in patients older than 12 years of age, those with chronic cutaneous or pulmonary disorders, or those receiving chronic therapy or short, intermittent courses of salicylates or corticosteroids (systemic or aerosolized). Acyclovir is most effective if initiated within the first 24 hours of the exanthem. (See the 1997 *Red Book* of the AAP for further details and specific recommendations regarding immunocompromised children and the role of varicella-zoster immune globulin.) A live attenuated varicella vaccine has been licensed for use in the United States since 1995, is available, and recommended for all nonimmune individuals (See Chapter 17, Immunizations).

Additional recommendations for children with varicella include keeping fingernails short in young children to prevent superinfection of lesions from scratching.

Children should drink plenty of fluids to avoid dehydration. Patients are considered contagious from 1–2 days prior to the onset of the rash until the lesions are all scabbed over (usually 5–7 days after the rash develops), at which time, children may return to school. In children with persistent or recurrent fever, secondary complications should be considered. A significant association between primary varicella injection and invasive group A beta-hemolytic streptococcal injection has been recognized and should be considered in the child with fever on or beyond the fourth day of the illness.

Treatment for zoster, or shingles, is primarily symptomatic and should consist of pain medications. Acyclovir can be considered if the eruption becomes generalized or affects immunocompromised patients. Herpetic whitlow, a HSV infection on the finger tip as a result of direct autoinoculation from oral lesions, and herpes gladiatorum, a cutaneous HSV infection on the skin seen in wrestlers, do not require treatment with antiviral agents such as acyclovir.

Bullous impetigo requires **oral antistaphylococcal therapy** with agents such as amoxicillin and clavulanate (Augmentin), erythromycin, or cefalexin (Keflex). Augmentin can be given two times a day for a total dose of 20–45 mg/kg/day. Diarrhea is the most common side effect and is dose dependent. The dose of either erythromycin or Keflex is 40 mg/kg/day and should be given four times daily. Erythromycin should be taken with meals or milk to lessen the likelihood of gastrointestinal upset.

For the treatment of tinea pedis, topical **antifungal agents,** such as 2% miconazole (Micatin), 1% tolnaftate (Tinactin), and undecylenate (Desenex), are available over the counter in powder form and can be applied twice daily. Antifungal creams (clotrimazole, ketoconazole), also available over the counter, can be used twice daily for four to six weeks. Vesicular lesions should be treated with wet compresses of Burow's solution, 1:80. The recommended application is 10–15 minutes three to four times a day for 3–5 days. In severe cases, an oral antifungal preparation, griseofulvin, may be prescribed for an extended period.

Tinea pedis can be difficult to control. Its treatment is centered around meticulous foot hygiene. Because careful foot care is often not a priority for most patients, complete eradication is not realistic. Patients should be instructed to wash and change their socks when they return from school, dry their feet completely, avoid occlusive shoes, and wear open-air shoes or sandals whenever possible. Cotton socks are recommended.

For the treatment of scabies, see Chapter 100, Papulosquamous Eruptions.

PROGNOSIS

Overall, the prognosis for vesicular exanthems is good, with most children recovering in 1–2 weeks, depending on the etiology. Secondary infections can occur with varicella, however, and should be suspected in children with persistent or recurrent fever. These complications include cellulitis, otitis media, pneumonia, and meningoencephalitis. Long-term sequelae associated with these secondary infections are rare. Reye syndrome, another complication of chickenpox, has an excellent prognosis when diagnosed early.

Case Resolution

In the case presented at the beginning of this chapter, the toddler has a classic presentation of primary varicella (chickenpox). Management should include symptomatic treatment with acetaminophen and antihistamines, along with topical preparations such as calamine lotion and oatmeal or Aveeno baths. The parent should be instructed regarding the natural course of this infection and be informed that the infection is highly contagious. In addition, symptoms indicating possible complications, such as persistent or recurrent fever, circumferential redness or swelling of the lesions, and shortness of breath, should be reviewed with the parents.

Selected Readings

American Academy of Pediatrics. Varicella-zoster infections. *In* Peter, G., (ed.). 1997 Red Book. Report of the Committee on Infectious Diseases, 24th ed. Elk Grove Village, IL, American Academy of Pediatrics, 1997:573–585.

Calvelli, F., and A. A. Gaspari. When the vesicles aren't chickenpox. Contemp. Pediatr. 10:48–62, 1993.

Eichenfield, L. F., and P. J. Honig. Blistering disorders in childhood. Pediatr. Clin. North Am. 38:959–976, 1991.

Freiden I. J., and S. D. Resnick. Childhood exanthems. Pediatr. Clin. North Am. 38:859–887, 1991.

Hurwitz, S. Clinical Pediatric Dermatology, 2nd ed. Philadelphia, W. B. Saunders, 1993.

Resnick S. D. New aspects of exanthematous diseases of childhood. Dermatol. Clin. 15:257–266, 1997.

THE NEW MORBIDITY

CHAPTER 103

ATTENTION DEFICIT/HYPERACTIVITY DISORDER

Iris Wagman Borowsky, M.D., Ph.D.

H$_x$ A 9-year-old boy is seen in the emergency department after nearly colliding with a car while riding his bicycle. He sustained only minor abrasions from a fall. The boy's mother states that her son is impulsive and frequently engages in risky behaviors. She reports that he is extremely active and has a short attention span. He is in the fourth grade and an average student, but he has a hard time following directions and is easily distracted in class. In addition, he tends to have trouble keeping friends.

In the examining room, the boy is quiet but answers questions appropriately. Except for a few scrapes, his physical examination is entirely normal.

Questions

1. What are the primary symptoms of attention deficit/hyperactivity disorder (ADHD)? What other conditions should be considered in the differential diagnosis of ADHD?
2. What other psychiatric disorders or neurodevelopmental disabilities commonly coexist with ADHD?
3. What is the appropriate evaluation of children with suspected ADHD?
4. What treatment modalities are useful in the management of ADHD?

Three major symptoms—inattention, impulsivity, and hyperactivity—are characteristic of ADHD. The *Diagnostic and Statistic Manual of Mental Disorders* (4th ed.) identifies three diagnostic subtypes of ADHD: (1) predominantly inattentive type, (2) predominantly hyperactive-impulsive type, and (3) combined type. Most children and adolescents with the disorder have the combined type, exhibiting symptoms of both inattention and hyperactivity-impulsivity.

Symptoms of ADHD must appear before 7 years of age and persist for at least 6 months before the disorder can be diagnosed. The behaviors are more frequent and severe than those typically seen in normal children at the same level of development and interfere with functioning in at least two settings (e.g., home and school).

EPIDEMIOLOGY

An estimated 3–5% of school-age children have ADHD. Boys are affected approximately six times as often as girls.

CLINICAL PRESENTATION

Children with ADHD have problems with selective attention. They may make careless mistakes or fail to pay attention to details. In addition, they are easily distracted and have difficulty concentrating on tasks long enough to complete them (D$_x$ Box). Difficulties following instructions and organizing tasks and activities are also characteristic of ADHD. Poor impulse control manifests as difficulty awaiting one's turn, frequently blurting out answers, and interrupting or intruding on others. Symptoms of hyperactivity include fidgetiness, difficulty remaining seated or playing quietly, and subjective feelings of restlessness in adolescents. Difficulties with social relationships and low frustration tolerance are also commonly seen in children with ADHD.

PATHOPHYSIOLOGY

The etiology of ADHD is unknown. Genetic, neurologic, and dietary factors may play a role.

Family studies indicate that **genetic factors** influence the development of ADHD. First-degree relatives of children with ADHD have a 25% risk of similar problems.

D$_x$ **Attention Deficit/Hyperactivity Disorder (Core Symptoms)**
• Inattention • Impulsivity • Hyperactivity

In addition, behavioral ratings and measures of attention are more alike in monozygotic twins than in same-sex dizygotic twins.

ADHD may be the result of **neurologic factors.** Patients with frontal lobe disorders exhibit inattention, impulsivity, and hyperactivity. The frontal and prefrontal regions of the brain appear to be involved in selective attention, distractibility, inhibition, planning, and organization. ADHD may be the result of neuroanatomic factors. Psychostimulants, the most effective pharmacologic therapy for ADHD, alter dopamine and catecholamine metabolism. Thus ADHD may have a neurochemical basis.

Various **dietary ingredients,** such as sugar, aspartame, food coloring, and food additives, have been implicated as a cause of hyperactivity and other behavioral problems in children. Many parents have put their children on special diets with no additives. Well-controlled studies have now shown that sugar and food additives have no adverse effects on behavior or cognitive function in children. Nevertheless, many parents believe that certain foods have negative effects on their children's behavior.

DIFFERENTIAL DIAGNOSIS

The symptoms of ADHD can be seen in a variety of conditions (Table 103–1). Developmental delay is frequently confused with ADHD. Sensory deficiencies, especially hearing impairment, can also imitate attention deficits. Inattention is often a component of autism, also called pervasive developmental disorder, but autistic children exhibit stereotyped behaviors and markedly impaired speech and social interactions. Iron deficiency anemia and low-level lead poisoning also may have detrimental effects on behavior and development. Seizure disorders, such as petit mal (absence) or partial complex seizures, may be misdiagnosed as ADHD. Possible side effects of certain medications, such as phenobarbital or theophylline, may mimic ADHD. Hy-

---

TABLE 103–1. Differential Diagnosis of Attention Deficit/Hyperactivity Disorder

Developmental delay
Learning disability
Language disorder
Sensory deficiencies (especially hearing impairment)
Autism
Seizure disorder
Iron deficiency
Environmental toxins (lead)
Side effects of medication (phenobarbital)
Hyperthyroidism
Congenital infection
In utero exposure to drugs or alcohol
Previous brain insult (trauma, infection)
Family stresses
Ineffective parenting
Psychiatric disorders
   Conduct disorder
   Oppositional disorder
   Anxiety disorders
   Affective disorders (depression, bipolar illness)
   Personality disorders (aggression, antisocial behavior)
   Substance abuse

Questions: Attention Deficit/Hyperactivity Disorder

- What are the problem behaviors?
- How old was the child when the behaviors began?
- Where do the behaviors occur (at home, at school, or in both settings)?
- Did the child's mother develop any infections during the pregnancy?
- Did the child's mother use alcohol, marijuana, or any other drugs during the pregnancy?
- Were there any perinatal complications?
- At what age did the child attain various developmental milestones?
- Does the child take any medications?
- Does the child have any history of trauma, seizures, meningitis, or recurrent OM?
- What is the child's temperament and personality?
- Does the family have a history of ADHD, learning disability, or substance abuse, or other psychiatric disorders?

---

perthyroidism can cause the symptoms of ADHD, but other signs of increased metabolism, such as elevated heart rate, tremors, or weight loss, should be apparent. Exposure to alcohol or drugs *in utero* has been associated with subtle difficulties with learning and attention at a later time. Congenital infections, CNS infections in early childhood, and traumatic brain injuries may produce behaviors similar to those seen in ADHD.

In addition, psychosocial problems, such as family stresses (e.g., marital discord, unemployment, poverty, substance abuse) or ineffective parenting (e.g., inconsistent discipline) must be considered in the differential diagnosis of ADHD. Comorbidity is extremely common in children with ADHD. Up to 44% of these children carry another psychiatric diagnosis, 32% carry two other diagnoses, and 11% carry three other diagnoses. Learning or language disabilities, conduct disorder, oppositional disorder, anxiety, depression, and bipolar illness commonly coexist with ADHD in children. In adolescents and young adults, personality disorders such as aggression and antisocial behavior and substance abuse are often seen together with attention deficits. These conditions can magnify the symptoms of children with ADHD or may explain the symptoms entirely.

EVALUATION

History

The diagnostic evaluation of ADHD should begin with a description by caregivers of the child's problem behaviors, including examples of situations in which the behaviors occur. A thorough history should be obtained (Questions Box). The physician should find out how parents handle their child's behavioral problems; this provides insight into their parenting style. Family stresses should be evaluated. Interviewing the child alone provides an opportunity for the child to describe his or her thoughts and feelings. The physician should ask what problems the child is having at home and at school and find out how the child is coping with these difficulties.

Copies of report cards and teachers' descriptions of children's behavior are extremely helpful in obtaining the school history. Speaking to children's current teachers directly may also be useful. In addition, many rating scales (e.g., Conners scales, child behavior checklist) have been developed to allow parents and teachers to report children's behavior in various domains (e.g., inattention, hyperactivity, anxiety, aggression). These scales are used to aid in the diagnosis of ADHD as well as to evaluate the effects of treatment.

Physical Examination

The physical examination should include an assessment of growth parameters and any minor congenital anomalies as well as a careful neurologic examination. The child's weight, height, and head circumference should be plotted on a growth curve and the pattern of growth evaluated. Children should be examined for dysmorphic features such as the facies associated with fetal alcohol syndrome. A neurologic examination should include an assessment of the child's affect, speech, hearing, and vision. Some children with ADHD exhibit indicators of neuromaturational delays, the so-called soft neurologic signs, such as choreiform movements, involuntary movements, and motor slowness.

Observing the child's behavior during the office visit is important, but most children with ADHD do not display hyperactivity in the office. Interaction between the child and his or her parents should be observed. The physician should note whether the child listens to parental instructions and how parents deal with any misbehavior. Does the child cooperate with the examination? How well does the child relate to adults? The physician should watch the child play (e.g., draw, play with toys) and note the child's organization of activities, attention span, distractibility, and motor activity.

Laboratory Tests

The history and physical examination should direct the laboratory evaluation. Referral for further evaluation of speech, hearing, and vision should be done if indicated. A hematocrit and lead level are useful to rule out iron deficiency anemia and lead intoxication. Thyroid function tests are appropriate if signs or symptoms of hyperthyroidism are present (e.g., increased appetite, hyperactive precordium).

Psychometric tests of intelligence (IQ) and academic achievement help identify learning disabilities. Tests designed specifically to measure attention and impulsivity can be helpful, particularly in assessing response to medication.

Diagnostic Studies

An EEG is indicated if absence or partial complex seizures are suspected.

MANAGEMENT

Treatment of ADHD must be multifaceted and long-term to be successful. Family education is essential, and counseling about ADHD should provide factual informa-

tion about the disorder, emphasize the strengths of children and families, and address parental concerns. The physician can ease parents' guilt by telling them that their children's problems are not the result of insufficient parenting. Children who discover that their problems are not their fault may feel that a heavy burden has been lifted from their shoulders. Both parents and children may find it difficult to accept that the child has a chronic disorder, however. The pediatrician can help by supporting families' efforts to seek treatment. Support groups for parents of children with ADHD can also provide assistance.

Behavior Management

The goals of behavior management include helping children learn to follow rules and complete important tasks, increasing children's self-control, and reducing stress within families. Management of overactive children who have difficulty focusing attention, following rules, and controlling impulses can be challenging for both parents and teachers. As often as possible, parents should give children positive feedback for good behavior and should set a good example for children. Parents should focus on one behavior at a time, such as doing homework, putting toys away, or completing chores.

Behavioral techniques include rewards for positive behaviors (e.g., verbal praise, hugs, points or stars on a chart that can be traded for material objects, special time with a parent or friend) and punishments for unacceptable behaviors (e.g., time out, loss of a privilege, extra chores, reduction in allowance). Acceptable and unacceptable behaviors should be clearly defined, and rewards and punishments should be spelled out in a contract drawn up with children. Because children with ADHD tend to lose interest in these behavioral programs over time, parents must be creative in periodically varying the rewards and penalties.

Educational Interventions

The pediatric practitioner can play an important role in optimizing each child's educational experience by keeping in contact with the child's teachers and attending school conferences where specific educational alternatives for the child with ADHD are discussed. Most children with ADHD can be managed in the regular classroom. If they are having behavioral or academic difficulties in the regular classroom, special educational placement in a smaller, more focused setting for part or all of the day may be indicated.

Teachers can help children with ADHD focus their attention and follow directions in the classroom in several ways (Table 103–2). Also, they should focus on and nurture children's strengths and provide children with many opportunities to experience success in the classroom. In addition, teachers should be supportive, try not to embarrass children but instead should foster their self-esteem. Positive reinforcement for good behavior as well as negative consequences for misbehavior should be addressed immediately. This can be achieved through a system in which points are gained or lost for specific behaviors. Accumulated points can be

TABLE 103–2. Strategies for Managing Children With ADHD in the Classroom

Seat children in the front of the classroom, where distractions can be minimized and teachers can see whether children are paying attention

Cue children secretly to remind them to refocus their attention

Give clear instructions and repeat them frequently

Shorten work periods by allowing children to get up and move around (e.g., handing out papers, cleaning chalkboard)

"cashed in" at the end of the day for a desired activity (e.g., playing a game). Teachers who are most successful in working with children with ADHD are able to set firm limits and discipline children without anger or frustration, while at the same time remaining flexible enough to recognize when a change in tactics is necessary.

Because children with ADHD are easily provoked into misbehavior and are prone to clashes with peers, they can also benefit from closer supervision in unstructured school areas such as the playground, cafeteria, halls, and bus. Programs designed to improve social competence and peer relationships (e.g., group social skills training, therapeutic recreational activities) may also be helpful.

Pharmacotherapy

Research has shown that medications produce short-term benefits for children with ADHDs, including longer attention span, better impulse control, and lower activity levels. Significant long-term effects such as improved social adjustment and school achievement have not been demonstrated. When used in combination with other treatment approaches, medications usually help school-age children. Children below 5 years of age are less likely to respond to drug therapy and are at greater risk of experiencing adverse effects.

Psychostimulants, the most commonly used agents for ADHDs, have an estimated response rate of 80%. The most commonly prescribed psychostimulants are methylphenidate (Ritalin), dextroamphetamine (Dexedrine), and pemoline (Cylert). Some children suffer adverse effects such as decreased appetite, insomnia, tics, headaches, and stomach aches. Methylphenidate, the most widely used and best studied of the psychostimulants, is usually prescribed first because it has minimal side effects. The usual effective dose is 0.3–0.7 mg/kg. An initial dose of 5–10 mg is typically given in the morning. If teachers report an improvement in morning classroom behavior, this dose can be continued; otherwise, it should be increased in increments of 2.5 or 5.0 mg per week until an effective level is reached. This dose can then be given two or three times a day. The third dose is given to help children complete homework assignments in the late afternoon. Weekend dosing is optional, depending on children's behavior and scheduled activities. Sustained-release methylphenidate is available to simplify dosing, but this form of the drug may not be as effective as the tablets.

A poor response to one stimulant does not predict a poor response to another. Dextroamphetamine and pemoline, which are both longer-acting than methylphenidate, may be appropriate if frequent dosing is a problem.

The physician should maintain close contact with children's teachers to monitor effects of medication, both positive and negative. Children who are doing well should have a brief examination approximately every 2 months, with particular attention to weight, height, and blood pressure. For children who are beginning to lose weight, the dose and schedule of medication can be changed to improve appetite at mealtimes. Because pemoline can be hepatotoxic, baseline and every-6-month monitoring of transaminase levels have been recommended with its use.

If psychostimulants are not effective or produce unacceptable side effects, clonidine or antidepressants (e.g., TCAs, monoamine oxidase inhibitors) may be introduced. These agents have some positive effects on the behavior of children with ADHDs.

Biofeedback

Studies suggest that some older children can learn to focus their attention through the use of biofeedback techniques. These techniques involve having children observe their EEG waves and selectively suppress certain waves. The technique is time and labor intensive and currently not readily available to all children.

PROGNOSIS

ADHD is a chronic condition, and over 50% of affected children continue to exhibit symptoms of ADHD into adulthood. Adults have an increased incidence of anxiety, low self-esteem, antisocial behavior, alcohol and drug abuse, interpersonal difficulties, and job changes. Poor outcomes are associated with lower intelligence, lower economic status, conduct problems, and family psychopathology (e.g., alcohol or drug abuse). Individual outcomes can be very good, however.

Case Resolution

In the case history presented at the beginning of this chapter, the boy's mother expresses concerns about her son's behavior. She describes symptoms of ADHD. The boy is referred to his primary care physician for diagnostic evaluation, which should include a full history, physical examination, and an assessment from his school.

Selected Readings

Altemeier, W. A., and Horwitz, E. The role of the school in the management of attention deficit hyperactivity disorder. Pediatr. Ann. 26:737–744, 1997.

American Psychiatric Association: Diagnostic and Statistical Manual of Mental Disorders, 4th ed. Washington, D.C., American Psychiatric Association, 1994.

Cantwell, D. P. Attention deficit disorder: A review of the past 10 years. J. Amer. Acad. Child Adolesc. Psychiatry 35:978–987, 1996.

Culbert, T. P., G. A. Banez, and M. I. Reiff. Children who have attentional disorders: Interventions. Pediatr. Rev. 15:5–14, 1994.

Current issues in attention deficit disorder. J. Clin. Psychiatry 59 (suppl. 7):1–82, 1998. (Entire issue on attention deficit disorder.)

Kelly, D. P., and G. P. Aylward: Attention deficits in school-aged children and adolescents: current issues and practice. Pediatr. Clin. North Am. 39:487–512, 1992.

Linden, M., Habib, T., and V. Radojevic. A controlled study of the effects of EEG biofeedback on cognition and behavior of children with attention deficit disorder and learning disabilities. Biofeedback Self Regul. 21:35–49, 1996.

National Institutes of Health. Diagnosis and treatment of attention deficit hyperactivity disorder. NIH Consensus Statement 1998 Nov. 16–18; 16(2).

Reiff, M. I., G. A. Banez, and T. P. Culbert. Children who have attentional disorders: diagnosis and evaluation. Pediatr. Rev. 14:455–464, 1993.

Soothill, J. F. Management of hyperactive inattentive children. Lancet 351:429–433, 1998.

Wolraich, M. L., et al. Effects of diet high in sucrose or aspartame on the behavior and cognitive performance of children. N. Engl. J. Med. 330:301–307, 1994.

Zametkin, A. J., and M. Ernst. Problems in the management of attention-deficit–hyperactivity disorder. N. Engl. J. Med. 340:40–46, 1999.

CHAPTER   1 0 4

PHYSICAL ABUSE

Carol D. Berkowitz, M.D.

H$_x$ A 6-month-old male infant arrives at the emergency department after becoming limp and nonresponsive at home. The mother states that her son was fine when she left him in the care of her boyfriend before going to the store for cigarettes. When she returned 1 hour later, he was asleep, but then he seized and stopped breathing. The infant is being ventilated by a bag.

On examination, the infant is pale and limp. The heart rate is 100 beats/min, and the blood pressure is 90/30. The only abnormality is the presence of bilateral retinal hemorrhages.

Questions

1. What are the major lethal injuries associated with physical abuse of children?
2. What are the types of injuries seen in physically abused children?
3. What are the presenting complaints of children with head injuries?
4. What are the legal obligations of physicians in the area of child abuse?

Physical child abuse was first described in the pediatric literature in 1962 by Kempe, et al in their classic paper on the battered child syndrome. Child abuse or maltreatment takes many forms, including physical abuse, FTT, sexual abuse, emotional abuse, prenatal exposure to substances such as drugs and alcohol, and Munchausen syndrome by proxy, a complex disorder in which parents confabulate or create a medical condition in their children

The nature and extent of inflicted injuries is variable and includes bruises, burns, fractures, lacerations, internal hemorrhage, and ruptures. Physicians must be aware of the legal obligations related to the suspicion of child abuse. They must assess the nature of the injuries, initiate appropriate medical therapy, and determine if the history offered is consistent with the medical findings.

EPIDEMIOLOGY

Over two million cases of child abuse are reported annually in the United States. Certain factors are associated with physical abuse. Most victims are young children; two-thirds are under the age of 3 years, and one-third are under the age of 6 months. Caring for young children is frequently demanding. Crying infants and toilet-training toddlers are particularly at risk for abuse. Factors such as lower socioeconomic class; substance abuse; poor parenting skills; and domestic violence, including spousal abuse, place children at risk for abuse.

CLINICAL PRESENTATION

Children who have been physically abused present with injuries that range from nonsevere to lethal (D$_x$ Box). Visible bruises, bites, and burns may be noted. Children may also have symptoms related to fractures, such as crying or refusal to walk or move an extremity. More severely injured children may present with seizures, apnea, shock, or cardiopulmonary arrest.

PATHOPHYSIOLOGY

Injuries in children who experience physical abuse are the result of direct trauma inflicted on the children. Head injuries, the most deadly form of abuse, may result from either a direct blow to the head or shaking. Classically, a crying infant is vigorously shaken and suffers acute axonal brain injury. This leads to "shaken

<table>
<tr><td>

Dx **Physical Abuse**

- Bruises
- Bites
- Burns
- Fractures
- Intracranial hemorrhage
- Intraabdominal hemorrhage
- Retinal hemorrhage
- History that changes
- Injuries not explained by history

</td></tr>
</table>

TABLE 104–1. Causes of Retinal Hemorrhages

Inflicted head trauma
Nonintentional head trauma (rare)
Birth trauma
Blood dyscrasias
Meningitis
Papilledema
Hypertension
Cytomegalovirus retinitis
High-altitude illness
Lead toxicity
Carbon monoxide toxicity
Methanol intoxication

baby syndrome" or "shaken impact syndrome." The infant stops crying and seems to fall asleep. Subdural bleeding occurs as bridging blood vessels are disrupted. In addition, brain swelling, apnea, and seizures result. The child may exhibit retinal hemorrhages as well as skeletal trauma. Such injuries are frequently associated with a fatal outcome or long-term damage to the CNS.

Circumstances surrounding other inflicted injuries is similar. Abusive parents often have unrealistic expectations of their children, especially around the time of toilet training. These parents have often been victims of abuse themselves. Corporal punishment is the only disciplinary modality they know. These parents also exhibit poor impulse control. Frequently they do not intend to harm their children but desire to alter children's behavior, and sometimes the outcome is unexpected.

DIFFERENTIAL DIAGNOSIS

When evaluating children with physical injuries, the major differentiation involves distinguishing between injuries that are intentional from those that are nonintentional. Practitioners should be suspicious of stories that change or are inconsistent with the injuries that children have sustained. Unwitnessed injuries in young children, particularly if they are preambulatory, should also be suspect.

Bruises, burns, and fractures may be intentional or nonintentional. Normal ambulatory children sustain bruises over bony prominences such as the shins with nonintentional trauma. Bruises over soft areas such as the thighs and cheeks or the pinnae of the ear suggest inflicted trauma. Injuries to the oral mucosa may result from efforts at forced feeding or occlusion of the mouth in an effort to silence crying. Retinal hemorrhages in infants most often result from intentional head trauma, such as shaking. They may also be due to other medical conditions that can usually be discerned from the history and physical examination (Table 104–1).

Children may be intentionally burned by being immersed in hot water or having hot objects such as irons or cigarettes held against them. Children who are immersed in hot water develop burns that may envelop an entire extremity, usually in a glove or stocking pattern, or form a doughnut pattern on the buttocks. These burns are distinct from splash or spill burns, which take on a drip pattern.

Long bone (especially humerus and femur) fractures should be suspect, particularly in preambulatory infants. Most falls do not result in fractures. Certain fractures, such as metaphysical chip fractures and rib, sternum, and scapula fractures, are highly suggestive of inflicted trauma.

Numerous medical conditions may mimic abuse. Bullous impetigo may resemble burns. A coagulopathy may lead to multiple bruises. Leukemia, thrombocytopenia, and aplastic anemia are also associated with bruises. Osteogenesis imperfecta may result in multiple fractures. Osteoporosis may be associated with meningomyelocele, and pathologic fractures of the long bones may occur as a result. Bone cysts may also lead to pathologic fractures.

EVALUATION

Children who present with injuries need to be evaluated with a careful history and complete physical examination. Infants with altered mental status should be evaluated in a similar manner, because their symptoms may be secondary to intracranial injury.

History

The history should focus on an explanation for the medical findings (Questions Box). Children should be interviewed alone if they are of an appropriate age. Physicians should determine if other risk factors, such as domestic violence or substance abuse, are present.

Questions: Physical Abuse

- What caused the injury?
- Was the child healthy until the injury occurred?
- Has the child sustained similar injuries in the past?
- Is there a family history of any conditions that would account for easy bruisability or fragility of the bones (e.g., von Willebrand's disease, osteogenesis imperfecta)?
- Is the child developmentally normal? Are the child's motor skills normal?
- Who was with the child when the injury occurred?
- What was done immediately after the injury? Was medical care sought?

Physical Examination

Children's state of hygiene and growth should be noted. The physical examination should be comprehensive. The location and color of bruises should be carefully recorded. Bruises tend to heal in distinctive patterns (Table 104–2). However, dating of bruises is imprecise because the degradation rate of hemoglobin within the bruise is influenced by the depth and extent of the bruise, and also the child's health and nutritional status. Large, blue spots, which are frequently apparent over the lower back in African-American, Hispanic, and Asian children, are referred to as Mongolian spots. These should not be mistaken for bruises.

Physicians should check for burns or other injuries, including pinch marks in the genital area, which may be inflicted on toddlers who have had a toilet-training accident.

In addition, physicians should look for any characteristic patterns that may have resulted from inflicted injuries, such as slap marks to the face or gag marks around the mouth. Belts, cords, and blunt instruments may also produce particular marks, referred to as patterned injuries (Fig. 104–1). Bite marks leave indentations of teeth that are unique to the perpetrator. Inflicted burns may also assume a characteristic pattern, such as a glove-stocking distribution (Fig. 104–2).

Practitioners should be aware that infants with injuries of the head and abdomen may present with no external signs of trauma but have seizures, apnea, or altered mental status, often with no explanation. The retina should be evaluated for hemorrhages.

Children with abdominal injuries may be in shock or have gastrointestinal symptoms such as vomiting, abdominal pain, or distention. Injuries may include hematomas of the bowel wall, perforations of the bowel, or trauma to solid organs such as the liver, spleen, pancreas, or kidneys. On physical examination, children may have signs of a surgical abdomen with rigidity, guarding, and diminished bowel sounds.

Laboratory Tests

Children who present with bruises should have a hematologic assessment, with a CBC and differential, including a platelet count, a PT, and a PTT. Cultures from lesions may help differentiate infection from burn injury.

Children with suspected abdominal trauma should be evaluated with a CBC, urinalysis, liver function studies, and amylase. These studies may demonstrate anemia secondary to hemorrhage, hematuria from renal injury, and elevated amylase from pancreatic trauma (see Chapter 43, Abdominal Trauma).

TABLE 104–2. Discoloration Caused by Healing Bruises

Color	Usual Healing Period
Swelling without discoloration	< 1 d
Purple color	1–5 d
Green color	5–7 d
Yellow color	7–10 d
Brown color	10–14 d

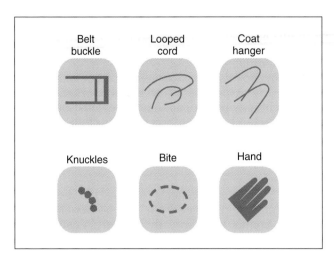

FIGURE 104–1. Patterned bruises associated with inflicted trauma.

Imaging Studies

Children with bruises should be evaluated with a skeletal survey to determine the existence of additional injuries or evidence of skeletal dysplasia. Scintigraphy is also useful in detecting occult fractures, such as those involving the ribs or scapulae.

Children with symptoms of head injury should be evaluated with CT scans and MRI studies. The combination of these two modalities is particularly useful in detecting hemorrhage in different areas and dating intracranial bleeding (see Chapter 44, Head Trauma).

Abdominal x-rays may demonstrate a disordered motility pattern with air-fluid levels or distended loops of bowel. Other imaging studies may show organ disruption or hemorrhage. Free air may be present under the diaphragm if there has been bowel perforation.

MANAGEMENT

The management of children who are suspected victims of abuse focuses on medical stabilization and psychosocial investigation. Injuries should be treated in the appropriate manner. Children with extensive inter-

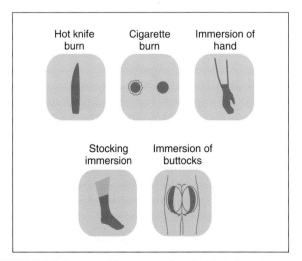

FIGURE 104–2. Patterned burns associated with inflicted trauma.

nal injuries frequently require admission to an intensive care unit. Consultation with appropriate surgical specialists in neurosurgery, orthopedics, or general surgery should be obtained.

The psychosocial assessment of the family often requires the expertise of a social worker. Further assessment may require an in-home evaluation such as that conducted by law enforcement or child protective services. All 50 states require that physicians who suspect child abuse report these suspicions to appropriate agencies. Physicians do not have to be certain of the abuse.

These mandated agencies pursue the evaluation. Children may be removed from their homes and placed in foster homes to ensure their safety. Cases of suspected abuse are usually evaluated in court to determine the safety of children's environment, the ability of parents to care for their children, and the criminal culpability of suspected perpetrators. Physicians may be expected to offer evidence in such hearings.

PROGNOSIS

The prognosis is variable. Some children succumb to inflicted injuries before coming to medical attention, and others sustain permanent neurologic damage. Even in cases in which the physical well-being of children is assured, their self-esteem has often been irreparably damaged.

Case Resolution

The opening vignette describes a classic case of shaken baby syndrome. The infant was left alone with an individual with limited parenting skills. Most likely, the crying infant was vigorously shaken, resulting in axonal injury, subdural hemorrhage, loss of consciousness, altered mental status, and seizures. The infant is intubated, given anticonvulsants, and admitted to a pediatric intensive care unit. Consultation with neurosurgery, ophthalmology, and social service is obtained. Appropriate imaging studies and skeletal surveys are performed when the infant is sufficiently stabilized.

Selected Readings

Chadwick, D. L. The diagnosis of inflicted injury in infants and young children. Pediatr. Ann. 21:477–483, 1992.

Davis, H. W., and B. J. Zitelli. Childhood injuries: accidental or inflicted? Contemp. Pediatr. 12:94–112, 1995.

Duhaime, A. C., et al. Head injury in very young children: mechanisms, injury types, and ophthalmologic findings in 100 hospitalized patients younger than 2 years of age. Pediatrics 90:179–185. 1992.

Feldman, K. W. Evaluation of physical abuse. In The Battered Child. Helfer, M. E., Kempe, R. S., and R. D. Krugman (eds.). Chicago, University of Chicago Press, pp. 175–220, 1997.

Johnson, C. F. Inflicted injury versus accidental injury. Pediatr. Clin. North Am. 37:791–814. 1990.

Kempe, C. H., et al: The battered child syndrome. JAMA 181:17–24, 1962.

Kleinman, P. R. Diagnostic Imaging of Child Abuse. St. Louis, Mosby, 1998.

Leventhal, J. M., et al. Fractures in young children: distinguishing child abuse from unintentional injuries. Am. J. Dis. Child. 147:87–92, 1993.

Monteleone, J. A., and A. E. Brodeur. Child Maltreatment. A Clinical Guide and Reference. St. Louis, G. W. Medical Publishing, Inc., 1994.

Reece, R. M. (ed.). Child Abuse: Medical Diagnosis and Management. Philadelphia, Lea & Febiger, 1994.

Schwartz, A. J., and L. R. Ricci. How accurately can bruises be aged in abused children? Literature review and synthesis. Pediatrics 97:254–257, 1996.

Sirontnak, A. P., and R. D. Krugman. Physical abuse of children: an update. Pediatr. Rev. 15:394–399, 1994.

CHAPTER 105

CHILD SEXUAL ABUSE

Carol D. Berkowitz, M.D.

H$_x$ A 4-year-old girl is brought to the emergency department with the complaint of vaginal itching and discharge. Her past health has been good, and she has no medical problems. She lives with her biologic parents and her 2-year-old brother.

On physical examination, the vital signs are normal, and the child is well except that the genital area is swollen and erythematous and a green vaginal discharge is present. The girl is interviewed briefly but denies that anyone has touched her. The mother states that she has never left her daughter unattended and is angered by the questions.

Questions

1. What are the anogenital findings in prepubescent and postpubescent children who may have experienced sexual abuse?
2. What behavioral problems are common in children who have been sexually abused?
3. What are the pitfalls in disclosure interviews of children who have been sexually abused?
4. What is the significance of sexually transmitted diseases in children who have been sexually abused?

Child sexual abuse is the involvement of children and adolescents in sexual activity that they cannot consent to because of their age and developmental level. An age disparity exists between the victims, who are younger, and the perpetrators, who are older. The intent of the abuse is the sexual gratification of the older individuals.

Sexual abuse has been recognized with increasing frequency since the 1980s, in part because medical knowledge about the anogenital anatomy in both normal and molested prepubescent children has expanded. Technical advances have altered the manner in which these children are evaluated. In particular, the colposcope, with its potential for magnification, and photographic or videotape documentation has been valuable. Parental awareness and school-based programs have led to increased disclosures about abuse as well as greater willingness on the part of adults to believe these disclosures.

Patient interviews are another key component of the assessment process. Nonleading, open-ended questions are asked by experts as few times as possible.

EPIDEMIOLOGY

Over two million cases of child abuse are reported annually in the United States. Between 20 and 40% of these cases involve allegations of child sexual abuse. Exact figures on the prevalence of child sexual abuse are not readily available, because they depend on reports of a condition that may not come to medical attention for many years, but data suggest that approximately 0.5–1% of children in the United States are sexually abused annually. Anonymous surveys indicate that about 20–25% of women and 10–15% of men have been sexually abused before reaching adulthood.

Victims of sexual abuse come from all socioeconomic and ethnic groups. Approximately 75% of victims who come to medical attention are girls and 25% are boys. Some investigators believe that the statistics for boys are falsely low because boys are generally reluctant to disclose their abuse. Girls are often victimized by male family members, such as fathers (biologic fathers and stepfathers), mothers' boyfriends, uncles, and grandfathers. Boys are more likely to be molested out of the home by nonrelatives, including coaches and teachers. Boys are more likely than girls to be abused by female perpetrators.

Frequently, the sexual abuse has been occurring for several years. The mean time from onset of abuse to disclosure is 3 years. Sometimes children are not ready to disclose but the abuse is discovered accidentally because the victims develop symptoms, such as vaginal discharge, or functional complaints. A routine or comprehensive physical examination may reveal anogenital abnormalities.

STDs, which vary in frequency in different geographic locations, are reported in between 2 and 28% of children who have been sexually abused (average estimated range: 10–15%). The incidence is higher in older children, particularly in adolescents.

CLINICAL PRESENTATION

Children may present with complaints related to the anogenital region such as bleeding, pain, swelling, dysuria, vaginal discharge, or difficulty stooling. More often, children have no specific anogenital symptoms. Instead, they have nonspecific complaints such as headache, abdominal pain, or vague systemic symptoms (e.g., fatigue). Behavioral changes may also be noted. These include sleep disturbances, hyperactivity, enuresis, encopresis, decreased appetite, and depression. Sexually abused adolescents manifest other behavioral problems such as school failure, delinquency, promiscuity, and suicide attempts. Some children may present with a history of sexually abusive experiences (D_x Box).

PSYCHOPHYSIOLOGY

Children suffer sexual abuse after becoming entrapped. Children may be enticed with promises of rewards or presents. They may be made to feel special or grown-up by being allowed to engage in adult behavior. Some children do not regard the sexual experiences as threatening but rather a means by which they can obtain the love they crave. Only when they grow older do they realize that these sexual relationships were not normal or appropriate.

Other children are coerced into sexual activity with threats of physical harm. Once they have acquiesced, they are maintained in the relationship with threats of reprisal if they disclose the abuse. Children feel both guilty and responsible for what has happened. This sense of responsibility is often perpetuated by the legal system, which may remove the children from their families and place them in a foster home or juvenile facility.

Lastly, some children enter into sexual relationships out of curiosity. They too become entrapped, particularly because they were so willing to participate.

Children who disclose the abuse often experience what has been referred to as the child abuse accommodation syndrome (Table 105–1). This syndrome attempts to explain how children adjust to abuse. A key component of the syndrome is the need for secrecy. Disclosures are often partial or incomplete, and they are frequently recanted as children are made to feel responsible for any resulting disruption of families.

D_x Child Sexual Abuse

- Anogenital erythema
- Anogenital bleeding
- Genital discharge
- Anogenital scarring
- Behavioral symptoms (e.g., encopresis, enuresis)
- Disclosure of abuse
- Somatic complaints (e.g., abdominal pain, headache)
- Sexually transmitted diseases
- Pregnancy (adolescents)
- Delinquency, promiscuity (adolescents)

TABLE 105–1. Child Abuse Accommodation Syndrome

Secrecy
Helplessness
Entrapment and accommodation
Delayed, unconvincing disclosure
Retraction

DIFFERENTIAL DIAGNOSIS

A number of medical conditions that involve the anogenital area may be mistaken for sexual abuse (Table 105–2).

Children may sustain accidental injuries to the genital area, usually straddle injuries that follow falls. Most often the labia majora, labia minora, or periurethral areas are affected. Bleeding and pain are presenting complaints; the hymen is unaffected.

Bleeding is also a frequent complaint in girls with urethral prolapse, a condition reported most often in prepubescent African-American girls between the ages of 4 and 8 years. These girls have a protuberant mass extruding from the urethra. The condition is of uncertain etiology but it is not related to abuse.

Lichen sclerosus et atrophicus, which is less common, is a dermatologic condition that may produce macules, papules, or hemorrhagic blisters in the anogenital area. The affected skin becomes atrophic, hypopigmented, and easily traumatized. The key to differentiating this condition from injuries related to sexual abuse is that the hymen is unaffected in lichen sclerosus et atrophicus.

Congenital malformations may also affect the anogenital area, particularly if tissues fail to fuse along the median raphe, which appears denuded as a consequence. Other congenital malformations include hemangiomas that may bleed and be mistaken for traumatized tissue. These tumors are most often noted in infants under 2–3 years of age, and they usually regress with time.

Medical conditions may also affect the perianal area and be mistaken for abuse. Crohn's disease may lead to fissures, fistulas, perirectal abscesses, or tags. In general, Crohn's disease affects older children and produces other symptoms such as fever, weight loss, and stooling problems, or extraintestinal symptomatology. Perirectal abscesses may occur in patients with neutropenia, sometimes as the presenting complaint of leuke-

TABLE 105–3. Conditions Associated With Vaginal Discharge

Sexually Transmitted Diseases
Gonorrhea
Chlamydial
Trichomonas
Bacterial vaginosis
Conditions That Are Not Transmitted Sexually
Candidiasis
Shigellosis
Group A beta-hemolytic streptococcus infection
Vaginal foreign body

mia. Hemorrhoids occur rarely in children, and their presence should raise concern about intra-abdominal venous congestion, as seen in portal vein thrombosis.

Vaginal discharges (Table 105–3) may be related to sexual abuse, particularly if they are secondary to STDs such as gonorrhea or *Chlamydia* infection. Other agents may produce similar symptoms, yet not be sexually related, including *Candida*, *Shigella*, and group A beta hemolytic streptococci. The streptococci may produce a painful erythematous rash in the perianal area, which is frequently misdiagnosed as secondary to trauma or sexual abuse.

EVALUATION

The extent and urgency of the evaluation is in part dependent on whether the allegations involve an acute abusive episode or one that occurred in the past. An acute abusive episode (one that has occurred within the previous 72 hours) warrants an immediate assessment.

History

In all cases, a careful, comprehensive medical history should be obtained, including allegations related to the abuse. A general medical history should be taken as well, with particular attention to prior trauma or operative procedures involving the anogenital area. A psychological history should also be obtained; certain behavioral problems may occur more frequently in children who have been abused (Table 105–4).

Children must also be interviewed. The interview is best accomplished by someone with professional expertise in the areas of interviewing and child sexual

TABLE 105–2. Conditions Mistaken for Sexual Abuse

Genital
Accidental trauma
Lichen sclerosus et atrophicus
Urethral prolapse
Congenital malformations
Hemangioma
Anal
Inflammatory bowel disease
Hemorrhoids
Anal abscess associated with neutropenia
Perirectal abscess
Perianal streptococcal infection

TABLE 105–4. Problems Reported in Sexually Abused Children

Enuresis
Encopresis
Sexualized behavior
Pseudomaturity
Recurrent urinary tract infections
Vaginal discharge
Sleep disturbances
Suicide
School failure
Delinquency (adolescents)
Promiscuity (adolescents)

abuse. This individual may be the physician, or a social worker, psychologist, or rape counselor. The interview should be structured to include open-ended questions, such as "Tell me what happened" (Questions Box). Ancillary methods, such as drawings or anatomically detailed dolls, may be used but are best left to experts with experience in these controversial modalities. Statements that children make should be recorded in the medical record as close to verbatim as possible. At some facilities interviews are videotaped or recorded on an audiotape. In addition, legal experts, such as individuals from the district attorney's office or law enforcement agency, may observe interviews through a one-way mirror.

Physical Examination

It is helpful for the examiner to be familiar with the normal anogenital anatomy of prepubescent children. The anatomy of boys remains constant throughout childhood, except for the increase in size of the penis and testes and the appearance of pubic hair during adolescence. Figure 105–1 shows the normal anogenital anatomy of girls, which changes from infancy through

adolescence. All girls are born with a hymen, which is thick and full and covers the hymenal orifice in newborns. As maternal hormones regress, the hymen becomes thinner and more translucent, frequently taking on a crescentic configuration. When puberty begins, the hymen once again becomes thickened, scalloped, and full. Careful examination of the hymen may involve positioning a child in not only the supine frog-leg position, but also the prone knee-chest position (Fig. 105–2). Penetration of the hymen in postpubescent adolescents may result in stretching without tearing of the tissue. In prepubescent children, transections may heal with little residual evidence. The physician must realize that a normal anogenital examination does not preclude sexual abuse. Many types of abuse (such as orogenital contact and fondling) are not expected to lead to any apparent changes.

In cases of acute molestation, evidence of injury may be readily apparent, particularly if the examination is performed with the assistance of magnification such as colposcopy, or enhancing agents such as toluidine blue, which is preferentially taken up by exposed endothelium. Injuries related to penile penetration usually involve the hymen in the six o'clock position and the area of the posterior fourchette (see Fig. 105–1).

The evaluation of children who have been molested in the past or on a chronic basis is more problematic. Many injuries heal with little residual scarring. Scarring that does occur may appear as disruptions in the hymenal contour, with notches or concavities. The pattern of blood vessels may also be interrupted, and areas of increased or decreased vascularity may be apparent. Sometimes marked reduction of the hymenal tissue is present.

Male genitalia are less often injured by sexual abuse. More often the injuries seen in prepubescent boys, as well as some girls, involve changes in the perianal area. The incidence of these changes in all children who have been sodomized is unknown but is believed to be low. When changes do occur, they may appear as scars, tags, or irregularities in anal contour and anal tone.

Laboratory Tests

When the molestation has occurred within 72 hours of the examination, forensic evidence should be collected, as required by law enforcement. This evidence usually involves samples of vaginal washings and dried secretions, which are evaluated for the presence of sperm or semen. In addition to confirming that sexual assault has occurred, presence of semen may help establish or eliminate an individual as a suspect. Forensic packages, which are referred to as rape kits, have specific instructions concerning the appropriate collection of samples.

A laboratory evaluation of any vaginal discharge is necessary. It is impossible to determine the etiology of the discharge accurately simply by its characteristics. In general, cultures of the vagina or urethra, rectum, and throat of children who have suffered sexual abuse should be assessed for the presence of *Neisseria gonorrhoeae*. These cultures should be evaluated in a reliable laboratory because of the legal implications of venereal infections in young children. Children who

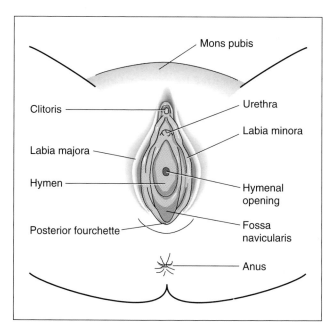

FIGURE 105–1. Normal anogenital anatomy of prepubescent girls.

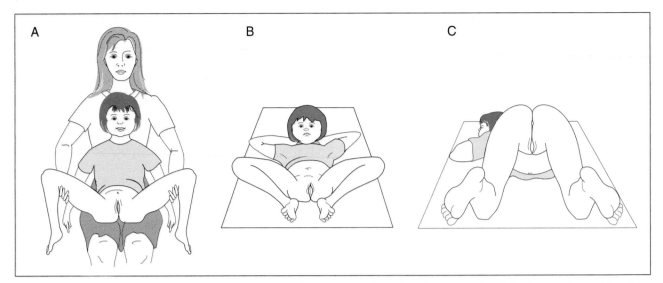

FIGURE 105–2. Various positions for an anogenital exam in a prepubescent girl. A. Seated on the mother's lap. B. Supine, frog-leg position. C. Prone, knee-chest position.

acquire these infections outside of the neonatal period are deemed to be victims of sexual abuse. Cultures to test for the presence of *Chlamydia* should be obtained. Rapid diagnostic studies, such as direct fluorescent antibodies, are not reliable in prepubescent children. Assessment for other STDs, such as herpes genitalis and condyloma acuminatum, should be based on clinical findings. Testing for syphilis should be performed if children have symptoms consistent with the diagnosis (e.g., condyloma latum, alopecia, rashes), if they have another STD, or if they live in a high prevalence area. Recommendations for testing for HIV are similar. The presence of disease in perpetrators also suggests the need for testing victims.

Other laboratory tests may be indicated if conditions other than sexual abuse are suspected. These include a CBC for leukemia or a barium enema for Crohn's disease.

MANAGEMENT

The management of children who have been sexually abused has three major components.

One, any medical problem sustained as a result of the abuse, such as traumatic injuries, must be addressed. In addition, STDs should be managed. The appropriate treatment of these conditions in pediatric patients is presented in Table 105–5. (See Chapter 76, Sexually Transmitted Diseases, for a more extensive discussion of STDs in adolescents.) Adolescents who have been the victims of an acute assault should be offered pregnancy counseling and STD prophylaxis.

Two, the emotional well-being of patients must be ensured. In cases of acute assault, crisis intervention is mandatory. If children have been the victims of chronic or prior sexual abuse, referral to appropriate counseling services should be implemented.

Three, the physician must report the incident of sexual assault or abuse to the appropriate agencies, as mandated by the laws of the locality in which the physician practices. The physician may be required to testify in court about particular findings and whether abuse occurred. Testifying may be intimidating. It is helpful for the physician to review the medical records ahead of time and to discuss this information with the attorney who issues the subpoena to the physician.

PROGNOSIS

Several factors influence the prognosis in cases of child sexual abuse, including relationship of the perpetrator to the child, chronicity of the abuse, support following the disclosure, and preexisting psychosocial conditions. Physical injuries are usually nonexistent or minor, and healing occurs with minimal residual evidence. In most cases, psychologic counseling is indicated. Such counseling is beneficial, and emotional recovery is not only possible but likely to occur in a supportive environment.

TABLE 105–5.   Management of Sexually Transmitted Diseases in Children

Infection	Medication	Dose
Neisseria gonorrhoeae	Ceftriaxone	125 mg IM
Chlamydia	Erythromycin	50 mg/kg/d for 10–14 days
	Azithromycin (> age 8 yr)	1 g PO in a single dose
	Doxycycline (> age 8 yr)	100 mg bid for 7 days
Herpes genitalis	Acyclovir	200 mg q4h for 10 days
Trichomonas	Metronidazole	30–50 mg/kg/d for 7 days divided (max: 250 mg tid)
Bacterial vaginosis	Metronidazole	15 mg/kg/d for 7 days (max: 500 mg bid)
Syphilis	Benzathine penicillin	50,000 units/kg, single IM dose (max: 2.4 million units)

Case Resolution

In the case history presented at the beginning of this chapter, the mother claims that no one has access to her child, but the girl's symptoms strongly suggest an infection with *N. gonorrhoeae.* Secrecy about abuse is very common. Both the child and the mother should be interviewed by a skilled person. Cultures for gonorrhea should be carefully collected and sent to the most reliable laboratory. Antibiotic therapy may be initiated if the child is symptomatic. The case may be referred immediately to social service and law enforcement agencies if there is a disclosure. Alternatively, if the child denies the abuse, the referral may be deferred pending laboratory confirmation of the diagnosis.

Selected Readings

American Academy of Pediatrics, Section on Child Abuse and Neglect. A Guide to References and Resources in Child Abuse and Neglect. 2nd ed. Elk Grove Village, IL. American Academy of Pediatrics, 1997.

Behrman, R. E. (ed.). The Future of Children: Sexual Abuse of Children. Palo Alto, CA, Center for the Future of Children, The David and Lucile Packard Foundation, 1994.

Berkowitz, C. D. Child sexual abuse. Pediatr. Rev. 13:443–452, 1992.

Chadwick, D. L., et al. Color Atlas of Child Sexual Abuse. Chicago, Year Book Medical Publishers, 1989.

Committee on Child Abuse and Neglect. Guidelines for the evaluation of sexual abuse of children. Pediatrics 103:186–191, 1999.

DeJong, A. R., and M. A. Finkel. Sexual abuse of children. Curr. Prob. Pediatr. 20:489–567, 1990.

Finkel, M. A., and A. R. DeJong. Medical findings in child sexual abuse. *In* R. M. Reece (ed.). Child Abuse: Medical Diagnosis and Management. Philadelphia, Lea & Febiger, 1994, pp. 185–247.

Heger, A. and S. J. Emans. Evaluation of the Sexually Abused Child. New York, Oxford University Press, 1992.

Holmes, W. C., and G. B. Slap. Sexual abuse of boys. JAMA 280: 1855–1862, 1998.

Jenny, C. Medical Evaluation of Physically and Sexually Abused Children. The Apsac Study Guides 3. Thousand Oaks, CA, Sage Publications, 1996.

Reichert, S. K. Medical evaluation of the sexually abused child. *In* Helfer, M. E., Kempe, R. S., and R. D. Krugman (eds.). The Battered Child. Chicago, The University of Chicago Press, 1997, pp. 313–328.

CHAPTER 106

FAILURE TO THRIVE

Carol D. Berkowitz, M.D.

H$_x$ A 2-year-old girl is brought to the office because of her small size. She was born at term but weighed only 2200 grams (less than fifth percentile) and measured 43 centimeters (less than fifth percentile). The mother is a 30-year-old gravida V para IV aborta I who smoked during pregnancy but denies using alcohol or drugs. She received prenatal care for only 2 weeks prior to delivery, and she claims to have felt well.

The child's physical health has been good. She is reported to be normal developmentally but speaks only four to five single words. She has not yet started toilet-training.

The family history for medical problems, including allergies, diabetes, and cardiac and renal disease, is negative. The mother is 5 feet (152 cm) tall, and the father is 5 feet, 4 inches (163 cm) tall. The girl has three siblings, aged 5 years, 4 years, and 3 years, who are all normal. The father is no longer in the household. The mother is not employed outside of the home, and she receives public assistance. She states that frequently there is not enough food in the home, although she receives food stamps.

On physical examination, the girl is less than the fifth percentile in height and weight. Although she is very active, she does not use any understandable words. The rest of the examination is normal.

Questions

1. What are the key prenatal factors that affect the growth of children?
2. How can caloric adequacy of a diet be assessed?
3. How do parental measurements affect their children's stature?
4. What are the behavioral characteristics of infants with environmental failure to thrive?
5. What are some strategies to increase caloric intake of infants and children?

Failure to thrive (FTT) can be defined as the failure of children to grow and develop at an appropriate rate. The term FTT first appeared in the pediatric literature in 1933. Previously, the condition was referred to as "cease to thrive." The terms "growth deficiency" or "growth impairment" are sometimes used. FTT is one way of consolidating two common pediatric problems, growth retardation and short stature, together.

Historically, FTT has been divided into two distinct categories, organic and nonorganic. In organic FTT, an underlying medical problem, such as cystic fibrosis or

---

D_x	**Failure to Thrive**

- Weight below fifth percentile
- Height below fifth percentile
- Weight for height below fifth percentile
- Rate of growth too slow
- Delayed developmental milestones
- Disturbed interactional skills

---

congenital heart disease, is believed to contribute to the failure to grow at an appropriate rate. In nonorganic FTT, also referred to as environmental deprivation, inadequate growth is attributed to lack of nourishment and a nonnurturing home environment. It is important to recognize that many children have growth problems with both organic and environmental components.

The diagnosis of FTT is made when the growth parameters of children as plotted on a standardized curve are below the fifth percentile in height or weight. Children who are above the fifth percentile may also be diagnosed with FTT if the rate of growth has decelerated and two major percentiles (e.g., decreased from the 75th percentile down to the 10th percentile) have been crossed within 6 months (D_x Box).

The challenge for the physician caring for the child with FTT is to determine the etiology of the problem, which may not be readily apparent. Nonspecific, nondirected laboratory tests are not helpful because their yield is low and their cost is high. The evaluation of small, underweight children requires a careful history and physical examination as well as an assessment of mother-infant interactions. A home visit helps because it permits evaluation of the mother-infant relationship in a more natural setting and an assessment of the family's economic and food resources.

EPIDEMIOLOGY

The prevalence of FTT varies in different segments of the population. Poverty puts children at risk for undernutrition, and 12% of Medicaid recipients are less than the third percentile in weight. Child neglect can lead to FTT but is not a necessary component; approximately 60% of cases of child abuse are reported for child neglect. Several other factors may contribute to variations in growth. All of these are not the result of a pathologic process but may reflect variations in individual genetic potential.

Environmental FTT occurs in three different family settings. In the type 1 family, an acute depressive episode in the mother is the key component. Family living conditions are good, and the educational background of the mother is adequate. The depressive episode is most commonly related to a loss that occurred during the pregnancy or shortly after delivery. The mother is too depressed to interact appropriately with her children. The type 2 family has marginal financial resources. The mother may be chronically depressed and the father involved in alcohol or sub-

stance abuse. Domestic violence frequently occurs. Spacing between children is less than 18 months, and the number of children is often the same as the age of the oldest child. The mother is too overwhelmed to meet the needs of the children. The type 3 family also involves a mother who is depressed and has experienced losses, usually of a chronic nature. Her financial and educational background are adequate, but she views one of her children (the one who now presents with FTT) as bad or evil and the source of all her problems. As a result, an individual child is singled out, and the neglect is intentional.

CLINICAL PRESENTATION

Children with FTT present with low weight, short stature, or poor appetite. Sometimes parents may express concern, and at other times teachers may detect children's growth problems. Some children with FTT are diagnosed during a health maintenance visit or when they are being evaluated for another medical problem, such as a febrile illness.

PATHOPHYSIOLOGY

The common pathway for the development of FTT in both organic and nonorganic cases is insufficient calories to sustain growth. Caloric intake may be inadequate for several reasons. Some factors are societal, specifically poverty and inadequate access to food. Other factors may involve increased caloric needs. Certain chronic conditions are characterized by increased caloric expenditure (e.g., some forms of chronic lung disease) or increased loss of ingested food (e.g., diarrhea).

In environmental FTT, a disturbed mother-infant interaction is believed to contribute to reduced caloric intake and any associated GI symptoms (i.e., vomiting). Although various disturbances in mother-FTT infant dyads have been described, maternal depression is the most common maternal feature noted in environmental FTT. Infants withdraw after unsuccessful attempts to interact with nonresponsive mothers, and infants become apathetic and disinterested in food. Alternatively, overactive mothers, some of whom have a bipolar (manic-depressive) disorder, are out of synchrony with their infants. The infants become agitated, especially during feedings, and cannot feed and frequently vomit. These infants, who may interact with persons other than their mothers, usually do well in other environments.

Older children with FTT have disturbed hypothalamic-pituitary functioning. The etiology of this dysfunction is uncertain but has been attributed to sleep disturbances.

DIFFERENTIAL DIAGNOSIS

The growth of children with FTT may be impaired with regard to weight, height, head circumference, or any combination of growth parameters. If weight is the only abnormal parameter, inadequate caloric intake is probably the major problem. If height is reduced and the weight is appropriate or high for height, the diagnosis may be short stature rather than FTT. Small head circumference in the face of low growth parameters suggests a central nervous system basis for the growth delay. It is important to determine if children's skills are developmentally appropriate when determining the etiology of FTT. Affect and interactional skills should also be noted. Environmentally deprived infants are apathetic and noninteractive. They may appear to have cerebral palsy or infantile autism, but their symptoms resolve with a change in surroundings.

The most common causes of short stature include familial short stature and constitutional delay. Children with familial short stature are small because the parents are short. Except for a deceleration in growth, which usually occurs between the ages of 6 and 18 months, children with constitutional delay appear healthy. They have a delayed bone age that is comparable to their height age (the age when their height is at the 50th percentile), however. In children with either familial short stature or constitutional delay, growth parameters at birth are usually normal.

Children with low growth parameters at birth may have been premature or have suffered from intrauterine growth restriction (IUGR). Most studies support the notion that well premature infants exhibit catch-up growth (head circumference by 18 months, weight by 24 months, and height by 40 months). Ill preterm infants may not demonstrate such catch-up growth either because of increased caloric needs related to residual medical problems (e.g., bronchopulmonary dysplasia) or impaired nutritional intake resulting from certain conditions (e.g., cerebral palsy).

Children who are small for gestational age may have suffered any of several *in utero* insults that affect postnatal growth, including exposure to cigarettes, alcohol, and illicit drugs. In addition, maternal infection with such diseases as rubella may result in a congenital infection in infants with subsequent growth impairment.

A number of other conditions may lead to disturbed growth, including endocrine disorders, skeletal dysplasias, food allergies, and malabsorption. These conditions occur less frequently and are usually more readily apparent as children undergo the evaluation for the growth problem.

EVALUATION

History

Careful questioning about certain topics provides clues to diagnosis in about 95% of cases. The physician should learn about the pregnancy and delivery, children's medical and dietary history, and the family history.

It is important to obtain a history of the pregnancy and delivery (Questions: Pregnancy and Delivery). Recurrent spontaneous abortions suggest that mothers may have an underlying problem such as a balanced chromosomal translocation that leads to fetal wastage. Mothers who have experienced repeated losses may have difficulty bonding with subsequent infants. The physician should determine whether mothers used cigarettes, alcohol, or drugs during the pregnancy by

---

> **Questions: Failure to Thrive (Pregnancy and Delivery)**
>
> - Was the pregnancy planned?
> - How did the mother feel when she learned that she was pregnant?
> - Was the infant wanted?
> - Was prenatal care obtained?
> - How many times has the mother been pregnant?
> - Is there a history of abortions, either spontaneous or therapeutic?
> - How much did the mother drink during the pregnancy, if at all?
> - How much did the mother smoke during the pregnancy, if at all?
> - How much did the mother use drugs (either prescribed or illicit) during the pregnancy, if at all? Which drugs did she use?
> - Did the mother take any medications during the pregnancy?
> - Did the mother have any rashes or illnesses during the pregnancy?
> - Was the infant term or premature?
> - How much did the infant weigh?

asking mothers questions beginning with the phrase "How much?" Any medications taken by the mother may affect the subsequent growth of their infants.

A review of children's medical history may also provide a clue to the etiology of FTT (Questions: Medical and Family History). It is essential that the physician obtain as many of the previous growth parameters as possible to determine whether children are small but growing at a normal rate or if their rate of growth is too slow. Previous illnesses should be assessed because these events may interrupt growth temporarily. Certain complaints may indicate underlying organic disorders, and recurrent infection raises the possibility of infection with HIV. A history of easy fatigability may be a clue to congenital heart disease. Although most children with congenital heart disease grow normally, growth problems may occur with congestive heart failure, some forms of cyanotic heart disease, and complex atrial septal defects, especially if associated with pulmonary hypertension. Children with urinary incontinence may have renal disease that interferes with their growth. The presence of seizures may be a sign of a CNS problem that makes it difficult to obtain adequate nutrition. Some children with seizures are heavily medicated and are too sleepy to eat.

A family history as well as a social history is important to obtain. Determination of parental heights, which is best accomplished by measuring the parents, is critical. This is particularly important in children with short stature. Specific mid-parental height curves allow the physician to determine if children's height is appropriate given the parental stature.

> **Questions: Failure to Thrive (Medical and Family History)**
>
> - Is the child's growth rate normal or slow?
> - Has the child had any previous illnesses (e.g., gastroenteritis, recurrent pneumonia)?
> - Does the child tire easily?
> - How tall are the parents?
> - Are there any medical problems that run in the family?

A nutritional assessment is an essential part of the history. The physician or another member of the health care team, such as a dietician, can perform this assessment. The dietary history can be determined either by using a 24-hour recall of children's intake during the previous day or a prospective 3-day diary, in which parents record the kinds and quantities of foods their children eat. This nutritional information can be used to find ways to alter children's diet to ensure adequate and balanced meals.

Physical Examination

The essential component of the physical examination is determination of growth parameters. Calculation of the body mass index (BMI = weight [kg] divided by height [m]^2) is useful. Children with a low BMI are suffering from undernutrition. Short children with a normal BMI are not. Children should also be evaluated for dysmorphic features. It is important to remember that children with Down syndrome grow at different rates than other children, and separate standardized curves for assessing these children are available (see Chapter 19, Well Child Care for Children with Trisomy 21). The presence of one major congenital anomaly or two minor anomalies suggests the existence of other anomalies. The incidence of growth hormone deficiency is reportedly higher in children with cleft lip and palate. Children with heart murmurs may have FTT related to congenital heart disease.

Infants with environmental FTT exhibit certain behavioral characteristics that are easy to recognize. They refrain from making eye contact and exhibit gaze avoidance. Infants are not cuddly and do not like being held. When held, they may arch their back in an effort to avoid the holder. Their muscles seem tense, and they are often considered to be hypertonic.

Psychosocial Assessment

The evaluation of children with FTT and their families entails a detailed psychosocial assessment to determine what environmental factors may be affecting children's growth. Such an assessment is helpful even if the FTT has an organic basis, because chronic disease has an effect on family functioning. This evaluation can be carried out by a primary care physician, social worker, or psychologist. The key is to query the caretaker about living conditions, adequacy of food supply, and economic resources.

Laboratory Tests

Routine laboratory tests appropriate for any pediatric health maintenance visit should be obtained in children with FTT if these studies have not been performed recently. Such tests include hematocrit, lead level (screening as determined by risk factors and geographic area), and urinalysis. Other laboratory tests should be determined by the findings on history and physical examination. Evaluation for endocrinopathies, such as hypothyroidism or growth hormone deficiency, should

be carried out in children whose bone age is less than their height age or who have symptoms of these disorders. Genetic consultation or chromosomal assessment should be performed in children with dysmorphic features or in families with a history of fetal wastage.

Imaging Studies

X-rays to determine bone age are useful in children with short stature that is not related to parental heights. Children with constitutional delay have a bone age that is consistent with their height age.

MANAGEMENT

Adequate Caloric Intake

Ensuring that children receive appropriate caloric intake is essential. The caloric intake, which averages 120–150 cal/kg/day for most infants, should be based on children's ideal rather than actual weight (see Chapter 11, Nutritional Needs). For infants on formula, the physician should review the exact preparation of formula with the mother. Overly diluted formula results in an unusually large intake volume with a lack of weight gain. For infants who are breast-fed, the physician should observe a feeding session to be certain that mothers have an adequate milk supply and infants are able to suck and swallow appropriately. Infants should be weighed before and after feeding. Some infants with FTT have neurologic problems that prevent them from sucking and swallowing consistently without becoming fatigued.

Children who are slow feeders may require formula concentration (Table 106–1). These infants may also receive added calories in the form of Polycose (glucose polymer) or oil such as medium-chain triglycerides mixed in the milk. Older children may be placed on supplemental feedings such as Pediasure or instant breakfast drinks. These drinks are a less expensive form of nutritional supplementation than Pediasure and are well tolerated. Up to 24 oz per day of the breakfast drinks can be consumed. They should be mixed with whole milk and given in addition to, not in place of, a balanced diet.

Mothers should be advised that many children preferentially tolerate six small meals a day rather than three large ones. In addition, parents should be told that access to nonnutritional foods such as cookies adversely affects children's appetites. Excess consumption of fruit juices should also be limited, since it

---

TABLE 106–1. Concentration of Infant Formula to Increase Caloric Intake

Concentrated Infant Formula (13 oz can)		
Formula (oz)	Water (oz)	Calories (cal/oz)
13	13	20
13	10	23
13	8	25
Powdered Formula		
Formula (scoops)	Water (oz)	Calories (cal/oz)
1	2	20
5	8	25

decreases the intake of other foods and may induce diarrhea. The physician should inform parents regarding foods that can be added to children's diets to increase caloric intake. These foods include powdered milk, cheese, sour cream, avocado, and peanut butter.

Parenting Issues

Some parents need more help about appropriate child-rearing practices than the physician can provide. They should be enrolled in parenting programs that address multiple aspects of the parenting process. Mothers with substance abuse problems may need to participate in drug treatment programs. Other caregivers may need individual counseling for depression or emotional problems.

In some middle-class families, meal time has evolved into a battle of control. Some children find that food is supplied in a manner more conducive to its consumption at school rather than at home. Parents should be counseled about avoiding conflicts about meals with children, because the children win simply by closing their mouths. Parents should be encouraged to allow toddlers independence around meal time.

Families may also require supplementary services to ensure that food supplies are adequate and financial resources are sufficient. Such services include food stamps, Supplemental Food Program for Women, Infants, and Children (WIC), and Temporary Assistance for Needy Families (TANF).

Home Visitation

Home visitation services provide useful diagnostic information and help parents implement advice. Such information may include lack of access to running water, overcrowding, and inadequate food resources. Home visitation may be available in the community through the use of public health nurses or private visiting nurse agencies. These nurses should interact with the primary care physician so that families' compliance with treatment recommendations can be determined.

Child Protective Services

Involvement by child protective services (CPS) may be necessary if parents are unable to comply with medical recommendations, if children do not grow, or if there is intentional neglect on the part of families. In some families with children with FTT, the home environment is not safe for the children, and they require placement elsewhere. Type 3 families need immediate referral to CPS, and some type 2 families also need such a referral (see Epidemiology).

Hospitalization

Hospitalization is occasionally necessary if infants with FTT are severely malnourished and food must be given in a controlled environment. These infants may also have intercurrent illnesses that require inpatient care. In addition, health care professionals may determine that the home environment is unsafe and that no other placement, such as foster care, is available.

Children with both organic and nonorganic FTT usually gain weight in the hospital. Thus, the hospitalization of children with FTT simply to demonstrate appropriate weight gain in a different environment is considered neither appropriate nor cost-effective. Some insurance companies will not reimburse hospitals for in-patient management of children with FTT. Additionally, some children with environmental FTT do not gain weight in the hospital because they are subjected to many diagnostic tests that interfere with nutritional intake (e.g., being NPO) and acquire nosocomial infections.

PROGNOSIS

Many children with FTT respond dramatically to change in diet or in environment. Improvement in affect and cognitive functioning frequently follows nutritional improvement. These children grow and achieve and maintain normal stature. With early intervention, cognitive abilities also can be fully realized. Even when intervention has been delayed, catch-up growth and development are expected, although 25–30% may have weight and occasionally height below the fifth percentile.

Continued monitoring for residual psychosocial or neurodevelopmental disabilities is appropriate even after growth has normalized.

Case Resolution

In the case scenario presented, the full-term infant had a low birth weight, which suggests IUGR. Although the mother reports using no alcohol or drugs, such denial is not uncommon. The child's growth pattern should be determined to see if the rate of growth has changed recently, and the BMI should be calculated to check for both undernutrition and short stature. A mid-parental height curve should be used to determine if the child's short stature is related to the parents' short stature. Intervention should involve mobilizing resources for the child and family to ensure adequate food and financial and emotional support.

Selected Readings

Bithoney, W. G., H. Dubowitz, and H. Egan. Failure to thrive/growth deficiency. Pediatr. Rev. 13:453–459, 1992.

Drotar, D. (ed.). New Direction in Failure to Thrive: Research and Clinical Practice. New York, Plenum Press, 1985.

Frank, D. A., and D. Drotar. Failure to thrive in child abuse: medical diagnosis and management. In Reece, R. M. (ed.). Child Abuse: Medical Diagnosis and Management. Philadelphia, Lea & Febiger, 1994, pp. 298–324.

Frank, D. A., M. Silva, and R. Needlman. Failure to thrive: mystery, myth, and method. Contemp. Pediatr. 10:114–133, 1993.

Helfer, R. E. The neglect of our children. Pediatr. Clin. North Am. 37:923–942, 1990.

Kessler, D. B., and P. Dawson. Failure to Thrive and Pediatric Undernutrition. A Transdisciplinary Approach. Baltimore, Paul H. Brookes Publishing Co., 1999.

McHugh, M. Child abuse in a sea of neglect: the inner-city child. Pediatr. Ann. 21:504–507, 1992.

Oates, R. K., and R. S. Kempe. Growth failure in infants. In The Battered Child. Helfer, M. E., Kempe, R. S., and R. D. Krugman (eds.). 5th ed. Chicago, The University of Chicago Press, 1997, pp. 374–391.

CHAPTER 107

INFANTS OF SUBSTANCE-ABUSING MOTHERS

Carol D. Berkowitz, M.D.

H_x An infant is born by emergency cesarean section because of abruptio placentae. The mother is a 29-year-old gravida VI para IV aborta II with a history of crack cocaine and heroin abuse during pregnancy. The infant is 36 weeks' gestation. The birth weight is 2400 g, and the length is 43 cm. The physical examination is normal.

The infant does well for the first 10 hours but then develops jitteriness, with irritability, diarrhea, sweating, and poor feeding. A urine toxicology test on the infant and mother are positive for cocaine.

Questions

1. What complications affect infants secondary to maternal substance abuse during pregnancy?
2. What withdrawal symptoms do newborn infants experience as a result of maternal substance abuse during pregnancy?
3. What typical behavioral and learning problems are found in infants and children whose mothers abused illicit substances during pregnancy?
4. What are the appropriate management strategies for infants who have experienced *in utero* drug exposure?

Maternal substance abuse during pregnancy places infants at risk for a number of medical as well as psychosocial and developmental problems. The particular problems experienced by infants depend on the drug (or drugs) to which they have been exposed. Many infants have been exposed to several drugs in addition to cigarettes and alcohol. The long-lasting effects of alcohol exposure are well-established, but the effect of newer drugs is less well-defined. Illicit drugs change in their popularity and availability at different points in time. Newborn nurseries can monitor the patterns of drug exposure in the local population.

The environment into which children are born also affects their health and and eventual development. Environments in which substance abuse is common are frequently suboptimal for normal growth and development for several reasons: (1) the impact of substance abuse on parenting; (2) fragmentation of families; (3) domestic violence; (4) incarceration of significant family members; (5) illnesses, including HIV infection, (6) limited financial resources; (7) homelessness or substandard housing; (8) unemployment; and (9) discrimination on the basis of race, gender, or culture. Because of these environmental problems, many drug-exposed infants are cared for by foster parents or nonparental family members. All these factors compound the assessment of problems related to drug exposure versus the accompanying environmental conditions. This differentiation is of less significance to the practitioner, who must anticipate and care for the multiple problems that drug-exposed children manifest, than to the researcher or epidemiologist.

EPIDEMIOLOGY

About 15% of the 56 million women between the ages of 15 and 44 years are substance abusers. An estimated 15% of infants who are born have been exposed to drugs or alcohol. Figures for inner city hospitals are different from those of small community hospitals in rural areas. In one high prevalence area, 70% of infants screened were positive for cocaine. A study in a suburban hospital revealed that 12% of infants tested positive for cocaine. Information gathered through the use of maternal questionnaires grossly underestimates the prevalence of substance abuse. For example, one study detected cocaine, heroin, or cannabinoids by meconium analysis in 42% of infants, but the maternal history was positive in only 10.5%. Meconium analysis has demonstrated not only extensive differences in the prevalence of *in utero* drug exposure in urban and rural hospitals, but also differences in the substances abused.

CLINICAL PRESENTATION

In utero growth restriction occurs frequently in drug-exposed infants. Neonates who have been exposed to drugs such as heroin and methadone may present with symptoms of drug withdrawal, such as tremors, sneezing, sweating, vomiting, diarrhea, poor appetite, irritability, and seizures. Symptoms usually occur within 72 hours of birth, but delayed effects of agitation, irritability, and poor socialization may persist for 4–6 months. Meconium aspiration is reported in heroin-exposed infants. Some cocaine-exposed infants have birth defects (e.g., absent limbs). Pre- and postnatal growth failure and microcephaly are associated with maternal alcohol abuse. Learning disabilities and ADHD are noted in older children who have been exposed *in utero* to alcohol and drugs. Oppositional and impulsive behavior may also be a presenting complaint. Facial dysmorphology with microphthalmia, microcephaly, and poorly developed philtrum with thin upper lip are other effects of alcohol abuse during pregnancy. Children who exhibit alcohol-related growth impairment, central nervous system dysfunction, and dysmorphic facies may have fetal alcohol syndrome (FAS).

PATHOPHYSIOLOGY

Drugs used by pregnant women may affect infants in three different ways. One, the drugs may be addictive and result in symptoms of withdrawal during the neonatal period; two, they may be toxic and lead to impaired functioning and neurodevelopmental problems; and three, they may be teratogenic and cause congenital anomalies and a dysmorphic appearance. The mechanism of action of the various substances on the developing fetus can be understood in terms of their biochemical properties.

In utero exposure to heroin and methadone results in physiologic addiction. These drugs are opiates that bind to opiate receptor sites in the brain and in the gut. When the opiates are no longer present, individuals experience withdrawal. *In utero* exposure is also believed to affect the respiratory center and may predispose infants to disturbed ventilatory control, and subsequent SIDS (see Chapter 39).

Cocaine is addictive, toxic, and teratogenic. It interacts with three receptor sites in the brain. One, cocaine blocks the reuptake of norepinephrine. Higher levels of norepinephrine are associated with an increased incidence of preterm labor. Heart rate and blood pressure rise, and vasoconstriction, diaphoresis, and tremors occur. Vasoconstriction may affect the placenta and lead to anomalies of placentation, such as placental infarcts or abruptio placentae. The fetus, who may also be affected by periods of vasospasm, hypoperfusion, and ischemia, may develop anomalies such as atresia of the GI tract, stroke, and absent limbs. In addition, cocaine-exposed infants have a higher incidence of cutaneous hemangiomas.

Two, cocaine decreases the reuptake of dopamine. This effect is apparent in cocaine-using mothers, who have decreased appetite, which affects maternal nutrition during pregnancy. Stereotypic behavior, hyperactivity, and sexual excitement may be associated with sexual promiscuity and the risk of HIV and STDs.

Three, cocaine decreases serotonin reuptake, leading to decreased sleep. The sleep cycle of cocaine-exposed infants is often disrupted.

Phencyclidine (PCP) has sympathomimetic effects, including increases in blood pressure, heart rate, respiratory rate, deep tendon reflexes, and tone. In addition, PCP has cholinergic effects, causing sweating, flushing, drooling, and pupillary constriction. Infants exposed to PCP *in utero* do not exhibit these symptoms, however, but display neurologic and developmental disorganization.

Alcohol has multiple teratogenic effects, including impairment of growth of the brain and the body. The impact on growth may be apparent at birth and continue after the newborn period. The disturbed neurologic development is also evidenced by microcephaly, microphthalmia, ptosis, mental retardation, and ADHD.

DIFFERENTIAL DIAGNOSIS

The major differential diagnoses relate to the symptomatology produced by the abused substance or substances (D_x Box). Infants exposed to addictive substances may present in the neonatal period with symptoms of withdrawal. Exposure to heroin and methadone is most commonly associated with this symptom pattern (Table 107–1). The irritability and jitteriness characteristic of *in utero* drug exposure may also be seen with hypoglycemia, hypocalcemia, and hypomagnesemia. These biochemical disturbances are often found in infants of diabetic mothers.

Sometimes the neurologic instability associated with drug withdrawal may progress to the point that infants experience a seizure. Seizures occur in 1–3% of heroin-exposed infants. Other causes of seizures, such as intraventricular hemorrhage or pyridoxine dependency, must be considered in the differential diagnosis. Sepsis, with or without fever, may also be associated with irritability. In addition, GI disturbances such as poor feeding, vomiting, or diarrhea in the newborn period are associated with drug withdrawal. Infectious gastroenteritis and formula intolerance are part of the differential diagnosis.

Specific syndromes of dysmorphic appearance may also be the result of alcohol or drug exposure. Fetal alcohol syndrome is the most comprehensive syndrome of dysmorphic appearance related to maternal substance abuse during pregnancy. Other causes of dysmorphic syndromes, such as gene and chromosome problems, must be ruled out.

In older children, presenting symptoms related to maternal substance abuse may take the form of neurobehavioral problems, such as impulsive behavior, antisocial behavior, and ADHD. It may not be readily apparent that the origin of children's difficulties lies in maternal substance abuse during pregnancy. Diagnosis is often difficult because of maternal denial and the many environmental factors that may be contributing to children's neurodevelopmental problems. A specific neurodevelopmental problem associated with maternal

---

D_x Infants of Substance-Abusing Mothers

- Symptoms of withdrawal (see Table 107–1)
- Growth retardation
- Developmental delay
- Sexually transmitted diseases
- Congenital anomalies

TABLE 107–1. Symptoms of Neonatal Withdrawal Syndrome

Irritability
Jitteriness
Tremors
Seizures
Sneezing
Hiccups
Vomiting
Diarrhea
Sweating
Poor feeding

cocaine abuse involves a hearing impairment and a disorder in which the processing of speech are affected. Delayed speech development may be noted.

FTT may also be a presenting complaint in infants or children who have been exposed to drugs or alcohol (see Chapter 106, Failure to Thrive, for a discussion of the differential diagnosis of FTT). It is important to consider maternal substance abuse in all patients who have been diagnosed with FTT, particularly if the affected children were small for gestational age.

Maternal substance abuse should be considered in all infants who present with certain infections such as STDs (most commonly hepatitis B, HIV, and syphilis).

EVALUATION

History

The possibility of maternal substance abuse should be considered in the face of certain maternal risk factors. These factors include the absence of prenatal care, evidence of poor maternal nutrition, poor maternal weight gain, presence of STDs, maternal hypertension and tachycardia, abruptio placentae, precipitous delivery, and a history of domestic violence.

Infants who manifest symptoms of withdrawal should be evaluated for the possibility of maternal substance abuse. This assessment involves an appropriate history as well as a toxicologic evaluation. Mothers disclose their drug history to varying extents, depending on the circumstances of the interview. If mothers are concerned about the health and well-being of their infants and do not fear legal repercussions, they are more likely to discuss their drug use. An appropriate drug history should be obtained in a nonjudgmental manner (Questions Box). Studies have shown that the use of a structured questionnaire rather than a cursory interview increases the incidence of reported substance abuse by 3- to 5-fold.

Physical Examination

Infants should be assessed for the common complications related to maternal substance abuse. They should undergo a full physical examination to check for the presence of any anomalies. Growth measurements should be noted, and physicians should determine if intrauterine growth restriction or microcephaly is evident. Premature infants should be monitored for all the problems related to prematurity, such as intraventricular hemorrhage and necrotizing enterocolitis. Signs of neonatal withdrawal syndrome should be assessed (see Table 107–1). Neurodevelopment status should be assessed and monitored at each visit. Neurologic abnormalities, particularly hypertonicity, coarse tremors, and extensor leg posture, are noted in the newborn period, and disturbances in both fine and gross motor coordination persist through the toddler years.

Laboratory Tests

In addition to obtaining a toxicologic history, screening for drugs should also be performed. The legal guidelines for screening mothers for drugs vary in different localities. In general, infants can be screened on medical grounds without parental consent because the information obtained is important in the care of the infant. Screening of the mother's urine without her consent is more problematic, however, because of the potential legal implications of a positive test.

Some centers have drug panels, which screen for the most commonly used substances, such as cocaine metabolites, opiates, amphetamines, barbiturates, and marijuana metabolites. Most of these tests, which utilize immunoassays, require 1–2 mL of infant urine. These tests are inexpensive and sensitive but not very specific. For example, antihistamines cross-react with amphetamines, and morphine (used during delivery) cannot be distinguished from heroin. Other tests using mass spectroscopy or gas chromatography are more expensive and require larger samples of urine.

Newer methods check for the presence of illicit drugs, particularly cocaine, in infant hair or meconium. These tests are able to document the presence of drugs in the time prior to delivery and may be positive even if urine screening is negative at the time of birth. The FDA has recently approved a drug testing kit that uses meconium to test for cocaine, opiate, and cannabinoid. Drugs to which the infant was exposed prepartum persist in meconium longer than they do in the urine. Additionally, meconium drug testing has a high sensitivity and specificity, and samples are easy to collect.

Further evaluation in the neonatal period should include an evaluation for the presence of STDs, particularly HIV, hepatitis B, and syphilis.

Imaging Studies

Some investigators recommend that cocaine-exposed infants be routinely evaluated with ultrasound for the presence of CNS hemorrhages. Other neuroimaging techniques should be used if infants appear lethargic in the nursery.

MANAGEMENT

In the neonatal period, the management of drug-exposed infants requires attention to medical condition,

---

Questions: Infants of Substance-Abusing Mothers

- Did the mother use any substances such as alcohol, cigarettes, marijuana, or prescription and illicit drugs during the pregnancy?
- Has she ever used these substances? Is she currently using these substances?
- If so, how much? How frequently? By what route? To what extent is she trying to abstain?
- Is the mother at risk for sexually transmitted diseases? Has she ever been tested?
- Did the mother have prenatal care? When did the care start?
- What is the status of other children in the family?
- Does the father abuse alcohol or drugs?

TABLE 107–2. Pharmacologic Management of Neonatal Drug Withdrawal

Medication	Dosage
Tincture of paregoric	1–4 drops/kg/dose PO q4–6h
Phenobarbital	1–3 mg/kg/dose PO or IM q6h
Methadone	0.1 mg/kg/dose PO q12h

such as prematurity, that may accompany drug exposure. Likewise, STDs such as congenital syphilis should be treated. Hepatitis B vaccine and hepatitis B immunoglobulin should be administered if appropriate.

Symptoms of neonatal substance withdrawal may also require treatment. Infants may respond to **swaddling** as a means of decreasing their increased irritability. In addition, they may require **medication.** Table 107–2 lists the substances commonly used to manage the symptoms of neonatal drug withdrawal. In general, these agents should be used in infants with vomiting, diarrhea, and marked irritability. Medications should be tapered over time, allowing infants to outgrow the dosage. Paregoric is particularly useful in opiate-exposed infants and is even noted to improve sucking coordination. Phenobarbital may be preferred in cases of polydrug abuse.

Social service is a key component of management. In many jurisdictions, child protective services must be notified about positive toxicologic tests on newborn infants or their mothers. Likewise, infants who display symptoms of neonatal drug withdrawal may also have to be reported to these agencies. These agencies are generally responsible for performing a home assessment and determining the adequacy of the environment. In some cases, infants may be assigned to foster homes. Parents may be ordered to participate in drug treatment programs and parenting classes.

After the newborn period the focus of management is provision of **well child care.** Infants who have been exposed to cocaine *in utero* should have BAER testing in early infancy to detect hearing impairment. Attention should be paid to physical growth and administration of immunizations. Monitoring of neurodevelopmental status should be carried out. If a sensory impairment or neurodevelopmental delay is apparent, children should be referred to appropriate community agencies. Federal programs that operate under the Individuals with Disabilities Education Act (IDEA) provide interventional services for disabled and at-risk children 6 years of age and younger.

Symptoms of ADHD in older children may require similar intervention, with recommendation for specific school programs as well as pharmacologic treatment.

Regular assessments of school performance should be obtained from children's teachers. Standardized neurodevelopment tests should be administered at periodic intervals to ensure appropriate progress.

PROGNOSIS

Many infants, particularly those exposed to alcohol *in utero,* suffer long-term sequelae such as neurodevelopmental disabilities. Remedial educational programs help, but do not cure, such disabilities. Initial reports suggested that the effects of *in utero* cocaine exposure were equally devastating. More recent studies show that a key factor determining the outcome in cocaine-exposed infants is the environment in which they are raised. A stable, nurturing environment minimizes the many adverse effects of drug exposure and promotes normal neurodevelopment by enforcing the acquisition of skills and knowledge.

Case Resolution

The case history presented highlights the typical features of the drug-exposed infant. Management includes testing for hepatitis B, syphilis, and HIV and administering medication such as phenobarbital if the irritability does not respond to swaddling or other measures. The situation should be reported to child protective services to ensure an assessment of the infant's home environment.

Selected Readings

Arendt, R., J. Angelopoulos, A. Salvator, and L. Singer. Motor development of cocaine-exposed children at age two years. Pediatrics 103:86–92, 1999.

Berlin, C. M. Effects of drugs on the fetus. Pediatr. Rev. 12:282–287, 1991.

Callahan, C. M., et al. Measurement of gestational cocaine exposure: sensitivity of infants' hair, meconium, and urine. J. Pediatr. 120:763–768, 1992.

Chirboga, C. A., Brust, J. C. M., Bateman, D., and W. A. Hauser. Dose-response effect of fetal cocaine exposure on newborn neurologic function. Pediatrics 103:79–85, 1999.

Dixon, S. D., K. Bresnahan, and B. Zuckerman. Cocaine babies. Meeting the challenge of management. Contemp. Pediatr. 7:70–92, 1990.

Fulroth, R., B. Phillips, and D.J. Durand. Neurologic manifestations of cocaine exposure in childhood. Pediatrics 93:557–560, 1994.

Ostrea, E. M., Jr. Testing for exposure to illicit drugs and other agents in the neonate: A review of laboratory methods and the role of meconium analysis. Curr. Prob. Ped. 29:37–60, 1999.

Siddiqi, T. A., and R. C. Tsang. Babies of substance-abusing mothers: an overview. Pediatr. Ann. 20:527–530, 1991.

Volpe, J. Effect of cocaine use on the fetus. N. Engl. J. Med. 326:399–407, 1992.

CHAPTER 108

SUBSTANCE ABUSE

Monica Sifuentes, M.D.

H$_x$ A 17-year-old adolescent male is brought to your office by his father with a chief complaint of chronic cough. You have followed this patient and his siblings for several years and know the family quite well. The father appears very concerned about "this cough that just won't go away." The adolescent is not concerned about the cough, however, and reports no associated symptoms such as fever, sore throat, chest pain, or sinus pain. You ask the father to step out of the room for the rest of the interview and the physical examination.

On further questioning, the patient reports that he smokes a few cigarettes a day and has tried marijuana as well as cocaine. He denies regular use of these substances, but reports exposure to these drugs at parties and when he hangs out with "certain friends." The adolescent is now in the eleventh grade, attends school regularly, and thinks school is "OK." His grades are average to above average, but he thinks he might fail history this semester. Although he used to play baseball, he dropped out last year. He hopes to get a part-time job at a local fast food restaurant this summer if his parents let him. Currently he is sexually active and uses condoms occasionally. He denies suicidal ideation and exposure to any firearms.

On physical examination, he appears well developed and well nourished with an occasional dry cough. He is afebrile, and his respiratory rate, heart rate, and blood pressure are normal. Pertinent findings on examination include slight conjunctival injection bilaterally and mild erythema of the posterior pharynx. No tonsillar hypertrophy is apparent. The rest of the examination is within normal limits.

Questions

1. What are the most common manifestations of substance use and abuse in adolescents?
2. What are the risk factors associated with substance abuse in adolescents?
3. What other conditions must be considered when evaluating adolescents with a history of chronic substance abuse?
4. What laboratory evaluation, if any, should be considered in adolescents with suspected substance use or abuse?
5. What are the specific consequences, if any, of short-term and long-term use or abuse of substances such as alcohol, marijuana, cocaine, opiates, and hallucinogens?

Primary care practitioners can become involved in adolescent substance abuse either through prevention and anticipatory guidance or through the identification and treatment of a substance abuse problem in their patients. Ideally, all adolescent patients should be questioned and counseled about the use of illicit drugs, alcohol, and tobacco at each health maintenance visit (see Chapter 18, Health Maintenance in Older Children and Adolescents, and Chapter 4, Talking to Adolescents). Unfortunately, this rarely occurs because most health care professionals often feel uncomfortable opening this "Pandora's box." Primary care practitioners thus lose a valuable opportunity to adequately assess adolescents for substance abuse.

Substance use can be defined as the use of or experimentation with illicit drugs, alcohol, or tobacco. Illicit drugs include marijuana; cocaine; amphetamines; hallucinogens such as lysergic acid diethylamide (LSD), mescaline, and psilocybin, which is found in *Psilocybe mexicana* mushrooms; opiates; and phencyclidine (PCP). **Substance abuse** refers to the chronic use of mind-altering drugs in spite of adverse affects. **Addiction** is the term applied to compulsive and continued use of a substance in the face of these adverse consequences. The substance may produce physical dependence or symptoms of withdrawal when it is discontinued.

EPIDEMIOLOGY

Current Trends and Prevalence Rates

A wide range of substances are currently being used by young adolescents in the United States. Alcohol, tobacco, and marijuana are clearly the more common and most popular substances.

In a recent survey of graduating high school seniors, approximately 90% admitted to **alcohol** use at some time. Just over half (51%) of students reported drinking alcohol during the month preceding the survey, and 3–5% admitted that they used alcohol daily. Binge drinking has probably contributed most to the overall morbidity and mortality associated with alcohol use in adolescents. Among high school seniors in the class of 1993, 30% reported having five or more drinks in a row at least once during the previous 2 weeks. By 1997, this figure rose to almost 40% of 12th graders who experienced episodic heavy drinking during the month preceding the survey.

Although **tobacco** use among adolescents decreased from 1975 to 1993, approximately 20% of teenagers still report smoking one or more cigarettes per day in the past month. Eleven percent of adolescents smoked a half a pack or more cigarettes per day in 1993 compared to 19% in 1977. Eight percent of eighth-graders were smoking on a daily basis. In 1997, frequent cigarette use was reported by almost 17% of high school students according to the CDC.

In 1995, almost 40% of high school seniors admitted to using an illicit drug during the previous 12 months. The overall lifetime prevalence was 50%, indicating that nearly one out of two graduating seniors has tried an illicit substance at some time in the past. It is important to remember that these statistics do not include the estimated 15–20% of students who drop out of school before their senior year.

Marijuana is the most commonly used illicit psychoactive substance. In 1993, 35% of high school seniors reported ever having used marijuana, and in 1997, this figure increased to over 50%. Nearly 27% reported some use in the past month. Daily use of marijuana has been reported in 5% of high school seniors.

The use of other substances amongst adolescents had generally taken a downward trend in the late 1980s and early 1990s; however, figures are increasing again. Reportedly, approximately 9% of high school graduates in 1997 tried cocaine, with approximately 4% having used it in the previous month. In addition, almost 5% reported ever having used "crack" or "freebase" (smoking cocaine). The 1991 prevalence rate for LSD usage was 5%, and its use has shown no appreciable decline in the past 10 years. In fact, LSD use among teens has increased significantly and may be more widespread than cocaine among high school students. According to a 1995 survey, almost 12% of high school seniors nationwide had tried LSD. Amphetamine use among 12th graders was comparable in 1993. Fifteen percent reported having tried amphetamines in their lifetime; 9% used them in the past year; and almost 4% in the past month.

Concurrently, the reported use of over-the-counter nonprescription stimulants that contain caffeine or phenylpropanolamine has increased. Other substances used to "get high," such as inhalants, are often used by younger students (preteens). Nineteen percent of ninth graders surveyed by the CDC in 1997 reported having sniffed or inhaled substances to become intoxicated.

Although not considered an illicit substance by some, anabolic steroids are abused by some adolescents, mostly males, to increase muscle size and strength. In 1997, approximately 3% admitted to using them at some time in their lives. Other studies indicate as many as 5.5% of high school students participating in sports use anabolic steroids (6.6% males, 3.9% females).

Demographics

In general, adolescent males use illicit drugs more than females do, with a few exceptions. Males are more likely to use anabolic steroids, but females reportedly use amphetamines, barbiturates, tranquilizers, and over-the-counter diet pills more than their male counterparts. In addition, although annual prevalence rates for overall alcohol use show little gender difference, adolescent males have a higher rate of heavy drinking. Tobacco usage is essentially the same for both sexes.

Non–college-bound adolescents are more likely to use illicit substances than their college-bound counterparts, and these adolescents are also more likely to use drugs more frequently. There is no difference, however, between the two groups in the rates of ever having tried illicit substances. The influence of parental education, socioeconomic status, and race or ethnicity on the use and abuse of illicit substances is difficult to determine.

Risk Factors and Risk Behaviors

The strongest predictor of drug use is having friends who use drugs regularly. In addition, it has been shown that the more risk factors identified, the greater the risk of substance abuse.

Several factors are important precursors (risk factors) to drug use during adolescence. These include association with drug-using peers; attitudinal factors, such as favorable attitudes regarding drug use and low religiosity; school failure, beginning in the late elementary years; young age of initiation of alcohol or drug use; environmental factors, such as the prevalence of drug use in a given community; a family history of alcoholism or drug use; poor parenting practices; high levels of conflict within the family; minimal bonding between parents and children; and early and persistent problem behaviors during childhood.

CLINICAL PRESENTATION

Adolescents who are involved in substance abuse may present to the physician in several different ways. Illicit substance use might be uncovered during the routine interview for an annual health maintenance visit or preparticipation sports physical. Alternatively, the adolescent might have physical complaints including chronic cough, persistent allergies, chest pain, and fatigue. They also may have recently been in a motor vehicle crash, or their parents may complain of frequent mood swings.

PATHOPHYSIOLOGY

Although several theories have been proposed to explain why casual substance use develops into abuse and addiction in some adolescents, the most critical factor seems to be the presence of underlying psychopathology. Adolescents who have major depressive disorders, attention deficit disorders and hyperactivity, or schizophrenia, for example, may use mood-altering substances to treat unpleasant feelings of dysphoria and low self-esteem. Although initially temporary, this method of self-medication makes chronic use with some substances likely.

DIFFERENTIAL DIAGNOSIS

The differential diagnosis for symptoms and behaviors associated with substance abuse includes underlying psychiatric disorders. Affective, antisocial, conduct, and attention deficit disorders can be the primary or secondary condition in adolescents who are abusing drugs. Like adults, adolescents may be using illicit drugs to self-medicate. The pharmacology and toxicity of the illicit substances most commonly used by adolescents are summarized in Table 108–1.

TABLE 108–1. Pharmacology and Toxicity of Substances Commonly Used by Adolescents*

Substance	Pharmacology	Toxic Effects	Toxicity
Nicotine	Potent psychoactive drug, acting on receptors in CNS to produce effects: stimulation, relaxation, focuses attention		Nontolerant individuals: Weakness Nausea Vomiting Feeling unwell
Marijuana	Active ingredient (delta-9-tetrahydrocannabinol) is rapidly absorbed into bloodstream from inhaled smoke	Euphoria, mood fluctuations, hallucinations	Acute: Panic attacks Psychosis (rare) Chronic: Short-term memory impairment Amotivational syndrome Reduced sperm counts
Alcohol	Causes nerve cell membranes to expand and become more "fluid"—interfering with neuronal conduction Interference of neurotransmitters	Mild: Disinhibition, euphoria, mild impaired coordincation Moderate: Increased sedation, slurred speech, ataxia	Severe: Confusion Stupor Coma Respiratory depression
Cocaine	Increased release and decreased reuptake of biogenic amines causing CNS stimulation Local anesthesia Vasoconstriction	Produces a sense of well-being and heightened awareness, decrease in social inhibition, intense euphoria	Delirium Confusion Paranoia Hypertension Tachycardia Hyperpyrexia Mydriasis
Stimulants Amphetamines Crystal methamphetamine	CNS stimulation (sympathomimetic)	Heightened awareness Restlessness and agitation Decreased appetite Low doses increase ability to concentrate	Hypertension Hyperthermia Seizures Stroke Coma Arrhythmias
Hallucinogens LSD Mescaline Mushrooms	Inhibits release of serotonin	Distortions of reality— "synesthesias" common ("hearing," smells)	Paranoia Flashbacks Psychosis Depression
Phencyclidine (PCP)	Dissociative anesthetic with analgesic, stimulant, depressant, and hallucinogenic properties	Dissociative anesthetic Dose-dependent euphoria, dysphoria, perceptual distortion	Psychoses Aggressive, violent behavior Depression Seizures Rhabdomyolysis
Opiates Opium Heroin Methadone	Binds to opioid receptors in CNS, causing CNS depression	Sedative analgesics Euphoria followed by sedation	Respiratory depression CNS depression Miosis Bradycardia, hypotension, arrhythmia Seizures, rhabdomyolysis
Sedatives Benzodiazepines Barbiturates	CNS depression, binds to specific receptor that potentiates GABA	Sedation Anxiety reduction	Similar to opioid intoxication
Anabolic steroids	Bind to androgen receptors at cellular level, stimulate production of RNA and protein synthesis	Euphoria Increased irritability and aggressiveness Induction of mental changes at high doses	Psychosis
Inhalants	CNS stimulation and excitement, progressing to depression	Euphoria Hallucinations Psychosis	Respiratory depression Arrhythmia Seizures "Sudden sniffing death syndrome" (Sudden death secondary to arrhythmia)

*Data from Schwartz, B. and E. M. Alderman. Substances of abuse. Pediatr Rev 18:206–214, 1997.

EVALUATION

History

The interview should be conducted in a private, quiet area with minimal chance of interruptions. If parents have accompanied adolescents, they should be politely asked to leave the room after issues of confidentiality are addressed in the presence of both parties. This avoids further awkward moments when parents ask what was disclosed during the interview with their children. After parents have left the room, issues regarding confidentiality and privacy should be reviewed once again with adolescents. Special circumstances, such as disclosures of sexual or physical abuse and possible suicide or homicide, that dictate that confidentiality be broken should also be discussed (see Chapter 4, Talking to Adolescents).

The interview should then proceed in a casual, nonpressured fashion. Initial inquiries should concern less threatening general topics such as school, home life, and outside activities, including activities with friends (Table 108–2). The acronym **HEADSSS** allows review of the essential components of the psychosocial history: **h**ome, **e**ducation or employment, **a**ctivities, **d**rugs, **s**exual activity, **s**uicide or depression, and **s**afety (see Chapter 4, Talking to Adolescents).

Some practitioners prefer to use questionnaires to obtain this background information. A questionnaire is given to patients to fill out while they are waiting to be seen, and the responses are reviewed by practitioners during the visit (see Table 108–2). Controversy exists regarding the role of such questionnaires, primarily concerning the truthfulness of answers.

Questions: Adolescent Substance Abuse

- Do any of the adolescent's friends drink alcohol, smoke marijuana or tobacco, or use any other drugs?
- What drugs, including alcohol and tobacco, are currently being used by the adolescent? For how long and how frequently?
- In what environments does the adolescent use these substances?
- Has the adolescent ever blacked out or been arrested while under the influence of drugs or alcohol?
- Has drug or alcohol use ever interferred with school, work, or other social activities?
- Has drug or alcohol use adversely affected relationships with family, friends, or romantic partners?
- Has the patient ever had sexual encounters while under the influence of drugs or alcohol?
- Does the adolescent ever use drugs or alcohol to feel better or to forget why he or she feels sad?
- Do the adolescent's parents use alcohol, tobacco, or illicit drugs?

More specific questions related to the use of alcohol and tobacco as well as illicit substances should be asked after general subjects have been discussed (Questions Box). If adolescents seem wary of answering these questions, it may be helpful to initially inquire about their friends. Questions should be phrased with the assumption that the responses will be affirmative (e.g., How many beers do you drink in a week?). It is hoped that this less threatening approach invites more honest answers. An assessment of the risk of suicidal behavior is also indicated. Further questions relevant to substance abuse are given in Table 108–3.

Physical Examination

Positive findings on physical examination are rare, especially in adolescents who use alcohol or other substances only occasionally. In adolescents with a

---

TABLE 108–2.   Questionnaire Items Relevant to Substance Abuse

		Y	N
1.	Do you smoke cigarettes?	Y_____	N_____
2.	Do you smoke marijuana?	Y_____	N_____
3.	Do you often feel "bummed out," down, or depressed?	Y_____	N_____
4.	Do you ever use drugs or alcohol to feel better?	Y_____	N_____
5.	Do you ever use drugs or alcohol when you are alone?	Y_____	N_____
6.	Do your friends get drunk or get high at parties?	Y_____	N_____
7.	Do you get drunk or get high at parties?	Y_____	N_____
8.	Do your friends ever get drunk or get high at rock concerts?	Y_____	N_____
9.	Do you ever get drunk or get high at rock concerts?	Y_____	N_____
10.	Have your school grades gone down recently?	Y_____	N_____
11.	Have you flunked any subjects recently?	Y_____	N_____
12.	Have you had recent problems with your coaches or advisers at school?	Y_____	N_____
13.	Do you feel that friends or parents just do not seem to understand you?	Y_____	N_____

Reproduced, with permission, from Schonberg, S.K. (ed.). American Academy of Pediatrics: Substance Abuse: A Guide for Professionals. American Academy of Pediatrics, Elk Grove, Il., 1988.

TABLE 108–3.   Open-ended Questions Intended to Provide a Basis for Further Exploration of Advanced Substance Abuse

1. What do your friends do at parties? Do you go to the parties? Do you drink? Get drunk? Get high?
2. Do you drive drunk? Stoned? Have you ridden with a driver who was drunk or stoned? Could you call home and ask for help? What would your parents say? Do?
3. Do you go to rock concerts? Do you drink there? Do you get high? Who drives after the concert?
4. After drinking, have you ever forgotten where you had been or what you had done?
5. Have you recently dropped some of your old friends and started going with a new group?
6. Do you feel that lately you are irritable, "bitchy," or moody?
7. Do you find yourself getting into more frequent arguments with your friends? Brothers and sisters? Parents?
8. Do you have a girlfriend/boyfriend? How is that going? Are you having more fights/arguments with him/her lately? Have you recently broken up?
9. Do you find yourself being physically abusive to others? Your brothers/sisters? Your mother/father?
10. Do you think your drinking/drug use is a problem? Why?

Reproduced, with permission, from Schonberg, S.K. (ed.). American Academy of Pediatrics: Substance Abuse: A Guide for Professionals. American Academy of Pediatrics, Elk Grove, Il., 1988.

history of chronic substance abuse, however, certain physical findings may be present.

All vital signs should be reviewed. Tachycardia and hypertension occur primarily with acute intoxication with cocaine or stimulants such as amphetamines. The current weight also should be recorded and compared to previous values, and any significant loss should be noted. The skin should be examined closely for track marks, skin abscesses, or cellulitis, especially if patients admit to using drugs intravenously. Findings consistent with hepatitis (hepatomegaly and jaundice) may also be present in these individuals. The presence of diffuse adenopathy, thrush, leukoplakia, seborrheic dermatitis, or parotitis should raise the suspicion of human immunodeficiency virus infection. Upper respiratory symptoms such as chronic nasal congestion, long-lasting "colds" and "allergies," and epistaxis can occur with chronic inhalation of cocaine. Signs of nasal congestion, septal perforation, and wheezing may be noted on examination. In addition, smoking crack cocaine can cause chronic cough, hemoptysis, and chest pain. Smoking marijuana over long periods of time can result in similar findings. Gynecomastia can be seen with use of anabolic steroids, marijuana, amphetamine, and heroin. In the adolescent female using anabolic steroids, there may be signs of virilization, such as a deep voice, hirsutism, and male pattern baldness.

The neurologic evaluation is probably the most important part of the examination. Any abnormalities in memory, cognitive functioning, or affect should be noted. Chronic marijuana use is sometimes accompanied by an amotivational syndrome.

Acute intoxication with some drugs such as cocaine may lead to delirium, confusion, paranoia, seizures, hypertension, tachycardia, arrhythmias, mydriasis, and hyperpyrexia. Acute PCP intoxication produces abnormal neurologic signs, tachycardia, and hypertension. Findings such as central nervous system and respiratory depression, miosis, and cardiovascular effects (e.g., pulmonary edema, orthostatic hypotension) are consistent with opiate overdose.

Laboratory Tests

Drug screening in the evaluation of possible substance abuse is usually not indicated. Specific laboratory studies should be performed only in patients who are known substance abusers and are enrolled in a treatment program or in patients with an acute presentation of altered mental status, intoxication, or abnormal neurologic findings. In the office setting, these symptoms are frequently absent, and urine or serum studies to "check" for drug use are not warranted. If these tests are performed, they require the adolescent's consent. They should not be performed simply to allay parental anxiety or confirm suspicions regarding possible substance abuse.

Urine testing is available to detect marijuana and its metabolites, cocaine, amphetamines, PCP, opiates, barbiturates, and benzodiazepines. Blood levels can be obtained for alcohol, marijuana, cocaine, amphetamines, barbiturates, and benzodiazepines. Although salivary or urinary concentrations of cotinine and nicotine concentrations can also be performed, these measurements are primarily used in research studies.

Testing for specific inhalants is not routinely done. The deleterious effects of these substances on the hematologic, liver, and renal systems can be evaluated by performing a complete blood count, liver function tests, prothrombin time and partial thromboplastin time, and blood urea nitrogen and creatinine.

MANAGEMENT

One of several approaches to the problem of substance abuse can be chosen depending on the degree of risk-taking behavior and drug involvement.

Anticipatory Guidance

If adolescents and their peers are not participating in any high-risk behaviors, pediatricians should provide patients with age-appropriate anticipatory guidance. This should include information regarding safety issues, consequences of alcohol and tobacco use, and exposures to illicit drugs. Adolescents should be encouraged to continue their current behavior but should be invited to return to the office if they have any questions or problems. This may be particularly helpful for adolescents whose daily environment exposes them to high-risk situations.

Early Intervention

Primary care practitioners should provide early intervention guidance to adolescents who are engaging in occasional high-risk behavior but whose substance use does not interfere with or disrupt their daily lives. Such use implies only occasional or casual use of illicit substances by patients or peers. Interventional guidance involves discussing potential risks created by adolescents' current behavior. For example, individuals who drink alcohol or smoke marijuana at parties have an increased risk of involvement in a motor vehicle crash afterward. Another common scenario involves alcohol intoxication and poor judgment with regard to sexual behavior.

Specialized Programs

Adolescents who are routinely using drugs but are clearly motivated to stop can often be managed by primary care physicians. Many of these teenagers began using illicit substances at an older age, have a fairly good relationship with their families, have supportive relationships with friends who do not use drugs, and have continued to do well in school and participate in other outside activities. At first, practitioners should identify the problem and establish that adolescents desire to change their behavior. Then they should meet with families, develop an appropriate strategy, and follow adolescents periodically in the office. Periodic reinforcement by physicians is necessary, especially in the beginning. Referral to outpatient programs, such as Alcoholics Anonymous or Narcotics Anonymous, may also be indicated.

Mental Health or Treatment Programs

Referral to a mental health or specialized treatment program is indicated for adolescents who continue to use drugs despite office treatment. In addition, those teenagers who have a suspected psychological or psychiatric condition should be referred immediately for evaluation. Other criteria for specialty treatment include a long history of drug abuse, a serious life-threatening event in conjunction with substance abuse (e.g., attempted suicide), familial strife, or persistent involvement with a drug-dependent crowd.

Primary care practitioners should become familiar with local inpatient programs and residential substance abuse treatment facilities in the community. Although the selection of a program is often dictated by financial resources, it is very important to select an appropriate one. Guidelines exist to aid practitioners in the selection process. These guidelines include total abstinence, appropriate professionals with expertise in drug abuse, familial involvement in the program, family therapy, and appropriate outpatient follow-up.

Prevention Programs

Prevention programs have been developed to assist and influence the decisions young people make about the use of illicit substances. Current programs focus on multiple aspects of the lives of children and adolescents. Programs may involve individual decision making, self-esteem, and basic education regarding drugs. They frequently emphasize communication skills, family values and dynamics, parenting skills, and positive peer associations. Structured curricula have also been created for use in the schools, and community outreach programs have been organized by groups such as local police departments. The actual effectiveness of each type of program is a subject of controversy, but they are all aimed at somehow preventing the initial or continued use of illicit substances.

PROGNOSIS

It is difficult to assess the outcome for adolescents who undergo treatment for substance abuse because definitions of success vary. For some teenagers, success implies periods of sobriety, for others it means complete abstinence, and for still others it is abstinence in addition to recovery from other contributing problems. Specific outcome data that are available, however, reveal that abstinence rates are positively correlated with regular attendance in a support group and parental participation in these groups. In addition, general success rates range from 15% to 45%, depending on

short- or long-term assessments. As expected, there is a lifetime potential for relapse among all substance abusers.

Case Resolution

In the case presented above, the adolescent is at high risk for substance abuse given his drug-using friends, tobacco use, possible school failure, and recent change in extracurricular activities (i.e., dropping out of baseball). The findings on physical examination are also consistent with his smoking history. The physician should review these risk factors with the teenager and acknowledge the difficulty in removing one's self from such an environment. The adolescent's motivation to change his behavior should be assessed and referrals to special intervention programs can be discussed. Regardless of the outcome, the physician should continue to see the teenager at an agreed-upon interval to monitor his behavior.

Selected Readings

American Academy of Pediatrics. Committee on Sports Medicine and Fitness. Adolescents and anabolic steroids: a subject review. Pediatrics 99:904–908, 1997.

American Academy of Pediatrics. Committee on Substance Abuse. Testing for drugs of abuse in children and adolescents. Pediatrics 98:305–310, 1996.

American Academy of Pediatrics. Committee on Substance Abuse. Tobacco, alcohol, and other drugs: The role of the pediatrician in prevention and management of substance abuse. Pediatrics 101:125–128, 1998.

American Academy of Pediatrics. Committee on Substance Abuse and Committee on Native American Child Health. Inhalant abuse. Pediatrics 97:420–423, 1996.

Brown, R. R., and S. A. Coupe. Illicit drugs of abuse. Adolesc. Med. State of the Art Rev. 4:321–340, 1993.

Comerci, G. D. Office assessment of substance abuse and addiction. Adolesc. Med. State of the Art Rev. 4:277–293, 1993.

Fishman, M., et al. Substance abuse among children and adolescents. Pediatr. Rev. 18:394–403, 1997.

Hawking, J. D., and Fitzgibbon. Risk factors and risk behaviors in prevention of adolescent substance abuse. Adolesc. Med. State of the Art Rev. 4:249–262, 1993.

Heyman, R. B., and H. Adger. Office approach to drug abuse prevention. Pediatr. Clin. North Am. 44:1447–1455, 1997.

Knight, J. R. Adolescent substance use: screening, assessment, and intervention. Contemp. Pediatr. 14:45–72, 1997.

MacKenzie R. G., and B. Heischober. Methamphetamine. Pediatr. Rev. 18:305–309, 1997.

Rodgers, P. D., and M. J. Werner (eds.). Substance Abuse. Pediatr. Clin. North Am. 42:241–490, 1995.

Schonberg, S. K. (ed.). American Academy of Pediatrics: Substance Abuse: A Guide for Professionals. American Academy of Pediatrics, Elk Grove, IL, 1988.

Schwartz, R. H. Adolescent heroin use: a review. Pediatrics 101:1461–1466, 1998.

Schwartz, R. H. LSD makes a comeback. Contemp. Pediatr. 13:71–81, 1996.

Takahashi, A., and J. Franklin. Alcohol abuse. Pediatr. Rev. 17:39–45, 1996.

Werner, M. J., and H. Adger. Early identification, screening, and brief intervention for adolescent alcohol use. Arch. Pediatr. Adol. Med. 149:1241–1248, 1995.

CHAPTER 109

EATING DISORDERS

Monica Sifuentes, M.D.

H$_x$ A 16-year-old adolescent female is brought to the office by her mother because she feels that her daughter is too thin. The mother complains that her daughter does not eat much at dinner and always says she is not hungry. Recently the girl bought diet pills that were advertised in a teen magazine. She claims that the pills are supposed to help her gain weight, so she doesn't understand why her mother is so upset. She says she feels fine and considers herself healthy.

The girl is a tenth grade student at a local public school and attends classes regularly, although her friends are occasionally truant. She is involved in the drill team, the swim team, and the student council. She has many friends who have "nicer" figures than she does. Neither she nor her friends smoke tobacco or use drugs, but they occasionally drink beer at parties. The girl is not sexually active and denies a history of abuse. Her menstrual periods are irregular; the last one was approximately 6 weeks ago.

She currently lives with her mother, father, and two younger siblings. Although things are "okay" at home, she thinks her parents are too strict and don't trust her. They have just begun to allow her to date.

Her physical examination is significant for a thin physique and normal vital signs. On the growth chart, her weight is at the 15th percentile and her height at the 75th percentile, giving her a body mass index (BMI) of 17 (10th percentile). The remainder of her physical examination is unremarkable.

Questions

1. What are the common characteristics of eating disorders in adolescents?
2. What are the important historical points to include when interviewing patients with suspected eating disorders?
3. How is the diagnosis of anorexia nervosa and bulimia nervosa made?
4. What is the treatment plan for adolescents with eating disorders?
5. What are the medical complications of anorexia and bulimia nervosa?
6. What is the prognosis for these conditions? How can primary care practitioners help improve the outcome?

Eating disorders are complex problems that are sometimes difficult to diagnose based on strict DSM-IV criteria (Table 109–1). Adolescents may have partial or atypical forms, a combination of both anorexia and bulimia nervosa, or an underlying affective component that confuses the issue. In addition, preoccupation with physical appearance and weight is not uncommon or necessarily pathologic in today's society. Both the fashion industry and media promote the idea that thinness and beauty are interrelated. Thus, average adolescents who long to be accepted by peers and who are learning to develop a sense of independence and control are prime targets for the development of eating disorders.

TABLE 109–1. Diagnostic Criteria for Anorexia and Bulimia Nervosa

Anorexia Nervosa

A. Refusal to maintain body weight at or above a minimally normal weight for age and height.
B. Intense fear of gaining weight or becoming fat, even though underweight.
C. Disturbance in the way in which one's body weight or shape is experienced, undue influence of body weight or shape on self-evaluation, or denial of the seriousness of the current low body weight.
D. In post-menarcheal females, amenorrhea, i.e., the absence of at least three consecutive cycles.

Bulimia Nervosa

A. Recurrent episodes of binge eating, characterized by the following:
  (1) eating, in a discrete period of time an amount of food that is definitely larger than most people would consume under similar circumstances and in the same period of time
  (2) a sense of lack of control over eating during the episode
B. Recurrent inappropriate compensatory behavior in order to prevent weight gain (self-induced vomiting, laxative, or diuretic use).
C. Criteria A and B both occur on average, at least twice a week for 3 months.
D. Self-evaluation is unduly influenced by body shape and weight.
E. The disturbance does not occur exclusively during episodes of anorexia nervosa.

Adapted and reproduced, with permission, from Diagnostic and Statistical Manual of Mental Disorders (DSM-IV). Washington, D.C., American Psychiatric Association, 1994.

EPIDEMIOLOGY

In general, eating disorders are most common among caucasian females and in more affluent communities. Although they occur in other settings, in previous years they were nearly unheard of in lower socioeconomic groups. Today, they can be seen in all ethnic, cultural, and social backgrounds. In addition, males make up an estimated 5–10% of all patients with eating disorders.

Although dieting behavior among adolescents and young adults is not uncommon, true anorexia nervosa has a prevalence of approximately 0.5–1% in these individuals. Estimates have ranged from 1% to 10% in high-risk groups such as upper and middle class white females. Fewer than 5% of these cases are males, with a female:male ratio of 9:1. The age of onset is usually during early or middle adolescence (age 12–16 years). However, anorexia has been reported to have a second peak later in adolescence.

The prevalence of bulimia nervosa is approximately 1–4%, although some studies report that as many as 8% of adolescents and college women and 0.4% of men are bulimic. The age of onset tends to be later than for anorexia, with symptoms beginning during late adolescence (age 17–20 years). Females outnumber males by a factor of five.

Several other behavioral and affective disorders have been associated with anorexia and bulimia nervosa. These include major depression in patients as well as first-degree relatives, alcoholism and substance abuse, other addictive behaviors (e.g., laxative abuse), poor impulse control and anxiety disorders, and obsessive-compulsive personality. In addition, suicidal behavior (attempts) is more likely in individuals with bulimia.

Mild variants of eating disorders, which do not meet full diagnostic criteria, occur in approximately 5–10% of post-pubertal females. Additionally, greater than half of junior high and high school girls have dieted at some time, many repeatedly.

PSYCHOBIOLOGY

ANOREXIA NERVOSA

Although several factors predispose individuals to the development of anorexia nervosa, this condition has no single cause. Longitudinal studies clearly point to a significant role of dieting behavior in the pathogenesis of an eating disorder. However, since not all dieters develop an eating disorder, other risk factors must be involved. Current theory suggests that a complex relationship among many factors may lead to anorexia.

Biologic Factors

It has been postulated that the normal increase in adipose tissue with the onset of puberty creates a special problem for some females. An eating disorder may develop as an attempt to control or combat this normal pubertal weight gain. Preexisting hypothalamic dysfunction has also been implicated as a contributing factor to anorexia. In addition, changes in neurotransmitter levels have been shown to occur with initial vomiting or dieting. These changes may then lead to specific psychiatric symptoms that may perpetuate eating disorders.

Genetic Factors

A possible genetic predisposition to anorexia has been shown in studies of monozygotic twins. The incidence of the disorder is increased in sisters and other female relatives of patients with anorexia.

Personal Characteristics

In general, patients with anorexia are described as obsessive-compulsive personality types, perfectionists, and overachievers. They also display low self-esteem and high anxiety levels despite their successes. They are the "model daughters" who have never caused any previous problems given their compliant, self-sacrificing, nonassertive nature.

Familial Influences

Researchers have noted that certain family dynamics may serve to initiate and perpetuate anorexia nervosa. Typically, the family is overprotective and rigid, with the mother often enmeshed in her daughter's life. Conflict resolution tends to be poor. An inability to express feelings within the family is often evident.

Social/Environmental Pressures

Both the media and societal standards are believed to play a role in "setting the stage" for an eating disorder. Affluent communities are especially at risk for this. Within these social circles, thinness, food, eating, and exercise can become the prime focus of daily activity.

In addition, young women become caught in what has been labeled a "slender trap" in which thinness is equivalent to attractiveness and success. Food restriction or purging are a means of attaining thinness. An inability to maintain thinness equals failure. Role models in the media, such as fashion models and actresses, also serve as ideals by which young people create their standards.

Other Influences

Involvement in particular extracurricular activities, such as ballet and gymnastics, may contribute to the development of anorexia in females. For male athletes, such influences include participation in sports such as wrestling, in which maintaining a given weight is important and dieting is used to achieve that weight. Chronic medical conditions, such as diabetes mellitus or inflammatory bowel disease (IBD), may also contribute to the development of an eating disorder.

BULIMIA NERVOSA

Several theories have been proposed to explain the etiology of bulimia nervosa. Most likely, multiple factors contribute to the development of this eating disorder.

Familial Influences

Family theory assumes that the eating disorder is a symptom of familial dysfunction and may be associated with physical or sexual abuse. With bulimia, unlike anorexia, conflict is discussed openly but negatively within the family. The relationship between mothers and daughters is distant rather than enmeshed. Parents and relatives have a high rate of depression as well as alcoholism.

Social/Environmental Influences

The sociocultural theory notes the influence of societal pressures to be thin. This thinness is synonymous with success. Thus, the binge-purge cycle is maintained as the adolescent attempts to become successful and avoid failure.

Cognitive-Behavioral Theory

This theory suggests that the eating disorder is a manifestation of irrational thoughts that adolescents have concerning weight, dieting, and self-esteem. Dieting and starvation result from cultural pressures and emotional instability. The binge-purge cycle develops as a coping mechanism for dealing with the disinhibition and guilt associated with these practices.

Psychodynamic Theory

This theory views bulimia as an attempt to control distressful feelings, such as depression, low self-esteem, and ineffectiveness. Adolescents may exhibit impulsive behaviors, including shoplifting and sexual activity. Treatment focuses on identifying these underlying processes.

Addiction Theory

This theory views binging and purging activity as an addictive behavior. Treatment stresses abstinence, support groups, and relapse prevention.

DIFFERENTIAL DIAGNOSIS

It is important to differentiate anorexia nervosa from bulimia nervosa. Differences between these two conditions are listed in Table 109–2. Occasionally, this distinction may be difficult to make, especially if patients display behavior consistent with both conditions. In addition, most patients with eating disorders have associated comorbid psychiatric disorders. Major

---

> **Questions: Eating Disorders**
>
> - Have there been any changes in the adolescent's weight?
> - What did he or she eat yesterday?
> - How does the adolescent and his or her friends handle weight control?
> - How much does the adolescent want to weigh?
> - How often does the adolescent weigh himself or herself?
> - How does the adolescent feel about how he or she looks?
> - Do any particular areas of the body, such as the thighs, lower abdomen, and buttocks, most concern the adolescent?
> - What does the adolescent do when he or she feels "fat"? Does the adolescent vomit to lose weight?
> - Has the adolescent or any of his or her friends ever used diuretics, ipecac, enemas or laxatives to lose weight or compensate for overeating?
> - How compulsive is the adolescent about exercise?
> - In what sports, if any, does the adolescent participate?
> - For females, are menstrual periods regular?
> - Does the adolescent have any other symptoms associated with complications of eating disorders?
> - Does the adolescent have any depressive symptoms, such as sleeping problems, that can accompany eating disorders?
>
> **For Patients With Bulimia Nervosa**
> - When do binges occur?
> - What are the precipitating factors?
> - What happens, specifically, during a typical episode?

---

affective disorders to consider include depression, bipolar disorder, and obsessive-compulsive disorder. Anxiety disorders and substance abuse also are commonly seen, although the latter is more strongly associated with bulimia nervosa.

Other diagnoses to consider when evaluating patients for anorexia include IBD, diabetes mellitus, malignancies, Addison disease, hyper- or hypothyroidism, hypopituitarism, tumors of the CNS, and substance abuse, particularly with amphetamines and crack cocaine.

EVALUATION

History

A complete medical history should be obtained from all adolescents with suspected eating disorders (Questions Box). Inquiries should focus on symptoms associated with complications such as dysphagia secondary to esophagitis from recurrent vomiting, constipation from fluid restriction, or muscle weakness associated with emetine toxicity from chronic ipecac use. A thorough psychosocial assessment should be performed. The **HEADSSS** format (**h**ome, **e**mployment and education, **a**ctivities, **d**rugs, **s**exual activity/sexuality, **s**uicide and depression, **s**afety) is useful to direct the psychosocial interview from general topics to more sensitive ones (see Chapter 4, Talking to Adolescents). The use of psychological testing/questionnaires to assess cognition and depression may be beneficial.

A dietary history should be taken as well. Direct questions regarding food intake and weight gain or loss should be asked. In addition, adolescents should be asked how they specifically maintain their weight.

TABLE 109–2. Differences Between Anorexia Nervosa and Bulimia Nervosa

Anorexia Nervosa	Bulimia Nervosa
Vomiting or diuretic or laxative abuse uncommon	Vomiting or diuretic or laxative abuse common
Severe weight loss	Less weight loss; avoidance of obesity
Slightly younger	Slightly older
More introverted	More extroverted
Hunger denied	Hunger pronounced
Eating behavior may be considered normal and a source of self-esteem	Eating behavior is ego-dystonic
Sexually inactive	Sexually active
Obsessional fears with paranoid features	Histrionic features
Amenorrhea	Menses irregular or absent
Death from starvation/suicide	Death from hypokalemia/suicide

Reproduced, with permission, from Shenker, I.R. Bulimia nervosa. In E.R. McAnarney et al. (eds.). Textbook of Adolescent Medicine. Philadelphia, W.B. Saunders, 1992.

A detailed menstrual history must also be obtained from females, because secondary amenorrhea is frequently present in patients with anorexia. Menses may be irregular or absent with bulimia as well. A family history of eating disorders, substance abuse, or psychiatric disease should also be addressed.

Physical Examination

In both conditions, the patient should undress, wearing only underwear, for the physical examination. This prevents any bulky clothes from hiding the true body habitus. The height and weight should be plotted on a growth chart, and the body mass index (BMI) should be calculated (BMI = weight [kg] ÷ height [m²]). Delayed growth or short stature should also be noted, because it can occur with severe malnutrition as well as other systemic conditions. Vital signs, including blood pressure, should also be recorded. The overall general appearance of patients must be noted. Adolescents with anorexia are often emaciated with an obvious loss of subcutaneous tissue. Patients with bulimia may be mildly obese or of normal weight with a full-appearing facies secondary to parotid and submaxillary swelling, a complication of frequent purging.

Physical findings in patients with **anorexia nervosa** are consistent with a "state of hibernation." Hypothermia, orthostatic hypotension, bradycardia, and lanugo (downy hair) on the arms and back are seen. The palms and soles may be yellow secondary to hypercarotenemia, and pigmentation of the chest and abdomen may be increased as a result of malnutrition. Loss of pubic and scalp hair as well as dry skin may also be seen. The breasts should be examined carefully for galactorrhea. The presence of galactorrhea, along with a history of amenorrhea, warrants further investigation for a prolactinoma.

The abdomen should be palpated for tenderness or masses. Bowel sounds are often decreased in patients with anorexia, and stool may be palpated secondary to constipation. A rectal examination should be performed for any evidence of bloody stool, which is a finding consistent with IBD. The extremities should be evaluated for coldness and mottling. Finally, a complete neurologic examination, including a mental status evaluation, should be performed to exclude any signs of a CNS lesion or endocrine disorder.

In patients with **bulimia nervosa,** specific physical findings, if any, are often associated with dehydration and electrolyte imbalances that occur as a result of chronic vomiting or laxative abuse. Vital signs should be reviewed for tachycardia and orthostatic hypotension; their presence indicates hemodynamic instability. The skin should be inspected on the dorsum of the hand over the knuckles for scratches, scars, or calluses from self-induced vomiting. Petechiae and subconjunctival hemorrhages may also be seen as a result of severe retching. The oropharynx should be inspected for dental caries, enamel erosion, or discoloration as well as for parotid hypertrophy. The abdomen should be palpated for epigastric tenderness or midabdominal pain. Positive findings may be due to esophagitis, gastritis, or pancreatitis.

From a musculoskeletal standpoint, any muscle weakness or cramping should be appreciated and may indicate an electrolyte abnormality. Edema of the extremities may be seen in laxative abusers and should be noted.

Laboratory Tests

Table 109–3 lists the laboratory studies necessary in the evaluation of patients with **anorexia nervosa.** A CBC may be helpful because leukopenia, anemia, and rarely, thrombocytopenia can be found with this disorder. Electrolytes (sodium, potassium, chloride, and carbon dioxide) and a BUN are important especially if patients use diuretics, laxatives, or ipecac. The ESR may be low with anorexia and high with IBD or some other inflammatory process. Normal liver function tests aid in excluding other causes of weight loss. Some endocrine tests help differentiate a hormonal problem from anorexia (see Table 109–3). An ECG allows practitioners to diagnose QT_c prolongation, heart block, and arrhythmias.

Laboratory abnormalities in **bulimia nervosa** reflect the type and extent of purging behavior of adolescents. Table 109–3 summarizes the necessary laboratory studies for patients with bulimia.

MANAGEMENT

It is the role of primary care practitioners to recognize when weight becomes an obsession for adolescents and when abnormal behaviors develop for maintenance of obvious malnutrition. When treating patients with eating disorders, physicians must first establish trust. Patients should be assured that practitioners are not attempting to remove all control. Next, a compromise must be reached between adolescents and pediatricians regarding the minimum acceptable weight given the

---

TABLE 109–3.   Laboratory Assessment of an Eating Disorder

Anorexia Nervosa
Complete blood count, erythrocyte sedimentation rate
Serum electrolytes (Na, K, Cl, CO_2)
Blood urea nitrogen/creatinine
Serum glucose
Serum calcium
Serum protein, albumin, cholesterol
Liver function tests
Endocrine labs:
  Follicle-stimulating hormone
  Luteinizing hormone
  Estradiol
  Thyroid function tests: $TSH/T_4/T_3$
  Cortisol
Urine pH and urinalysis
Electrocardiogram

Bulimia Nervosa
Serum electrolytes (Na, K, Cl, CO_2)
Serum glucose
Serum calcium, phosphorous, magnesium, zinc
Blood urea nitrogen/creatinine
Serum amylase
Urine pH and urinalysis
Electrocardiogram

patient's height. A contract that describes goals of treatment should then be established. Weight gain should be the initial priority, especially in adolescents with anorexia.

Family and individual counseling is often indicated. Patients must acknowledge the problem and their need for assistance before a referral can be made. This allows them to assert themselves and remain in control. Support groups may also be beneficial.

Numerous studies have shown that eating disorders are best treated by an interdisciplinary professional team experienced in the care of adolescents. This team should consist of the primary care provider, an adolescent medicine specialist, a psychologist or psychiatrist, a nutritionist, and a social worker. Ideally, the team is available to offer both inpatient as well as outpatient services. Criteria for inpatient admission should be established by the team and reviewed with patients and their families. Treatment for depression or any other affective disorder must be provided by a member of the team.

Inpatient treatment is required for weight loss greater than 30% below normal or a BMI less than 16; continued weight loss while on outpatient treatment; or a history of rapid weight loss over 3 months. Other indications include cardiovascular compromise, such as bradycardia (< 50 beats/min), orthostatic hypotension, or altered mental status; evidence of persistent hypothermia (< 36° C); suicidal or out-of-control behavior; electrolyte disturbances or uncompensated acid-base abnormalities; and significant dehydration. Rarely does confirmation of the diagnosis warrant an inpatient stay.

PROGNOSIS

Overall, the outcome for patients with eating disorders is variable, with the recovery of some patients after minimal intervention and the development of more chronic problems in others. Binge eating, for example, may replace food restriction. The prognosis is more favorable if the patient's condition is identified early and treated aggressively. Predictors of poor outcome for anorexia nervosa include very low body weight, long duration of illness, a concomitant personality disorder, a dysfunctional parent-child relationship, and vomiting. For bulimia nervosa, factors found to be predictive of poor outcome include severity of eating pathology and frequency of vomiting, extreme weight fluctuations, associated comorbid disorders, impulsivity, low self-esteem, and suicidal behavior.

The mortality rate for anorexia nervosa is less than 5%. Exact figures for bulimia have not been determined. The most common cause of death in both disorders is suicide. Medical causes are less common but are often due to cardiac arrhythmias from electrolyte abnormalities.

Case Resolution

In the case history presented at the beginning of this chapter, the girl does not meet the strict criteria for the diagnosis of anorexia nervosa, but her preoccupation with weight is worrisome. Concerns about her behavior should be discussed with the girl and her family. If she and her family agree, she should be referred to a psychologist and nutritionist for further evaluation, with the continued support and involvement of the primary care physician.

Selected Readings

Fisher, M., Golden, N. H., Katzman, D. K., et al. Eating disorders in adolescents: a review. J. Adolesc. Health 16:420–437, 1995.

Fisher, M. Medical complications of anorexia and bulimia nervosa. Adolesc. Med. State Art Rev. 3:487–502, 1992.

Harper, G. Eating disorders in adolescence. Pediatr. Rev. 15:72–77, 1994.

Joffe, A. Too little, too much: eating disorders in adolescents. Contemp. Pediatr. 7:114–135, 1990.

Kreipe, R. E. Eating disorders among children and adolescents. Pediatr. Rev. 16:370–379, 1995.

Kreipe, R. E., and M. Uphoff. Treatment and outcome of adolescents with anorexia nervosa. Adolesc. Med. State Art Rev. 3:519–540, 1992.

Shenker, I. R., and D. W. Bunnell. Bulimia nervosa. In McAnarney, E. R., et al. (eds.). Textbook of Adolescent Medicine. Philadelphia, W. B. Saunders, 1992.

Stashwick, C. When you suspect an eating disorder. Contemp. Pediatr. 13:124–153, 1996.

Steiner, H., and J. Lock. Anorexia nervosa and bulimia nervosa in children and adolescents: a review of the past 10 years. J. Am. Acad. Child. Adolesc. Psychiatry 37:352–359, 1998.

Tofler, I. R., et al. Physical and emotional problems with elite female gymnasts. N. Engl. J. Med. 335:281–283, 1996.

Yager, J. (guest ed.). Eating disorders. Psychiatr. Clin. North Am. 19:639–859, 1996.

Zerbe, K. J. Eating disorders: the apple doesn't fall far from the tree. Contemp. Pediatr. 13:65–78, 1996.

CHILDHOOD OBESITY

Charlotte W. Lewis, M.D., R.D.

Hx   An 11-year-old girl is brought to your office by her mother to discuss their concerns about the child's weight, which is 59 kg (130 lb). Her height is 140 cm (55 in) giving her a body mass index (BMI) of 30 kg/m² (>95th percentile for age). The rest of the physical examination, including vital signs, is normal. The mother, who also is overweight, says she doesn't want her daughter to "end up like me." The patient says she would like to lose weight because she is tired of the other children at school making fun of her for being fat. The history reveals that this patient is an only child who lives with her single mother in low-income housing in a large urban city. The mother works the day shift as a nurse's aide at a nearby nursing home. Because the mother is often tired, meals are simple and often consist of prepackaged foods such as Danish pastry for breakfast and frozen dinners for supper. At school, the girl buys her lunch, which usually consists of whole milk, a bag of chips, and a cookie. After school, the girl goes home, where she watches television and snacks on chips and soda until her mother arrives home from work. The mother does not allow her daughter to play outside because the neighborhood is unsafe.

Questions

1. How is obesity defined and measured?
2. How does genetic susceptibility influence a person's risk for obesity?
3. What is the relationship between childhood and adult obesity?
4. What are the complications of obesity?
5. How can obesity be treated?

Childhood obesity is of significant concern because overweight children are more likely to be overweight in adulthood and at increased risk for a number of chronic conditions. In addition, the psychosocial toll that being obese exacts on overweight adults and children cannot be overemphasized. Obese children are often shunned by their peers at school and have difficulty making friends, while obese adolescents complete less schooling, go on to have lower household incomes, and are more likely to live in poverty than non-obese counterparts. The primary care provider is in the ideal position to counsel families whose children are at risk for obesity and to assist children who are obese.

Defining obesity presents certain challenges. Ideally, a measure of obesity would correlate with adiposity and predict morbidity and mortality. Unfortunately, an inexpensive and widely available method that meets these criteria is not available. Body mass index (BMI; weight

Dx   Obesity

- BMI ≥ 95th percentile for age (> 85th percentile = at risk)
- Weight-for-height ≥ 95th percentile
- >120% of ideal body weight for height and age

in kilograms/[height in meters]²) is the best and most widely used surrogate measure for obesity in adults. New standards for adults have established a BMI of 25 or greater as overweight based on the increased risk of morbidity and mortality above this level. There are fewer data about the interpretation of BMI in children. However, BMI is the preferred method for assessing degree of obesity in children, although other criteria are also used (Dx Box). The BMI changes with age as a child matures and changes in proportion, bone mass, and lean-to-fat tissue composition. Ideally Tanner stage–specific standards will be developed. Interpretation of the BMI in children is somewhat controversial. Most experts define children at the 85th–95th percentile for age as **at risk for becoming overweight** and children at greater than 95th percentile for age as **overweight** (in the technical definition, the term "overweight" rather than "obese" is used because BMI is not a direct measure of adiposity; however, "obese" and "overweight" are used interchangeably in this chapter and elsewhere). Other methods that attempt to estimate fat mass directly include skin-fold measurements, hydrostatic weighing, bioelectrical impedance, and dual-energy x-ray absorptiometry (DEXA). These technologies are not widely available to the primary care practitioner, however.

EPIDEMIOLOGY

The prevalence of obesity among both adults and children is on the rise in developed countries. Approximately one-third of adults and 14% of children in the United States are significantly overweight. Over the last 30 years the percentage of young people who are overweight has more than doubled. Certain subpopulations, notably Hispanic children and African American girls, seem to be at particularly high risk for obesity. Prevention and treatment of obesity is important to avoid health risks that affect the individual and are costly to society as a whole. Health care expenses directly attributable to obesity account for $68 billion dollars per year in the United States.

CLINICAL PRESENTATION

Obese children usually present to the physician in one of two ways. The parents or the child may come in concerned that the child is overweight. The physician then must make a determination based on evaluation of growth parameters. Alternatively, the family may have little concern that their child is overweight, and in fact some parents believe that a "pudgy" child is a healthy child. However, measurement of the child's weight and height during the physical examination indicates that the child is overweight or is gaining weight more rapidly than expected and will soon be overweight.

PATHOPHYSIOLOGY

Our understanding of the exact pathophysiologic mechanisms responsible for obesity is incomplete. Multiple hormones and neurotransmitters have been identified in obese animal models. In recent years, investigative interest has focused on the role of leptin, a hormone produced in adipose tissue, in the regulation of obesity. Circulating leptin levels are increased in obese children and adults. Leptin production is mediated through the *ob* gene, and its role is to modulate the body's nutritional status through the control of appetite and energy expenditure. In the final common pathway, energy intake exceeds expenditure and excess energy is stored in the form of adipose tissue. However, obesity is a complex disease with multiple determinants influencing this final step. It is known from twin and other studies that susceptibility to obesity is influenced to a large extent by **genetics.** Parental obesity more than doubles the risk of adult obesity among both obese and non-obese children less than 10 years of age. Yet, the magnitude of recent increases in obesity rates suggests the importance of **behavioral** and **environmental** factors as well. National surveys indicate that Americans are consuming more calories now than they were 30 years ago. This trend can likely be attributed to the increasingly widespread availability of calorically dense food. Results of this survey also demonstrate that Americans of all ages are less physically active. The reasons for this are many and include changes in transportation patterns and household work and shifts in the workforce from primarily manufacturing to more sedentary service-oriented industries. Children have decreased opportunities for activity owing to safety concerns, parental work habits, the availability of television and other electronic toys, and decreases in physical education and after-school recreation programs.

DIFFERENTIAL DIAGNOSIS

The vast majority, greater than 95%, of children who present to the physician as overweight have primary obesity (resulting from excessive caloric intake and/or decreased activity). A small proportion of overweight children will have an organic cause. A thorough history, physical examination, and evaluation of growth parameters will help differentiate primary from organic obesity. While children with primary obesity tend to have normal or increased height for age, children with an organic etiology, such as hypothyroidism, are shorter than normal or have a delayed rate of growth. Certain genetic syndromes are associated with obesity but affected children usually are short, developmentally delayed, and have dysmorphic features such as polydactyly and hypogonadism that are readily identifiable during the physical examination. These genetic disorders include Prader-Willi syndrome, pseudohypoparathyroidism, and Laurence-Moon-Biedl syndrome.

EVALUATION

History

The history should include the age of the child, parental weights, and lifestyle information (Questions Box). Obtaining an in-depth diet history is critical (Box 110–1). In addition, a history of signs or symptoms of complications of obesity should be elicited. For example, a teen may complain of hip pain suggestive of slipped capital femoral epiphyses (SCFE), or there may be a history of snoring and daytime sleepiness necessitating further evaluation for obstructive sleep apnea (OSA).

Physical Examination

The accurate measurement of height and weight and plotting of growth parameters on a growth curve are essential components of well-child care. In addition to allowing assessment of the child's height, weight, and rate of growth relative to other children, the revised growth curves will enable the physician to plot weight and height to determine a child's BMI and percentile

---

Questions: Obesity

- Is there a family history of obesity, hypertension, diabetes, or hyperlipidemia?
- Where does the child live? With whom does the child live?
- Are there kitchen facilities in the home (e.g., refrigerator, microwave, hot plate, stove, and oven)?
- How often does the child/family go to fast-food or other restaurants?
- Who does the shopping and food preparation? Are there financial problems, time limitations?
- What are the child's usual daily activities?
  —How does the child get to/from school?
  —What does the child do at recess, lunch, physical education class?
  —What does the child do after school?
  —What activities does the child do on the weekend?
  —What activities are participated in as a family?
- How much time does the child spend watching TV? Playing with video games or on the computer?
- Who gives the parents advice on how to feed the child?
- What does parent/child think about child's weight? What do other family members think of child's weight?
- Does child get teased or ostracized because of weight?
- Has the child tried to lose weight before? How?
- Some additional questions for older children/adolescents include
  —Has the child/teen participated in fad dieting? Fasting? Laxative use? Diuretic use?
  —Has the child/teen used drugs to lose weight (illicit, OTC or prescription)?
  —Has the child/teen used nutritional supplements for weight loss?
  —Has the child/teen ever binged? Purged?
  —Does the child/teen use tobacco? Alcohol?

relative to other children of the same age and sex. The child should be examined for any dysmorphic features suggestive of a genetic syndrome.

The clinician should assess for potential complications of obesity when examining an overweight child. While many complications of obesity do not manifest until adulthood, overweight children are at increased risk for a number of conditions such as hypertension, hyperlipidemia, type II diabetes, OSA, and orthopedic problems such as Blount's disease and SCFE. The physician should be alert for additional physical findings. The skin should be examined for acanthosis nigricans, which is associated with insulin resistance in obese children, and for hirsutism, which, in an obese adolescent girl, may indicate the presence of polycystic ovary disease. These conditions may occur together in the HAIR-AN syndrome (*h*yper*a*ndrogenism, *i*nsulin *r*esitance, *a*canthosis *n*igricans). The musculoskeletal examination should focus on assessment for Blount's disease, SCFE, or other degenerative joint disease. The cardiopulmonary system should be examined for evidence of hypertension, congestive heart failure, or cor pulmonale.

Laboratory Studies

Except for the rare case where an organic etiology of obesity is suspected, laboratory studies are of limited usefulness in the initial evaluation of the obese child. Chromosomal analysis using fluorescent in situ hybridization (FISH) may detect syndromal disorders with obesity. Thyroid function studies or cortisol levels may be assessed if hormonal disorders are suspected. More often, laboratory studies may be needed to evaluate for a potential complication of primary obesity. It is recommended that adolescents with a BMI greater than the 85th percentile be assessed for fasting glucose and lipid profile. Clinicians may want to consider these laboratory studies in younger obese children with a family history of type II diabetes or hyperlipidemia. Children with histories suggestive of OSA should receive a sleep study and may require a cardiovascular evaluation to rule out cor pulmonale.

Imaging Studies

Radiologic studies are indicated to detect orthopedic complications of obesity such as SCFE or Blount's disease.

MANAGEMENT

The treatment of obesity is one of the most challenging areas in medicine today. Planning intervention strategies is complicated because it is not only an individual's intake, physical activity level, and genetic endowment that influence the development of obesity. Family beliefs and behaviors as well as community attitudes, practices, priorities, and resources also play a critical and often underappreciated role. These many factors must be considered as we plan prevention and treatment programs. Interventions done on an individual basis are unlikely to be successful if the effect of the family and community on eating and activity level are not also addressed. Traditionally, treatment for obesity has been directed only to the obese individual in the form of "dieting." However, dieting, or temporarily restricting one's intake as a means to lose weight, has proven to be a dismal failure. More than 90% of patients who lose weight through dieting will ultimately regain this weight. Surgical and medical (medications, very low calorie diets) treatments for obesity are fraught with risks of complications and side effects.

The care of the obese *child* adds an additional dimension to the formidable task of individual obesity treatment. Efforts to alter the intake of a child, if not done carefully, may interfere with normal growth and development. Many children who are obese in childhood will not go on to be obese adults, providing another reason that treatment must be approached with caution. The pediatrician's first task is to assess a child's future risk. This is largely determined by the age of the child and history of parental obesity. Obese children less than 3 years old are at low risk for future obesity. These children should be monitored but, for the most part, do not require treatment. Between the ages of 3 and 5, a history of obesity in the parents substantially increases the odds of a child becoming obese as an adult. The chance of adult obesity in an obese 3- to 5-year-old child with at least one obese parent is 62%. As the child ages, the child's obesity status becomes a more important predictor of future obesity. The probability that an overweight child over the age of 6 will be obese as an adult is 50%. Children who are at such high risk for adult obesity clearly require close attention and active intervention by the clinician.

The practitioners' goal in caring for obese children may not be weight loss *per se* but rather normal growth in height while slowing weight gain or maintaining weight at a constant level. The only effective and safe means of obesity treatment available is **behavior and lifestyle modification.** The aims of behavior and lifestyle modification are to promote a change to a healthier lifestyle that includes healthful eating, increased physical activity, and development of healthy body image and self-esteem. Consideration of these goals is especially important given that increasing numbers of teenagers and even younger children are participating in unhealthy weight loss practices including laxative, diuretic, and diet pill use and induced vomiting and fasting (see Chapter 109, Eating Disorders). In doing so, children and teens are potentially compromising their health and nutritional status to meet unrealistic goals for body image.

Behavior and lifestyle modification efforts must be tailored for the individual child, family, and community. Before any intervention will be successful, the child and the family must be ready to make a change. They must be willing to accept that these changes are not a temporary fix but are meant to be adopted as a permanent part of the patient's and family's lifestyle. Because it is difficult for individuals to modify ingrained behaviors and habits related to food and activity, patients will require ongoing follow-up from their clinician throughout the process. Family and patient support groups and organized programs for overweight children may be helpful as well. Families should be counseled that setbacks are to be expected and should not discourage them from further efforts.

Ways in which the clinician can help families toward a more healthful lifestyle are listed in Box 110–2. Some items on this list address changes in single aspects of the diet, such as decreasing intake of juice. Juice is largely a source of empty calories, and excessive juice consumption has been associated with risk of obesity. Other items are more complex such as providing a family with a guide for healthy eating. Many people understand that good nutrition is important but do not know how to translate this into healthy food choices. For example, a person might know to limit fat, cholesterol, and sodium but not know which foods are high in these ingredients. Guides to healthy eating may take the form of the Food Pyramid (Figure 110–1) or an individualized plan. A dietitian can assist the practitioner in developing a plan and counseling a family.

The lifestyle history (Questions Box) will identify potentially modifiable factors; however, changes need to be negotiated and acceptable to the patient and their family. Changes that are inconsistent with a patient's and family's values, culture, and resources are unlikely to be adopted. For example, participation in after-school sports may not be a realistic option for a child if the family cannot afford fees or equipment or there is no transportation for the child to get to and from the program.

PREVENTION

Taken together, poor diet and inadequate physical activity are responsible for 300,000 deaths per year in the United States and are second only to tobacco use as a leading contributor to preventable premature death. Most diet and activity related habits and behaviors that originate in childhood and adolescence are difficult to change when an individual is older. Prevention of obesity is our best option for reversing the trend toward obesity in this country, and therefore prevention of obesity needs to be a priority for all clinicians who care for children. Efforts should focus on three areas: (1) anticipatory guidance starting at a young age on the importance of healthful eating and regular physical activity, (2) reinforcement with families of the importance of developing a healthy attitude toward food and eating and of promoting positive self-esteem and reasonable expectations for body image, and (3) advocacy for public health measures aimed at increasing opportunities for healthful eating and regular physical activity within our communities.

PROGNOSIS

Unfortunately, obese children who remain obese into adulthood are at greatly increased risk for certain complications including hypertension, coronary artery disease, gallbladder disease, diabetes, some types of cancer, and obstructive sleep apnea.

BOX 110–2. Ten Ways to Help Families Toward a Healthier Lifestyle

1. Learn as much as you can about the child and family's usual diet and activity pattern so that you can negotiate changes which will be acceptable.
2. Provide families with a guide for healthy eating. Educate families on interpretation of nutrition information on food labels.
3. Educate families on foods which are high in fat and calories. Have them try alternative methods of food preparation (e.g., baking or broiling rather than frying).
4. Encourage intake of "unprocessed" foods such as fresh fruits and vegetables and whole-grain products. Limit processed and prepackaged foods and snacks, and keep these out of the house as much as possible.
5. Help families come up with low-fat, nutritious snacks they can keep on hand.
6. After a year of age, switch from a bottle to a cup.
7. For children older than 2 years of age, change to low-fat or fat-free milk. Limit milk to 16–24 oz per day after the first year of life.
8. Limit juice to less than 8 oz per day. Limit soda to special occasions.
9. Limit TV to less than 1 hour per day. Limit other sedentary activities such as playing video and computer games.
10. Incorporate physical activity into the child's and family's daily routine. Find a sport that the child can master and enjoys.

Case Resolution

The opening vignette describes an overweight girl. She is at substantial risk for remaining obese into adulthood based on her present weight and her mother's history of obesity. Working with a dietitian, the mother and her daughter learn about the components of a healthy diet. They plan meals and snacks that are healthy and easily prepared in advance. The girl begins to make her own lunch each night before school. Rather than whole milk, the mother buys nonfat milk and no longer keeps juice, cookies, chips, or soda around the house. A social worker helps find an after-school program at the nearby YMCA. The patient starts attending and with some special attention from the coach finds she enjoys basketball and would like to try out for the junior high school team next year. The mother wants to exercise more, and so the girl and her mother go for nightly walks around the track at the local high school.

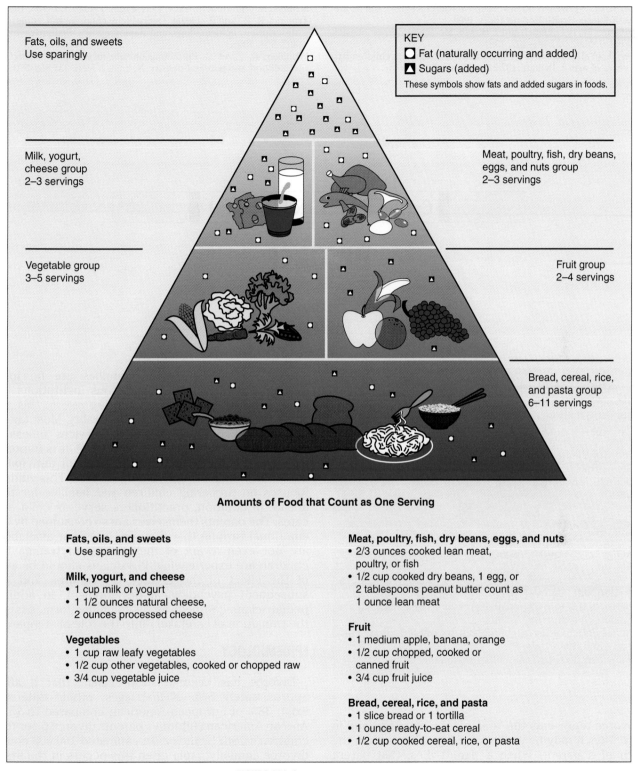

Amounts of Food that Count as One Serving

Fats, oils, and sweets
- Use sparingly

Milk, yogurt, and cheese
- 1 cup milk or yogurt
- 1 1/2 ounces natural cheese,
  2 ounces processed cheese

Vegetables
- 1 cup raw leafy vegetables
- 1/2 cup other vegetables, cooked or chopped raw
- 3/4 cup vegetable juice

Meat, poultry, fish, dry beans, eggs, and nuts
- 2/3 ounces cooked lean meat,
  poultry, or fish
- 1/2 cup cooked dry beans, 1 egg, or
  2 tablespoons peanut butter count as
  1 ounce lean meat

Fruit
- 1 medium apple, banana, orange
- 1/2 cup chopped, cooked or
  canned fruit
- 3/4 cup fruit juice

Bread, cereal, rice, and pasta
- 1 slice bread or 1 tortilla
- 1 ounce ready-to-eat cereal
- 1/2 cup cooked cereal, rice, or pasta

FIGURE 110–1. Food Guide Pyramid

Over the next 6 months, you follow the girl and her mother closely. The most recent growth parameters show that the girl has maintained her weight at 59 kg but has grown 5 cm to 145 cm, giving her a BMI of 28. The mother has lost 5 lb over this time period, and both are excited about continuing their new lifestyle.

Selected Readings

Barlow, S. E., and W. H. Dietz. Obesity evaluation and treatment: expert committee recommendations. Pediatrics 102:e29, 1998.

Gortmaker, S. L., et al. Social and economic consequences of overweight in adolescence and young adulthood. N. Engl. J. Med. 329:1008–1012, 1993.

Kreipe, R. E. Overweight adolescents: clinical challenges and strategies. Adolesc. Health Update 10(2), 1998.

Rosenbaum, M., R. L. Leibel, and J. Hirsch. Medical progress: obesity. N. Engl. J. Med. 337:396–407, 1997.

Rosner, B., et al. Percentiles for body mass index in U. S. children 5 to 17 years of age. J. Pediatr. 132:211–222, 1998.

Strauss, R. Childhood obesity. Curr. Probl. Pediatr. 29:1–36, 1999.

Troiano, R. P., and K. Flegal. Overweight children and adolescents: description, epidemiology, and demographics. Pediatrics 101(3S): 497–504, 1998.

Whitaker, R. C., et al. Predicting obesity in young adulthood from childhood and parental obesity. N. Engl. J. Med. 337:869–873, 1997.

CHAPTER 111

DIVORCE

Carol D. Berkowitz, M.D.

H$_x$ A 7-year-old girl who has been your patient for 5 years is brought in by her mother with abdominal pain that occurs on a daily basis and is not associated with any other symptoms. The pain is periumbilical. In obtaining the history, you learn that the father has moved out of the home and the parents are planning a divorce. The mother believes that her daughter's symptoms may relate to the impending divorce, and she wants to know what else to expect.

Questions

1. What are the problems faced by children whose parents are undergoing divorce?
2. What are the age-related reactions of children in families undergoing divorce?
3. What is the role of pediatricians in counseling families undergoing divorce?
4. What anticipatory guidance can be offered about custody and remarriage?
5. How can pediatricians help step-families adjust?

Divorce represents the "death" of a marriage, and in some ways it may be even worse for children than the death of a parent. When a parent dies, that parent becomes idealized in the mind of children, but when parents divorce, the noncustodial parent is devalued. In fact, each parent is often devalued by the other. For children, parents are no longer the idealized figures that they once were. The challenge for pediatricians is to maintain a neutral position. This may be particularly difficult because much of the contact has been with one parent rather than the other, usually the mother.

Pediatricians play a specific role in managing children going through a parental divorce because other re-sources are few. Extended families are no longer available to provide help. Religious institutions have often failed to assume a counseling role in this area; some religions view divorce unfavorably. Most families do not seek out mental health services unless the problems are overwhelming. Therefore, it is important for pediatricians to become involved in anticipatory guidance of families undergoing divorce. This guidance focuses on preparing children and families for times ahead. In addition, practitioners serve as child advocates. The parents themselves are so consumed by their emotional turmoil that they are often not available or are not even aware of the stress and trauma their children are experiencing. Physicians should be aware of the effect of the divorce on children and their subsequent psychological development. In addition, pediatricians can help as new families form, assisting the transition of caretakers into the role of stepparents.

EPIDEMIOLOGY

Divorce has become so prevalent that it affects approximately 50% of marriages. Ethnic differences exist; 38% of European American compared to 75% of African American children's parents divorce prior to the children's 18th birthday. An estimated 100,000 couples divorce annually; most often this occurs in the first 14 years of marriage (mean: 7.1 years). Approximately one million children per year are affected by divorce. In 1990, 30% of all children lived in households in which parents were divorced or remarried. Children between the ages of 3 and 8 years are the major age group affected. Children involved with parental divorce take 2½–3 years to regain their equilibrium and master a sense of control. Divorce usually results in a decline of economic resources to mothers and children. In the first year after divorce, income is reduced to 58% of the pre-divorce level. Even after 5 years, income for mothers and children is only 94% of the pre-divorce amount; for intact couples, income has risen to 130% during that time period.

Types of custody include single parent custody, joint custody, joint legal custody, and joint physical custody, where parents have physical access to the child with equal frequency. Birds-nest custody is joint custody where children remain in the home and parents take turns moving in and out. Many states now allow for joint custody. Issues of remarriage and stepsiblings are also important. Eighty percent of divorced men and 75% of divorced women remarry, and 40% of these remarriages end in divorce. As a result of the high rate of remarriage, one in six children in the United States has a stepparent. Such children often have to readjust to differing roles in differing households and differing relationships between their biologic parents, stepparents, biologic siblings, and stepsiblings.

PSYCHOPHYSIOLOGY

The reaction to divorce that children experience depends, to a large extent, on the age of the child (Table 111–1). In general, children do not have the cognitive ability to understand the meaning of divorce until they are 9 or 10 years of age.

Children up to the age of 2 years experience sleeping and feeding disturbances, as well as spitting up and clinginess. Between the ages of 2½–4 years, children usually manifest regressive behavior. They become needy and dependent, and their behavior is characterized by irritability, whining, crying, fearfulness, increased separation anxiety, and sleep problems. Both aggression and regression, particularly in the area of toilet training, may develop. One third of children in this age group continue to exhibit regressive behavior 1 year after divorce.

Preschool-age children between the ages of 3½–5 years often show more aggressive patterns of behavior with hitting, biting, and temper tantrums. Regressive behavior may also be seen. Young children feel particularly responsible for their parents' divorce (i.e., the parents are divorcing the child). At this point in development, children experience what Piaget has referred to as an egocentric way of thinking. Self-blame, decreased self-esteem, and a high level of fantasy, particularly about parental reunion, are apparent. Approximately 1 year after divorce, 65% of these children still show decreased levels of functioning.

Children who are 5–6 years of age are often depressed and may exhibit immature behavior. Girls in this age group seem to handle a divorce more poorly than boys. Two thirds of girls are less well adjusted 1 year after the divorce, as opposed to only about one fourth of boys. These children appear moody and daydream. They may also be whiny and have temper tantrums.

School-age children between the age of 6 years and adolescence seem to experience profound disequilibrium with feelings of shame, anger, and loneliness. This anger may be manifested by antisocial behavior. Older children also talk about an overwhelming feeling of sadness and grief. Their somatic complaints include headache, abdominal pain, and an increase in symptoms of preexisting medical conditions such as asthma. Sometimes the somatic complaints of children, particularly those in the school-age group, are attributed by one parent to the poor living conditions at the other parent's household.

It is important for physicians to anticipate that 50% of children involved in parental divorce show a deterioration in their school performance. Therefore, the school should be notified about the divorce and changes in family structure. Decreased school performance is attributed to decreased ability to concentrate, sadness, and depression.

Parental divorce is particularly difficult for adolescents, who describe it as "extraordinarily painful." The experience is worse for younger adolescents. During the first stages of divorce, they experience a personal sense of abandonment and a loss of parental love. Older adolescents are concerned about their future potential as marital partners. They also feel anxious about financial security, especially money for college. De-idealization of both parents is precipitous. Adolescent girls do better than boys early on, but this reverses with time. This pattern is referred to as a "sleeper effect" or "delayed effect," with girls subsequently feeling rejected and unattractive. Divorce during adolescence sometimes leads to "precocious sexual activity" or risk- or thrill-seeking behavior. In addition, the adolescent may turn to alcohol or drug use to help cope with the stress of parental divorce. Boys may engage in illegal activities such as burglary.

DIFFERENTIAL DIAGNOSIS

Children who present with complaints including headache, abdominal pain, enuresis, and poor school performance should always be assessed for environmental factors that may be contributing to their symptomatology. Interestingly, many parents who are undergoing a divorce do not appreciate the impact the divorce is having on their children. They are often caught up in their own personal feelings and are not aware of their children's symptomatology. It is appropriate to consider organic etiologies for any somatic complaint.

EVALUATION

The focus of the evaluation should be on the interviewing process. Determination of the full extent of the

TABLE 111–1. Children's Reaction to Divorce	
Age	Symptoms
2½–4 yr	Regressive behavior
3½–5 yr	Aggressive behavior
5–6 yr	Whiny, immature behavior
6–adolescence	Disequilibrium
	Depression
	Somatic complaints
	Poor school performance

impact of the home factors on children's symptomatology may take several visits. It is not appropriate to pursue extensive laboratory tests without first adequately determining what changes are occurring within the household.

History

The medical evaluation of children undergoing a parental divorce should include a review of the medical history and a discussion with the child of factors of change (Questions Box). This may help open up a discussion that reveals that the parents are in the process of divorce or that the father has moved out of the household.

Physical Examination

Any symptom or specific complaint, such as headache or abdominal pain, should also be addressed (see Chapter 91, Abdominal Pain, and Chapter 95, Headaches). Depression and the risk for suicide should also be evaluated (see Chapter 113, Adolescent Depression and Suicide). A complete physical examination is usually warranted because children who are experiencing stress may also develop stress-related medical problems.

Laboratory Tests

Some simple baseline laboratory studies may be warranted, particularly in children who have complaints such as abdominal pain or enuresis. These tests may include a CBC or urinalysis.

MANAGEMENT

Management of children whose family is undergoing divorce is complex. In addition to treating any somatic complaints that may be related to the divorce, physicians play a key role in anticipatory guidance. Physician involvement before parents actually separate helps. Initially, physicians should advise parents about how to talk to children and what to expect in terms of their reaction. It is important for parents to tell children that they are separating from one another and not from the children. As stated above, parents undergoing a divorce are in so much turmoil that they themselves may not see their children's problems. In addition, their parenting skills may suffer, and routine procedures such as meals and bedtime may become disrupted, sporadic, and irregular.

Table 111–2 summarizes advice to parents. "When," "how," "who," and "what" to tell should be discussed. Generally, children should be told of impending divorce by both parents with support from the extended family. Unfortunately, studies report that 80% of preschoolers were told by one parent.

The "when" to tell depends on children's age. Younger children should be told a few days before the actual separation. Older children should be told at least several weeks before. Practitioners should advise parents about "how" to tell. Displays of emotion are permissible. Parents should be encouraged to show their emotions, but not to the extent that they appear overwhelmed or uncontrollable.

The "who" to tell includes not only the children but also the neighbors and the school, so that the feeling of shame or secrecy is less. The "what" to tell involves freeing the children of any blame for the divorce and answering their questions.

It is important for physicians not to become involved in custody disputes, but if they are asked to give an opinion, they should try to evaluate the parenting skills of both parents. In the past, custody was given to the mother in 90% of cases, but this is now decreasing. Questions that physicians should ask themselves when advising about custody include: What are the emotional ties between parents and children? Do children indicate a preference for one parent? Children may be overwhelmed by feelings of loyalty and be torn if asked to choose one parent over the other, which makes this a difficult problem. What is the capacity of each parent to provide emotional and physical support for children? It is important to consider a need for continuity, and it is vital to keep conditions as close as possible to the predivorce situation. Children should not have to move. Living arrangements need to be reassessed on a periodic basis.

Physicians should be aware of the factors that support joint custody. Joint custody tends to maintain

---

TABLE 111–2.   Talking to Children About Divorce

Who
Who tells?   Both parents
Who is told?   Children, physicians, teachers, neighbors

When
Before either parent leaves
Age-dependent
  Older children: weeks ahead
  Younger children: days ahead

How
Calmly, with emotional control

Where
Privately, in the home

What
Stress that children are not to blame; that the divorce is between parents, not between parents and children; it is the parents who cannot get along
Explain expected living arrangements

a parent-child attachment, and children experience less of a sense of loss. They have more cognitive and social stimulation. Joint custody relieves the burden of single parenthood, and parents who have joint custody are less likely to use children as bargaining tools. Parents themselves are freer to enter into different relationships and are less emotionally dependent on their children.

Although physicians should not become involved in monetary issues, concerns related to payment and cost of medical care are appropriate to discuss. Practitioners should consider involving noncustodial parents in children's health care. Such parents could be notified if medical problems occur.

Pediatricians may also be helpful in counseling noncustodial parents about interacting with children. In general, visitation should reflect previous relationships as closely as possible. Noncustodial parents should be advised not to become camp counselors who focus on fun and games but to be influential figures who help the children meet the challenges of normal living such as completing homework and doing chores and tasks. It is also important for noncustodial parents to be consistent. If a meeting is planned, the parents must show up. Although a couple are no longer married, they can still be coparents rather than rivals. Noncustodial parents should be encouraged to participate in school and sports activities.

Custodial parents may attribute children's somatic complaints to poor care while under visitation with noncustodial parents. Allegations related to abuse, most often sexual abuse, may also arise. These allegations should be taken seriously. An appropriate medical and psychological evaluation is necessary (see Chapter 105, Child Sexual Abuse). The most difficult situations involve allegations of sexual abuse of preverbal children, where conclusions may be contingent on the physical findings, which are usually nonconclusive.

Issues related to parental dating and remarriage should be addressed at an early stage. Parents should be advised that pediatricians may be a resource in helping families readjust. Remarriage is often a difficult time for children because they experience feelings of rejection secondary to displacement by stepparents. Grandparents may also be a source of support.

The pediatrician can also serve as a resource for stepparents. Although stepparents do not have legal rights to consent for medical care of their stepchildren, they should become familiar with the children's medical history. Stepparents grow into their parenting role, and it takes 2–7 years for families to become blended. The pediatrician can help families adjust by recommending books such as *Talking about Stepfamilies* by M. Rosenberg or giving referrals to organizations such as Stepfamily Association of America at 800-735-0329.

PROGNOSIS

The prognosis for children undergoing a parental divorce depends, in part, on the degree of dysfunction that existed in the family before separation and the ability of the children to communicate their concerns. Supportive intervention by family, friends, and physicians is key to facilitating the necessary adjustment. Being a child of divorced and remarried parents has been likened to having dual citizenship. The experience is rewarding if the countries are not at war with one another.

Case Resolution

The case history shows that functional somatic complaints are not uncommon, especially in school-age children of divorced parents. The mother and her daughter should be advised about how stressful divorce is for children. A careful medical examination may reassure both the mother and child about the child's physical well-being. Issues related to custody, financial responsibility, and the need for consistency should all be addressed. In addition, the pediatrician should refer the family to outside agencies if necessary.

Selected Readings

Baris, M. A., and C. B. Garrity. Children of Divorce. Dekalb, IL, Psytec, 1988.

Behrman, R. E. (ed.). Children and divorce: overview and analysis. Future Child. 4(1):4–14, 1994.

Dell, M. L. Divorce—are you ready to help? Contemp. Pediatr. 12:57–68, 1995.

Emery, R. E., and M. J. Coiro. Divorce: Consequences for children. Pediatr. Rev. 16:306–310, 1995.

Green, M. Reaching out to children of divorce. Contemp. Pediatr. 5:22–42, 1988.

Long, N., and R. Forehand. The effects of parental divorce and parental conflict on children: an overview. J. Dev. Behav. Pediatr. 8:292–296, 1987.

Schmitt, B. D. Helping children cope with divorce. Contemp. Pediatr. 9:81–86, 1992.

Visher, J. S., and E. B. Visher. Beyond the nuclear family: Resources and implications for pediatricians. Pediatr. Clin. North Am. 42:31–43, 1995.

Wallerstein, J. S. The long-term effects of divorce on children: a review. J. Am. Acad. Child Adolesc. Psychiatry 30:349–360, 1991.

Wallerstein, J. S., and J. R. Johnston. Children of divorce: recent findings regarding long-term effects and recent studies of joint and sole custody. Pediatr. Rev. 11:197–203, 1990.

CHAPTER 112

VIOLENCE

Carol D. Berkowitz, M.D.

H$_x$ You are asked to talk to the students of an elementary school where an on-campus shooting of one student by another, older student has occurred. The shooting took place in the school yard at lunchtime and was directly witnessed by over 40 students. Since the episode a week earlier, school absenteeism and disruptive classroom behavior have increased.

Questions

1. In what settings are children exposed to violence?
2. What is the prevalence of violence in these various settings?
3. What is the impact of violence on students' academic performance?
4. What can physicians do to counteract violence in society?
5. What is the impact of gangs in a community?

Violence is the actual or threatened use of physical force against an individual or group that may or does result in injury or death. Children are exposed to violence in various settings. In the home, violence may be between parents, between parents and children, and between siblings. In the schools, violence has escalated in recent years. This is particularly worrisome because the violence has become more lethal with the increase in the number of guns. Corporal punishment may occur at home as well as in school. In the community, violence involves gangs and criminal acts. The large number of innocent bystanders who are shot during gang conflicts makes some neighborhoods especially unsafe.

Concern has also been expressed about exposure to violence through the media, including television and interactive videogames. It is believed that violence in the media has contributed to an acceptance of violence in society, where violence has become an expected phenomenon.

EPIDEMIOLOGY

In 1933, natural causes accounted for more than three times as many deaths as violent incidents or injuries in adolescents. By 1985, natural causes accounted for only 27% of all adolescent deaths. Homicide is presently the second leading cause of death in children and adolescents and the principal cause of death for African Americans and Hispanics 15–24 years of age. The United States has the highest teenage homicide rate in the industrialized world. The rate is four times that of the 20 other Western nations combined.

Males and African Americans are more likely to die by homicide. If current trends continue, five of every 1000 African American males who turn 15 this year will die by homicide before age 25. Nonfatal violence is even more prevalent and results in long-term neurologic and physical disabilities.

A survey of 1035 youngsters in Chicago's South Side found that by age 11, four of five children had witnessed a beating either at home or in the street. One of three children had seen a shooting or stabbing, and one of four had seen a murder committed.

Violence in the school is equally pervasive. The late 1990s witnessed a number of mass slayings on school campuses across the United States. In 1989, the National Adolescent School Health Survey reported the following data:

1. Fifty percent of boys and about 33% of girls participated in at least one fight during the year. These once trivial quarrels now frequently escalate to lethal confrontations because of the ready availability of guns.
2. About 14% of boys and 13% of girls were robbed at least once in school, and a similar proportion were robbed on their way to or from school.
3. Seventeen percent of boys and 9% of girls were attacked at least once in school, and 20% of boys and 20% of girls were attacked in the vicinity of school.
4. Weapons frequently accompany youngsters to school. At one school in New York City, 2669 weapons were confiscated from students during the 1988–89 school year. A 1990 report noted that 50% of the boys at one Baltimore high school had brought a gun to school at least once. A Youth Risk Behavior Survey conducted that same year indicated that approximately one of every five high school students carried a firearm, knife, or club to school during the preceding month. Over 200 million firearms, including 50 million handguns, are privately owned in the United States. Nearly half of all U.S. homes contain firearms, and 25 million households have handguns. The average age of acquisition of a gun is 12.5 years, usually as a gift from an older male relative. Access to handguns is simple. When questioned, 41% of boys and 21% of girls said that they could get a handgun if they wanted. It has been said that adolescents find it easier to obtain a handgun than a driver's license.

The number of children who witness violence exceeds the number who are victims of violence. A 1993 study of school children in Washington, D.C., by the National Institutes of Mental Health reported that 19% of first and second graders had been victimized but 61% had witnessed violence to someone else; for fifth and sixth graders, the figures were 32% and 72%, respectively.

CLINICAL PRESENTATION

Children who are affected by violence may have various symptoms. Physical evidence of victimization, including bruises or wounds from stabbing or gunshots, may be apparent. Children who are emotionally traumatized often present with somatic complaints such as abdominal pain, headache, or vomiting. These children may also have symptoms consistent with depression such as poor appetite and sleep disturbances. They may re-experience the traumatic event or persistently avoid places or people connected with the event. These symptoms are part of the diagnostic criteria of post-traumatic stress disorder.

Children who have witnessed violence in school settings may exhibit school refusal behavior or apparent school phobia because of fears for their safety within the school setting. Poor school performance may also follow a violent episode in the school or be related to an inability to concentrate because of fear in the school setting. Domestic violence and child abuse may lead to symptoms of low self-esteem, poor school performance, and acting-out behavior.

PSYCHOPHYSIOLOGY

Violence that affects children and adolescents has several facets. In violent situations, children fit into one of three categories: aggressors, victims, or bystanders. Aggressors are the initiators of violence, victims are the targets of violence, and bystanders are the observers of violence. Bystanders are often characterized as "innocent," but they can contribute to violent behavior by instigating as well as endorsing it. What are some of the factors that encourage children to participate in anti-social behavior?

Peer group influence is particularly strong, especially in individuals with low self-esteem. The concepts of identity (the "macho" image) and rite of passage—becoming an adult—relate to peer pressure. In addition, teenagers feel invincible, and this contributes to their risk-taking behavior. They wish to assert independence and autonomy from adult authority figures. Learning disabilities, a history of physical abuse, and school or athletic failure, are additional factors contributing to low self-esteem. Some children are felt to have biologic risk factors for violence. They often manifest aggressive behavior including shoving and starting fights. Studies suggest a link between head injury, lead poisoning, epilepsy, and birth trauma and subsequent violent and aggressive behavior. The relationship between dopamine, serotonin, and androgen and violent behavior is being evaluated.

Although the majority of teenage homicides are not related to gang activity, the presence of gangs in a community has a deleterious effect on the community and its sense of safety and well-being. Los Angeles, which has 100,000 gang members, is reported to be the gang capital of the United States. Studies suggest that about one-fifth of adolescent males in communities of 10,000 or more belong to gangs. Participation in a delinquent peer group is a strong predictor of later delinquent behavior. Teenage gangs are of two types. The first type are loosely organized "crews" or "posses" whose members tend to "hang out" together, drink and use drugs together, and engage in vandalism or petty theft. The second type are gangs organized to sell drugs. Gang membership is associated with high morbidity and mortality. In addition, gangs are also responsible for the deaths of uninvolved individuals who are gunned down during drive-by shootings. Such shootings are often adjacent to school grounds and not infrequently occur during school hours.

Substance abuse is another factor associated with violence and violent death. Alcohol and drug use increase risk-taking behavior and impulsiveness. Approximately 50% of all homicide victims have elevated blood alcohol levels. The medical examiner of Washington, D.C., once reported that 80% of homicide victims had cocaine in their bodies.

Although the role of the media in contributing to violence is more controversial, more than 200 studies have reported some link between viewing violence on television and the subsequent development of violent behavior. These data come from naturalistic field studies, longitudinal studies, and population-based studies. The National Institutes of Mental Health has concluded that heavy exposure to violence on television is significantly related to subsequent aggressive behavior among children and adolescents. Additional concern relates to the violence against individuals that is portrayed in interactive videogames.

EVALUATION

The evaluation of children to determine the risk of their becoming perpetrators or victims of violence is challenging. Ideally, all children should be assessed at each health maintenance visit. Risk factors for aggressive behavior should be identified. Children at greater risk for antisocial behavior include those who have experienced neurologic injuries and those who have been prenatally exposed to certain drugs such as opiates, cocaine, or alcohol. It is also suggested that lead poisoning may increase the risk for aggressive behavior. In addition, certain psychological attributes, including hyperactivity, impulsivity and cognitive deficit associated with low intelligence, and poor concentration, may also place children at higher risk. Poor bonding between children and parents has been associated with subsequent aggressive behavior patterns.

Children should be questioned about being victimized or witnessing violence either in their school, community, or home environment or viewing violence on television. Statements such as "There seems to be a lot of fighting going on in schools and homes, and I'd like to talk to you about it" facilitate the discussion.

In addition, children should be questioned specifically about their involvement as aggressors in violent acts. They should then be asked about the number of fights they have engaged in. Appropriate questions are: "How many shoving fights have you had in the last month?," "What were they about?," "Did you or anyone else get hurt?," "How did you get out of the fight?,"

"Have you ever been threatened with a gun?," and "Have you ever carried a gun?"

Parents should also be asked about violent acts within the home. They should routinely be questioned about the presence of guns in the home, whether the guns are kept unloaded and locked up, and whether ammunition is stored in the home, and if so, where. Parenting skills and parental approach to discipline should be determined. Violence in the home is an independent risk factor for perpetration of violence. Children who have witnessed violence should be evaluated to determine the effect of such exposure on their day-to-day functioning and school performance. Children should be assessed for their ability to eat and sleep normally and perform daily activities.

Neither physical examination nor laboratory assessment is helpful unless children have sustained specific physical injuries.

MANAGEMENT

Pediatricians can deal with violence in several ways. They can work with aggressors in an effort to reduce violent behavior, treat victims and help them recover from physical as well as emotional injuries, assist schools and communities with violence reduction programs, and advocate for legislation concerning gun control and gun safety and portrayals of violence by the media, including television. Practitioners can work with numerous groups and organizations, such as law enforcement agencies and the American Bar Association, to structure programs and lobby for change.

When dealing one-on-one with aggression-prone children, pediatricians should strive to assist children with their development of nonviolent problem-solving skills such as articulating anger and frustration or enlisting the aid of an adult to resolve conflicts. Conflict resolution strategies can be discussed by pediatricians with parents and patients. In addition, families should be instructed to prohibit their access to guns, thereby diminishing the lethality of children's aggressive behavior.

The American Academy of Pediatrics has defined an age-related stepwise approach for families to foster a nonviolent environment during childhood and adolescence. The components of this approach include early nurturing, limit setting, safety and screening, and treatment and referral.

Victims of violence need emotional support. These individuals may develop isolated or multiple somatic complaints. Alternatively, they may manifest symptoms of posttraumatic stress disorder, experiencing depression, anxiety, and sleep and eating disruptions. Children may need referral to mental health counselors to assist them in restoring a sense of control over their lives. Pediatricians as well as mental health specialists may assist schools where an episode of violence has occurred. Sessions for students allow them to articulate their fears and reactions. There are established techniques such as Mitchell's Critical Incident Stress Debriefing to assist physicians working with youths traumatized by having witnessed violence. Intervention by physicians helps prevent the development of posttraumatic stress disorder.

Several interventional strategies may be employed through the schools to reduce violence. Early intervention during grade and middle school is important. Just as drug prevention programs are geared toward younger children, programs to deglorify violence should also be instituted. This is one of the goals of the U.S. Public Health Service for the year 2000. Strategies for achieving this objective include the following actions:

1. Counteracting the cultural acceptance of violence.

2. Decreasing aggressive behavior between parents and their children through child abuse prevention programs. The Healthy Start program in Hawaii which offers prenatal training in parental skills is credited with decreasing infant abuse in a high-risk population.

3. Reducing the exposure of children and adolescents to violence in the media by helping parents select appropriate television programs to watch.

4. Improving the recognition, management, and treatment of adolescent victims and those at high risk for assault.

Schools can use educational interventions that stress nonviolent conflict resolution and teach such skills. One such educational intervention is the Violence Prevention Project of the Health Promotion Program for Urban Youth. This program, which consists of 10 sessions, teaches that anger is normal and uses videotapes and role playing to teach students how to channel anger in a constructive manner. The STAR (Straight Talk About Risks) program utilizes a curriculum developed by the Center to Prevent Handgun Violence to educate students from kindergarten through 12th grade about firearms.

Schools may also have to use additional means, including metal detectors and campus police, to ensure the safety and well-being of students. School attendance should be enforced, and parents should be called when students are absent. Students who are found to be off campus should be returned to the school and their presence enforced on school grounds.

Concerned parents can use schools to mobilize their efforts. Grass roots organizations similar to Mothers Against Drunk Drivers (MADD) are emerging to address the problem of adolescent violence. Save Our Sons and Daughters (SOSAD), founded over 15 years ago in Detroit, is now a national organization. Other groups include New York City's Mothers Against Violence and Parents of Murdered Children and Atlanta's Mothers of Murdered Sons (MOMS). A novel approach to reducing handguns in the United States is modeled after efforts to reduce smoking by holding tobacco companies liable for illnesses related to cigarettes. Recent civil action has awarded money to shooting victims and found gun companies liable and negligent.

Pediatricians can also serve as leaders to encourage the community, through schools, to develop quality youth programs. These programs should provide the following services:

1. Address various needs: remedial services, crisis intervention programs, and enrichment activities.

2. Be open year round with long hours.

3. Serve a wide range of age groups, so youths can interact with people of various ages.

4. Allow for continuity, with no age-based mandatory termination.

5. Provide contact with adults who can serve as role models.

6. Provide opportunities for youths to practice leadership.

7. Do outreach and case management.

PROGNOSIS

The prognosis varies with the nature of children's involvement in the violence. Some children sustain significant physical injuries such as neurologic impairment or disfigurement. Other children are emotionally traumatized, and even with psychological counseling, they have difficulty with the normal tasks of childhood such as attending school. Long-term involvement by primary care physicians is needed by children who are the physical or emotional victims of violence.

Case Resolution

In the case history presented at the beginning of this chapter, the physician should discuss the fears and feelings of the students to help facilitate their coping with the violence. Safety should also be discussed to empower the students to avoid violent situations. The use of teaching tapes and role playing helps the students think of solutions to dangerous situations before these conditions develop.

Selected Readings

Christoffel, K. K. Pediatric firearm injuries: time to target a growing population. Pediatr. Ann. 21:430–436, 1992.

Cohall, A. T., et al. Teen violence: the new mortality. Contemp. Pediatr. 8:76–86, 1991.

Deutsch, M., and E. Brickman. Conflict resolution. Pediatr. Rev. 15:16–22, 1994.

Gellert, G. A. Confronting Violence. Boulder, CO, Westview Press, 1997.

Hennes, H., and A. D. Calhoun (ed.). Violence among children and adolescents. Pediatr. Clin. North Am. 45:269–467, 1998 [entire].

Hutson, H. R., D. Anglin, and M. J. Pratts. Adolescents and children injured or killed in drive-by shootings in Los Angeles. N. Engl. J. Med. 330:324–327, 1994.

Role of the pediatrician in violence prevention. Pediatrics 94:577–651, 1994 [entire suppl].

Role of the pediatrician in youth violence prevention in clinical practice and at the community level: AAP Task Force on Violence. Pediatrics 103:173–181, 1999.

Ropp, L., et al. Death in the city: an American childhood tragedy. JAMA 267:2905–2910, 1992.

Schwarz, D. F. Violence. Pediatr. Rev. 17:197–201, 1996.

Senturiam Y., K. K. Christoffel, and M. Donovan. Children's household exposure to guns: a pediatric practice-based survey. Pediatrics 93:469–475, 1994.

CHAPTER 113

ADOLESCENT DEPRESSION AND SUICIDE

Monica Sifuentes, M.D.

H$_x$ A 15-year-old girl is brought to your office by her mother with the chief complaint of easy fatigability. The mother is concerned because her daughter is always tired, although several other physicians have told her that the girl is healthy. The adolescent, who states no complaints or concerns, appears very shy. She is currently in the tenth grade, likes school, receives average grades, and speaks both English and Spanish. She says she has a few friends at school and adamantly denies any drug, alcohol, or tobacco use. She has never been sexually active and reports no history of sexual or physical abuse.

The mother, a single parent, moved to the United States from El Salvador approximately 2 years ago with her two daughters. They are currently living with relatives in a two-bedroom apartment. The mother is employed as a housekeeper, and the patient and her sister help their mother clean homes on weekends. During the week they make dinner for the rest of the family as a means of contributing to the rent.

The girl's physical examination is entirely normal, although her affect appears flat.

Questions

1. What is the significance of nonspecific symptoms, such as fatigue, during adolescence?

2. What factors contribute to depression in adolescents?

3. What are the classic signs and symptoms of depression in adolescents?

4. What are some important historical points to cover when interviewing adolescents with suspected depression?

5. How is the risk of suicide assessed in adolescent patients?
6. How should suicidal behavior (i.e., suicide attempts) be managed in adolescents?

Depression has been identified as one of the multiple risk factors that predispose adolescents to suicide. However, not all teenagers who try to take their own lives are depressed, and conversely, not all depressed adolescents attempt suicide. This distinction is important to keep in mind when evaluating adolescents for either depression or suicidal behavior.

EPIDEMIOLOGY

Depression

The exact prevalence of depression in adolescents is difficult to determine because depression is both an illness and a symptom. Depressive symptoms have been reported in as many as 47.7% of girls and 41.7% of boys in the 14- to 15-year age group. The overall prevalence of depression as an illness is approximately 5%; mild depression is reported in 13–28% of teens, moderate depression in 7%, and severe depression in 1.3%. Depression occurs more commonly in adolescents than in prepubertal children and is more frequent in females than males after puberty.

Several risk factors contribute to the development of depressive disorders in adolescents (Table 113–1). Certain psychiatric conditions are also associated with depression, including anxiety disorders, eating disorders, substance abuse, conduct disorders, and borderline personality disorders.

Suicide and Suicidal Behavior

Suicide is the third leading cause of death in the United States in individuals 10–24 years of age; only accidents and homicides result in more deaths in young people. In 1960 the annual suicide rate in this age group was 5.2/100,000, and by 1990 it had more than doubled to 13.2/100,000. In particular, the 1990 suicide rate for 15- to 19-year-old adolescents was 11.1/100,000, triple that of 1960. For every suicide that is completed successfully, 15–20 suicides are attempted.

According to the 1997 Youth Risk Survey of the Centers for Disease Control and Prevention, 20.5% of all students in grades 9–12 had thought of attempting suicide during the previous 12 months. Approximately

---

TABLE 113–1.   Risk Factors Associated With Depressive Disorders in Adolescents

Family history of psychiatric illness (e. g., parent with an affective condition or another family member with a bipolar or recurrrent unipolar disorder). The age of onset of depression in the affected parent is important; the earlier the age of onset, the greater the likelihood of depression in the children.
History of environmental trauma (e.g., sexual or physical abuse, loss of a loved one)
Chronic illness
Certain medications (e.g., propranolol, phenobarbital)

TABLE 113–2.   Risk Factors Associated With Suicide in Adolescents

History of a previous suicide attempt (most important)
Preexisting psychiatric condition
Alcohol and illicit substance abuse
Family history of psychiatric disorders, especially depression, substance abuse, and suicidal behavior
Family disruption, including violence, divorce, or the death of a loved one
Exposure to an unexpected suicide in the school or community
Chronic debilitating illness
Anxiety about sexual identity (homosexuality or bisexuality)
History of physical or sexual abuse
Availability of firearms in the home

16% of these students had made specific suicide plans; about 50% of those students with suicide plans reported attempting to take their lives. Almost 3% of the individuals who attempted suicide required medical attention. Overall, female students were much more likely than male students to have considered attempting suicide (27% vs. 15%).

Several risk factors associated with adolescent suicide have been identified (Table 113–2). Adolescent females are more likely to attempt suicide than males, but males are more likely to succeed (ratio of 4:1 boys to girls). This fact may result from the lethality of the methods, such as firearms or hanging, that males usually choose. While females are more likely to ingest pills, the role of firearms is increasing. The availability of firearms and alcohol, which varies from state to state, greatly contributes to the occurrence of suicide. Up to 45% of individuals who have committed suicide show some evidence of intoxication at the time of death. Although most suicide attempts are impulsive, studies have shown that adolescents often have communicated their suicidal intent or ideation to someone before the attempt. Fifty percent of adolescents who attempt suicide have sought medical care within the preceding month and 25% within the preceding week. In contrast, only one-third have received previous mental health care.

CLINICAL PRESENTATION

Depressed or suicidal adolescents may visit physicians for a variety of reasons. They may present with seemingly nonemergent complaints and a flat affect or with multiple concerns and an anxious appearance. Sometimes adolescents are accompanied by family or friends, and they are often reticent to discuss psychosocial issues. Occasionally, they are referred by school officials for educational problems.

PATHOPHYSIOLOGY

Although depression does not necessarily have one single etiology, three primary theories to explain depression have been proposed. A combination of genetic, biochemical, and psychosocial/environmental factors probably contribute to depression.

The **psychoanalytic hypothesis** proposes that low self-esteem, which is the result of a critical and punitive childhood, leads to self-destructive anger. This self-destructive thinking and behavior then results in depression.

The **biologic explanation** includes dysregulation of specific neurotransmitters such as norepinephrine, serotonin, and dopamine. Antidepressant compounds induce noradrenergic and serotoninergic responses. The **genetic basis** of depression is supported by statistics that indicate that 25% of children who take their own lives have a family member or close relative who has committed suicide. Similarly, a family history of major depression is a significant risk factor for the development of depression in children. Recent studies suggest the incomplete penetrance of a dominant gene as a possible etiology.

The hypothesis known as **"the final common pathway"** states that depression is caused by a number of factors (see Table 113–1) that interact and lead to one common outcome. Specific behaviors triggered by a biochemical alteration, an infectious agent, or an environmental experience may result in depression and self-deprecation.

DIFFERENTIAL DIAGNOSIS

The differential diagnosis of depression includes any condition that may affect the patient's nutritional status and lead to malnourishment (D_x Box). Examples include cancer, tuberculosis, and eating disorders such as anorexia nervosa. In addition, endocrine disorders such as hypothyroidism, hyperthyroidism, and Addison's disease can mimic depression. CNS pathology, although rare, includes postconcussive syndromes and cerebrovascular accidents. Illicit substance abuse and alcoholism should also be investigated. Side effects of both prescribed and over-the-counter medications may also produce depressive symptoms. Psychological disorders that include depressive symptoms must also be considered. These include adjustment disorders, uncomplicated bereavement, separation anxiety, and dysthymia, which is more chronic and less severe than major depression.

EVALUATION

History

The assessment of an adolescent for depression is an important part of any routine encounter, but the diagnosis of depression is difficult to make after just one interview. Initially, a complete **HEADSSS** assessment

---

Questions: Adolescent Depression

- Does the adolescent occasionally feel sad and not know why?
- Does the adolescent have unexplained crying spells?
- Does the adolescent feel "mad," "bored," or "grouchy"?
- Does the adolescent seem inappropriately jovial?
- Have there been any recent losses in the adolescent's life that may explain his or her feelings?
- Is the adolescent having trouble with concentration or memory?
- Does the adolescent have trouble falling asleep at night or with early morning awakening?
- Has the adolescent lost weight recently or shown any disinterest in food?
- Does the adolescent have feelings of hopelessness and have any desire to hurt himself or herself? Has the adolescent made any previous suicide attempts?
- Do the parents or siblings have a history of drug or alcohol use?
- Is there a family history of affective disorders?
- Is there a history of family violence?

(**h**ome, **e**mployment and education, **a**ctivities, **d**rugs, **s**exual activity/sexuality, **s**uicide and depression, **s**afety) should be performed on all adolescents (see Chapter 4, Talking to Adolescents). A thorough history should be obtained (Questions Box: Adolescent Depression). Mood changes should be noted; a labile affect can be a symptom of ongoing depression. Physicians should remember that patients who are malnourished for any reason can have a depressed affect.

To identify youths at risk for suicide, practitioners must inquire about specific areas of adolescents' lives. Adolescents who are suspected of being at risk for suicide must be questioned directly about suicide ideation. Initially questions should be nonspecific and become more specific as the interview proceeds, especially if answers to the initial questions are positive (Questions Box: Adolescent Suicide).

Questions: Adolescent Suicide

- Does the adolescent have any chronic medical problems (e.g., epilepsy)?
- Is the adolescent on any medications (e.g., phenobarbitol)?
- Is the adolescent experiencing any psychiatric difficulties, social maladjustments, or family or environmental challenges (e.g., recent parental divorce, school expulsion)?
- Does the adolescent have a history of symptoms of depression, conduct problems, or psychosis?
- Does the adolescent have a history of substance abuse?
- How is the adolescent progressing in school?
- Does the adolescent have any legal problems?
- Does the adolescent suffer any social isolation or have interpersonal conflicts with family or friends?
- Has the adolescent suffered any personal losses recently?
- Are there any family problems such as abuse or neglect?
- Is the adolescent at risk for suicide?
  - Has the adolescent ever thought that life was not worth living?
  - Does the adolescent ever feel hopeless?
  - Does the adolescent have a previous history of suicide attempts?
  - Does the adolescent presently have a plan for suicide?
  - Does the adolescent have access to a firearm?
  - Has there recently been a suicide in the school or community?

D_x Adolescent Depression

- Depressed or irritable mood
- Decreased interest in most activities, including school
- Significant weight changes
- Sleeping problems
- Psychomotor agitation or retardation
- Fatigue
- Feelings of worthlessness or guilt
- Diminished ability to concentrate or think
- Preoccupation with death or suicide

Promises to maintain confidentiality with adolescents considered at risk for suicide are discouraged because parental involvement is strongly advised. Precipitating and motivating factors for any previous suicide attempts should be determined prior to the development of a treatment plan. The lethality of previous attempts should be evaluated.

Physical Examination

A thorough physical examination and a review of systems should be completed to rule out a chronic medical condition or an organic etiology for nonspecific complaints. If patients have a history of sexual abuse or assault or a history of sexual activity, a genital examination should be performed to check for STDs. Otherwise, the physical examination is of little help in adolescent patients with a true affective disorder.

Laboratory Tests

No routine laboratory studies are recommended, although some authors advocate screening tests to rule out organic etiologies for depression. A complete blood count with differential, electrolytes, blood urea nitrogen, creatinine, liver function tests, and thyroid function tests may be considered. Psychometric testing may help rule out a concommitant learning disability or ADHD. A dexamethasone suppression test or other neuroendocrine evaluation is not necessary to diagnose depression. Before a tricyclic antidepressant (TCA) is prescribed, a baseline ECG should be performed to rule out conduction defects. The ECG should be repeated as the TCA dose is increased. In addition, liver function tests should be obtained and followed while on therapy.

MANAGEMENT

Depression

If depressive symptoms are associated with an adjustment disorder and if family, peers, or school factors are involved, **supportive counseling** is indicated. The duration and depth of counseling depends, in part, on how comfortable primary care practitioners feel performing this task. Identification of the problem and development of a reasonable solution with adolescents often helps. **Psychological referral** may be initiated if patients require more prolonged treatment.

If family difficulties are the major problem, family members and physicians or counselors should meet to assess the magnitude of the problem and the motivation required to address it. Physicians should use this opportunity to educate both adolescents and families about depression. The need for individual as well as family therapy should be discussed and the appropriate referrals should be made at the end of the meeting.

Immediate **psychiatric referral** is indicated if adolescents have severe depressive features that interfere with daily functioning or if they are suicidal, homicidal, or psychotic. Such management is also appropriate if supportive counseling has been ineffective. Psychiatric

intervention may include **pharmacotherapy** (e.g., TCAs, selective serotonin reuptake inhibitors [SSRIs]), as well as psychotherapy. TCAs prevent reuptake of catecholamines at the synaptic level and therefore increase serotonin, norepinephrine, or dopamine levels (depending on the particular TCA). The efficacy of TCAs in the treatment of adolescent depression, however, is controversial. Anticholinergic side effects also are not uncommon and may limit the usefulness of some medications. There have been more promising results with the use of SSRIs such as fluoxetine (Prozac) in adolescents. An advantage of these medications is that they are nonlethal if ingested impulsively.

Suicide and Suicidal Behavior

Adolescents who are considered at risk for suicide must be asked directly if they are, in fact, suicidal (Questions: Adolescent Suicide). Response to this inquiry determines whether adolescents should be treated on an inpatient or outpatient basis. Adolescents with no previous suicide attempts, ambivalence regarding suicidal thoughts, no real intent to die, and a good family support system may be managed as **outpatients.** In patients who deny current suicidal ideation, a no-suicide agreement must be made between the physician or psychologist and the adolescent. At this time the precipitants for possible suicidality must be reviewed and alternative methods for coping should be rehearsed. In addition, all potential means of suicide, particularly firearms, must be removed from the home or place of residence. It is not enough to "secure" firearms; they must be removed. Referral to a therapist is recommended as soon as possible. Preferably, this should be arranged while adolescents are in the office, and they should be given a definite time and date for the appointment. Ideally, the therapist should meet with the family before the first appointment. Detoxification from drugs or alcohol, if necessary, should also be addressed.

All suicidal threats or ideations by adolescents should be taken seriously, and psychiatric referral is required. Adolescents judged to be at serious risk for suicide should be managed as **inpatients.** Patients who have attempted to take their own lives should be admitted to a pediatric or adolescent unit for 24–48 hours. The purpose of hospitalization is threefold: (1) to stabilize patients medically, if necessary; (2) to observe and evaluate patient-family dynamics; and (3) to impress on patients and families that the attempt has been recognized and taken seriously. Intervention requires the involvement of mental health professionals in addition to social services. Transfer to an inpatient psychiatric treatment center is indicated for those adolescents who are judged by mental health consultants to have serious suicidal intentions or an underlying psychiatric illness.

PROGNOSIS

The risk of recurrence of major depression in adolescents who have recovered is substantial. A recent study reports that 5% of patients relapse within 6 months of recovery, 12% within 1 year, and an estimated 33%

within 4 years. Prepubertal-onset depression is associated with an approximately 30% risk of developing future bipolar disorder or mania.

The risk of repeated suicidal behavior appears to be greatest within the first 3 months following the initial attempt. Reported reattempt rates are 6–15% in the first 1–3 years following the initial attempt.

Case Resolution

In the case history presented at the beginning of this chapter, the girl's symptoms may be indicative of depression because she seems to have insufficient time for friends and just recently moved to the United States. She appears to be at low risk for suicide, however. The physician should nonetheless inquire about suicidality and then make arrangements to follow the girl's condition closely. If depression is confirmed at future visits or if she becomes suicidal, both she and her family should be referred to a mental health professional for intervention.

Selected Readings

Adler, R. S., and M. S. Jellinek. After teen suicide: issues for pediatricians who are asked to consult to schools. Pediatrics 86:982–987, 1990.

Bell, C. C., and D. C. Clark. Adolescent suicide. Pediatr. Clin. North Am. 45:365–380, 1998.

Brown-Jones, L. C., and D. P. Orr. Enlisting parents as allies against depression. Contemp. Peds. 13:67–86, 1996.

Centers for Disease Control and Prevention. CDC Surveillance Summaries. Youth Risk Surveillance—United States, 1997. MMWR 47(SS-3), 1998.

Centers for Disease Control and Prevention. Programs for the prevention of suicide among adolescents and young adults. MMWR 43(RR-6):3–17, 1994.

Crumley, F. E. Substance abuse and adolescent suicidal behavior. JAMA 263:3051–3056, 1990.

Hodgman, C. H. Adolescent depression and suicide. Adolesc. Med. State of the Art Rev. 1:81–95, 1990.

Jellinek, M. S., and J. B. Snyder. Depression and suicide in children and adolescents. Pediatr. Rev. 19:255–264, 1998.

Lewisohn, P. M., et al. Major depression in community adolescents: age at onset, episode duration, and time to recurrence. J. Am. Acad. Child Adolesc. Psychiatry 33:809–818, 1994.

Lopez, R. I. Role of the primary care pediatrician in adolescent psychosocial assessment and intervention. Adolesc. Med. State of the Art Rev. 3:147–160, 1992.

Shrand, J. A., and M. S. Jellinek. Psychopharmacology in mood and anxiety disorders. Contemp. Peds. 12:21–48, 1995.

Slap, G. B., et al. Adolescent suicide attempters: do physicians recognize them? J. Adolesc. Health 13:286–292, 1992.

Tishler, C. L. Adolescent suicide: assessment of risk, prevention, and treatment. Adolesc. Med. State of the Art Rev. 3:51–59, 1992.

Woods, E. R., et al. The associations of suicide attempts in adolescents. Pediatrics 99:791–796, 1997.

CHRONIC DISEASES OF CHILDHOOD AND ADOLESCENCE

C H A P T E R   1 1 4

CANCER IN CHILDREN

Pamela S. Cohen, M.D. and Pamelyn Close, M.D., M.P.H.

H$_x$ A 10-year-old boy has a history of intermittent fevers of 102.2° F (39.0° C) for 1 month. For 2 days, he has experienced increasing shortness of breath with rapid respirations. His face is dusky and plethoric, and the veins in his neck are prominent. The remainder of the examination is normal.

The blood count is normal, but the ESR is 110. A chest x-ray reveals a large mediastinal mass.

Questions

1. What signs and symptoms are associated with malignant conditions in children?
2. What oncologic emergencies require immediate attention?
3. What factors correlate with the development of cancer in children?

EPIDEMIOLOGY

Cancer accounts for 10.4% of deaths from all causes in children under 15 years of age in the United States, second only to accidents (43.9%). By the year 2000, approximately 12,500 cases per year of cancer in young people less than 20 years of age will be diagnosed. This reflects an increase in incidence of about 1% per year. Although acute leukemia has been the most common cancer diagnosis, with brain tumors second, a change downward in the occurrence of acute lymphocytic leukemia (ALL) and an increase in the incidence of brain tumors have shifted the distribution of diagnoses as follows: acute leukemia (25–30%), brain tumors (25–30%), lymphomas (13%), neuroblastoma (8%). The remaining diagnoses are scattered among several less common pediatric solid tumors. (Fig. 114–1.)

Case-control epidemiology studies looking for the causes of pediatric cancer have evaluated foods, prena-tal exposures of parents and affected offspring, electromagnetic fields, radon, and various other environmental factors with no conclusive evidence of causality to date. Although many environmental factors are known to induce carcinogenesis, including ionizing and ultraviolet radiation, stilbestrol, and androgen, these agents do not appear to play a significant role in childhood cancer. Infectious agents such as EBV, papillomavirus type 5, and hepatitis B are associated with the development of certain types of cancer, but they too appear to play a minimal role in the initiation events that trigger childhood malignancy. Inheritance of mutations in tumor suppressor genes such as the retinoblastoma gene or the p53 gene predispose affected children in families with these mutations to particular malignancies at a greater frequency and earlier age than in unaffected individuals.

Although the macroscopic causes of pediatric cancer are not well elucidated, significant research progress has been made in determining some of the cellular and subcellular events that either actively trigger or fail to prevent malignancy. Most malignant cells have a genetic makeup that differs from the constitutional karyotype of the host. Thus, while most cancers are not heritable, they appear to result from a genetic error or abnormality that occurs in the process of normal growth and development. An initiation event appears to alter or knock out one allele of a gene pair, and a second event results in loss of heterozygosity for that genetic locus. A good example is the p53 tumor suppressor gene mentioned above. p53 is a recessive gene whose protein product acts to induce cell cycle arrest or apoptosis in response to DNA damage. Either an inherited abnormality of p53 or a serendipitous accident to p53 can cause heterozygosity for that gene. If a second event knocks out complete function of p53, a DNA-damaged cell can escape the signal to arrest its growth or to undergo apoptosis. The result can be a malignant transformation that allows the abnormal cell to grow unchecked.

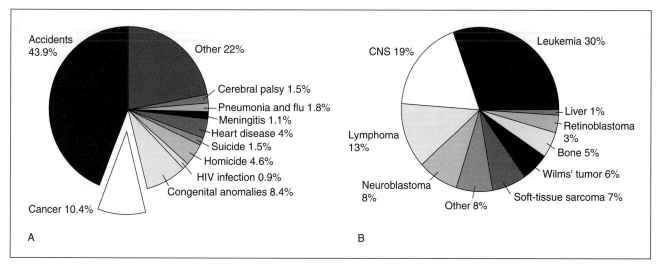

FIGURE 114-1. Leading causes of death in children between the ages of 1 and 14 years A. (Adapted from U. S. Vital Statistics.) **Distribution of cancers in children less than 15 years of age B.** (Reproduced, with permission, from Pizzo, P. C., and D. A. Pollack. Principles and Practice of Pediatric Oncology. Philadelphia, J. B. Lippincott, 1993, p. 4; adapted from Surveillance, Epidemiology and End Results Program.)

CLINICAL PRESENTATION (Table 114-1)

Children with **leukemia,** whether acute or chronic, commonly complain of diffuse bone pains and can present with symptoms related to anemia, thrombocytopenia, or neutropenia. Mucosal bleeding, particularly from the gums, is commonly seen in children with acute myeloblastic leukemia (AML). Frank DIC is characteristic of AML, especially acute promyelocytic leukemia. Children with leukemia often also have hepatosplenomegaly, lymphadenopathy, or mediastinal masses.

Superior vena cava (SVC) syndrome, seen primarily in ALL, may occur in children with such masses. Children with SVC syndrome have respiratory difficulties and are plethoric and cyanotic due to compression of the mediastinal mass on the trachea and blockage of venous return and lymphatic drainage. Symptoms of SVC syndrome sometimes rapidly progress over a period of hours to pleural or pericardial effusion and respiratory arrest. Involvement of the CNS by leukemia can result in signs of increased ICP (e.g., headache, vomiting, hypertension, seizures, cranial neuropathies). In advanced situations with tumor cell lysis, the products of dead tumor cells can cause renal sludging and ultimate shutdown. In such situations, patients with leukemia may present in renal failure with hyperkalemia, hyperphosphatemia, hypocalcemia, and hyperuricemia (tumor lysis syndrome).

Children with **brain tumors** can present with diverse signs and symptoms, depending on the anatomic location of the tumor (infratentorial, supratentorial, or brain stem), age of the child (e.g., infants with open sutures) and presence and degree of ICP. Infratentorial tumors (more common in children) commonly present with gaze palsies, cerebellar signs (especially truncal ataxia), dysmetria, or vomiting. Supratentorial tumors can cause seizures, upper motor neuron signs (e.g., hemiparesis, asymmetric hyperreflexia, clonus), sensory changes, behavioral changes, decreased school performance, and disorders of the midbrain (Parinaud's syndrome—paralysis of upward gaze). Signs and symptoms of ICP are often in the forefront of complaints with both infra- and supratentorial tumors. Headaches, morning or persistent vomiting, lethargy and loss of developmental milestones in infants, and change in school performance in older children all warrant close evaluation.

Children with spinal cord involvement from a primary spinal tumor (or an axial sarcoma or neuroblastoma with cord compression) may present with persistent back pain, sometimes intense radicular pain, local bony tenderness of the affected vertebrae, weakness, abnormal reflexes, abnormal dermatomal sensory exam, and subtle symptoms of bowel or bladder dysfunction. Suspicion of a spinal neurologic deficit constitutes a true oncologic emergency for which timely, appropriate consultation must be sought.

Lymphomas in children can be divided pathologically into either Hodgkin's or non-Hodgkin's types. Children with **Hodgkin's lymphoma** classically have a protracted history (often at least 2–3 months) of enlarging lymphadenopathy, sometimes in association with constitutional symptoms (i.e., "B" symptoms) that include fever, night sweats, and weight loss greater than 10% of body weight. **Non-Hodgkin's lymphoma** often can be subdivided into two categories: lymphoblastic and nonlymphoblastic. Children with **lymphoblastic lymphoma** often present with supradiaphragmatic disease and may have cervical or supraclavicular lymphadenopathy, sometimes in association with a mediastinal mass or SVC syndrome. Central nervous system disease in such children is associated with signs of increased ICP. Patients with small, noncleaved, **nonlymphoblastic lymphoma** of the Burkitt's or non-Burkitt's type often present with intra-abdominal disease, intussusception, abdominal obstruction, hepatosplenomegaly, and obstructive jaundice. Children with Burkitt's lymphoma may also present with isolated jaw tumors. In

TABLE 114–1. Signs and Symptoms of Childhood Cancer

Disease	Symptoms	Signs
Leukemia	Fatigue	Anemia
	Fever, infection	Neutropenia
	Petechiae, purpura, bleeding	Thrombocytopenia
		Lymphadenopathy
	Disseminated intravascular coagulation	Hepatosplenomegaly
		Mediastinal mass
	Superior vena cava (SVC) syndrome	Papilledema
		Cranial neuropathies
	Headache	Renal failure
	Seizures	
	Oliguria/anuria	
Brain tumors	Supratentorial tumors	
	Seizures	Upper motor neuron signs
	Visual dysfunction	Marcus Gunn pupils
	Unilateral motor dysfunction	Parinaud's syndrome
		Diabetes insipidus
	Infratentorial tumors	
	Deficits of balance	Appendicular dysmetria
	Difficulty breathing	Sixth nerve palsy
		Cranial neuropathies
		Horner's syndrome
	Increased intracranial pressure	
	Headache	Papilledema
	Vomiting	Systemic hypertension
	Diplopia	Sixth nerve palsy
	Motor weakness	"Setting sun" sign
	Loss of developmental milestones	Large head size
Lymphoma	Supradiaphragmatic (lymphoblastic):	
Non-Hodgkin's lymphoma	Respiratory difficulty, cough	Mediastinal mass +/– effusions
	SVC syndrome	Lymphadenopathy
	Enlarged/enlarging lymph nodes	
	Infradiaphragmatic (small, noncleaved):	
	Abdominal obstruction	Abdominal mass
	Intussception	Hepatosplenomegaly
	Abdominal distension	Obstructive jaundice
Hodgkin's lymphoma	Constitutional symptoms (fever, weight loss, pruritis)	Lymphadenopathy +/– matted nodes
Neuroblastoma	Abdominal mass	Hypertension
	Skin nodules	Hepatosplenomegaly
	Proptosis, "racoon eyes"	Horner's syndrome
	Nystagmus	
	Diarrhea	
	Spinal cord compression symptoms	
Rhabdomyosarcoma	Related to primary site	
Wilms' tumor	Rapid development of abdominal swelling	Abdominal mass
		Hypertension
	Painless hematuria	Associated congenital anomalies:
		Aniridia
		Hemihypertrophy
		Urogenital anomalies
Ewing's sarcoma	Painful swelling of bone	
	Constitutional symptoms (fever, fatigue)	
Osteosarcoma	Painful swelling of bone	

addition, patients with lymphoma can manifest any of a number of paraneoplastic syndromes. These include idiopathic thrombocytopenic purpura, autoimmune hemolytic anemia, nephrotic syndrome, and peripheral neuropathies, which may be mediated by abnormal and lymphoma-driven humoral or cell-mediated processes. In general, patients may either have entirely normal blood counts or a mild anemia, but occasionally their bone marrow may be infiltrated, giving a clinical picture consistent with leukemia with anemia, thrombocytopenia, or neutropenia.

Neuroblastoma, the most common soft tissue tumor aside from brain tumors, is of sympathetic ganglionic cell origin, and as such, can present as intra-adrenal or extra-adrenal (paraspinal) abdominal masses, posterior (paraspinal) mediastinal masses, cervical masses, or in some cases with disseminated disease of the liver, spleen, skin, and bone and bone marrow. Because these tumors produce excess catecholamine analogs, children may have hypertension, diarrhea, nystagmus, opsomyoclonus (random dysconjugate eye movements), and cerebellar ataxia. Proptosis and hemorrhage due to metastases behind the orbit can result in "raccoon eyes." A mediastinal tumor may be associated with unilateral Horner's syndrome due to compression of cranial nerve VII. Children with widespread disease, especially those over the age of 2 years, may have infiltration of the bone marrow leading to pancytopenia and severe bony pain.

Rhabdomyosarcoma, another soft tissue sarcoma of childhood, presents primarily with signs and symptoms related to whether the tumor has developed in the head and neck, chest, abdomen/pelvis, or extremities. One classic presentation, sarcoma botryoides, occurs when the tumor is located in the vagina or uterus. **Wilms' tumor,** which arises in the kidney, usually appears as an abdominal mass that sometimes rapidly enlarges as the result of hemorrhage. Painless hematuria may be present, even in the absence of an abdominal mass. Children may have hypertension and associated congenital anomalies including aniridia, hemihypertrophy, and various urogenital conditions.

The **bone sarcomas** that occur in children include Ewing's sarcoma, osteosarcoma, and other rarer sarcomas. All bone tumors appear as growing, painful swellings of bone; patients with Ewing's sarcoma may also have associated constitutional symptoms such as low-grade fever, fatigue, and weight loss.

PATHOPHYSIOLOGY

As described in the epidemiology section, the pathophysiology of carcinogenesis has its origins in genetic mutation. The complete process of cancer development is incompletely understood but begins with a series of sequential genetic mutations that affect the complex processes that control cell growth, differentiation, and death. Figure 114–2 outlines the pathway of cell proliferation. Growth factors are often responsible for exogenous stimulation of proliferation, and growth factor receptors transduce this signal into the cell via cytoplasmic second messengers such as protein kinase C and activated *ras* proteins, which in turn transmit the signal

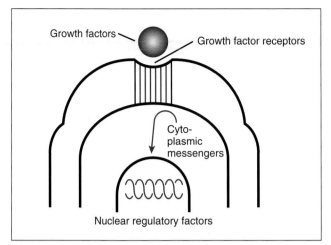

FIGURE 114–2. Pathway of stimulated cell proliferation. Cellular proliferation can be modified by extracellular signals, such as growth factors, that interact with receptors on the surface membrane. These receptors can be transmembrane proteins that transduce the regulatory signal through the membrane, which initiates an intracellular cascade of molecular messages that culminates in the alteration of nuclear proteins. This regulates the expression of genes important for cellular proliferation and tumorigenesis. (Reproduced, with permission, from Pizzo, P. C., and D. A. Pollack. Principles and Practice of Pediatric Oncology. Philadelphia, J. B. Lippincott, 1993, p. 64.)

to nuclear regulatory factors. These factors ultimately regulate transcription of new RNA and protein, resulting in the desired cellular response of either stimulation or inhibition of growth. Dysregulation of growth via mutations in genes controlling all of these steps has been identified in tumors (Table 114–2). Similar aberrations in genes regulating differentiation and cell death have also been described.

Cancer's threat to a living organism lies in its uncontrolled growth. By growing unchecked and invading, compressing, and metastasizing to vital organs, malignant cells threaten normal life functions and cause symptoms specific to the affected area of the body.

TABLE 114–2.   Types of Genes Altered During Carcinogenesis

Gene Type	Selected Examples
Potential cancer genes	
Dominant oncogenes	c-src, N-ras
Recessive cancer genes	Retinoblastoma gene, p53
Growth regulators	
Growth factors	PDGF, TGF-α, NGF, EGF
Growth factor receptors	EGF receptor, insulin receptor
Cytoplasmic messenger protein	
G proteins	c-ras, G protein subunit of adenylate cyclase
Cyclic-AMP-dependent protein kinases	Protein kinase A
Nuclear regulatory factors	
Transcription factors	c-myc, c-fos

Adapted from Pizzo, P.A., and D.G. Poplack. Principles and Practice of Pediatric Oncology. Philadelphia, J.B. Lippincott, 1993, p. 62.
Abbreviations: PDGF, platelet-derived growth factor; TGF-α, transforming growth factor-alpha; NGF, nerve growth factor; EGF, epidermal growth factor.

Questions: Cancer

- How long has the child had the symptoms?
- Does the child have a family history of cancer?
- Does the child have a history of constitutional symptoms (e.g., fever, weight loss)?
- Does the child have a history of recent onset of pallor, fever, bleeding, pain, swelling, hematuria, or malaise?
- Has the child been attending school or participating in routine activities?
- Has the child been exposed to any environmental toxins?

DIFFERENTIAL DIAGNOSIS

The symptoms of cancer may be varied and mimic common pediatric conditions. Lymphadenopathy, which is associated with leukemia, lymphoma, and metastatic disease, is more frequently due to infection (see Chapter 65, Lymphadenopathy). Not all masses noted on physical examination are tumors; they may represent infection, trauma, or physical anomalies (see Chapter 59, Neck Masses). CNS symptomatology may be related to tumor, infections, hemorrhage, or problems such as seizures or migraine.

EVALUATION

History

The history should focus on the duration and evolution of symptoms, associated systemic complaints (e.g., anorexia, fever, night sweats), relevant family history, and unusual environmental exposures (e.g., ionizing radiation) (Questions Box). The impact of the symptoms on daily activities (e.g., school attendance, sports) should be determined.

Physical Examination

A full physical examination should be performed, with particular attention paid to symptomatic areas (see Table 114–1). In general, the lymph nodes should be carefully assessed for enlargement, and the abdomen for organomegaly. Neurologic symptoms, including headache, vomiting, or focal complaints, warrant a full neurologic examination. Increased ICP may manifest as papilledema, sixth nerve palsy, or systemic hypertension. In infants, increased ICP can manifest with the "setting sun" sign (eyes deviated downward), large head size, or full fontanelles. Both supratentorial and infratentorial tumors can in some situations metastasize to the spinal cord (see Chapter 45, Increased Intracranial Pressure).

Laboratory Tests (Table 114–3)

Children with nonspecific symptoms are usually evaluated with a CBC, ESR, and chemical panels that assess electrolytes and renal and liver function. Certain tumors secrete or synthesize characteristic markers and metabolites that are pathognomonic for their diagnosis. For example, elevated levels of the sympathetic neuro-

TABLE 114–3. **Diagnostic Tests and Imaging Studies Used in the Evaluation of Childhood Cancer**

Disease	Diagnostic Tests	Imaging Studies
Leukemia	Bone marrow aspirate and biopsy Cytogenetic analysis of bone marrow CBC with platelet count, differential PT, PTT, fibrinogen Serum electrolytes, Ca, PO$_4$ BUN, creatinine, uric acid, LDH CSF cell count, cytology	Chest x-ray (look for mediastinal mass)
Brain tumors	(None usually indicated except in case of suspected teratoma: serum and CSF α-fetoprotein, β-human chorionic gonadotropin, carcinoembryonic antigen)	MRI of brain with gadolinium MRI of spine for selected tumors
Lymphoma	Bone marrow aspirate and biopsy CSF cell count and cytology Serum LDH, electrolytes, Ca, PO$_4$ ESR	Gallium scan CT chest, abdomen, pelvis
Neuroblastoma	Serum ferritin CBC with platelet count Serum electrolytes, liver and renal panel Serum LDH Bone marrow aspirate and biopsy	CT or MRI of primary tumor site CT of chest, abdomen, pelvis, (+/– head) with contrast Bone scan MIBG scan
Rhabdomyosarcoma	CBC with platelet count Liver and renal panel Bone marrow aspirate and biopsy CSF cell count and cytology (head and neck primary tumors only)	CT or MRI of primary tumor site CT of chest, abdomen, pelvis Bone scan
Wilms' tumor	Urinalysis	CT of primary tumor site Ultrasound of inferior vena cava CT of chest Bone scan
Ewing's sarcoma	ESR CBC with platelet count Bone marrow aspirate and biopsy Serum LDH	CT or MRI of primary tumor site CT of chest Bone scan
Osteosarcoma		MRI of primary tumor site CT of chest Bone scan

Abbreviations: CBC, complete blood count; PT, prothrombin time; PTT, partial thromboplastin time; BUN, blood urea nitrogen; CSF, cerebrospinal fluid; CT, computed tomography; LDH, lactate dehydrogenase; MRI, magnetic resonance imaging; ESR, erythrocyte sedimentation rate; MIBG, metaiobenzylguanidine; Ca, calcium; PO$_4$, phosphate.

transmitter metabolites vanillylmandelic acid and homovanillic acid are found in the urine of individuals with neuroblastoma or pheochromocytoma. The substances α-fetoprotein, β-human chorionic gonadotropin, and carcinoembryonic antigen are sometimes secreted in the blood, urine, or CSF of patients with malignant teratomas. Detection of these proteins in body fluids can also be an indicator of response to therapy and can predict relapse.

Imaging Studies (Table 114–3)

The MRI scan is a valuable tool in the diagnosis and staging of tumors. When performed using contrast with gadolinium, MRI is far more powerful than the CT scan even with contrast, particularly for visualizing lesions in the brain and brainstem areas. MRI of the spine with gadolinium contrast has largely replaced myelography without the additional morbidity of the latter. This technique is especially good for visualizing sarcomas (e.g., neuroblastoma, rhabdomyosarcoma, Ewing's sarcoma).

Once the diagnosis of malignancy is made, children should receive the appropriate imaging studies to assess the local and metastatic spread of the disease before the initiation of therapy. Every malignancy has specific areas to which it is more likely to metastasize.

The initial diagnosis of a malignancy or its relapse, regardless of clinical likelihood, *must* be documented pathologically before treatment is initiated. The only exception to this rule is radiologic evidence of a brainstem tumor, which for all intents and purposes is consistent with the diagnosis of brainstem glioma. Even when a child is in respiratory distress (e.g., with SVC syndrome secondary to a mediastinal mass), coordinated efforts must be made by the pediatrician, oncologist, intensivist, pathologist, and surgeon to obtain pathology specimens before the initiation of therapy. In less emergent situations, children with suspected malignancies should, when at all possible, be referred to an experienced pediatric surgeon associated with a children's cancer center for evaluation of biopsy versus surgery.

MANAGEMENT

Because the management of malignancies in children is a large topic, this discussion will touch on basic principles of oncologic management in pediatrics.

Four basic therapeutic modalities for the treatment of malignant disease are available; these are **surgery, chemotherapy, radiation therapy,** and **stem cell** or **bone marrow transplantation.** Depending on the particular diagnosis, children with malignancies may require treatment with one or more of these modalities, singly or in combination. The reader should refer to a textbook on pediatric oncology to obtain further details concerning "standard of care" treatments for individual tumor types.

The surgeon should utilize the best surgical approach to minimize "tumor spill" and should be familiar with any intraoperative sampling requirements that may be necessary to stage the cancer adequately for further adjuvant therapy postoperatively (e.g., lymph node sampling in neuroblastoma). **Collection of fresh tissue** at biopsy for specialized genetic tests and tumor banking can contribute significantly to a complete pathologic diagnosis. In addition, in some situations (e.g., a hepatoblastoma that is initially unresectable),

an initial biopsy is the appropriate management. Chemotherapy to shrink the tumor to a point at which complete surgical resection is possible should follow.

If the index of suspicion for malignancy is very high, affected children should be transferred to a pediatric cancer center if possible. Optimal outcome depends on several factors: **correct pathologic diagnosis; careful medical management,** including administration of chemotherapy and monitoring of side effects; **precision customization of radiation fields** if radiation therapy is necessary; **optimal surgical resection,** if indicated; and **therapeutic ability and experience** with administration of treatment to small children. Centers that specialize in the treatment of pediatric cancer are experienced in the diagnosis and treatment of rare malignancies and are thus best equipped to treat affected children. Post-treatment analysis of children treated on protocols at specialized pediatric cancer centers have 4-year disease-free survival rates that are significantly better than those of children treated outside this setting.

In the interest of cost-containment and convenience as well as children's well-being, it is often more feasible for children to be closer to home between chemotherapy cycles. Primary care physicians should be familiar with the management of various infectious complications to which children undergoing cancer therapy are prone. Recent technological advances have made home administration of chemotherapy and selected supportive care therapies possible.

Fever in children with neutropenia (absolute neutrophil count $< 500/cm^3$) requires a different therapeutic approach than fever in otherwise normal children. Until proven otherwise, children with fever and neutropenia (usually induced by chemotherapy, sometimes in combination with radiation therapy) must be assumed to have a serious bacterial infection. They should be treated accordingly, with hospitalization, intravenous antibiotics, thorough examination for site of infection and careful hemodynamic monitoring. Initial treatment consists of antibiotic coverage for *Staphylococcus aureus,* gram-negative enteric organisms, and *Pseudomonas aeruginosa* (e.g., ceftazidime with or without gentamicin). Additional coverage for anaerobic infection (e.g., mucositis), viral infection (e.g., herpes stomatitis, varicella) and other pathogens (e.g., fungi) depends on the child's treatment history and clinical findings.

The placement of indwelling venous catheters has revolutionized cancer therapy in pediatrics, making frequent venous access for both diagnostic and therapeutic purposes more easily tolerated by children. Broviac, Hickman, and Port-A-Caths, some of the indwelling catheters used by pediatric oncologists, are all associated with a finite incidence of catheter infections, which can result either from contamination of blood (line infections) or infections around the catheter site itself (tunnel infection). *Staphylococcus epidermidis* and *S. aureus,* the pathogens generally involved in catheter-related infections, can sometimes be cultured from blood drawn from the line; these infections are usually treatable with intravenous vancomycin.

PROGNOSIS

The prognosis for children with all forms of cancer has dramatically and steadily improved over the last 30 years. Almost three-quarters of children diagnosed with cancer can look forward to being cured owing largely to the efforts of national collaborative group science and treatment protocols. Figure 114–3 shows the improvement in cure rates for the most common pediatric cancers. By the year 2000, it is estimated that 1:1000 adults will be a survivor of childhood cancer. This increased survival affects the natural history of these diseases; some survivors will go on to develop second

FIGURE 114–3. Percentage of children surviving common pediatric cancers between 1960 and 1991. (Data from Parker, S. L., et al. Cancer statistics, 1996. CA Cancer J Clin 46:5–27, 1996.)

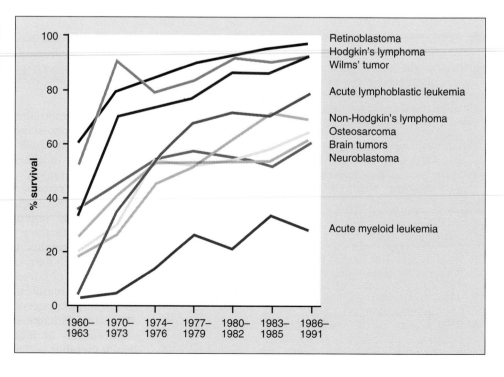

malignancies either as a result of their chemotherapy or radiation treatment or as a result of having inherited mutant tumor suppressor genes (e.g. Li-Fraumeni syndrome, familial retinoblastoma) that predispose them to tumor development. As cure rates improve, efforts are being made to reduce the radiation and chemotherapy doses known to be associated with both second malignancies and other significant long-term side effects that challenge survivors' quality of life. Continued multidisciplinary surveillance of children known to be at risk for treatment or disease-related long term effects should help to optimize a favorable outcome.

Case Resolution

In the case history, the boy undergoes a mediastinoscopic biopsy of the mediastinal mass, which reveals lymphoblastic lymphoma. No evidence of disease in the bone marrow or spinal fluid is present, which would indicate a worse prognosis. Treatment involves chemotherapy, and the prognosis is quite good. Symptoms of SVC due

to obstruction from the tumor resolve with shrinkage of the tumor secondary to therapy.

Selected Readings

Brodeur, A. E., and G. M. Brodeur. Abdominal masses in children: neuroblastoma, Wilms' tumor, and other considerations. Pediatr. Rev. 12:196–206, 1991.

Donaldson, S. S., and M. P. Link. Hodgkin's disease: treatment of the young child. Pediatr. Clin. North Am. 38:457–474, 1991.

Lamkin, B. C., et al. Biologic characteristics and treatment of acute nonlymphocytic leukemia in children. Pediatr. Clin. North Am. 35:743–764, 1988.

Packer, R. J. Childhood tumors. Curr. Opin. Pediatr. 9(6):551–557, 1997.

Pediatric brain tumors. Semin. Pediatr. Neurol. 4:254–272, 273–281, 282–291, 292–303, 304–319, 320–332, 333–339, 1997.

Pizzo, P. A. Cancer and the pediatrician: an evolving partnership. Pediatr. Rev. 12:5–6, 1990.

Pizzo, P. A., et al. The child with cancer and infection. I. Empiric therapy for fever and neutropenia, and preventive strategies. J. Pediatr. 119:679–694, 1991.

Poplack, D. G. Acute lymphoblastic leukemia. In Pizzo, P. A., and D. G. Poplack (eds.). Principles and Practice of Pediatric Oncology, 2nd ed. Philadelphia, J. B. Lippincott, 1993, pp. 431–483.

CHAPTER 115

PEDIATRIC HIV

Carol D. Berkowitz, M.D.

Hx A 6-month-old girl who was born to a substance-abusing mother is brought in by the maternal grandmother for increasing respiratory distress of 2 days' duration. The infant has been with the grandmother since 2 weeks of age, when her mother abandoned her. The infant has had poor growth, two ear infections, and thrush, which has not responded to treatment with nystatin. On physical examination, the weight is at the tenth percentile, and the length is at the 25th percentile. Thrush is apparent in the mouth, and rales are found in the lungs. The infant is hypoxic, with a pulse oximeter reading of 85%. A chest x-ray reveals diffuse alveolar filling.

Questions

1. What are the risk factors for HIV infection in children?
2. What can be done to prevent the perinatal transmission of HIV from a mother to her infant?
3. What are the pitfalls associated with diagnosing HIV infection in children?
4. What are the usual manifestations of HIV infection in children?
5. What methods are available for treatment of HIV infection in children?

Human immunodeficiency virus (HIV) may produce a chronic, progressive disease. In the United States, approximately 7000 infants are born each year to HIV-infected mothers. Identification of these mothers and the initiation of antiviral therapy significantly reduce the rate of perinatal transmission. Although many HIV-infected children are managed by subspecialists, such as immunologists and infectious disease experts in tertiary care centers, the primary care physician remains in a unique position to provide routine health care and anticipatory guidance for these HIV-infected children.

Currently, many HIV-infected newborns are identified as a result of maternal screening and are asymptomatic at the time of diagnosis. Older asymptomatic infants and children may be identified serologically when another family member is diagnosed with HIV infection. Others

may be symptomatic and present with an assortment of medical problems related to the HIV infection. HIV infection is protean in its manifestations and may be mistaken for many other illnesses. It is important for physicians to be aware of the prevalence of HIV infection in their geographic location to help assess the patients' potential risk.

EPIDEMIOLOGY

Pediatric HIV, which is defined as infection between birth and 13 years, accounts for about 2% of the total number of cases of HIV infection in the United States. Annually, 40,000 new cases of HIV infection are identified in the United States. Approximately 2000 new cases are in individuals under age 25. Seventy-five percent of pediatric HIV cases involve minority populations, particularly African-American and Hispanic groups. In addition, approximately 75% of the cases come from specific geographic areas, namely New York, New Jersey, Florida, California, and Puerto Rico.

In over 80% of the pediatric cases, transmission has been vertical (Table 115–1). Children have acquired the infection from HIV-infected mothers. The overall rate of vertical transmission in the absence of maternal treatment or medical intervention is estimated to be about 25–30% in the United States. This rate varies geographically. In Scandinavia, it is reported to be 15%, whereas in Africa, it is reported to be as high as 40%. The current rate of vertical transmission in the United States has been reduced to 8% with the advent of aggressive prenatal and peripartum treatment of the mother and infant.

Intravenous drug abuse, sexual activity with intravenous drug abusers, or any high-risk sexual behavior are risk factors for HIV infection in females. It is estimated that about one-third of infected women have acquired the infection through heterosexual contact with HIV-infected males. In addition, up to one-third of mothers in some areas in the United States have acquired HIV through blood transfusion.

Mother-infant transmission may occur at three different times: (1) *in utero,* (2) at birth, or (3) during breast-feeding. Transmission at the time of birth involves exposure of infants to maternal genital secretions or blood. Studies to assess the impact of cesarean section have reported divergent results regarding a lower

---

D_x Pediatric HIV

- Recurrent bacterial infections
- Opportunistic infections (thrush, *P. carinii*)
- Anemia
- Thrombocytopenia
- Neutropenia
- Failure to thrive
- Diarrhea
- Wasting
- Fever
- Lymphadenopathy
- Parotitis
- Lymphoid interstitial pneumonia
- Hepatosplenomegaly
- Xeroderma
- Neurodevelopmental abnormalities
- Malignancies

---

rate of transmission in infants delivered by this method. As noted above, zidovudine treatment of mothers during pregnancy and at the time of delivery and of their infants after birth reduces the rate of transmission. Transmission during breast-feeding occurs because breast milk is rich in lymphocytes, which may contain viral particles.

In approximately 20% of cases, children have been infected with HIV as a result of transfusion, either for hemophilia or for other conditions. Prior to 1985, blood was not screened routinely for the presence of HIV. In countries where routine screening does not occur, children as well as adults may be infected through transfusions.

Children may also acquire HIV if they are the victims of sexual abuse by infected perpetrators. Adolescents acquire HIV infection in a manner similar to adults (i.e., homosexual or heterosexual activity, intravenous drug abuse, transfusion).

CLINICAL PRESENTATION

Following infection with the HIV virus, usually within 4–6 weeks of exposure, patients experience a flulike illness, with fever and myalgia. These symptoms are often attributed to influenza. Patients regain a sense of well-being within several days, and further symptoms of HIV infection may not appear for many years. There appears to be a bimodal pattern of HIV in children who acquire their infection perinatally. Rapid progressors (10–30%) develop AIDS during their first year of life. Most children do not develop symptoms for 4–6 years, and some do not become symptomatic for at least 8–9 years.

Children who are infected with HIV may present with an assortment of symptoms, depending on their age and method of acquisition of the virus (D_x Box). Children often develop recurrent bacterial infections, including sepsis, meningitis, and recurrent otitis media. These illnesses are similar to those in non–HIV-infected children, but symptoms tend to be more severe, last longer,

---

TABLE 115–1.   Acquisition of Human Immunodeficiency Virus Infection in Children

Infants and Children
Vertical transmission
   Maternal intravenous drug abuse
   Maternal sexual activity
   Maternal transfusion
Transfusion
Breast-feeding
Sexual abuse

Adolescents
Sexual activity
Intravenous drug abuse
Transfusion

and recur more frequently. HIV-infected infants not under treatment may also present with FTT, which reportedly affects 50–90% of untreated infants infected with HIV. The etiology of the impaired growth is unclear but appears to relate to decreased nutrition and increased caloric needs.

Other symptoms include infection with opportunistic organisms such as *Candida* (recurrent thrush or esophagitis) or *Pneumocystis carinii.* Almost any organ system can be affected in HIV-infected children, and other presenting problems include anemia, thrombocytopenia, lymphadenopathy, hepatosplenomegaly, cardiomyopathy, and tumors.

PATHOPHYSIOLOGY

HIV, an RNA retrovirus, synthesizes DNA through reverse transcription after cell invasion. HIV attaches to receptors on CD4 cells and other cells (e.g., monocytes, microglia cells). Following attachment, the viral envelope glycoprotein, gp120, interacts with a cell receptor. This then leads to cell invasion and ultimately cell death. By invading CD4 cells, HIV diminishes CD4 cell numbers. CD4 cells are important for cell-mediated immune function, and a reduction in their number makes patients particularly susceptible to infection with a host of organisms. Invasion of the microglia cells in the brain results in impaired neurologic function. Any body organ can be infected. Infection of the heart leads to the development of cardiomyopathy, and infection of the kidneys results in symptoms of nephritis.

DIFFERENTIAL DIAGNOSIS

The presence of repeated bacterial infections or certain other infections should suggest the need for an assessment for either congenital or acquired immunodeficiency disorders. Differentiating between these conditions is usually contingent upon the detection of antibodies to HIV or detection of viral DNA or RNA. HIV-infected children are prone to **bacterial illnesses** caused by common pathogens such as *Streptococcus pneumoniae.* In addition, these children are also susceptible to opportunistic infections. ***P. carinii* pneumonia (PCP)** is the most common opportunistic infection. Additional organisms causing opportunistic infections include *Candida,* particularly involving the esophagus and lower respiratory tract; *Cryptosporidium,* causing a chronic, watery diarrhea; CMV, although this is not uncommon in non–HIV-infected children under the age of 6 months; and *Mycobacterium,* involving both *M. tuberculosis* and *M. avium intracellulare. M. avium intracellulare,* which usually develops late in the course of HIV infection, results in anemia, fever, and diarrhea.

HIV-infected children may also develop **lymphoid interstitial pneumonia (LIP).** This disorder involves the appearance of multiple nodule-like lesions throughout the lungs. Biopsy of these lesions demonstrates the presence of lymphocytes. Although affected children may be relatively asymptomatic, they may experience hypoxia, cough, and occasional wheezing. An association between LIP and parotitis appears to exist. Parotid enlargement is reported in about 15% of symptomatic children infected with HIV. X-ray as well as laboratory evaluations reveal differences between LIP and PCP. Children with PCP are more symptomatic and often experience acute respiratory distress.

Some presenting complaints are directly related to the HIV infection. Such conditions include hematologic disorders, such as anemia, neutropenia, and thrombocytopenia; skin problems, including dry and itchy skin; and developmental delay, or loss of milestones. Malignancies, particularly lymphoma, may develop. However, malignancies are much less common in children than in adults.

HIV-infected children are categorized according to both their clinical and their immunologic status. Immunologic categories include no evidence of suppression, evidence of moderate suppression, and evidence of severe suppression, based on levels of age-specific CD4 cell count. Similarly, clinical categories for signs and symptoms are none, mild, moderate, and severe. Asymptomatic children under the age of 18 months may have antibodies that have been passively acquired from their infected mother.

EVALUATION

History

Infants or children who present with signs or symptoms of HIV infection should be evaluated for risk factors, including maternal factors (see Table 115–1), prior transfusion, or the possibility of sexual abuse. In addition, adolescents should be assessed for high-risk behavior, including unprotected sexual intercourse and intravenous drug abuse. A complete medical and social history should be obtained in all children and adolescents who may be infected with HIV (Questions Box).

The health status of parents should also be ascertained, especially if children have acquired the infection vertically. Parents who are ill may have a difficult time tending to the needs of infected children.

Physical Examination

A complete physical examination should be performed. Growth parameters should be plotted on a growth curve, and children's nutritional status should be assessed.

> **Questions: Pediatric HIV**
>
> - What types of infections has the child had in the past?
> - How frequent were these infections?
> - How did the child respond to medications? Did the infections resolve rapidly?
> - What organs and organ systems were involved in these infections?
> - Besides the infections, is the child ill in any other way?
> - Has the child's growth been normal?
> - Has the child's development been normal?
> - Did the child acquire the infection from the mother? What are her risk factors?
> - Has the child ever had a blood transfusion?
> - Is the child now taking any medications?
> - Has the child received any immunizations?

The skin should be assessed for dryness or rashes. The extent and location of any lymphadenopathy and the presence of organomegaly should be noted. Evidence of infection, including thrush and otitis media, should be determined. The lungs should be carefully examined for the presence of abnormal breath sounds such as rales or wheezes. A neurodevelopmental assessment should be undertaken to detect neurologic impairment or developmental delay.

Laboratory Tests

HIV infection is usually diagnosed by the detection of HIV antibodies. Such testing is done using an ELISA assay. If the assay is positive, a Western blot test is routinely done. A positive Western blot is evidence of HIV infection in children over the age of 18 months.

Diagnosis of HIV in infants under 18 months of age cannot be based solely on the presence of HIV antibodies since such antibodies are passed transplacentally from mother to infant. Currently, the presence of both viral DNA and viral RNA can be measured using PCR. PCR positivity is interpreted as evidence of infection. HIV can also be detected by viral culture.

To help evaluate the HIV status of patients, the number of CD4 cells should be determined. Table 115–2 lists the normal CD4 cell numbers by age. It is important to note that children maintain higher levels of CD4 cells than adults. In addition, CD8 cell levels should be assessed, and the CD4:CD8 cell ratio should be determined. Periodic reassessment of CD4 and CD8 cells, liver function studies, and complete blood counts is recommended to monitor disease progression. Disease progression is also assayed by monitoring quantitative RNA PCR. Quantitative RNA PCR is used to determine treatment strategies. These values reflect the viral burden in the peripheral blood.

Another useful laboratory test in HIV-infected children is the quantitative immunoglobulin assay. Circulating gamma globulin is markedly elevated, reflecting abnormal B cell activity. The gamma globulin is often not specific and not functional, and children may fail to develop specific antibodies in response to vaccines or infections, an important consideration when determining a management plan.

If symptoms of infection, such as fever, otorrhea, and dysuria, are present, appropriate specimens (e.g., blood, ear, urine) for culture should be collected. Blood cultures should be obtained if fever without a known source is present. Specimens should also be submitted for opportunistic pathogens such as *P. carinii* if pulmonary symptoms are present.

TABLE 115–2. CD4 Cell Numbers (cells/mL) by Age in Children

Age	Normal Level
	(mean)
0–1 yr	3200
1–2 yr	2500
2–6 yr	1700
>6 yr	1000

Evidence of organ impairment may be noted by other laboratory tests. HIV-positive children are often anemic and have mildly decreased platelet levels. They should be evaluated with a CBC and platelet count. Neurodevelopmental testing should be used to determine children's neurologic status as well as their developmental level.

Most HIV-infected children are currently managed with poly-drug therapy. Appropriate laboratory tests should be obtained to determine if adverse drug reactions or side effects are occurring.

Imaging Studies

If impairment in the neurodevelopmental level is apparent, children should be evaluated using CT scanning or MRI, which may show cerebral atrophy and calcification of the basal ganglia as well as ventriculomegaly. Chest x-rays should be obtained in children who are experiencing pulmonary symptoms. These x-rays may show evidence of LIP, with a diffuse nodular pattern, or evidence of PCP, as demonstrated by marked alveolar filling.

MANAGEMENT

The management of children who are infected with HIV has several components. Key to appropriate management is delivery of **routine well child care,** particularly immunizations. HIV-infected children can receive their routine immunizations except for oral polio vaccine. Children with HIV should be immunized with an inactive polio vaccine to make certain that they are not infected by the vaccine strain of polio, which can revert in the gastrointestinal tract to a more virulent strain. HIV-infected children should receive influenza vaccine, once they are older than six months of age, and pneumococcal vaccine, once they are over the age of two years.

Antiretroviral therapy is now routinely given to HIV-infected children, even if they are asymptomatic. Treatment is guided more by quantitative viral burden than by patient symptomatology. The current management approach is referred to as **HAART: h**ighly **a**ctive **a**ntiretroviral **t**herapy. The premise of this approach is that if HIV infected children are treated early and effectively with HAART, before their immune system is damaged, the immune system will probably recover. There are three major categories of antiretroviral agents: **nucleoside analogues** that inhibit reverse transcriptase, **non-nucleoside reverse transcriptase inhibitors,** and **protease inhibitors.** Table 115–3 lists the medications now available for the management of HIV infection. Recommendations currently call for the combined use of two or more of these medications as opposed to monotherapy. Monotherapy with zidovudine is still administered to newborns of HIV-infected mothers for a period of 6 weeks. Careful monitoring for reduction of viral burden as well as presence of side effects and drug interactions is critical to insure a safe but optimal therapeutic response. The CD4 count should also be followed on a regular basis since it is affected by the success of the therapy and is associated with the risk of opportunistic infection.

TABLE 115–3. Antiretroviral Agents for HIV

Nucleoside Analogs: Incorporated into Viral DNA and Block Reverse Transcriptase
Zidovudine (ZDV or AZT, Retrovir)
Stavudine (d4T, Zerit)
Zalcitabine (ddC, Hivid)
Didanosine (ddI, Videx)
Lamivudine (3TC, Epivir)

Nonnucleoside Reverse Transcriptase Inhibitors: Bind Directly to Reverse Transcriptase and Prevent Conversion of RNA to DNA
Nevirapine (Viramune)
Delavirdine mesylate (Rescriptor)

Protease Inhibitors: Prevent Assemblage and Release of HIV from Infected CD4 Cells
Saquinavir (Fortovase)
Nelfinavir mesylate (Viracept)
Ritonavir (Norvir)
Indinavir (Crixivan)

In addition to antiretroviral therapy, children with HIV should receive prophylaxis against potential opportunistic infections. The decision to initiate such therapy should be based on the CD4 count, disease prevalence, and past infection. In children, therapy is often instituted to prevent infection with *Pneumocystis carinii*, *Mycobacterium avium-intracellulare*, and *Candida*. Medications available to help prevent these infections are listed in Table 115–4.

Intravenous gamma globulin is used in some patients, particularly those who appear to have recurrent bacterial infections or those who fail to mount specific antibody responses to antigens. Infections should be managed with the appropriate antibiotic therapy. Children who develop anemia may require transfusion or erythropoietin, and those who develop neutropenia from disease or zidovudine may need granulocyte-stimulating factor.

The nutritional needs of children should be met. This may require the use of supplemental agents (see Chapter 106, Failure to Thrive). In addition, children's emotional and social needs should be addressed. Because society still stigmatizes HIV-infected individuals, HIV-infected children are frequently cautioned against disclosing their HIV status to their friends. Such secrecy may make them feel isolated from their peers. This isolation can be lessened by involving these children in groups or camps with other HIV-infected

TABLE 115–4. Prophylaxis for Common Opportunistic Infections in Children

Pneumocystis Carinii
Trimethoprim-sulfamethoxazole
Dapsone
Pentamidine (IV or aerosolized)
Mycobacterium Avium Intracellulare
Clarithromycin
Azithromycin
Rifabutin
Candida
Nystatin
Clotrimazole
Fluconazole

children. If well enough, HIV-infected children should attend regular school. Federal law prohibits discrimination on the basis of handicapping conditions. Some HIV-infected children are in foster care, which raises other concerns about the emotional strain on the foster parents. Both foster parents and biologic parents who care for HIV-infected children should also be encouraged to join support groups.

PROGNOSIS

The prognosis for individuals infected with HIV has changed dramatically in the past 5 years. The aggressive use of antiretroviral therapy during pregnancy, labor, and in the newborn period has reduced the rate of perinatal transmission to about one-third of its previous rate. In addition, HAART, and aggressive prophylaxis of opportunistic infections has significantly reduced mortality and improved the quality of life of infected infants, children, and adults. At this time, it is uncertain whether HIV can ever be eradicated from a patient, but the viral burden can be reduced to the point that the virus can often not be detected by current methodologies.

Case Resolution

The infant in the case history has recurrent thrush and has had two episodes of otitis. The past history of maternal substance abuse is a risk factor for HIV. The acute symptoms suggest an acute respiratory infection, and the x-ray findings of diffuse alveolar filling are consistent with *P. carinii* infection. The infant should be admitted to the hospital. Aggressive antiretroviral and antipneumocystis therapy must be instituted immediately to ensure a good outcome. The hypoxia should also be managed with oxygen administration.

Selected Readings

Antiretroviral therapy and medical management of pediatric HIV infection and 1997 USPHS/IDSA report on the prevention of opportunistic infections in persons infected with human immunodeficiency virus. Pediatrics (suppl)102:1005–1085, 1998.

Centers for Disease Control and Prevention; 1994 revised classification system for human immunodeficiency virus infection in children less than 13 years of age. MMWR 43:1–11, 1994.

Connor, E. M., et al. Reduction of maternal-infant transmission of human immunodeficiency virus type 1 with zidovudine treatment. N. Engl. J. Med. 331:1173–1180, 1994.

Cunningham, C. K., et al. Comparison of human immunodeficiency virus 1 DNA polymerase chain reaction and qualitative and quantitative RNA polymerase chain reaction in human immunodeficiency virus1-exposed infants. Pediatr. Infec. Dis. J. 18:30–35, 1999.

Flexner, C. HIV-Protease inhibitors. N. Engl. J. Med. 338:1281–1292, 1998.

Guidelines for the use of antiretroviral agents in pediatric HIV infection. MMWR 47:1–43(suppl), 1998.

Kline, M. W., et al, and the AIDS Clinical Trials Group 240 Team. A randomized comparative trial of stavudine (d4T) versus zidovudine (ZDV, AZT) in children with human immunodeficiency virus infection. Pediatrics 101:214–220, 1998.

McKinney, R. E., and C. M. Wilfert. Treatment of pediatric HIV infection. HIV Adv. Res. Ther. 4:22–29, 1994.

Mofenson, L. M. A critcal review of studies evaluating the relationship of mode of delivery to perinatal transmission of human immunodeficiency virus. Pediatr. Infect. Dis. J. 14:169–176, 1995.

Oleske, J. M. The many needs of the HIV-infected child. Hosp. Pract. 29:63–69, 1994.

Pizzo, P. A., and C. M. Wilfert (eds.). Pediatric AIDS. The Challenge and Practice of HIV Infection in Infants, Children, and Adolescents, 3rd ed. Baltimore, Lippincott Williams & Wilkins, 1998.

Rand, T. H., and A. Meyers. Role of the general pediatrician in the management of human immunodeficiency virus infection in children. Pediatr. Rev. 14:371–379, 1993.

Spector, S. A., et al. A controlled trial of intravenous immune globulin for the prevention of serious bacterial infections in children receiving zidovudine for advanced human immunodeficiency virus infection. N. Engl. J. Med. 331:1181–1187, 1994.

Wiznia, A. A., et al. Virlogic, immunologic, and clinical evaluation of human immunodeficiency virus antibody status of symptom-free children born to infected mothers. J. Pediatr. 125:352–355, 1994.

CHAPTER 116

CHRONIC RENAL FAILURE

Cheryl P. Sanchez, M.D. and Isidro B. Salusky, M.D.

H$_x$ A previously healthy 6-year-old boy was diagnosed with chronic renal failure after his pediatrician noted that he was "falling off" his growth curve. His appetite is fair, but his activity levels have declined over the last few months. His past history is remarkable for recurrent urinary tract infections, polyuria, and intermittent enuresis.

Physical examination reveals his height and weight to be less than the fifth percentile for his age. His blood pressure is more than the 95th percentile for age. He is pale, short in stature, and appears to have genu valgum ("knock knees").

Questions:

1. What are the relevant questions to ask about past and family history in children who present with CRF?
2. What laboratory studies should be obtained during the initial assessment of children with CRF?
3. What additional diagnostic tests should be performed to determine the etiology of the renal failure?
4. What are the approaches to the management of children with CRF?

Chronic renal failure (CRF) is defined as the irreversible reduction in glomerular filtration rate (GFR) below 25% of normal for more than 3 months. Early recognition of children with CRF is important in order to prevent the complications associated with the progressive decline in renal function. The signs and symptoms of CRF in children are nonspecific; thus, it is vital that the primary medical caretaker, usually the pediatrician or family practitioner, recognize the earliest signs and symptoms and institute proper medical care. Prompt referral to a pediatric nephrologist must be made, and follow-up consultations by both physicians should be performed to optimize the management of these children.

Acknowledgment: This work has been partially supported by U.S. Public Health Service grants DK-35423, RR-00865, and MO1-RR00865, and by the Casey Lee Ball Foundation.

EPIDEMIOLOGY

The incidence of CRF in children is unknown. Current estimates are based on the number of children accepted for dialysis and renal transplantation; however, some children do not require dialysis or transplantation until adulthood.

The incidence of CRF varies considerably in children of different age groups in different geographic locations. According to the North American Pediatric Renal Transplant Cooperative Study Group (NAPRTCS), approximately 35% of children with CRF are between the ages of 6 and 12 years, 17% are less than 2 years of age, and only 3.5% are greater than 18 years of age. Two-thirds of these children have a structural anomaly, and children less than 6 years of age have a higher incidence of congenital urinary tract malformations. Some geographic locations report an increased prevalence of certain renal diseases (e.g., hemolytic-uremic syndrome in Argentina).

CLINICAL PRESENTATION

Children with CRF are often asymptomatic, and the abnormality is detected during routine health examinations or screening. For a small percentage of these children, CRF is inadvertently discovered when they present with another illness. Patients may be referred to the physician because of growth retardation, hypertension, or anemia. Frequently, a history of recurrent UTIs secondary to undiagnosed vesicoureteral reflux, or bladder abnormalities is uncovered. Children may complain of vague generalized symptoms, including malaise, anorexia, and vomiting, which may be associated with advanced renal failure. Currently, children do not usually develop advanced kidney disease without previous medical contact.

Growth Failure

Failure to thrive (FTT) is one of the most frequent clinical presentations of children afflicted with CRF.

Maximum growth occurs during the early years in life, and children with congenital renal problems are most affected. In the NAPRTCS study, height deficits were greatest for children less than 5 years of age, with nearly 50% below the third percentile for age and sex. In addition, children with worse renal function tended to have greater height deficits. Children with CRF often present with anorexia, feeding difficulties, and vomiting. Sexual development is often delayed in affected children.

Anemia

The anemia of CRF is normochromic and normocytic. Insufficient erythropoietin production occurs when the glomerular filtration rate (GFR) is below 30 mL/min/$1.73m^2$. Anemia is frequently accompanied by decreased serum iron levels, increased total iron binding capacity, and low reticulocyte counts. Uremic patients are predisposed to develop bleeding tendencies because of platelet dysfunction.

Metabolic and Electrolyte Abnormalities

Children with congenital renal abnormalities, especially obstructive uropathies, may develop polyuria owing to inability to concentrate urine, and salt-wasting may be a prominent feature. Conversely, children with advanced renal failure may have impaired sodium excretion leading to water retention and, consequently, fluid overload and hypertension.

Hyperkalemia is not an unusual component of CRF, and it becomes evident when the GFR falls below 10 mL/min/1.73 m^2. Hypokalemia is a less common problem and may be secondary to excessive diuretic use or strict dietary restriction.

Metabolic acidosis ensues when the GFR is below 50% of normal. The acidosis of CRF, irrespective of etiology, is mainly caused by the overall decrease in ammonia excretion. In patients with proximal renal tubular acidosis (e.g., Fanconi's syndrome), bicarbonate wasting may be a prominent feature.

Glucose intolerance may occur in some children with CRF despite elevated insulin levels.

Cholesterol and triglycerides are often elevated with CRF. The characteristic plasma lipid abnormality is a moderate hypertriglyceridemia. More than 50% of children develop hyperlipidemia by the time they reach end-stage renal disease.

Renal Osteodystrophy

The development of bone disease occurs invariably in children with CRF. Several factors are involved in the genesis of bone disease in children with chronic renal failure. Clinical manifestations include growth retardation and skeletal deformities including genu valgum, ulnar deviation of the hands, pes varus, and slipped capital femoral epiphyses.

Hypertension

The incidence of hypertension in children varies from 38–78%. Prolonged hypertension may accelerate deterioration of renal function. An acute rise in blood pressure usually results in seizures in children. Other manifestations include headache, congestive heart failure, nerve palsies, and not uncommonly, cerebral hemorrhage. Hypertension is frequently seen in children with CRF secondary to polycystic kidney disease or chronic glomerulonephritis.

Cardiac Dysfunction

Congestive heart failure may be a prominent clinical finding in children with fluid overload, uncontrollable hypertension, or presence of uremic cardiomyopathy.

Neurologic Dysfunction

Children with CRF may have impaired neurodevelopment. Memory deficits, lack of concentration, depression, and weakness may occur. In smaller children, microcephaly, hypotonia, and lack of maturation on EEG may be apparent. Younger children (<6 years of age) are most affected, since significant brain growth and maturation occur during the early years in life. Children who are severely uremic may suffer from global developmental retardation and seizures. Unless neurodevelopmental delays are recognized promptly and early intervention is instituted, problems are most often progressive.

PATHOPHYSIOLOGY

The progressive decline in renal function leads to impairment of both excretory and endocrine functions of the kidney. The body is unable to excrete water, electrolytes, and "uremic toxins," and the kidney is incapable of producing erythropoietin and 1,25-dihydroxyvitamin D.

Growth retardation in children with CRF is multifactorial; inadequate nutrition, metabolic acidosis, secondary hyperparathyroidism, insensitivity to growth hormone, and inadequate levels of 1,25-dihydroxyvitamin D may all play a role in the impairment of linear growth. Serum levels of growth hormone are normal to high. However, several investigators have shown decreased production of insulin-like growth factor I (IGF-I) and accumulation of its binding proteins, resulting in reduced levels of unbound IGF-I.

The development of renal osteodystrophy has been associated with the following factors: phosphorus retention, decreased production of 1,25-dihydroxyvitamin D, abnormal parathyroid gland function, hypocalcemia, skeletal resistance to the action of parathyroid hormone (PTH), and abnormalities in the calcium-sensing receptor. All these factors contribute to the development

---

D$_x$ Chronic Renal Failure

- Growth retardation/growth failure
- Anemia
- Bone disease
- Metabolic acidosis

of secondary hyperparathyroidism which is frequently associated with high levels of serum PTH and increased bone remodeling. With the advent of the radioimmuno-assay to measure the intact molecule of the PTH, and the availability of various forms of vitamin D, the diagnosis and management of patients with renal osteodystrophy have changed over the last decade.

When the glomerular function starts to decline, metabolic acidosis and accumulation of nitrogenous wastes occur. Fluid and electrolyte imbalance, especially hyperkalemia, may accompany this problem. Excessive fluid and salt accumulation and increased renin production secondary to a poorly functioning kidney often lead to severe hypertension requiring immediate intervention. Chronic fluid overload and poorly controlled hypertension contribute to the development of cardiac dysfunction.

Several uremic toxins have been identified (e.g., PTH), although no specific cause has been associated with delays in neurodevelopment. Previously, developmental delay was attributed to aluminum toxicity secondary to the widespread use of aluminum-containing agents as phosphate binders. However, with the advent of the use of calcium-containing salts, developmental delay is still prevalent.

Delays in sexual development are frequently seen in adolescents; this problem has been attributed to several factors including primary gonadal dysfunction, insufficient production of gonadal steroids associated with pituitary dysfunction, and elevated gonadotropin concentration. In addition, pulsatile hormone secretion is frequently impaired in children with CRF.

Decrease in erythropoietin production occurs in the kidney once the GFR falls below 25% of normal.

DIFFERENTIAL DIAGNOSIS

It is necessary to differentiate between acute and chronic renal failure in children who present with impairment of kidney function for the first time, since therapeutic strategies may differ. Patients with CRF usually present with retarded linear growth and signs of clinical and radiographic evidence of renal osteodystrophy. Renal ultrasound frequently reveals small, shrunken kidneys, reflecting the chronicity of the disease. Anemia, hypertension, fluid and electrolyte abnormalities are often associated with either chronic or acute renal failure.

A variety of kidney problems, whether congenital, hereditary, acquired, or metabolic, may result in CRF. In infants and children, congenital and anatomic malformations account for the largest percentage of patients who progress to chronic renal failure; more than 50% of these children require kidney transplantation. These malformations include hypoplastic/dysplastic kidneys, obstructive uropathy, and reflux nephropathy. The hereditary diseases most commonly encountered are hereditary nephritis (Alport's syndrome), brachio-oto-renal syndrome (BOR), and juvenile nephronophthisis. Acquired diseases such as chronic glomerulonephritis, membranoproliferative glomerulonephritis, and focal and segmental glomerulosclerosis affect a large percentage of older children who progress to CRF.

Although specific cures are not available for most of these renal conditions, it is essential to perform a complete diagnostic workup to determine the etiology of the renal problem. Such information may identify the presence of an inherited problem that may require genetic counseling and, in some cases, anticipation of problems associated with renal transplantation. Some renal diseases may recur immediately in the allograft (e.g., focal segmental glomerulosclerosis); parents and children must be informed early about this possibility in preparation for renal transplantation.

EVALUATION

Complete evaluation of children presenting with renal failure must be performed in order to differentiate whether the condition is acute or chronic, since management strategies may differ in these two conditions.

History

A thorough history must be obtained, including a complete and detailed family history that may provide some clues to the diagnosis of the patient's condition (Questions Box).

Physical Examination

A complete physical examination is required. Height and weight must be measured accurately. Blood pressure, using the appropriate cuff size, must be taken by the primary physician. The presence of heart murmurs or adventitious heart sounds that may indicate cardiac or pericardial involvement must be noted. Gross eye examination should be performed, including fundal examination, to assess for evidence of chronic hypertension. In addition, macular abnormalities and hearing problems may provide clues to a heritable disease (e.g.,

---

Questions: Chronic Renal Failure

- Does the child have a history of prolonged illness, pallor, weakness, vomiting, or loss of appetite?
- Does the child have any history of headaches, visual or hearing problems?
- Does the child have any history of hematuria, proteinuria, or urinary tract infections?
- How is the child's growth and development (compared to siblings and other children)?
- Does the child have any problems with micturition (e.g., dribbling, weak stream)?
- Does the child have polyuria or polydipsia?
- Does the child have daytime or nighttime enuresis?
- What is the child's dietary history?
- Have any family members (immediate or distant) had kidney diseases (including hematuria, proteinuria, cysts in the kidney, UTIs) or undergone any form of urologic surgery?
- Have any family members ever been on dialysis or undergone kidney transplantation?
- Do any family members have any ear/hearing or eye abnormalities?
- Did the mother have any problems during pregnancy (e.g., polyhydramnios or oligohydramnios)?

Alport's syndrome). Any ear abnormalities (e.g., preauricular pits or ear tags) accompanied by hearing deficits are usually associated with some form of renal disease (e.g., branchio-oto-renal syndrome). Undescended testes may be evident in some children with urogenital problems.

Laboratory Tests

For the initial laboratory workup, CBC, electrolytes, urea nitrogen, creatinine, calcium, phosphorus, and urinalysis must be obtained (Fig. 116–1). Glomerulonephritides usually present with numerous RBCs, WBCs, proteinuria, and a variety of casts in the urine. If nephrotic range proteinuria is suspected (protein excretion >40 mg/m^2/hour), a 24-hour urine collection may be indicated. In infants and children, however, urine collection may be difficult. Thus, a urine protein/creatinine ratio >0.2 is a good predictor of the magnitude of proteinuria; these methods are highly correlated in children. Immunologic studies including C3, C4 antinuclear antibody, and anti-double-stranded DNA (anti-ds-DNA) should be obtained if the renal disease suggests the presence of an immune complex mediated nephritis (e.g., systemic lupus erythematosus, postinfectious glomerulonephritis, or membranoproliferative glomerulonephritis).

Imaging Studies

Ultrasound is by far one of the best radiographic tools in the assessment of patients with CRF. Renal ultrasound yields important information (e.g., kidney size, echogenecity, presence of hydronephrosis or stones) that may help establish the diagnosis of the renal disease. The presence of small kidneys usually indicates chronic disease that may date back to fetal development. Increased echogenecity with normal kidney size indi-

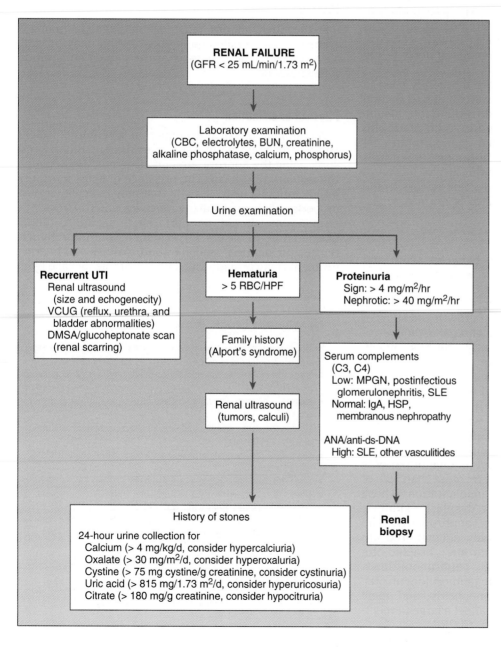

FIGURE 116–1. Initial diagnostic workup of a pediatric patient with chronic renal failure. ANA, antinuclear antibodies; BUN, blood urea nitrogen; CBC, complete blood count; DMSA, dimercaptosuccinic acid; ds, double-stranded; GFR, glomerular filtration rate; HPF, high-power field; HSP, Henoch-Schönlein purpura; MPGN, membranoproliferative glomerulonephritis; SLE, systemic lupus erythematosis; UTI, urinary tract infection; VCUG, voiding cystourethrogram.

cates the presence of medical renal disease in more than 90% of cases.

Renal ultrasound does not yield much information in patients with recurrent UTIs unless the infections have caused major parenchymal kidney damage. A voiding cystourethrogram (VCUG) is indicated in these patients to be able to diagnose vesicoureteral reflux and evaluate the anatomy of the bladder and any obstructions in the lower urinary tract. An intravenous pyelogram (IVP) is done infrequently in children with recurrent UTIs unless the anatomy of the upper urinary tract including the kidneys need to be evaluated. The use of the spiral CT scan in the evaluation of patients with renal failure has increased over the last few years. This procedure requires relatively less time than the standard CT scan and can be used to evaluate the kidney parenchyma, and the upper and lower urinary tract.

Nuclear imaging of the kidneys has provided vital information in the workup of children with CRF. In general, nuclear studies are not routinely done unless specifically indicated. Measurement of the GFR may be helpful, although it does not have a significant impact on the long-term management of children with chronic renal failure. GFR measurements can be performed using technetium-99m-DTPA which yields an estimate of the GFR within 5% of the true value. In some centers, the newer Tc-99m-MAG$_3$ is being used to evaluate effective renal plasma flow, whereas, Tc-99m-DMSA is currently done to assess renal parenchymal involvement in both acute pyelonephritis and recurrent UTIs. This nuclear imaging study provides an excellent image of the renal parenchyma, and is frequently utilized in the detection of renal scars in patients with recurrent UTIs. Significant renal parenchymal scars portend the development of hypertension later in life.

MANAGEMENT

The management of children with CRF has improved over the last decade. Newer modes of treatment and early intervention have made great improvements in the lifestyles and psychological well-being of affected children.

Dietary management remains an important and challenging part in the overall management of children with CRF. Frequently, these children are anorectic and require supplementation with fat, carbohydrate, and protein. Some patients, especially younger children, may require tube feedings in order to meet their daily nutritional requirements. Children with CRF should receive the recommended daily allowance for protein and calories according to age and sex; adjustments need to be made depending on the child's weight gain. Protein restriction is not advised; studies have shown that restriction of protein intake does not retard the progression of renal failure in these patients. In patients with hypertension, appropriate salt intake must be given. Infants and children with congenitally obstructed and dysplastic kidneys often have polyuria, salt-wasting, and acidosis. Sodium chloride or sodium bicarbonate must be administered to these children, and their required daily fluid intake may be higher to maintain normal intravascular volume.

Recombinant human growth hormone (rhGH) therapy has revolutionized the management of growth retardation in children with CRF. Growth velocity has been shown to increase significantly after 12 months of rhGH therapy. Although growth response diminishes after the first year of rhGH treatment, there is continued improvement in the standard deviation scores for height in children with CRF.

The use of recombinant human erythropoietin in children with CRF has become a standard of treatment. The correction of anemia results in improved appetite, increased physical activity, and more importantly, avoidance of the risks associated with blood transfusion. Prior to the availability of erythropoietin, most patients received frequent blood transfusions, increasing their risks of infection, transfusion reaction, and development of antibodies. Erythropoietin therapy must be accompanied by aggressive iron supplementation to maintain normal iron stores.

Most children with CRF do not become hyperkalemic unless their renal function falls below 10 mL/min/1.73 m^2. Initially, dietary intervention may be sufficient, but this is difficult in infants and small children whose diet is limited to formula and only a few solid foods. Pharmacologic interventions (i.e., diuretics, polystyrene sulfone) are used to manage hyperkalemia in these children. In situations where there is an acute rise in serum potassium level, emergent measures must be implemented (Table 116–1). Intravenous and inhaled β$_2$-agonists (e.g., salbutamol) acutely decrease serum potassium level by facilitating intracellular potassium uptake. If hyperkalemia is unresponsive to conservative medical measures, dialysis must be performed immediately.

Diuretic use in children with CRF should be individualized. Indications include fluid overload and hyperkalemia (potassium sparing diuretics such as aldactone should not be used). Diuretic therapy should not be used in patients with disturbed concentrating and diluting mechanisms, since some of these children may have polyuria and develop dehydration on diuretic therapy.

Antihypertensive medications should be started in children who fail to respond to conservative therapy, those with end-organ damage, and those who are symptomatic. Drugs currently used to treat hypertension in children with CRF include angiotensin converting enzyme (ACE) inhibitors, diuretics, adrenergic blockers, adrenergic agonists, peripheral vasodilators, and calcium channel blockers. Treatment with ACE inhibitors has been shown to be beneficial in slowing kidney dam-

---

TABLE 116–1.   Treatment of Hyperkalemia

Calcium gluconate, 0.5 ml/kg of 10% solution, or calcium chloride, 0.2 mL/kg of 10% solution (intravenous)
Sodium bicarbonate, 2 mEq/kg/dose (intravenous)
Glucose-insulin solution, 0.5 g/kg glucose with 0.25 units of insulin per gram of glucose (intravenous, monitor serum glucose closely)
Diuretics (loop diuretics; do not use potassium-sparing diuretics): furosemide, 1 mg/kg/dose (intravenous)
Polystyrene sulfonate (Kayexalate), 1 g/kg/dose orally (if awake) or rectally (do not use in patients with any gastrointestinal problems or anomalies)
Dialysis (if hyperkalemia persists despite the above measures)

age in patients with proteinuria and CRF. Caution must be exercised when ACE inhibitors are used in patients with a solitary kidney and in those with renal artery stenosis, since these medications can acutely decrease kidney function and precipitate hyperkalemia in patients with renal failure. Calcium channel blockers, especially nifedipine, have been used in cases of severe hypertension because of their rapid onset of action. However, great caution must be exercised, since blood pressure may acutely decline in these patients. Intravenous antihypertensive medications (e.g., labetalol, hydralazine) are recommended in patients with hypertensive crisis because dose titration is easier to achieve. For patients with poor compliance to daily oral medications, clonidine is currently available in the form of transdermal patches. However, patients should be warned of rebound hypertension and CNS side effects if the patch is removed abruptly.

Patients with long-standing hypertension must have regular echocardiograms to evaluate left ventricular hypertrophy, and serial ophthalmologic examination to follow eye-ground changes. If hypertension is secondary to fluid overload and salt retention, aggressive fluid removal with diuretic therapy must be used to achieve good control of blood pressure. Pericarditis, on the other hand, is usually a manifestation of severe uremia and may require pericardiocentesis. In some instances, the lack of response to medical management may be used as an additional criterion for the initiation of dialysis therapy (Table 116–2).

Several studies are currently being done to assess the effects of pharmacologic treatment on lipid and cholesterol abnormalities in children with CRF. At present, no recommendations have been made regarding the use of lipid-lowering agents in children with hypercholesterolemia and hypertriglyceridemia because of reported liver and muscle toxicity associated with some of these medications. Further studies are warranted to test the efficacy and safety of these medications in the pediatric population.

Treatment with phosphate-binding agents and vitamin D sterols (e.g., calcitrol, dihydrotachysterol) are primarily used in the management of renal osteodystrophy. Dietary phosphorus restriction (i.e., less than 800 mg/d) is reinforced in children with CRF but generally

is not well-followed because of unpalatability of food. As such, calcium-containing phosphate-binding medications have become integral in the management of these patients. Aluminum-containing phosphate-binding agents are infrequently used today because of aluminum toxicity. Precautions must be taken in children who are concomitantly treated with citrate-containing medications (e.g., sodium citrate), because citrate enhances the absorption of aluminum, increasing the risk of aluminum intoxication.

Recent developments in the understanding of the interaction between vitamin D, parathyroid hormone, and the calcium-sensing receptor have led to novel treatment modalities for patients with CRF. Vitamin D in the form of calcitriol, dihydrotachysterol, or alfacalcidiol has been used in the treatment of children with CRF. Earlier studies with vitamin D therapy demonstrated increases in linear growth in children with CRF; however, recent studies have not shown the same findings. In addition, concerns about a more rapid deterioration of renal function have also been addressed in these patients. To avoid these complications, certain biochemical markers including calcium, phosphorus, alkaline phosphatase, and parathyroid hormone levels (intact assay) must be followed closely in any child being treated with any vitamin D preparation and calcium-containing salts.

PROGNOSIS

The prognosis of children with CRF has changed in the last decade. Options for dialysis (hemodialysis or peritoneal dialysis) and kidney transplantation (cadaveric or living-related) must be discussed prior to occurrence of end-stage renal disease. Technical advances in dialysis allow the pediatric nephrologist to offer dialysis options to children of any age and have made long-term survival possible while children await renal transplantation.

Kidney transplantation is the ultimate treatment for children with CRF. Improvements in immunosuppressive medications and availability of other therapeutic strategies have considerably increased patient and graft survival after kidney transplantation. Full rehabilitation should be achieved after these children have undergone successful renal transplantation.

TABLE 116–2. Indications for Initiation of Dialysis

Severe fluid overload
    Congestive heart failure
    Uncontrollable hypertension
Uremic neuropathy
    Paresthesia
Electrolyte abnormalities unresponsive to medical management
    Intractable metabolic acidosis
    Hyperkalemia
Pericarditis
Severe renal osteodystrophy
    Metastatic calcification
    Severe skeletal deformities
Progressive malnutrition and severe growth retardation, especially in the first year of life
Severe anemia or bleeding diathesis

Case Resolution

In the case history presented at the beginning of this chapter, the initial evaluation of the young boy reveals anemia (hematocrit 30%), low serum bicarbonate (17 meq/L), slightly elevated serum creatinine (1.0 mg/dL), mildly elevated serum phosphorus level (6.0 mg/dL), and normal serum calcium level. Diagnostic workup shows bilateral ureteral reflux, worse on the right side, and the presence of only a small rim of kidney parenchyma on the right side.

Long-term management involves dietary intervention, treatment of metabolic acidosis, anemia, hyperphosphatemia, and hypertension. The patient also needs to be maintained on daily antibiotic prophylaxis therapy to prevent further urinary tract infections, and to be referred to a pediatric urologist. Since the patient is growth retarded, his daily caloric intake needs to be evaluated closely by a dietician, and growth hormone therapy may be started if the patient does not grow despite maximum caloric intake.

Selected Readings

Chan, J. C. M., et al. A prospective, double-blind study of growth failure in children with chronic renal insufficiency and the effectiveness of treatment with calcitriol versus dihydrotachysterol. J. Pediatr. 124:520–528, 1994.

Fine, R. N., et al. Long-term treatment of growth retarded children with chronic renal insufficiency, with recombinant human growth hormone. Kidney Int. 49:781–785, 1996.

Fivush, B. A., et al. Chronic renal insufficiency in children and adolescents: the 1996 annual report of NAPRTCS. Pediatr. Nephrol. 12:328–337, 1998.

Ismail, N. Use of erythropoietin, active vitamin D_3 metabolites, and alkali agents in predialysis patients. Am. J. Kidney Dis. 17(4):270–284, 1997.

Sanchez, C. P., W. G. Goodman, and I. B. Salusky. Prevention of renal osteodystrophy in predialysis patients. Am. J. Med. Sci. 317:398–404, 1999.

Sedman, A., et al. Nutritional management of the child with mild to moderate chronic renal failure. J. Pediatr. 129:S13–S18, 1996.

CHAPTER 117

DIABETES MELLITUS

Elizabeth A. Edgerton, M.D., M.P.H. and Helen DuPlessis, M.D., M.P.H.

H$_x$ A 7-year-old girl presents with a 3-week history of nocturnal polyuria. Her mother reports that her daughter seems to have lost weight in the past 2 months although she has had a good appetite. Laboratory tests reveal that the girl's serum sodium level is 130 mEq/L; potassium, 3.2 mEq/L; glucose, 324 mg/dL; and 1+ ketones. Urinalysis reveals specific gravity of 1.025 and moderate glucose and ketones. Her height and weight are slightly below normal for her age and the remainder of her physical examination is unremarkable.

Questions

1. What is the pathology of type 1 and type 2 diabetes?
2. What are diagnostic criteria for differentiating type 1 and type 2 diabetes?
3. What are the objectives of therapeutic interventions in children with diabetes?
4. What diagnostic evaluations are used in the ongoing management of diabetes?
5. What are the acute and chronic complications associated with diabetes?
6. What is the role of "tight glycemic control" in children and adolescents?

Diabetes mellitus is the second most common chronic illness after asthma among children in developed countries. Diabetes mellitus is a metabolic imbalance that results from insulin deficiency, impairment of insulin action, or both. Advancement in the knowledge about the pathophysiology supports the assessment that diabetes is a heterogeneous disease involving immune, environmental, and genetic factors. This has lead to a categorization of diabetes based on its pathophysiology rather than the therapeutic intervention. Diabetes associated with absolute insulin deficiency is called **type 1** (previously, juvenile onset or insulin-dependent), and diabetes associated with impaired insulin action is called **type 2** (previously, adult-onset or non-insulin-dependent).

EPIDEMIOLOGY

In the past, over 97% of children with diabetes presented with type 1 diabetes, with an overall incidence of 18:100,000 cases per year. Recently, two population-based studies showed a dramatic increase in the number of older children and adolescents presenting with type 2 diabetes. One study reviewed newly diagnosed cases of diabetes over a 12-year period and found that type 2 made up 4% of such cases before 1992 and 16% in 1994 in one Midwestern metropolitan area. Among adolescents, the incidence of type 2 diabetes increased from 3–10% before 1992 to 33% in 1994. In addition, the populations affected by type 1 and type 2 diabetes seem to differ. Type 1 diabetes is seen equally among girls and boys with the highest incidence among Caucasian youth. Type 2 diabetes is more prevalent among girls and has the highest incidence among African American, Mexican American, and Native American populations. The peak age of presentation for type 1 is between 5 and 15 years of age. Less is known about type 2 diabetes in children, but previous studies show a mean age of 13.8 years at presentation.

Dx Diabetes Mellitus

- Symptoms (polydipsia, polyuria, and polyphagia) together with a random plasma glucose over 200 mg/dL
- Fasting blood glucose over 126 mg/dL (confirmed on a subsequent day)
- Oral glucose tolerance test with 2-hour peak plasma glucose over 200 mg/dL

CLINICAL PRESENTATION

Children can vary in their clinical presentation from being asymptomatic to having fulminate metabolic imbalance (Dx Box). **Type 1 diabetes** commonly presents with a classic triad of polydipsia, polyuria, and polyphagia. The most consistent presenting complaint is increased urinary frequency, manifested as nighttime polyuria or secondary enuresis. Alterations in appetite and thirst are most commonly recognized when disease onset occurs in the preschool years (probably because parents are most able to monitor eating and drinking behaviors during the first few years of life). Weight loss can be variable but is more common in type 1 than type 2 diabetes. Ketoacidosis occurs in up to 45% of type 1 diabetics and 14% of type 2 diabetics and presents with vomiting, polyuria, dehydration, and Kussmaul respirations. **Type 2 diabetics** also report having the classic triad of symptoms, but are more often identified through screening urinalysis. Type 2 diabetes is highly associated with obesity (BMI ≥ 85th percentile [see Chapter 110, Childhood Obesity]), acanthosis nigricans, and having a first-degree relative with type 2 diabetes.

PATHOPHYSIOLOGY

Type 1 diabetes affects patients with an absolute insulin deficiency due to autoimmune destruction of the beta cells of the pancreas. The disease process is thought to be triggered by an environmental factor such as a virus or toxin in genetically susceptible individuals. The exposure occurs in early childhood, but disease progression can be variable. Over 90% of affected individuals carry either human leukocyte antigen DR3 or DR4. Discordance of disease among twins supports the theory that type 1 diabetes involves an environmental exposure in genetically susceptible individuals. Twin studies show evidence of a preclinical autoimmune process, which also has predictive value in identifying susceptible individuals at risk for developing type 1 diabetes. Immune changes include an increase in activated T-cells expressing HLA-DR, islet cell antibodies (ICA), insulin autoantibodies (IAA), and glutamic acid decarboxylase antibodies (GAD) (Table 117–1).

Disordered immune function, in which some antigenic components of pancreatic islet cells are not recognized as self, appears to be the pathogenic mechanism for the development of type 1 diabetes. It is generally believed that at least 90% of beta cell mass must be destroyed before problems with glycemic regulation are manifest. Endogenous insulin deficiency, occurring as a natural consequence of islet cell destruction, results in the inappropriate utilization of carbohydrate. Cellular uptake of glucose by liver, muscle, and adipose tissue is blocked. Synthesis of glycogen, protein, and fat is reduced, and a catabolic state marked by lipolysis, proteolysis, and ketone body formation ensues. Increased serum glucose and ketones present an overwhelming osmotic load to the kidneys, resulting in urinary losses of volume and cations (Na^+, K^+, NH_4).

The autoimmune phenomena described above are not evident in type 2 diabetes as demonstrated by the absence of islet cell antibodies. This disease, which is characterized by resistance to insulin, may assume different presentations in childhood. The more traditional form of type 2 diabetes presents in older children and adolescents and is highly associated with obesity and having a first-degree relative with type 2 diabetes.

DIFFERENTIAL DIAGNOSIS

The diagnosis is usually straightforward given the symptomatology, except in children who present at a very young age. Although the onset of diabetes is rare before 1 year of age, the disease does occur but with nonspecific symptoms (e.g., irritability, vomiting, tachypnea, and poor weight gain). Chemotherapeutic agents (e.g., L-asparaginase) and a variety of medications (e.g., corticosteroids, diuretics, oral contraceptives, diphenylhydantoin, epinephrine) may induce glucose intolerance. Glycosuria without evidence of ketosis or elevated blood glucose occurs in certain renal conditions (e.g., Fanconi's syndrome, carbohydrate malabsorption syndromes, heavy metal intoxication). Transient hyperglycemia, with or without glycosuria, may occur in response to physiologic stress (e.g., burns, trauma, hyperosmolar dehydration). In most of these cases, glucose regulation returns to normal within several days.

EVALUATION

Evaluation should focus both on the diagnosis of diabetes (hyperglycemia) and the category, since type 1 or type 2 diabetes can have different treatment modalities and disease course.

TABLE 117–1. Predictive Tests for Individuals Susceptible to Type 1 Diabetes*

Immunologic Marker(s)	Risk of Developing Type 1 Diabetes (within 5 to 8 years)
Islet cell antibodies (ICA)	25–70%
Insulin autoantibodies (IAA)	Variable (may not be specific to islet cell tissue)
Reduced first-phase insulin release (FPIR)	100%
ICA IAA	90%
Human leukocyte antigen with index case	25–30%

*Individuals with first-degree relative with type 1 diabetes.

History

The history should focus both on classic symptomatology and whether there is a family history of diabetes. Up to 80% of type 2 diabetics will report a positive family history of diabetes, compared to 20% of type 1 diabetics. In addition, exogenous causes of diabetes should be ruled out. Obtaining a history of viral infections or chemical exposures during early childhood may be useful (Questions Box).

Physical Examination

Growth parameters should be measured and plotted on standard growth curves. Obesity is present in 96% of type 2 diabetics, compared to 24% of type 1 diabetics. Even when obese, patients with diabetes may lose weight at the time of presentation. Uncomplicated type 1 diabetics may have an unrevealing physical examination, while type 2 diabetics may have physical findings associated with obesity. One study demonstrated that 60% of adolescent type 2 diabetics had acanthosis nigricans and 32% had hypertension at presentation. An intercurrent infection may trigger the symptomatology and should always be sought in cases of ketoacidosis. Children who present with ketoacidosis may have evidence of vomiting, dehydration, Kussmaul respirations, and, in severe cases, altered mental status.

Laboratory Tests

Initial laboratory tests should include evaluation of the serum and urine for glucose and ketones. For patients presenting in diabetic ketoacidosis (DKA), evaluation should also include a full chemistry panel to assess for metabolic acidosis, hypokalemia, and serum osmolality. Once the diagnosis of diabetes is suspected, further testing can assist in categorizing the type of diabetes. Tests include insulin levels and C-peptide (a marker of insulin levels). Both insulin and C-peptide levels are usually higher in patients with type 2 diabetes since they have insulin resistance rather than an absolute insulin deficiency. Insulin reserve can be measured by determining the basal and stimulated levels of C-peptide (> 0.6ng/mL basal level, > 1.5ng/mL 90 minutes after nutritional supplement such as Sustacal). In categorizing diabetics, it is important to note that some type 1 diabetics can have insulin reserves up to 2 years after diagnosis.

Oral glucose tolerance tests are rarely necessary to confirm the diagnosis of diabetes. Two-hour postprandial values in excess of 200 mg/dL or fasting glucose ≥ 126 mg/dL are evidence of diabetes. The introduction of the intravenous glucose tolerance test with measurement of first phase insulin release (FPIR) has allowed early diagnosis of individuals at risk for the disease prior to development of symptoms.

MANAGEMENT

Early diagnosis together with a comprehensive program of education and aggressive management are essential to prevent acute and long-term complications. Long-term objectives of therapeutic intervention in children with diabetes are (1) to facilitate normal physical growth and psychological and sexual maturation, (2) to promote normoglycemia through regulation of glucose metabolism, (3) to prevent acute complications (i.e., hypoglycemia, ketoacidosis), (4) to prevent or delay long-term sequelae, and (5) to accommodate physiologic changes that alter therapeutic needs (e.g., exercise, adolescence, intercurrent illness).

Effective management necessitates a multidisciplinary team of professionals skilled in handling the myriad issues that arise for families and children with diabetes. Most clinics specializing in the care of children with diabetes include a nurse educator, dietician, social worker, psychologist or therapist, and a pediatric diabetologist. In settings where such special care centers are available, the primary care physician serves as a key adjunct, underscoring the importance of ongoing patient-family involvement in disease management and ensuring optimal growth, development, and nutrition. In the absence of special care centers, the primary care physician assumes responsibility for all aspects of management, including the treatment of acute complications, monitoring compliance and control, and surveillance for long-term complications.

Effective therapeutic intervention is based on individual needs for energy, insulin, and exercise. A number of factors, including physical growth, insulin requirement, glycemic control, and activity level, influence those needs and must be assessed on a regular basis. For type 1 diabetics, insulin therapy is the mainstay of management, whereas for type 2 diabetes therapeutic options include weight control through diet and exercise (see Chapter 110, Childhood Obesity), oral hypoglycemic agents, and insulin. Oral hypoglycemic agents can lower blood glucose by increasing insulin secretion, increasing insulin action, decreasing hepatic glucose output, or decreasing nutrient absorption. These agents include sulfonylureas, metformin, and acarbose. Because of their limited use in the pediatric population and associated risk of hypoglycemia, type 2 diabetics may initially be managed with exogenous insulin.

Insulin

The purpose of insulin therapy is to enable children to approach normoglycemia in response to adequate amounts of food, insulin, and exercise. The amount of daily insulin required is dependent on the child's age,

---

Questions: Insulin-Dependent Diabetes Mellitus

- Is the child having increased urination (e.g., nighttime urination, unusual bed-wetting)?
- Is the child drinking or eating more than usual?
- Has the child experienced any weight loss?
- Has the child been taking or had access to any kind of medications (e.g., corticosteroids, L-asparaginase, diuretics ["water pills"], birth control pills)?
- Are there any family members with diabetes (first- or second-degree relatives)?

weight, and development. On average for type 1 diabetics, children less than 5 years of age require 0.6–0.8 units/kg, children between 5–11 years of age require 0.75–0.9 units/kg, and 12–18 year olds require 0.8–1.5 units/kg in a 24-hour period. Within 3–4 months of diagnosis, most individuals experience a partial remission, or "honeymoon" phase, during which time their insulin requirements decline dramatically. Conversely, illness, anxiety, and adolescence (i.e., pubertal changes) may cause the insulin requirement to increase. Even under conditions of increased need, reported daily insulin dosages in excess of two units per kilogram of body weight should stimulate investigations into patient compliance.

A number of insulin regimens currently in use take advantage of the variable onset of action of the different insulin preparations (Table 117–2). The new insulin analogs are monomers of insulin rather than insulin aggregates. They provide a rapid onset and a shorter duration of action. This allows for easier adjustment of insulin dose depending on the child's appetite, since the injection can be given directly before the meal. While these new forms of insulin have not yet been approved for the pediatric population, they may serve an important role in managing pediatric diabetes in the future. Children with newly diagnosed diabetes should use semisynthetic or recombinant human insulin preparations to minimize the possibility of allergic reactions. Any change in insulin preparation should be undertaken cautiously and only under medical supervision, because brands vary in strength, purity, and glycemic response.

Morning hyperglycemia may result from one of two phenomena, which must be distinguished, because the appropriate therapeutic responses are opposite. The **dawn phenomenon** probably involves a nocturnal surge of growth hormone, resulting in hyperglycemia that is present during the night (2:00 to 4:00 AM) and is sustained until morning. The treatment involves increasing the evening dose of intermediate-acting insulin. In the **Somogyi phenomenon,** morning glucose is high as a physiologic response to nighttime hypoglycemia. Treatment of this condition requires decreasing the evening intermediate-acting insulin or increasing the carbohydrate content of a bedtime snack.

Adolescents require special consideration. The sexual maturation process occurs in the setting of relative insulin resistance, other hormonal alterations, and a burden of developmental tasks, which make glycemic control problematic at best. Daily insulin requirements may increase to 1.5–2 units/kg during adolescence, but return to prepubertal levels at the end of the teenage years. Particular efforts must be made to ensure physical and psychological growth in the context of these special tasks. Dietary manipulation and consideration of alternative (usually more intensive) insulin and monitoring regimens is critical for successful glycemic control during this challenging period.

External infusion pumps are not widely used in young children because of the danger of mechanical malfunction (leading to hypo- or hyperglycemia). Their use may be considered, however, in children with unstable diabetes or severe, chronic, intercurrent illness.

Glucose Monitoring

Self-monitoring of glycemic response through the in-home assessment of blood glucose levels is critical to effective therapy. The introduction of reflectance meters (glucometers) has obviated the need for inaccurate, visually read strips of glucose-sensitive paper. Some protocols for home blood monitoring involve a single morning test, whereas others measure glucose three to four times daily. Most diabetologists advocate testing before each meal and at bedtime during the first year after diagnosis. Depending on the age of the child, an acceptable range for glycemic control is 80–150 mg/dL. Patients also need to monitor their urine for ketones whenever their blood glucose readings exceed 240 mg/dL.

Glycosylated hemoglobin (HbA_{1C}) measurements reflect glucose control over the preceding 2–3 months. The normal value is 4–6% of total hemoglobin. HbA_{1C} values <8% are excellent, between 8–10% are average, and >10% are poor. The Diabetes Control and Complications Trial (DCCT) studied the effect of different levels of glycemic control on the complications of diabetes. Although the study only included pediatric patients 13 years or older, the study did show that patients with "tight glycemic control" had lower HbA_{1C} levels and fewer long term complications than patients not tightly controlled. Adolescents with "tight control" had a greater risk of hypoglycemic events than the control group, a fact that must be taken into consideration in determining the ideal glycemic control for a child. In general, tight glycemic control is not recommended for children less than 5 years of age; for older children, glycemic control should be individually tailored. Whenever children's routines undergo dramatic change, stepped-up home monitoring and medical consultation are advisable. Caution should be used in interpreting HbA_{1C} values in infants and others in whom fetal hemoglobin is present, because fetal hemoglobin may falsely elevate the value of glycosylated hemoglobin. Although compliance with intensive regimens is an indisputable challenge (particularly as responsibility for management shifts from parent to child), increasing evidence underscores the importance of "tight control."

TABLE 117–2. Commonly Used Insulin Preparations*

Type	Onset of Action	Duration of Effect
Insulin analog Lispro	0–1 hr	2 hr
Short-acting Regular	0.5 hr	5–12 hr

Intermediate-acting
   (zinc or protamine)
   Lente
   NPH
	1.5–2.5 hr	18–24 hr

Long-acting Ultralente	2–4 hr	20–28 hr

*Twice daily injections: One half of the total daily dose before breakfast and dinner. Each dose should be made up of intermediate- and short-acting insulin in 2:1 ratio.
  Basal bolus: Intermediate/long-acting insulin at bedtime with regular insulin before each meal.

Nutrition

The timing, amount, and types of foods eaten for meals and snacks should be relatively consistent from one day to the next to match the relative constancy of the exogenous insulin. Daily caloric requirements should be distributed in the following way: carbohydrate, 50% (<10% in the form of sucrose); protein, 20–25%; fat, 25–30% (6–8% polyunsaturated, <10% saturated). The distribution of these calories should be approximately 25% for breakfast and lunch, 30% for dinner, and 20% for snacks. Snacks are an important part of the nutrition regimen for children with diabetes. Most nutritionists recommend three snacks for young children (between meals and at bedtime) and two for older children. Some investigators promote the ingestion of cornstarch at bedtime as a means of stabilizing the serum glucose. Dietary discipline is a tremendous challenge for many children. Introducing one change at a time may make such dietary manipulations more acceptable over the long run.

Exercise

Exercise contributes to glucose control by facilitating the utilization of glucose without the assistance of insulin. If not carefully undertaken on a regular basis, exercise can precipitate acute hypoglycemia. Physical activity enhances the body's sensitivity to insulin and can even decrease the daily insulin requirement. Thoughtful planning of exercise involves compensatory changes in food intake and insulin doses. For example, extra energy intake at bedtime may offset the nighttime hypoglycemia that accompanies late afternoon exercise. Seasonal physical activities may necessitate an adjustment in the insulin regimen at certain times of the year.

Education

The role of education is pivotal to the successful management of diabetes in childhood and throughout life. During childhood, educational efforts must be focused on the entire family unit. Affected children must be involved as early as possible and in ways that are developmentally appropriate. The process should involve the early introduction of basic survival information, such as insulin therapy and management of complications. This can be followed by more detailed information, including strategies to reduce long-term sequelae.

PROGNOSIS

Diabetic ketoacidosis is the major cause of morbidity and mortality in children and adolescents, followed by **hypoglycemia.** Clinical signs of hypoglycemia in older children include shakiness, blurred vision, and dysarthria. Concerns about the neurodevelopmental impact of hypoglycemia in young children have led to the recommendation of more liberal glycemic control in early onset disease. Diabetic ketoacidosis, precipitated by an intercurrent infection or poor compliance, is a metabolic derangement that always requires urgent medical attention and often necessitates hospitalization. Replacement of fluids, attention to electrolyte abnormalities, and insulin therapy are the mainstays of treatment in the face of this complication.

Long-term complications include **proliferative retinopathy, nephropathy, peripheral and autonomic neurologic impairment,** and **early onset of cardiovascular disease.** Ophthalmologic evaluation, overnight urine protein measurement, and a detailed neurologic examination should occur once or twice each year depending on the duration of disease. Intensive therapeutic intervention results in significant reduction in retinopathy, nephropathy, and cardiac and peripheral vascular disease. Preliminary evidence warrants consideration of such therapy with the expectation of benefit in long-term outcomes.

Case Resolution

The girl in the opening case history is admitted to the hospital to help determine appropriate insulin dosing. She and her family require ongoing education. Careful management is necessary to optimize normal growth and development as well as delay or prevent long-term sequelae.

Selected Readings

Charron-Prochownik, D., T. Maihle, L. Siminerio, and T. Songer. Diabetes Care 20:657–660, 1997.
Chua, S. C. and R. L. Leibel. An ounce of prevention. J. Pediatr. 128:591–593, 1996.
Glaser, N., and K. L. Jones. Non-insulin-dependent diabetes mellitus in children and adolescents. In Adv. Pediatr. 43:359–396, 1996.
Kaufman, F. R. Diabetes in children and adolescents. Med. Clin. North Am. 43:721–738, 1998.
Kaufman, F. R. Diabetes mellitus. Pediatr. Rev. 18:383–393, 1997.
Leslie, R. D. G. and R. B. Elliott. Early environmental events as a cause of IDDM: Evidence and implications. Diabetes 43:843–850, 1994.
Pinhas-Hamiel, O., et al. Increased incidence of non-insulin-dependent diabetes mellitus among adolescents. J. Pediatr. 128:608–615, 1996.
Report of the expert committee on the diagnosis and classification of diabetes mellitus. Diabetes Care 20:1183–1197, 1997.
Scott, C. R., et al. Characteristics of youth-onset non-insulin-dependent diabetes mellitus and insulin-dependent diabetes mellitus at diagnosis. Pediatrics 100:84–91, 1997.
Sheild, J. P. H., and J. D. Baum. Advances in childhood onset diabetes. Arch. Dis. Child. 78:391–394, 1998.
Tamborlane, W. V., and J. Ahern. Implications and results of the diabetes control and complications trial. Pediatr. Clinics. North Am. 44:285–300, 1997.

CHRONIC LUNG DISEASE

Elizabeth A. Edgerton, M.D., M.P.H. and Helen DuPlessis, M.D., M.P.H.

H$_x$ A 3-month-old male infant is seen for routine health maintenance after discharge from the neonatal intensive care unit. He was born by emergent cesarean section after a precipitous labor at 30 weeks' gestation. Symptoms of respiratory distress were present in the delivery room and the newborn was treated with surfactant, endotracheal intubation, and mechanical ventilation for the first 15 days of life. The course was complicated by the discovery of a grade I intraventricular hemorrhage on day 3 of life, apnea of prematurity, and slow feeding until approximately 1 week ago. The infant received a 6-day course of corticosteroids prior to extubation and is currently maintained on 0.5 L of oxygen, theophylline, spironolactone, iron, and vitamins.

On physical examination, the infant is small but well-nourished and has nasal cannulae in place. Auscultation of the lungs reveals occasional expiratory wheezes in both lung fields.

Questions

1. What monitoring is appropriate in the outpatient care of infants who required intubation in the newborn period?
2. What considerations should be made for the routine health care needs of children with chronic lung disease?
3. What are the long-term sequelae associated with bronchopulmonary dysplasia? Cystic fibrosis?
4. What medical advances have affected the natural history of bronchopulmonary dysplasia? Cystic fibrosis?

Chronic lung diseases in the pediatric population are associated with significant morbidity and mortality. Missed school days, developmental and emotional difficulties, and superimposed acute respiratory illnesses and premature death are among the many serious sequelae experienced by children with these diseases. Asthma, bronchopulmonary dysplasia (BPD), and cystic fibrosis (CF) can be characterized as chronic lung diseases. For a complete discussion of asthma in children, see Chapter 61, Wheezing and Asthma. This chapter includes a separate discussion of the evaluation and management considerations unique to BPD and CF, followed by discussion of the common preventive and health maintenance measures with which the primary care physician should be familiar.

EPIDEMIOLOGY

Bronchopulmonary Dysplasia

Approximately 15–47% of neonates weighing less than 1500 g admitted to a neonatal intensive care unit (tertiary level nurseries) in the United States will develop BPD. The incidence is greatest for neonates weighing between 500–699 g: as many as 85% of them will develop BPD. Over the last 30 years, there has been an overall increase in the incidence of BPD. This may be due to the increased survival of very low birth-weight infants (<750 g) and the increased sensitivity of diagnosis.

Cystic Fibrosis

The incidence of CF is 1:2500 among Caucasians, with a carrier rate of 5%, but drops to 1:17,000 in African Americans. The condition is inherited in an autosomal recessive manner, and girls and boys are equally affected.

CLINICAL PRESENTATION

Bronchopulmonary Dysplasia

BPD is a disorder seen in infants who meet the following criteria: (1) supplemental oxygen required at 36 weeks postconceptional age, (2) radiographic findings characteristic of BPD, (3) clinical symptoms of respiratory disease (e.g., tachypnea, retractions, increased work of breathing), and (4) history of assisted ventilation (D_x: Bronchopulmonary Dysplasia Box).

Cystic Fibrosis

Most children with CF present during the first year of life with symptoms related to pancreatic insufficiency or pulmonary disease. FTT, steatorrhea, and obstructive liver disease are common indications of the malabsorption that affect 80% of patients (D_x: Cystic Fibrosis Box). Children may present with wheezing, airway hyperreactivity, and frequent lower respiratory tract infections, often with unusual organisms such as *Pseudomonas*, *Klebsiella*, and *Staphylococcus*.

D$_x$ **Bronchopulmonary Dysplasia**

- Supplemental oxygen requirement to maintain PaO_2 above 50 mm Hg
- Radiographic findings consistent with BPD (e.g., hyperinflation, fibrotic changes)
- Clinical symptoms of respiratory distress (e.g., tachypnea, retractions, increased work of breathing)
- History of assisted ventilation

D$_x$ Cystic Fibrosis

- Evidence of exocrine glandular dysfunction (e.g., pancreatic insufficiency, chronic pulmonary disease, intestinal malabsorption) *plus*
- Sweat chloride content greater than 60 mEq/L *or*
- Definitive genetic screening

PATHOPHYSIOLOGY

Bronchopulmonary Dysplasia

Although the pathophysiology of BPD is not fully understood, it appears that three processes contribute to its development. Immaturity of the lung is the first process as evidenced by the presence of respiratory distress syndrome (RDS), most commonly associated with prematurity. The second contributory process is barotrauma and oxygen toxicity as a result of assisted ventilation. This iatrogenic injury leads to an immune response resulting in pulmonary inflammation, the third contributory process. Other factors associated with BPD include the administration of excessive colloid or the presence of a pulmonary infection with *Ureaplasma urealyticum*.

Cystic Fibrosis

CF is a disorder of exocrine glandular dysfunction characterized by severe pulmonary disease, pancreatic insufficiency, and intestinal malabsorption. The basic defect in CF involves malfunction of chloride transport through the chloride channel. Sodium accompanies the chloride. The recessive mutation responsible for 70% of cases is a chromosomal deletion on the long arm of chromosome 7. The cystic fibrosis transmembrane regulator gene (CFTR) codes for a protein involved in the regulation of chloride transport. This mutation leads to an accumulation of thick mucus that results in obstruction, scarring, and ultimate destruction of the excretory glands.

DIFFERENTIAL DIAGNOSIS

Bronchopulmonary Dysplasia

Pulmonary infections, congenital heart disease, and congenital lung malformation (e.g., bronchogenic cysts, adenomatoid malformations) may all result in symptoms of respiratory distress. The history and classic radiographic findings usually distinguish BPD from other diseases.

Cystic Fibrosis

In the absence of family history or neonatal screening programs, children with CF may go undiagnosed for years until the severity and multiplicity of exocrine dysfunction is recognized. Children who present with acholic or "fatty" stools (i.e., steatorrhea) may undergo diagnostic evaluation for the myriad causes of intestinal malabsorption. Wheezing and recurrent pulmonary infections may prompt diagnostic considerations of asthma (or reactive airway disease), congenital lung malformation, α_1-antitrypsin deficiency, or an immunodeficiency. Children who present with FTT may be suspected of having endocrinologic, genetic, or environmental disorders (see Chapter 106, Failure to Thrive).

EVALUATION

BRONCHOPULMONARY DYSPLASIA

History

The history should focus on respiratory events in the neonatal period as well as on the severity of pulmonary disease since discharge from the nursery (Questions: Bronchopulmonary Dysplasia Box). In addition, a review of the patient's most recent radiographs is essential to facilitate accurate interpretation of any future x-rays, because chronic scarring may be present.

Physical Examination

The physical examination should focus on growth, development, nutritional, and respiratory status. Growth parameters and anthropometric measurements should be obtained regularly. A careful lung examination should be part of every assessment. Because steroid therapy is associated with biventricular hypertrophy and systemic hypertension, monitoring blood pressure on a regular basis is necessary.

Laboratory Tests

In infants with BPD, pulse oximetry should be performed and the usefulness of supplemental oxygen should be evaluated. Oxygen saturation should be measured at times when oxygenation is expected to fall (e.g., while feeding and sleeping). Regular chemistries such as serum electrolytes are indicated for infants with BPD before they are given diuretics and other medications that may cause electrolyte and acid-base disturbances.

Imaging Studies

Pulmonary function should be assessed frequently. These children are at risk for excessive and unnecessary

---

Questions: Bronchopulmonary Dysplasia

- Was the infant delivered prematurely? If so, how may weeks before term?
- Did the mother take any medications or receive antenatal steroids?
- How much did the infant weigh at birth?
- Did the infant ever require mechanical ventilation or oxygen in the newborn period? If so, for how long?
- Has the child had frequent respiratory infections or problems?
- How many times has he or she been to the emergency department or spent a night in the hospital as a result of respiratory illness?
- Does the child currently require oxygen during feeding?
- Is the child taking any medications?

Questions: Cystic Fibrosis

- Did the child have any GI problems in the newborn period?
- What is the pattern and appearance of the child's stool?
- Does the child have a good appetite?
- How has the child been growing?
- Has the child ever had any respiratory problems or infections requiring a visit to the emergency department or a stay in the hospital?
- Has the child ever had polyps in the nose?
- Does anyone else in the family have similar problems?
- Are the parents related?

radiation exposure. Radiographs are probably not indicated for minor infections; much more can be gained from microbiologic evaluations of sputum and blood and from objective evaluations of pulmonary function (e.g., spirometry, oximetry, blood gas).

CYSTIC FIBROSIS

History

The history should focus on nutritional symptoms and intestinal and respiratory function in children with CF (Questions: Cystic Fibrosis Box).

Laboratory Tests

The clinical test accepted as the "gold standard" for the diagnosis of CF is the quantitative pilocarpine iontophoretic sweat test. Sweat glands in the skin of the forearm are stimulated using topical pilocarpine gel and a measured electrical current. Premeasured filter paper is utilized for the collection of sweat, which is then analyzed for chloride concentration.

The sweat test is sometimes problematic in children under 3 months of age. Stool trypsinogen has been of some use in small infants. For patients with a negative sweat chloride test but clinical symptoms consistent with cystic fibrosis, genotyping is indicated. Clinical laboratories usually test for 15–30 mutations, yielding a diagnostic sensitivity of 90%. Although prenatal genetic screening is available for at-risk pregnancies, population-based testing has not been recommended because screening does not diagnose approximately 25–30% of cases.

Imaging Studies

Radiographs should be used as they are for children with BPD (see Bronchopulmonary Dysplasia: Imaging Studies). In addition, children with CF may require a CT of the sinuses to aid in the diagnosis and management of recurrent sinus infections.

MANAGEMENT

BRONCHOPULMONARY DYSPLASIA

Respiratory support and pharmacologic therapy are the mainstays of treatment of BPD.

Inpatient Therapy

Supplemental oxygen is required by most premature infants, regardless of the presence of neonatal respiratory distress syndrome. The route of delivery and concentration varies among institutions. Some neonatologists promote the early use of continuous positive airway pressure via nasal cannulae as an effective method of preventing alveolar collapse while minimizing potential barotrauma to premature lungs. This method has been effective in some institutions, but it has not been successful in others. Most neonatologists strive to minimize the duration of mechanical ventilation in an effort to reduce barotrauma, although intubation of the smallest premature infants is routine in many nurseries. The application of high-frequency ventilatory techniques may potentially decrease the amount of barotrauma to which infants are exposed. The use of these techniques is too new to allow evaluation of the possible impact on the incidence of chronic lung damage.

A variety of **pharmacologic agents,** most notably bronchodilators, diuretics, and corticosteroids, have been used in the treatment of BPD. The rationale for using **bronchodilators** was questioned for many years until researchers demonstrated that even very premature infants have sufficient bronchial smooth muscle to respond to a variety of agents. Indeed, smooth muscle may undergo hyperplasia during the development of BPD. Although multiple effects are attributed to methylxanthines (e.g., diuretic action, facilitation of cyclic AMP metabolism, respiratory stimulant), the relatively weak impact of these drugs on bronchial smooth muscle and potential for erratic metabolism results in their infrequent use as a primary therapy for BPD. However, methylxanthines are still used in the treatment of apnea of prematurity, which often complicates the course of infants who go on to develop BPD. Beta-adrenergic agents such as albuterol and metaproterenol can be quite effective in treating the acute episodes of bronchospasm, which makes them ideal for intermittent therapy. Reports do not support their use in long-term therapy of BPD. The results of studies of cromolyn sodium have been mixed.

Diuretics are frequently used in the management of BPD in premature infants both for treatment and prevention. Although well-controlled clinical trials are limited, many researchers believe that fluid restriction and diuresis decrease the likelihood of chronic lung damage through some mitigating effect on the development of pulmonary edema. The use of loop and thiazide diuretics improves short-term oxygen exchange and lung function. The mechanism of action is uncertain. The use of several other diuretics, including antioxidants and pulmonary vasodilators, is still experimental.

Corticosteroids are used for both prevention and treatment of BPD. Use of antenatal corticosteroids can decrease the incidence of neonatal respiratory distress syndrome and the need for assisted ventilation. Thus, antenatal corticosteroids should be considered for all fetuses between 24 and 34 weeks of gestation for whom delivery is imminently expected. The postnatal use of steroids is associated with decreased pulmonary resistance, increased lung compliance, and decreased oxygen requirements, and it can facilitate extubation. Most of these benefits are short-term. A meta-analysis of the effects of steroid use implemented prior to 8 days of age for ventilator-dependent infants showed some decrease in incidence of BPD and the relative risk of death. Large controlled studies are needed to better understand the outcomes of long-term steroid therapy. Currently, steroids are primarily used prior to extubation and during an acute exacerbation of BPD.

Surfactant is widely used for both the prevention and treatment of RDS. Its use has led to decreased mortality and improved quality of life for premature infants. Unfortunately, the incidence of chronic lung disease among neonates has not had the same drop. Why this discordant relationship exists is still under investigation. Current research is studying the role of cell adhesion molecules in the inflammatory process of BPD and may lead to new interventions.

Discharge Planning

Discharge planning for neonates with pulmonary problems requires the mobilization of a multidisciplinary team including social service workers, representatives of developmental/rehabilitation centers, health educators, and primary providers, all of whom participate in health care on discharge. Caregivers often need time to become accustomed to the special needs of chronically ill infants and their impact on other members of the household. Ongoing support for both psychosocial and physical stressors should be available.

Providing in-home care for infants with chronic lung disease should be encouraged, not only as an appropriate and cost effective use of scarce health care resources, but as the ultimate fulfillment of the attachment process between caregivers and children. Judicious determination of when infants are ready for discharge goes a long way toward ensuring the success of in-home care. Needs of infants for pulmonary support and physiotherapy should be minimal. Infants should have a well-established and consistent growth trajectory after attaining a reasonable postconceptual age and weight. Caregivers must be trained in basic life support and feel confident about the use of any special equipment such as apnea monitors, suction devices, and oxygen tanks.

Outpatient Management

Management of infants with BPD following discharge focuses on **health maintenance** as well as on any residual problems related to prematurity (see Chapter 20, Well Child Care for Preterm Infants).

Chronic lung disease and the alterations in respiratory dynamics affect nonrespiratory systems. The increased work of breathing raises metabolic demands. Children with BPD often require more than 180–200 kcal/kg of body weight/day to maintain acceptable growth. Intercurrent illnesses, posttussive emesis, and bronchospastic episodes challenge even those metabolic requirements. **Nutritional supplements** such as energy-dense formulas (i.e., 24 kcal/oz) and fat-soluble vitamins may be necessary to sustain adequate growth and nutrition. The cardiovascular system may be challenged by the respiratory requirements or by medications. Chronic hypoxemia leads to hypertrophy of smooth muscle in the pulmonary vasculature, which can progress to pulmonary hypertension and cor pulmonale. To prevent these complications, infants should maintain a baseline pulse oximetry ≥92%.

Infants with BPD have increased airway reactivity, decreased lung compliance, and increased number of upper respiratory tract infections. These altered lung dynamics and decreased pulmonary reserve underscore the need for early medical attention in the face of respiratory infections. **Pulmonary toilet** and early, judicious use of **antibiotic and antiviral therapies** can prevent further lung damage and allow the reparative process to proceed.

CYSTIC FIBROSIS

The management of CF focuses on the maintenance of adequate growth and development and the minimization of progressive lung disease (Table 118–1). **Adequate nutrition** is critical. Although children with CF often have substantial appetites, recurrent pulmonary infections, increased energy requirements, and malabsorption may result in a negative energy balance. One study demonstrated that 50% of patients in the cystic fibrosis registry were below the 10th percentile for height, weight, or both. Pancreatic insufficiency can be documented through quantitative fecal fat analysis, and enzyme replacement can be started early in life. Dietary intake and an assessment of basal caloric requirements should occur annually along with evaluation of serum protein, electrolytes, and fat-soluble vitamins (especially A and E). Anthropometric measurements (e.g., height, weight, head circumference, and triceps skinfold thickness) should be recorded quarterly so that growth failure can be recognized early and appropriate intervention undertaken. Ongoing **education of children and families** is an important process that facilitates compliance and improves the quality of patients' lives.

Respiratory hyperreactivity, pulmonary obstruction, and frequent infections inevitably lead to fibrotic lung

TABLE 118–1. Management of Cystic Fibrosis

Clinical Complication	Diagnostic Evaluation	Therapy
Growth and nutrition	Frequent assessment of basal caloric requirements	Caloric supplements and dietary adjustments
Pancreatic insufficiency	Fecal fat analysis	Pancreatic enzyme replacement Fat-soluble vitamins (A, D, E, K) replacement
Pulmonary disease	Pulmonary function tests (every 3 mo)	Routine percussion and postural drainage (P and PD) Appropriate antibiotic or antiviral therapy

disease and cor pulmonale. The early and judicious use of **antibiotics, antiviral agents** (e.g., ribavirin), **mucolytics** (e.g., acetylcysteine), and **bronchodilators** may halt this progression but cannot prevent it. The development of effective **antipseudomonal treatments** (quinolones) has improved the outlook for adolescents with CF, but the potential musculoskeletal morbidity associated with these drugs makes their use in younger patients controversial. **Lung transplants** are used with increasing frequency in this population, with good pulmonary outcomes and two-year survival rates in excess of 60%. At present transplants are by no means optimal therapies because of the morbidity and mortality associated with lifelong immunosuppression. New therapies under investigation include recombinant generated human DNAse and amiloride for the reduction of sputum viscocity, and the use of gene replacement for the overall treatment of cystic fibrosis.

Health Maintenance and Prevention

Although specific therapies for BPD and CF and their complications may differ, some basic health practices are common to both diseases. These children deserve the protection of active immunization at least as much as well children, and full doses should be administered at ages recommended for nonaffected children. In addition, children over 6 months of age should receive an annual influenza vaccination. Children with BPD or CF have no inherent increased susceptibility to pneumococcal or meningococcal infection, and vaccines against these infections are probably not necessary. Conversely, children with either lung disease should receive early consideration for antiviral therapy in the face of infections with respiratory syncytial virus or varicella. Infants with BPD are also candidates for monthly injections of palivizumab (Synagis, 15 mg/kg/month) during RSV season.

PROGNOSIS

The long-term outcome of children with BPD still leaves much to be desired. Although repair of chronic lung injury occurs with time, the mortality from BPD ranges from 10% to 73%. Of those who do survive, many will go on to have neurologic sequelae. Hospitalizations are significantly increased in infants with BPD.

Advancements in therapeutic modalities and lung transplantation have improved survival of individuals with CF (the median survival age is well into the late 20's), but the morbidity associated with the disease and these therapies results in a shortened lifespan. Once the biochemical basis of CF is better understood, biomolecular intervention may be effective in the treatment of this disease.

Case Resolution

The infant in the case scenario will benefit most from a well-informed, methodical, well-coordinated approach to preventive and primary health care. His growth and neurodevelopment should be monitored, and his serum electrolytes should be assessed periodically. He should receive appropriate immunizations for age.

Selected Readings

Abman, S. H., and J. R. Groothius. Pathophysiology and treatment of bronchopulmonary dysplasia: Current issues. Pediatr. Clin. North Am. 41:277–315, 1994.

Bancalari, E. Neonatal chronic lung disease. In Farnaroff, A. A., and R. J. Martin (eds.). Neonatal-Perinatal Medicine: Diseases of the Fetus and Infant, 6th ed., Vol. 2, St. Louis, Mosby, 1997, pp. 1074–1089.

Barrington, K. J., and N. N. Finer. Treatment of bronchopulmonary dysplasia: a review. Clin. Perinatology 25:177–202, 1998.

Colten, H. R. Cystic fibrosis. Curr. Pediatr. Ther. 15:155–157, 1996.

Dusick, A. M. Medical outcomes in preterm infants. Semin. Perinatol. 21:164–177, 1997.

FitzSimmons, S. C. The changing epidemiology of cystic fibrosis. Curr. Probl. Pediatr. 24:171–179, 1994.

Klein, R. B., and B. W. Huggins. Chronic bronchitis in children. Semin. Respir. Infect. 9:13–22, 1994.

McColley, S. A. Bronchopulmonary dysplasia: Impact of surfactant replacement therapy. Pediatr. Clin. North Am. 45:573–586, 1998.

Ramsay, P. L., et al. Early clinical markers for the development of bronchopulmonary dysplasia: Soluble E-Selectin and ICAM-1. Pediatrics 102:927–932, 1998.

Ramsey, B. W., and T. F. Boat. Outcome measures for clinical trials in cystic fibrosis. J. Pediatr. 124:177–192, 1994.

Ryan, C. A., and N. N. Finer. Antenatal corticosteroid therapy to prevent respiratory distress syndrome. J. Pediatr. 126:317–319, 1995.

Shalon, L. B., and J. W. Adelson. Cystic fibrosis. Gastrointestinal complications and gene therapy. Pediatr. Clin. North Am. 43:157–196, 1996.

Wilmott, R. W., and M. A. Fiedler. Recent advances in the treatment of cystic fibrosis. Pediatr. Clin. North Am. 41:431–452, 1994.

Wagner, M. H., and J. M. Sherman. Cystic fibrosis and the general pediatrician. Contemp. Pediatr. 14:89–112, 1997.

Zimmerman, J. J., and P. M. Farrell. Advances and issues in bronchopulmonary dysplasia. Curr. Probl. Pediatr. 24:159–170, 1994.

OSTEOMYELITIS

Elizabeth A. Edgerton, M.D., M.P.H. and Helen DuPlessis, M.D., M.P.H.

H$_x$ A 2-year-old boy is evaluated for refusing to walk. He has been in good health and his immunization status is appropriate for age. He has been walking normally since 12 months of age. Three days before presentation, the boy began to favor his left leg when he walked and played, and this morning he refused to put any weight on the leg. He had a tactile temperature last evening. The boy fell from a playground slide 2 weeks before his current symptoms began.

His physical examination is remarkable for a temperature of 100.4° F (38.0° C) and tenderness in the left lower leg that is poorly localized.

Questions

1. What pathogens are most commonly responsible for bone infections?
2. What is the appropriate evaluation for children with suspected osteomyelitis?
3. What therapeutic regimens are appropriate for the treatment of osteomyelitis?
4. When is surgical intervention indicated in children with osteomyelitis?
5. When is outpatient management appropriate for children with osteomyelitis?

Osteomyelitis is an infection of bone, most commonly of bacterial origin. The diagnosis and management of osteomyelitis may be problematic because of the nature of the clinical presentation and the lack of well-controlled, prospective studies of diagnosis and treatment. Despite the paucity of extensive scientific data, progress has been made in the radiographic diagnosis, antimicrobial treatment, and outpatient management. As with most serious health problems, a high index of suspicion leading to early diagnosis and prompt initiation of therapy can prevent the serious morbidity that may befall children with this condition.

EPIDEMIOLOGY

Osteomyelitis affects individuals of all ages, but half the cases occur in children less than 5 years of age. The duration of symptoms is short (2–7 days), and bone destruction at the time of presentation is minimal or nonexistent. Good epidemiologic data are not available, but many large centers report 5–10:10,000 cases of acute osteomyelitis each year. Peaks in the incidence are noted in the late summer and early fall in all areas of the world. Chronic osteomyelitis refers to bone infections presenting after a long duration of symptoms

(> 3 months) or after failure of previous antimicrobial therapy. Although acute osteomyelitis may become chronic in some children, the majority of chronic cases occur in adults.

CLINICAL PRESENTATION

Depending on the child's age, the presenting symptoms of osteomyelitis may vary. Neonates frequently present with pseudoparalysis and may even appear "toxic" or "septic." Toddlers are more likely to present with refusal to bear weight, while older children or adolescents may only have point tenderness over the bone. Fever is sometimes present but may be absent in as many as 50% of cases (D$_x$ Box). Late signs include erythema, warmth (calor), and induration overlying the infected part.

PATHOPHYSIOLOGY

Osteomyelitis results from infection of the bone and may be attributed to certain predisposing factors in addition to various bacteria. The microorganisms responsible for most cases of osteomyelitis are those implicated in other serious childhood infections. However, the success of the *Haemophilus influenzae* type B vaccine program has all but eliminated this organism as a significant pathogen in invasive diseases such as osteomyelitis.

Staphylococcus aureus is the most common organism to infect bone from birth through adulthood, reported as the causitive agent in as many as 89% of osteomyelitis cases. Streptococci and other gram-positive bacteria, followed by gram-negative organisms, are second in frequency to *S. aureus*. Some studies indicate that specific gram-negative bacteria, particularly *Pseudomonas aeruginosa*, have accounted for an increased percentage of cases of osteomyelitis in the last 25 years. *Salmonella* is the most common causative pathogen in osteomyelitis in patients with hemoglobinopathies,

---

D$_x$ Osteomyelitis (two or more of the listed findings)

- Tenderness to palpation over bone
- Erythema, swelling, or warmth over affected extremity (late)
- Fever, leukocytosis, or elevated sedimentation rate
- Positive culture (blood, bone, or subperiosteal aspiration)
- Scintigraphic or radiologic changes

such as sickle cell anemia. Other gram-negative bacteria that should be considered in these patients include *Shigella sonnei*, *Escherichia coli*, and *Serratia* spp.

Seeding of skeletal tissue with microorganisms can occur by three primary mechanisms. Blood-borne dissemination is by far the most common route of bone infection in children, giving rise to the term acute hematogenous osteomyelitis. In adults with skeletal infections, direct inoculation of bone with bacteria frequently occurs as a consequence of trauma (e.g., penetrating injuries, compound fractures), invasive orthopedic procedures, or contiguous spread of infections in joint spaces or soft tissues. In bacteremic animals, bone infections have readily been established following blunt trauma involving the skeleton, which has led to speculation about the role of nonpenetrating trauma in osteomyelitis in humans.

The predilection for infection of long bones to occur through the hematogenous route can be explained by developmental changes in the skeleton and the associated vasculature. The vasculature at the ends of long bones is composed of tiny capillaries through which blood flow is sluggish. It is postulated that blood-borne bacteria coursing slowly through these capillaries may exit the vessels and inoculate surrounding bone, particularly if the vessels have been traumatized. In newborns, tiny vessels traverse the metaphysis, cross the growth plate, and penetrate the epiphysis. This anatomy may explain the relatively high incidence of contiguous joint and soft tissue infection in neonates (as high as 70%). These vessels involute toward the end of the first year of life, after which time metaphyseal capillaries end in blind loops and the growth plates serve as a barrier to the egress of infected material. In toddlers and older children, infection is often confined to the metaphysis. Furthermore, if the infection has been present for more than a few days, decompression of the purulent material may progress underneath the periosteum or, in rare instances, lead to the formation of a sequestrum, a piece of necrotic bony material that has been separated from surrounding healthy bone and vascular supply.

DIFFERENTIAL DIAGNOSIS

Osteomyelitis must be differentiated from trauma, inflammation of the joint (e.g., infectious or rheumatologic disease), infection of the skin (cellulitis), malignancies affecting bone, leukemic bone involvement, myositis, diskitis, and age-related orthopedic abnormalities such as Legg-Calvé-Perthes disease and slipped capital femoral epiphyses (see Chapter 84, Evaluation of Limp).

The organisms responsible for osteomyelitis may be influenced by a number of factors related to host defenses and the particular circumstances of infection. The age and the immune status of the host and the mechanism of infection may all be associated with peculiar microbiology.

Osteomyelitis is an uncommon infection in the neonatal period, and morbidity and mortality are high when diagnosis and treatment is delayed. The clinical features, causative organisms, and long-term outcome vary dramatically when compared to bone infections at other periods of childhood.

In the majority of affected neonates, osteomyelitis has a benign course characterized by absent or low-grade fever. Swelling or decreased mobility near the affected site is difficult to detect without a high index of suspicion and a focused examination. Consequently, most infections with this indolent presentation are diagnosed after a delay of 5–10 days. In 15–25% of neonates with bone infections, the illness is acute. Septic emboli seed the bone during an episode of serious bacteremia. The presence of transphyseal vessels results in a much larger incidence of contiguous spread to joints and soft tissues in infants. In addition, multiple bony foci may be present in up to 50% of cases.

S. aureus is the most common etiologic agent in all age groups. Group B streptococcus (GBS) and enteric gram-negative rods (GNRs) are also significant causal microorganisms in neonates. Long-term morbidity is relatively uncommon with GBS infections, although infection with other organisms, including *S. aureus* and GNRs, may result in residual deformities as a consequence of growth plate disruption.

Bone infections with mycobacteria and fungi are uncommon in all age groups and almost impossible to diagnose without a high index of suspicion. Skeletal infection with tubercle bacilli is primarily a disease of older children and adults who were never or inadequately treated for their primary infection. Vertebral body involvement (Pott's disease), the most common form of mycobacterial osteomyelitis, is characterized by spinal rigidity secondary to paraspinous muscle spasm. Nighttime pain is a common complaint occurring when the protective spasms relax. Ultimately, destruction of the vertebral body results in a wedge-shaped collapse called a gibbus deformity. The current epidemic of tuberculosis along with the increasing number of individuals with HIV or otherwise compromised immune systems may make chronic infections from mycobacteria and fungi more prevalent.

Much has been written about the association of *Pseudomonas* osteomyelitis with puncture wounds through tennis shoes. Although no well-controlled studies of puncture wound infections have been conducted, provocative evidence exists to warrant consideration of infection by *P. aeruginosa* in certain situations. Apparently the bacteria reside in the foam of tennis shoes, and puncture wounds through this colonized material into the forefoot may result in deep infection because of the propensity of *Pseudomonas* to infect cartilaginous structures. Comprehensive management of puncture wound infections should include tetanus prophylaxis, wound cleansing, diagnostic radiography, and an aggressive search for a retained foreign body when appropriate.

No evidence indicates that prophylactic antipseudomonal therapy is warranted for these puncture wounds. However, afebrile, apparently healthy children who present with localized pain, swelling, and decreased ability to bear weight 1–3 weeks after a puncture wound should stimulate an aggressive search for bone infection. If the workup indicates an underlying bone infection, surgical debridement should be considered in addition to postoperative antibiotic regimens to cover both *Staphylococcus* and *Pseudomonas* (ceftazidime, gentamicin).

Bone pain in children with sickle-cell disease requires the physician to distinguish between infarctions due to vaso-occlusive phenomena and true osteomyelitis. The initial clinical presentation may differ only in the degree of fever or the unusual severity of pain. More commonly, however, osteomyelitis should be seriously suspected when pain symptoms fail to respond to conventional treatment for sickle crises such as rest, analgesia, and hydration.

Salmonella is clearly an important infective agent. It is speculated that the integrity of the intestinal mucosa is regularly compromised by microinfarcts in individuals with sickle cell anemia. *Salmonella* use this route to invade the blood stream, where they ultimately reach metaphyseal vessels in which blood flow is possibly even more sluggish than in hematologically normal persons. Faulty splenic clearance mechanisms also may contribute to the risk of infection. *Salmonella* osteomyelitis is often multifocal and sometimes symmetrical.

In general, radiographic diagnosis of osteomyelitis in patients with hemoglobinopathies is difficult because of the similar pathophysiologic changes of bone infarcts and bone infection. Hyperemia and osteoclastic activity are characteristic of both infarcts and infection, rendering most nuclear medicine imaging techniques ineffective in distinguishing between these two conditions. Gadolinium-enhanced magnetic resonance imaging (MRI) also has limited ability to distinguish between acute infarction and osteomyelitis. Gallium 67 scans which use technetium Tc 99m sulfur colloid to image the marrow, show improved sensitivity over other methods in distinguishing infection from infarct, possibly because its uptake is less dependent on blood flow.

EVALUATION

History

Most cases of osteomyelitis come to medical attention during the first week of illness. A thorough history should be taken (Questions Box).

Physical Examination

Localized findings may be missed on physical examination even in the most systematic evaluation. Refusal to move an extremity may be found. Tenderness to palpation is often elicited in older children in the early stages of infection. Fever and localized swelling or erythema are late findings.

Questions: Osteomyelitis

- Has the child suffered any recent trauma?
- Has the child ever had any of the following symptoms: fever, weight loss, rashes, joint swelling?
- How long have the symptoms been present?
- Does the child have a hematologic disorder such as sickle cell anemia?

Laboratory Tests

Routine laboratory evaluation should include CBC, ESR, C-reactive protein (CRP), and cultures of blood or bone. Leukocytosis is present in as few as 35% of cases, and ESR and CRP are elevated in 92% and 98% of cases, respectively. Both ESR and CRP are nonspecific indicators of inflammation but vary temporally during the course of the infection, normalizing when the process resolves. CRP can be elevated as quickly as 6 hours after a triggering stimulus, usually peaks at 2 days, and with appropriate therapy normalizes after 1 week. ESR may not peak until 3 days after a stimulus and on average normalizes after 3 weeks. Therefore, both ESR and CRP are useful in diagnosing osteomyelitis and monitoring response to therapy.

Imaging Studies

Radiographic findings on plain films are not usually evident before 10–14 days, and as a result they are useful only for eliminating other entities that may be considered in the early stages of disease or as a baseline for future studies. Radionucleotide imaging techniques can be extremely helpful in the early diagnosis of osteomyelitis. Technetium-99m, which localizes in areas of increased vascularity or osteoblastic activity, is very sensitive in diagnosing osteomyelitis outside of the newborn period. Gallium- or leukocyte-labeled indium scans are useful adjuncts if the results of Tc-99m scans are equivocal or when infection is superimposed on conditions characterized by increased turnover of bone (e.g., trauma).

The use of CT and MRI is still being studied. These techniques give much better anatomic detail, which often helps determine the extent of abscesses that require surgical intervention. They may also be useful in the diagnosis and management of chronic osteomyelitis.

MANAGEMENT

Management involves **antibiotic therapy,** which must be tailored to age and situation-specific pathogens; when symptoms persist or pus or devitalized bone is present, **surgical intervention** may be necessary. The initial choice of antibiotics must be sufficiently broad to cover the predominant pathogens under specific prevailing conditions. In all cases of suspected osteomyelitis, coverage for *Staphylococcus* and other gram-positive organisms is necessary (neonates: nafcillin and a third-generation cephalosporin or aminoglycoside; infants and children: cefuroxime or nafcillin and chloramphenicol) (Table 119–1).

The route, duration, and location of antibiotic therapy are constantly reconsidered as new antimicrobial agents become available and the pressures for cost-effective treatment increases. At this time, therapy for acute osteomyelitis should be initiated with parenteral antibiotics in an inpatient setting. Once acute signs and symptoms have resolved, and children are able to bear weight, consideration should be given to outpatient management. Depending on the causal organism and the availability of effective oral antibiotics, this may be

TABLE 119–1. Antibiotic Treatment for Children With Osteomyelitis

Likely Organisms	Recommended Antibiotics
Neonates	
Group B streptococcus	Nafcillin and third-generation
Staphylococcus aureus	cephalosporin or amino-
Coliform bacteria	glycoside
Other gram-negative bacteria	
Infants and Children	
S. aureus	Cefuroxime or nafcillin and
Haemophilus influenzae type B	chloramphenicol
Group A streptococcus	
Streptococcus pneumoniae	
Pseudomonas	Ceftazidime and amino-
	glycosides
Patients with Hemoglobinopathies	
Salmonella	Ampicillin, chloramphenicol,
Other gram-negative bacteria	or third-generation
S. aureus	cephalosporin
	Nafcillin

undertaken with either parenteral or oral medication. Intramuscular ceftriaxone, administered once daily, has also been used, but its effectiveness must be documented in cases of staphylococcal infections.

Regardless of the route, serum bactericidal concentrations (peak >1:8; trough >1:4) and ESR should be followed to document treatment effectiveness. Therapy for less than 35 days has been associated with treatment failures in infections with staphylococci or GNRs. Shorter treatment courses may be undertaken in the face of uncomplicated infections with *H. influenzae* type B or streptococcus. Some investigators suggest the continuation of therapy for 1 week beyond the point at which the ESR returns to normal.

Although antibiotic therapy is curative in most cases of acute osteomyelitis, surgical intervention may be critical when the diagnosis occurs late in the course of the disease. In these instances, abscesses and sequestra form, which antibiotics are incapable of penetrating. Bacteremia and constitutional symptoms (e.g., fever and pain) that persist 72 hours after the initiation of antimicrobial therapy may be an indication for either diagnostic or therapeutic surgical intervention. Because neonatal osteomyelitis may result in growth plate disruption, some institutions advocate aggressive surgical drainage and debridement. Surgery is also indicated in the face of sinus tract formation and other signs of chronic osteomyelitis.

PROGNOSIS

Although mortality from osteomyelitis is rare, delays in diagnosis or inadequate treatment of skeletal infections can result in significant morbidity because of the proximity of the infection to growth plates of long bones. Abscess formation, recurrent infections, and contiguous joint involvement are much more common when adequate treatment is begun more than four days after the onset of clinical symptoms. Leg-length discrepancies, resulting from delayed or inadequate therapy, may occur years after the initial infection. Children who have had osteomyelitis need long-term follow-up.

Chronic osteomyelitis may exist as a complicated or recurrent infection of the original organism, or as an infection with unusual pathogens—mycobacteria or fungi—that resists surgical and antimicrobial therapy. Unifocal recurrences uncomplicated by additional organisms frequently respond to appropriate combinations of surgery and antimicrobial agents.

Multifocal and culture-negative cases of chronic osteomyelitis may wax and wane for months following aggressive antimicrobial and surgical treatment, however. Girls are more often affected by chronic multifocal disease than boys and often present with weeks to months of malaise, pain, loss of function, and swelling of adjacent joints. Therapy beyond adequate surgical drainage and a 6-week regimen of antibiotics rarely affect the course of these cases; they eventually resolve spontaneously.

Case Resolution

In the case scenario, a high index of suspicion leads to the early diagnosis of osteomyelitis using a bone scan, with subsequent confirmation by blood cultures positive for *S. aureus*. The toddler receives a short course of parenteral antibiotics in the hospital during which time the CRP and ESR normalize. The child demonstrates appropriate antibiotic serum levels and is able to complete his total course of 6-weeks of antibiotics as an outpatient. At follow-up, he had no residual orthopedic deformity.

Selected Readings

Jaramillo, D., et al. Osteomyelitis and septic arthritis in children: Appropriate use of imaging to guide treatment. AJR 165:399–403, 1995.

Krogstad, P., and B. L. Smith. Osteomyelitis and septic arthritis. *In* Feigin, R. D., and J. D. Cherry (eds.). Textbook of Pediatric Infectious Diseases, 4th ed. Philadelphia, W. B. Saunders, 1998, pp. 683–698.

Lew, D. P., and F. A. Waldvogel. Osteomyelitis. N. Engl. J. Med. 336:999–1006, 1997.

Nelson, J. D. Bone and joint infections. Curr. Pediatr. Ther. 15:492–494, 1996.

Sonnen, G. M., and N. K. Henry. Pediatric bone and joint infections: diagnosis and management. Pediatr. Clin. North Am. 43:933–947, 1996.

Unkila-Kallio, L., et al. Serum C-reactive protein, erythrocyte sedimentation rate, white blood cell count in acute hematogenous osteomyelitis of children. Pediatrics 93:59–62, 1994.

JUVENILE RHEUMATOID ARTHRITIS

Elizabeth A. Edgerton, M.D., M.P.H. and Helen DuPlessis, M.D., M.P.H.

H$_x$ A 4-year-old girl is evaluated for pain in the legs and arms of 6–8 months' duration. Symptoms began with pain and swelling in the left elbow that lasted for approximately 2½ months. After an initial evaluation, including radiographs, the girl was diagnosed with a "bad sprain" and was treated with a 2-week course of an NSAID. The elbow improved, but it still caused discomfort occasionally. About 5 months ago, the child was evaluated for painful knees and diagnosed with "growing pains." She has had no trauma, fevers, or rashes, but her activity level has decreased since the symptoms began. The mother has noted swelling in all three of the joints at one time or another but reports no erythema. On physical examination the vital signs are normal. Both knees are swollen but not erythematous. Range of motion in the knees and left elbow is decreased.

Questions

1. What findings are indicative of juvenile rheumatoid arthritis (JRA)?
2. What is the role of diagnostic imaging in the diagnosis and treatment of JRA?
3. Are any prognostic factors associated with JRA?
4. What are the indications for orthopedic intervention in children with JRA?
5. What medical therapies are currently used in the management of JRA?

Juvenile rheumatoid arthritis (JRA) is a diagnostic term applied to a specific collection of disorders characterized by a chronic inflammatory process of joints, specifically chronic synovitis. JRA initially affects children under the age of 16 years but can be seen into early adulthood. The diagnosis is particularly difficult to make because of the tremendous variability in clinical presentation, unpredictable disease course, and limited laboratory findings. A number of terms other than JRA have been proposed to describe the broad spectrum of arthropathies affecting children. These include juvenile arthritis, juvenile chronic arthritis, and juvenile chronic polyarthritis. Conditions other than JRA included in these diagnostic categories are mentioned briefly in Differential Diagnosis.

EPIDEMIOLOGY

Any discussion of the epidemiology of JRA is imprecise at best for the reasons stated above. JRA represents the most common form of rheumatic disease in children, with a reported incidence of 9.5–25/100,000 in children 16 years of age or less. African American and Asian populations are much less likely to suffer from JRA, whereas Native Americans are more frequently affected. The age at presentation has a bimodal distribution, with an initial peak in the preschool age range (1–4 years) and a second peak before puberty (8–12 years). Overall, girls are affected two to three times more often than boys, but this varies with disease subtype and age of onset. In prepubertal children the sex distribution is relatively equal.

CLINICAL PRESENTATION

Swelling and inflammation (i.e., warmth) of joints is present in all cases of JRA, although the timing, location, and number of joints involved may vary with the stage of disease and specific type of JRA (D$_x$ Box). Young children may have decreased activity, inability or refusal to bear weight, or exhibit behaviors that appear to be developmentally regressive before joint effusion and inflammation is appreciated.

Fever (temperature: >100.4° F [38.0° C]) may be present in either the systemic or polyarticular subtype, but additional symptoms are more common in systemic JRA. In systemic JRA, fever spikes occur once or twice each day, and are usually accompanied by a characteristic ephemeral rash that occurs in discrete, small (< 1 cm) macules on the trunk or extremities. The rash may be missed because it usually occurs in the evening hours and is quite transient.

PATHOPHYSIOLOGY

A precise etiology for JRA has not been fully elucidated, but it does involve the combined interaction of immunologic, genetic, and environmental factors. Alterations in the production of autoantibodies, abnormalities in the cytokine network, and response to infectious agents play a significant role in the development of the disease. Genetic factors are also evident. Studies of

D$_x$ Juvenile Rheumatoid Arthritis

- Joint swelling
- Joint pain
- Limitation of motion of joints
- Fever
- Iridocyclitis
- Limitation of ability to open mouth (temporomandibular joint involvement)

twins and family clusters demonstrate increased incidence and strong concordance of onset, subtype, and course. In addition, the recent advances in immunogenetics have uncovered striking associations between certain human leukocyte antigen (HLA) genes and particular subtypes of JRA, providing evidence for a genetic component to JRA.

DIFFERENTIAL DIAGNOSIS

The diagnosis of JRA is primarily based on clinical features, which may evolve over a period of weeks to months. During the early stages of JRA, associated clinical symptoms may be similar to those in infective arthritis, Lyme disease, and a variety of orthopedic conditions such as Legg-Calvé-Perthes disease, slipped capital femoral epiphyses, and Osgood-Schlatter disease. The distinction between JRA and other forms of childhood arthritis such as SLE, juvenile ankylosing spondylitis (JAS), and arthritis associated with immune deficiencies, in particular, is the most difficult to make. SLE is a multisystem disease, and as organ systems other than the musculoskeletal system become involved, the diagnosis becomes more apparent. JAS may be distinguished from JRA by the presence of characteristic sacroiliac joint involvement and the frequent presence of the HLA B27 antigen. Children with immunologic deficiencies may present with joint symptoms, like children with JRA, but an evaluation of immunoglobulins and complement usually indicates the deficiency.

Children under 16 years of age with persistent arthritis (≥ 6 weeks) who do not meet the criteria for other types of arthritides may be considered for the diagnosis of JRA (Table 120–1). The particular clinical manifestations evident within 3–6 months of initial presentation often allow the disease to be classified into one of three subtypes.

Pauciarticular JRA, the most common type, accounting for more than 50% of all cases of JRA, is characterized by involvement of four or fewer joints during the early stages. Girls are most frequently affected, and those with positive antinuclear antibody (ANA) are at significant risk of developing chronic uveitis. Immunogenetic studies indicate an association with HLA alleles

Questions: Juvenile Rheumatoid Arthritis

- Has the child ever had any swelling, warmth, or redness of joints?
- Does the child have any difficulty walking or running? If so, does this occur at any particular time of the day?
- Have the parents ever noticed any type of skin rash? If so, are the rashes temporally related to the joint swellings?
- Has the child ever had any serious eye problems?
- Has the child had any other health problems (e.g., kidney, lung, or brain diseases)?
- Has the child traveled recently or been bitten by a tick?

DR8, DR5, and to a lesser extent, DR6. Systemic symptoms of pauciarticular disease are rare, but after the first 6–12 months the disease pattern may become polyarticular.

Polyarticular JRA, accounting for 10–25% of cases, involves five or more joints during the first 6 months of illness. This subtype can be divided into two categories based on laboratory findings and clinical course. Children with positive rheumatoid factor (RF) who account for 10–15% of all cases of JRA make up the first group. They are primarily adolescent females whose clinical course more nearly resembles adult rheumatoid arthritis, with severe erosion and degeneration of joints. Furthermore, there is a strong association between RF-positive JRA and the DR4 antigen, which is the predominant HLA association in adult rheumatoid arthritis. Children with negative RF, the second group, have variable clinical manifestations. Although seronegative, they may have an increased prevalence of the DR4 antigen and develop severe erosive disease. Alternatively, they may manifest a pauciarticular pattern with uveitis and an association with the pauciarticualr HLA antigens.

Systemic onset arthritis, often referred to as Still's disease, accounts for 10% of all cases of JRA. The hallmark of this subtype is the presence of systemic features such as fever, which can be quite elevated (temperature: 102.2° F [39.0° C]), hepatosplenomegaly, and rash. Joint involvement may be variable, as in RF-negative polyarthritis. HLA associations seem to fall into the two patterns indicated above; children with severe disease are more likely to have the DR4 antigen, and others may have DR5 or DR8.

EVALUATION

History

The history should focus on joint symptoms (arthritis rather than arthralgias), specific extra-articular manifestations such as uveitis, and systemic signs such as fever and skin rashes (Questions Box).

Physical Examination

A thorough physical examination should be performed, with special attention paid to the assessment of all joints and extremities. The examiner should also look

---

**TABLE 120–1. Criteria for the Classification
of Juvenile Rheumatoid Arthritis***

Age of onset < 16 years
Arthritis in one or more joints defined as swelling or effusion or presence of two
   or more of the following signs:
     Limitation of range of motion
     Tenderness or pain on motion
     Increased heat
Duration of disease for 6 weeks or more
Type of disease during the first 6 months classified as:
   Polyarthritis (≥ 5 joints)
   Pauciarticular disease (oligoarthritis) (≤ 4 joints)
   Systemic disease (Still's disease): arthritis with intermittent fever
Exclusion of other forms of juvenile arthritis

*Reproduced, with permission, from Cassidy J. T., and R. E. Petty. Juvenile rheumatoid arthritis. *In* Textbook of Pediatric Rheumatology, 3rd ed. New York, W. B. Saunders, 1995, p. 133.

for evidence of skin rashes, lymphadenopathy, or organomegaly. Although joint involvement in JRA may be variable, swelling and inflammation, rather than simple arthralgias, are present in all cases. Larger joints (e.g., wrists, ankles, knees, shoulders, elbows) are usually involved. The pattern of arthritis is often symmetric, except in pauciarticular JRA. In the polyarticular subtype, smaller joints including the phalanges and temporomandibular joints may also be affected.

Because of their ephemeral nature, skin rashes may not be evident during an office visit. Nevertheless, a careful inspection of the skin of a completely unclothed child in a well-lighted room should still be performed.

Laboratory Tests

Laboratory studies are more often useful in ruling out other causes of arthritis than in specifically diagnosing JRA. Unlike adults with rheumatoid arthritis, fewer than 10% of children will be positive for rheumatoid factor (RF), making this a poor screening test. ANA may be positive in pauciarticular JRA. The pattern of ANA immunofluorescence and the presence of multisystem disease distinguishes SLE from JRA. An ESR is a nonspecific finding of inflammation and is elevated in only 50% of cases.

Analysis of joint fluid aspirates may distinguish infectious arthritis from JRA. At present, serologic titers against *Borrelia burgdorferi* (the infectious agent in Lyme disease) are frequently uninterpretable. The physician should rely on the clinical pattern of disease progression to rule out this entity.

Imaging Studies

Plain radiography is a useful adjunct in making the diagnosis of JRA because the resulting synovial proliferation may destroy articular surfaces, leading to erosion and ankylosis of bone. However, such studies may actually underestimate the extent of joint damage. The earliest radiographic findings in JRA are soft tissue swelling, periarticular osteopenia, and periosteal new bone formation. As increasing amounts of cartilage are destroyed, joint space narrowing occurs. The most severe cases progress to bony erosion and other evidence of joint destruction. These changes can lead to either bone overgrowth or growth retardation secondary to early fusing of the epiphysis.

MRI has proven to be much more useful in identifying early cartilage loss, changes due to avascular necrosis, and other intra-articular pathology. The increased sensitivity of MRI may prove useful in guiding medical and orthopedic interventions.

MANAGEMENT

The management of children with JRA necessitates a multidisciplinary approach designed to address not only the progression of inflammatory joint symptoms but also children's functional, nutritional, and emotional well-being. Specific functional status instruments are available to aid the clinician in assessing subtle changes in children's activities and quality of life. These instruments can also be helpful in longitudinal assessment of each child's clinical course. If possible, children should receive care where such support is readily available. The primary care physician can best serve the patient by overseeing the coordination of health care activities, providing routine preventive care, and treating minor illness or flare-ups in close communication with the rheumatologist. In settings where access to subspecialists is limited, the primary care physician must accept a much more active role in the ongoing assessment and management of children with JRA. Affected children and their families must be kept informed of the child's condition and appropriate therapies. In addition, they must be counseled about the unpredictable nature of JRA, advances and controversies in therapies, and the importance of their participation in treatment decisions.

Physical and Occupational Therapy

Children are most likely to maintain their normal routine when adaptations and interventions that address their limitations, maximize their functional status, and minimize their deformities are used. Carefully selected **physical activities,** such as swimming and bicycling, interspersed with periods of rest, decrease the incidence of bone demineralization, muscle atrophy, contractures, and advanced joint damage. For children who are unable to bear weight, **range-of-motion exercises** are necessary substitutes. **Splints** and other orthotics are useful to prevent contractures and maximize the functional status of joints.

Medical Treatment

Currently, all treatment protocols for JRA are targeted at controlling the inflammatory process, and to date are not viewed as curative. NSAIDs (Table 120–2) are the mainstay for treatment. Children may have varied responses to the different classes of NSAIDs, therefore it is important to try more than one class before classifying children as refactory. Up to two-thirds of children will require additional treatment with **slow-acting antirheumatic drugs** (SAARD). These second-line drugs include penicillamine, hydroxychloroquine, gold, sulfasalazine, and methotrexate. In random placebo-controlled trials of second-line drugs, methotrexate was the only drug to be shown more effective than placebo, but controversy still exists over its long-term toxicity. **Corticosteroids** are primarily used for extraarticular complaints such as uveitis and systemic symptoms but also can be used for intraarticular injections in cases of severe joint inflammation.

The approach to medical therapy for JRA may change significantly in the future as the merits of the traditional approach are questioned. Some rheumatologists argue that reliance on the least toxic pharmaceuticals as the mainstay of therapy may result in missed opportunities to modify or curtail disease progression. Data from

TABLE 120–2. Medical Therapy for Juvenile Rheumatoid Arthritis

Drug	Dosage	Toxicities	Comments
NSAIDs			
Aspirin	60–100 mg/kg/d	GI effects, Reye's syndrome	Salicylate level (20–25 mg/dL)
Various NSAIDs	Dosage varies with product	GI, renal effects; platelets, anemia	Urinalysis, CBC; indomethacin, naprosyn, ibuprofen available in liquid formulations
SAARDs			
Methotrexate	10 mg/m²/wk	GI effects, oral ulcers, hepatotoxicity, bone marrow suppression	Supplemental folic acid may minimize toxicities, monitor liver function tests
Steroids			
Oral	Dosage varies with drug	GI effects, infection, growth retardation, glaucoma, osteoporosis, endocrine derangements	Ongoing ophthalmologic care; infection surveillance
Ophthalmic	1–2 drops 4–6 times daily		
Intraarticular	10–40 mg (prednisolone)		

longitudinal studies of JRA combined with the increased sensitivity of diagnostic imaging techniques appear to indicate that (1) joint damage occurs more readily than previously thought and (2) children once believed to be in remission have ongoing inflammation and joint destruction as they enter into adulthood. To date, no convincing studies prove the existence of so-called disease-modifying antirheumatic drugs, but this an active area of research.

Orthopedic Intervention

Orthopedic procedures play a critical role in the management of JRA. Although **soft tissue releases, tendon lengthening,** and **synovectomies** do not alter the course of the disease, they do much to improve function and relieve pain. **Reconstructive surgery** is sometimes necessary for joints that have been destroyed by severe erosive disease. Collaboration between the surgeon, the medical team, and physical or occupational therapists lead to optimal functional outcomes for children with JRA.

PROGNOSIS

Mortality is not increased in children with JRA, but morbidity affecting growth, emotional well-being, and functional capacity may be high. Progressive joint destruction and pharmacologic therapy, especially steroids, may adversely affect the linear growth rate and final adult height. Disease progression may severely limit children's ability to perform self-care activities and participate in age-appropriate physical activities. These and other factors related to chronic disease may also threaten their sense of emotional well-being.

Certain attributes such as the presence of RFs or ANAs in the serum have universally well-delineated prognostic implications. Progression from a pauciarticular or systemic presentation to polyarticular involvement indicates a worse prognosis. Severe joint destruction is more likely to occur in children with the systemic subtype of JRA who have persistent fevers and thrombocytosis.

Case Resolution

The girl in the case scenario has both signs and symptoms of pauciarticular JRA. Three joints (both knees and left elbow) are involved. Initial laboratory evaluation should include a CBC, ESR, RF, and ANA. The absence of fever eliminates an infectious etiology for the symptoms. X-rays of the affected joints are also appropriate, as is consultation with a pediatric rheumatologist.

Selected Readings

Ansell, B. M. Juvenile chronic arthritis: Special problems and presentations in children. *In* Klippel, J. H., and P. A. Dieppe, (eds.). Rheumatology, 2nd ed. St. Louis, Mosby, 1998, 5. 19.1–19.4

Bywaters, E. G. L. Juvenile chronic arthritis: History. *In* Klippel, J. H., and P. A. Dieppe, (eds.). Rheumatology, 2nd ed. St. Louis, Mosby, 1998, 5. 17.1–17.4.

Cassidy, J. T., and L. S. Hillman. Abnormalities in skeletal growth in children with juvenile rheumatoid arthritis. Rheum. Dis. Clin. North Am. 23:499–521, 1997.

Giannini, E. H., and G. D. Cawkwell. Drug treatment with juvenile rheumatoid arthritis: past, present, and future. Pediatr. Clin. North Am. 42:1099–1125, 1995.

Murry, K. J. and M. H. Passo. Functional measures in children with rheumatic disease. Pediatr. Clin. North Am. 42:1127–1154, 1995.

Murray, K., S. D. Thompson, and D. N. Glass. Pathogenesis of juvenile chronic arthritis: genetic and environmental factors. Arch. Dis. Child. 77:530–534, 1997.

Prieur, A. M. Juvenile chronic arthritis: Management. *In* Klippel, J. H., P. A. Dieppe, (eds.). Rheumatology, 2nd ed. St. Louis, Mosby, 1998, 5. 21.1–21.10.

Shaller, J. G. Juvenile rheumatoid arthritis. Pediatr. Rev. 18:337–349, 1997.

Singsen, B. H., and R. Goldbach-Mansky. Methotrexate in the treatment of juvenile rheumatoid arthritis and other pediatric rheumatic and nonrheumatic disorders. Rheum. Clin. North Am. 23:811–840, 1997.

White, P. H. Juvenile chronic arthritis: Clinical features. *In* Klippel, J. H., and P. A. Dieppe, (eds.). Rheumatology, 2nd ed. St. Louis, Mosby, 1998, 5. 18.1–18.10.

CHAPTER 121

NEPHROTIC SYNDROME

Elaine S. Kamil, M.D.

Hx   A 2-year-old boy is brought to the office because of abdominal distention. He has just recovered from a runny nose that lasted a week, with no fever or change in activity. His mother complains that his eyelids were very swollen that morning, and she says that his thighs look "fat." She has noticed that he has fewer wet diapers. He has always been a healthy child, and his immunizations are up-to-date. The family has a history of asthma and allergic rhinitis.

Physical examination shows an active 2-year-old boy. Head and neck examination is clear, except for a few shotty anterior cervical lymph nodes and some minimal periorbital edema. Chest examination reveals some decreased breath sounds at the bases. The abdomen is moderately distended; bowel sounds are active and a fluid wave is detectable. There is 2+ pitting edema of the lower legs, extending up to the knees. The urine has a specific gravity of 1.030; pH 6; 4+ protein; and trace, nonhemolyzed blood. Microscopic examination shows 4–6 RBCs per high-power field and 10–20 hyaline and fine granular casts per low-power field.

Questions

1. What is the differential diagnosis of edema and ascites in previously healthy young children?
2. What criteria are used to determine if children require hospitalization or can be managed as outpatients?
3. What laboratory evaluation and therapy are instituted initially?
4. What are the important issues to address in parent education?
5. What is the prognosis of young children with nephrotic syndrome?

Although nephrotic syndrome is not a common childhood disease, every pediatrician can expect to care for at least one nephrotic child at some time. Nephrotic syndrome may have serious or even fatal complications, and the disease tends to follow a chronic, relapsing course. Thus, it is important for the pediatrician to become familiar with the signs and symptoms of the disease and with the most current treatment modalities aimed at keeping affected children healthy and active.

Nephrotic syndrome occurs when an individual excretes a sufficient quantity of plasma proteins, primarily albumin, in the urine to cause hypoalbuminemia. Substantial urinary protein losses, hypercholesterolemia, and hypoalbuminemia characterize nephrotic syndrome. The condition is usually accompanied by obvious edema, but occasionally edema is not clinically detectable (D$_x$ Box).

D$_x$ Nephrotic Syndrome

- Heavy proteinuria (> 40 mg/m^2/h or 50 mg/kg/24 h in children)
- Hypoalbuminemia
- Hypercholesterolemia
- Edema

In children, proteinuria of more than 40 mg/m^2/h (> 50 mg/kg in 24 h) is considered nephrotic range proteinuria. (In adult-sized patients, proteinuria of more than 3.5 g in 24 hours is associated with nephrotic syndrome.) Collection of a 24-hour urine sample is cumbersome in children, and the urinary total protein/creatinine ratio (U TP/CR) done on a random urine sample is a useful alternative. Whereas a ratio greater than 3.5 is considered nephrotic range proteinuria in adults with normal renal function, a ratio greater than 1.0 is considered diagnostic in children (see Chapter 73, Proteinuria). Twenty-four hour urine protein losses (g/m^2/d) in children can be estimated by multiplying the U TP/CR by 0.63.

EPIDEMIOLOGY

Minimal change disease (MCD) is the most common form of nephrotic syndrome in childhood. The annual prevalence of new cases of nephrotic syndrome is 2–3:100,000 children in the population less than 16 years of age. The cumulative prevalence of this chronic disease is 16:100,000. Ninety percent of childhood cases are not associated with any systemic disease, and two-thirds of cases of childhood nephrotic syndrome present before age 5 years. The ratio of boys to girls with nephrotic syndrome is 2:1. By late adolescence, both sexes are equally affected.

CLINICAL PRESENTATION

Typical children with nephrotic syndrome are preschool-aged boys who usually present because they appear swollen to the parents. Some children are active and relatively asymptomatic despite the edema, whereas others may be very uncomfortable, with markedly swollen eyelids, abdominal discomfort, scrotal or labial edema, and even respiratory compromise. Usually children have a history of preceding infection, most typically a URI. Occasionally children develop diarrhea secondary to edema of the bowel wall.

Occasionally children with nephrosis are critically ill due to peritonitis, bacteremia, or (rarely) a major thrombotic episode. Because their immune state is compromised, rapid evaluation and treatment of children with these complications of nephrotic syndrome are essential for survival. The primary peritonitis associated with nephrotic syndrome may be confused with an acute abdomen, such as may be seen with appendicitis. Some children who are experiencing a severe relapse have hypotensive symptoms secondary to intravascular volume reduction.

PATHOPHYSIOLOGY

The exact cause of MCD and focal segmental glomerulosclerosis (FSGS) is not known. Although this is controversial, many nephrologists consider FSGS to result from severe, treatment-resistant MCD. The best current theory postulates that some stimulus (usually infectious) causes a clone of lymphocytes or monocytes to proliferate and produce one or more cytokines that are toxic to the glomerular epithelial cells or the glomerular basement membrane. This cytokine induces a reduction in the net negative charge across the glomerular basement membrane. The constituents of this membrane and of the chemicals coating the glomerular epithelial and endothelial cells normally bear a net negative charge. The presence of these negatively charged chemicals creates a charge-selective barrier to filtration. This barrier plays a significant role in the ultrafiltration of macromolecules present in the plasma, enhancing the filtration of molecules bearing a positive electrical charge and retarding the filtration of molecules bearing a negative electrical charge. During episodes of relapse, patients with MCD show a breakdown in the normal charge-selective barrier to filtration, often resulting in massive proteinuria. Kidney biopsies from patients with nephrotic syndrome demonstrate a net reduction in anionic sites during periods of relapse.

Evidence indicating that the proteinuria may be due to some soluble factor is threefold. (1) Some patients who develop end-stage renal disease from idiopathic nephrotic syndrome (particularly FSGS) have experienced a relapse of the nephrotic condition with massive proteinuria immediately after transplantation of a normal kidney. (2) Infusion of peripheral blood mononuclear cell products from nephrotic children induces albuminuria in rats. (3) Removal of serum proteins by adsorption to a protein A Sepharose column has led to remission of proteinuria in some patients who have experienced a recurrence of nephrotic syndrome after transplantation. The remission of the proteinuria after treatment with immunosuppressive medication provides further evidence that the nephrotic syndrome is mediated in some way by the immune system.

Normal adults are able to synthesize 12 g of albumin per day in the liver, and adults with nephrotic syndrome may synthesize 14 g of albumin per day. Therefore the **hypoproteinemia** characteristic of nephrotic syndrome cannot be explained completely by measured amounts of urinary protein losses (about 3.5 g/d). The difference between the hepatic synthetic capacity for albumin and the measured urinary losses can be explained by protein catabolism in the kidney. Renal tubular epithelial cells reabsorb filtered plasma proteins and catabolize them to amino acids, which then reenter the amino acid pool of the body. Thus, the magnitude of losses of plasma proteins at the glomerular level is far greater than the amount measured in a 24-hour urine sample.

The **hypoalbuminemia** seen in nephrotic syndrome is a result of the massive proteinuria, and the **hypercholesterolemia** occurs as a consequence of the hypoalbuminemia. The hyperlipidemia is partially the result of a generalized increase in hepatic protein synthesis that also involves the overproduction of lipoproteins. In addition, less lipid is transported into the adipose tissue, because the activity of lipoprotein lipase is reduced in adipose tissue during active nephrotic syndrome. Hyperlipidemia is most pronounced in children with MCD. Serum albumin and serum cholesterol are generally inversely correlated.

DIFFERENTIAL DIAGNOSIS

Nephrotic syndrome is considered either primary or secondary. Primary nephrotic syndrome is not associated with a systemic disease. Secondary nephrotic syndrome is a feature of a systemic disease such as anaphylactoid purpura or SLE. Most children with nephrotic syndrome have the primary form of the disease.

Children with primary nephrotic syndrome are also classified according to their response to steroid therapy. Affected individuals may be categorized as steroid-sensitive, steroid-dependent, or steroid-resistant. Typically, children who are steroid-sensitive and remain so have MCD, although strictly speaking, a renal biopsy must be performed before the diagnosis of MCD is made. Sensitivity to or dependence on corticosteroids is a critical factor in determining children's prognosis.

Nephrotic syndrome is also classified by the appearance of the glomeruli on renal biopsy. A summary of the histologic lesions causing nephrotic syndrome appears in Table 121–1. About 95% of young children with nephrotic syndrome have MCD. In these children, light microscopy shows normal-appearing glomeruli. Immunofluorescent microscopy is generally negative but may show some mesangial IgM deposits, and electron microscopy simply shows foot process effacement of the visceral epithelial cells. In individuals with FSGS, light microscopy may show enlarged glomeruli and glomeruli

TABLE 121–1.   Distribution of Histologic Type by Age of Onset in Children With Nephrotic Syndrome

Age (years)	MCD*	FSGS	MN	MPGN	Other GN
1–4	95%	3%	2%	—	—
4–8	75%	15%	1%	7%	2%
8–16	52%	15%	2%	25%	6%

*MCD remains the dominant histologic type through midadolescence but becomes relatively less important in later childhood and adolescence.

Abbreviations: MCD, minimal change disease; FSGS, focal segmental glomerulosclerosis; MN, membranous nephropathy; MPGN, membranoproliferative glomerulonephritis; other GN, other forms of glomerulonephritis.

with segments of sclerosis. Immunofluorescence may reveal some IgM and complement in the sclerotic segments, and electron microscopy shows areas of foot process effacement of glomerular epithelial cells. Biopsies performed later in the disease course show some totally sclerotic glomeruli, areas of interstitial fibrosis, and atrophy.

Other primary renal diseases that can cause nephrotic syndrome in children include membranous nephropathy, membranoproliferative glomerulonephritis, IgA nephropathy and other forms of chronic glomerulonephritis, congenital nephrotic syndrome, and diffuse mesangial proliferative glomerulonephritis. Chronic hepatitis B infection may cause membranous nephropathy or membranoproliferative glomerulonephritis. Rarely, poststreptococcal acute glomerulonephritis and other forms of postinfectious acute glomerulonephritis may also cause nephrotic syndrome. With the exception of congenital nephrotic syndrome, all of these diseases show (1) the presence of immune deposits in the glomerular mesangial regions or along the glomerular basement membrane and (2) some element of cellular proliferation, which may be severe. In these disease states, the presence of nephrotic syndrome is indicative of marked injury to the glomerular capillary wall. Infants with congenital nephrotic syndrome have been found to have diminished numbers of anionic sites along the glomerular basement membrane, suggesting that the biochemical composition of the membrane is abnormal.

Because of the varying distribution of edema fluid, nephrotic syndrome may be confused with sinusitis or an allergic reaction (periorbital edema), obesity (ascites), or an abdominal mass (ascites). Other causes of generalized edema such as congestive heart failure or liver disease can be easily excluded.

EVALUATION

History

The clinical evaluation should include a careful history (Questions Box).

Physical Examination

A complete physical examination is necessary. Blood pressure should be monitored because hypertension or hypotension may occur. The extent of the peripheral and central edema, including swelling of the eyelids, should be assessed. The physician should obtain a reliable, overall impression of the child's level of comfort and activity. The examination should also include a careful search for infection, particularly life-threatening infections such as pneumonia or peritonitis. Examination of the head and neck should focus on signs of recent infection such as otitis media. The presence of dullness to percussion at the bases of the thorax is consistent with large pleural effusions. Ascites may be minimal or massive. With severe ascites, scrotal or labial edema may occur. If the child has a history of abdominal pain, a careful check for signs of peritoneal irritation should be made. The skin should be inspected for infection and rashes.

Laboratory Tests

The laboratory evaluation of children with nephrotic syndrome begins with a urinalysis. The dipstick shows 3+ or 4+ protein, although a dilute urine may be only 2+. Microscopic hematuria may be present in up to 25% of children with MCD. The presence of associated glycosuria in a nephrotic child who is not on steroid therapy raises a concern for FSGS. Careful microscopic examination is necessary. Casts are seen frequently because urinary proteins precipitate in the tubules. The casts are hyaline, fine, and coarse granular. WBC casts are sometimes seen because some children with nephrotic syndrome also have increased amounts of leukocytes in their urine. Large amounts of RBCs and RBC casts are not seen in uncomplicated MCD and, if present, indicate another cause for the nephrotic syndrome. If RBC casts are seen together with substantial hematuria, an antistreptolysin-O titer should be added to the preliminary evaluation. A random U TP/CR should be done to determine whether children have nephrotic range proteinuria.

If the urine shows only proteinuria, with perhaps some microscopic hematuria, blood tests should include a CBC, serum creatinine and BUN, serum albumin, cholesterol, C3, and antinuclear antibody (ANA). The CBC may show a high hematocrit from hemoconcentration, because many children experience volume contraction as a complication of hypoproteinemia. Children may also have very high platelet counts (sometimes > 1,000,000/μL). The BUN and creatinine help assess renal function. The serum albumin and cholesterol are required to differentiate nephrotic syndrome from other edematous states. A low level of C3 is associated with other renal diseases such as membranoproliferative glomerulonephritis, acute postinfectious glomerulonephritis, and SLE. The ANA is useful in screening for SLE and other collagen vascular diseases. Hepatitis B serology is helpful in children who come from a population at risk for hepatitis B infection, such as recent immigrants from Southeast Asia or children of intravenous drug abusers. Although not part of the routine laboratory evaluation, measurement of quantitative immunoglobulins often shows low IgG levels and elevated IgM levels.

Questions: Nephrotic Syndrome

- Has the child recently had any infections, such as pharyngitis or a URI?
- Are the child's eyelids swollen? Do they look more or less puffy at other times during the day, especially on awakening or after crying?
- Does the child have a history of rashes characteristic of diseases that are associated with nephrotic syndrome?
- Is there a history of fever, oliguria, or abdominal pain?
- Is the child playful and active, or is the edema so significant that movement is uncomfortable?
- Are the ascites and pleural effusions so severe that some respiratory compromise is evident?

Imaging Studies

Chest x-rays help assess the severity of pleural effusions in children with marked ascites and respiratory compromise.

MANAGEMENT

Hospitalization

The decision to admit a child with nephrotic syndrome to the hospital is determined by the child's functional status. All children with severe edema compromising ambulation or respiration should be admitted. Other indications for admission include unstable vital signs, fever, marked oliguria, and severe hemoconcentration (hematocrit > 48–50%).

Most children with nephrotic syndrome are hospitalized for control of edema or treatment of a complication such as infection. The management of children in relapse is aimed at minimizing edema and preventing complications until the disease can be controlled with immunosuppressive therapy. Intake, output, and weight need to be closely monitored. Blood pressure should be followed, although hypertension is uncommon.

If children have a fever (temperature: > 100.7° F [38.2° C]), blood and urine cultures should be obtained and antibiotics started pending culture results. If signs of peritoneal inflammation are evident, paracentesis should also be performed to obtain samples of the ascites fluid for Gram stain, cell count, and culture. Broad-spectrum antibiotics should be given to cover respiratory pathogens, especially pneumococcus, and enteric pathogens. All children who are newly diagnosed with nephrotic syndrome should have a purified protein derivative (PPD) test, because immunosuppression associated with steroid therapy may facilitate reactivation of tuberculosis infection.

Intravenous albumin (25%) should be used selectively because albumin infusions are very expensive, and the infused albumin is excreted very rapidly in the urine. Infusions are indicated in children with marked ascites, scrotal or labial edema, or significant pleural effusions. They are also helpful in maintaining blood pressure and renal perfusion in septic children with nephrotic syndrome. The usual dose is 1 g/kg, up to 25 g, infused over 60 minutes, with close monitoring of blood pressure. Furosemide (1 mg/kg intravenously) is usually administered postinfusion. The albumin infusions may be repeated every 6–12 hours as necessary. If children with oliguria fail to increase their urine output after the first or second albumin infusion, they need to be evaluated immediately for the presence of acute renal failure (see Chapter 47, Acute Renal Failure). Mobilization of edema fluid in children with acute tubular necrosis precipitates pulmonary edema.

Supportive Therapy

Diet

Because sodium plays a key role in edema formation, children with nephrotic syndrome should be placed on a no-added-salt diet that limits dietary sodium to 3 g/d. Technically, sodium restriction is indicated only during times of relapse, but a constant no-added-salt diet helps entire families maintain a consistent regimen. In general, fluid restriction is not necessary except in unusual circumstances (e.g., a steroid-resistant patient with severe fluid retention problems). Although earlier teachings recommended the use of high-protein diets, newer research has shown that these diets increase urinary protein losses.

Activity

In the past, children with nephrotic syndrome were treated with bed rest, because the supine position reduces urinary protein losses somewhat. No evidence shows that bed rest has a significant impact on children's clinical state, however. Therefore most pediatric nephrologists recommend that children be allowed full activity. Boys with marked scrotal edema may be more comfortable resting in bed while diuresis is being initiated. Children with nephrotic syndrome should not be isolated from other children and should be allowed to attend school.

Diuretics

Diuretics are often helpful in children in relapse, particularly in children with steroid-resistant disease. Serum potassium levels, as well as clinical signs of intravascular volume, should be monitored. If children have moderate intravascular volume contraction, the injudicious use of diuretics could precipitate hypotension and increase the risk of thrombosis and acute tubular necrosis. The most commonly used diuretic is furosemide (1–2 mg/kg per dose given orally or intravenously). Spironolactone is sometimes added to the diuretic regimen for its potassium-sparing effect.

Long-term Management

The goal of long-term management is induction and maintenance of remission from active nephrotic syndrome. At the same time, the side effects of medications should be minimized. Spontaneous remission eventually occurs in children with MCD, but the 70% historical mortality rate makes waiting for a spontaneous remission unacceptable. Remissions are induced and maintained with the use of immunosuppressive medications. Figure 121–1 summarizes an approach to the overall management of nephrotic syndrome with these agents. A list of commonly used medications and dosages appears in Table 121–2.

Corticosteroids and Alkylating Agents

Over 90% of children with primary nephrotic syndrome respond to corticosteroid therapy. Steroids are therefore both diagnostic and therapeutic, because failure to respond to steroids can be a marker for disease other than MCD. Even so, some children with MCD are steroid-resistant at some time in their disease. Steroids can be started in children who are newly diagnosed with nephrotic syndrome if they have no signs of systemic disease, no more than microscopic hematuria, a normal C3 (or results pending), and normal

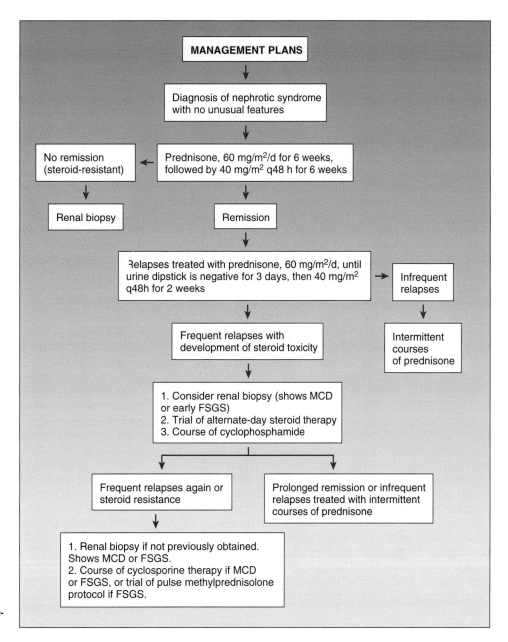

FIGURE 121-1. Management of nephrotic syndrome in children.

renal function. Acute infection should be managed with specific antimicrobial therapy to avoid infection-related steroid resistance.

Prednisone is usually started at 60 mg/m²/d. It can either be given once a day, in the morning, or divided into two or three daily doses. If first episodes of nephrotic syndrome are treated with a prolonged course of corticosteroids (60 mg/m²/d for 6 weeks followed by 40 mg/m²/48 h), the children are subsequently less likely to follow a frequently relapsing course. Proteinuria resolves within 2 weeks in many children with MCD and by 4 weeks in more than 90%. Serum albumin normalizes soon after proteinuria clears, but hypercholesterolemia may take many weeks to return to normal.

The pediatrician can easily manage steroid-sensitive children, but children with more difficult nephrotic syndrome should be managed in conjunction with the pediatric nephrologist. Children with relapses are treated with daily prednisone (60 mg/m²) until the urine is protein-free for three days. This regimen is followed by two weeks of 40 mg/m² every other morning. An increased incidence of side effects (e.g., cushingoid appearance, hypertension, obesity, glucose intolerance, cataracts, osteopenia, decreased growth rate) occurs

TABLE 121-2.   Treatment Options in Childhood Nephrotic Syndrome

Medication	Dose	Length of Therapy
Prednisone	60 mg/m²/d	Varies
Cyclophosphamide	2–3 mg/kg/d (cumulative dose < 200 mg/kg)	12 weeks
Chlorambucil	0.15–0.2 mg/kg/d (cumulative dose ≤ 8.2 mg/kg)	8 weeks
Cyclosporine	3 mg/kg/q12h	Varies
Levamisole	2.5 mg/kg qod	Varies

when children require frequent courses of prednisone therapy. In frequently relapsing children, a chronic course of alternate-day steroid therapy may eliminate relapses and reduce steroid toxicity. Usually prednisone 60 mg/m^2 is given every other morning initially. The dose is then gradually tapered over several months to the lowest dose that keeps the child in remission.

If alternative-day steroid therapy fails to maintain remission, cyclophosphamide or chlorambucil is administered. Both these alkylating agents may induce long-lasting remission in children with steroid-dependent or frequently relapsing nephrotic syndrome. Either agent is started while children are on steroid therapy, and the steroids are gradually tapered during the course of treatment with the alkylating agent. In the past a diagnostic renal biopsy was routine prior to starting an alkylating agent. Many pediatric nephrologists now consider such therapy in steroid-sensitive or steroid-dependent children without a biopsy, however, provided that renal function is normal. Initially a daily dose of cyclophosphamide 2 mg/kg was recommended for 8 weeks. However, a 12-week course is more likely to induce prolonged remission and still be safe.

Potential toxicities of cyclophosphamide include bone marrow suppression with increased risk of infection, alopecia, hemorrhagic cystitis, gonadal toxicity, and a small but indeterminately increased risk of developing a malignancy at some time. CBCs should be monitored weekly, and parents should be cautioned about the increased risk of overwhelming varicella infections in children who have not yet had a varicella infection or vaccination. The dose should be withheld if the WBC count falls below 4000/μL and restarted when the WBC returns or exceeds 4000/μL. Alopecia and hemorrhagic cystitis are rare when the recommended dose is used. A 12-week course of cyclophosphamide (2 mg/kg/d) does not appear to increase the risk of infertility, but longer courses are associated with oligospermia, aspermia, and ovarian dysfunction. Postpubertal individuals may be at greater risk for gonadal toxicity than prepubertal children.

When steroid-sensitive or steroid-dependent children have failed to achieve prolonged remission after cyclophosphamide therapy, a diagnostic renal biopsy should be performed. Renal biopsy is indicated early in the course of illness for steroid-resistant children. If FSGS is identified on biopsy, treatment involves a prolonged course of intravenous methylprednisolone therapy or cyclosporine. Therapeutic options for children with MCD who continue to be steroid-dependent after a course of cyclophosphamide include treatment with cyclosporine or levamisole. Although cyclosporine is more likely to induce prolonged remission, it only maintains remission while being administered. Children trade steroid dependence for cyclosporine dependence. Nevertheless, for children with steroid toxicity, a 6- to 12-month course of cyclosporine allows resolution of the adverse effects of steroids and is generally well tolerated when administered by the experienced physician. Side effects such as hirsutism and gingival hyperplasia are frequent at the onset of therapy. These effects regress as the dose is decreased or the drug is dis-

continued, however. Hypertension is not uncommon. The most common metabolic abnormality seen with cyclosporine use is hypomagnesemia. Long-term therapy may lead to significant nephrotoxicity, and rarely patients experience liver toxicity.

Because of potential toxicity, cyclosporine should only be prescribed by a physician familiar with the drug. Cyclosporine requirements may change with remission and relapse, and the family and physician should be aware of several drug interactions. Any medication interfering with the cytochrome P-450 enzyme system in the liver, such as erythromycin, greatly increases cyclosporine levels and should be used only under extraordinary circumstances. Children who require prolonged treatment with cyclosporine should have follow-up kidney biopsies performed after a year of therapy to assess for any nephrotoxicity.

Immunization Issues

Because of the unusual susceptibility to pneumococcal infections, children with nephrotic syndrome over the age of 2 years should receive the pneumococcal vaccine. The vaccine is best administered while the children are in remission, but it produces protective titers even in children who are on alternate-day steroid therapy at the time of immunization. Patients on multiple immunosuppressives should have their pneumococcal antibody titers measured, and a second dose of vaccine should be administered if they fail to seroconvert. Influenza vaccine should be administered each fall to children with nephrotic syndrome using the age-appropriate schedule and dosage.

Some of the routine childhood immunizations (diphtheria-tetanus-pertussis, *Haemophilus influenzae* type B, hepatitis B) should be administered by the usual schedule but while children are in remission (see Chapter 17, Immunizations). Some controversy exists concerning the use of live virus vaccines in children who require long-term immunosuppressive therapy. No vaccines should be administered if children are currently being treated with an alkylating agent. The parenteral polio vaccine (IPV) may be substituted for the oral vaccine, and IPV may be used for "boosters." Because they may secondarily expose the nephrotic child to the OPV virus, siblings of nephrotic children should receive IPV instead of OPV. The measles-mumps-rubella (MMR) vaccine could potentially cause a relapse. Based on the limited data on the use of varicella vaccine in nephrotic children, it is probably safe to administer varicella vaccine while the children are in remission, and not on immunosuppressive medications.

Parent Education

Because nephrotic syndrome follows a chronic, relapsing course, parent education is essential for effective long-term management. Parents need to be instructed about using urinary dipsticks (Albustix) to monitor protein excretion. Generally urine dipsticks should be used daily during periods of active relapse and when medication is being tapered. Otherwise, the dipstick should be checked whenever children have infections, including URIs, or whenever they look "puffy," and weekly when asymptomatic.

Weight should also be monitored, especially during relapse. Children should be weighed each morning when they awaken. Urine output should be measured in more difficult cases. As parents become more familiar with the nephrotic syndrome, they may contact the physician about medication changes. Parents should also contact the physician about "danger signs" such as fever (temperature: > 100.7° F [38.2° C]), significant abdominal pain, or exposure to varicella. If children do not have protective antibodies against varicella and if they are taking any immunosuppressive medication (including prednisone), the varicella-zoster immune globulin should be administered within 72 hours of exposure to varicella. If varicella infection develops, intravenous acyclovir should be instituted.

PROGNOSIS

In the preantibiotic era, nephrotic syndrome was frequently fatal, usually because of overwhelming infection. After the introduction of antibiotics, the mortality rate fell. The use of corticosteroids has led to a further reduction in mortality. Currently, the mortality rate is about 5%, almost exclusively due to infections from encapsulated organisms or from thrombosis. The greatest risk of death in children with nephrotic syndrome is among the children with resistance to corticosteroid therapy.

The long-term outlook for the majority of children with nephrotic syndrome is favorable, particularly for steroid-sensitive patients. Relapses often disappear by the completion of puberty. Occasionally children continue to have relapses into adulthood. Approximately 20% of children with steroid-sensitive MCD still experience relapses 15 years after the onset of their disease. Disease recurrence is highly unlikely if 8 years pass without a relapse. Less than 10% of initially steroid-

sensitive children with nephrotic syndrome develop end-stage renal disease. This occurs almost exclusively in children with FSGS. FSGS may recur after kidney transplants, particularly in young children with aggressive FSGS.

Case Resolution

In the opening scenario, the child most likely has MCD. He appears stable enough to be managed as an outpatient and should be placed on a salt-restricted diet and prednisone. The overall prognosis depends on a close interaction among the parents, pediatrician, and consulting pediatric nephrologist.

Selected Readings

Arbeitsgemeinschaft Für Pädiatrische Nephrologie. Short versus standard prednisone therapy for initial treatment of idiopathic nephrotic syndrome in children. Lancet I:380–383, 1988.

Bernard, D. B. Extrarenal complications of the nephrotic syndrome. Kidney Int. 33:1184–1202, 1988.

Brodehl, J. Conventional therapy for idiopathic nephrotic syndrome in children. Clin. Nephrol. 35:S8–15, 1991.

Eddy, A. A., and H. W. Schnaper. The nephrotic syndrome: From the simple to the complex. Semin. Nephrol. 18:304–316, 1998.

International Study of Kidney Disease in Children. Minimal change nephrotic syndrome in children: deaths during the first 5 to 15 years' observation. Pediatrics 73:497–501, 1984.

Kher, K. K., M. Sweet, and S. P. Makker. Nephrotic syndrome in children. Curr. Prob. Pediatr. 18:203–251, 1988.

Lewis, M. A., et al. Nephrotic syndrome: from toddlers to twenties. Lancet I:255–259, 1989.

Mendoza, S. A., et al. Treatment of steroid-resistant focal segmental glomerulosclerosis with pulse methylprednisolone and alkylating agents. Pediatr. Nephrol. 4:303–307, 1990.

Niaudet, P., M. F. Gagnadoux, and M. Broyer. Treatment of childhood steroid-resistant idiopathic nephrotic syndrome. Adv. Nephrol. 28:43–61, 1998.

Quien, R. M., B. A. Kaiser, A. Deforest, et al. Response to the varicella vaccine in children with nephrotic syndrome. J. Pediatr. 131:688–690, 1997.

Thabet, M. A. E. H., J. R. Salcedo, and J. C. M. Chan. Hyperlipidemia in childhood nephrotic syndrome. Pediatr. Nephrol. 7:559–566, 1993.

CHAPTER 122

SEIZURES AND EPILEPSY

Kenneth R. Huff, M.D.

H$_x$ A 6-year-old boy is evaluated for unusual episodic behaviors. The previous week his mother was awakened by the boy's brother and found her son lying in bed unresponsive and drooling, with his head and eyes averted to the right, his right arm slightly raised, and his body stiff. His face was jerking intermittently. When the paramedics arrived, the boy's posturing and movements had stopped. After the event he could speak but was somewhat incoherent. He was taken to the local emergency department, where his examination and mental status were normal. Screening blood and urine tests were normal, and he was discharged. His family was instructed to see his pediatrician for further recommendations.

His father remembers two or three other episodes of a somewhat different nature in the past month. These occurred as the boy was being put to bed. They involved some body stiffening and facial grimacing, with the mouth slightly open and the tongue twisted and deviated to one side. The child could not speak but appeared to be trying to talk. The episodes lasted 20–30 seconds. Afterwards the boy was his usual self and could tell his father what had been said to him.

The child has had no intercurrent illnesses or abnormal behavior apart from these "spells," and he has lost no abilities. A paternal cousin and grandfather had seizures during childhood but "grew out of them." The examination is completely normal.

Questions

1. Is it likely that the episodic behavior was a seizure?
2. What historical data about an event support the diagnosis of a seizure disorder?
3. How does the EEG help in classifying the type of seizure disorder?
4. What rationale should be used to formulate short-term and long-term treatment plans?

Seizures are a common medical problem in children. Diagnosing an episode that does not contain generalized convulsing movements as a seizure is sometimes problematic. Seizures are defined as episodic, stereotypic behavior syndromes of abrupt onset that result in loss of responsiveness and that generally are not provoked by external stimuli. Frequently, this behavior correlates with brain electrical discharges on EEG.

A detailed history of the nature of the episodic behavior from an eyewitness is paramount both in making the diagnosis of a seizure disorder and in elucidating the type of seizure problem. The EEG is most often an adjunct to diagnosis. It is abnormal in many individuals who do not have clinical seizures and it may be normal interictally in many patients with clinical seizures, because of its sampling limitations. Special techniques can sometimes help alleviate these limitations.

The type of seizure problem is important information in devising the management plan. Seizures can simply be classified as primary generalized seizures or partial seizures. However, some partial seizures can secondarily generalize, thereby clinically mimicking primary generalized seizures. Making this latter distinction illustrates the importance of eyewitness information. Many treatment options are available, but the therapeutic plan must be individualized to the child's seizure type to optimize seizure control and minimize side effects. With appropriate treatment, the majority of children with seizure disorders are handicapped neither scholastically nor socially and can enjoy normal lives.

EPIDEMIOLOGY

About 0.5–1.0% of all children experience at least one afebrile seizure. Recurrent seizures can occur as a component of a static encephalopathy after brain malformation or dysgenesis, encephalitis or meningitis, metabolic disorder, hypoxic/ischemic injury, or severe head trauma. Such secondary or symptomatic seizures make up approximately one-third of childhood epilepsies. The remaining two-thirds of epileptic seizures occur presumably as part of a genetic epileptic syndrome without the presence of encephalopathy between seizures. Most often seizures occur in children without any known cause or association.

CLINICAL PRESENTATION

Children present with a history of an episode of abrupt onset characterized by a loss of ability to respond to external stimuli (D_x Box). They may experience various sensory phenomena before losing consciousness and may feel sleepy following the period of unconsciousness. During the seizure, observers may note only an akinetic or staring spell or dramatic, rhythmic spasms of the face, extremities, or torso, depending on the type of seizure. Major motor seizures are frequently associated with autonomic system changes, including skin vasculature, sweating, saliva production, and sphincter control. Most seizure episodes are not provoked or attenuated by environmental factors (except for the provocative factors of fever and intercurrent illness). Between episodes, children's general physical and neurologic examination may be entirely normal.

PATHOPHYSIOLOGY

A seizure represents a sudden, synchronous depolarizing change in the electrical activity of a network of neurons that becomes widely propagated over the cortex, affecting awareness, responsiveness to external stimuli, and motor control. Partial seizure disorders may result from a focal cortical lesion, such as a glial scar or dysplasia caused by a remote insult (e.g., an infarct) or dysgenesis that disrupts the electrical organization and allows for periodic, abnormal transmission of impulses.

Exactly what produces the synchronous depolarization of the neurons and the propagation is not well

---

D_x Seizures

- Abrupt loss of responsiveness
- Rhythmic clonic movements
- Sustained changes in posture or tone
- Simple automatic movements
- Staring without change in tone
- Simultaneous change in cerebral electrical activity (repetitive discharges)

understood. Several physiologic mechanisms, including neuronal circuitry, membrane ion channel abnormalities, and glial transmitter precursor metabolism or uptake, are probably involved. An understanding of the mechanism involved in familial epilepsy syndromes awaits the definition of the various gene products.

Seizure Types

Seizures can be simply classified as either **primary-generalized seizures,** which include grand mal, generalized tonic-clonic convulsions, and petit mal (absence) seizures (so named because of the child's complete loss of awareness at the outset of the episode), or **partial seizures,** which include focal motor, psychomotor, and other partial disorders (Table 122–1). The examples presented here should not be considered an exhaustive list of seizure syndromes but some of the more important types encountered in practice.

The majority of all seizures in older children result from a partial seizure disorder. **Psychomotor seizures** are partial seizures that have a wide range of ictal (seizure) behaviors, including focal clonic jerking, aversive or asymmetric hypertonic posturing, and more complex stereotypic fumbling or fingering behaviors. The seizures are usually preceded by a sensory aura or emotional manifestations and may be followed by postictal drowsiness. In some instances, children have partial sensory awareness during seizures. In other cases, however, they are completely unconscious, and the initial partial motor manifestations can rapidly generalize, sometimes without being observed. Partial seizures are more often associated with focal brain pathologic processes, including traumatic lesions, infarcts, malformations, infections (e.g., viral infections or cerebral cysticercosis), and hippocampal sclerosis (seen on MRI).

Rolandic seizures are a relatively common partial seizure syndrome that sometimes is familial and has a good prognosis. These episodes commonly occur when children are drowsy or awakening. Sensory auras precede the motor manifestations, which involve the tongue, mouth, or face and which can partially or completely generalize to the rest of the body. The clinical syndrome is accompanied by a characteristic focal EEG discharge over the central temporal region of the scalp.

TABLE 122–1.   Classification of Epileptic Seizures

Partial seizures (seizures beginning locally)
    Elementary symptoms: focal seizures
    Complex symptoms: psychomotor seizures
    Partial seizures evolving secondarily to generalized seizures
Generalized seizures (bilaterally symmetric; onset not local)
    Absence seizures (petit mal): typical and atypical
    Tonic-clonic seizures
    Tonic seizures
    Clonic seizures
    Myoclonic seizures (minor motor)
    Atonic seizures (drop attacks)
    Infantile spasms
Unclassified seizures (includes neonatal "subtle" seizures)

TABLE 122–2.   Partial Complex Versus Absence Seizures

	Partial Complex	Absence
Aura	Frequent	None
Loss of consciousness	Sometimes partial	Complete
Motor movements	Sometimes complex	Blinking
Postictal state	Frequent	None
Duration	> 30 seconds	< 15 seconds
Frequency	Few per day	Many per hour or day
Hyperventilation provoked	No	Yes
EEG	Variable or normal	3/sec spike-wave
Prognosis past adolescence	Frequently persists	Rarely occurs

An **absence seizure** may sometimes be difficult to distinguish from a partial seizure (Table 122–2). The absence spell is a brief (2–15 seconds) loss of consciousness without loss of tone. Staring and minor movements such as lip smacking or licking or semipurposeful-appearing movements of the hands are often the only observed behaviors. There is no postictal period. Because absence seizures occur multiple times a day and children are often unaware of them, parents may dismiss the subtle behavior change and inattention as daydreaming. However, these seizures may adversely affect learning. Hyperventilation, a useful diagnostic test that can be performed in the office, may provoke absence seizures. The EEG is confirmatory and distinguishes classic petit mal seizures with 3-second spike-wave discharges from variant syndromes. The classic petit mal is more often familial with dominant gene transmission, age-specific manifestation between 4 and 16 years, and sensitivity to ethosuximide; the atypical variant has a poorer prognosis for early resolution and is more resistant to anticonvulsant therapy.

A number of age-related seizure syndromes exist perhaps related to maturational events in brain circuitry. Although the appearance of these syndromes is stereotypic, in most cases the prognosis depends on the etiologic diagnosis.

Neonatal seizures may be tonic, focal clonic, or multifocal clonic. A vigorous search for etiology of the seizure is often successful. Problems commonly leading to neonatal seizures include hemorrhage (germinal matrix in the premature infant or subarachnoid space from trauma in older neonates); hypoxic ischemic damage from asphyxia; infections producing sepsis/meningitis postnatally or prenatal encephalitis; drug withdrawal in the infant of a substance-abusing mother; metabolic problems including hypoglycemia, hypocalcemia, or hypomagnesemia in the infant of a diabetic mother; amino or organic acidopathies occurring a few days after feedings have begun; and congenital brain malformations.

Infantile spasms are an age-related seizure syndrome with typical movements of flexion contraction of the trunk with the head bowed or sudden raising of the arms sometimes accompanied by a cry. These behaviors often occur several times in succession in a series. This syndrome occurs in infants between 3 months and 2 years of age. Another perhaps related syndrome of serial spasms, **Ohtahara's syndrome,** occurs at a younger age and is characterized by a different EEG pattern but carries a similar ominous prognosis for impaired intellectual development. A third syndrome in older children that is also associated with a different EEG pattern, Lennox-Gastaut syndrome, has the same poor prognosis for seizure control and cognitive development but produces several different seizure types, including tonic, absence, and drop attacks, which are equally difficult to control. Different types of brain lesions in these age groups (including focal lesions) can result in the same generalized seizure syndromes. Examples include tuberous sclerosis; neonatal ischemia, hemorrhage, or meningitis; and major malformations. These disorders most often present in the context of a moderate to severe learning disability.

DIFFERENTIAL DIAGNOSIS

Seizures are distinguished from nonepileptic paroxysmal disorders on the basis of history. The circumstances of place and time as well as details about the nature of the behavior are important pieces of data. **Syncope** is often preceded by symptoms of lightheadedness, nausea, tinnitus, and eventually a gradual darkening of vision sometimes without loss of auditory perception. The syncopal episode is also frequently situational, unlike a seizure. It occurs when children are in hot, stuffy environments; when they have been standing in one place for a long time; or when they see or experience a painful or traumatic event such as an injection or phlebotomy. Boys may experience syncope during early morning micturition.

Breathholding spells are characterized by apnea and loss of responsiveness accompanied by either cyanosis or pallid skin. Breathholding spells are also "situational." Infants or children are often upset and often are crying just before such spells. They may be frightened by a seemingly minor injury or angry after a toy is taken away or a disciplinary action is administered. Children may then throw themselves backward and stiffen, and they may even have a few clonic jerks. (See Chapter 30, Breath-Holding Spells.)

Selective attention is frequently mistaken for minor motor or absence seizures. This behavior often occurs when children are involved in passive activities (e.g., watching television, playing a video game, or daydreaming) and do not respond to verbal stimuli such as hearing their own name. Generally, attention lapses do not occur during talking or eating; electrically generated brain discharges (seizures) occur however even during these activities.

Epileptic seizures must also be differentiated from **pseudoseizures,** which actually occur most often in patients who have true seizures. Such episodes may resemble true seizures very well, the psychodynamics of secondary gain or other motivation for the behavior may not be apparent and the "need" for attention may have some legitimacy, and the standard EEG is not helpful. Pseudoseizures should be suspected in children who have witnessed seizures in relatives or close friends, who have seizures that recur in the same situations, who do not experience a change in seizure frequency with therapeutic levels of anticonvulsants, and whose seizures appear "suggestible." Diagnosis can often be supported in the most complicated cases by provocatory testing by suggestion, with the caretaker's consent. The child is told that an intravenous placebo injection will produce the "seizure," and simultaneous video EEG monitoring of a subsequent episode will confirm at least suggestibility and support a pseudoseizure diagnosis. Serum prolactin level determination can be adjunctive, and psychological assessment may detect underlying problems that require specific treatment (e.g., sexual abuse or other major psychological trauma). The prognosis of pseudoseizures in children is better than in adults and relates to the psychosocial genesis of the problem in most children.

EVALUATION (Table 122–3)

History

The history should determine the exact events surrounding the seizure episode. A detailed history of the nature of the behavior from an eyewitness is extremely important (Questions Box). The physician should determine whether children experienced any loss of their normal level of responsiveness. Most often this change in mental status is abrupt, although a warning behavior or aura that lasts for a few seconds may precede complete loss of responsiveness. The warning behavior or aura may be a cry, an expression of fear, or irritability. If children are articulate, they may be able to describe a sensory phenomenon or relate an indescribable sensation.

A change in muscle tone and activity is frequently associated with the abrupt change in mental status unless the spell is an absence seizure. Most often, the tone is increased with general extensor posturing, more focal hypertonicity, or more complex torsion or "aversive" upper body posturing. The patient may fall if not supported. Rhythmic jerking or clonic movements (focal or general), including the trunk, limbs, face, and eyes, may occur concomitantly. Respirations may involve rhythmic grunting or nearly imperceptible movements. Swallowing may not occur, so that saliva pools or forms at the lips. Autonomic changes including skin color change (circumoral cyanosis), increased pulse, and loss of sphincter control frequently occur with

---

TABLE 122–3.   Initial Evaluation of Seizure Patients

Eyewitness account of the episode

Description of children's own experiences before, during, and after the episode if they are articulate

Past history from caregiver concerning remote injuries to the nervous system, progressive neurologic symptoms, or intercurrent illness

Careful neurologic examination looking for signs of cerebral hemisphere lateralization

Brain imaging study when a partial seizure is observed, a crescendo history of neurologic symptoms is obtained, or focal neurologic signs are found on interictal examination

Waking and sleep electroencephalogram with hyperventilation

major motor spells. The ictal period generally lasts 30 seconds to 2 minutes, although observers frequently overestimate this time. Postictal periods of sleepiness or lethargy may occur. Their length is often correlated with the length or intensity of the seizure.

Children and those around them are often unaware of the occurrence of minor motor or absence seizures. Often an observant teacher brings a child's problem to a physician's attention. During a spell, a child has no change in tone or clonic movements and may have only subtle facial or hand movements. The episode lasts only a few seconds, and there are no preictal or postictal behaviors.

Historical information can help determine potential etiologies of the seizure problem. A distant brain insult or hereditary disposition may be the cause. A progressive encephalopathy indicates a need for degenerative disease investigation.

Physical Examination

Children should be examined carefully for focal neurological signs, particularly asymmetries. The examination should include a developmental assessment and mental status examination. The physician should look for signs of potential genetic problems, such as dysmorphic features or organ malformations, which often correlate with cerebral dysgenesis; abnormal skin pigmentation or vessels, suggesting a neurocutaneous disorder; and organomegaly or bony abnormalities indicating the possibility of a storage disorder. Children who are old enough to cooperate should be asked to hyperventilate to provoke an absence spell if the history is suggestive of this type of seizure.

Laboratory Tests

An EEG should be requested to help with the diagnosis of the type of seizure disorder. In children with

partial seizure disorders, the interictal discharge is helpful in localizing the site of genesis of abnormal electrical activity. Sleep is often essential to observing abnormalities. If a normal waking EEG is obtained and seizures continue to recur, it is sometimes useful to increase the likelihood of sleep during the record by prior sleep deprivation. Special techniques (e.g., prolonged monitoring with telemetry or special anatomic electrode placements) can sometimes help overcome standard EEG limitations of sample time and inaccessible areas of cerebral cortex. It should be noted, however, that the standard EEG is rarely normal in typical or atypical petit mal disorders.

Historical information can frequently guide the need for metabolic tests. A blood sugar determination is useful acutely, but electrolytes are rarely abnormal in older children who have been well prior to the seizure. Neonates and infants with recurrent unexplained seizures should have metabolic screening including organic acid and amino acid levels and a therapeutic trial of pyridoxine. Tissue biopsy histologic analysis and specific assays may be indicated for diagnosis when physical signs suggest possible specific etiologies.

Imaging Studies

The quality and variety of data gathered by brain neuroimaging modalities have increased markedly. MRI scans are particularly helpful if a progression in neurologic symptoms or signs has occurred, if there is a history of prior neurologic insult, if an asymmetry of strength or tone is noted on examination, or if signs of dysgenesis are present in other parts of the body. Even in the absence of these factors, partial or focal seizures have a higher yield of abnormal imaging results than do febrile seizures or petit mal disorders, which have a low yield. Acutely, intravenous contrast should generally be given because loss of focal blood-brain barrier with inflammatory or neoplastic lesions can lead to seizures. Children with recurrent or resistant seizures should be imaged particularly when surgical treatment is under consideration. Helpful modalities in studying such children include positron emission tomography (PET), single photon emission computerized tomography (SPECT), functional MRI, and physiologic MRI. These studies help define the nature of damaged or epileptic cortex and differentiate it from normal cortex.

MANAGEMENT

Anticonvulsants are the mainstay of management of seizure disorders (Table 122–4). Anticonvulsants are prescribed if the risk of recurrence of seizures is significant based on seizure classification and individual factors. A structural lesion seen on imaging studies or the clinical situation and EEG may suggest a high recurrence risk. The choice of anticonvulsant depends on age, neurologic diagnosis, other conditions or medications, and social factors. The dose and number of anticonvulsants prescribed for children reflect a balance of seizure resistance, risk of recurrence, and potential toxicity of medication.

TABLE 122–4. Drugs Useful for Treating Seizures

Seizure Type	Dose (mg/kg/d)	Toxic Symptoms
Partial seizures		
Carbamazepine	approx. 30	Gastrointestinal distress, headache
Phenytoin	4–8	Ataxia, nystagmus
Primidone	12–25	Drowsiness, ataxia
Newer medications		
Lamotrigine	4–7	Dizziness, sedation
Gabapentin	4–8	Somnolence, ataxia
Vigabatrin	15–50	Drowsiness, behavioral disturbances
Topiramate	8–10	Weight loss, speech disturbance
Neonatal seizures		
Phenobarbital	5	Lethargy, irritability
Generalized seizures		
Valproic acid	30–60	Tremors, sedation
Felbamate	45	Insomnia, anorexia
Topiramate	8–10	Weight loss, speech disturbance
Myoclonic seizures		
Clonazepam	0.15	Drowsiness, ataxia
Absence seizures		
Ethosuximide	30	Nausea, hiccups
Valproic acid	30–60	Tremors, sedation
Infantile spasms		
Adrenocorticotropic hormone	40 units/m^2	Increased appetite, acne
Valproic acid	30–60	Tremors, sedation
Vigabatrin	15–50	Drowsiness, behavioral disturbances

Carbamazepine is often recommended for partial seizures. Toxicity is generally mild or nonexistent; adverse events include gastrointestinal upset, dizziness, and headache. Phenytoin is also effective for these types of seizures. It can be given intravenously for status epilepticus. Phenobarbital is effective in neonatal seizures but may have deleterious effects on behavior and learning in older children. Ethosuximide is used for classical petit mal seizures. Valproic acid is used for atypical petit mal and other seizure disorders resistant to other anticonvulsants. Felbamate is also effective in many difficult-to-treat epilepsy syndromes although a low incidence of severe bone marrow suppression has limited its use. Newer anticonvulsants including gabapentin, lamotrigine, vigabatrin, and topiramate have proven effective. Gabapentin is useful as an adjunctive agent because of its lack of interaction with other anticonvulsants. Lamotrogine is useful in both partial and primary generalized seizure disorders. Vigabatrin is useful in infantile spasms. Topiramate is effective in partial seizures, generalized seizures, and Lennox-Gastaut syndrome.

Periodic monitoring of efficacy and side effects is essential in children who take medication daily on a long-term basis. A log of seizure frequency helps assess medication efficacy. Gastrointestinal and neurologic symptoms (sedation and ataxia) are the most common side effects. The perception by the child or parent of symptoms being related to the medication as well as the actual presence of side effects or toxicity contribute to the complex issue of compliance. Drug levels are useful in monitoring dosage, compliance, and the likelihood that symptoms are the result of drug side effects. Organ toxicity (bone marrow, liver, and pancreas) must be considered and monitored with many medications. Hypersensitivity reactions and Stevens-Johnson syndrome usually occur within 2 months of beginning the medication. Drug interactions can be important and can include the liver cytochrome P450-inducing potential of barbiturates and the potential of other medications such as erythromycin antibiotics to inhibit carbamazepine metabolism and produce acute toxicity.

Surgery for epilepsy in childhood is developing fast. Children with seizure syndromes including Sturge-Weber syndrome, Rasmussen's encephalitis, catastrophic seizure disorders of early childhood such as infantile spasms related to a localized zone of epileptogenic cerebral tissue, and hamartomatous cortex–producing seizures have benefitted most. Extensive presurgical imaging and physiologic monitoring are necessary for surgery candidates.

PROGNOSIS

In general, approximately two-thirds of children who have experienced a tendency for seizure recurrence have a good prognosis for prevention of further recurrence and little or no problem with side effects of medication. They can lead normal lives without handicap. The etiologic diagnosis is the most important prognostic factor. The type of epilepsy, EEG findings, child's age, difficulty of initial seizure control, and time since the last seizure are also important.

Some seizure types have intrisically poor prognoses. For example, infantile spasms are prognostically ominous because even in the absence of a metabolic diagnosis, children frequently suffer head growth and developmental arrest unless the seizures are controlled with medication. Partial complex disorders and the atypical variant of petit mal syndrome sometimes have a poorer prognosis for early resolution and may be more resistant to treatment with anticonvulsants. However, some of the seizure syndromes with a familial tendency such as rolandic seizures and typical petit mal seizures have a relatively good prognosis for both control by medication and ultimate complete resolution.

The individualized decision to discontinue medication is often complex. The prognosis for recurrence of seizures, the parents' and children's reactions to seizures and to the prospect of their recurrence, and social factors such as school participation may all contribute to the decision. Children and parents must be aware that none of the prognostic factors, whether considered individually or in combination, are absolute predictors of seizure recurrence in a given child.

Case Resolution

The boy described in the case history at the beginning of the chapter had a generalized seizure when he was taken to the emergency room. The previous episodes recalled by thefather had characteristics of partial seizures. The tonic-clonic seizure was probably a secondary generalized rather than a primary generalized seizure. The possibility of sylvian seizures is suggested by the circumstances of the prior episodes, which occurred when the boy was drowsy; their "facial" symptomatology; and the family history. This diagnosis was confirmed by EEG. Carbamazepine was prescribed. The boy experienced no side effects or seizure recurrences and was successfully able to discontinue the medication 3 years later.

Selected Readings

Armstrong, D. and E. Mizrahi, Pathologic basis of the symptomatic epilepsies in childhood. J. Child Neurol. 13:361–371, 1998.

Brunquell, P. Psychogenic seizures in children. Int. Pediatr. 10(Suppl 1):47–54, 1995.

Camfield, P., and C. Camfield, (eds.). Management issues in pediatric epilepsy. Semin. Pediatr. Neurol. 1:71–143, 1994.

Donat, J. The age-dependent epileptic encephalopathies. J. Child Neurol. 7:7–21, 1992.

Guarino, E., and M. Morrell, Management of the adolescent with epilepsy: hormones, antiepileptic drugs, and reproductive health. Int. Pediatr. 10(Suppl 1):66–71, 1995.

Haslam, R.H.A. Nonfebrile seizures. Pediatr. Rev. 18:39–49, 1997.

Holmes, G. L. Diagnosis and Management of Seizures in Children. Major Problems in Pediatrics, vol. 30. Philadelphia, W. B. Saunders, 1987.

Neville, B. Evaluation of children for epilepsy surgery. Int. Pediatr. 10(Suppl 1):78–80, 1995.

Pellock, J. (ed.). New antiepileptic drugs in childhood epilepsy. Semin. Pediatr. Neurol. 4:1–67, 1997.

Scheuer, M. L., and T. A. Pedley. Current concepts: the evaluation and treatment of seizures. N. Engl. J. Med. 323:1468–1474, 1990.

Shields, W. D. Anatomic and functional imaging in epilepsy. Int. Pediatr. 10(suppl 1):72–77, 1995.

Terndrup, T. Clinical issues in acute childhood seizure management in the emergency department. J. Child Neurol. 13(Suppl 1):S7–S10, 1998.

Wyllie, E. The Treatment of Epilepsy: Principles and Practice. Philadelphia, Lea & Febiger, 1993.

INDEX

Note: Page numbers in *italics* refer to illustrations; page numbers followed by t refer to tables.